Radiographic Positioning AND Related Anatomy Workbook AND Laboratory Manual

VOLUME 2

FIFTH EDITION

Radiographic Positioning AND Related Anatomy

Workbook AND Laboratory Manual

VOLUME 2
Chapters 14-24

Kenneth L. Bontrager, MA, RT(R)
John P. Lampignano, M.Ed., RT(R) (CT)

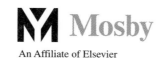

Mosby

An Affiliate of Elsevier

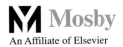

Mosby

An Affiliate of Elsevier

Executive Editor: Jeanne Wilke
Developmental Editor: Jennifer Moorhead
Project Manager: Linda McKinley
Production Editor: Rich Barber
Designer: Julia Ramirez
Cover Art: Amy Buxton

5th EDITION
Copyright © 2001 by Mosby, Inc.

Previous edition copyrighted 1997

NOTICE

Pharmacology is an ever-changing field. Standard safety precautions must be
followed, but as new research and clinical experience broaden our knowledge,
changes in treatment and drug therapy may become necessary or appropriate. Readers
are advised to check the most current product information provided by the
manufacturer of each drug to be administered to verify the recommended dose, the
method and duration of administration, and contraindications. It is the responsibility
of the treating physician, relying on experience and knowledge of the patient, to
determine dosages and the best treatment for each individual patient. Neither the
publisher nor the editor assumes any liability for any injury and/or damage to persons
or property arising from this publication.

Permissions may be sought directly from Elsevier's Health Sciences
Rights Department in Philadelphia, USA: phone: (+1)215-238-7869,
fax: (+1)215-238-2239, email: healthpermissions@elsevier.com. You may
also complete your request on-line via the Elsevier Science homepage
(http://www.elsevier.com), by selecting 'Customer Support' and then
'Obtaining Permissions'.

Mosby

11830 Westline Industrial Drive
St. Louis, Missouri 63146

Printed in the United States of America

International Standard Book Number
0-323-0143-64

04 GW/KPT 9 8 7 6 5 4

Acknowledgments

I am pleased to acknowledge and recognize those persons who have made significant contributions to the fifth edition of this student workbook and laboratory manual.

I first want to thank **John P. Lampignano,** MS, RT(R) (CT), who as coauthor expanded the objectives for each chapter and submitted first drafts of additional questions for the new sections of the textbook. John is a very qualified and effective educator and has put a lot of effort and energy into this project. Thank you, John, for your excellent contributions.

I want to thank **David Hall,** MS, RT(R) for his careful and meticulous review and proofing of all chapters of this manuscript. Not only did he make corrections, but he also made valuable suggestions for improving the clarity of the information being presented.

I also thank **Jeanne Rowland, Jennifer Moorhead,** and **Rich Barber** of the Mosby staff for their help and support in the preparation of this manuscript.

David Hall and **Cindy Murphy,** ACR, also reviewed, made suggestions, and proofed the more than 1200 questions in the computerized test bank, which is available as an ancillary to these workbooks and the textbook. Thank you, Dave and Cindy, for the significant time and effort you invested in this project. Both John Lampignano and I greatly appreciate your valuable contributions.

Last and most important, I want to thank my wife, **Mary Lou,** for organizing our rough composition of questions and answers, along with the associated illustrations, into an orderly and easy-to-follow format.

KLB

I would like to thank **Ken Bontrager** for his patience and dedication in developing my skills as a writer. I've been honored to work with him over the past two editions. **Jennifer Moorhead,** our developmental editor, deserves praise for her dedication and vision in coordinating this project. She kept us on task and focused but always with a smile and a gentle word.

I would like to thank the diagnostic medical imaging faculty and clinical instructors at GateWay Community College who provide a shining example of excellence each and every day for our students and community. To my students—past, present, and future—you have made teaching a rewarding experience! Without you, I would never have had the courage to write a single word. Finally, to my close friend, **Jerry Olson,** who taught me everything about radiography and many things about life—you have made my life richer and more worthwhile.

My family—**Deborah, Daniel,** and **Molly**—provide me with the greatest joy of all. I look at each of you and realize that I'm the luckiest person alive. Thank you for your love and support for the past 25 years. This book is dedicated to each of you.

JPL

Preface

The success of the first four editions of this workbook and the accompanying textbook, along with the associated audiovisual materials, is demonstrated by the many schools of radiologic technology throughout the United States, Canada, and other countries that have been using all or parts of these instructional media for more than 25 years.

New to This Edition

New illustrations and **expanded questions** have been added to reflect all the new content added to the fifth edition of *Textbook of Radiographic Positioning and Related Anatomy*. The use of visuals in these review exercises not only increases comprehension but also increases retention, because most individuals retain information most effectively through visual images.

The **detailed laboratory activities** have been updated, and the positioning question and answer exercises have been expanded with less emphasis on rote memory recall. More **situational questions** involving **clinical applications** have been added. These questions aid in the understanding of positioning principles and of which anatomical structures are best demonstrated on which projections. The clinical situational questions added to each chapter require students to think through and understand how application of this positioning information relates to specific clinical examples.

Pathology questions have been added to help students understand why they are performing specific exams and how exposure factors may be affected.

Critique exercises have been reorganized to be consistent with the new format of radiographic critique descriptions in the textbook.

Included in the positioning chapters of both the textbook and these workbooks are new sections on **geriatric** and **pediatric considerations, alternative modalities and procedures,** and **pathologic indications.** As in the textbook, entirely new sections added to the workbook include **venipuncture, digital radiography, bone densitometry, sialography,** and **hysterosalpingography.** Introductions to **nuclear medicine, radiation oncology,** and **ultrasound imaging** have also been added.

How to Work with the Textbook and the Workbook and Laboratory Manuals

This fifth edition of the student workbook and laboratory manual is organized to be in complete agreement with the fifth edition of the *Textbook of Radiographic Positioning and Related Anatomy*. Each chapter in the textbook has a corresponding chapter in the workbook-manuals to reinforce and supplement the information presented in the main text.

The most effective way to use this workbook-manual is for the student to complete the workbook chapter exercises immediately after reading and studying corresponding chapters in the textbook. To use both the student's and the instructor's time most effectively, this study should be done **before** the classroom presentation. The instructor can therefore spend more time in both the classroom and laboratory on problem areas and answering questions and less time on the fundamentals of anatomy and positioning, which students should already have learned.

Ancillaries

A **computerized test bank** (CTB) is available to instructors who use the textbook in their classrooms. The test bank features more than 1200 questions and 60 images. Some of these questions originally appeared as the Final Evaluation Exams in the Instructor's Manual in previous editions, but they have been expanded and fully revised into registry-type questions for the test bank. These questions can be used as final evaluation exams for each chapter, or they can be used to create custom exams.

Also available for the first time is an **electronic image collection** (EIC), which features more than 2000 images that are fully coordinated with the fifth edition textbook and workbooks. The fourth edition slide set contains 1780 slides and includes the two-volume Instructor's Manual with lecture notes and thumbnail prints of each slide.

Contents

Volume 2

Volume 1

Student Instructions

The following information will show you how correctly using this workbook and the accompanying textbook will help you master radiographic anatomy and positioning.

This course becomes the core of all your studies and your work as a radiographer. **This is one course that you must master.** You cannot become a proficient radiographer by marginally passing this course. Therefore please read these instructions carefully **before** beginning Chapter 1.

Objectives

Study the list of objectives carefully so that you will understand what you must know and be able to do after you complete each chapter.

Learning Exercises

These exercises are the focal point of this workbook-laboratory manual. Using them correctly will help you learn and remember the important information presented in each chapter of the textbook. To maximize the benefits from each exercise, **follow the correct six-step order of activities** as outlined next:

Chapter 1   Textbook and Workbook

Chapter 1 is a comprehensive introduction that prepares you for the remaining chapters of this positioning course. It is divided into six sections in both the textbook and this workbook. Your instructor may assign specific sections of this chapter at various times during your study of radiographic positioning and/or procedures. Read and study these sections in the textbook first, and then complete the corresponding review exercise in this workbook before taking that portion of the self-test.

Chapters 2 to 24

PART I

Step 1.   A. **Textbook:** Carefully read and learn the **radiographic anatomy** section of each chapter. Include the anatomic reviews on labeled radiographs provided in each chapter of the textbook. Pay particular attention to those items in **bold type** and to the **summary review boxes** where provided.

Step 2.   B. **Workbook:** Complete **Part I** of the review exercises on **radiographic anatomy.** Do **not** look up the answers in the textbook or look at the answer sheet until you have answered as many of the questions as you can. Then refer to the textbook and/or the answer sheet and correct or complete those questions you missed. Reread those sections of the textbook in which you could not answer questions. Textbook page numbers are provided next to each review exercise in this workbook.

PART II

Step 3. **A. Textbook:** Carefully read and study Part II on **radiographic positioning.** Note the general **positioning considerations, alternate modalities,** and **pathologic indications** for each chapter. This is followed by the specific positioning pages, which include **pathology demonstrated; technical factors;** and the **dose ranges** of skin, midline, and specific organ doses where provided. Pay particular attention to dose comparisons between different techniques, or anteroposterior (AP) versus posteroanterior (PA) projections. Learn the **specific positioning steps,** the **central ray location and angle,** and the four-part **radiographic criteria** for each projection or position.

Step 4. **B. Workbook:** Complete **Part II** of the review exercises, which include **technical considerations and positioning.** Also included is a section on **problem solving for technical and positioning errors.** As before, complete as many of the questions as you can before looking up the answers in the textbook or checking the answers on the answer sheet.

The last review exercise covers **radiographic critique questions** in the workbook. This challenging section is based on the critique radiographs at the end of chapters in the textbook. These important exercises will help you make the transition from factual knowledge to application and will help you prepare for clinical experience. **Compare each critique radiographs that demonstrate errors with correctly positioned radiographs in that chapter of the textbook** and see if you can determine which radiographic criteria points could be improved and which are repeatable errors. Students who complete these exercises successfully will be ahead of those students who don't attempt them before coming to the classroom. The instructor will then explain and clarify those repeatable and nonrepeatable errors on each radiograph.

PART III

Step 5. **Workbook – Laboratory Activity:** These exercises must be performed in a radiographic laboratory using a phantom and/or a student (without making exposure) with an energized radiographic unit and illuminators for viewing radiographs. Arrange for a time when you can use your radiographic laboratory or a diagnostic radiographic room in a clinic setting.

This is one of the most important aspects of this learning series and should not be neglected or underemphasized. Students frequently have difficulty transferring the information they have learned about positioning to effective use in a clinical setting. Therefore you must carry out the laboratory activities as described in each chapter. Your instructors and/or lab assistants will assist you as needed in these exercises.

Each radiograph taken of the phantom and/or other radiographs provided by your instructor should be evaluated as described in your lab manual. Critique and evaluate each radiograph for errors of less-than-optimal positioning or exposure factors based on radiographic criteria provided in the textbook. Also, with the help of your instructor, learn how to discriminate between less-than-optimal, but passable radiographs, and those that need to be repeated. This generally requires additional experience and practice before you can make these judgments without assistance from a supervising technologist or radiologist.

Step 6. Self-Test

You should **take the self-test only after you have completed all of the preceding steps.** Treat the self-test like an actual exam. After you have completed it, compare your answers with the answer sheet at the end of this workbook. If your score is less than 90% to 95%, you should go back and review the textbook again; pay special attention to the areas you missed before you take the final chapter evaluation exam provided by your instructor.

Warning: Statistics prove that students who diligently complete all the exercises described in this section will invariably get higher grades in their positioning courses and will perform better in the clinical setting than those who don't. **Avoid the temptation of taking shortcuts.** If you bypass some of these exercises or just fill in the answers from the answer sheets, your instructors will know by your grade and by your clinical performance that you have taken these shortcuts. Most importantly, you will know that you are not doing your best and you will have difficulty competing with better prepared technologists in the job market when you graduate.

Go to it and enjoy the feeling of satisfaction and success that only comes when you know you're doing your best!

CHAPTER 14

Upper Gastrointestinal System

Radiographic procedures involving the administration of some form of contrast medium are described in the next four chapters. These include common procedures, which may comprise 20% to 30% of the radiology department case load. You will likely be performing these examinations early in your clinical training. If you learn and understand the fundamentals provided in these next four chapters, combined with clinical experience, you will soon become a proficient radiographer of these organ systems.

CHAPTER OBJECTIVES

After you have completed **all** the activities of this chapter, you will be able to:

- _____ 1. List the major organs of the upper gastrointestinal system and specific accessory organs.
- _____ 2. List the three primary functions of the digestive system.
- _____ 3. List three divisions of the pharynx.
- _____ 4. Identify the anatomic location, function, and features of the esophagus, stomach, and duodenum.
- _____ 5. Identify the effect of body position on the distribution of air and contrast media in the stomach.
- _____ 6. Describe the impact of body habitus on the position and shape of the stomach.
- _____ 7. Using drawings and radiographs, identify specific anatomy of the upper gastrointestinal system.
- _____ 8. Identify differences between mechanical digestion and chemical digestion.
- _____ 9. Identify the contrast media, patient preparation, room preparation, and the fluoroscopic procedure for an esophagram and an upper gastrointestinal series.
- _____ 10. List and define the specific pathologic indications and contraindications for an esophagram and upper GI series.
- _____ 11. Match specific types of pathology to the correct radiographic appearances and signs.
- _____ 12. Describe specific breathing maneuvers and positioning techniques used to detect esophageal reflux.
- _____ 13. List the basic and special positions or projections for the esophagram and upper gastrointestinal (GI) series to include, size and type of image receptor, central ray location, direction and angulation of the central ray, and anatomy best demonstrated.
- _____ 14. Identify which anatomy is best demonstrated with specific projections of an esophagram and upper GI series.
- _____ 15. List patient dose ranges for skin, midline, and gonads for specific projections of an esophagram and upper GI series.
- _____ 16. Given various hypothetical situations, identify the correct modification of a position and/or exposure factors to improve the radiographic image.

POSITIONING AND FILM CRITIQUE

- _____ 1. Using a peer, position for basic and special projections for the esophagram and upper GI series.
- _____ 2. Critique and evaluate esophagram and upper GI series radiographs based on the four divisions of radiographic criteria: (1) structures shown, (2) position, (3) collimation and CR, and (4) exposure criteria.
- _____ 3. Distinguish between acceptable and unacceptable esophagram and upper GI series radiographs that result from exposure factors, motion, collimation, positioning, or other errors.

Learning Exercises

Complete the following review exercises after reading the associated pages in the textbook as indicated by each exercise. Answers to each review exercise are given at the end of the review exercises.

PART I: Radiographic Anatomy, Digestion, and Body Habitus

REVIEW EXERCISE A: Radiographic Anatomy of the Upper Gastrointestinal System
                      (see textbook pp. 442-448)

1. List the seven major components of the alimentary canal:

    A. _____   E. _____

    B. _____   F. _____

    C. _____   G. _____

    D. _____

2. List the four accessory organs of digestion:

    A. _____   C. _____

    B. _____   D. _____

3. What are the three primary functions of the digestive system?

    A. _____

    B. _____

    C. _____

4. What two terms refer to a radiographic examination of the pharynx and esophagus?

    _____ or _____

5. Which term describes the radiographic study of the distal esophagus, stomach, and duodenum?

    _____

6. The three pairs of salivary glands that are accessory organs of digestion associated with the mouth are:

    A. _____

    B. _____

    C. _____

7. The act of swallowing is called _____ .

8. List the three divisions of the pharynx:

    A. _____   B. _____   C. _____

9. What structures create the two indentations seen along the lateral border of the esophagus?

    A. _____   B. _____

10. List the three structures that pass through the diaphragm.

    A. _____   B. _____   C. _____

11. What part of the upper GI tract is a common site for ulcer disease? _____

12. What term describes the junction between the duodenum and jejunum? _____
    (This is a significant reference point in small bowel studies.)

13. The C-loop of the duodenum and pancreas are _____ (intraperitoneal or retroperitoneal)
    structures?

14. Name the following structures of the mouth and pharynx (Fig. 14-1):

    A. _____

    B. _____

    C. _____

    D. _____

    E. _____

    F. _____

    G. _____

    H. _____

    I. _____

    J. _____

    K. _____

    L. _____

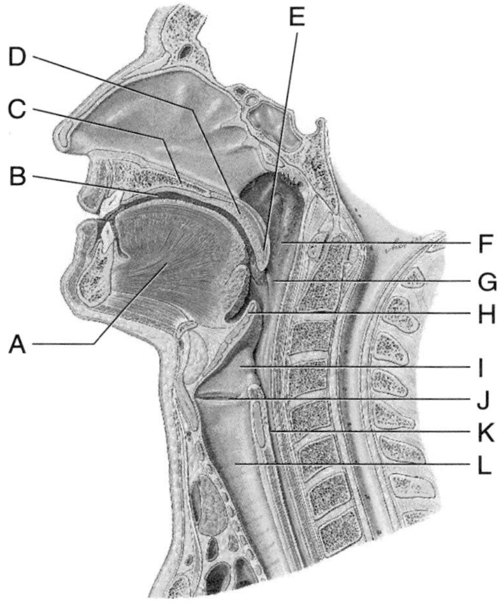

Fig. 14-1 Structures of the mouth and pharynx.

15. Identify the correct body position for each of the following drawings of the stomach filled with air and barium (Fig.
    14-2) (erect, prone, or supine) Barium = white, Air = black.

    A. _____   B. _____   C. _____

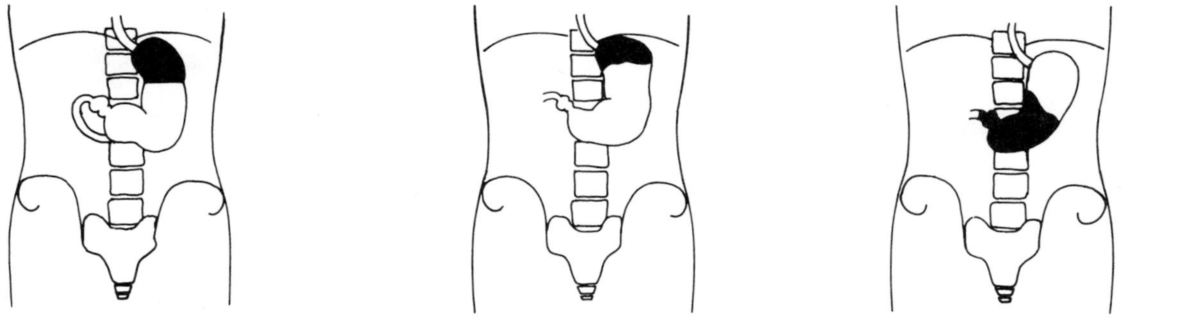

Fig. 14-2 Body position identification based on stomach filled with air or barium.

16.   True/False: The body of the stomach curves inferiorly and posteriorly from the fundus.

17.   Identify the parts labeled on Fig. 14-3:

A.   _____

B.   _____

C.   _____

D.   _____
      (formed by rugae along lesser curvature)

E.   _____

F.   _____

G.   _____

H.   _____

I.   _____

J.   _____
      (abdominal segment of esophagus)

K.   _____

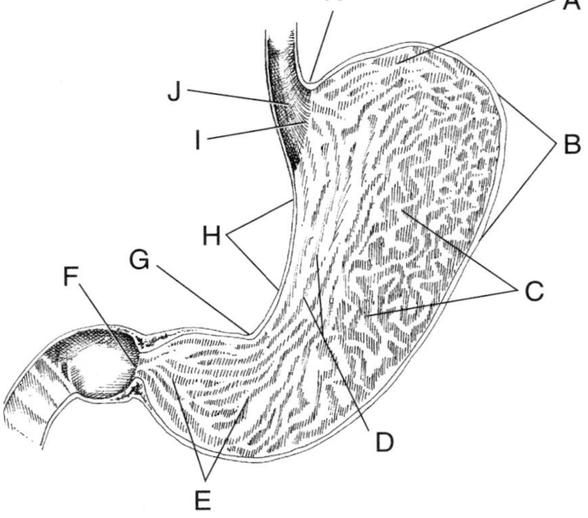

Fig. 14-3 Sectional anatomy of the stomach.

18.   The three main subdivisions of the stomach are:

A.   _____   B.   _____   C.   _____

19.   The division of the stomach labeled "E" is divided into two parts, which are _____ and

      _____ .

20.   The correct term for "gastric folds" of the stomach is _____ .

21.   Identify the parts labeled on Fig. 14-4:

A.   _____

B.   _____

C.   _____

D.   _____

E.   _____

F.   _____

G.   _____

H.   Region of _____

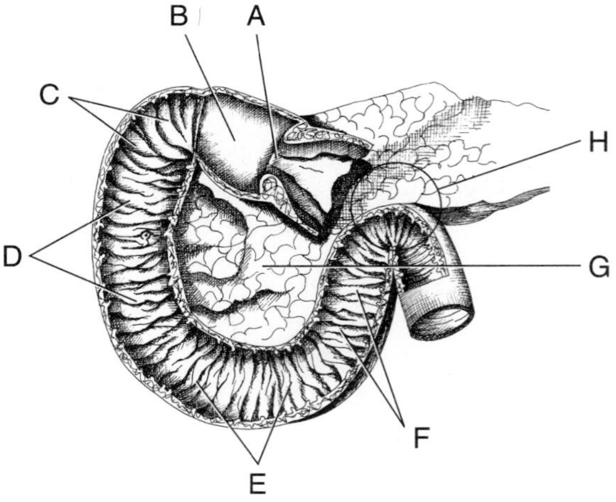

Fig. 14-4 Anatomy of the duodenum and pancreas.

22. Name the two anatomic structures implicated in the phrase "romance of the abdomen" illustrated in Fig. 14-4.

   A. _____   B. _____

23. Identify the gastrointestinal structures labeled on Fig. 14-5:

   A. _____

   B. _____

   C. _____

   D. _____

   E. _____

   F. _____

   G. _____

   H. _____

   I. _____

   J. _____

   K. _____

   L. _____

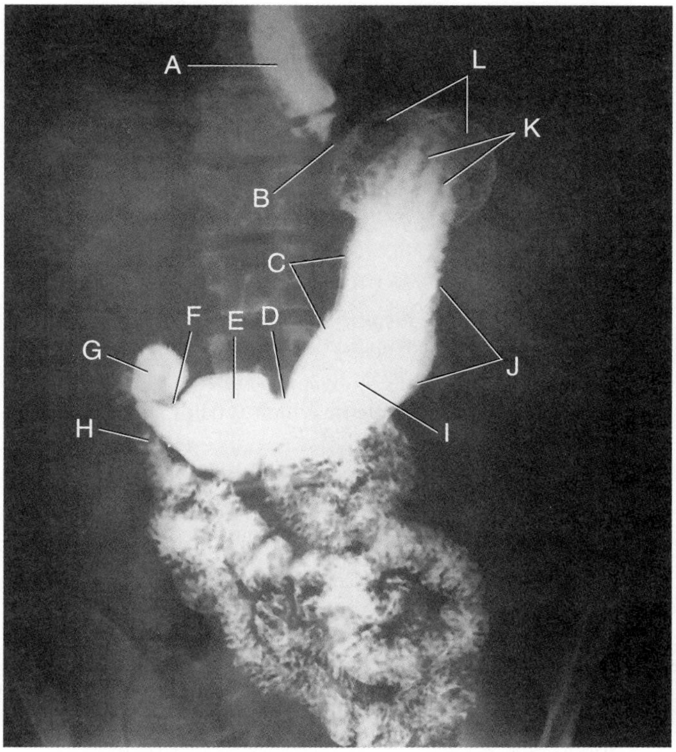

Fig. 14-5 Radiograph of gastrointestinal structures.

REVIEW EXERCISE B: Mechanical and Chemical Digestion and Body Habitus (see textbook pp. 419-421)

1. True/False: Mechanical digestion includes movements of all the gastrointestinal tract.

2. Peristaltic activity is *not* found in the following structure:

   A. Pharynx   C. Stomach

   B. Esophagus   D. Small intestine

3. Stomach contents are churned into a semifluid mass called _____ .

4. A churning or mixing activity present in the small bowel is called _____ .

5. List the three classes of substances that are ingested and need to be chemically digested.

   A. _____   B. _____   C. _____

6. Biological catalysts that speed up the process of digestion are called _____ .

7. List the end products of digestion of the following classes of foods:

   A. Carbohydrates _____

   B. Lipids _____

   C. Proteins _____

8. List the liquid substance that aids in digestion and is manufactured in the liver and stored in the gallbladder.

   _____

9. Absorption primarily takes place in the (A), _____ although some substances are absorbed

   through the lining of the (B) _____ .

10. _____ is a substance that is not an enzyme but serves to emulsify fats.

11. Of the three primary food substances listed in question 7, the digestion of which one begins in the mouth?

   _____

12. Any residues of digestion or unabsorbed digestive products are eliminated from the _____
    as a component of feces.

13. Peristalsis is an example of which type of digestion? _____

14. Which term describes food once it is mixed with gastric secretions in the stomach? _____

15. A high and transverse stomach would be found in a(n) _____ patient.

    A. Hypersthenic   C. Hyposthenic

    B. Sthenic   D. Asthenic

16. A J-shaped stomach more vertical and lower in the abdomen with the duodenal bulb at the level of L3-4 would be

    found in a _____ patient.

    A. Hypersthenic   C. Hyposthenic/asthenic

    B. Sthenic   D. None of the above

17. On the average, how much will abdominal organs drop in the erect position? _____

18. Name the two abdominal organs most dramatically affected, in relation to location, by body habitus:

    A. _____   B. _____

19. Would the fundus of the stomach be more superior or more inferior when one takes in a deep breath?

    _____ Why? _____

20. Match the types of mechanical digestion that occur in each of the following anatomical sites (each anatomical site may
    have more than one type of digestion).

	ANATOMICAL SITES		TYPES OF MECHANICAL DIGESTION
_____	1. Oral cavity	A.	Mastication
_____	2. Pharynx	B.	Deglutition
_____	3. Esophagus	C.	Peristalsis
_____	4. Stomach	D.	Mixing
_____	5. Small intestine	E.	Rhythmic segmentation

PART II: Radiographic Positioning

REVIEW EXERCISE C: Contrast Media, Fluoroscopy, and Pathologic Indications and Contraindications for
Upper Gastrointestinal Studies (see textbook pp. 452-468)

1. True/False: With the use of digital fluoroscopy, the number of post-fluoroscopy radiographs ordered has greatly diminished.

2. What is the most common form of positive contrast medium used for studies of the gastrointestinal system?

    _____

3. Another term for a negative contrast medium is _____ .

4. What types of crystals are most commonly used to produce carbon dioxide gas as a negative contrast medium for

    gastrointestinal studies? _____

5. Is a mixture of barium sulfate a suspension or a solution? _____

6. True/False: Barium sulfate never dissolves in water.

7. True/False: Certain salts of barium are poisonous to humans, so barium contrast studies require a pure sulfate salt of
    barium for human consumption during GI studies.

8. What is the ratio of water to barium for a thin mixture of barium sulfate? _____

9. What is the chemical symbol for barium sulfate? _____

10. When is the use of barium sulfate contraindicated? _____

11. What patient condition would prevent the use of a water-soluble contrast media for an upper GI?

    _____

12. What is the major advantage for using a double-contrast media technique for esophagrams and upper GIs?

    _____

13. The speed with which barium sulfate passes through the GI tract is called gastric _____ .

14. What is the purpose of the gas with a double contrast media technique?

    _____

15. Image intensification:

    A. The photospot or cine images, such as recorded on 105 mm film, are taken from the _____
        (input or output) side of the image intensifier?

    B. Conventional spot cassette taken on 18 x 24 cm (8 x 10 in.) cassettes are taken from the _____
        (input or output) side of the image intensifier?

    C. Which of the images in A or B above is the brighter image? _____

    D. How many times brighter is the fluoro image when enhanced or brightened by the image intensifier? _____

16. What device found beneath the radiographic table when correctly positioned greatly reduces scatter from the fluoro-scopic x-ray tube?

   A. Lead skirt   B. Lead drape   C. Bucky slot shield   D. Fluoroscopy tube shield

17. How is the device referred to in question 16 activated or placed in its correct position for fluoroscopy?

   _____

18. What is the major benefit in using a compression paddle during an upper GI study?

   A. Reduces exposure to the patient   C. Reduces exposure to arms and hands of radiologist

   B. Reduces exposure to the eyes of radiologist   D. Reduces exposure to the torso of radiologist

19. During an upper GI fluoroscopy procedure, if the technologist stands directly beside the radiologist next to the pa-tient's head and shoulders (see textbook, p. 56, zone C in Fig. 166), how much radiation would the technologist re-ceive to the lead apron at waist level during each fluoro exam if the radiologist averaged 5 minutes of fluoroscopy exposure per patient? (Hint: determine exposure dose range in mR/min in zone C and multiply by 5 minutes.)

   _____

20. Where is the best place for the technologist to stand during an upper GI procedure, and how much exposure would he or she receive in that position with 5 minutes of fluoroscopy?

   _____

21. List the six advantages or unique features and capabilities of digital fluoroscopy over conventional fluoro recording systems:

   A. _____

   B. _____

   C. _____

   D. _____

   E. _____

   F. _____

22. What is another term describing intermittent "road mapping" when used in digital fluoroscopy?

   _____

23. Match the following definitions or statements to the correct pathologic indication for the esophagram:

   _____ A. Difficulty in swallowing   1. Achalasia

   _____ B. Replacement of normal squamous epithelium with columnar   2. Zenker's diverticulum
              -epithelium
   _____ C. May lead to esophagitis   3. Esophageal varices

   _____ D. May be secondary to cirrhosis of the liver   4. Carcinoma of esophagus

   _____ E. Large outpouching of the esophagus   5. Barrett's esophagus

   _____ F. Also called *cardiospasm*   6. Esophageal reflux

   _____ G. Most common form is adenocarcinoma   7. Dysphagia

24. Match the following definitions or statements to the correct pathologic indication for the upper GI series:

    ——— A. Blood in vomit   1. Hiatal hernia

    ——— B. Inflammation of lining of stomach   2. Gastric carcinoma

    ——— C. Blind outpouching of the mucosal wall   3. Bezoar

    ——— D. Undigested material trapped in stomach   4. Hematemesis

    ——— E. Synonymous with gastric or duodenal ulcer   5. Gastritis

    ——— F. Portion of stomach protruding through diaphragmatic opening   6. Perforating ulcer

    ——— G. Only 5% of ulcers lead to this form of ulcer   7. Peptic ulcer

    ——— H. Double contrast upper GI is the gold standard for diagnosing this condition   8. Diverticulae

25. Match the following pathologic conditions or diseases to the correct radiographic appearance:

    ——— A. Its presence indicates a possible sliding hiatal hernia   1. Ulcers

    ——— B. Speckled appearance of gastric mucosa   2. Hiatal hernia

    ——— C. "Wormlike" appearance of esophagus   3. Achalasia

    ——— D. Stricture of esophagus   4. Zenker's diverticulum

    ——— E. Gastric bubble above diaphragm   5. Schatzke's ring

    ——— F. Irregular filling defect within stomach   6. Gastritis

    ——— G. Enlarged recess in proximal esophagus   7. Esophageal varices

    ——— H. "Halo" sign during upper GI   8. Gastric carcinoma

REVIEW EXERCISE D: Patient Preparation and Positioning for Esophagram and Upper Gastrointestinal Study (see textbook pp. 427-445)

1. What does the acronym NPO stand for and what does it mean?

    _____

2. True/False: The patient must be NPO 4 to 6 hours before an esophagram.

3. True/False: The esophagram usually begins with fluoroscopy with the patient in the erect position.

4. What materials may be used for swallowing to aid in the diagnosis of radiolucent foreign bodies in the esophagus?

    _____

5. List the four tests that may be performed to detect esophageal reflux:

    A. _____   C. _____

    B. _____   D. _____

6. A breathing technique in which the patient takes in a deep breath and bears down is called the

   _____

7. What position is the patient usually placed in during the water test? _____

8. The compression paddle is sometimes used by the radiologist during an esophagram to better visualize the

   _____ region.

9. What type of contrast media should be used if the patient has a history of bowel perforation?

   _____

10. What is the minimum amount of time that the patient should be NPO before an upper GI?

    _____

11. Why should cigarette and gum chewing be restricted before an upper GI?

    _____

12. Why should the technologist review the patient's chart before the beginning of an upper GI?
    A. Identify any known allergies   C. Look for pertinent clinical history
    B. Ensure that the proper study has been ordered   D. All of the above

13. In which hand does the patient usually hold the barium cup during the start of an upper GI? _____

14. List the recommended dosages of barium sulfate during an upper GI for each of the following pediatric age groups:

    Newborn to 1 year: _____

    1 to 3 years: _____

    3 to 10 years: _____

    Over 10 years: _____

15. What is the name of the special adapter attached to a syringe to deliver contrast media through a nasogastric tube?

    _____

16. Which one of the following imaging modalities is an alternative to an esophagram in detecting esophageal varices?
    A. Nuclear medicine   C. Sonography
    B. Computed tomography   D. None of the above

17. Gastric emptying studies are performed using:
    A. Intraesophageal sonography   C. Magnetic resonance
    B. Radionuclides   D. Computed tomography

18. Why is the RAO preferred over the LAO for an esophagram?

    _____

19. How much obliquity should be used for the RAO projection of the esophagus?

   _____

20. Which optional position should be performed to demonstrate the upper esophagus located between the shoulders?

   _____

21. Which aspect of the GI tract is best demonstrated with an RAO position during an upper GI?

   A. Fundus of stomach   C. Body of stomach
   B. Pylorus of stomach and C-loop   D. Fourth (ascending) portion of duodenum

22. How much obliquity should be used for the RAO position during an upper GI?

   A. 30 to 35°   C. 40 to 70°
   B. 15 to 20°   D. 10 to 15°

23. What is the average kVp range for an esophagram and upper GI when using barium sulfate (without double-contrast study)?

   _____

24. Which aspect of the upper GI tract will be filled with barium with the PA projection (prone position)?

   _____

25. What is the purpose of the PA axial projection for the hypersthenic patient during an upper GI?

   _____

26. What CR angle is used for the PA axial projection?

   A. 10 to 15° caudad   C. 35 to 45° cephalad
   B. 20 to 25° cephalad   D. 60 to 70° cephalad

27. Which projection taken during an upper GI will best demonstrate the retrogastric space?

   A. RAO   C. LPO
   B. Lateral   D. PA

28. A double contrast upper GI requires a slightly **higher** or **lower kVp** compared with a single contrast medium study?

   _____

29. The female gonadal dose range for a well-collimated RAO projection of the upper GI procedure is:

   A. 10 to 15 mrad   C. 200 to 500 mrad
   B. 50 to 100 mrad   D. 600 to 1000 mrad

30. The upper GI series usually begins with the table and patient in the _____ position.

31. The five most common basic or routine projections for an upper GI series are (not counting a possible AP scout image):

   A. _____   C. _____   E. _____

   B. _____   D. _____

32. The three most common basic or routine projections for an esophagram are:

   A. ———————————— B. ———————————— C. ————————————

33. The major parts of the stomach on an average patient are usually confined to which abdominal quadrant?

   _____

34. Most of the duodenum is usually found to which side of the midline on an average patient? Right or left?

   _____

35. True/False: Respiration should be suspended during inspiration for upper GI radiographic projections.

REVIEW EXERCISE E: Problem Solving for Technical and Positioning Errors (see textbook pp. 461-478)

1. **Situation:** A radiograph of an RAO projection taken during an esophagram demonstrates incomplete filling of the esophagus with barium. What can the technologist do to ensure better filling of the esophagus during the repeat exposure?

   _____

   _____

2. **Situation:** A series of radiographs taken during an upper GI reveal that the stomach mucosa is not well visualized. The following factors were used during this positioning routine: high-speed screens, Bucky, 40 in. (102 cm) SID, 80 kVp, 30 mAs, and 300 ml of barium sulfate ingested during the procedure. Which exposure factor should be changed to produce a more diagnostic study?

   _____

   _____

3. **Situation:** A radiograph taken during an upper GI reveals that the anatomical side marker is missing. The technologist is unsure whether it is a recumbent AP or PA projection. The fundus of the stomach is filled with barium. Which position does this radiograph represent?

   _____

   _____

4. **Situation:** A radiograph of an RAO projection taken during an upper GI reveals that the duodenal bulb is not well demonstrated and not profiled. The RAO was a 45° oblique performed on a hypersthenic-type patient. What positioning modification needs to be made to produce a better image of the duodenal bulb?

   _____

   _____

5. **Situation:** A radiograph of an upper GI was taken, but the student technologist is unsure of the position. The radiograph demonstrates that the fundus is filled with barium, but the duodenal bulb is air-filled and seen in profile. Which position does this radiograph represent?

   _____

   _____

6. **Situation:** A patient with a clinical history of hiatal hernia comes to the radiology department. Which procedure should be performed on this patient to rule out this condition?

_____

7. **Situation:** A patient with a possible lacerated duodenum enters the emergency room. The physician orders an upper GI to determine the extent of the injury. What type of contrast media should be used for this examination?

_____

_____

8. **Situation:** A patient with a fish bone stuck in his esophagus enters the emergency room. What modification to a standard esophagram may be needed to locate the foreign body?

_____

_____

9. **Situation:** An upper GI is being performed on a thin, asthenic-type patient. Due to room scheduling conflicts, this patient was brought into your room for the overhead follow-up images after the upper GI fluoro is completed. Where would you center the CR and the 11 x 14 in. (30 x 35 cm) image receptor to ensure that you included the stomach and duodenal regions?

_____

_____

10. **Situation:** A patient with a clinical history of a possible bezoar comes to the radiology department. What is a bezoar, and what radiographic study should be performed to demonstrate this condition?

_____

_____

11. **Situation:** A radiograph of an RAO position taken during an esophagram reveals that the esophagus is superimposed over the vertebral column. What positioning error led to this radiographic outcome?

_____

_____

12. **Situation:** A PA projection taken during an upper GI series performed on an infant reveals that the body and pylorus of the stomach are superimposed. What modification needs to be employed during the repeat exposure to separate these two regions?

_____

_____

_____

PART III: Laboratory Exercises (see textbook pp. 469-478)

You must gain experience in positioning each part of the esophagram and upper GI procedures before performing the following exams on actual patients. You can get experience in positioning and radiographic evaluation of these projections by performing exercises using radiographic phantoms and practicing on other students (although you will not be taking actual exposures).

LABORATORY EXERCISE A: Radiographic Evaluation

1. Evaluate and critique the radiographs produced during the previous experiments, additional radiographs of esophagrams, and upper GI procedures provided by your instructor. Evaluate each position for the following points. (Check off when completed.):

_____ Evaluate the completeness of the study. (Are all the pertinent anatomic structures included on the radiograph?)

_____ Evaluate for positioning or centering errors (e.g., rotation, off centering).

_____ Evaluate for correct exposure factors and possible motion. (Are the density and contrast of the images acceptable?)

_____ Determine whether markers and an acceptable degree of collimation and/or area shielding are visible on the images.

LABORATORY EXERCISE B: Physical Positioning

On another person, simulate performing all basic and special projections of the upper GI as follows: (Check off each when completed satisfactorily.) Include the following six steps as described in the textbook.

Step 1. Appropriate size and type of image receptor holder with correct markers
Step 2. Correct CR placement and centering of part to CR and/or image receptor
Step 3. Accurate collimation
Step 4. Area shielding of patient where advisable
Step 5. Use of proper immobilizing devices when needed
Step 6. Approximate correct exposure factors, breathing instructions where applicable, and "making" exposure

Projections	Step 1	Step 2	Step 3	Step 4	Step 5	Step 6
• RAO esophagram	____	____	____	____	____	____
• Left lateral esophagram	____	____	____	____	____	____
• AP (PA) esophagram	____	____	____	____	____	____
• LAO esophagram	____	____	____	____	____	____
• Soft tissue lateral esophagram	____	____	____	____	____	____
• RAO upper GI	____	____	____	____	____	____
• PA upper GI	____	____	____	____	____	____
• Right lateral upper GI	____	____	____	____	____	____
• LPO upper GI	____	____	____	____	____	____
• AP upper GI	____	____	____	____	____	____

Answers to Review Exercises

Review Exercise A: Radiographic Anatomy of the Upper Gastrointestinal System

1. A. Mouth
   B. Pharynx
   C. Esophagus
   D. Stomach
   E. Small intestine
   F. Large intestine
   G. Anus
2. A. Salivary glands
   B. Pancreas
   C. Liver
   D. Gallbladder
3. A. Intake and digestion of food
   B. Absorption of digested food particles
   C. Elimination of solid waste products
4. Esophagram or barium swallow
5. Upper gastrointestinal series (UGI) or upper GI
6. A. Parotid
   B. Sublingual
   C. Submandibular
7. Deglutition
8. A. Nasopharynx
   B. Oropharynx
   C. Laryngopharynx
9. A. Aortic arch
   B. Left primary bronchus
10. A. Esophagus
    B. Inferior vena cava
    C. Aorta
11. Duodenal bulb or cap
12. Duodenojejunal flexure (suspensory ligament or ligament of Trietz)
13. Retroperitoneal or behind peritoneum
14. A. Tongue
    B. Oral cavity (mouth)
    C. Hard palate
    D. Soft palate
    E. Uvula
    F. Nasopharynx
    G. Oropharynx
    H. Epiglottis
    I. Laryngopharynx
    J. Larynx
    K. Esophagus
    L. Trachea
15. A. Erect
    B. Prone
    C. Supine
16. False (inferiorly and anteriorly)
17. A. Fundus
    B. Greater curvature
    C. Body
    D. Gastric canal
    E. Pyloric portion
    F. Pyloric orifice (or just pylorus)
    G. Angular notch (incisura angularis)
    H. Lesser curvature
    I. Esophagogastric junction (cardiac orifice)
    J. Cardiac antrum
    K. Cardiac notch (incisura cardiaca)
18. A. Fundus (labeled A)
    B. Body or corpus (labeled C)
    C. Pyloric (labeled E)
19. Pyloric antrum and pyloric canal
20. Rugae.
21. A. Pylorus (pyloric sphincter)
    B. Bulb or cap of duodenum
    C. First (superior) portion of duodenum
    D. Second (descending) portion of duodenum
    E. Third (horizontal) portion of duodenum
    F. Fourth (ascending) portion of duodenum
    G. Head of pancreas
    H. Suspensory ligament of duodenum or ligament of Treitz
22. A. Head of pancreas
    B. C loop of duodenum
23. A. Distal esophagus
    B. Area of esophagogastric junction
    C. Lesser curve of stomach
    D. Angular notch-incisura angularis
    E. Pyloric region of stomach
    F. Pyloric valve or sphincter
    G. Duodenal bulb
    H. Second-descending portion of duodenum
    I. Body of stomach
    J. Greater curvature of stomach
    K. Gastric folds or rugae of stomach
    L. Fundus of stomach

Review Exercise B: Mechanical and Chemical Digestion and Body Habitus

1. True
2. A. Pharynx
3. Chyme
4. Rhythmic segmentation
5. A. Carbohydrates
   B. Proteins
   C. Lipids (fats)
6. Enzymes
7. A. Simple sugars
   B. Fatty acids and glycerol
   C. Amino acids
8. Bile
9. A. Small intestine
   B. Stomach
10. Bile
11. Carbohydrates
12. Large intestine
13. Mechanical
14. Chyme
15. A. Hypersthenic

16. C. Hyposthenic/asthenic
17. 1 to 2 in. (2.5 to 5 cm)
18. A. Stomach
    B. Gall bladder
19. Inferior, because of its proximity to the diaphragm
20. 1. A, B
    2. B
    3. B, C
    4. C, D
    5. C, E

Review Exercise C: Contrast Media, Fluoroscopy, and Pathologic Indications and Contraindications for Upper Gastrointestinal Studies

1. True
2. Barium sulfate
3. Radiolucent contrast medium
4. Calcium carbonate
5. Suspension
6. True
7. True
8. One part water to one part barium sulfate (1:1)
9. BaSO4
10. When the mixture may escape into the peritoneal cavity (p. 424)
11. Sensitivity to iodine
12. Better coating and visibility of the mucosa. Polyps, diverticulae, and ulcers are better demonstrated
13. Motility
14. It forces the barium sulfate against the mucosa for better coating
15. A. Output
    B. Input
    C. A. Photospot or cine images are brighter
    D. 1000 to 6000 times
16. C. Bucky slot shield
17. By moving the Bucky all the way to the end of the table
18. C. Reduces exposure to arms and hands of radiologist
19. 1.7 − 3.3 × 5 = 8.5 − 16.5 mRad
20. Away from the patient and table and/or behind the radiologist. (Zone F) Would receive less than 2.0 mrad (0.4 x 5 = 2.0 mrad)
21. A. No cassettes are required for filming
    B. Optional post-fluoroscopy overhead images
    C. Multiple frame formatting and multiple original films
    D. Cine loop capability
    E. Image enhancement and manipulation (by computers)
    F. Reduced patient exposure (of 30 to 50%)

22. "Frame hold" capability of specific fluoroscopy images
23. A. 7, B. 5, C. 6, D. 3, E. 2, F. 1, G. 4
24. A. 4, B. 5, C. 8, D. 3, E. 7, F. 1, G. 6, H. 2
25. A. 5, B. 6, C.7, D. 3, E. 2, F. 8, G. 4, H.1

Review Exercise D: Patient Preparation and Positioning for Esophagram and Upper Gastrointestinal Study

1. "Non Per Os," Latin for "nothing by mouth" (pg. 466)
2. False (8 hours NPO for upper GI but not for an esophagram)
3. True
4. Barium soaked cotton balls, barium pills or marshmallows followed by thin barium
5. A. Breathing exercises
   B. Water test
   C. Compression technique
   D. Toe-touch maneuver
6. Valsalva maneuver
7. LPO
8. Esophagogastric junction
9. Oral, water-soluble iodinated contrast media
10. Eight hours
11. Both activities tend to increase gastric secretions
12. D. All of the above
13. Left hand
14. Newborn to 1 year: 2 to 4 ounces
    1 to 3 years: 4 to 6 ounces
    3 to 10 years: 6 to 12 ounces
    Over 10 years: 12 to 16 ounces
15. Christmas tree or tapered adapter
16. C. Sonography
17. B. Radionuclides

18. Places the esophagus between the vertebral column and heart
19. 35 to 40°
20. Optional swimmer's lateral
21. B. Pylorus of stomach and C-loop
22. C. 40 to 70°
23. 100 to 125 kVp
24. Body and pylorus of stomach and duodenal bulb
25. To prevent superimposition of the pylorus over the duodenal bulb, and to better visualize the lesser and greater curvatures of the stomach
26. C. 35 to 45° cephalad
27. B. Lateral
28. Lower
29. A. 10 to 15 mrad
30. Upright (erect)
31. A. RAO
    B. PA
    C. Right lateral
    D. LPO
    E. AP
32. A. RAO
    B. Left lateral
    C. AP
33. Left Upper Quadrant (LUQ)
34. Right
35. False (expiration)

Review Exercise E: Problem Solving for Technical and Positioning Errors

1. When using thin barium, have the patient drink continuously during the exposure. With thick barium, have the patient hold two or three spoonfuls in the mouth and make the exposure immediately after swallowing.
2. When using barium sulfate as a contrast media, 110 to 125 kVp should be used to ensure proper penetration of the contrast filled stomach and visualize the mucosa. 80 to 100 kVp would be adequate for a double contrast study.
3. AP. Since the fundus is more posterior than the body or pylorus, it will fill with barium when the patient is in a supine (AP) position.
4. With a hypersthenic patient, more rotation of up to 70° may be required to better profile the duodenal bulb. (Note: the radiologist under fluoro will frequently oblique the patient as needed for the overhead oblique to best profile the duodenal region.)
5. The LPO position (recumbent) will produce an image where the fundus and body is filled with barium but the duodenal bulb is airfilled.
6. Upper GI series
7. An oral, water-soluble contrast media should be used for an upper GI when ruptured viscus or bowel is suspected (not barium sulfate, which is not water-soluble).
8. With radiolucent foreign bodies in the esophagus, shredded cotton soaked in barium sulfate may be used to help locate it. Marshmallows with barium or a barium capsule may also be used.
9. Would center lower than usual, to the mid L3-4 region or about 1½ to 2 in. (4 to 5 cm) above the level of the iliac crest
10. A mass of undigested material that gets trapped in the stomach-a rare condition, but it can be diagnosed with an upper GI study.
11. Under-obliquity or rotation of the body into the RAO position led to the esophagus being superimposed over the vertebral column
12. Angle the CR 20 to 25° cephalad to open up the body and pylorus of the stomach

SELF-TEST

My Score = _____ %

Directions: This self-test should be taken only after completing **all** of the readings, review exercises, and laboratory activities. The purpose of this test is not only to provide a good learning exercise but also to serve as a good indicator of what your final evaluation grade will be. It is strongly suggested that if you do not get at least a 90% to 95% grade on this self-test, you should review those areas where you missed questions **before** going to your instructor for the final evaluation exam.

1. Which one of the following is **not** a function of the gastrointestinal system?

   A. Intake and digestion of food   C. Production of hormones

   B. Absorption of nutrients   D. Elimination of waste products

2. Which one of the following is **not** a salivary gland?

   A. Parotid   C. Pineal

   B. Sublingual   D. Submandibular

3. What is another term for an esophagram? _____

4. What is the name of the condition that results from a viral infection of the parotid gland? _____

5. The act of chewing is termed:

   A. Mastication   C. Aspiration

   B. Deglutition   D. Peristalsis

6. Which structure in the pharynx prevents aspiration of food and fluid into the larynx:

   A. Uvula   C. Soft palate

   B. Epiglottis   D. Laryngopharynx

7. The esophagus extends from C5-6 to:

   A. T9   C. T10

   B. L1   D. T11

8. Which one of the following structures does not pass through the diaphragm?

   A. Trachea   C. Aorta

   B. Esophagus   D. Inferior vena cava

9. Wavelike involuntary contractions that help propel food down the esophagus are called _____.

10. The Greek term *gaster,* or *gastro,* means _____.

11. Which one of the following aspects of the stomach is defined as an indentation between the body and pylorus?

    A. Cardiac antrum   C. Incisura cardiaca

    B. Pyloric antrum   D. Incisura angularis

12. Which aspect of the stomach will fill with air when the patient is prone?

    A. Fundus   C. Duodenal bulb

    B. Body   D. Pylorus

13. True/False: The numerous mucosal folds found in the small bowel are called *rugae.*

14.   True/False: The lateral margin of the stomach is called the *lesser curvature.*

15.   Which aspect of the stomach will barium gravitate to when the patient is in the supine position?

      _____

16.   Which two structures create the "romance of the abdomen?"

      _____

17.   Match the following aspects of the upper gastrointestinal system with the correct definition.

      _____   1. Pyloric orifice   A. Middle aspect of stomach

      _____   2. Cardiac notch   B. Horizontal portion of duodenum

      _____   3. Fundus   C. Rugae

      _____   4. Fourth portion of duodenum D. Opening between esophagus and stomach

      _____   5. Gastric folds   E. Opening leaving the stomach

      _____   6. Body   F. Found along superior aspect of fundus

      _____   7. Esophagogastric junction   G. Indentation found along lesser curvature

      _____   8. Angular notch   H. Ascending portion of duodenum

      _____   9. Third portion of duodenum   I. Most posterior aspect of stomach

18.   Identify the structures labeled on Fig. 14-6:

      A. _____

      B. _____

      C. _____

      D. _____

      E. _____

      F. _____

      G. _____

      H. _____

      I. _____

      J. _____

      K. _____

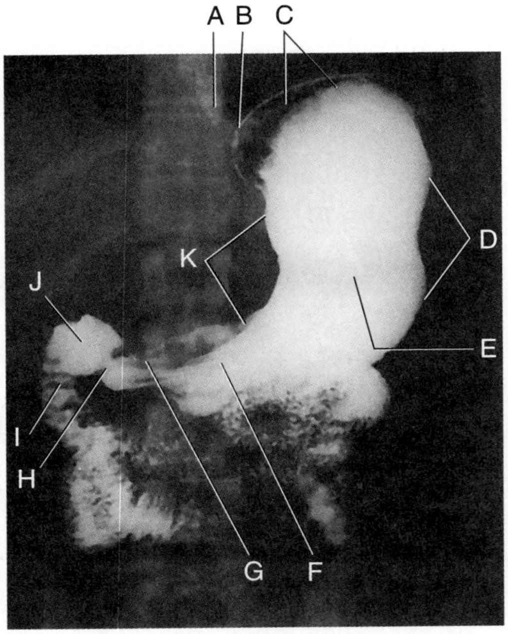

Fig. 14-6 Radiograph of gastrointestinal structures, demonstrating body position.

19.   A.   Which body position does Fig. 14-6 represent? _____

      B.   How could you determine this? _____

20. Which body position does Fig. 14-7 represent? _____

21. A.   Which body position does Fig. 14-8 represent? _____

    B.   How could you determine this? _____

22. A.   Which oblique (anterior or posterior) does Fig. 14-9 represent? _____

    B.   How could you determine this _____

    C.   Which specific oblique does Fig. 14-10 represent? _____

    D.   How could you determine this? _____

23. Which term describes food once it enters the stomach and is mixed with gastric fluids? _____

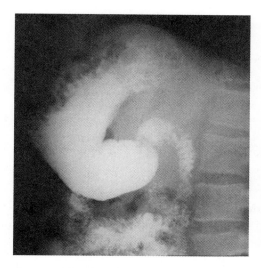

Fig. 14-7 Gastrointestinal radiograph demonstrating body position.

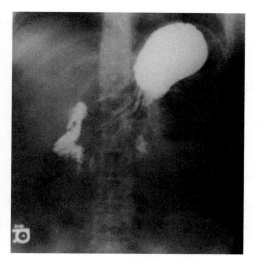

Fig. 14-8 Gastrointestinal radiograph demonstrating body position.

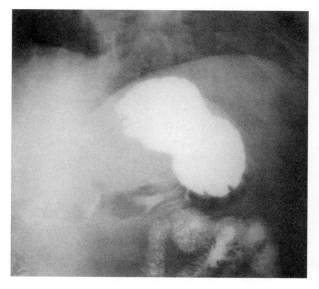

Fig. 14-9 Oblique radiograph of gastrointestinal structures.

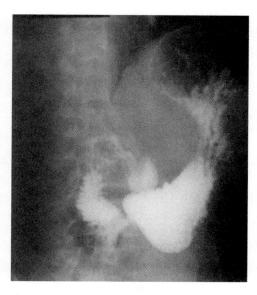

Fig. 14-10 Oblique radiograph of gastrointestinal structures.

24. Which one of the following nutrients is not digested?

    A. Vitamins   C. Carbohydrates

    B. Lipids   D. Proteins

25. The churning or mixing activity of chyme in the small intestine is called:

    A. Peristalsis   C. Rhythmic segmentation

    B. Deglutition   D. Digestion

26. A _____ or _____ type of body habitus will usually have a low

    and vertical stomach with the pyloric portion of the stomach at the level of _____.

27. A high and transverse stomach indicates a _____ body type with the pyloric portion at the

    level of _____.

28. What is the most common radiopaque contrast media used in the gastrointestinal system?

    _____

29. What type of radiolucent contrast medium is most commonly used for double-contrast gastrointestinal studies?

    _____

30. A. What is the ratio of barium to water for a thick mixture of barium sulfate? _____

    B.   What is the ratio for a thin barium mixture? _____

31. When should a water-soluble contrast media be used during an upper GI rather than barium sulfate?

    _____

32. Cinefluorography cameras record the image from the _____ (input or output) side of the
    image intensifier?

33. Image intensified fluoroscopy is _____ brighter than older conventional fluoroscopy with-
    out intensifiers.

    A. 100 times   C. 1000 to 6000 times

    B. 10 times   D. 10,000 to 60,000 times

34. True/False: Digital fluoroscopy does not require the use of image receptor cassettes.

35. Digital fluoroscopy leads to 30% to 50% _____ (higher or lower) patient dose as com-
    pared with conventional fluoroscopy.

36. Protective aprons of _____ mm lead equivalency must be worn during fluoroscopy.

    A. 1.0   C. 0.25

    B. 0.50   D. 0.15

37. A large, outpouching of the upper esophagus is:

    A. Zenker's diverticulum   C. Barrett's esophagus

    B. Achalasia   D. Esophageal varices

38. Other than the esophagram, what other imaging modality is used to diagnose Barrett's esophagus?

   A. Computed tomography   C. Magnetic resonance

   B. Nuclear medicine   D. Sonography

39. A phytobezoar is:

   A. Outpouching of the mucosal wall   C. Rare tumor

   B. Trapped mass of hair in the stomach   D. Trapped vegetable fiber in the stomach

40. What is the reason that the patient may be asked to swallow a mouthful of water drawn through a straw during an esophagram?

   _____

41. How much obliquity should be used for the RAO esophagram projection? _____

42. Why is an RAO rather than an LAO preferred for an esophagram?

   _____

43. Why is the AP projection of the esophagus not a preferred projection for the esophagram series?

   _____

44. What can be added to the barium sulfate and swallowed to detect a radiolucent foreign body lodged in the esopha-

   gus? _____

45. Which upper GI position will best demonstrate the retrogastric space? _____

46. An upper GI series is performed on an asthenic patient. A radiograph of the RAO position reveals that the duodenal bulb and C-loop are not in profile. The technologist obliqued the patient 50 degrees. What modification of the position is required during the repeat exposure?

   _____

47. A radiograph taken during a double-contrast, upper GI demonstrates that the fundus is barium-filled, and the duodenal bulb is air-filled. This was either an AP or a PA radiograph, which needs to be repeated. Which specific position does this radiograph represent?

   _____

48. **Situation:** A patient with a clinical history of cirrhosis of the liver with GI bleeding comes to the radiology department. What may be the most likely reason that an esophagram was ordered for this patient?

   _____

49. During an esophagram, the radiologist asks the patient to try to bear down as if having a bowel movement. What is the maneuver called and why did the radiologist make such a request?

   _____

50. During an upper GI, the radiologist reports that she sees a "halo" sign in the duodenum. What form of pathology did the radiologist observe?

   _____

CHAPTER 15

Lower Gastrointestinal System

CHAPTER OBJECTIVES

After you have completed **all** the activities of this chapter, you will be able to:

_____ 1. List three divisions of the small intestine and the major parts of the large intestine.

_____ 2. Identify the function, location, and pertinent anatomy of the small and large bowel.

_____ 3. Differentiate between the terms *colon* and *large intestine*.

_____ 4. Identify on drawings and radiographs, specific anatomy of the lower gastrointestinal canal from the duodenum through the anus.

_____ 5. Identify the sectional differences that differentiate the large intestine from the small intestine.

_____ 6. List specific pathologic indications and contraindications for a small bowel series and for a barium enema examination.

_____ 7. Match specific types of pathology to the correct radiographic appearances and signs.

_____ 8. Identify patient preparation for a small bowel series and for a barium enema.

_____ 9. List five safety concerns that must be followed during a barium enema procedure.

_____ 10. Identify the radiographic procedure and sequence for a small bowel series.

_____ 11. Identify the purpose, pathologic indications, and the methodology for the enteroclysis and the intubation method procedures.

_____ 12. Identify the patient preparation, room preparation, and the fluoroscopic procedure for a barium enema.

_____ 13. Identify the purpose, clinical indications, and methodology for an evacuative proctogram.

_____ 14. Identify the correct procedure for inserting a rectal tube.

_____ 15. List specific information related to the basic positions or projections of a small bowel series and barium enema examination to include size and type of, image receptor, central ray location, direction and angulation of the central ray, and the anatomy best demonstrated.

_____ 16. Identify the advantages, procedure, and positioning for an air contrast barium enema.

_____ 17. Identify patient dose ranges for skin, midline, and gonads for each small bowel and barium enema projection.

_____ 18. Given various hypothetical situations, identify the correct modification of a position and/or exposure factors to improve the radiographic image.

POSITIONING AND FILM CRITIQUE

_____ 1. Using a peer, position for basic and special projections for the small bowel and barium enema series.

_____ 2. Critique and evaluate small bowel and barium enema series radiographs based on the four divisions of radiographic criteria: (1) structures shown, (2) position, (3) collimation and CR, and (4) exposure criteria.

_____ 3. Distinguish between acceptable and unacceptable small bowel and barium enema series radiographs resulting from exposure factors, motion, collimation, positioning, or other errors.

Learning Exercises

Complete the following review exercises after reading the associated pages in the textbook as indicated by each exercise. Answers to each review exercise are given at the end of the review exercises.

PART I: Radiographic Anatomy

Review Exercise A: Radiographic Anatomy and Function of the Lower Gastrointestinal System (see textbook pp. 480-485)

1. List the three divisions of the small bowel in descending order starting with the widest division:

   A. _____   B. _____   C. _____

2. Which division of the small bowel is the shortest? _____

3. Which division of the small bowel is the longest? _____

4. Which division of the small bowel has a feathery or coiled-spring appearance during a small bowel series?

   _____

5. A. If removed and stretched out during autopsy, how long is the average small bowel? _____

   B. In a person with good muscle tone, the length of the entire small bowel is _____

   C. The average length of the large intestine is _____

6. In which two abdominal quadrants would the majority of the jejunum be found?

   _____

7. Which muscular band marks the junction between the duodenum and jejunum?

   _____

8. Which two aspects of the large intestine are **not** considered part of the colon?

   _____

9. The colon consists of _____ sections and _____ flexures.

10. List the two functions of the ileocecal valve: A. _____

                                                  B. _____

11. What is another term for the appendix? _____

12. Match the following aspects of the small and large intestine to the following characteristics:

     _____ 1. Jejunum   A. Longest aspect of the colon

     _____ 2. Duodenum   B. Widest portion of the colon

     _____ 3. Ileum   C. A blind pouch inferior to the ileocecal valve

     _____ 4. Cecum   D. Aspect of small intestine that is the smallest in diameter but longest in length

     _____ 5. Appendix   E. Distal part; also called the _iliac colon_

     _____ 6. Ascending colon   F. Shortest aspect of small intestine

     _____ 7. Descending colon   G. Lies in pelvis but possesses a wide freedom of motion

     _____ 8. Transverse colon   H. Makes up 40% of the small intestine

     _____ 9. Sigmoid colon   I. Found between the cecum and transverse colon

13. A. What is the term for the three bands of muscle that pull the large intestine into

     pouches? _____

    B. These pouches or sacculations, seen along the large intestine wall, are called _____.

14. The part of the large intestine directly anterior to the coccyx is the _____

15. Identify the labeled structures demonstrated on Fig. 15-1 and Fig. 15-2. Include secondary names where indicated.

Fig. 15-1

A. _____ (_____)

B. _____

C. _____

D. _____

E. _____ (_____) _____

F. _____

G. _____ (_____) _____

H. _____

I. _____

J. _____

K. _____

L. _____

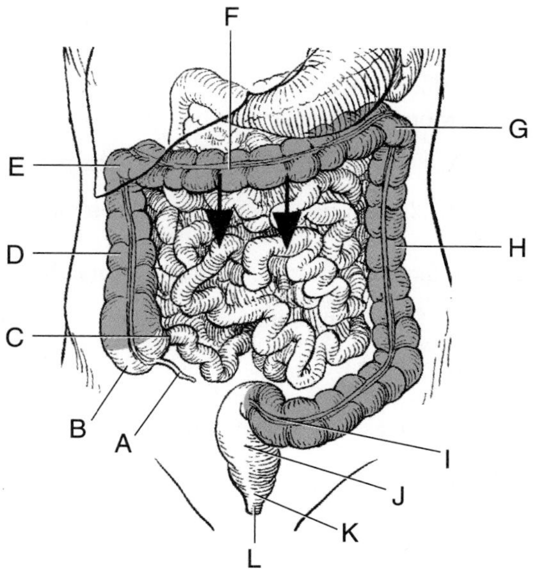

Fig. 15-1 Structures of the lower gastrointestinal tract, anterior view.

Fig.   15-2

M. _____

N. _____

O. _____

P. _____

Q. _____

R. _____

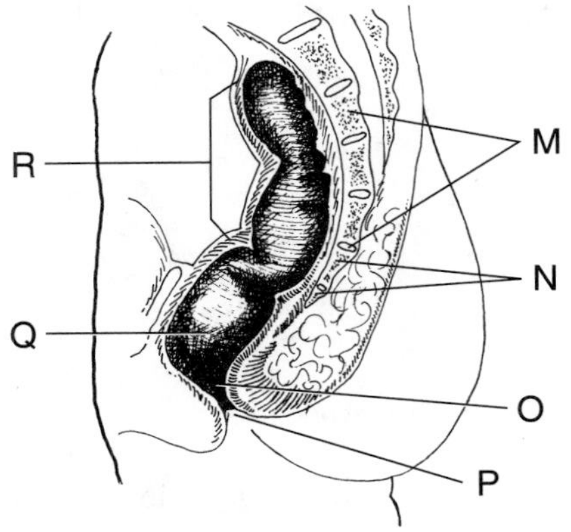

Fig. 15-2 Structures of the lower gastrointestinal tract, lateral view.

16. Which portion of the small intestine is located **primarily** to the left of the midline? _____

17. Which portion of the small intestine is located **primarily** in the RLQ? _____

18. Which portion of the small intestine has the smoothest internal lining and does **not** present a feathery appearance when barium filled? _____

19. Which aspect of the small intestine is **most fixed** in position? _____

20. In which quadrant does the terminal ileum connect with the large intestine? _____

21. The widest portion of the large bowel is the _____.

22. Which flexure of the large bowel usually extends more superiorly? _____

23. Inflammation of the appendix is called _____.

24. Which of the following structures will fill with air during a barium enema with the patient supine? (More than one answer may be correct.)

    A. Ascending colon   C. Rectum   E. Descending colon
    B. Transverse colon   D. Sigmoid colon

25. Which aspect of the GI tract is primarily responsible for digestion, absorption, and reabsorption?

    A. Small intestine   C. Large intestine
    B. Stomach   D. Colon

26. Which aspect of the GI tract is responsible for the synthesizing and absorption of vitamins B and K, and amino acids?

    A. Duodenum   C. Large intestine
    B. Jejunum   D. Stomach

27. Four types of digestive movements occurring in the large intestine are listed below as A through D. Which one of these movement types also occur in the small intestine? _____

    A. Peristalsis   C. Mass peristalsis
    B. Haustral churning   D. Defecation

28. Identify the gastrointestinal structures labeled on Fig. 15-3.

A. _____

B. _____

C. _____

D. _____

E. _____

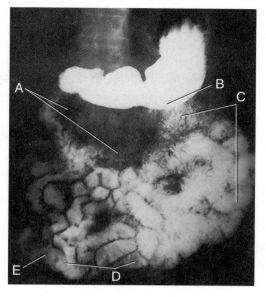

Fig. 15-3 Structure identification on a PA, 30-minute small bowel radiograph.

29. Identify the gastrointestinal structures labeled on Fig. 15-4.

A. _____

B. _____

C. _____

D. _____

E. _____

F. _____

G. _____

H. _____

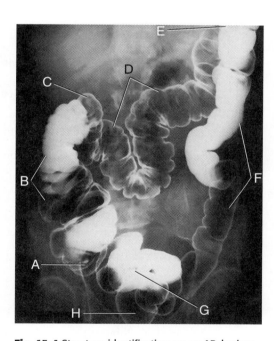

Fig. 15-4 Structure identification on an AP, barium enema radiograph.

PART II: Radiographic Positioning

Review Exercise B: Pathologic Indications and Radiographic Procedures for the Small Bowel Series and Barium Enema (see textbook pp. 486-504)

1. Which of the following conditions relate to a radiographic study of the small bowel?

    A. May perform as a double-contrast media study

    B. An enteroclysis procedure

    C. Timing of the procedure is necessary

    D. All of the above

2. Match the following definitions or statements to the correct pathologic indication for the small bowel series:

    _____ A. Common birth defect found in the ileum   1. Ileus

    _____ B. Common parasitic infection of the small intestine 2. Neoplasm

    _____ C. Obstruction of the small intestine   3. Meckel's diverticulum

    _____ D. Patient with lactose or sucrose sensitivities   4. Malabsorption syndrome

    _____ E. New growth   5. Enteritis

    _____ F. A form of sprue   6. Celiac disease

    _____ G. Inflammation of the intestine   7. Regional enteritis

    _____ H. Chronic inflammatory disease of the GI tract   8. Giardiasis

3. Match the following pathologic conditions or diseases to the correct radiographic appearance:

    _____ A. Circular staircase or herringbone sign   1. Adenocarcinoma

    _____ B. Cobblestone appearance   2. Meckel's diverticulum

    _____ C. Napkin ring sign   3. Ileus

    _____ D. Dilatation of the intestine with thickening   4. Giardiasis of circular folds

    _____ E. Large diverticulum of the ileum   5. Regional enteritis

4. Giardiasis is a condition acquired through:
    A. Contaminated food   C. Person-to-person contact
    B. Contaminated water   D. All of the above

5. Meckel's diverticulum is best diagnosed with which imaging modality
    A. Small bowel series   C. Magnetic resonance imaging
    B. Enteroclysis   D. Nuclear medicine

6. Whipple's disease is a disorder of the:
    A. Distal small intestine   C. Proximal large intestine
    B. Proximal small intestine D. Distal large intestine

7. List the two conditions that may prevent the use of barium sulfate during a small bowel series?
    A. _____   B. _____

8. What type of patients should be given extra care when using a water-soluble contrast media?

    _____

9. How much barium sulfate is generally given to an adult patient for a small-bowel-only series? _____

10. When is a small bowel series deemed completed?

    _____

11.   How long does it usually take to complete a small bowel series? _____

12.   When is the first radiograph generally taken during a small bowel series? _____

13.   True/False: Fluoroscopy is sometimes used during a small bowel series to visualize the ileocecal valve.

14.   True/False: It takes approximately 12 hours for barium sulfate, given orally, to reach the rectum.

15.   The term *enteroclysis* describes what type of a small bowel study? _____

16.   Which two clinical conditions are best evaluated through an enteroclysis procedure?

_____

17.   What type of contrast media is used for an enteroclysis?

_____

18.   The tip of the catheter is advanced to the _____ during an enteroclysis.

   A.   Duodenojejunal flexure (suspensory ligament)   C.   Pyloric sphincter

   B.   C-loop of duodenum   D.   Ileocecal sphincter

19.   A procedure to alleviate postoperative distention of a small intestine obstruction is called:

   A.   Diagnostic intubation   C.   Therapeutic intubation

   B.   Enteroclysis   D.   Small bowel series

20.   What is the recommended patient preparation before a small bowel series?

_____

21.   Which position is recommended for small bowel radiographs? Why?

_____

22.   Match the following definitions or statements to the correct pathologic indication for the barium enema:

   _____   A.   A twisting of a portion of the intestine on its own mesentery   1.   Polyp

   _____   B.   Outpouching of the mucosal wall   2.   Diverticulum

   _____   C.   Inflammatory condition of the large intestine   3.   Intussusception

   _____   D.   Severe form of colitis   4.   Volvulus

   _____   E.   Telescoping of one part of the intestine into another   5.   Ulcerative colitis

   _____   F.   Inward growth extending from the lumen of the intestinal wall   6.   Colitis

23.   Which type of patient usually experiences intussusception? _____

24.   A condition of numerous herniations of the inner wall of the colon is called _____

25.   Which one of the following pathologic indications may produce a "tapered or corkscrew" radiographic sign during a
barium enema?

   A.   Diverticulosis   C.   Volvulus

   B.   Ulcerative colitis   D.   Diverticulitis

26. Which one of the following conditions may produce the "stove pipe" radiographic sign during a barium enema?

    A. Ulcerative colitis   C. Diverticulosis

    B. Appendicitis   D. Adenocarcinoma

27. True/False: The barium enema is a commonly recommended procedure for diagnosing possible acute appendicitis.

28. Which four conditions would prevent the use of a laxative cathartic before a barium enema procedure?

    A. _____   C. _____

    B. _____   D. _____

29. True/False: Any stool retained in the large intestine may require cancellation of a barium enema.

30. True/False: An example of an irritant cathartic is magnesium citrate.

31. True/False: Synthetic latex enema tips or gloves do not cause problems for latex-sensitive patients.

32. List the three types of enema tips commonly used (all are considered single-use and disposable):

    A. _____   B. _____   C. _____

33. What water temperature is recommended for barium enema mixtures? _____

34. To minimize spasm during a barium enema, _____ can be added to the contrast media mixture.

    A. Glucagon   C. Saline

    B. Lidocaine   D. Valium

35. What is the name of the patient position recommended for insertion of the rectal enema tip?

    _____

36. The initial insertion of the rectal enema tip should be pointed toward the:

    A. Symphysis pubis   C. Umbilicus

    B. Bladder   D. Tip of coccyx

37. Which one of the following procedures is most effective to demonstrate small polyps in the colon?

    A. Single-contrast barium enema   C. Enteroclysis

    B. Double-contrast barium enema   D. Evacuative proctogram

38. Which one of the following procedures uses the thickest mixture of barium sulfate?

    A. Single-contrast barium enema   C. Evacuative proctogram

    B. Double-contrast barium enema   D. Enteroclysis

39. Which one of the following clinical conditions is best demonstrated with evacuative proctography?

    A. Intussusception   C. Rectal prolapse

    B. Volvulus   D. Diverticulosis

40. Which aspect of the large intestine must be demonstrated during evacuative proctography?

    A. Sigmoid colon   C. Anorectal angle

    B. Haustra   D. Rectal ligament

41. Into which position is the patient placed for imaging during the evacuative proctogram?

    A. AP spine   C. Ventral decubitus

    B. Left or right lateral decubitus   D. Lateral

42. True/False: A special tapered enema tip is inserted into the stoma before a colostomy barium enema.

43. True/False: The enema bag should not be more than 36 in. (90 cm) above the table-top before the beginning of the procedure.

44. True/False: The technologist should review the patient's chart before a barium enema to determine if a sigmoidoscopy or colonoscopy was performed recently.

45. True/False: Both computed tomography and sonography may be performed to aid in diagnosing appendicitis.

REVIEW EXERCISE C: Positioning of the Lower Gastrointestinal System (see textbook pp. 505-517)

1. Why is the Chassard-Lapine position not commonly performed as part of a barium enema routine?

    A. Produces a poor image of the rectosigmoid colon   C. Requires the use of a 14 × 17 in.   cassette

    B. High gonadal dose and difficult position for patients   D. Must use a long SID (>72 in)

2. Which two alternate special projections, other than the Chassard-Lapine position, demonstrate the rectosigmoid region as commonly performed by 40% or more of clinical institutions.

    _____

3. The _____ projection is a recommended alternate projection for the lateral rectum with a double-contrast BE exam.

4. Where is the CR centered for the 15-minute radiograph during a small bowel series?

    A. Iliac crest   C. 2 inches (5 cm) above iliac crest

    B. Xiphoid process   D. ASIS

5. What kVp is recommended for a small bowel series (with barium)? _____

6. What are the breathing instructions for a PA projection during a small bowel series?

    _____

7. Once the small bowel procedure has gone beyond 2 hours, radiographs are taken generally every

    _____.

8. Which ionization chambers should be activated for both PA small bowel and AP and oblique barium enema projections?

    A. All three chambers   C. Left and right upper chambers

    B. Center chamber only   D. AEC should not be used for barium procedures

9. How much midline dose (also female gonadal dose) is acquired for a PA small bowel or barium enema projection of a small to average-size patient?

    A. 5 to 10 mrad   C. 100 to 200 mrad

    B. 30 to 50 mrad   D. 400 to 500 mrad

10. Which type of patient may require two 35 x 43 cm (14 x 17 in.) crosswise cassettes for an AP barium enema projection?

    A. Hypersthenic   C. Hyposthenic

    B. Sthenic   D. Asthenic

11. Which position(s) taken during a barium enema will best demonstrate the right colic flexure?

    _____

12. How much rotation is required for oblique barium enema projections? _____

13. Which position should be taken if the patient cannot lie prone on the table for the anterior oblique to visualize the

    left colic flexure? _____

14. Which of the following barium enema positions provides the greatest amount of skin dose?

    A. Decubitus position (AP)   C. Obliques

    B. Lateral   D. AP axial

15. Which projection, taken during a double-contrast barium enema, will produce an air-filled image of the right colic

    flexure, ascending colon, and cecum? _____

16. Where is the CR centered for a lateral projection of the rectum? _____

17. True/False: If a retention-type enema tip is used, it should be removed after fluoroscopy is completed before overhead filming to better visualize the rectal region.

18. Which aspect of the large intestine is best demonstrated with an AP axial projection? _____

19. What is the advantage of performing an AP axial oblique projection rather than an AP axial?

    _____

20. A. What is another term describing the AP and PA axial projections? _____

    B. What CR angle is required for the AP axial? _____

    C. What CR angle is required for the PA axial? _____

21. Which projection for a double-contrast barium enema series best demonstrates the descending colon for possible

    polyps? _____

22. Which one of the following substances can be given to the patient to help stimulate evacuation following a barium enema?

    A. Milk   C. Wine or beer

    B. Coffee or hot tea   D. Garlic bread

23. What kVp range is recommended for a postevacuation projection following a barium enema? _____

24. A. What is the recommended kVp for a single-contrast barium enema study? _____

    B. What is the recommended kVp for a double-contrast study? _____

REVIEW EXERCISE D: Problem Solving for Technical and Positioning Errors (see textbook pp. 486-517)

1. **Situation:** A radiograph of a double-contrast barium enema projection reveals an obscured anatomical side marker. The technologist is unsure whether it is an AP or PA recumbent projection. The transverse colon is primarily filled with barium, with the ascending and descending colon containing a lesser amount. Which position does this radiograph represent?

    _____

    _____

2. **Situation:** A radiograph of a lateral decubitus projection taken during an air-contrast barium enema reveals that the upside aspect of the colon is overpenetrated. The following factors were used during this exposure: 120 kVp, 30 mAs, 40 in. (102 cm) SID, high-speed screens, and compensating filter for the air-filled aspect of the large intestine. Which one of these factors must be modified during the repeat exposure?

    _____

    _____

3. **Situation:** A radiograph of an AP axial barium enema projection of the rectosigmoid segment reveals that there is considerable superimposition of the sigmoid colon and rectum. The following factors were used during this exposure: 120 kVp, 20 mAs, 40 in. (102 cm) SID, 35° caudad CR angle, and collimation. Which one of these factors must be modified or corrected for the repeat exposure?

    _____

    _____

4. **Situation:** A barium enema study performed on a hypersthenic patient reveals that the majority of the radiographs demonstrate that the left colic flexure was cut off. What can be done during the repeat exposures to avoid this problem?

    _____

    _____

    _____

5. **Situation:** A technologist has inserted an air-contrast retention tip for a double-contrast BE study. He is not sure how much to inflate the retention balloon. Should he inflate it as much as the patient can tolerate, or is there a better alternative?

    _____

    _____

    _____

6. **Situation:** A student technologist is told to place the patient onto the x-ray table in a Sims position in preparation for the tip insertion for a barium enema. Describe how the patient should be positioned.

    _____

    _____

    _____

7. **Situation:** A patient with a clinical history of regional enteritis comes to the radiology department. What type of procedure would be most diagnostic for this condition?

    _____

    _____

8. **Situation:** A patient is referred to the radiology department for a presurgical, small bowel series. What modification to the standard study needs to be made for this particular patient?

    _____

    _____

9. **Situation:** A patient comes to the radiology department for a small bowel series. However, due to a stroke, the patient is unable to swallow the contrast media. What type of study should be performed for this patient?

    _____

    _____

10. **Situation:** A young infant with a possible intussusception is brought to the emergency room. Which radiographic procedure may serve a therapeutic role for correcting this condition?

    _____

    _____

11. **Situation:** Before a barium enema, the technologist experienced difficulty in inserting the enema rectal tip (without causing significant pain for the patient). What should the technologist do to complete this task?

    _____

12. **Situation:** During the fluoroscopy aspect of a barium enema, the radiologist detects an unusual defect within the right colic flexure. She asks that the technologist provide the best images possible of this region. Which two projections will best demonstrate the right colic flexure?

    _____

13. **Situation:** A patient with a clinical history of possible enteritis comes to the radiology department. Which type of radiographic GI study would most likely be indicated for this condition. (Of course, this would have to be requested by the referring physician.)

    _____

14. **Situation:** A patient's clinical history includes possible giardiasis. What radiographic procedures would likely be indicated for this condition?

    _____

15. **Situation:** A patient came to the radiology with a request for a small bowel series. The patient's chart indicates a possible large bowel obstruction.

    _____

    What radiographic exams and/or projections should be performed first before giving the patient barium to ingest for a small bowel series?

    _____

PART III: Laboratory Activities (see textbook pp. 505-517)

You must gain experience in positioning each part of the lower GI procedures before performing the following exams on actual patients. You can get experience in positioning and radiographic evaluation of these projections by performing exercises using radiographic phantoms and practicing on other students (although you will not be taking actual exposures).

LABORATORY EXERCISE A: Radiographic Evaluation

1.　Evaluate and critique the radiographs produced during the previous experiments, additional radiographs of esophagrams, and lower GI procedures provided by your instructor.　Evaluate each position for the following points. (Check off when completed.):

_____　Evaluate the completeness of the study.　(Are all of the pertinent anatomic structures included on the radiograph?)

_____　Evaluate for positioning or centering errors (e.g., rotation, off centering)

_____　Evaluate for correct exposure factors and possible motion.
(Are the density and contrast of the images acceptable?)

_____　Determine whether markers and an acceptable degree of collimation and/or area shielding are visible on the images.

LABORATORY EXERCISE B: Physical Positioning

On another person, simulate performing all basic and special projections of the lower GI as follows.　(Check off each when completed satisfactorily.) Include the following six steps as described in the textbook.

Step 1. Appropriate size and type of film holder with correct markers
Step 2. Correct CR placement and centering of part to CR and/or film
Step 3. Accurate collimation
Step 4. Area shielding of patient where advisable
Step 5. Use of proper immobilizing devices when needed
Step 6. Approximate correct exposure factors, breathing instructions where applicable, and "making" exposure

	Step 1	Step 2	Step 3	Step 4	Step 5	Step 6
• PA 15- or 30-minute small bowel	_____	_____	_____	_____	_____	_____
• PA 1- or 2-hour small bowel	_____	_____	_____	_____	_____	_____
• PA or AP barium enema	_____	_____	_____	_____	_____	_____
• RAO and LAO barium enema	_____	_____	_____	_____	_____	_____
• LPO and RPO barium enema	_____	_____	_____	_____	_____	_____
• Right and left lateral decubitus	_____	_____	_____	_____	_____	_____
• AP and LPO axial	_____	_____	_____	_____	_____	_____
• PA and RAO axial	_____	_____	_____	_____	_____	_____
• Lateral rectum	_____	_____	_____	_____	_____	_____
• Ventral decubitus lateral rectum	_____	_____	_____	_____	_____	_____

Answers to Review Exercises

Review Exercise A: Radiographic Anatomy and Function of the Lower Gastrointestinal System

1. A. Duodenum
   B. Jejunum
   C. Ileum
2. Duodenum
3. Ileum
4. Jejunum
5. A. 23 feet or 7 meters
   B. 15 to 18 feet or 4.5 to 5.5 meters
   C. 5 feet or 1.5 meters
6. LUQ and LLQ
7. Suspensory ligament of the duodenum or ligament of Treitz (this site is a reference point for certain small bowel exams because it remains in a relatively fixed position).
8. Cecum and rectum
9. 4 sections, 2 flexures
10. A. Prevents contents from the ileum to pass too quickly into cecum
    B. Prevents reflux back into the ileum
11. Vermiform appendix
12. 1. H, 2. F, 3. D, 4. B, 5. C,
    6. I, 7. E, 8. A, 9. G
13. A. Taeniae coli
    B. Haustra
14. Rectal ampulla
15. A. Appendix (vermiform process)
    B. Cecum
    C. Ileocecal valve
    D. Ascending colon
    E. Right colic (hepatic) flexure
    F. Transverse colon
    G. Left colic (splenic) flexure
    H. Descending colon
    I. Sigmoid colon
    J. Rectum
    K. Anal canal
    L. Anus
    M. Sacrum
    N. Coccyx
    O. Anal canal
    P. Anus
    Q. Rectal ampulla
    R. Rectum
16. Jejunum
17. Ileum
18. Ileum
19. Duodenojejunal junction
20. Right lower quadrant (RLQ)
21. Cecum
22. Left colic (splenic)
23. Appendicitis
24. B. Transverse colon
    D. Sigmoid colon

25. A. Small intestine
26. C. Large intestine
27. A. Peristalsis
28. A. Duodenum
    B. Area of suspensory ligament/ duodenojejunal junction
    C. Jejunum
    D. Ileum
    E. Area of ileococal valve
29. A. Cecum
    B. Ascending colon
    C. Right colic (hepatic) flexure
    D. Transverse colon
    E. Left colic (splenic) flexure
    F. Descending colon
    G. Sigmoid colon
    H. Rectum

Review Exercise B: Pathologic Indications and Radiographic Procedures for the Small Bowel Series and Barium Enema

1. D. All of the above
2. A. 3
   B. 8
   C. 1
   D. 4
   E. 2
   F. 6
   G. 5
   H. 7
3. A. 3
   B. 5
   C. 1
   D. 4
   E. 2
4. D. All of the above
5. D. Nuclear medicine
6. B. Proximal small intestine
7. A. Possible perforated hollow viscus
   B. Large bowel obstruction
8. Young and dehydrated
9. 2 cups or 16 ounces
10. When the contrast medium passes through the ileocecal valve
11. 2 hours
12. 15 to 30 minutes after ingesting the contrast medium
13. True
14. False (24 hours)
15. Double-contrast method
16. Regional enteritis (Crohn's disease) and malabsorption syndromes
17. High-density barium sulfate and air or methylcellulose
18. A. Duodenojejunal flexure (suspensory ligament)
19. C. Therapeutic intubation

20. NPO for at least 8 hours before procedure; no smoking or gum chewing
21. Prone. To separate the loops of bowel
22. A. 4
    B. 2
    C. 6
    D. 5
    E. 3
    F. 1
23. Infants
24. Diverticulosis
25. C. Volvulus
26. A. Ulcerative colitis
27. False
28. A. Gross bleeding
    B. Severe diarrhea
    C. Obstruction
    D. Inflammatory lesions
29. True
30. False (castor oil is an irritant cathartic)
31. True
32. A. Plastic disposable
    B. Rectal retention
    C. Air-contrast retention
33. Room temperature (85 to 90 degrees)
34. B. Lidocaine
35. Sims position
36. C. Umbilicus
37. B. Double contrast barium enema
38. C. Evacuative proctogram
39. C. Rectal prolapse
40. C. Anorectal angle
41. D. Lateral
42. True
43. False (not more than 24 in. (60 cm) above tabletop when beginning the procedure)
44. True
45. True

Review Exercise C: Postioning of the Lower Gastrointestinal System

1. B. High gonadal dose and difficult position for patients
2. AP or PA axial (butterfly)
3. Ventral decubitus
4. C. 2 inches (5 cm) above iliac crest
5. 100 to 125 kVp
6. Make exposure on expiration
7. Hour
8. A. All three chambers
9. B. 30 to 50 mrad
10. A. Hypersthenic
11. RAO or LPO

12. 35 to 45°
13. RPO
14. B. Lateral
15. Left lateral decubitus
16. Level of ASIS at the midcoronal plane
17. False (generally should not be removed until after overhead filming is completed unless directed to do so by the radiologist)
18. Rectosigmoid segment
19. Creates less superimposition of the rectosigmoid segments
20. A. Butterfly projections
    B. AP: CR angled 30 to 40° cephalad C. PA: CR 30 to 40° caudad
21. Right lateral decubitus (left side up)
22. B. Coffee or hot tea
23. 80 to 90 kVp
24. A. 100 to 125 kVp
    B. 80 to 90 kVp

Review Exercise D: Problem Solving for Technical and Positioning Errors

1. PA prone. Since the transverse colon is an intraperitoneal aspect of the large intestine located more anteriorly, it will fill with barium in the PA prone position.

2. Even with the use of a compensating filter, a reduction in kVp is required. Since less barium sulfate is used during an air-contrast procedure, the kVp range should be 80 to 90.
3. The CR was angled in the wrong direction. The AP axial projection requires a 30 to 40° cephalad angle.
4. Use two 14 x 17 in. (35 x 43 cm) crosswise cassettes for the AP/PA and oblique projections, one centered higher and one lower. Since hypersthenic patients have a wider distribution of the large intestine, two crosswise-placed cassettes will ensure that all of the pertinent anatomy is demonstrated.
5. Retention catheters should only be fully inflated by the radiologist under fluoroscopic control.
6. Lay on left side and flex head and upper body forward, drawing the right leg up above the partially flexed left leg.
7. Enteroclysis, a double-contrast small bowel procedure. A basic small bowel series may also demonstrate this condition, but the enteroclysis with double contrast is more effective in demonstrating mucosal changes.

8. Since the patient is having surgery soon after the small bowel series, a water-soluble, iodinated contrast media should be used. Barium sulfate should not be given to presurgical patients.
9. A diagnostic, intubation small bowel series would be preferred. A nasogastric tube would be passed into the small intestine, allowing the contrast media to be instilled. This procedure is effective for patients who can't swallow.
10. A barium enema or air enema often leads to re-expansion of the telescoped aspect of the large intestine (see textbook, p. 659).
11. Inform the radiologist and have him or her insert it under fluoroscopy guidance
12. RAO or LPO projections
13. A small bowel series (enteritis is an inflammation or infection of the small intestine)
14. An upper GI, small bowel combination series (gastroenteritis is an inflammation or infection of both the stomach and small intestine)
15. An acute abdominal series and a barium enema to rule out a possible large bowel obstruction. (Barium by mouth is contraindicated with a possible large bowel obstruction.)

SELF-TEST

Directions: This self-test should be taken only after completing all of the readings, review exercises, and laboratory activities for a particular section.   The purpose of this test is not only to provide a good learning exercise but also to serve as a good indicator of what your final evaluation grade will be. It is strongly suggested that if you do not get at least a 90% to 95% grade on each self-test, you should review those areas in which you missed questions before going to your instructor for the final evaluation exam for this chapter. (There are 78 questions or blanks—each is worth 1.3 points.)

1. During life, how long is the entire small intestine?

   A. 15 to 18 feet (4.5 to 5.5 meters)   C.   5 to 10 feet (1.5 to 3 meters)

   B.   20 to 25 feet (6 to 7.5 meters)   D.   30 to 40 feet (9 to 12 meters)

2. Which aspect of the small intestine is considered the longest?

   A.   Duodenum   C.   Ileum

   B.   Jejunum   D.   Cecum

3. What is the name for the band of muscular tissue found at the junction of the duodenum and jejunum?

   A.   Valvulae conniventes   C.   Duodenal flexure

   B.   Haustra   D.   Suspensory ligament of the duodenum

4. Which aspect of the small intestine possesses the smallest diameter?

   A.   Ileum   C.   Cecum

   B.   Duodenum   D.   Jejunum

5. The part of the intestine with a "feathery" and "coiled spring" appearance when filled with barium is the:

   A.   Ileum   C.   Jejunum

   B.   Duodenum   D.   Cecum

6. List the two aspects of the large intestine not considered part of the colon.

   A. _____   B. _____

7. What is another term for the appendix ? _____

8. True/False: The rectum possesses two anteroposterior curves that have a direct impact on rectal enema tip insertions.

9. True/False: The small sacculations found within the jejunum are called *haustra.*

10. Which colic flexure (right or left) is located 1 to 2 inches (2.5 to 5 cm) higher or more superior in the abdomen?

11. Identify the labeled structures on the following radiographs (Fig. 15-5 and Fig. 15-6). Include secondary names where indicated by parentheses.

Fig.15-5:

A. _____

B. _____

C. _____

D. _____

E. _____

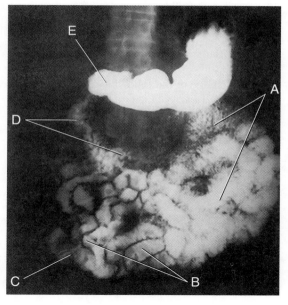

Fig. 15-5 Structure identification on a gastrointestinal radiograph.

Fig.15-6:

F. _____ (_____) _____

G. _____

H. _____

I. _____

J. _____

K. _____

L. _____ (_____) _____

M. _____

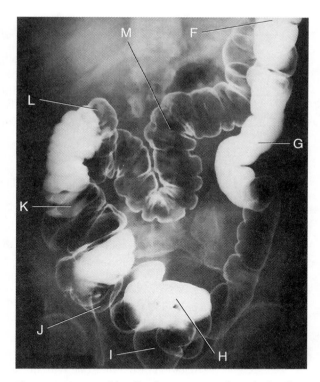

Fig. 15-6 Structure identification on a gastrointestinal radiograph.

12. Which one of the following structures is considered to be most anterior?

A. Cecum   C. Transverse colon

B. Rectum   D. Ascending colon

13. Where does the reabsorption of inorganic salts occur in the gastrointestinal tract?

    A. Duodenum   C. Stomach

    B. Large intestine   D. Jejunum

14. Which one of the following digestive movements occurs in the small intestine?

    A. Haustral churning   C. Mass peristalsis

    B. Rhythmic segmentation   D. Mastication

15. Match the following pathologic indications to their correct definition:

    _____ 1. Meckel's diverticulum   A. Telescoping of the bowel into another

    _____ 2. Diverticulosis   B. A new growth extending from mucosal wall

    _____ 3. Enteritis   C. A twisting of the intestine on its own mesentery

    _____ 4. Whipple's Disease   D. Caused by an outpouching of the intestinal wall

    _____ 5. Polyp   E. Chronic inflammatory condition of small intestine

    _____ 6. Malabsorption syndrome   F. Outpouching located in distal ileum

    _____ 7. Diverticulitis   G. Unable to process certain nutrients

    _____ 8. Volvulus   H. May be caused by cutting off blood supply to it or infection

    _____ 9. Intussusception   I. Inflammation of the small intestine

    _____ 10. Regional enteritis   J. Inflammation of small herniations in the intestinal wall

    _____ 11. Ulcerative colitis   K. Caused by a flagellate protozoan

    _____ 12. Giardiasis   L. Disorder of proximal small intestine

    _____ 13. Appendicitis   M. Chronic inflammatory condition of the large intestine

16. Match the following radiographic appearances to the correct pathologic indication:

    _____ 1. A tapered or corkscrew appearance seen during a barium enema   A. Ulcerative colitis

    _____ 2. Apple-core lesion   B. Diverticulosis

    _____ 3. String sign   C. Intussusception

    _____ 4. Dilatation of the intestine with thickening of the circular folds   D. Volvulus

    _____ 5. Stovepipe appearance of colon   E. Regional enteritis

    _____ 6. Mushroom-shaped dilatation with a small amount of barium passing beyond it   F. Polyp

          G. Neoplasm

    _____ 7. Jagged or sawtooth appearance of the intestinal mucosa   H. Giardiasis

    _____ 8. Inward growth from intestinal wall

17. Which of the following imaging modalities/procedures is performed to diagnose an intussusception?

    A. Barium enema   C. Nuclear medicine scan

    B. Enteroclysis   D. CT

18. True/False: The barium enema is recommended to diagnose appendicitis.

19. What breathing instructions should be given to the patient during insertion of the enema tip?

    _____

20. Why is the PA rather than an AP position recommended for a small bowel series?

    _____

21. What is the minimum amount of time a patient needs to remain NPO before a small bowel series?

    _____

22. What is another term for a laxative? _____

23. Which type of rectal enema tip is ideal for the patient with a relaxed anal sphincter? _____

24. What is the name of the drug that can be given to help control spasm during a barium enema?

    _____

25. What drug can be added to the barium sulfate mixture to minimize spasm during a barium enema?

    _____

26. Which one of the following pathologic indications is best diagnosed during an evacuative proctogram?

    A. Regional enteritis   C. Volvulus

    C. Diverticulosis   D. Prolapse of rectum

27. Which region of the large intestine must be visualized during an evacuative proctogram study?

    A. Cecum   C. Ileocecal valve

    B. Anorectal angle   D. Left colic flexure

28. True/False: A small balloon retention catheter may be placed within the stoma of the colostomy to deliver contrast media during a barium enema.

29. Which oblique position, the LAO or RAO, best demonstrates the ascending colon and cecum? _____

30. What is the average length of time in a routine small bowel series for the barium to reach the large intestine?

    _____

31. Which one of the following commercial contrast media would be used during an evaluative proctogram?

    A. Hypaque   C. Gastroview

    B. Gastrographin   D. Anatrast

32. Which ionization chambers should be activated for a lateral barium enema projection of the rectum?

    A. All three chambers   C. Center chamber only

    B. Right and left upper chambers   D. Right upper chamber only

33. How much obliquity of the body is required for the LAO barium enema projection? _____

34. The CR and film should be centered about _____ higher for the 15- or 30-minute small bowel image than for the later images.

35. The term *evacuative proctography* is sometimes used for a lower GI tract procedure may also be commonly called

    _____.

36. A patient is unable to lie prone on the radiographic table during a barium enema. Which specific position will best

    demonstrate the right colic flexure? _____

37. **Situation:** A patient is scheduled for an air-contrast barium enema. During the fluoroscopy phase of the study, the radiologist detects a possible polyp in the lower descending colon. Which specific position will best demonstrate this region of the colon?

    _____

    _____

38. **Situation:** A patient with a clinical history of a rectocele comes to the radiology department. Which radiographic procedure will best diagnose this condition?

    _____

39. True/False: A PA axial oblique (RAO) barium enema projection is an optional projection to demonstrate the right colic flexure.

40. True/False: On a hypersthenic-type patient, a 35 x 43 cm (14 x 17 inches) film placed lengthwise centered correctly will generally include the entire barium-filled large intestine on one film.

41. True/False: The female gonadal dose for a lateral barium enema projection is approximately 15 to 20 times greater than for a lateral decubitus (AP) projection.

42. The skin dose range for a lateral rectum position on an average size patient is:

    A. 50 to 100 mrad   C. 500 to 1000 mrad

    B. 200 to 400 mrad   D. 2000 to 3000 mrad

43. A. The RAO position best demonstrates the _____ (right or left) colic flexure with the

        CR and image receptor centered to the level of _____.

    B. The LAO position best demonstrates the _____ (right or left) colic flexure with the CR

        and image receptor centered to the level of _____.

CHAPTER 16

Gallbladder and Biliary Ducts

CHAPTER OBJECTIVES

After you have completed **all** the activities of this chapter, you will be able to:

_____ 1. Identify specific anatomy and functions of the liver, gallbladder, and biliary ductal system.

_____ 2. Describe the production, storage, and purpose of bile.

_____ 3. On drawings and radiographs, identify specific anatomy of the biliary system.

_____ 4. Describe the impact of body habitus on the position of the gallbladder.

_____ 5. Define specific terms related to conditions and procedures of the biliary system.

_____ 6. Define specific pathologies of the biliary system.

_____ 7. Match specific biliary pathologies to the correct radiographic appearances and signs.

_____ 8. Identify special and alternative radiographic procedures of the biliary system.

_____ 9. List the advantages of ultrasound of the gallbladder as compared to the oral cholecystogram.

_____ 10. List information related to the operative, percutaneous transhepatic, T-tube, and laproscopic cholangiogram and endoscopic retrograde cholangiopancreatogram procedures, including purpose of study, contraindications, imaging, and post-procedure care.

_____ 11. List information related to the basic and special projections for an oral cholecystogram, including size and type of image receptor, central ray location, direction and angulation of the central ray, and anatomy best visualized.

_____ 12. Identify the patient dose ranges for skin, midline, and gonads for various oral cholecystogram projections.

_____ 13. Given various hypothetical situations, identify the correct modification of a position and/or exposure factors to improve the radiographic image.

POSITIONING AND FILM CRITIQUE

_____ 1. Using a peer, position for basic and special projections for an oral cholecystogram procedure.

_____ 2. Critique and evaluate oral cholecystogram and cholangiogram radiographs based on the four divisions of radiographic criteria: (1) structures shown, (2) position, (3) collimation and CR, and (4) exposure criteria.

_____ 3. Distinguish between acceptable and unacceptable biliary study radiographs resulting from exposure factors, motion, collimation, positioning, or other errors.

Learning Exercises

Complete the following review exercises after reading the associated pages in the textbook as indicated by each exercise. Answers to each review exercise are given at the end of the review exercises.

PART I: Radiographic Anatomy

Review Exercise A: Radiographic Anatomy of the Gallbladder and Biliary System (see textbook pp. 520-522)

1. What is the average weight of the adult human liver? _____

2. Which abdominal quadrant contains the gallbladder? _____

3. What is the name of the soft tissue structure that separates the right from the left lobe of the liver?

    _____

4. Which lobe of the liver is larger, the right or left? _____

5. List the other two lobes of the liver (in addition to right and left lobes):

    A. _____   B. _____

6. True/False: The liver performs over 100 functions.

7. True/False: The average healthy adult liver produces 1 gallon, or 3000 to 4000 ml, of bile per day.

8. List the three primary functions of the gallbladder:

    A. _____

    B. _____

    C. _____

9. What is the name of the hormone that causes the gallbladder to contract? _____

10. True/False: The hormone identified in question 9 is secreted by the liver.

11. True/False: Concentrated levels of cholesterol in bile may lead to gallstones.

12. What is a common site for impaction, or lodging, of gallstones? _____

13. True/False: In about 40% of individuals, the hepatopancreatic ampulla is totally separated into two ducts rather than the one enlarged ampulla.

14. True/False: An older term for the main pancreatic duct is *the duct of Vater.*

15. The gallbladder is located more (posteriorly or anteriorly) within the abdomen? _____

16. Match the following structures to their primary location within the abdomen.

——— 1. Liver   A. Near midsagittal plane

——— 2. Gallbladder on asthenic patient   B. To left of midsagittal plane

——— 3. Gallbladder on hypersthenic patient   C. To right of midsagittal plane

——— 4. Gallbladder on hyposthenic patient

17. Identify the major components of the gallbladder and the biliary system on Fig. 16-1:

A. _____

B. _____

C. _____

D. _____

E. _____

F. _____

G. _____

H. _____

I. _____

J. _____

K. _____

L. _____

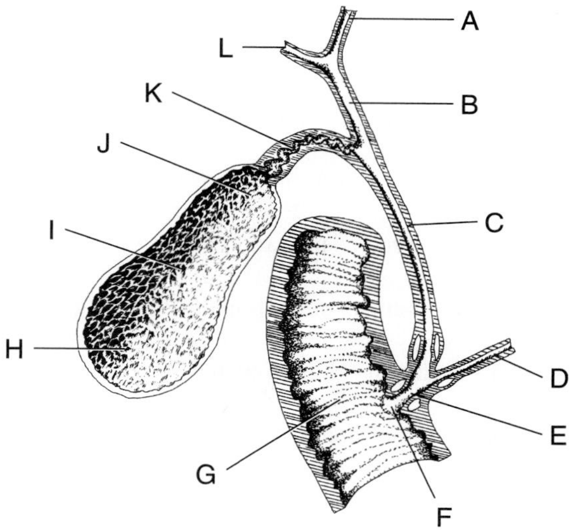

Fig. 16-1 Components of the gallbladder and biliary system.

18. Identify the labeled structures on this sagittal view of the abdomen (Fig. 16-2):

A. _____

B. _____

C. _____

D. _____

E. _____

F. _____

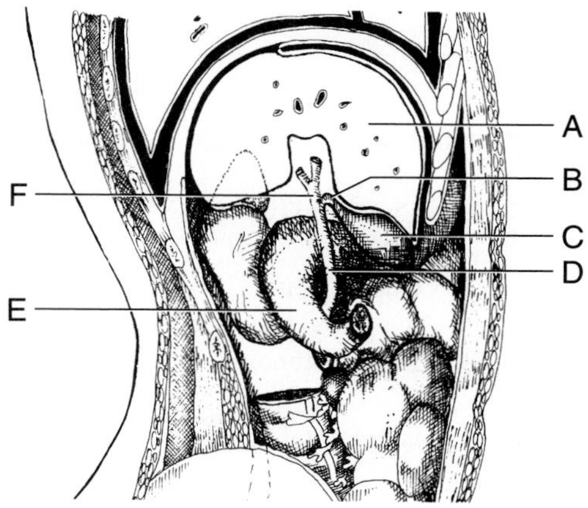

Fig. 16-2 Lateral, cut-away view of components of the gallbladder and biliary system.

19. What position should the patient be placed in if the primary purpose is to drain the gallbladder into the duct system?

_____

20. Which projection (AP or PA) would place the gallbladder closest to the image receptor for the best visualization?

    _____

21. Which radiographic oblique position will project the gallbladder away from the spine? _____

PART II: Radiographic Positioning

REVIEW EXERCISE B: Radiographic Procedures and Positioning of the Gallbladder and Biliary Ducts (see textbook pp. 523-538)

1. The prefix *chole* refers to _____ .

2. The prefix *cysto* refers to _____ .

3. Radiographic examination of the gallbladder is called _____ .

4. Radiographic examination of the biliary ducts is called _____ .

5. Radiographic examination of both the gallbladder and biliary ducts is called _____ .

6. The acronym *OCG* refers to _____ .

7. Oral types of contrast media designed to visualize the gallbladder are called _____ .

8. List the three biliary functions measured during an OCG

    A. _____

    B. _____

    C. _____

9. In addition to hypersensitivity to iodinated compounds, what are the three other contraindications for an OCG?

    A. _____   C. _____

    B. _____

10. Match the following pathologic indications with their correct definition:

    _____ 1. Cholelithiasis   A. Defects present at birth

    _____ 2. Cholecystitis   B. Emulsion of biliary stones

    _____ 3. Biliary stenosis   C. Condition of having gallstones

    _____ 4. Congenital anomalies   D. Inflammation of the gallbladder

    _____ 5. Neoplasm   E. Benign or malignant tumors

    _____ 6. Milk calcium bile   F. Narrowing of the biliary ducts

11. True/False: Most gallstones contain enough calcium to be at least minimally visualized on a plain abdomen radiograph.

12. True/False: Chronic cholecystitis is usually associated with gallstones.

13. True/False: Acute cholecystitis may produce a thickened gallbladder wall.

14. True/False: A nonvisualized gallbladder is always the result of a pathologic condition.

15. True/False: The patient must take laxatives 8 hours before an OCG to ensure that the colon is free of feces, which may obscure the gallbladder.

16. True/False: The evening meal before an OCG should contain a slight amount of fat.

17. True/False: Most disorders of the gallbladder and biliary duct are caused by gallstones.

18. How many hours before an OCG should the cholecystopaques be taken? _____

19. What is the optimal kVp range for an OCG? _____

20. What five questions should a patient be asked before taking the cholecystogram scout?

   A. _____

   B. _____

   C. _____

   D. _____

   E. (Female) _____

21. What is the purpose of the fatty meal or CCK study? _____

22. List four advantages of a gallbladder ultrasound instead of the conventional OCG:

   A. _____

   B. _____

   C. _____

   D. _____

23. What special imaging equipment is required if the surgeon desires a real-time image during an operative cholangiogram?

   _____

24. Why will the surgeon sometimes dilute the contrast media with saline before an operative cholangiogram?

   _____

25. List the three advantages to a laparoscopic cholangiogram as compared to the conventional operative cholangiogram:

    A. _____

    B. _____

    C. _____

26. Postoperative (T-tube) cholangiograms are generally performed in (surgery or in the radiology department)

    _____ .

27. Which one of the following procedures may be performed during a postoperative (T-tube) cholangiogram?

    A. Remove the gallbladder   C. Remove a biliary stone

    B. Remove a liver cyst   D. Catheterize the hepatic portal vein

28. Which one of the following clinical conditions is best suited for a percutaneous cholangiogram (PTC)?

    A. Obstructive jaundice   C. Liver hemorrhage

    B. Ascites   D. Cholelithiasis

29. Why is a chest radiograph commonly ordered following a PTC? _____

30. Which one of the following is not an expected risk associated with a PTC?

    A. Liver hemorrhage   C. Escape of bile

    B. Pneumothorax   D. Cholecystitis

31. A radiographic procedure of examining the biliary and main pancreatic ducts is called a(n):

    A. (write out full term) _____

    B. What initials are commonly used for this procedure? _____

    C. What type of special endoscope is commonly used for this procedure? _____

    D. Which member of the health care team usually performs this procedure? _____

    E. Why should a patient remain NPO at least 1 hour following this procedure? _____

32. Match the following biliary procedures with the means of introducing the contrast media during these procedures:

    _____ 1. ERCP   A. Direct injection through a catheter placed during an endoscopic process

    _____ 2. PTC   B. No contrast media required

    _____ 3. T-tube cholangiogram   C. Oral ingestion

    _____ 4. Immediate cholangiogram   D. Direct injection by a needle

    _____ 5. OCG   E. Direct injection through indwelling drainage tube puncture

    _____ 6. Cholecystosonography   F. Direct injection through catheter during surgery

33. True/False: Conditions such as sickle cell anemia may produce gallstones in pediatric patients

34. True/False: A HIDA nuclear medicine scan is intended to diagnose cirrhosis of the liver.

35. Which imaging modality/procedure is recommended for a gallbladder study on a pediatric patient?
    A. OCG   C. MRI
    B. Sonography   D. CT

36. True/False: Gallbladder projections result in approximately equal amounts of gonadal dose for males and females.

37. True/False: The right upper AEC pickup cell is recommended for gallbladder projections.

38. The gallbladder is usually found on the sthenic patient at the level of _____ .
    A. T12   B. L4   C. T10   D. L2

39. Centering for a PA scout projection on a hypersthenic patient is usually _____ as compared with a sthenic patient.
    A. Lower and more midline   C. Higher and midline
    B. About the same location   D. Higher and more lateral

40. Which oblique position will project the gallbladder away from the spine? _____

41. How much obliquity is required for this projection taken on (A) an asthenic patient? _____

    (B) a hypersthenic patient? _____

42. Which two possible positions during an OCG will stratify any possible gallstones? _____

43. Which specific decubitus position should be performed to demonstrate possible stratification (layering out) of gallstones? _____

44. What is the gonadal dose given to a female patient with a decubitus projection during an OCG?
    A. Not measurable   C. 50 to 100 mrad
    B. 5 to 10 mrad   D. 200 to 400 mrad

45. How much lower should centering be for an erect gallbladder projection as compared with a recumbent projection?

REVIEW EXERCISE C: Problem Solving for Technical and Positioning Errors (see textbook pp. 523-538)

1. **Situation:** An asthenic-type patient comes to the radiology department for an oral cholecystogram. The PA scout film fails to reveal the location of the gallbladder. The following factors were used during the initial exposure: 10 x 12 lengthwise cassette, 70 kVp, 30 mAs, 40 in. (102 cm) SID, Bucky, CR centered to the level of L2. Which of these factors can be modified to increase the chances of locating the gallbladder?

2. **Situation:** A radiograph of a PA scout projection for the gallbladder reveals that the gallbladder is only faintly visible. The patient assures the technologist that she had taken all the required tablets. The following factors were used during the exposure: 85 kVp, AEC with center cell, Bucky, CR centered to the level of L2. Which of these factors can be modified to improve the visibility of the gallbladder?

3. **Situation:** A radiograph of an LAO projection reveals that the gallbladder is superimposed over the spine. What type of positioning modification is needed to prevent this superimposition during the repeat exposure?

    _____

    _____

4. **Situation:** During an operative cholangiogram, the resultant radiograph reveals that the biliary ducts are superimposed over the spine. As requested by the surgeon, the initial projection was taken AP in the supine position. What can be done to shift the biliary ducts away from the spine during the repeat exposure?

    _____

    _____

5. **Situation:** A patient with right upper quadrant pain enters the emergency room. The physician is concerned about gallstones, but the patient states that he is hypersensitive to iodine. Which procedure of the biliary system would be ideal for this patient?

    _____

    _____

6. **Situation:** A patient with signs of obstructive jaundice enters the emergency room.   The patient's skin has a yellow tinge to it. Which radiographic study of the biliary system would be recommended for this patient?

    _____

    _____

7. **Situation:** During an OCG, the patient's gallbladder is well-visualized with contrast media. But the radiologist is concerned about the function of the gallbladder. Which particular study would evaluate the function of the gallbladder?

    _____

    _____

8. **Situation:** A patient who may have a stone in the main pancreatic duct enters the emergency room. Which procedure would be ideal to demonstrate this duct and determine if a stone is present?

    _____

    _____

9. **Situation:** A patient with a history of acute cholecystitis comes to the radiology department for an OCG. The scout image does not demonstrate an opacified gallbladder. What other procedure (s) can be ordered to visualize the gallbladder and biliary ducts?

    _____

    _____

10. **Situation:** A patient who may have a neoplasm of the gallbladder comes to the radiology department. Which imaging modalities or procedures would best diagnose this condition?

    _____

    _____

PART III: Laboratory Exercises (see textbook pp. 533-538)

Although it is impossible to duplicate many aspects of biliary studies on a phantom in the lab, evaluation of actual radiographs and physical positioning is possible. You can get experience in positioning and radiographic evaluation of these projections by performing exercises using radiographic phantoms and practicing on other students (although you will not be taking actual exposures). Technologists must learn the positioning routine, room setup, and fluoroscopy procedure for their particular facility.

LABORATORY EXERCISE A: Radiographic Evaluation

Using actual radiographs of OCG and cholangiogram procedures provided by your instructor, evaluate and critique each position for the following points.   (Check off when completed.):

_____   Evaluate the completeness of the study. (Are all of the pertinent anatomic structures included on the radiograph?)

_____   Evaluate for positioning or centering errors (e.g., rotation, off centering)

_____   Evaluate for correct exposure factors and possible motion. (Is the contrast media properly penetrated?)

_____   Determine whether patient obliquity is correct for specific positions.

_____   Determine whether markers and an acceptable degree of collimation and/or area shielding are visible on the images.

LABORATORY EXERCISE B: Physical Positioning

On another person, simulate performing all basic and special projections of an OCG as follows.   (Check off each when completed satisfactorily.) Include the following six steps as described in the textbook.

Step 1.   Appropriate size and type of image receptor with correct markers
Step 2.   Correct CR placement and centering of part to CR and/or image receptor
Step 3.   Accurate collimation
Step 4.   Area shielding of patient where advisable
Step 5.   Use of proper immobilizing devices when needed
Step 6.   Approximate correct exposure factors, breathing instructions where applicable, and "making" exposure

Projections	Step 1	Step 2	Step 3	Step 4	Step 5	Step 6
• PA scout	____	____	____	____	____	____
• LAO	____	____	____	____	____	____
• Right lateral decubitus	____	____	____	____	____	____
• PA erect	____	____	____	____	____	____

Optional:

• RPO for biliary ducts	____	____	____	____	____	____

Answers to Review Exercises

Review Exercise A: Radiographic Anatomy of the Gallbladder and Biliary System

1. 3 to 4 pounds (1.5 kg) or $\frac{1}{60}$ of total body weight
2. Right upper quadrant
3. Falciform ligament
4. Right
5. A. Quadrate
   B. Caudate
6. True
7. False (1 qt or 800 to 1000 ml)
8. A. Store bile
   B. Concentrate bile
   C. Contract to release bile into duodenum
9. Cholecystokinin (CCK)
10. False (by the duodenal mucosa)
11. True
12. Duodenal papilla
13. True
14. False (duct of Wirsung)
15. Anteriorly
16. 1. C, 2. A, 3. C, 4. C
17. A. Left hepatic duct
    B. Common hepatic duct
    C. Common bile duct
    D. Pancreatic duct
    E. Hepatopancreatic ampulla (ampulla of Vater)
    F. Duodenal papilla
    G. Duodenum
    H. Fundus of gallbladder
    I. Body of gallbladder
    J. Neck of gallbladder
    K. Cystic duct
    L. Right hepatic duct
18. A. Liver
    B. Cystic duct
    C. Gallbladder
    D. Common bile duct
    E. Duodenum
    F. Common hepatic duct
19. Supine
20. PA
21. LAO

Review Exercise B: Radiographic Procedures and Positioning of the Gallbladder and Biliary Ducts

1. Bile
2. Bladder or sac
3. Cholecystography
4. Cholangiography
5. Cholecystocholangiography
6. Oral cholecystogram
7. Cholecystopaques
8. A. Functional ability of the liver to remove contrast media
   B. Patency and condition of the biliary ducts
   C. Concentrating and contracting ability of the gallbladder
9. A. Advanced hepatorenal disease
   B. Active gastrointestinal disease
   C. Pregnancy
10. 1. C, 2. D, 3. F, 4. A, 5. E, 6. B
11. False (only about 15 % are visualized)
12. True
13. False (may be other reasons)
14. False (may be other reasons)
15. False (only NPO 8 hrs)
16. True
17. True
18. 10 to 12 hours before the procedure
19. 70 to 80 kVp
20. A. How many pills were taken and at what time?
    B. Any reaction from the pills?
    C. Did you have breakfast?
    D. Do you still have your gallbladder?
    E. Is there a possibility of pregnancy?
21. Measure the function of the gallbladder
22. A. No ionizing radiation
    B. Better detection of small calculi
    C. No contrast media is required
    D. Is a less time-consuming procedure
23. Mobile digital C-arm fluoroscopy
24. Reduce the risk of spasm of the biliary ducts
25. A. It can be performed as an outpatient procedure
    B. It is a less invasive procedure
    C. Reduced hospital time and cost
26. In the radiology department
27. C. Remove a biliary stone
28. A. Obstructive jaundice
29. Rule out a possible pneumothorax
30. D. Cholecystitis

31. A. Endoscopic retrograde cholangio-pancreatogram
    B. ERCP
    C. Duodenoscope or video endoscope
    D. Gastroenterologist
    E. Prevent aspiration of food or liquid into the lungs
32. 1. A, 2. D, 3. E, 4. F, 5. C, 6. B
33. True
34. False (HIDA scans are a study of the gallbladder and biliary ducts)
35. B. Sonography
36. False (female ≈6 mrad; males 0.1 mrad)
37. False (the center cell should be used)
38. D. L2
39. D. Higher and more lateral
40. LAO (or RPO if the patient cannot lie supine)
41. A. 40°
    B. 15°
42. Erect or right lateral decubitus
43. Right lateral decubitus (PA)
44. B. 5 to 10 mrad
45. 1 to 2 in (2.5 to 5 cm)

Review Exercise C: Problem Solving for Technical and Positioning Errors

1. Center the CR lower and more midline for an asthenic patient. Also, using a 14 x 17 in. (35 x 43 cm) cassette for the scout, instead of a 10 x 12 in. (24 x 30 cm), will provide greater coverage of the abdomen.
2. Lower the kVp to the 70 to 76 range
3. Increase obliquity to project the gallbladder away from the spine
4. Request that the patient be rotated into a 15 to 25° RPO position
5. Ultrasound of the gallbladder. It does not require any contrast media
6. Percutaneous transhepatic cholangiogram (PTC) (The PTC may also be preceded by an ultrasound study.)
7. Fatty meal or CCK study
8. ERCP
9. Sonography or nuclear medicine-HIDA scan
10. Sonography or computed tomography

SELF-TEST

My Score = _____ %

Directions: This self-test should be taken only after completing **all** of the readings, review exercises, and laboratory activities for a particular section. The purpose of this test is not only to provide a good learning exercise but also to serve as a good indicator of what your final evaluation grade will be. It is strongly suggested that if you do not get at least a 90% to 95% grade on each self-test, you should review those areas in which you missed questions **before** going to your instructor for the final evaluation exam for this chapter. (There are 70 questions or blanks—each is worth 1.4 points.)

1. The gallbladder is located in the _____ margin of the liver.

   A. Anterior inferior   C. Mid aspect

   B. Posterior superior   D. Anterior superior

2. Which one of the following is **not** a major lobe of the liver?

   A. Caudate   C. Inferior

   B. Quadrate   D. Left

4. What is the name of the soft-tissue structure that divides the liver into left and right lobes?

_____

5. What is the primary function of bile? _____

6. Which duct is formed by the union of the left and right hepatic ducts? _____

7. What is the average capacity of the gallbladder? _____

8. Which chemical process leads to concentration of bile within the gallbladder? _____

9. Which hormone leads to contraction of the gallbladder to release bile? _____

10. Which duct carries bile from the cystic duct to the duodenum? _____

11. Match the following biliary structures to their correct description or definition:

   _____ 1. Pancreatic duct   A. Series of mucosal folds in cystic duct

   _____ 2. Fundus   B. A protrusion into the duodenum

   _____ 3. Hepatopancreatic ampulla   C. Middle aspect of gallbladder

   _____ 4. Spiral valve   D. Duct connected directly to gallbladder

   _____ 5. Hepatopancreatic sphincter   E. Narrowest portion of gallbladder

   _____ 6. Duodenal papilla   F. Broadest portion of gallbladder

   _____ 7. Cystic duct   G. Enlarged chamber in distal aspect of common bile duct

   _____ 8. Neck   H. Duct of Wirsung

   _____ 9. Body   I. Circular muscle

12. Which general body position will encourage drainage of bile/contrast media from the gallbladder?

    _____

    Why? _____

13. Identify the labeled parts and/or structures on the radiograph of an OCG (Fig. 16-3) and of biliary ducts from two
    different operative cholangiogram procedures (Fig. 16-4).

    Fig.   16-3

    A. _____

    B. _____

    C. _____

    D. _____

    Fig. 16-4

    E. _____

    F. _____

    G. _____

    H. _____

    I. _____

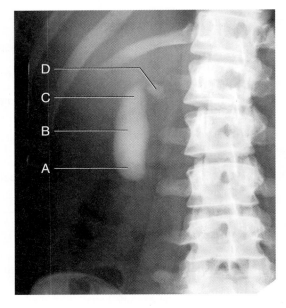

Fig. 16-3 Radiograph of an OCG and of biliary ducts.

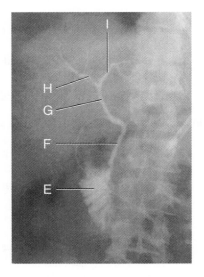

Fig. 16-4 Radiograph of an operative
cholangiogram procedure.

14.   Match the prefixes and terms on the left with the correct description on the right.

      _____ 1.   Cysto-   A.   Radiographic study of gallbladder and biliary ducts

      _____ 2.   Chole-   B.   Radiographic study of gallbladder

      _____ 3.   Cholecystocholangiogram   C.   Radiographic study of biliary ducts

      _____ 4.   Cholecystogram   D.   Condition of having gallstones

      _____ 5.   Cholangiogram   E.   Inflammation of gallbladder

      _____ 6.   Cholecystopaque   F.   Oral contrast media for gallbladder

      _____ 7.   Cholecystitis   G.   OCG

      _____ 8.   Oral cholecystogram   H.   Denotes sac or bladder

      _____ 9.   Cholelithiasis   I.   Denotes bile

15.   True/False: Drugs have been developed that will dissolve gallstones and may avoid the need to have surgery in select cases.

16.   True/False: Gallbladders with acute cholecystitis rarely become radiopaque during an OCG.

17.   Match the following pathologic indications with the correct definition and/or statement:

      _____ 1.   Biliary stenosis   A.   Emulsion of biliary stones

      _____ 2.   Congenital anomalies   B.   May be caused by bacterial infection or ischemia of the gallbladder

      _____ 3.   Chronic cholecystitis   C.   Narrowing of one of the biliary ducts

      _____ 4.   Choledocholithiasis   D.   Although benign, they may affect production, storage, or release of bile

      _____ 5.   Acute cholecystitis   E.   Signs may include calcification of the gallbladder wall

      _____ 6.   Milk calcium bile   F.   Approximately 80% of the patients with this condition have gallstones

      _____ 7.   Carcinoma of gallbladder G.   Stones in the biliary ducts

18.   How long should a patient remain NPO before an OCG? _____

19.   How far in advance should the oral contrast media be taken for an OCG? _____

20.   Which kVp range is ideal for an OCG? _____

21.   Why is a patient placed into the RPO position during a fatty meal or CCK procedure?

      _____

22.   How long does it take the gallbladder to begin to contract after an injection of CCK? _____

23.   True/False: Ultrasound of the gallbladder requires that the patient be NPO for at least 8 hours before the study.

24. True/False: Ultrasound of the gallbladder is considered a noninvasive procedure.

25. How is the contrast media instilled into the biliary ducts during an operative cholangiogram?

   _____

26. On average, how much contrast media is injected during an operative cholangiogram?

   _____

27. What must the technologist do with respect to the grid-image receptor if the OR table is tilted during an operative

   cholangiogram? _____

   _____

28. Why is a laparoscopic cholecystectomy considered less invasive as compared with traditional cholecystectomy?

   _____

29. What is the most common clinical reason for performing a T-tube cholangiogram?

   _____

30. Which one of the following conditions is a pathologic indication for a percutaneous transhepatic cholangiogram
    (PTC)?
    A. Chronic cholecystitis   C. Neoplasm of the gallbladder
    B. Obstructive jaundice   D. Cholelithiasis

31. What type of needle is most often used for a PTC?
    A. 6-inch spinal needle   C. 18-gauge angiocath
    B. 18-gauge butterfly   D. Skinny needle

32. Match the following by indicating which procedure is performed in the operating room by a surgeon and which is per-
    formed in the radiology department by a radiologist.

    _____ A. T-tube cholangiogram   S. In operating room by a surgeon

    _____ B. Operative cholangiogram   R. In radiology department by a radiologist

    _____ C. Percutaneous transhepatic cholangiogram

33. True/False: An ERCP can be considered both a diagnostic and therapeutic procedure.

34. True/False: A percutaneous transhepatic cholangiogram (PTC) is generally performed in the radiology department
    and involves placing a needle through the liver directly into a biliary duct.

35. True/False: A pediatric patient with hemolytic anemia may develop gallstones.

36. True/False: A HIDA scan is a special MRI study of the liver using a contrast agent.

37. True/False: CT is an excellent imaging modality for demonstrating tumors of the liver, gallbladder, or pancreas.

38. Which ionization chamber needs to be activated for an LAO projection of the gallbladder?

   _____

39. What is the primary difference between the operative cholangiogram and the T-tube cholangiogram? (Both are performed to visualize possible choleliths.)

_____

_____

40. **Situation:** A radiograph of an LAO projection reveals that the gallbladder is superimposed over the spine. What modification is needed during the repeat exposure to avoid this problem?

_____

41. Why is the erect gallbladder projection preferred as a PA rather than an AP projection?

_____

42. **Situation:** During an OCG, the radiologist believes that stones may be present in the gallbladder. She requests that the technologist provide a projection to stratify any possible stones. Which two projections may accomplish this goal?

_____

43. **Situation:** A patient scheduled for an OCG complains that she can't lie prone or on her right side due to recent surgery. Which position could be performed to ensure that the gallbladder will not be superimposed over the spine?

_____

44. **Situation:** A patient with a history of possible gallstones is scheduled for an OCG. During the patient interview, she states that she had a piece of bacon before coming into the hospital. When the scout image is taken, the gallbladder is not visualized. What other imaging options can the radiologist order to determine if there are gallbladder stones?

_____

45. Which one of the following studies is considered an invasive procedure?

A. OCG   C. Sonography of the gallbladder

B. CT of the gallbladder   D. PTC

17

Urinary System

CHAPTER OBJECTIVES

After you have completed **all** the activities of this chapter, you will be able to:

_____ 1. Identify the location and pertinent anatomy of the urinary system to include the adrenal glands.

_____ 2. Identify specific structures of the macroscopic and microscopic anatomy and physiology of the kidney.

_____ 3. Identify the orientation of the kidneys, ureters and urinary bladder with respect to the peritoneum and other structures of the abdomen.

_____ 4. List the primary functions of the urinary system.

_____ 5. Describe the spatial relationship between the male and female reproductive system and the urinary system.

_____ 6. On drawings and radiographs, identify specific anatomy of the urinary system

_____ 7. Identify key lab values and drug concerns that must be verified prior to intravenous injections of contrast media.

_____ 8. Identify characteristics specific to either ionic or nonionic contrast media.

_____ 9. Differentiate between mild, moderate, and severe reactions and from side effects to injected contrast media. List several examples of each.

_____ 10. Identify the steps and safety measures to be observed during a venipuncture procedure.

_____ 11. List safety measures to be followed before and during the injection of an iodinated contrast media.

_____ 12. Define specific urinary pathologic terminology and indications.

_____ 13. Match specific types of urinary pathology to the correct radiographic appearances and signs.

_____ 14. List the purpose, contraindications, and six high-risk patient conditions for intravenous urography.

_____ 15. Identify two methods utilized to enhance pelvicalyceal filling during intravenous urography and contraindications for their use.

_____ 16. Identify the purpose of the nephrogram and nephrotomogram.

_____ 17. Identify specific aspects related to the retrograde urogram and how this procedure differs from an intravenous urogram.

_____ 18. Identify specific aspects related to the retrograde cystogram.

_____ 19. Identify specific aspects related to the retrograde urethrogram.

_____ 20. List specific information related to the basic and special projections for excretory urography, retrograde urography, cystography, urethrography, and voiding cystourethrography to include size and type of image receptor, central ray location, direction and angulation of central ray, and anatomy best visualized.

_____ 21. Identify the patient dose ranges for skin, midline, and gonads for specific urinary system projections.

_____ 22 Given various hypothetical situations, identify the correct modification of a position and/or exposure factors to improve the radiographic image.

POSITIONING AND FILM CRITIQUE

_____ 1. Using a peer, position for basic and special projections for an intravenous urogram procedure.

_____ 2. Critique and evaluate urinary study radiographs based on the four divisions of radiographic criteria: (1) structures shown, (2) position, (3) collimation and CR, and (4) exposure criteria.

_____ 3. Distinguish between acceptable and unacceptable urinary study radiographs due to exposure factors, motion, collimation, positioning, or other errors.

Learning Exercises

Complete the following review exercises after reading the associated pages in the textbook as indicated by each exercise. Answers to each review exercise are given at the end of the review exercises.

PART I: Radiographic Anatomy

REVIEW EXERCISE A: Radiographic Anatomy of the Urinary System (see textbook pp. 540-546)

1. The kidneys and ureters are located in the _____ space.

   A. Intraperitoneal   C. Extraperitoneal

   B. Infraperitoneal   D. Retroperitoneal

2. The _____ glands are located directly superior to the kidneys.

3. Which structures create a 20° angle of the upper pole of the kidney in relation to the lower pole?

   _____

4. What is the specific name for the mass of fat that surrounds each kidney? _____

5. What degree of rotation from supine is needed to place the kidneys parallel to the film?

   _____

6. Which two bony landmarks can be palpated to locate the kidneys? _____

7. Which term describes an abnormal drop of the kidneys when the patient is placed erect?

   _____

8. List the three functions of the urinary system.

   A. _____

   B. _____

   C. _____

9. A buildup of nitrogenous waste in the blood is called:

   A. Hemotoxicity   C. Sepsis

   B. Uremia   D. Renotoxicity

10. The longitudinal fissure, found along the central medial border of the kidney, is called the _____ .

11. The peripheral or outer portion of the kidney is called the _____ .

12. The term that describes the total functioning portion of the kidney is _____ .

13. The microscopic function and structural unit of the kidney is the _____ .

14. Which structure of the medulla is made up of a collection of tubules that drain into the minor calyx?

_____

15. What is another name for the glomerular capsule? _____

16. True/False: The glomerular capsule and proximal and distal convoluted tubules are located in the medulla of the kidney.

17. True/False: The efferent arterioles carry blood to the glomeruli.

18. Identify the renal structures labeled on Fig. 17-1:

A. _____

B. _____

C. _____

D. _____

E. _____

F. _____

G. _____

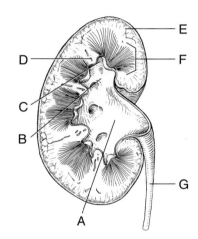

Fig. 17-1 Cross-section of a kidney.

19. Identify the structures making up a nephron and collecting duct (Fig. 17-2). With each structure, check whether it is located in the cortex or medulla portion of the kidney.

	STRUCTURE	CORTEX	MEDULLA
A.	_____	____	____
B.	_____	____	____
C.	_____	____	____
D.	_____	____	____
E.	_____	____	____
F.	_____	____	____
G.	_____	____	____
H.	_____	____	____
I.	_____	____	____

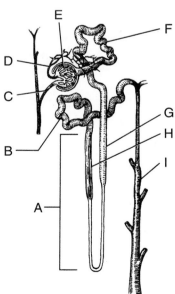

Fig. 17-2 Structures of a nephron and collecting duct.

20. Which two processes move urine through the ureters to the bladder?

A. _____   B. _____

21. Which one of the following structures is located most anterior?

A. Proximal ureters   C. Urinary bladder

B. Kidneys   D. Suprarenal glands

22. What is the name of the junction found between the distal ureters and urinary bladder? _____

23. What is the name of the inner posterior region of the bladder formed by the two ureters entering and the urethra exiting?

_____

24. What is the name of the small gland found just inferior to the male bladder? _____

25. The total capacity for the average adult bladder is:

A. 100 to 200 milliliters   C. 350 to 500 milliliters

B. 200 to 300 milliliters   D. 500 to 700 milliliters

26. Which one of the following structures is considered to be most posterior?

A. Ovaries   C. Vagina

B. Urethra   D. Kidneys

27. Identify the urinary structures labeled on Fig.17-3.

A. _____

B. _____

C. _____

D. _____

E. _____

F. _____

G. _____

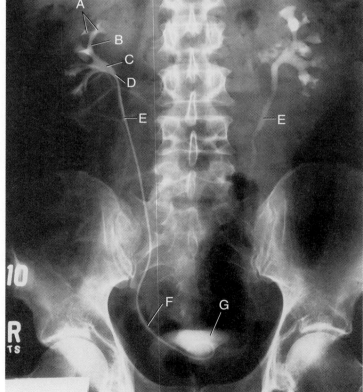

Fig. 17-3 AP retrograde pyelogram radiograph.

PART II: Radiographic Positioning, Contrast Media, and Pathology

REVIEW EXERCISE B: Contrast Media, Contrast Media Reactions, and Venipuncture (see textbook pp. 547-554)

1. List the two ways contrast media are administered in urography.

   A. _____   B. _____

2. The two major types of iodinated contrast media used for urography are ionic and nonionic. For each of the following characteristics, indicate which apply to ionic (I) and which to nonionic (N) contrast media:

   _____   1.   Uses a parent compound of a benzoic acid

   _____   2.   Will not significantly increase the osmolality of the blood plasma

   _____   3.   Incorporates sodium or meglumine to increase solubility of the contrast media

   _____   4.   Creates a hypertonic condition in the blood plasma

   _____   5.   Is more expensive

   _____   6.   Produces less severe reactions

   _____   7.   Is a near-isotonic solution

   _____   8.   Greater risk of disrupting homeostasis

   _____   9.   Uses a parent compound of an amide or glucose group

   _____   10. May increase the severity of side effects

3. Which one of the following compounds is a common **anion** found in ionic contrast media?

   A. Diatrizoate or iothalamate   C.   Benzoic acid

   B. Sodium or meglumine   D.   None of the above

4. Any disruption in the physiological functions of the body that may lead to a contrast media reaction is

   called _____ .

   A. Homeostasis   C.   Vasovagal

   B. Anaphylactoid   D.   Chemotoxic

5. The normal creatinine level for an adult should range between: _____

6. Normal BUN levels for an adult should range between: _____

7. A. Glucophage is a drug that is taken for the management of _____

   B. The American College of Radiology recommends that Glucophage be withheld _____

   hours before a contrast media procedure and not taken for _____ hours following a

   contrast media procedure.

8. List the six conditions that may place a patient at greater risk of a contrast media reaction:

   A. _____

   B. _____

   C. _____

   D. _____

   E. _____

   F. _____

9. True/False: Mild contrast media reactions are usually self-limiting and do not require medication.

10. True/False: Urticaria is the formal term for excessive vomiting.

11. The leakage of contrast media from a vessel into the surrounding soft tissues is called _____

12. A reaction, based upon fear or anxiety, is called _____ .

13. An expected outcome to the introduction of contrast media is described as a _____ .

14. Indicate whether the following symptoms denote a side effect (SE), mild reaction (Mi R), moderate reaction (Mo R), or severe reaction (SR).

   _____ 1. Convulsions   _____ 10. Extravasation

   _____ 2. Metallic taste   _____ 11. Excessive urticaria

   _____ 3. Cyanosis

   _____ 4. Giant hives

   _____ 5. Itching

   _____ 6. Vasovagal response

   _____ 7. Temporary hot flash

   _____ 8. Difficulty in breathing

   _____ 9. Laryngeal spasm

15. What should the technologist do first when a patient is experiencing either a moderate or a severe contrast media reaction? _____

16. Intravenous contrast media may be administered by either:

   A. _____

   B. _____

17. True/False: The patient (or legal guardian) must sign an informed consent form before a venipuncture procedure.

18. For most IVUs, veins in the _____ are recommended for venipuncture.

    A. Iliac fossa   C. Axillary fossa

    B. Anterior, carpal region   D. Antecubital fossa

19. The most common size of needle used for bolus injections of contrast media is:

    A. 23 to 25 gauge   C. 18 to 20 gauge

    B. 14 to 16 gauge   D. 28 gauge

20. The two most common types of needles used for bolus injection of contrast media are

    _____ and _____

21. In the correct order, list the four primary steps followed during a venipuncture procedure as listed and described in the textbook:

    1. _____

    2. _____

    3. _____

    4. _____

22. True/False: The bevel of the needle needs to be facing downward during the actual puncture into a vein.

23. True/False: If extravasation occurs during the puncture, the technologist should slightly retract the needle and then push it forward again.

24. True/False: If unsuccessful during the initial puncture, a new needle should be used during the second attempt.

25. True/False: The radiologist is responsible for documenting all aspects of the venipuncture procedure in the patient's chart.

REVIEW EXERCISE C: Radiographic Procedures, Contraindications, Pathologic Terminology, and Indications (see textbook pp. 555-565)

1. A. Why is the term *IVP* incorrect in describing a radiographic exam of the kidneys, ureters, and bladder following intravenous injection of contrast media?

    _____

    B. What is the correct term and correct initials for this exam? _____

2. Which specific aspect of the kidney is visualized during an IVU? _____

3. Which one of the following conditions is a common clinical indication for an IVU?

    A. Sickle cell anemia   C. Hematuria

    B. Multiple myeloma   D. Anuria

4. Which one of the following conditions is described as a rare tumor of the kidney?

    A. Pheochromocytoma   C. Melanoma

    B. Multiple myeloma   D. Renal cell carcinoma

5. Match the following urinary pathologic terms to the correct definition:

_____ A. Pneumouria   1. Passage of large volume of urine

_____ B. Urinary reflux   2. Presence of glucose in urine

_____ C. Uremia   3. Excess in the blood of urea and creatinine

_____ D. Anuria   4. Diminished amount of urine being excreted

_____ E. Polyuria   5. Presence of gas in urine

_____ F. Micturition   6. Indicated by presence of uremia, oliguria, or anuria

_____ G. Retention   7. Constant or frequent involuntary passage of urine

_____ H. Oliguria   8. Backward return flow of urine

_____ I. Glucosuria   9. Absence of a functioning kidney

_____ J. Urinary incontinence   10. Complete cessation of urinary secretion

_____ K. Renal agenesis   11. Act of voiding

_____ L. Acute renal failure   12. Inability to void

6. Match the correct pathologic indication to the following definitions:

_____ A. Age-associated enlargement of the prostate gland   1. Vesicorectal fistula

_____ B. Fusion of the kidney during the development of the fetus   2. Renal hypertension

_____ C. Inflammation of the capillary loops of the glomeruli of the kidneys   3. Ectopic kidney

_____ D. Artificial opening between the urinary bladder and aspects of the large intestine   4. Horseshoe kidney

_____ E. A large stone that grows and completely fills the renal pelvis   5. Staghorn calculus

_____ F. Increased blood pressure to the kidneys due to atherosclerosis   6. Polycystic kidney disease

_____ G. Normal kidney that fails to ascend into the abdomen but remains in the pelvis   7. Benign Prostatic Hyperplasia

_____ H. Multiple cysts in one or both kidneys   8. Glomerulonephritis

7. Match the following radiographic appearances to the correct pathologic indication:

   _____ A. Rapid excretion of contrast media   1. Malrotation

   _____ B. Mucosal changes within bladder   2. Vesicorectal fistula

   _____ C. Bilateral, small kidneys with blunted calyces   3. Renal cell carcinoma

   _____ D. Irregular appearance of renal parenchyma or collecting system   4. BPH

   _____ E. Signs of abnormal fluid collections   5. Renal hypertension

   _____ F. Abnormal rotation of the kidney   6. Renal calculi

   _____ G. Elevated or indented floor of bladder   7. Cystitis

   _____ H. Signs of obstruction of urinary system   8. Chronic Bright's disease

8. True/False: If an IVU and barium enema are both scheduled, the IVU should always be performed first.

9. True/False: The patient should void before an IVU to prevent possible rupture of the bladder if compression is applied.

10. What is the primary purpose of ureteric compression? _____

11. List the six conditions that could contraindicate the use of ureteric compression:

    A. _____   D. _____

    B. _____   E. _____

    C. _____   F. _____

12. When does the timing for and IVU exam start? _____

13. List the basic five-step timed imaging sequence for a routine IVU.

    A. _____   D. _____

    B. _____   E. _____

    C. _____

14. What is the primary difference between a standard and a hypertensive IVU?

    _____

15. In what department are most retrograde urograms performed? _____

16. True/False: A retrograde urogram examines the anatomy and function of the pelvicalyceal system.

17. True/False: The Brodney clamp is used for male and female retrograde cystourethrograms.

18. Which of the following involves a direct introduction of the contrast media into the structure being studied?

    A. Retrograde urogram   C. Retrograde urethrogram

    B. Retrograde cystogram   D. All of the above

19. Which of the following alternative imaging modalities is NOT being utilized to diagnosed renal calculi?

   A. Nuclear medicine   C. Magnetic resonance imaging

   B. Sonography   D. Computed tomography

20. True/False: Urinary studies on pediatric patients should be scheduled early in the morning to minimize the risk of dehydration.

REVIEW EXERCISE D: Radiographic Positioning of the Urinary System (see textbook pp. 566-574)

1. What are the three reasons a scout projection is taken before an injection of contrast media for an IVU?

   A. _____   C. _____

   B. _____

2. What kVp range is recommended for an IVU? _____

3. Which ionization chambers should be activated for an AP scout projection? _____

4. True/False: Both the female midline dose and the female gonadal dose for an average unshielded AP projection for an IVU are in the 100 to 200 mrad range.

5. True/False: Male and female patients should have the gonads shielded for an AP scout projection.

6. True/False: Tomograms taken during an IVU with an exposure angle of 10° or less are called *zonography.*

7. How many tomograms (zonograms) are usually produced during an IVU? _____

8. At what stage of an IVU is the renal parenchyma best seen?

   A. 5 minutes following injection   C. During the post-void film

   B. 10 minutes following injection   D. Within 1 minute following injection

9. Where is the CR centered for a nephrotomogram?

   A. At xiphoid process   C. At iliac crest

   B. Midway between xiphoid process and iliac crest   D. At axillary costal margin

10. Which specific position, taken during an IVU, will place the left kidney parallel to the film?

   _____

11. How much obliquity is required for the LPO/RPO projections taken during an IVU? _____

12. Which position will best demonstrate possible nephroptosis? _____

13. How will an enlarged prostate gland appear on a post-void radiograph taken during an IVU?

   _____

14. Where should the pneumatic paddle be placed for the ureteric compression phase of an IVU?

   _____

15. What can be done to enhance filling of the calyces of the kidney if ureteric compression is contraindicated?

   _____

16. What specific anatomy is examined during a retrograde ureterogram?

    A. Primarily the ureters   C. Entire urinary system

    B. Primarily the renal pelvis and calyces   D. Urinary bladder

17. A retrograde pyelogram is primarily a nonfunctional study of the _____.

18. What CR angle is utilized for the AP projection taken during a cystogram?

    A. 20 to 25° caudad   C. 10 to 15° caudad

    B. 5 to 10° cephalad   D. 30 to 40° caudad

19 True/False: For a lateral cystogram, both the male and female dose are in the 100 (±50) mrad range.

20. Which specific position is recommended for a male patient during a voiding cystourethrogram?

_____

REVIEW EXERCISE E: Problem Solving for Technical and Positioning Errors (see textbook pp. 566-574)

1. **Situation:** A radiograph of an AP scout projection of the abdomen, taken during an IVU, reveals that the symphysis pubis is slightly cut off. The patient is too large to include the entire abdomen on a 35 x 43 cm (14 x 17 in.) IR. What should the technologist do in this situation?

_____

_____

2. **Situation:** A nephrogram is ordered as part of an IVU study. When the nephrogram image is processed, there is a minimal amount of contrast media within the renal parenchyma, and the calyces are beginning to fill with contrast media. What specific problem led to this radiographic outcome?

_____

_____

3. **Situation:** A 45° RPO radiograph taken during an IVU reveals that the left kidney is foreshortened. What modification is needed to improve this image during the repeat exposure?

_____

_____

4. **Situation:** An AP projection taken during the compression phase of an IVU reveals that the majority of the contrast media has left the collecting system. The technologist placed the pneumatic paddles near the umbilicus and ensured that they were inflated. What can the technologist do to ensure better retention of contrast media in the collecting system during the compression phase of future IVUs?

_____

_____

5. **Situation:** An AP projection radiograph taken during a cystogram reveals that the floor of the bladder is superimposed over the symphysis pubis. What can the technologist do to correct this problem during the repeat exposure?

_____

_____

6. **Situation:** A patient comes to the radiology department for an IVU. While taking the clinical history, the technologist learns the patient has renal hypertension. How must the technologist modify the IVU imaging sequence to accommodate this patient's condition?

_____

_____

7. **Situation:** A patient comes to the radiology department for an IVU. The AP scout reveals an abnormal density near the lumbar spine that the radiologist suspects is an abdominal, aortic aneurysm. What should the technologist do about the ureteric compression phase of the study that had been ordered?

_____

_____

8. **Situation:** A patient comes to the radiology department for an IVU. The patient history indicates that he may have an enlarged prostate gland. Which projection will best demonstrate this condition?

_____

9. **Situation:** A patient with a history of bladder calculi comes to the radiology department. A cystogram has been ordered. During the interview, the patient reports that he had a severe reaction to contrast media in the past. What other imaging modality (or modalities) can be performed to best diagnose this condition?

_____

10. **Situation:** The same patient described in question 9 may also have calculi in the kidney. What is the preferred imaging modality for this situation when iodinated contrast media cannot be used?

_____

PART III: Laboratory Exercises (see textbook pp. 555-574)

Although it is impossible to duplicate many aspects of urinary studies on a phantom in the lab, evaluation of actual radiographs and physical positioning is possible. You can get experience in positioning and radiographic evaluation of these projections by performing exercises using radiographic phantoms and practicing on other students (although you will not be taking actual exposures). Technologists must learn the positioning routine, room setup, and fluoroscopy procedure for their particular facility.

LABORATORY EXERCISE A: Radiographic Evaluation

1. Using actual radiographs of IVU, cystogram and retrograde urogram procedures provided by your instructor, evaluate each position for the following points (check off for each radiograph when completed):

   _____ Evaluate the completeness of the study. (Are all pertinent anatomic structures included on the radiograph?)

   _____ Evaluate for positioning or centering errors (e.g., rotation, off centering)

   _____ Evaluate for correct exposure factors and possible motion. (Is the contrast media properly penetrated?)

   _____ Determine whether patient obliquity is correct for specific positions.

   _____ Determine whether markers and an acceptable degree of collimation and/or area shielding are visible on the images.

LABORATORY EXERCISE B: Physical Positioning

On another person, simulate performing all basic and special projections of the IVU as follows. (Check off each when completed satisfactorily.) Include the following six steps as described in the textbook.

Step 1. Appropriate size and type of image receptor with correct markers
Step 2. Correct CR placement and centering of part to CR and/or image receptor
Step 3. Accurate collimation
Step 4. Area shielding of patient where advisable
Step 5. Use of proper immobilizing devices when needed
Step 6. Approximate correct exposure factors, breathing instructions where applicable, and "making" exposure

Projections	Step 1	Step 2	Step 3	Step 4	Step 5	Step 6
• AP scout	____	____	____	____	____	____
• LPO and RPO	____	____	____	____	____	____
• AP cystogram	____	____	____	____	____	____
• Lateral cystogram	____	____	____	____	____	____

Answers to Review Exercises

Review Exercise A: Radiographic Anatomy of the Urinary System

1. D. Retroperitoneal
2. Suprarenal glands
3. Psoas muscles
4. Perirenal fat, or adipose capsule
5. 30°
6. Xiphoid process and iliac crest
7. Nephroptosis
8. A. Remove nitrogenous waste
   B. Regulate water levels
   C. Regulate acid-base balance
9. B. Uremia
10. Hilum
11. Cortex
12. Renal parenchyma
13. Nephron
14. Renal pyramids
15. Bowman's capsule
16. False (located in the cortex)
17. False (afferent)
18. A. Renal pelvis
    B. Major calyx
    C. Minor calyx
    D. Renal sinuses
    E. Cortex
    F. Medulla
    G. Ureter
19. A. Loop of Henle, medulla
    B. Distal convoluted tubule, cortex
    C. Afferent arteriole, cortex
    D. Efferent arteriole, cortex
    E. Glomerular capsule, cortex
    F. Proximal convoluted tubule, cortex
    G. Descending limb, medulla
    H. Ascending limb, medulla
    I. Collecting tubule, medulla
20. A. Peristalsis
    B. Gravity
21. C. Urinary bladder
22. Ureterovesical junction
23. Trigone
24. Prostate gland
25. C. 350 to 500 milliliters
26. D. Kidneys
27. A. Minor calyces
    B. Major calyces
    C. Renal pelvis
    D. Ureteropelvic junction (UPC)
    E. Proximal ureter
    F. Distal ureter
    G. Urinary bladder

Review Exercise B: Contrast Media, Contrast Media Reactions, and Venipuncture

1. A. Intravenous injection
   B. Catheterization
2. 1. I, 2. N, 3. I, 4. I, 5. N, 6. N, 7. N, 8. I, 9. N, 10. I
3. A. Diatrizoate or Iothalmate
4. A. Homeostasis
5. 0.6 to 1.5 mg/dl
6. 8 to 25 mg/100 ml
7. A. Diabetes mellitus
   B. 48 hours, 48 hours
8. A. Hypersensitivity toward iodinated contrast media
   B. Diabetes mellitus
   C. Asthma or other respiratory conditions
   D. Multiple myeloma
   E. Severe dehydration
   F. Chronic or acute renal failure or hepatic disease
9. True
10. False (it's the term for hives)
11. Extravasation
12. Vasovagal response
13. Side effect.
14. 1. SR, 2. SE, 3. SR, 4. Mo R, 5. Mi R, 6. Mi R, 7. SE, 8. SR, 9. SR, 10. Mi R, 11. Mo R
15. Call for medical assistance
16. A. Bolus injection
    B. Drip infusion
17. True
18. D. Antecubital fossa
19. C. 18 to 20 gauge
20. Butterfly and over-the-needle catheter
21. 1. Wash hands and put on gloves
    2. Select site and apply tourniquet
    3. Confirm puncture site and cleanse
    4. Initiate puncture
22. False (facing upward)
23. False (needle should be withdrawn and pressure applied)
24. True
25. False (technologist or the one doing the venipuncture is responsible)

Review Exercise C: Radiographic Procedures, Contraindications, Pathologic Terminology and Indications

1. A. An IVP implies a study of the renal pelvis (pyelo) (Intravenous Pyelogram)
   B. Intravenous urogram (IVU)
2. The collecting system of the kidney
3. C. Hematuria
4. A. Pheochromocytoma
5. A. 5
   B. 8
   C. 3
   D. 10
   E. 1
   F. 11
   G. 12
   H. 4
   I. 2
   J. 7
   K. 9
   L. 6
6. A. 7
   B. 4
   C. 8
   D. 1
   E. 5
   F. 2
   G. 3
   H. 6
7. A. 5
   B. 7
   C. 8
   D. 3
   E. 2
   F. 1
   G. 4
   H. 6
8. True
9. True
10. To enhance filling of the pelvicalyceal system with contrast media
11. A. Possible ureteric stones
    B. Abdominal mass
    C. Abdominal aortic aneurysm
    D. Recent abdominal surgery
    E. Severe abdominal pain
    F. Acute abdominal trauma
12. At start of injection of contrast media
13. A. 1-minute nephrogram or nephrotomography
    B. 5-minute full KUB
    C. 15-minute full KUB
    D. 20-minute posterior R and L obliques
    E. Post-void (prone PA or erect AP)
14. A hypertensive IVU requires a shorter span of time between projections
15. In surgery
16. False (nonfunctional exam)
17. False (used for males only)
18. D. All of the above
19. C. Magnetic resonance imaging
20. True

Review Exercise D: Radiographic Positioning of the Urinary System

1. A. Verify patient preparation
   B. Determine if exposure factors are correct
   C. Detect any abnormal calcifications

2. 65 to 75 kVp
3. Upper right and left ionization chambers
4. False (in the 30 to 50 mrad range)
5. False (not female; would obscure essential anatomy)
6. True
7. Three
8. D. Within 1 minute following injection
9. B. Midway between xiphoid process and iliac crest
10. RPO
11. 30°
12. Erect position
13. The prostate gland will indent the floor of the bladder
14. Just medial to the ASIS
15. Place the patient in a 15° Trendelenburg position
16. A Primarily the ureters
17. Renal pelvis, major and minor calyces of the kidneys
18. C. 10 to 15° caudad

19. True
20. 30° RPO

Review Exercise E: Problem Solving for Technical and Positioning Errors

1. A second, smaller IR of the bladder should be taken placed crosswise to include this region. The larger IR should be centered 1 or 2 in. (2 to 5 cm) higher to include the upper abdomen.
2. Too long of a delay between the injection of contrast media and the filming of the nephrogram. The nephrogram needs to be taken close to 60 seconds following injection.
3. Decrease the obliquity of the RPO to no more than 30°.
4. Place the pneumatic paddles just medial to the ASIS to allow for compression of the distal ureters against the pelvic brim.

5. Increase caudad angulation of the central ray to project the symphysis pubis below the bladder.
6. Decrease the span of time between projections to capture all phases of the urinary system. (Take images at 1, 2, and 3 minutes rather than 1, 5, and 15 minutes.)
7. The technologist should not perform the compression phase of the study. Ureteric compression is contraindicated when an abdominal aortic aneurysm is suspected. (The technologist should consult with the radiologist or physician.)
8. The erect pre-void AP projection will best demonstrate an enlarged prostate gland.
9. Ultrasound or CT
10. CT is preferred but a nuclear medicine procedure could also be performed.

SELF-TEST

My Score = _____%

Directions: This self-test should be taken only after completing **all** of the readings, review exercises, and laboratory activities for a particular section. The purpose of this test is not only to provide a good learning exercise but also to serve as a good indicator of what your final evaluation grade will be. It is strongly suggested that if you do not get at least a 90% to 95% grade on this self-test, you should review those areas in which you missed questions *before* going to your instructor for the final evaluation exam for this chapter. (There are 62 questions or blanks—each is worth 1.6 points.)

1. The kidneys are _____ structures.

   A. Retroperitoneal   B. Intraperitoneal   C. Infraperitoneal   D. Extraperitoneal

2. The ureters enter the _____ aspect of the bladder.

   A. Lateral   B. Anterolateral   C. Posterolateral   D. Superolateral

3. The kidneys lie on the _____ (anterior or posterior) surface of each psoas major muscle.

4. The kidneys lie at a _____ angle in relation to the coronal plane.

5. The three constricted points along the length of the ureters where a kidney stone is most likely to lodge are:

   A. _____   C. _____

   B. _____

6. An abnormal drop of more than _____ inches or _____ cm in the position of the kidneys when the patient is erect indicates a condition termed nephroptosis.

7. The buildup of nitrogenous waste in the blood creates a condition called _____ .

8. How much urine is normally produced by the kidneys in 24 hours?

   A. 2.5 liters   B. 180 liters   C. 0.5 liter   D. 1.5 liters

9. The renal veins connect directly to the:

   A. Abdominal aorta   C. Azygos vein

   B. Superior mesenteric vein   D. Inferior vena cava

10. The 8 to 18 conical masses found within the renal medulla are called the _____ .

11. The major calyces of the kidney unite to form the _____ .

12. The microscopic unit of the kidney (of which there are over a million in each kidney) is called the

    _____ .

13. True/False: The loop of Henle and collecting tubules are located primarily in the medulla of the kidney.

14. True/False: About 50% of the glomerular filtrate processed by the nephron is reabsorbed into the kidney's venous system.

15. The inner, posterior triangular aspect of the bladder that is attached to the floor of the pelvis is called the:

    _____ .

16. Identify the structures labeled on this
     radiograph (Fig. 17-4):

     A. _____

     B. _____

     C. _____

     D. _____

     E. _____

     F. _____

17. The term describing the radiographic
     procedure demonstrated on Fig. 17-4
     radiograph is:

     _____

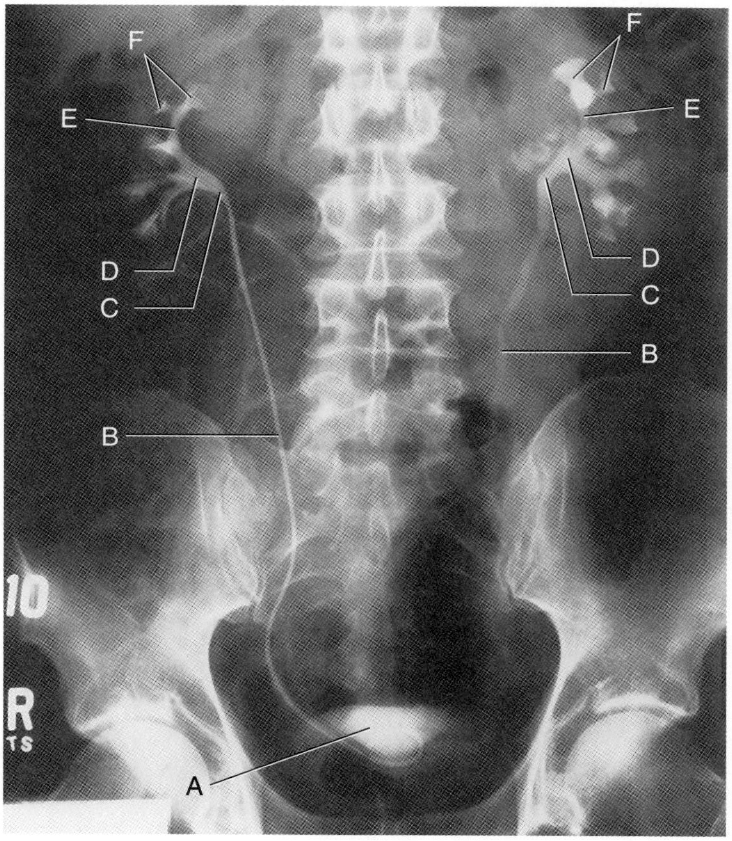

Fig. 17-4 Radiograph of the urinary system.

18. Under what circumstances should a pregnant patient have an IVU performed?

     _____

19. List the two types of iodinated contrast media used for urinary studies? _____

     _____

20. Match the following characteristics to the correct type of iodinated contrast media:

     _____ 1. Dissociates into two separate ions once injected   I. Ionic

     _____ 2. Possesses low osmolality   N. Nonionic

     _____ 3. Uses a salt as its cation

     _____ 4. Parent compound is a carboxyl group

     _____ 5. Less expensive as compared to the other type

     _____ 6. Produces a less severe contrast media reaction

     _____ 7. Diatrizoate is a common anion

     _____ 8. Does not contain a cation

     _____ 9. Creates a hypertonic condition in blood plasma

     _____ 10. Creates a near isotonic solution

21. The normal range of creatinine in an adult is:

  A. 2.0 to 3.4 mg/dl   C. 8 to 25 mg /100 ml

  B. 0.6 to 1.5 mg /dl   D. 0.1 to 1.25 mg /dl

22. How long must a patient be withheld from Glucophage before having an iodinated contrast media procedure?

  A. 48 hours   C. 24 hours

  B. 2 hours   D. 72 hours

23. Which one of the following conditions is considered high risk for an iodinated contrast media procedure?

  A. Hematuria   C. Diabetes mellitus

  B. Renal failure   D. Hypertension

24. What is the best course of action for a patient experiencing a mild contrast media reaction?

  A. Observe and reassure patient   C. Inform your supervisor

  B. Call for immediate medical attention D. Inform the referring physician

25. A vasovagal reaction is classified as:

  A. Side effect   C. Moderate reaction

  B. Mild reaction   D. Severe reaction

26. Extravasation is classified as a:

  A. Side effect   C. Moderate reaction

  B. Mild reaction   D. Severe reaction

27. Profound shock is classified as a:

  A. Side effect   C. Moderate reaction

  B. Mild reaction   D. Severe reaction

28. Tachycardia is classified as a:

  A. Side effect   C. Moderate reaction

  B. Mild reaction   D. Severe reaction

29. Which one of the following veins is NOT normally selected for venipuncture during an IVU?

  A. Basilic   C. Axillary

  B. Cephalic   D. Radial

30. At what angle is the needle advanced into the vein during venipuncture? _____

31. The complete cessation of urinary secretion is called: _____

32. A technique of using acoustic waves to shatter large kidney stones is called: _____

33. The most common reason for urinary tract infection is:

  A. Renal calculi   C. Urinary incontinence

  B. Uremia   D. Vesicourethral reflux

34. Which one of the following conditions may produce hydronephrosis?

    A. Renal obstruction   C. Renal hypertension

    B. Glomerulonephritis   D. BPH

35. Which one of the following pathologic indications is an example of a congenital anomaly of the urinary system?

    A. Ectopic kidney   C. Polycystic kidney disease

    B. Pyelonephritis   D. BPH

36. True/False: The patient should void before the IVU to prevent dilution of the contrast media in the bladder.

37. True/False: The patient should complete a bowel cleansing procedure before the IVU.

38. Which one of the following conditions would contraindicate the use of ureteric compression?

    A. Hematuria   C. Hematuria

    B. Ureteric calculi   D. Multiple myeloma

39. Typically, at what timing sequence during an IVU are the oblique projections taken? _____

40. Which projection(s) best demonstrate the renal parenchyma, and when are they taken?

    _____

41. Which procedure may use a Brodney clamp? _____

42. Which specific body position will place the right kidney parallel to the film? _____

43. True/False: The gonadal dose for the AP post-void projection is higher for male patients than for female patients.

44. True/False: The retrograde ureterogram will demonstrate the ureters, renal pelvis, and major and minor calyces.

45. **Situation:** An AP projection taken during a retrograde cystogram reveals that the symphysis pubis is superimposed over the floor of the bladder. What can be done during the repeat exposure to correct this problem?

    _____

CHAPTER 18

Mammography

After you have completed **all** the activities of this chapter, you will be able to:

_____ 1. On drawings and radiographs, identify specific anatomy of the mammary glands.

_____ 2. Identify specific regions of the breast using the quadrant and the clock systems.

_____ 3. List the three general categories of breasts according to their tissue composition, age of the patient, and radiographic density.

_____ 4. List the technical considerations and equipment essential for quality images of the breast.

_____ 5. Identify the purpose of breast compression and the average pounds of force used when applying compression.

_____ 6. Identify alternative imaging modalities available to study the breast. Include advantages and disadvantages of each system.

_____ 7. Define specific types of breast pathology.

_____ 8. List the American College of Radiology (ACR) nomenclature of terms and abbreviations for mammographic positioning.

_____ 9. Describe the basic and special projections most commonly performed in mammography; include patient positioning, CR placement, and structures best seen.

_____ 10. Describe the Eklund technique for imaging breasts with implants.

_____ 11. List the average skin dose and mean glandular dose (MGD) range for each projection of the breast as described in the textbook.

_____ 12. Given mammographic images, identify specific positioning and exposure factor errors.

POSITIONING AND FILM CRITIQUE

_____ 1. Using a peer in a simulated setting, position for basic and special mammographic projections.

_____ 2. Using appropriate radiographic phantoms, produce satisfactory radiographs of specific positions (if equipment is available).

_____ 3. Critique and evaluate mammographic images based on the four divisions of radiographic criteria: (1) structures shown, (2) position, (3) collimation and CR, and (4) exposure criteria.

_____ 4. Distinguish between acceptable and unacceptable mammographic images due to exposure factors, motion, collimation, positioning, or other errors.

Learning Exercises

Complete the following review exercises after reading the associated pages in the textbook as indicated by each exercise. Answers to each review exercise are given at the end of the review exercises.

PART I: Mammography Quality Standards, Anatomy, and Technical Considerations

REVIEW EXERCISE A: Mammography Quality Standards Act, Anatomy of the Breast, and Technical Considerations (see textbook pp. 576-584)

1. Radiographic examination of the mammary gland or breast is called _____.

2. In 1992 the American Cancer Society recommended that women over the age of _____ should have a screening mammogram performed.

   A. 35   C. 45

   B. 40   D. 50

3. The Mammographic Quality Standards Act (MQSA), which went into effect on October 1, _____, was passed to ensure high-quality mammography service requiring certification by the secretary of the Department of Health and Human Services (DHHS).

   A. 1992   C. 1994

   B. 1993   D. 1995

4. Women between the age of 40 and 49 years old should have a mammogram at least every:

   A. 1 year   C. 5 years

   B. 2 years   D. 6 months

5. As stated in the textbook, breast cancer accounts for _____ of all new cancers detected in women.

   A. 12%   C. 32%

   B. 15%   D. 50%

6. In Canada, mammography guidelines are set by the _____ .

7. The junction of the inferior part of the breast with the anterior chest wall is called the _____ .

8. The pigmented area surrounding the nipple is the _____ .

9. Breast tissue extending into the axilla is called the tail of the breast or the _____ .

10. In the average female breast, the _____ (craniocaudad or mediolateral) diameter is usually greater.

11. Five o'clock in the right breast would be in what quadrant? _____

12. Based on the clock system method, a suspicious mass at 2 o'clock on the right breast would be at _____ o'clock if it were in a similar position on the left breast.

13. What is the large muscle commonly seen on a mammogram that is located between the bony thorax and the mammary gland? _____

14. Two fibrous sheets of tissue join together just posterior to the breast to form the _____ space.

15. What is the function of the mammary gland?

_____

16. What are the three tissue types found in the mammary gland?

A. _____   B. _____   C. _____

17. Various small blood vessels, fibrous connective tissues, ducts, and other small structures seen on finished mammo-

grams are collectively called _____ .

18. Bands of connective tissue passing through the breast tissue are known as _____ .

19. Classify the following types of breasts into one of the three general categories: fibro-glandular (FG), fibro-fatty (FF),
or fatty (F).

_____ 1. 20 years, no children   _____ 5. 50 years, two children

_____ 2. 35 years, no children   _____ 6. Male

_____ 3. 35 years, three children   _____ 7. 35 years, lactating

_____ 4. 25 years, pregnant   _____ 8. 10 years

20. Which is the least dense of the following tissues: fibrous, glandular, or adipose? _____

21. Identify the labeled parts on this sagittal section drawing (Fig. 18-1):

A. _____

B. _____

C. _____

D. _____

E. _____

F. _____

G. _____

H. _____

I. _____

J. _____

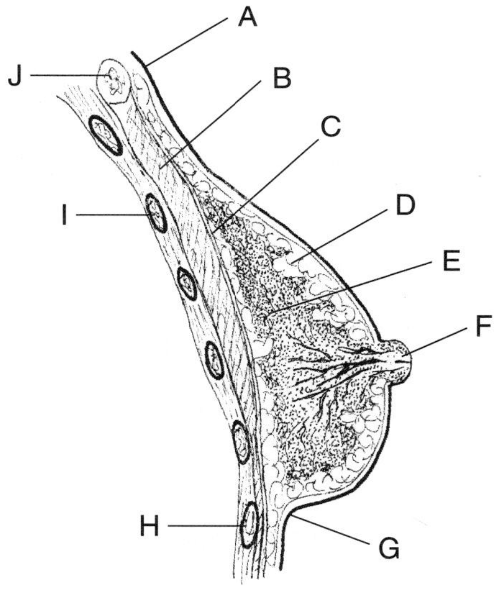

Fig. 18-1 Sagittal section of the breast.

22. Identify the labeled parts on Fig. 18-2:

    A. _____

    B. _____

    C. _____

    D. _____

    E. _____

    F. _____

    G. _____

    H. _____

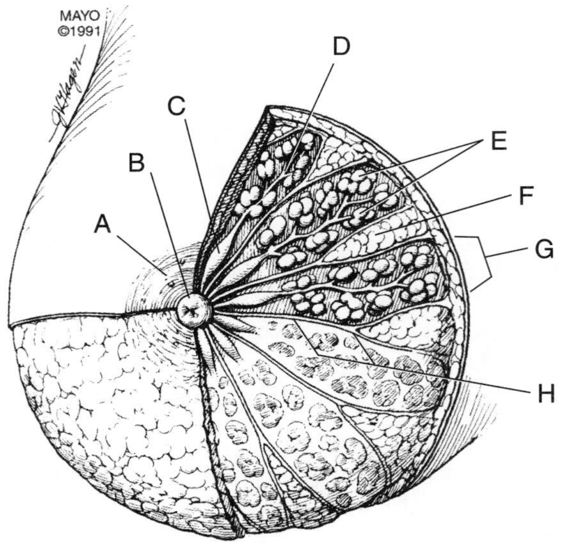

Fig. 18-2 Cutaway anterior view of the breast.

23. The glandular tissue of the breast is divided into _____ lobes.

24. Which portion of the breast is nearest to the chest wall (apex or base)? _____

25. Which portion of the breast is nearest to the nipple (apex or base)? _____

26. The central ray is usually directed through the _____ of the breast.

27. The ideal kilovoltage for mammography is between _____ and _____ kVp.

28. Name the target material used in mammography x-ray tubes. _____

29. The focal spot size on a dedicated mammography unit should be _____ mm or less.

30. Typically, compression applied to the breast is _____ to _____ pounds of pressure.

31. List the two functions of compression during mammography:

    A. _____

    B. _____

32. What is the primary advantage of decreasing the thickness of the breast with compression?

    _____

33. The average required mAs range in mammography using 25 to 28 kVp is:

    A. 10 to 15   C. 40 to 60

    B. 20 to 30   D. 75 to 85

34. What is the typical skin dose for a mammographic projection?

    A. 100 to 200 mrad   C. 800 to 1000 mrad

    B. 400 to 600 mrad   D. 1200 to 1500 mrad

35. To minimize patient dose, the American College of Radiology (ACR) recommends a repeat rate of less than _____ .

   A. 2%   C. 10%

   B. 5%   D. 15%

36. True/False: MGD, as used in patient dose measurements in mammography, refers to mean gonadal dose.

37. True/False: Grids and AEC are used for most mammograms.

38. Which three image qualities need to be present in a good film mammogram?

   A. _____   B. _____   C. _____

39. What type of pathology is best diagnosed with ultrasound of the breast?

   _____

40. Which imaging modality is most effective in diagnosing problems related to breast implants?

   _____

41. True/False: Automatic exposure control cannot be used with breast implants.

42. List the two advantages of digital mammography over conventional film-screen systems:

   A. _____

   B. _____

43. Mammoscintigraphy utilizes the radionuclide called:

   A. Sulphur colloid   C. Technetium

   B. Iodine 131   D. Sestimibi

44. The most common form of benign tumor of the breast is:

   A. Fibroadenoma   C. Fibrocystic lesion

   B. Adenocarcinoma   D. Adenosarcoma

45. List the correct positioning term description for the following ACR abbreviations:

   A. MLO _____   F. LM   _____

   B. SIO _____   G. XCCL _____

   C. AT   _____   H. LMO   _____

   D. CC   _____   I. ID   _____

   E. RL   _____   J. CV   _____

PART II: Radiographic Positioning

REVIEW EXERCISE B: Positioning of the Breast (see textbook pp. 585-590)

1. What are the two basic projections performed for screening mammograms?

    A. _____   B. _____

2. What landmark determines the correct height for placement of the image receptor for the craniocaudad projection?

    _____

3. Anatomical markers and patient identification information need to be placed near the _____ side of the breast.

4. In the craniocaudad projection, what structure must be in profile? _____

5. In the craniocaudad projection, the head should be turned _____ (toward or away) from the side being radiographed.

6. Which basic projection will demonstrate more of the pectoral muscle? _____

7. How much CR/image receptor angulation is utilized for an average-size breast for the mediolateral oblique projection?

    _____

8. The patient with a small, thin breast would require _____ (more or less) CR angulation with the mediolateral oblique projection as compared with the average-size breast.

9. For the mediolateral oblique projection, the arm of the side being examined should be placed:

    A. On the hip   C. Resting on top of the head

    B. Forward, toward the front of the body   D. Behind the back, palm out

10. Which special projection is usually requested when a lesion is seen on the mediolateral oblique but not on the craniocaudad projection? _____

11. In both the craniocaudad and the mediolateral projections, the central ray is always directed to the

    _____ of the breast.

12. What is the most commonly requested special projection of the breast? _____

13. Which projection will most effectively show the axillary aspect of the breast? _____

14. How much is the CR/ image receptor angled from vertical for the mediolateral, true lateral projection?

    _____

15. Mark the following statements: **T** for True, **F** for False.

    _____ 1. It is important for all skin folds to be smoothed out and all wrinkles and pockets of air removed on each projection for the breast.

    _____ 2. Since the base of the breast is well-shown on the craniocaudad projection, this area does not need to be shown on the mediolateral oblique projection.

    _____ 3. The axillary aspect of the breast is usually well-visualized on the craniocaudad projection.

    _____ 4. Mammography is usually done in the standing position.

    _____ 5. Because of a short exposure time, the patient does not need to be completely motionless during the exposure.

    _____ 6. Use of AEC would result in underexposed films with breast implants.

    _____ 7. In the craniocaudad projection, the chest wall must be pushed firmly against the image receptor.

    _____ 8. Standard CC and MLO projections should be performed on patients who have implants.

    _____ 9. Firm compression should not be used on patients with breast implants.

    _____ 10. The patient skin dose for a true mediolateral projection is approximately 30% less than for the mediolateral oblique projection.

16. Which technique (method) is commonly used for the breast with an implant? _____

17. During the procedure mentioned in question 16, what must be done to allow the anterior aspect of the breast to be compressed and properly visualized? _____

18 If a lesion is too deep toward the chest wall and cannot be visualized with a laterally exaggerated craniocaudal projection, a _____ projection should be performed.

    A. Mediolateral oblique   C. Mediolateral
    B. Craniocaudal   D. Axillary tail

19. Telemammography is performed primarily to:

    A. Send digital images to remote locations   C. Reduce dose per projection
    B. Magnify specific regions of interest   D. Demonstrate the deep chest wall

20. What is the average mean glandular dose (MGD) dose for projections of the breast?

    A. 100 to 150 mrad   C. 500 to 700 mrad
    B. 200 to 400 mrad   D. 900 to 1000 mrad

REVIEW EXERCISE C: Critique Radiographs of the Breast (see textbook p. 591)

These questions relate to the radiographs found at the end of Chapter 18 of the textbook. Evaluate these radiographs for positioning accuracy as well as exposure factors, collimation, and correct use of anatomical markers. Describe the corrections needed to improve the overall image. The major, or "repeatable," errors imply that these specific errors require a repeat exposure regardless of the nature or degree of the other errors. Answers to each critique are given at the end of this chapter.

A. CC Projection (Fig. C18-35)   *Description of possible error:*

  1. Structures shown: _____

  2. Part positioning: _____

  3. Collimation and central ray: _____

  4. Exposure criteria: _____

  5. Markers: _____

  Repeatable error(s): _____

B . MLO Projection (Fig. C18-36)   *Description of possible error:*

  1. Structures shown: _____

  2. Part positioning: _____

  3. Collimation and central ray: _____

  4. Exposure criteria: _____

  5. Markers: _____

  Repeatable error(s): _____

C. CC Projection (Fig. C18-37)   *Description of possible error:*

  1. Structures shown: _____

  2. Part positioning: _____

  3. Collimation and central ray: _____

  4. Exposure criteria: _____

  5. Markers: _____

  Repeatable error(s): _____

D. MLO Projection (Fig. C18-38)   *Description of possible error:*

   1. Structures shown: _____

   2. Part positioning: _____

   3. Collimation and central ray: _____

   4. Exposure criteria: _____

   5. Markers: _____

   Repeatable error(s): _____

E. CC Projection (Fig. C18-39)   *Description of possible error:*

   1. Structures shown: _____

   2. Part positioning: _____

   3. Collimation and central ray: _____

   4. Exposure criteria: _____

   5. Markers: _____

   Repeatable error(s): _____

F. CC Projection (Fig. C18-40)   *Description of possible error:*

   1. Structures shown: _____

   2. Part positioning: _____

   3. Collimation and central ray: _____

   4. Exposure criteria: _____

   5. Markers: _____

   Repeatable error(s): _____

PART III: Laboratory Exercises

This part of the learning activity exercise needs to be carried out in the radiology department where the mammography machine is located. Part B can be carried out in a classroom or any room where illuminators are available.

LABORATORY EXERCISE A: Positioning

For this section you need another person to act as your "patient." Male and female students should be separated for this exercise, and students can be fully clothed for the simulated positioning. A clinical instructor must be present.
Include each of the following during this exercise. (Check off when completed.)

_____   Manipulate the x-ray machine into all the positions and become familiar with the locks and devices.

_____   Place or exchange the cone on the machine.

_____   Place a cassette into the cassette holder.

_____   Place a fist on the image receptor tray and compress it by using the compression device.
          (This should be performed so the student can sense the pressure of the device.)

_____   Place another student in position and *simulate* the CC, MLO, XCCL, and ML positions.

_____   **Optional:** If the department or school possesses a breast phantom, perform the basic and special mammogram positions.

LABORATORY EXERCISE B: Film Critique and Evaluation

Your instructor will provide various breast radiographs for these exercises.   Some will be optimal quality radiographs that meet all or most of the evaluation criteria described for each projection in the textbook. Others will be less than optimal quality, and others will be unacceptable, requiring a repeat exam. You should evaluate each radiograph as specified below.

Radiographs

1	2	3	4	5	6	
_____	_____	_____	_____	_____	_____	a. Correct alignment and centering of part
_____	_____	_____	_____	_____	_____	b. Pectoral muscle is included
_____	_____	_____	_____	_____	_____	c. Tissue thickness is distributed evenly
_____	_____	_____	_____	_____	_____	d. Optimal compression is noted
_____	_____	_____	_____	_____	_____	e. Dense areas are adequately penetrated
_____	_____	_____	_____	_____	_____	f. High tissue contrast and optimal resolution noted
_____	_____	_____	_____	_____	_____	g. Absence of artifacts
_____	_____	_____	_____	_____	_____	h. Marker is in proper position; patient identification, including date, is accurate
_____	_____	_____	_____	_____	_____	i. Based on acceptable variances to criteria factors, determine which of these radiographs are acceptable and which are unacceptable and should have been repeated. (Place a check if the radiograph needs to be repeated.)

Answers to Review Exercises

Review Exercise A: Mammography Quality Standards Act, Anatomy of the Breast, and Technical Considerations

1. Mammography
2. B. 40
3. C. 1994
4. B. 2 years
5. C. 32%
6. Canadian Association of Radiologists
7. Inframammary crease
8. Areola
9. Axillary prolongation
10. Mediolateral
11. Lower inner quadrant (LIQ)
12. 10 o'clock
13. Pectoralis major muscle
14. Retromammary
15. Lactation or secretion of milk
16. A. Glandular
    B. Fibrous or connective
    C. Adipose (fatty)
17. Trabeculae
18. Cooper's ligaments
19. 1. FG, 2. FG, 3. FF, 4. FG, 5. F, 6. F, 7. FG, 8. F
20. Adipose
21. A. Skin
    B. Pectoralis major muscle
    C. Retromammary space
    D. Adipose (fatty) tissue
    E. Glandular tissue
    F. Nipple
    G. Inframammary crease
    H. 6th rib (lower breast margin - varies among individuals)
    I. 2nd rib (upper breast margin)
    J. Clavicle
22. A. Areola
    B. Nipple
    C. Ampulla
    D. Ducts
    E. Alveoli
    F. Mammary fat
    G. Lobe
    H. Cooper's ligament
23. 15 to 20
24. Base
25. Apex
26. Base
27. 25 and 28 kVp
28. Molybdenum
29. 0.3 mm
30. 25 to 40
31. A. Decrease thickness of breast
    B. Bring breast structures closer to IR
32. Reducing the amount of scatter radiation produced from the breast
33. D. 75 to 85
34. C. 800 to 1000 mrad
35. B. 5%
36. False (mean glandular dose)
37. True
38. A. Fine detail
    B. Edge sharpness
    C. Soft tissue visibility
39. Distinguishing a cyst from a solid mass
40. Magnetic resonance imaging (MRI)
41. True
42. A. Mammographic images can be digitally enhanced, modified, or enlarged without additional exposure
    B. Digital mammographic images can be sent to remote locations by telephone or satellite
43. D. Sestimibi
44. A. Fibroadenoma
45. A. Mediolateral oblique
    B. Superolateral-inferomedial oblique
    C. Axillary tail view
    D. Craniocaudal
    E. Rolled lateral
    F. Lateromedial
    G. Laterally exaggerated craniocaudal
    H. Inferolateral-superomedial
    I. Implant displaced
    J. Cleavage view

Review Exercise B: Positioning of the Breast

1. A. Craniocaudal (CC)
   B. Mediolateral oblique (MLO)
2. Inframammary crease
3. Axillary
4. Nipple
5. Away
6. Mediolateral oblique (MLO) projection
7. 45 degrees from vertical
8. More
9. B. Forward, toward front of body
10. Laterally exaggerated craniocaudal (XCCL) projection
11. Base
12. Laterally exaggerated craniocaudal (XCCL) projection
13. Laterally exaggerated craniocaudal (XCCL) projection
14. 90°
15. 1. T, 2. F, 3. F, 4. T, 5. F, 6. F, (overexposed) 7. T, 8. T, 9. T, 10. F (is the same)
16. Ecklund technique
17. The breast implant needs to be "pinched" or pushed posterior toward the chest wall out of the exposure field

18. D. Axillary tail
19. B. Magnify specific regions of interest
20. A. 100 to 150 mrad

Review Exercise C: Critique Radiographs of the Breast

A. CC projection (Fig. C18-36)
1. *Folds of fatty tissue superimpose breast tissue
2. Breast not pulled away from chest wall and folds of tissue not pulled back
3. Collimation not applicable for mammography. CR centering is acceptable
4. Exposure factors are acceptable
5. Anatomical side marker visible
   Repeatable error(s): Criteria #1

B. MLO projection (Fig. C18-37)
1. *Pertinent muscle not seen to nipple level, and outer tissue is not compressed
2. Lower part of breast not pulled away from chest wall onto film sufficiently
3. Collimation not applicable for mammography. CR centering is acceptable
4. Exposure factors are acceptable
5. Anatomical side marker visible
   Repeatable error(s): Criteria #1

C. CC projection (Fig. C18-37)
1. *Part of lateral posterior breast is cut off
2. *Medial posterior breast not included, and shoulder is superimposed over the lateral posterior tissue
3. Collimation not applicable for mammography. CR centering is acceptable
4. Exposure factors are acceptable
5. Anatomical side marker visible
   Repeatable error(s): Criteria #1 and #2

D. MLO projection (Fig. C18-38)
1. *Posterior medial breast cut off, no pectoral muscle visible. (White specks are calcium; they are not dust artifacts.)
2. *Breast not pulled out away from chest wall
3. Collimation not applicable for mammography. CR centering is acceptable
4. Exposure factors are acceptable
5. Anatomical side marker visible
   Repeatable error(s): Criteria #1 and #2

E. CC projection (Fig. C18-39)
   1. *Motion is present, which obliterates all detail
   2. Acceptable (dark half circle indicates posterior breast is included)
   3. Collimation not applicable for mammography. CR centering is acceptable
   4. Exposure factors are acceptable
   5. Anatomical side marker visible
      Repeatable error(s): Criteria #1

F. CC projection (Fig. C18-40)
   1. *Hair artifacts evident on posterior breast tissue, obscures breast tissue detail
   2. Acceptable
   3. Collimation not applicable for mammography. CR slightly off-centered toward medial side
   4. Exposure factors are acceptable
   5. Anatomical side marker visible
      Repeatable error(s): Criteria #1

SELF-TEST

Directions: This self-test should be taken only after completing **all** of the readings, review exercises, and laboratory activities for a particular section.   The purpose of this test is not only to provide a good learning exercise but also to serve as a good indicator of what your final evaluation grade will be. It is strongly suggested that if you do not get at least a 90% to 95% grade on this self-test, you should review those areas in which you missed questions *before* going to your instructor for the final evaluation exam for this chapter. (There are 58 questions or blanks—each is worth 1.7 points.)

1. What does the acronym *MQSA* represent, and what year did it go into effect? _____

2. Which health facilities (if any) are exempt from the MQSA requirements? _____

3. In 1992, the American Cancer Society recommended that all women over age _____ undergo screening mammography.

4. Currently, 1 in _____ American women develops breast cancer sometime in her life.

5. The junction between the inferior aspect of the breast and chest wall is called the _____ .

6. In which quadrant of the breast would the tail or axillary prolongation be found? _____

7. One o'clock in the left breast would relate to _____ in the right breast using the clock system.

8. Which large muscle is directly located posterior to the mammary gland? _____

9. What is the function of the mammary gland? _____

10. Name the bands of connective tissue passing through the breast tissue to provide support.

    _____

11. Which of the three breast tissues is radiographically the least dense? _____

12. What is the term used by radiologists for various small structures seen on the mammogram?

    _____

13. Which term describes the thickest portion of the breast near the chest wall? _____

14. Which one of the following tissue types would be found in the breasts of a 25-year-old pregnant female?

    A. Fibro-glandular   C. Fatty

    B. Fibro-fatty   D. Cystic

15. Which one of the following tissue types would be found in the breasts of a 35-year-old female who has borne two children?

    A. Fibro-glandular   C. Fatty

    B. Fibro-fatty   D. Cystic

16. The male breast would be classified as:

    A. Fibro-glandular   C. Fatty

    B. Fibro-fatty   D. Cystic

17. Which one of the following tissue types requires more compression during mammography as compared with the others?

   A. Fibro-glandular   C. Fatty

   B. Fibro-fatty   D. Cystic

18. Identify the anatomy on Fig. 18-3:

   A. _____

   B. _____

   C. _____

   D. _____

   E. Which basic mammogram projection is demonstrated

      in Fig. 18-3? _____

   F. The right marker on this mammogram is correctly placed on

      the _____ side of the breast.

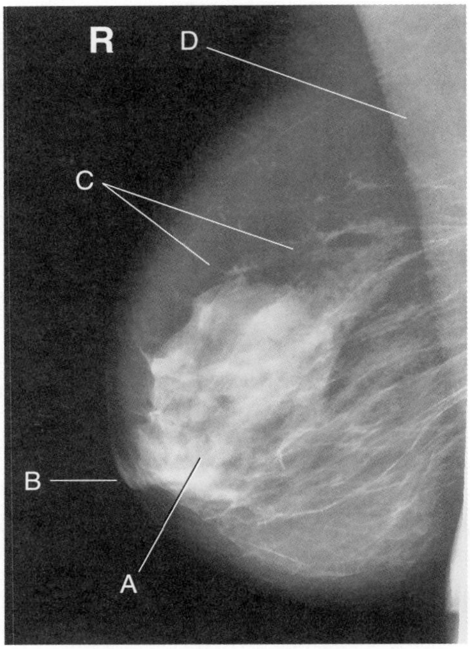

Fig. 18-3 Breast anatomy on a mammogram.

19. The target material used in mammography x-ray tubes is _____ .

20. To utilize the maximum advantage of the anode-heel effect, the anode side of the x-tube should be over the

    _____ (base or apex) of the breast.

21. True/False: Automatic exposure control (AEC) can be used for most mammographic projections.

22. True/False: Compression of the breast will improve image quality by reducing scatter radiation.

23. True/False: A grid is generally not used for mammography.

24. What size focal spot should be used for telemammography of small breast nodules or tissue samples?

    _____

25. What is the magnification factor for an exposure with a source-object distance (SOD) of 20 inches and source

    image-receptor distance (SID) of 40 inches? _____

26. The average MGD (mean glandular dose) received by the patient during a basic two-projection mammogram exami-

    nation is in the _____ range.

   A. 50 to 150 mrad   C. 400 to 600 mrad

   B. 200 to 300 mrad   D. 800 to 1100 mrad

27. Which imaging modality is best suited to distinguish a cyst from a solid mass within the breast?

_____

28. Which imaging modality is best suited to diagnose an extracapsular rupture of a breast implant?

_____

29. True/False: A radiolucent breast implant is being designed that will permit AEC to be used with these devices.

30. True/False: The principal way to reduce patient dose during mammography is to use higher kVp techniques.

31. True/False: One reason that mammoscintigraphy is not ordered more frequently is the high number of false positives reported with this procedure.

32. Which one of the following radionuclides is used for sentinal node studies?

   A. Sulphur colloid   C. Technetium

   B. Sestimibi   D. Iodine 131

33. Carcinoma of the breast is divided into two categories: _____ and _____ .

34. Which one of the following ACR abbreviations refers to the _laterally exaggerated craniocaudal_ projection?

   A. LECC   C. LCC

   B. LXCC   D. XCCL

35. What is the ACR abbreviation for a _mediolateral oblique_ projection? _____

36. List the two basic projections taken during a screening mammogram:

   A. _____   B. _____

37. Which of the basic projections taken during a mammogram will best demonstrate the pectoral muscle?

_____

38. The typical kVp range for mammography is _____ .

39. Which projection best demonstrates the axillary aspect of the breast? _____

40. What are the ACR abbreviations for the special projection, inferolateral-superomedial, used with a pacemaker?

_____

41. The use of automatic exposure control (AEC) when performing a projection with a breast implant in place can lead

   to _____ (over or under) exposure of the breast.

42. A. The technique of "pinching" the breast to push an implant posteriorly to the chest wall is known as the

      _____ technique.

   B. What is the correct ACR term and abbreviation for this technique? _____

43. What other special projection can be taken if a lesion is too deep into the axillary tail aspect of the chest wall to be seen with an XCCL, laterally exaggerated craniocaudal projection? (Include the correct ACR term and abbreviation.)

_____

44. Identification markers should always be placed near the _____ .

45. How is the opposite breast prevented from superimposing the breast being examined on the MLO projection?

_____

46. With a large breast, which of the two basic projections is most likely to require two images to include all the breast tissue?

_____

47. Which projection is usually requested when a lesion is seen on the MLO (mediolateral oblique) but not on the CC (craniocaudad) projection?

_____

48. What landmark determines the correct height for placement of the image receptor for the CC (craniocaudad) projection?

_____

49. Which one of the following projections is recommended for demonstrating inflammation of the breast?

    A. Craniocaudal   C. Mediolateral (true lateral)

    B. Mediolateral oblique   D. Laterally exaggerated craniocaudal

50. **Situation:** A mammogram is performed for a patient with breast implants. The resultant images are overexposed. The following factors were used: 28 kVp, AEC, grid, and gentle compression. Which one of the following modifications would produce more diagnostic images during the repeat study?

    A. Lower kVp   C. Use manual exposure factors

    B. Do not use a grid   D. Do not use breast compression

CHAPTER 19

Trauma and Mobile Radiography

This chapter has been divided into the following four main sections:

1. **Trauma and Fracture Terminology.** Radiographers should know the more common fracture terms included in this chapter to better understand patient histories and to ensure that the most appropriate projections are taken to demonstrate these fracture sites.
2. **Positioning Principles and Grid Use.** Understanding certain positioning principles, including correct use of portable grids, is essential in trauma and mobile radiography as it is described in this section.
3. **Mobile X-ray Equipment and Radiation Protection.** Understanding the various types of mobile x-ray and fluoroscopy equipment used in trauma radiography (including use in surgery) is essential for radiographers. Knowing and following safe radiation protection practices for workers around mobile equipment is especially important due to the unshielded environments where mobile equipment is generally used (such as in the emergency room, surgery, or in patients' rooms.
4. **Trauma and Mobile Positioning and Procedures.** This section describes specific positioning for each body part in which the patient cannot be moved from the supine position. Adaptation of CR angles and film placement as required is demonstrated and described for each body part.

CHAPTER OBJECTIVES

After you have completed **all** the activities of this chapter, you will be able to:

_____ 1. Define and apply terms for specific types of fractures and soft-tissue injuries.

_____ 2. List the projections taken for a post-reduction study of the limbs, including open and closed reductions.

_____ 3. Explain the two positioning principles that must be observed during trauma radiography.

_____ 4. List the three grid use rules to prevent grid cutoff.

_____ 5. Describe the two primary types of mobile radiographic units and their operating principles.

_____ 6. Explain the features, operating principles, and uses of mobile fluoroscopy units.

_____ 7. List the three methods for maintaining a sterile field with C-arm type equipment.

_____ 8. List the three cardinal rules of radiation protection as they apply to trauma and mobile radiography.

_____ 9. Describe the difference in exposure field levels with different orientations of the x-ray tube and intensifiers with the C-arm.

_____ 10. Explain why the AP projection orientation of the C-arm is not recommended.

_____ 11. List projections for trauma and mobile procedures of the chest, bony thorax, and abdomen.

_____ 12. List projections for trauma and mobile procedures for various parts of the upper and lower limbs.

_____ 13. List projections for trauma and mobile procedures of the cervical, thoracic, and lumbar spine.

_____ 14. List trauma and mobile procedures for the skull and facial bones.

Learning Exercises

The following review exercises should be completed only after careful study of the associated pages in the textbook as indicated by each exercise.

After completing each of these individual exercises, check your answers with the answer sheets that follow before continuing to the next exercise.

REVIEW EXERCISE A: Radiographic Trauma and Fracture Terminology (see textbook pp. 595-600)

1. True/False: Mobile CT units are available for use in emergency and surgical situations.

2. True/False: Nuclear medicine is effective in diagnosing certain emergency conditions such as pulmonary emboli.

3. True/False: For trauma patients who cannot be moved for conventional diagnostic imaging, other modalities, such as ultrasound or nuclear medicine, may be used rather than trying to move the patient into specific positions.

4. List the two terms for describing displacement of a bone from a joint:

   A. _____   B. _____

5. List the four regions of the body most commonly dislocated during trauma:

   A. _____   C. _____

   B. _____   D. _____

6. What is the correct term for a partial dislocation? _____

7. A forced wrenching or twisting of a joint that results in a tearing of supporting ligaments is a

   _____.

8. An injury in which there is no fracture or breaking of the skin would describe a _____.

9. What is the correct term that describes the relationship of the long axes of fracture fragments?

   _____

10. Which term describes a type of fracture in which the fracture fragment ends are overlapped and not in contact?

    _____

11. A. Which term describes the angulation of a distal fracture fragment toward the midline? _____

    B. Would this fracture angulation be described as a medial or lateral apex? _____

12. What is the primary difference between a simple and compound fracture?

    _____

13. List two types of incomplete fractures:

    A. _____   B. _____

14. Which type of comminuted fracture produces several wedge-shaped separate fragments? _____

15. What is the name of the fracture in which one fragment is driven into the other? _____

16. List the secondary name for the following fractures:

    A. Hutchinson's fracture: _____

    B. Baseball fracture: _____

    C. Compound fracture: _____

    D. Depressed fracture: _____

    E. Simple fracture: _____

17. True/False: An avulsion fracture is the same as a chip fracture.

18. What type of reduction fracture does *not* require surgery? _____

19. Match the following types of fractures to the correct definition (use each choice only once):

    _____ 1. Greenstick   A. Fracture of proximal half of ulna with dislocation of radial head

    _____ 2. Comminuted   B. Fracture of the base of the 1st metacarpal

    _____ 3. Monteggia's   C. Fracture of the pedicles of C2

    _____ 4. Boxer's   D. Fracture of distal radius with anterior displacement

    _____ 5. Smith's   E. Complete fracture of distal fibula, frequently with fracture of medial malleolus

    _____ 6. Hutchinson's   F. Fracture of lateral malleolus, medial malleolus, and distal posterior tip of tibia

    _____ 7. Bennett's   G. Incomplete fracture with broken cortex on one side of bone only

    _____ 8. Avulsion   H. Fracture resulting in multiple (two or more) fragments

    _____ 9. Depressed   I. Fracture of distal 5th metacarpal

    _____ 10. Stellate   J. Intra-articular fracture of radial styloid process

    _____ 11. Trimalleolar   K. Fracture of distal radius with posterior displacement

    _____ 12. Compression   L. Indented fracture of the skull

    _____ 13. Pott's   M. Fracture due to a severe stress to a tendon

    _____ 14. Colles'   N. Fracture with fracture lines radiating from center point

    _____ 15. Hangman's   O. Fracture producing a reduced height of the anterior vertebral body

20. A. Fig. 19-1 illustrates which specific "named fracture?"

_____

   B. Which bone is most commonly fractured, and which displacement commonly occurs with this fracture?

_____

   C. Describe the type of injury or fall that commonly results

   in this type of fracture? _____

_____

21. A. Fig. 19-2 illustrates which specific "named" fracture?

_____

   B. Which bone(s) is(are) commonly fractured with this

   type of fracture? _____

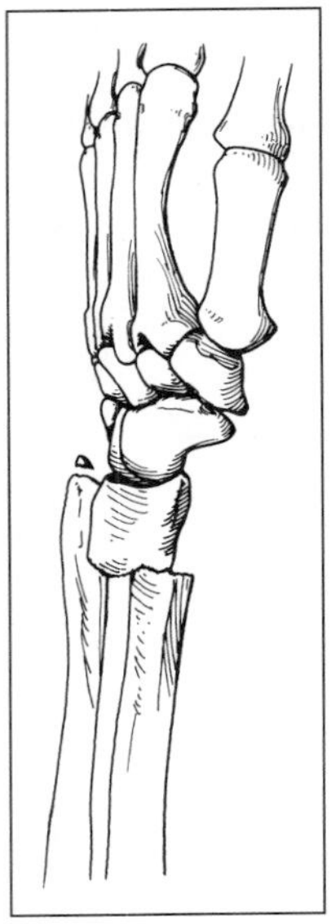

Fig. 19-1 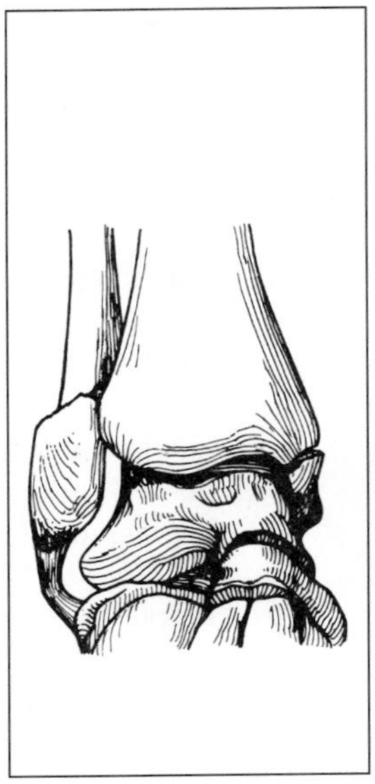   **Fig. 19-2**

REVIEW EXERCISE B: Positioning Principles and Grids (see textbook pp. 600-602)

1. Which single term best describes the primary difference between trauma positions and standard positioning?

_____

2. What should be done to achieve specific projections if the patient cannot move due to trauma?

_____

3. What is the minimum number of projections generally required for any trauma study? _____

4. How many joints must be included for an initial study of a long bone? _____

5. True/False: A follow-up post reduction radiograph of the middle portion of long bones should be collimated closely to the fracture region.

6. Grids are required for any body part measuring greater than _____ cm.

7. List the three factors that must be met to avoid grid cutoff (three limitations or rules to prevent grid cutoff):

   A. _____   B. _____   C. _____

8. True/False: Lead grid lines usually run parallel to the centerline of the long axis of the grid.

9. True/False: To avoid grid cutoff, the angulation of the CR must be perpendicular to the length of the grid.

10. What does "grid focal range" mean? _____

11. What is the preferred grid ratio for a grid used for portable procedures? _____

12. What is considered to be a medium grid focal range? _____

13. A typical long focal range portable grid has a focal range of _____ .

14. What happens to the radiographic image if the SID exceeds a grid's focal range? _____

15. True/False: One particular surface of a focused grid must always be facing the x-ray tube to prevent grid cutoff.

16. A common grid ratio used for mobile work is:

    A. 4:1   B. 6:1 or 8:1   C. 10:1 or 12:1   D. 16:1

REVIEW EXERCISE C: Mobile X-ray Equipment and Radiation Protection (see textbook pp. 603-606)

1. List the two primary types of mobile x-ray units:

   A. _____   B. _____

2. Which type of mobile unit is lighter in weight? _____

3. With battery-powered types, how long does recharging take if the batteries are fully discharged?

   _____

4. True/False: A fully charged battery-powered mobile unit has a driving range of up to 10 miles on level ground.

5. What is the common term for a mobile fluoroscopy unit? _____

6. What are the two primary components of a mobile fluoroscopy unit (located on each end of the structure from which it gets its name)?

   A. _____   B. _____

7. Why shouldn't the mobile fluoroscopy unit be placed in the AP projection ("tube on top" position)?

   _____

8. With the tube and intensifier in a horizontal position, at which side of the patient should the surgeon stand if he or she must remain near the patient—the x-ray tube side or the intensifier side? _____ .

   Why? _____

9. Of the two monitors found on most mobile fluoroscopy units, which one is generally considered the "active" monitor—the right or the left? _____

10. True/False: Image orientation on the mobile fluoroscopy monitors must be determined by the operator *before* the patient is brought into the room.

11. True/False: All mobile digital type fluoroscopy units have the ability to magnify the image on the monitor during fluoroscopy.

12. True/False: The pulse mode with mobile fluoroscopy units is helpful during procedures to produce brighter images, but it results in significantly increased patient exposure.

13. True/False: Standard cassettes with conventional single-exposure radiographs can be used with most mobile fluoroscopy units.

14. True/False: AEC exposure systems are not feasible with mobile fluoroscopy.

15. Name the feature that allows an image to be held on the monitor while also providing continuous fluoroscopy imaging?

    _____

16. List the three methods for maintaining a sterile field with the mobile fluoroscopy unit.

    A. _____   C. _____

    B. _____

17. List the three terms describing the cardinal rules of radiation protection:

    A. _____   B. _____   C. _____

18. Which cardinal rule is *most* effective in reducing occupational exposure? _____

19. Which one of the following measures is most effective (and practical) in limiting exposure with mobile fluoroscopy?

    A. Limit C-arm procedures to surgery cases only

    B. Prevent non-radiologists from using the C-arm

    C. Use intermittent or "foot-tapping" fluoroscopy

    D. Limit all fluoroscopy procedures to no more than 10 minutes

For Questions 20 to 24, review exposure field information on Figs. 19-3 and 19-4. Also see the textbook, p. 606.

20. **Situation:** The C-arm is in position for a PA projection. What exposure field range would the operator receive at waist level standing 3 feet from the patient?

    A. 20 to 25 mR/hr   C. 50 to 100 mR/hr

    B. 25 to 50 mR/hr   D. 100 to 300 mR/hr

21. Approximately how much exposure at waist level would the operator receive with 5 minutes of fluoroscopy exposure standing 3 feet from the patient? (Hint: first convert mR/hr to mR/min by dividing by 60, then multiply by minutes of fluoroscopy time.)

    A. 5 mR   C. 25 mR

    B. 60 mR   D. 2 mR

22. If a radiographer receives 50 mR/ hr standing 3 feet from the mobile fluoroscopy unit, what would be the exposure rate if he or she moved back to a distance of 4 feet?

    A. 10 mR/hr

    B. 25 mR/hr

    C. 100 mR/hr

    D. No significant difference

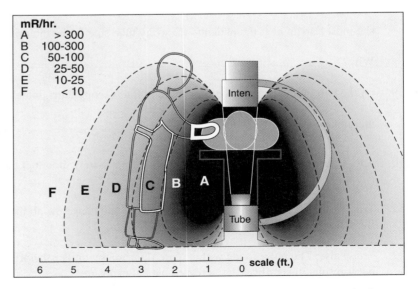

mR/hr.	
A	> 300
B	100-300
C	50-100
D	25-50
E	10-25
F	< 10

Fig. 19-3 Occupational exposure during mobile fluoroscopy, PA projection.

23. A radiographer standing 1 foot from a mobile fluoroscopy unit is receiving approximately 400 mR/hr. What is the *total* exposure to the radiographer if the procedure takes 10 minutes of fluoroscopy time to complete?

_____

24. **Situation:** An operator receives 25 mR/hr to the facial and neck region with the C-arm in position for a PA projection (intensifier on top). Approximately how much would the operator receive at the same distance if the C-arm were reversed to an AP projection position (tube on top)?

    A. 25 to 50 mR/hr

    B. 50 to 100 mR/hr

    C. 100 to 300 mR/hr

    D. 300 to 500 mR/hr

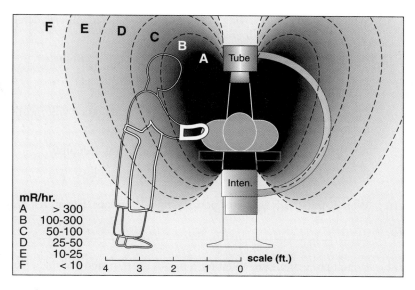

mR/hr.
A   > 300
B   100-300
C   50-100
D   25-50
E   10-25
F   < 10

Fig. 19-4 Occupational exposure during mobile fluoroscopy, AP projection.

25. A 30° C-arm tilt from the vertical perspective will increase exposure to the head and neck regions of the operator by a factor of _____ .

REVIEW EXERCISE D: Trauma and Mobile Positioning and Procedures (see textbook pp. 607-628)

1. How is the CR centered and aligned in relationship to the sternum for an AP portable projection of the chest?

_____

2. True/False: Focused grids are recommended for mobile chest projections.

3. Which way (crosswise or lengthwise) should a 35 x 43 cm (14 x 17 in.) IR be placed for an AP portable chest on an average or large patient? _____ Why? _____

_____

4. What specific position should be performed to demonstrate a possible pneumothorax in the left lung for a patient who cannot stand or sit erect? _____

5. Which position can be used to replace the RAO of the sternum for the patient who cannot lie prone on the table but can be rotated into a semi-supine position? _____

6. How must the grid be aligned to prevent grid cutoff when angling the CR mediolaterally for an oblique projection of the sternum when the patient cannot be rotated or moved at all from the supine position?

_____

7. Other than the straight AP, what other projection of the ribs can be taken for the supine immobile patient who cannot be rotated into an oblique position?_____

8. Which one of the following positions or projections will best demonstrate free intra-abdominal air on the patient who cannot stand or sit erect?

   A. Left lateral decubitus   C. Right lateral decubitus

   B. AP KUB   D. Dorsal decubitus

9. Which one of the following projections of the abdomen will most effectively demonstrate a possible abdominal aortic aneurysm?

   A. Left lateral decubitus   C. Right lateral decubitus

   B. AP KUB   D. Dorsal decubitus

10. What is the disadvantage of performing a PA rather than an AP projection of the thumb?

    _____

11. Which projections are taken for a post-reduction study of the wrist?

    _____

12. **Situation:** A study of a fractured wrist was taken with the following exposure factors: 60 kVp, 10 mAs, detail screens. A fiberglass cast is placed on the wrist and a post-reduction study is ordered. Which one of the following techniques would be ideal for the post-reduction study?

    A. 70 kVp and 10 mAs   C. 65 kVp and 10 mAs

    B. 80 kVp and 10 mAs   D. 55 kVp and 15 mAs

13. True/False: A PA horizontal beam projection of the elbow can be taken for a patient with multiple injuries.

14. True/False: For a trauma lateral projection of the elbow, the CR must be kept parallel to the interepicondylar plane.

15. **Situation:** A patient with a possible fracture of the proximal humerus enters the emergency room. Because of multiple injuries, the patient is unable to stand or sit erect. What positioning routine should be performed to diagnose the extent of the injury?

    _____

16. **Situation:** A patient with a possible dislocation of the proximal humerus enters the emergency room. Because of multiple injuries, the patient is unable to stand or sit erect. In addition to a basic AP projection, what second projection will demonstrate whether it is an anterior or posterior dislocation?

    _____

17. How much CR angulation should be used for an AP axial projection of the clavicle on a hypersthenic patient?

    A. 10°   B. 15°   C. 20°   D. 25°

18. A lateral "Y" projection taken AP for a trauma patient usually requires a _____ degree rotation of the body away from the image receptor.

    A. 20 to 30   B. 45   C. 50 to 60   D. 70

19. To ensure that the joints are opened up for an AP projection of the foot, how is the CR aligned?

    A. Perpendicular to the long axis of the tibia

    B. Perpendicular to the plantar surface

    C. 10° posteriorly from perpendicular to plantar surface

    D. 10° posteriorly from perpendicular to dorsal surface

20. **Situation:** An orthopedic surgeon orders a mortise projection of the ankle, but the patient has a severely fractured ankle and cannot rotate the ankle medially for the mortise projection. What can the radiographer do to provide this projection without rotating the ankle?

_____

21. **Situation:** A patient with a possible dislocation of the patella enters the emergency room. What type of positioning routine should be performed on this patient that would safely demonstrate the patella?

_____

22. **Situation:** A patient with a possible fracture of the proximal tibia and fibula enters the emergency room. The basic AP and lateral projections are inconclusive. Because of severe pain, the patient is unable to rotate the leg from the AP position. What position or projection could be performed that would provide an unobstructed view of the fibular head and neck?

_____

23. Which one of the following positions would be performed on a trauma patient to provide a lateral view of the proximal femur?

   A. Danelius-Miller method   C. Waters method

   B. Fuchs method   D. Ottonello method

24. Which lateral projection can be taken of the proximal femur without having to abduct or flex the unaffected limb?

_____

25. How is the CR aligned for the method identified in question 24?

_____

26. **Situation:** A patient with injuries suffered in a motor vehicle accident enters the emergency room. The ER physician orders a lateral C-spine projection to rule out a fracture or dislocation. Because of the thickness of the shoulders, C6-7 is not visualized. What additional projection can be taken safely to demonstrate this region of the spine?

_____

27. **Situation:** A patient with a possible C2 fracture enters the emergency room on a backboard. The AP projection does not demonstrate C2. In addition, the patient cannot open his mouth because of a mandible fracture. Which projection can be performed safely to demonstrate this region of the spine?

   A. Fuchs   C. Vertebral arch projection

   B. Judd   D. 35 to 40° cephalad axial projection

28. Which projection will best demonstrate (with only minimal distortion) the pedicles of the cervical spine on a severely injured patient?

_____

29. Identify the two CR angles for the double angle Method Two for the oblique cervical spine.

   A. _____° medial   B. _____° cephalad

30. When using the Method Two, double angle technique, how is the cassette positioned for an oblique cervical spine to minimize distortion?

_____

31. **Situation:** A patient with a possible basilar skull fracture enters the emergency room. The ER physician wants a projection that best demonstrates a sphenoid effusion. The patient cannot stand or sit erect. Which one of the following projections would achieve this goal?

    A. AP skull
    B. Lateral recumbent skull
    C. Horizontal beam lateral skull
    D. Modified Waters projection

32. Which one of the following projections of the skull would project the petrous ridges in the lower one third of the orbits on a supine trauma patient?

    A. AP skull, CR 0° to OML
    B. AP skull, CR 15° caudad to OML
    C. AP skull, CR 15° cephalad to OML
    D. AP skull, CR 30° caudad to OML

33. True/False: AP projections of the skull and facial bones will increase exposure to the thyroid gland as compared to PA projections.

34. True/False: The CR should not exceed a 30° caudad angle for the AP axial projection of the cranium to avoid excessive distortion of the cranial bones.

35. How is the CR angled and where is it centered for the AP acanthioparietal (reverse Waters) projection of the facial bones?

    _____

36. What type of CR angulation is required for the trauma version of an axiolateral projection of the mandible?

    _____

37. **Situation:** A patient with a Monteggia's fracture enters the emergency room. Which one of the following positioning routines should be performed on this patient?

    A. AP and lateral thumb
    B. PA and horizontal beam lateral wrist
    C. AP and horizontal beam lateral lower leg
    D. PA or HP and horizontal beam lateral forearm

38. **Situation:** A patient with a possible Greenstick fracture enters the emergency room. What age group does this type of fracture usually affect?

    A. Pediatric
    B. Young adult
    C. Middle age
    D. Elderly

39. **Situation:** A patient with a possible Pott's fracture enters the emergency room. Which one of the following positioning routines should be performed on this patient?

    A. AP and horizontal beam lateral lower leg
    B. PA and horizontal beam lateral wrist
    C. AP and lateral thumb
    D. Three projections of the hand

40. **Situation:** A patient is struck directly on the patella with a heavy object, shattering it. The resultant fracture most likely would be described as a:

    A. Burst fracture
    B. Compression fracture
    C. Stellate fracture
    D. Smith's fracture

Answers to Review Exercises

Review Exercise A: Radiographic Trauma and Fracture

1. True
2. True
3. False. It is important to rotate the x-ray tube and image receptor around patients if they are unable to move.
4. A. Dislocation
   B. Luxation
5. A. Shoulder
   B. Fingers or thumb
   C. Patella
   D. Hip
6. Subluxation
7. Sprain
8. Contusion
9. Apposition
10. Bayonet apposition
11. A. Varus (deformity) angulation
    B. Lateral apex
12. A simple fracture does not break through the skin, but a compound fracture protrudes through the skin.
13. A. Torus fracture
    B. Greenstick fracture
14. Butterfly fracture
15. Impacted fracture
16. A. Chauffeur's
    B. Mallet
    C. Open
    D. Ping-pong
    E. Closed
17. False. (A chip fracture involves an isolated fracture not associated with a tendon or ligament.)
18. Closed reduction
19. 1. G, 2. H, 3. A, 4. I, 5. D, 6. J, 7. B, 8. M, 9. L, 10. N, 11. F, 12. O, 13. E, 14. K, 15. C
20. A. Colles' fracture
    B. Distal radius, posterior displacement of distal fragment
    C. Fall on outstretched arm
21. A. Pott's fracture
    B. Distal fibula and occasionally the distal tibia or medial malleolus

Review Exercise B: Positioning Principles and Grids

1. Adaptation
2. Move the CR and IR around the patient to produce similar projections rather than moving the patient
3. Two. Two projections should be taken 90° to each other
4. Two. Both joints must be included on the initial study
5. False (must include at least one joint nearest injury)
6. 10
7. A. Correct CR centering
   B. Correct CR angling
   C. Correct grid focal range
8. True
9. False (parallel to)
10. The SID range in which the x-ray beam can pass through the grid without excessive absorption
11. 6:1 or 8:1 grid ratio
12. 34 to 46 in. (86 to 117 cm)
13. 48 to 72 in. (122 to 183 cm)
14. It will create "off-distance" grid cut-off
15. True
16. B. 6:1 or 8:1

Review Exercise C: Mobile X-ray Equipment and Radiation Protection

1. A. Battery powered, battery driven type
   B. Standard AC power source, non-motor drive
2. Standard power source, non-motor drive
3. 8 hours
4. True
5. C-arm
6. A. X-ray tube
   B. Image intensifier
7. Because it results in a significant increase in exposure to the head and neck region of the operator
8. Intensifier side; the radiation field pattern extends out farther on the x-ray tube side
9. Left monitor
10. True
11. True
12. False (reduces exposure to patient)
13. True
14. False (can be used)
15. Roadmapping
16. A. Draping the total C-arm, tube, and intensifier
    B. Draping the patient
    C. Using a "shower curtain" type arrangement to maintain a sterile field
17. A. Time
    B. Distance
    C. Shielding
18. Distance
19. C. use intermittent or "foot-tapping" fluoroscopy
20. C. 50 to 100 mR/hr

21. A. 5 mR (60 mR ÷ 60 min = 1 mR × 5 min = 5)
22. B. 25 mR/hr
23. 67 mR (400 ÷ 60 x 10 = 67)
24. C 100 to 300 mR/hr
25. Four

Review Exercise D: Trauma and Mobile Positioning and Procedures

1. Centered 3 to 4 in. (7 to 10 cm) below jugular notch, angled caudad so as to be perpendicular to sternum
2. False (not recommended due to probable grid cutoff)
3. Crosswise, to prevent side cutoff of the right or left lateral margins of the chest. More important with portable chests due to increased divergence of x-ray beam at the shorter SID.
4. Right lateral decubitus
5. 15 to 20° LPO
6. Crosswise
7. 30 to 40° cross-angled mediolateral projection (Note: This results in image distortion and should be done as a last resort)
8. A. left lateral decubitus
9. D. dorsal decubitus
10. Increase OID of the thumb (increases distortion)
11. PA and lateral projections
12. C. 65 kVp and 10 mAs
13. True
14. True
15. AP and horizontal beam, transthoracic lateral
16. A horizontal beam transthoracic lateral
17. B. 15°
18. A. 20 to 30
19. C. 10° posteriorly from perpendicular to plantar surface (Note: This would also be 10° posteriorly from plane of IR)
20. Angle the CR 15 to 20° lateromedially to the long axis of the foot
21. AP and horizontal beam lateral with no flexion of knee
22. 45° lateromedial cross-angle AP projection of the knee and proximal tibia/fibula
23. A. Danelius-Miller method
24. Mediolateral (Sanderson) projection
25. Cross-angled mediolaterally to be near perpendicular to the long axis of the foot
26. Swimmer's lateral using a horizontal beam CR

27. D. 35 to 40° cephalad axial projection
28. 45° oblique using the double-angle method with IR perpendicular to CR
29. A. 45° medial
    B. 15° cephalad
30. Cassette placed on a stool under the table and patient, set at a 45° angle, perpendicular to CR

31. C. horizontal beam lateral skull
32. C. AP skull, CR 15° cephalad to OML
33. True
34. False (should not exceed 45°)
35. Parallel to the mentomeatal line, centered to acanthion
36. 25 to 30° cephalad and possibly 5 to 10° posterior to clear the shoulder

37. D. PA or AP and horizontal beam lateral forearm
38. A. Pediatric
39. A. AP and horizontal beam lateral lower leg
40. C. Stellate fracture

SELF-TEST

My Score = _____%

Directions: This self-test should be taken only after completing **all** of the readings, review exercises, and laboratory activities for a particular section.   The purpose of this test is not only to provide a good learning exercise but also to serve as a strong indicator of what your final evaluation grade will be. It is strongly suggested that if you do not get at least a 90% to 95% grade on this self-test, you should review those areas in which you missed questions before going to your instructor for the final evaluation exam for this chapter. (There are 68 questions or blanks—each is worth 1.5 points.)

1. From the list of possible fracture types on the left, indicate which fracture is represented on each drawing or radiograph by writing in the correct term where indicated (A through I):

   • Single (closed) fracture

   • Compound (open) fracture

   • Torus fracture

   • Greenstick fracture

   • Plastic fracture

   • Transverse fracture

   • Oblique fracture

   • Spiral fracture

   • Comminuted fracture

   • Impacted fracture

   • Baseball (mallet) fracture

   • Barton's fracture

   • Bennett fracture

   • Colles' fracture

   • Monteggia's fracture

   • Nursemaid's elbow fracture

   • Pott's fracture

   • Avulsion fracture

   • Chip fracture

   • Compression fracture

   • Stellate fracture

   • Tuft fracture

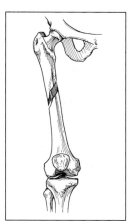

A. _____

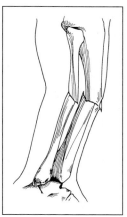

B. _____

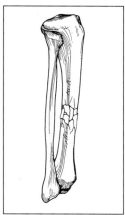

C. _____

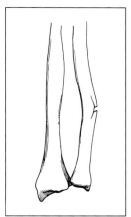

D. _____

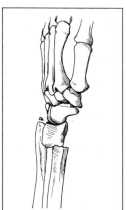

E. _____

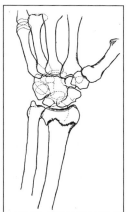

F. _____

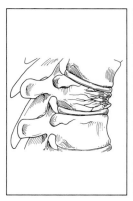

G. _____

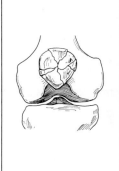

H. _____

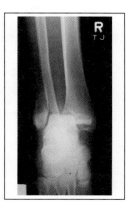

I. _____

2. A. What is the correct term for the displacement of a bone from a joint? _____

    B. What is the correct term for a partial displacement? _____

3. What region of the body encounters partial dislocations most frequently? _____

4. Which one of the following terms describes a poor alignment between the ends of a fractured bone?
    A. Dislocation   C. Apex angulation
    B. Lack of apposition   D. Anatomical apposition

5. Which one of the following terms describes a bending of a distal fracture away from the midline?
    A. Valgus angulation   C. Apex angulation
    B. Varus angulation   D. Bayonet apposition

6. Match the following definitions to the correct type of fracture (use each answer only once):

    _____ 1. Fracture through the pedicles of C2   A. Nursemaid's elbow

    _____ 2. Fracture of proximal half of ulna with dislocation of radial head   B. Bennett's

    _____ 3. Fracture due to a disease process   C. Baseball

    _____ 4. Fracture resulting in an isolated bone fragment   D. Pathological

    _____ 5. Subluxation of the radial head of a child   E. Hangman's

    _____ 6. Fracture along base of 1st metacarpal   F. Hutchinson's

    _____ 7. Fracture of distal phalanx with finger extended   G. Stress or fatigue

    _____ 8. Also called a *March fracture*   H. Chip

    _____ 9. Also called a *Chauffeur's fracture*   I. Monteggia's

7. True/False: Any trauma study requires at least two projections as close to 90° opposite from each other as possible.

8. True/False: On an initial study of a long bone, both joints should be included for each projection.

9. Which one of the following projections (on a sthenic adult) would require the use of a grid?
    A. AP leg (tibia-fibula)   C. Lateral elbow
    B. Lateral ankle   D. AP shoulder

10. What is the preferred grid ratio for trauma radiography?
    A. 5:1   C. 10:1 to 12:1
    B. 6:1 to 8:1   D. 16:1

11. List the two factors that determine a grid's focal range:

    A. _____   B. _____

12. True/False: Using an SID greater than the established focal range will produce grid cutoff.

13. Which type of mobile radiography x-ray unit is self-propelled? _____

14. Which type of mobile x-ray unit is lighter weight? _____

15. True/False: C-arms are most generally stationary fluoroscopy units used in surgery.

16. True/False: The C-arm fluoroscopy unit can be rotated 180°.

17. True/False: The AP projection during a C-arm procedure is recommended to minimize OID.

18. True/False: Digital C-arm units can store images on video tape or computer hard disk memory.

19. What is the term for the process of holding one image on the C-arm monitor while also providing continuous fluo-

    roscopy? _____

20. What is the primary benefit of the "pulse mode" on a digital C-arm unit? _____

21. List the three cardinal rules of radiation protection:

    A. _____   B. _____   C. _____

22. Which one of the cardinal rules is most effective in reducing occupational exposure?

    _____

23. **Situation:** A radiographer using a C-arm fluoroscope receives 125 mR/hr standing 2 feet from the patient. What is
    the exposure rate if the radiographer moves to a distance of 6 feet?

    A. Less than 10 mR/hr   C. 30 to 50 mR/hr

    B. 15 to 30 mR/hr   D. 50 to 75 mR/hr

24. **Situation:** A radiographer receives 30 mR/hr during a C-arm fluoroscopic procedure. What is the *total* exposure

    dose if the procedure takes 8 minutes of fluoroscopy time? _____

25. True/False: The exposure dose is greater on the image intensifier side as compared with the x-ray tube side with the
    C-arm in the horizontal configuration.

26. True/False: A 30° tilt of C-arm from the vertical perspective will increase the dose by a factor of three to the head
    and neck region.

27. **Situation:** A patient with a possible pleural effusion in the right lung enters the emergency room. The patient is un-
    able to stand or sit erect. What position would best demonstrate this condition?

    A. Right lateral decubitus   C. Dorsal decubitus

    B. AP supine   D. Semi-erect AP

28. Where is the CR centered for an AP semi-erect projection of the chest? _____

29. **Situation:** A patient with a crushing injury to the thorax enters the emergency room. The patient is on a backboard
    and cannot be moved. Which projections can be performed to determine if the sternum is fractured?

    _____

30. **Situation:** A patient with possible ascites (fluid accumulation in peritoneal cavity of the abdomen) enters the emergency room. The patient is unable to stand or sit erect. Which one of the following positions would best demonstrate this condition?

    A. AP supine KUB   C. Left lateral decubitus

    B. Dorsal decubitus   D. Prone KUB

31. How many projections are required for a post-reduction study of the wrist? _____

32. How is the CR aligned for a trauma lateral projection of the elbow? _____

33. Which lateral projection would best demonstrate the mid-to-distal humerus without rotating the limb?

    _____

34. How much obliquity of the body is generally required for a lateromedial scapula projection with a trauma patient

    who can be turned up partially on her side? _____

35. To ensure that the CR is aligned properly for an AP trauma projection of the foot, the CR is angled:

    _____ .

36. **Situation:** A patient with a possible fracture of the ankle enters the emergency room. The patient cannot rotate the lower limb. What can be done to provide the orthopedic surgeon with a mortise projection of the ankle?

    _____

37. Which one of the following statements is *not* true about the Sanderson method?

    A. The unaffected leg does not need to be moved at all.

    B. The patient is obliqued into a 15 to 20° posterior oblique position.

    C. The affected leg is rotated 10 to 15° internally if possible.

    D. The CR is angled to be perpendicular to the long axis of the foot of the affected limb.

38. Which one of the following projections will demonstrate the C1-2 vertebra if the patient cannot open his mouth?

    A. 35 to 40° cephalad, AP axial projection   C. 15 to 20° cephalad, AP axial projection

    B. Swimmer's lateral   D. Articular pillar projection

39. **Situation:** A patient with a possible fracture of the cervical spine pedicles enters the emergency room. Which one of the following projections will best demonstrate this region of the spine with the least distortion without moving the patient?

    A. Perform a Swimmer's lateral

    B. Perform an articular pillar projection

    C. Perform a double angle oblique projection with IR perpendicular to CR

    D. Perform a 45° CR oblique projection with IR flat on table-top

40. What are the two advantages of angling the cassette 45° for the trauma oblique cervical, which also results in a long OID for the Method Two double angle projection?

    A. _____

    B. _____

41. Which one of the following facial bone projections will best demonstrate air-fluid levels in the maxillary sinuses for a patient unable to stand or sit erect?

    A. AP acanthioparietal   C. AP modified acanthioparietal

    B. Trauma, horizontal beam lateral   D. AP axial

42. A. On a horizontal beam lateral trauma skull projection, should the cassette be placed lengthwise or crosswise to

    the patient? _____

    B. Where should the CR be centered for this lateral skull projection? _____

43. **Situation:** A patient with a possible compression fracture of the lumbar spine enters the emergency room. Which specific position of the lumbar spine series would best demonstrate this?

    A. AP   C. Lateral

    B. LPO and RPO   D. AP L5-S1 projection

44. **Situation:** A patient with a possible Barton's fracture comes to the radiology department. Which one of the following positioning routines would best demonstrate this?

    A. AP or PA and lateral wrist   C. AP and lateral foot

    B. AP, mortise, and lateral ankle   D. AP and lateral lower leg

45. Radiologists often use the Salter-Harris system to classify _____ fractures.

    A. Pathologic   C. Stellate

    B. Trimalleolar   D. Epiphyseal

CHAPTER 20

Pediatric Radiography

Positioning considerations are unique to pediatric radiography and present a definite challenge for all radiographers. Children cannot be handled and positioned like miniature adults. They have special needs and require patience and understanding. Their anatomical makeup is vastly different from that of adults, especially the skeletal system. The bony development (ossification) of children goes through specific growth stages from infancy to adolescence. These need to be understood by radiographers so that the appearance of the normal growth stages can be recognized. Examples of normal bone development patterns at various ages are included in this chapter and in the textbook.

The basic and optional projections and positions are much different for children than for adults. You need to know and understand these differences to be able to visualize the essential anatomy on children of various ages.

The most obvious differences for children when compared with adults are the methods of positioning and immobility. Small children cannot just be instructed to hold still in certain positions or to hold their breath during the exposure. You will need to learn how to relate to children and communicate with them to get their cooperation without forceful immobilization.

Special immobilization techniques need to be learned along with the use of various types of commonly available immobilization paraphernalia. Specialized restraining devices available in many departments will be explained and demonstrated in this chapter.

Radiation protection for these small patients must also be a major concern, because the younger the child, the more sensitive that child's tissues are to radiation. Thus **accurate collimation and gonadal shielding** are absolutely essential. High-speed screens and films should also be used, and **repeats must be minimized.** Specific patient doses in icon boxes for each projection are not provided in this chapter because of the many variables involved. However, **keeping all child doses as low as possible** is even more important than in adult radiography. Therefore, careful study of this chapter and related clinical experience are essential **before** you attempt a radiographic examination on a small child or infant. As a student, you may have limited opportunity to observe and assist with pediatric patients during your training. This makes learning and mastering the information provided in this chapter of the textbook and this workbook-laboratory manual even more important.

CHAPTER OBJECTIVES

After you have completed **all** the activities of this chapter, you will be able to:

_____ 1. List the steps and process of the technologist's introduction to the child and parent and the potential role of the parent during the child's examination.

_____ 2. Define the term *nonaccidental trauma (NAT)* and describe the role of technologists if they suspect child abuse based on individual state guidelines.

_____ 3. Identify the more common commercial immobilization devices and explain their function.

_____ 4. List the most common types of paraphernalia used for immobilization.

_____ 5. List the six steps of "mummifying" an infant. Perform this procedure on a simulated patient.

_____ 6. Define terms relating to bone development or ossification and identify the radiographic appearance and the normal stages of development of secondary growth centers.

_____ 7. Identify methods of reducing patient and parent doses and repeat exposures during pediatric procedures.

_____ 8. Identify alternative imaging modalities and procedures performed on pediatric patients.

_____ 9. List the common pathologic indications for radiographic examinations of the chest, upper and lower limbs, pelvis and hips, skull, and pediatric abdomen procedures.

_____ 10. For select forms of pathology of the pediatric skeletal system, determine whether manual exposure factors would increase, decrease, or remain the same.

_____ 11. Describe positioning, technical factors, shielding requirements, and immobilization techniques for procedures of the chest, skeletal system, and abdomen.

_____ 12. List general patient preparation requirements for procedures of the pediatric abdomen, including specific minimum patient preparation requirements for the upper GI, lower GI, and IVU procedures.

_____ 13. List the types and quantities of contrast media based on age as recommended for upper GI, lower GI, and IVU procedures.

_____ 14. Using an articulated pediatric mannequin, correctly immobilize and position a patient.   Using gonadal shielding, perform examinations of the chest, abdomen, upper limb, lower limb, pelvis and hips, and skull.

_____ 15. According to established evaluation criteria, critique and evaluate radiographs provided by your instructor for each of the previously mentioned examinations.

_____ 16. Discriminate between acceptable and unacceptable radiographs and describe how positioning or technical errors can be corrected.

Learning Exercises

Complete the following review exercises after reading the associated pages in the textbook as indicated by each exercise. Answers to each review exercise are given at the end of the review exercises.

PART I: Introduction to Pediatric Radiography

REVIEW EXERCISE A: Immobilization, Ossification, Radiation Protection, Pre-examination Preparation, and Pathologic Indications (see textbook pp. 630-639)

1. List the two important general factors that produce a successful pediatric radiographic procedure:

    A. _____

    B. _____

2. List the three possible roles for the parent during a pediatric procedure.

    A. _____

    B. _____

    C. _____

3. True/False: Parents should never be in the radiographic room with their child.

4. True/False: Battered child syndrome (BCS) is the acceptable term for child abuse.

5. True/False: The technologist is responsible for reporting potential signs of child abuse to the police.

6. True/False: The technologist should always use as short an exposure time as possible during pediatric procedures.

7. List the correct term for the following pediatric immobilization devices:

    A. A piece of Plexiglas with short Velcro straps for immobilization of upper and lower limbs: _____

    B. A device used to hold down upper or lower limbs without obscuring essential anatomy: _____

    C. A device with an adjustable-type bicycle seat and two clear plastic body clamps: _____

8. Which of the immobilization devices just mentioned is most commonly used for erect chests and abdomens?

   _____

9. True/False: Sandbags completely filled with fine sand should be used to immobilize pediatric patients.

10. If stockinettes are used for immobilization, what size should be used for a larger pediatric patient?

    A. 1 inch   C. 3 inch

    B. 2 inch   D. 4 inch

11. Which type of tape is *not* recommended for immobilization purposes on children (because it may create an artifact on the radiograph when placed over the region being radiographed)?

    _____

12. When adhesive tape is used to immobilize (if not placed directly over parts to be radiographed), what two methods are used to prevent the adhesive tape from injuring the fragile skin of infants?

    A. _____

    B. _____

13. A. If Ace bandages are used for immobilization of the legs, which size should be used on infants and smaller chil-

        dren: 3 inch, 4 inch, or 6 inch? _____

    B. What size should be used on older children? _____

14. Briefly describe the six steps for "mummifying" a child.

    1. _____

        _____

    2. _____

        _____

    3. _____

        _____

    4. _____

        _____

    5. _____

        _____

    6. _____

        _____

15. Primary centers of bone formation (ossification) involving the midshafts of long bones are called

    _____ .

16. Secondary centers of ossification of the long bones are called _____.

17. The spaces between the primary and secondary areas of ossification are called _____.

18. At approximately what age does the epiphysis of the fibular apex first become clearly visible (see textbook, p. 634)?

    A. 1 or 2 years old   C. 5 or 6 years old

    B. 3 or 4 years old   D. Teens

19. At approximately what age does the skeleton reach full ossification?

    A. 12 years old   C. 25 years old

    B. 18 years old   D. 40 years old

20. List three safeguards to help reduce repeat exposures during pediatric procedures:

    A. _____   C. _____

    B. _____

21. List three safeguards to reduce the patient dose during pediatric procedures (in addition to gonadal shielding):

    A. _____   C. _____

    B. _____

22. When two technologists are working together, match the following duties with the primary or assisting technologist:

    _____ 1. Makes exposures   A. Primary technologist

    _____ 2. Positions the patient   B. Assisting technologist

    _____ 3. Processes the images

    _____ 4. Positions the tube and collimates

    _____ 5. Sets exposure factors

    _____ 6. Instructs the parents

23. True/False: Clothing, bandages, and diapers generally do not need to be removed from the regions being radiographed on pediatric patients since they do not cause artifacts on the radiographs (if metallic fasteners are not present).

24. Which one of the following imaging modalities is most effective in diagnosing pyloric stenosis in children?

    A. Sonography   C. Functional MRI

    B. Spiral/helical CT   D. Nuclear medicine

25. Functional MRI may be used to detect disorders in all the following conditions *except:*

    A. Autism   C. Hydrocephalus

    B. Tourette's syndrome   D. Attention deficient hyperactivity disorder

26. Match the following pathologic indications of the pediatric chest with the best definition and/or statement (use each choice only once):

    _____ A.   Meconium aspiration   1.   Bacterial infection can lead to closure of the upper airway

    _____ B.   Hyaline membrane disease   2.   Also known as *respiratory distress syndrome*

    _____ C.   Neonate Graves' disease   3.   Inherited disease leading to clogging of bronchi

    _____ D.   Epiglottitis   4.   Condition may develop during stressful births

    _____ E.   Cystic fibrosis   5.   Viral infection leading to labored breathing and dry cough

    _____ F.   Croup   6.   Coughing up blood

    _____ G.   Hemoptysis   7.   A form of hyperthyroidism

27. Match the following pathologic indications of the pediatric skeletal system to the best definition and/or statement:

    _____ A.   Meningocele   1.   Most common form of short-limbed dwarfism

    _____ B.   Kohler's bone disease   2.   Hereditary disorder characterized by soft and fragile bones

    _____ C.   Legg-Calve-Perthes disease   3.   Congenital defect where the spinal cord protrudes through an opening in the vertebral column

    _____ D.   Talipes equinus   4.   A common lesion at the hip

    _____ E.   Osteogenesis imperfecta   5.   Group of diseases affecting the epiphyseal plates of long bones

    _____ F.   Achondroplasia   6.   Congenital defect in which the meninges of the spinal cord protrude through an opening in the vertebral column

    _____ G.   Myelocele   7.   Inflammation of the navicular bone in the foot

    _____ H.   Osteochondroses   8.   Congenital deformity of the foot involving plantar flexion

28. Match the following pathologic indications of the pediatric abdomen to the best definition and/or statement:

    _____ A.   Hydronephrosis   1.   May result in repeated, forceful vomiting

    _____ B.   Pyloric stenosis   2.   Rhythmic contractions of large intestine are absent

    _____ C.   NEC   3.   Condition characterized by absence of on opening in an organ

    _____ D.   Atresias   4.   Condition resulting from an allergic reaction to gluten

    _____ E.   Hypospadias   5.   Enlarged renal collection system due to obstruction

    _____ F.   Hirshsprung's disease   6.   Inflammation of the inner lining of the intestine

    _____ G.   Celiac disease   7.   Congenital defect in male urethra

29. Indicate whether the following pathologic conditions require that manual exposure factors be increased (+), decreased (−), or remain the same (0):

   A. Pneumonia _____

   B. Pneumothorax _____

   C. Osteogenesis imperfecta _____

   D. Legg-Calve- Perthes disease _____

   E. Osteomalacia _____

   F. Osteopetrosis _____

   G. Volvulus _____

30. True/False: Malignant bone tumors are rare in young children.

PART II: Radiographic Positioning

REVIEW EXERCISE B: Pediatric Positioning of the Chest, Skeletal System, and Skull (see textbook pp. 641-652)

1. Complete the following technical factors for an AP or PA pediatric chest:

   A. Grid or non-grid: _____   D. SID, AP supine chest: _____

   B. kVp range: _____   E. SID, PA erect chest: _____

   C. Image receptor lengthwise or crosswise: _____

2. What kVp range is generally used for a lateral chest? _____

3. Should a grid be used for a lateral chest (yes or no)? _____

4. The Pigg-O-Stat can be used effectively for an erect PA and lateral chest from infancy to approximately age

   _____.

5. When should a chest exposure be made for a crying child?

   _____

6. Which radiographic structures are evaluated to determine rotation on a PA projection of the chest?

   _____

7. How is the x-ray tube aligned for a lateral projection of the chest if the patient is on a Tam-em board?

   _____

8. True/False: If available, the Pigg-O-Stat should be used rather than relying on parental assistance during a pediatric chest examination.

9. True/False: A well-inspired, erect chest radiograph taken on a young pediatric patient will visualize only six to seven ribs above the diaphragm.

10. True/False: The entire upper limb is commonly included on an infant rather than individual exposures of specific parts of the upper limb.

11. True/False: Except for survey exams, individual projections of the elbow, wrist, and shoulder should generally be taken on older children rather than including these regions on a single projection.

12. Match the following pathologic indicators with the correct radiographic procedure:

_____   1. Atelectasis   A. Chest

_____   2. Kohler's disease   B. Upper or lower limb

_____   3. Cystic fibrosis

_____   4. Talipes

_____   5. RDS

13. Which single radiographic position will provide a lateral projection of bilateral lower limbs for the nontraumatic pediatric patient?

_____

14. Which radiographic projections (and method) are performed for the infant with congenital club feet?

_____

15. True/False: It is important to place the foot into true AP and lateral positions when performing a clubfoot study.

16. True/False: It is possible to provide gonadal shielding for both male and female pediatric patients for AP and lateral projections of hips.

17. What size image receptor should be used for a skull routine on a 6-year-old patient? _____

18. Which one of the following CR angulations will place the petrous ridges in the lower one third of the orbits with an AP reverse Caldwell projection of the skull?

A. 15° cephalad to OML   C. CR perpendicular to OML

B. 15° caudad to OML   D. 30° cephalad to OML

19. Which one of the following pathologic indicators would apply to a pediatric skull series?

A. Osteomyelitis   B. CHD   C. Mastoiditis   D. Hyaline membrane disease

20. Which skull positioning line is placed perpendicular to the film for an AP Towne 30° caudal projection of the skull?

A. IOML   B. OML   C. MML   D. AML

21. True/False: Parental assistance for skull radiography is preferred rather than using head clamps and a mummy wrap on a pediatric patient.

22. True/False: Children more than 5 years old can usually hold their breath after a practice session.

23. Correct centering for the following can be achieved by placing the central ray at the level of which structure or landmark?

A. AP, PA, or lateral chest _____

B. AP abdomen (infants and small children) _____

C. AP supine abdomen (older children) _____

D. AP skull _____

REVIEW EXERCISE C: Positioning of the Pediatric Abdomen and Contrast Media Procedures (see textbook pp. 653-662)

1. True/False: The chest and abdomen are generally almost equal in circumference in the newborn.

2. True/False: Bony landmarks in infants are easy to palpate and locate.

3. True/False: It is difficult to distinguish the small bowel from the large bowel on a plain abdomen on an infant.

4. True/False: The radiographic contrast on a pediatric abdominal radiograph is high compared with that of an adult abdominal radiograph.

5. Complete the recommended NPO fasting before the following pediatric contrast media procedures:

   A.   Infant to 1-year-old upper GI: _____   C.   Infant lower GI _____

   B.   1 year and older upper GI: _____   D.   Pediatric IVU _____

6. List five conditions that contraindicate the use of laxatives or enemas in preparation for a lower GI study:

   A. _____

   B. _____

   C. _____

   D. _____

   E. _____

7. Indicate which of the following pathologic indicators apply for an AP abdomen (KUB) by placing an X in the corresponding column. Place an X by only those indicators that apply to the abdomen.

   _____ A. Croup   _____ E. Mastoiditis

   _____ B. NEC   _____ F. Hepatomegaly

   _____ C. Intussusception   _____ G. Appendicitis

   _____ D. Foreign body localization _____ H. Hydrocephalus

8. Where is the CR centered for a small child erect abdomen? _____

9. A.   What is the minimum kVp for an AP abdomen projection of a newborn without a grid? _____

   B.   A grid is recommended for a pediatric AP abdomen if the abdomen measures more than _____ cm.

10. Which one of the following projections of the abdomen will best demonstrate the prevertebral region?

    A. AP supine KUB   B. PA prone KUB   C. Dorsal decubitus abdomen   D. AP erect abdomen

11. Which one of the following conditions is caused by inflammation of the inner lining of the large or small bowel, resulting in tissue death?

    A. NEC   B. CHD   C. Intussusception   D. Meconium ileus

12. Which of the following procedures or projections should be performed for a possible meconium ileus?

    A. IVU procedure   B. Barium enema   C. AP supine abdomen   D. AP erect abdomen

13. List the amount of barium that should be given to the following patients for an upper GI series:

    A.   Newborn to 1 year old: _____   C.   3 to 10 years old: _____

    B.   1 to 3 years old: _____   D.   Over 10 years old: _____

14. What is the only recourse if a pediatric patient refuses to drink barium for an upper GI series?

    _____

15. True/False: A piece of lead vinyl should be placed beneath the child's lower pelvis during conventional fluoroscopy to reduce the gonadal/mean bone marrow dose.

16. True/False: The transit time of the contrast media for reaching the cecum during a pediatric small bowel series is approximately 2 hours.

17. True/False: Latex enema tips should be used for barium enemas for children under the age of 1 year.

18. True/False: Small retention enema tips can be used on infants during a barium enema to help barium retention.

19. What type of contrast media is recommended for reducing an intussusception? _____

20. What is the maximum height of the barium enema bag before the beginning of the procedure? _____

21. A backward flow of urine from the bladder into the ureters and kidneys is called _____ .

22. A malignant tumor of the kidney common in children under the age of 5 years is:

    A.   Wilms' tumor   B.   Adenocarcinoma   C.   Ewing's sarcoma   D.   Teratoma

23. What is the most common pathologic indication for a voiding cystourethrogram? _____

24. True/False: A radionuclide study for vesicourethral reflux provides a smaller patient dose compared to a fluoroscopic voiding cystourethrogram.

25. Indicate the suggested contrast media dosages for IVU procedures for the following weight categories of pediatric patients:

    A.   0 to 12 lb   _____

    B.   13 to 25 lb   _____

    C.   26 to 50 lb   _____

    D.   51 to 100 lb   _____

    E.   >100 lb   _____

26. What are the suggested contrast media dosages for the following metric weight measurements?

    A.   0 to 11 kg   _____

    B.   12 to 23 kg   _____

    C.   24 to 45 kg   _____

    D.   >45 kg   _____

27. True/False: The lower abdomen can be shielded for the 3-minute film taken during an IVU for both males and females.

28. True/False: To help depress the large bowel and create a radiolucent window to better visualize the kidneys, a carbonated drink should be given to pediatric patients before an IVU.

29. True/False: Most radiologists prefer their pediatric patients to be dehydrated before an IVU.

30. True/False: Since allergic reactions to iodinated contrast agents are rare in pediatric patients, the use of ionic contrast media is recommended for IVUs.

PART III: Laboratory Exercises (see textbook pp. 630-662)

Exercises A and B need to be carried out in a radiographic laboratory or a general diagnostic room in the radiology department. General immobilization paraphernalia need to be available (i.e., tape, sheets or large towels, sandbags, various sizes and shapes of positioning sponge blocks, retention bands, head clamps, stockinettes, and Ace bandages). More common commercial immobilization devices such as the Tam-em Board or the Pigg-O-Stat (or similar devices) are optional if such are available. However, at least one of these devices should be made available for student use.

Exercise C can be carried out in a classroom or any room where illuminators (view boxes) are available.

LABORATORY EXERCISE A: Immobilization

For this section you will need some type of large articulate doll mannequin to use as your patient. The doll should have arms and legs that are flexible (similar to that of a child). This does not need to be a phantom-like doll since radiographs will not be taken, but it will be used to simulate immobilization techniques and positioning for various body parts.

Check each of the following as you complete that activity.

_____ 1. Complete the six steps of "mummifying."

_____ 2. Use a tubular-type stockinette of appropriate size to immobilize the "patient's" arms and hands placed above and behind the head.

_____ 3. Use the appropriate size Ace bandage to immobilize the lower limbs by wrapping with appropriate tension from the hips to the ankles.

_____ 4. Apply a retention band correctly across the abdomen and upper and lower limbs to completely immobilize these parts of the "patient."

_____ 5. Use sandbags under and over the legs and over each arm to immobilize for an AP abdomen.

_____ 6. Apply tape correctly in combination with sandbags to immobilize the head and the upper and lower limbs.

_____ 7. Apply head clamps to immobilize the head in combination with mummification of the patient and the use of sandbags or a retention band to prevent limb or body movement.

Tam-em Board if available:

_____ 8. Immobilize your patient correctly with the Velcro straps to restrain the upper and lower limbs and across the pelvic region.

Pigg-O-Stat if available:

_____ 9. Immobilize your "patient" correctly with the arms above the head using the plastic side body clamps to restrain the arms and head.

LABORATORY EXERCISE B: Physical Positioning

This section again requires the use of a large articulated doll mannequin. Practice the following projections or positions until you can perform them accurately and without hesitation. Place a check by each when you have achieved this.

Include the following details as you simulate the basic projections for each exam as follows. Assume the patient will not cooperate and that forceful immobilization is required. Use suggested immobilization techniques.

_____ Correct size and type of image receptor (appropriate for size of "patient")

_____ Correct centering of part to image receptor

_____ Correct SID, and location and angle of central ray

_____ Selection of appropriate restraining devices and application of the same

_____ Correct placement of markers

_____ Correct use of contact gonadal shield

_____ Accurate collimation to body part of interest

_____ Approximate correct exposure factors

	EXAMINATION	*IMMOBILIZATION*
_____ 1.	AP chest, supine	Tam-em-Board or sand bags and/or stockinette and "Ace" bandages
_____ 2.	Lateral chest, patient recumbent in lateral position	Sandbags and tape, or retention band

If Tam-em Board is available:

_____ 3.	Lateral chest, patient supine, horizontal beam CR	Tam-em Board (see textbook, p. 631)

If Pigg-O-Stat is available:

_____ 4.	PA chest erect, 72 in. (180 cm) SID	Pigg-O-Stat (see textbook, p. 642)
_____ 5.	Lateral chest erect, 72 in. (180 cm) SID	Pigg-O-Stat (see textbook, p. 644)
_____ 6.	AP abdomen, erect	Pigg-O-Stat (see textbook, p. 655)
_____ 7.	AP abdomen, supine	Tam-em Board, or tape, sandbags and retention band (see textbook, p. 654)
_____ 8.	AP and lateral upper limb (from shoulder to hand)	Tape, sandbags and/or retention band (see textbook, p. 645)
_____ 9.	AP and lateral lower limb (from hips to feet)	Tape, sandbags and/or retention band (see textbook, p. 647)
_____ 10.	AP and lateral feet (such as follow-up exams for clubfeet)	Sitting on pad using tape (see textbook, p. 648)
_____ 11.	AP pelvis and hips	Tape and sandbags and/or retention band (see textbook, p. 649)
_____ 12.	Lateral hips	Tape and sandbags and/or retention band (see textbook, p. 652)
_____ 13.	AP skull, 15° AP and 30° Towne	Head clamps or tape for head. Mummification and sandbags or retention band for limbs and body (see textbook, p. 651)
_____ 14.	Lateral skull, turned into lateral position	Head clamps or tape for head. Mummification and sandbags or retention band for limbs and body (see textbook, p. 652)
_____ 15.	Lateral skull, horizontal beam in supine position	Tam-em Board and tape for head (see textbook, p. 652)

LABORATORY EXERCISE C: Anatomy Review and Critique Radiographs of the Abdomen

Use those radiographs provided by your instructor. These should include optimal-quality and less-than-optimal quality radiographs of each of the following: chest, supine and erect abdomen, AP and lateral upper limb, AP and lateral pelvis and hips, AP and lateral lower limb, and AP and lateral skull radiographs.

Radiographs of the pelvis and upper and lower limbs of patients of various ages should be included to demonstrate the normal ossification or growth stages from infancy to adolescence.

Place a check by each of the following when completed.

    _____   1.   Examine normal stages of growth by the appearance of the epiphyses in the pelvis and the long bones of the upper and lower limbs. Estimate the approximate age of the patient by the appearance of such epiphyses.

    _____   2.   Critique each radiograph based on evaluation criteria provided for each projection in the textbook. Pediatric radiographs require a wider range of acceptable positioning criteria than for adults. Part centering and specific central ray locations are not as critical for pediatric radiographs because multiple anatomical parts or bones are included on one film. This is possible because detailed views of joint areas are not as important since these secondary growth areas are not yet fully developed. Thus complete limbs can be included on one film.

The following criteria guidelines can be used and checked as each radiograph is evaluated. Determine the corrections or adjustments in positioning or exposure factors necessary to bring those less-than-optimal radiographs up to a more desirable standard.

       Radiographs   *Criteria Guidelines*

1	2	3	4	5	6		
___	___	___	___	___	___	a.	Correct image receptor size as appropriate for age and size of patient?
___	___	___	___	___	___	b.	Correct orientation of part to image receptor?
___	___	___	___	___	___	c.	Acceptable alignment and/or centering of part to image receptor?
___	___	___	___	___	___	d.	Correct collimation and correct CR angle where appropriate (such as for an AP skull)?
___	___	___	___	___	___	e.	Evidence of gonadal shield correctly placed (if this should be visible)?
___	___	___	___	___	___	f.	Pertinent anatomy well visualized?
___	___	___	___	___	___	g.	Evidence of motion?
___	___	___	___	___	___	h.	Optimal exposure (density and/or contrast)?
___	___	___	___	___	___	i.	Patient ID with date and side markers visible without superimposing essential anatomy?

Answers to Review Exercises

Review Exercise A: Introduction, Immobilization, Ossification, Radiation Protection, Pre-exam Preparation, and Pathologic Indications

1. A. Technologist's attitude and approach to a child
   B. Technical preparation of the room
2. A. Serve as an observer in the room to lend support and comfort to their child
   B. Serve as a participator to assist with immobilization
   C. Remain in the waiting room, and do not accompany the child into the room
3. False (may be permissible with proper lead shielding if not pregnant)
4. False (correct term is *nonaccidental trauma, NAT*)
5. False (should report to radiologist or superior)
6. True
7. A. Tam-em board
   B. Plexiglass hold-down paddle
   C. Pigg-o-stat
8. Pigg-o-stat
9. False (should not be overfilled so as to be soft and pliable)
10. D. 4 inch
11. Adhesive
12. A. Twisting the tape so the adhesive surface is not against the skin
    B. Placing a gauze pad between the tape and the skin
13. A. 4 in.
    B. 6 in.
14. 1. Place the sheet on the table folded in half or thirds lengthwise
    2. Place patient in middle of sheet with the right arm down to the side. Fold sheet across the patient's body and pull sheet across the body keeping the arm against the body.
    3. Place the patient's left arm along the side of the body and on top of the sheet. Bring the free sheet over the left arm to the right side of the body. Wrap the sheet around the body as needed.
    4. Pull the sheet tightly so the patient cannot free arms.
    5. Place a long piece of tape from the right to the left wrapped arm to prevent the patient from breaking out of the sheet.
    6. Place a piece of tape around the patient's knees.
15. Diaphysis
16. Epiphyses

17. Epiphyseal plates
18. C. 5- or 6-year-old
19. C. 25 years old
20. A. Proper immobilization
    B. Short exposure times
    C. Accurate technique charts
21. A. Close collimation
    B. Low-dosage techniques
    C. Minimum number of images
22. 1. B, 2. A, 3. B, 4. A, 5. B, 6. A
23. False (Should be removed, may cause artifacts)
24. A. Sonography
25. C. Hydrocephalus
26. A. 4, B. 2, C. 7, D. 1, E. 3, F. 5, G. 6
27. A. 6, B. 7, C. 4, D. 8, E. 2, F. 1, G. 3, H. 5
28. A. 5, B. 1, C. 6, D. 3, E. 7, F. 2, G. 4
29. A. (+), B. (-), C. (-), D. (0), E. (-), F. (+), G. (-)
30. True

Review Exercise B: Pediatric Positioning of the Chest, Skeletal System, and Skull

1. A. Non-grid
   B. 70 to 80 kVp
   C. Crosswise
   D. 50 to 60 in. (127 to 212 cm)
   E. 72 in. (180 cm)
2. 75 to 80 kVp
3. No
4. Two
5. As the child fully inhales and holds his or her breath
6. The sternoclavicular joints and lateral rib margins should be equidistant from the vertebral column
7. Horizontally
8. True
9. False (9 or 10)
10. True
11. True
12. 1. A, 2. B, 3. A, 4. B, 5. A
13. Bilateral frogleg
14. AP and lateral feet, Kite method
15. False (Take two projections 90° from each other)
16. True (if correctly placed)
17. 10 x 12 in. (24 x 30 cm) (a child's skull is near adult size)
18. A. 15° cephalad to OML
19. C. Mastoiditis
20. B. OML
21. False
22. True
23. A. Mammillary (nipple) line
    B. 1 in. (2.5 cm) above umbilicus
    C. At level of iliac crest
    D. Glabella

Review Exercise C: Positioning of the Pediatric Abdomen and Contrast Media Procedures

1. True
2. False (most bony landmarks are nonexistent in infants)
3. True
4. False (contrast is low)
5. A. 4 hours
   B. 6 hours
   C. No prep required
   D. 4 hours
6. A. Hirschsprung's disease
   B. Extensive diarrhea
   C. Appendicitis
   D. Obstruction
   E. Dehydration (patients who cannot withstand fluid loss)
7. B, C, D, F, G
8. One inch (2.5 cm) above the umbilicus
9. A. 65
   B. 9 cm
10. C. dorsal decubitus abdomen
11. A. NEC
12. D. AP erect abdomen
13. A. 2 to 4 ounces
    B. 4 to 6 ounces
    C. 6 to 12 ounces
    D. 12 to 16 ounces
14. Insert a nasogastric tube into the stomach
15. True
16. False (usually 1 hour)
17. False (latex tips should not be used because of possible allergic response to latex)
18. False (retention tips should not be used on small children)
19. Air for the pneumatic reduction of intussusception
20. 3 feet
21. Vesicoureteral reflux
22. A. Wilms' tumor
23. Urinary tract infection (UTI)
24. True
25. A. 2 cc/lb
    B. 25 cc
    C. 1 cc/lb
    D. 50 cc
    E. 1/2 cc/lb
26. A. 3 ml/kg
    B. 2 ml/kg
    C. 50 ml
    D. 1 ml/kg
27. True
28. False (not recommended by pediatric radiologists)
29. False (should *not* be dehydrated)
30. False (not recommended)

SELF-TEST

Directions: This self-test should be taken only after completing all of the readings, review exercises, and laboratory activities for a particular section. The purpose of this test is not only to provide a good learning exercise but also to serve as a good indicator of what your final evaluation grade will be. It is strongly suggested that if you do not get at least a 90% to 95% grade on this self-test, you should review those areas where you missed questions before going to your instructor for the final evaluation exam for this chapter. (There are 73 questions or blanks—each is worth 1.4 points.)

1. At what age can most children be talked through a radiographic examination without forceful immobilization?

    A. 1 year   C. 3 years

    B. 2 years   D. 5 years

2. At the first meeting between the technologist and the patient (accompanied by an adult), which of the following generally should *not* be done?

    A. Introduce yourself

    B. Take the necessary time to explain what you will be doing

    C. Discuss the possible forceful immobilization that will be needed if the child will not cooperate

    D. Describe the total amount of radiation the patient will receive with that specific exam if it has to be repeated because of a lack of cooperation

    E. All of the above should be done

3. If child abuse is suspected by the technologist, he or she should:

    A. Ask the parent when the abuse occurred

    B. Report the abuse immediately to the necessary state officials as required by the state

    C. Refuse to do the examination or to touch the child until a physician has examined the patient

    D. Do none of the above

4. The following is *not* the name of a known commercially available immobilization device

    A. Posi-Tot   C. Pigg-O-Stat

    B. Tam-em Board   D. Hold-em Tiger

5. The most suitable immobilization device for erect chests and/or the abdomen is:

    A. Posi-Tot   C. Pigg-O-Stat

    B. Tam-em Board   D. Hold-em Tiger

6. List the three factors that will reduce the number of repeat exposures with pediatric patients.

    A. _____   C. _____

    B. _____

7. What important question should a female parent be asked before allowing her to assist with holding her child during an exposure? _____

8. Which immobilization device or method should be used for an erect 1-year-old chest procedure? Assume these devices are available.

    A. Tam-em board   C. Pigg-O-Stat

    B. Hold- down paddle   D. Parent holding child

9. Which one of the following procedures can be performed to diagnose possible genetic fetal abnormalities?

    A. Nuclear medicine fetal scan   C. Functional MRI

    B. Spiral/helical CT   D. 3-D ultrasound

10. Which of the procedures can be performed to evaluate children for attention deficient hyperactivity disorder?

    A. Spiral/helical CT   C. 3-D ultrasound

    B. Functional MRI   D. Nuclear medicine

11. Match the following conditions to the correct definition or statement (use each choice only once):

    _____ A. Croup   1. Due to an allergic reaction to gluten

    _____ B. Respiratory distress syndrome   2. Group of diseases affecting the epiphyseal growth plates

    _____ C. Epiglottitis   3. Abnormally enlarged ventricles in brain

    _____ D. Osteochondroses   4. A common condition in children between the ages of 1 to 3 due to a viral infection

    _____ E. Osteogenesis imperfecta   5. Enlargement of the liver

    _____ F. Hydrocephalus   6. Second most common form of cancer in children under 5 years of age

    _____ G. Osteomalacia   7. Bacterial infection of the upper airway that may be fatal if untreated

    _____ H. Hirschsprung's disease   8. Congenital defect in which an opening into an organ is missing

    _____ I. Celiac disease   9. Condition where the alveoli and capillaries of the lungs are injured or infected

    _____ J. Neuroblastoma   10. Bacterial infection of the kidney

    _____ K. Pyelonephritis   11. Also known as *congenital megacolon*

    _____ L. Atresia   12. Also known as *rickets*

    _____ M. Hepatomegaly   13. Inherited condition that produces very fragile bones

12. Indicate whether the following pathologic conditions require that manual exposure factors be increased (+), de-creased (-), or remain the same (0):

A.   Cystic fibrosis _____

B.   Hyaline membrane disease _____

C.   Osteogenesis imperfecta _____

D.   Hydrocephalus _____

E.   Idiopathic juvenile osteoporosis _____

F.   Osteopetrosis _____

G.   Volvulus _____

13. Which one of the following techniques will help remove the scapulae from the lung fields during chest radiography?

A.   Make exposure upon the second inspiration   C.   Extend arms upward

B.   Extend the chin   D.   Place arms behind the patient's back

14. What is the typical kVp range for a pediatric study of the upper limb? _____

15. True/False: A hand routine for a 7-year-old would be the same as for an adult patient.

16. True/False: For a bone survey of a young child, both limbs are commonly radiographed for comparison.

17. Which technique or method is performed to radiographically study congenital clubfoot?

_____

18. Where is gonadal shielding placed for a bilateral hip study on a female pediatric patient?

_____

19. Complete the following related to ossification by matching the correct term with the description.   More than one choice per blank is possible.

E = Epiphysis, **D** = Diaphysis, **EP** = Epiphyseal plate.

_____   1.   Primary centers

_____   2.   Secondary centers

_____   3.   Space between primary and secondary centers

_____   4.   Occurs before birth

_____   5.   Continues to change from birth to maturity

20. Match the examination in the right column most likely associated with the pathologic indicators in the left column. Answers may be used more than once.

_____ 1. Intussusception		A. Chest
_____ 2. NEC		B. Abdomen
_____ 3. Hydrocephalus		C. Upper and lower limbs
_____ 4. Atelectasis		D. Pelvis and hips
_____ 5. Premature closure of fontanelles		E. Skull
_____ 6. CHD		
_____ 7. Cystic fibrosis		
_____ 8. Meconium ileus		
_____ 9. Legg-Calve-Perthes disease		
_____ 10. Hemoptysis		
_____ 11. Shunt check		
_____ 12. Bronchiectasis		
_____ 13. Hyaline membrane disease		

21. How much is the CR angled from the OML for an AP Towne projection of the skull?

A. 15°   C. 25°

B. None   D. 30°

22. Where is the CR centered for a lateral projection of the skull?

A. At the EAM

B. Midway between the glabella and inion

C. 1 in. (2.5 cm) above the EAM

D. 3/4 in. (2 cm) anterior and superior to EAM

23. The NPO fasting period for a 6-month-old before an upper GI is:

A. 4 hours   C. 1 hour

B. 6 hours   D. 8 hours

24. Other than preventing artifacts in the bowel, what is the other reason that solid food is withheld for 4 hours before a pediatric IVU?

_____

25. Which one of the following conditions would contraindicate the use of laxatives before a contrast media procedure?

A. Gastritis   C. Appendicitis

B. Blood in stool   D. Diverticulosis

26. Where is the CR centered for a KUB on:

A. An 8-year-old child? _____

B. A 1-year-old child? _____

27. At what level is the CR centered for a PA and lateral pediatric chest? _____

28. What is the recommended amount of barium for an 8-year-old child having an upper GI?

_____

29. How is barium instilled into the large bowel for a barium enema study on an infant?

_____

30. What is the bowel prep for a pediatric voiding cystourethrogram (VCUG)? _____

31. When is urinary reflux most likely to occur during a VCUG? _____

32. For a pediatric small bowel study, the barium normally reaches the ileocecal region in_____
     hour(s).

33. A VCUG on a child is most commonly performed to evaluate for (A) _____ and is gener-

     ally scheduled to be completed (B) _____ (before or after) an IVU or ultrasound study of

     the kidneys.

34. True/False: Gonadal shielding should only be used in supine positions due to the difficulty in keeping the shield in
     place.

35. True/False: There should be no attempt to straighten out the abnormal alignment of the foot during a clubfoot study.

Angiography and Interventional Procedures

This chapter, which includes extensive detailed and somewhat complex anatomy and procedural information, is an excellent introduction to angiography. It provides effective preparation for the additional clinical training and experience that a special procedures technologist will need.

After you have completed **all** the activities of this chapter, you will be able to:

_____ 1. List the divisions and components of the circulatory system.

_____ 2. List the three functions of the cardiovascular system.

_____ 3. On drawings, identify the components of the pulmonary and general systemic circulation.

_____ 4. Identify the four chambers of the heart, associated valves, and coronary circulation.

_____ 5. List and identify the four arteries supplying blood to the brain and the three branches arising from the aortic arch.

_____ 6. List the major branches of the external and internal carotid arteries and the primary divisions of the brain supplied by each.

_____ 7. On drawings, identify the major veins of the neck draining blood from the head and neck region.

_____ 8. List the major venous sinuses found in the cranium.

_____ 9. List the four segments of the thoracic aorta and describe the three common variations of the aortic arch.

_____ 10. List and identify the five major branches of the abdominal aorta.

_____ 11. List and identify the major abdominal veins.

_____ 12. List and identify the major arteries and veins of the upper and lower limbs.

_____ 13. List four functions of the lymphatic portion of the circulatory system.

_____ 14. Identify the six steps related to the Seldinger technique

_____ 15. Identify the equipment generally found in a neuroangiographic room.

_____ 16. Identify the pathologic indications, contraindications, and general procedure for cerebral angiography.

_____ 17. Identify the indications, catheterization technique, and general procedure for thoracic and abdominal aortography.

_____ 18. Identify the pathologic indications, contraindications, and general procedure for peripheral angiography.

_____ 19. Identify specific examples of vascular and nonvascular interventional procedures.

132 REVIEW EXERCISE A: Radiographic Anatomy of Cardiovascular System, Pulmonary and Systemic Circulation, and Cerebral Arteries and Veins

CHAPTER 21

Learning Exercises

Complete the following review exercises after reading the associated pages in the textbook as indicated by each exercise. Answers to each review exercise are given at the end of the review exercises.

REVIEW EXERCISE A: Radiographic Anatomy of Cardiovascular System, Pulmonary and Systemic Circulation, and Cerebral Arteries and Veins (see textbook pp. 666-672)

1. List the two major divisions or components of the circulatory system:

   A. _____ B. _____

2. List the body system or part supplied by the following four divisions of the circulatory system:

   A. Cardio _____ C. Pulmonary _____

   B. Vascular _____ D. Systemic _____

3. List the three functions of the cardiovascular system:

   A. _____

   B. _____

   C. _____

4. Identify the major components of the general cardiovascular circulation as labeled on this drawing (Fig. 21-1):

   A. _____

   B. _____

   C. _____

   D. _____

   E. _____

   F. _____

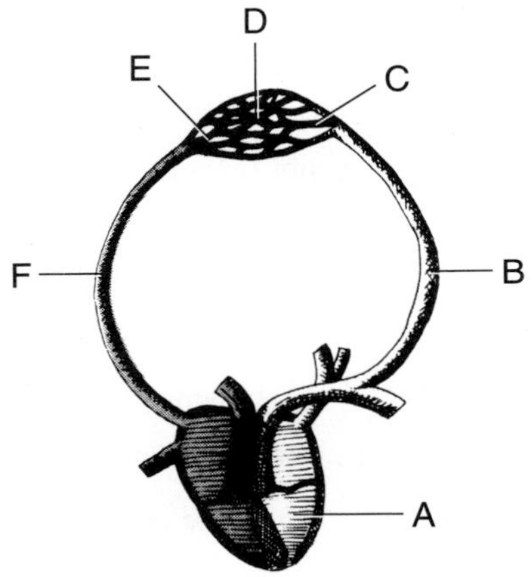

Fig. 21-1 Components of cardiovascular circulation.

5. Which of the six general components of the circulatory system, identified in question 4 above, carry oxygenated blood to body tissue?

   _____

6. Which of the six general components of the circulatory system carry deoxygenated blood?

   _____

CHAPTER 21 REVIEW EXERCISE A: Radiographic Anatomy of Cardiovascular System, Pulmonary and Systemic Circulation, and Cerebral Arteries and Veins

133

7. List the common term (where indicated) and the function for the following three blood components:

		COMMON TERM		FUNCTION
1.	Erythrocytes	A. _____	B. _____
2.	Leukocytes	A. _____	B. _____
3.	Platelets	A. (No other term given)	B. _____

8. Plasma, the liquid portion of blood, consists of (A) _____% water and (B) _____% plasma protein and salts, nutrients, and oxygen.

9. Identify the chambers of the heart and the associated blood vessels (arteries and veins) as labeled on Fig. 21-2.

A. _____ (chamber)

B. _____ (chamber)

C. _____ (chamber)

D. _____

E. _____

F. _____

G. _____

H. _____

I. _____

J. _____ (chamber)

K. _____

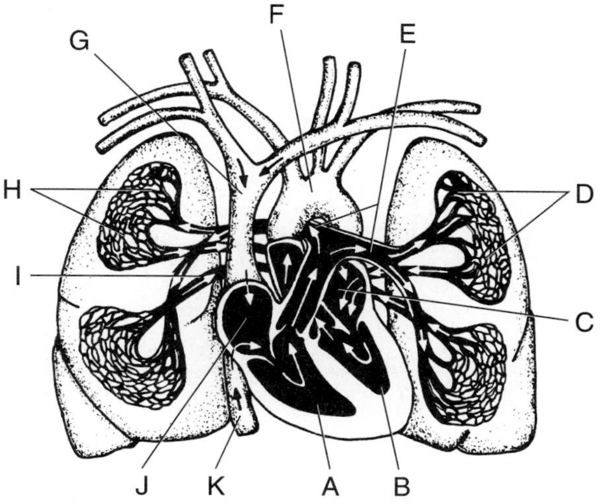

Fig. 21-2 Heart and pulmonary circulation (frontal view).

Questions 10 and 11 relate to Fig. 21-2

10. In general, arteries carry oxygenated blood, and veins carry deoxygenated blood. The exceptions to these are:

A. The _____ , which carry deoxygenated blood to the lungs.

B. The _____ , which carry oxygenated blood back to the atrium of the heart.

11. A. Blood from the upper body returns to the heart through the _____ .

B. Blood from the abdomen and the lower limbs returns through the _____ .

C. Both of these major veins enter the _____ of the heart.

12. Identify the four major valves between the following heart chambers and associated vessels.

A. Between right atrium and right ventricle: _____

B. Between right ventricle and pulmonary arteries: _____

C. Between left atrium and left ventricle: _____

D. Between left ventricle and aorta: _____

134 REVIEW EXERCISE A: Radiographic Anatomy of Cardiovascular System, Pulmonary and Systemic Circulation, and Cerebral Arteries and Veins

CHAPTER 21

13. A. The arteries that deliver blood to the heart muscle are the _____ .

    B. These arteries originate at the _____ .

14. List the three major branches of the coronary sinus:

    A. _____   C. _____

    B. _____

15. Identify the labeled arteries on this drawing (Fig. 21-3):

    A. _____

    B. _____

    C. _____

    D. _____

    E. _____

    F. _____

    G. _____

    H. _____

    I. _____

    J. _____

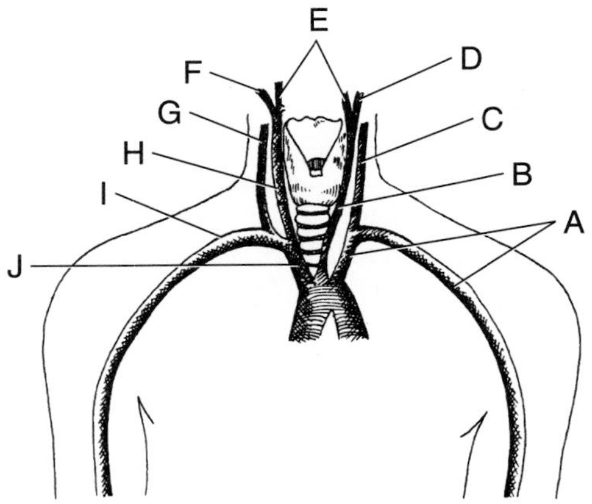

Fig. 21-3 Arterial branches of the aortic arch.

16. List the three major branches of arteries arising from the arch of the aorta that supply the brain with blood:

    A. _____   C. _____

    B. _____

17. List the four major arteries supplying blood to the brain (important radiographically on a four-vessel angiogram).

    A. _____   C. _____

    B. _____   D. _____

18. True/False: The brachiocephalic artery bifurcates to form the right common and right vertebral arteries.

19. True/False: The level for bifurcation of the common carotid artery into the internal and external carotid arteries is at the level of C3-4.

20. Any injection of the common carotid inferior to the bifurcation would result in filling both the

    _____ and _____ arteries.

21. What is the name of the "S-shaped" portion of the internal carotid artery near the petrous portion of the temporal bone?

    A. Carotid sinus   C. Carotid body

    B. Carotid canal   D. Carotid siphon

CHAPTER 21   REVIEW EXERCISE A: Radiographic Anatomy of Cardiovascular System, Pulmonary and Systemic Circulation, and Cerebral Arteries and Veins

135

22. List the two end branches of the internal carotid artery:

    A. _____   B. _____

23. The _____ artery supplies much of the forebrain with blood.

24. The _____ supply the posterior circulation of the brain.

25. The two vertebral arteries unite to form the single _____ artery.

26. Which of the two major branches of each internal carotid artery (anterior cerebral or middle cerebral) supply the lateral aspects of the cerebral hemispheres? _____

27. The anterior and middle cerebral arteries superimpose one another to a greater extent on the

    _____ (lateral or frontal) view.

28. Identify which one of the following four drawings (Fig. 21-4) demonstrate the following:

    1. Middle cerebral artery and branches of the internal carotid artery   _____

    2. Anterior cerebral artery and branches of the internal carotid artery   _____

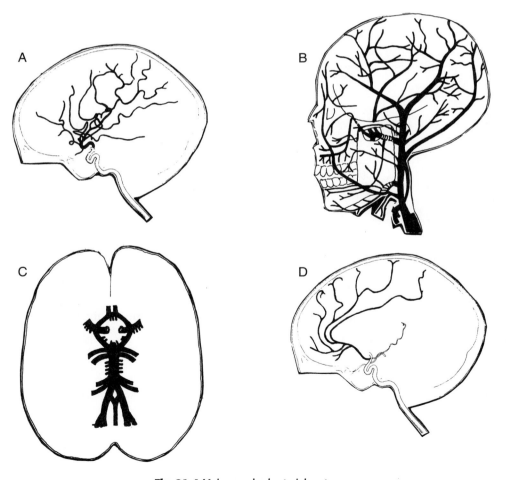

Fig. 21-4 Major cerebral arterial systems.

29. The posterior brain circulation communicates with the anterior circulation at the base of the brain in an arterial circle configuration called the circle of Willis (Fig. 21-5). Identify the five arteries or branches that make up the circle of Willis, the left half of which are labeled on this drawing.

1. _____

2. _____

3. _____

4. _____

5. _____

6. A. Identify the major structure (labeled A) that would be located in the center of the circle of Willis.

_____

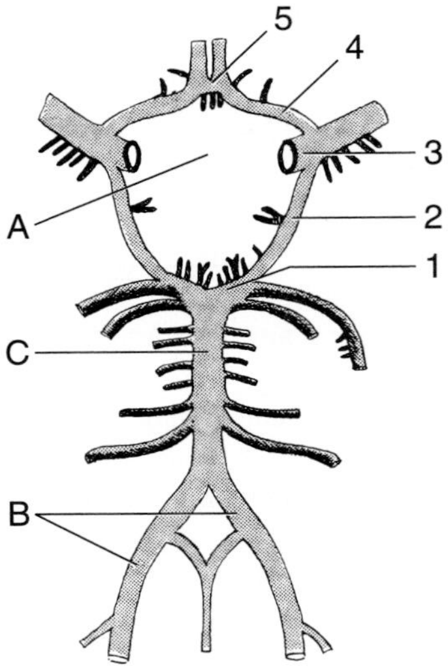

Fig. 21-5 Structure identification of the Circle of Willis.

B. The right and left _____ enter the cranium through the foramen magnum.

C. They then unite to form this single _____ artery.

30. List the three pairs of major veins draining the head, face, and neck region:

A. _____

B. _____

C. _____

31. A. The three pairs of major veins, described in question 30, join the subclavian vein to form the

_____ vein.

B. This vein joins the equivalent vein on the other side to form the _____, which returns

blood to the _____ of the heart.

32. True/False: The sinuses found in the brain are situated between layers of the dura mater.

33. True/False: All veins found in the brain possess no valves and are extremely thin.

34. Which one of the following dura mater sinuses is located in the superior portion of the falx cerebri?
   A. Superior sagittal sinus   C. Straight sinus
   B. Inferior sagittal sinus   D. Sigmoid sinus

35. Which bony landmark signifies the location of the confluence of venous sinuses?
   A. Foramen magnum   C. Internal occipital protuberance
   B. Petrous portion of temporal bone   D. Sella turcica

REVIEW EXERCISE B: Radiographic Anatomy of Thoracic and Abdominal Arteries and Veins, Portal System, Upper and Lower Arteries and Veins, and Lymphatic System (see textbook pp. 673-677)

1. List the four segments of the aorta as labeled on Fig. 21-6.

    A. _____

    B. _____

    C. _____

    D. _____

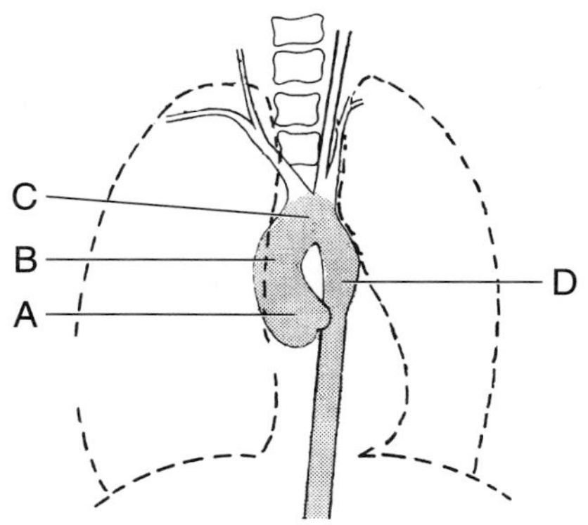

Fig. 21-6 Four segments of the aorta.

2. List the three common variations of the aortic arch that may be visualized on aortograms and are demonstrated in Fig. 21-7.

    A. _____

    B. _____

    C. _____

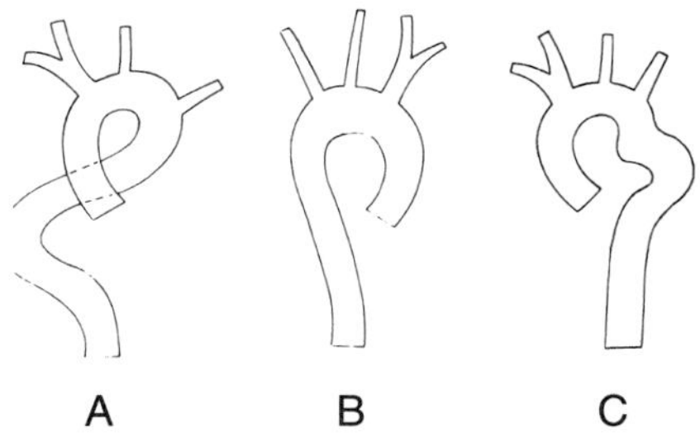

Fig. 21-7 Variations of the aortic arch.

3. Which one of the following veins receives blood from the intercostal, bronchial, esophageal, and phrenic veins?

    A. Pulmonary veins   B. Azygos vein   C. Inferior vena cava   D. Superior vena cava

4. List the five major branches of the abdominal aorta as labeled 1 through 5 on this drawing (Fig. 21-8):

    They are listed in order from the top down.

    1. _____

    2. _____

    3. _____

    4. _____

    5. _____

5. List the three branches of the celiac artery labeled A-C.

    A. _____

    B. _____

    C. _____

    List the divisions of the abdominal aorta as it enters the pelvic region labeled D-F.

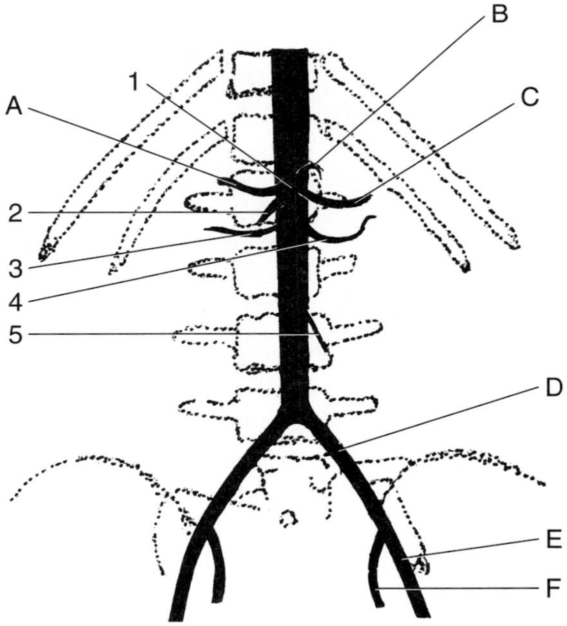

Fig. 21-8 Branches and divisions of the abdominal aorta.

    D. _____

    E. _____   F. _____

138 REVIEW EXERCISE B: Radiographic Anatomy of Thoracic and Abdominal Arteries and Veins, Portal System, Upper and Lower
Arteries and Veins, and Lymphatic System
CHAPTER 21

6. At what level does the descending aorta pass through the diaphragm to become the abdominal aorta?

   A. T10   C. L1

   B. T12   D. L2

7. The distal abdominal aorta bifurcates at the level of _____ vertebra.

8. Venous blood is returned to the heart from structures below the diaphragm through the inferior vena cava. Identify the major venous tributaries to the inferior vena cava as labeled on Fig. 21-9:

   A. _____

   B. _____

   C. _____

   D. _____

   E. Inferior vena cava

   F. _____

   G. _____

   H. _____

   I. _____

   J. _____

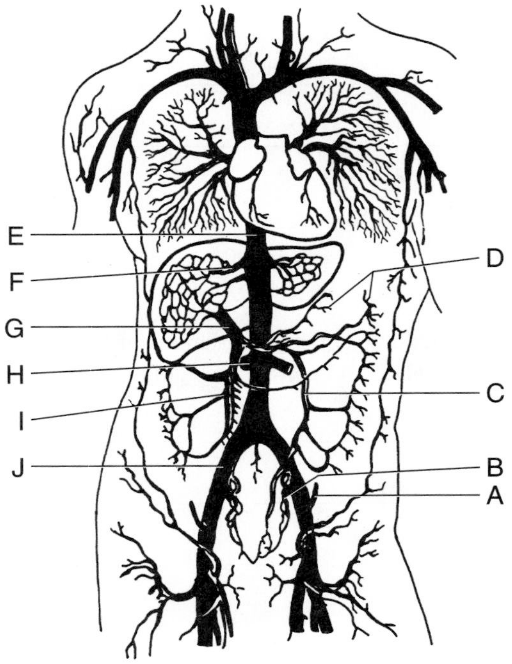

Fig. 21-9 Tributaries to the inferior vena cava.

9. Identify the following veins (A, B, D, and E) that make up the portal system as labeled on Fig. 21-10:
   Hint: A and B are the two major veins that unite to form the hepatic portal vein (C).

   A. _____

   B. _____

   C. Hepatic portal vein

   D. _____ drain "filtered" blood from the liver and return it to the

   E. _____

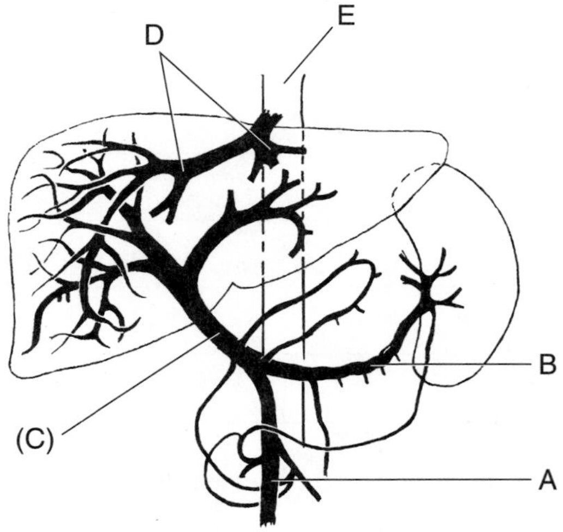

Fig. 21-10 Portal system.

10. Identify the following upper limb arteries (Fig. 21-11):

On the right side of the body, the *"A"* _____

artery gives rise to the *"B"* _____ artery.

Identify the following primary arteries of the upper limb labeled *C-F.*

C. _____

D. _____

E. _____

F. _____

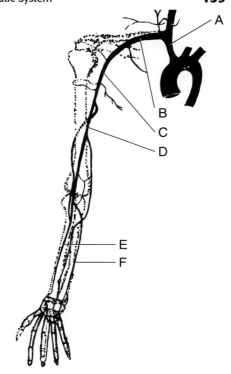

Fig. 21-11 Upper limb arteries.

11. Identify the following upper limb veins (Fig. 21-12):

The venous system of the upper and lower limbs may be divided into two sets. For the upper limb these begin with:

A. _____ and

B. _____ , which

form two parallel drainage channels.

Label the veins *C-G* returning blood to the heart:

C. _____

D. _____

E. _____

F. _____

G. _____

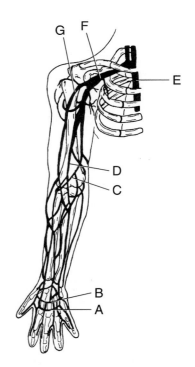

Fig. 21-12 Upper limb veins.

12. The vein most commonly used to draw blood at the elbow is

the _____ .

(Hint: This is one of the veins *[A-G]* as identified in Fig. 21-12.)

140 REVIEW EXERCISE B: Radiographic Anatomy of Thoracic and Abdominal Arteries and Veins, Portal System, Upper and Lower
Arteries and Veins, and Lymphatic System
CHAPTER 21

Lower Limb Arteries (Fig. 21-13)

13. Identify the following: The lower limb arterial system begins at the

"A" _____ artery and continues as the

"B" _____ artery until it divides into the

"C" _____ and "D" _____

arteries in the area of the proximal and mid femur. At the knee this becomes the

"E" _____ artery, which continues into the foot as the

"F" _____ artery.

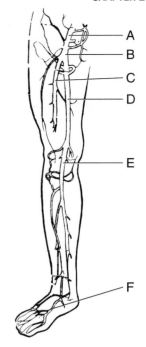

Fig. 21-13 Lower limb arteries.

Lower Limb Veins (Fig. 21-14)

14. Identify the following labeled veins of the lower limb:

A. _____

B. _____

C. _____

D. _____

E. _____

F. _____

G. _____

H. _____

I. _____

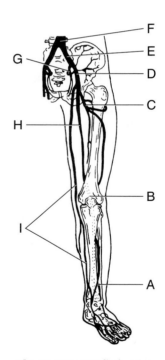

Fig. 21-14 Lower limb veins.

15. The longest vein in the body is the _____ of the lower limb. (Hint: This is one of the labeled veins in Fig. 21-14.)

16. Which duct in the lymphatic system receives interstitial fluid from the left side of the body, lower limbs, pelvis and abdomen and drains this fluid into the left subclavian vein?

17. List the four functions of the lymphatic system:

    A. _____

    B. _____

    C. _____

    D. _____

18. The general term describing radiographic examination of the lymphatic **vessels and nodes** following injection of

    contrast media is _____.

19. The term frequently used to study the lymph **vessels** specifically following injection of contrast media is

    _____.

20. True/False: It may take up to 24 hours following injection of the contrast medium to visualize the lymph nodes during a lymphogram.

21. True/False: Oil-based contrast media should never be used during a lymphogram.

REVIEW EXERCISE C: Cerebral Angiographic Procedures and Equipment and Supplies (see textbook pp. 678-685)

1. True/False: Computed tomography angiography (CTA) does not require the use of iodinated contrast media to demonstrate vascular structures.

2. True/False: Magnetic resonance angiography (MRA) does not require the use of any type of contrast media or vessel puncture.

3. True/False: Rotational angiography units move around the anatomy up to 360° during the procedure.

4. True/False: Nuclear medicine complements other angiographic modalities even though it provides little anatomical detail.

5. True/False: Most pediatric angiographic procedures require patient sedation.

6. Which of the following individuals is (are) not part of the angiographic team?

    A. Scrub nurse   C. Technologist

    B. Respiratory therapist   D. Radiologist

7. A common method or technique of introducing a needle and/or catheter into the blood vessel for angiographic pro-

    cedures is called the _____ .

8. List the six steps to the previously mentioned technique (in the correct order).

    A. _____   D. _____

    B. _____   E. _____

    C. _____   F. _____

9. Other than the method listed above, what are two other techniques for accessing a vessel during angiography?

    A. _____

    B. _____

10. Which one of the following is not a common risk or complication of angiography?

    A. Embolus formation   C. Hypertension

    B. Dissection of a vessel   D. Contrast media reaction

11. Which one of the following vessels is preferred for arterial vessel access during angiography?

    A. Femoral artery   C. Axillary artery

    B. Brachial artery   D. Common carotid artery

12. True/False: Angiographic rooms need to be considerably larger than conventional radiographic rooms.

13. The purpose of the heating device on an electromechanical injector is _____.

14. Outlets for _____ and _____ should be located on the room walls
    near the work area.

15. True/False: The use of digital and/or digital subtraction angiography (DSA), as part of a PAC system, can eliminate
    the need for hard-copy images.

16. True/False: The older photographic image subtraction method resulted in superior quality images compared to the
    newer digital subtraction system but was too time consuming to be used for most procedures.

17. List three post processing options with digital imaging to improve or modify the image:

    A. _____

    B. _____

    C. _____

18. True/False: Magnetic resonance angiography requires the use of special contrast media to demonstrate vasculature.

19. True/False: Carbon dioxide can be used instead of iodinated contrast media during angiography when iodinated
    agents are contraindicated.

20. List the five common pathologic indicators for cerebral angiography.

    A. _____

    B. _____

    C. _____

    D. _____

    E. _____

21. The point of bifurcation is of special interest to the radiologist and at this point, the internal carotid artery is more

    _____ (medial or lateral) when compared with the external carotid on an AP projection.

22. List those vessels commonly demonstrated during cerebral angiography:

A. _____

B. _____

C. _____

D. _____

REVIEW EXERCISE D: Radiographic Procedures and Positioning for Thoracic, Angiocardiography, Abdominal, Peripheral, and Interventional Angiography (see textbook pp. 685-697)

1. List specific pathologies that are common indications for thoracic and pulmonary angiography.

A. _____

B. _____

C. _____

D. _____

E. _____

2. The most common pathologic indicator for **pulmonary** arteriography is _____.

3. The preferred puncture site for a thoracic aortogram is the:

A. Femoral vein   C. Pulmonary artery

B. Pulmonary vein   D. Femoral artery

4. The preferred puncture site for a pulmonary arteriogram is:

A. Femoral vein   C. Pulmonary artery

B. Pulmonary vein   D. Femoral artery

5. What is the average amount of contrast media injected during a thoracic angiogram?

A. 5 to 8 ml   C. 20 to 25 ml

B. 10 to 15 ml   D. 30 to 50 ml

6. To prevent superimposition of the aortic arch with surrounding structures during a thoracic aortogram, a _____ degree RPO is often performed.

A. 5 to 10   C. 45

B. 15 to 20   D. 60

7. Coronary angiography is typically a study of the:

A. Coronary arteries   C. Coronary veins

B. Aortic arch   D. Chambers of the heart

8. What type of catheter is typically used for a left ventriculogram? _____

9. The average imaging rate during angiocardiography is:

   A.   2 to 3 frames per second   C.   15 to 30 frames per second

   B.   8 to 10 frames per second   D.   45 to 60 frames per second

10. Which one of the following terms describes the pumping efficiency of the left ventricle?

    A.   Ejection fraction   C.   Ejection coefficient

    B.   Systolic contraction ratio   D.   Myocardial perfusion ratio

11. List five common pathologic indicators for abdominal angiography.

    A.   _____

    B.   _____

    C.   _____

    D.   _____

    E.   _____

12. The common puncture site for selective abdominal angiography is the _____ artery using
    the Seldinger technique.

13. Selective abdominal angiography can be performed to visualize specific branches (and associated organs) of the ab-
    dominal aorta.   Which three branches are most commonly catheterized for this purpose?

    A.   _____   C.   _____

    B.   _____

14. List the term for an angiographic study of the superior and inferior vena cava. _____

15. True/False: Venograms are rarely performed today due to increased use of color duplex ultrasound.

16. To study the left upper limb arteries, the catheter is passed from the aortic arch into the:

    A.   Left common carotid   C.   Left vertebral artery

    B.   Left brachiocephalic vein   D.   Left subclavian artery

17. True/False: Lymphography can be performed to diagnose Hodgkin's lymphoma.

18. Which one of the following conditions may contraindicate a lymphogram?

    A.   Advanced pulmonary disease   C.   Cervical cancer

    B.   Prostate cancer   D.   Peripheral swelling

19. What type of contrast agent is most often used for a lymphogram?

    A.   Water-soluble iodinated-nonionic C.   Oil-based

    B.   Water-soluble iodinated-ionic   D.   Negative-CO_2

20. Why is a blue dye injected subcutaneously at the beginning of a lower limb lymphogram?

    A.   Helps to identify lymph vessels   C.   Anesthetizes lymph vessels

    B.   Increases transit time of contrast media   D.   Reduces risk of contrast media reaction

21. Indicate whether the following interventional procedures are vascular or nonvascular procedures.

——— 1. Percutaneous transluminal angioplasty (PTA)   A. Vascular procedure

——— 2. Infusion therapy   B. Nonvascular procedure

——— 3. Percutaneous biliary drainage (PBD)

——— 4. Percutaneous gastrostomy

——— 5. Stent placement

——— 6. Embolization

——— 7. Percutaneous abdominal drainage

——— 8. Nephrostomy

——— 9. Thrombolysis

——— 10. Percutaneous needle biopsy

——— 11. Percutaneous vertebroplasty

——— 12. Transjugular intrahepatic portosystemic shunt (TIPS)

22. What vasoconstrictor is commonly given during infusion therapy to control bleeding?

_____

23. What type of catheter is often used to retrieve urethral stones? _____

24. What type of catheter is used for transluminal angioplasty? _____

25. What is the correct term describing the interventional procedure for dissolving a blood clot?

_____

26. Which one of the following pathologic indications is most common for performing a percutaneous biliary drainage (PBD)?

   A. Biliary obstruction   C. Posttraumatic biliary leakage

   B. Suppurative cholangitis   D. Unresectable malignant disease

27. True/False: Percutaneous abdominal drainage procedures have a success rate of only 50%.

28. True/False: Percutaneous gastrostomy is performed primarily for patients who are unable to eat orally.

29. True/False: Interventional angiographic procedures are used primarily for providing diagnostic information and secondarily for treatment of disease.

30. True/False: Interventional imaging procedures are most commonly performed by technologists in surgery with the assistance of a radiologist.

Answers to Review Exercises

Review Exercise A: Radiographic Anatomy of Cardiovascular System, Pulmonary and Systemic Circulation, and Cerebral Arteries and Veins

1. A. Cardiovascular
   B. Lymphatic
2. A. Heart
   B. Blood vessels
   C. Heart to lungs
   D. Throughout the body
3. A. Transportation of oxygen, nutrients, hormones, and chemicals
   B. Removal of waste products
   C. Maintenance of body temperature, water, and electrolyte balance
4. A. Heart
   B. Artery
   C. Arteriole
   D. Capillary
   E. Venule
   F. Vein
5. B (artery) and C (arteriole)
6. E (venule) and F (vein)
7. 1. A. Red blood cells
      B. Transports oxygen
   2. A. White blood cells
      B. Defends against infection and disease
   3. A. (No other term given)
      B. Repairs tears in blood vessels and promotes blood clotting
8. (A) 92, (B) 7
9. A. Right ventricle
   B. Left ventricle
   C. Left atrium
   D. Capillaries of left lung
   E. Pulmonary arteries
   F. Aorta (arch)
   G. Superior vena cava
   H. Capillaries of right lung
   I. Pulmonary veins
   J. Right atrium
   K. Inferior vena cava
10. A. Pulmonary arteries
    B. Pulmonary veins
11. A. Superior vena cava
    B. Inferior vena cava
    C. Right atrium
12. A. Tricuspid valve
    B. Pulmonary (pulmonary semilunar) valve
    C. Mitral (bicuspid) valve
    D. Aortic (aortic semilunar) valve
13. A. Right and left coronary arteries
    B. Aortic bulb
14. A. Great cardiac vein
    B. Middle cardiac vein
    C. Small cardiac vein

15. A. Left subclavian
    B. Left common carotid
    C. Left vertebral
    D. Left internal carotid
    E. Right and left external carotids
    F. Right internal carotid
    G. Right vertebral
    H. Right common carotid
    I. Right subclavian
    J. Brachiocephalic
16. A. Brachiocephalic artery
    B. Left common carotid artery
    C. Left subclavian artery
17. A. Right common carotid artery
    B. Left common carotid artery
    C. Right vertebral artery
    D. Left vertebral artery
18. False (right common carotid and right subclavian)
19. True
20. Internal and external carotid
21. D carotid siphon
22. A. Anterior cerebral artery
    B. Middle cerebral artery
23. Anterior cerebral
24. Vertebrobasilar arteries
25. Basilar
26. Middle cerebral arteries
27. Lateral
28. 1. A
    2. D
29. 1. Posterior cerebral arteries
    2. Posterior communicating arteries
    3. Internal cerebral arteries
    4. Anterior cerebral arteries
    5. Anterior communicating artery
    6. A. Hypophysis (pituitary) gland
       B. Vertebral arteries
       C. Basilar
30. A. Right and left internal jugular veins
    B. Right and left external jugular veins
    C. Right and left vertebral veins
31. A. Brachiocephalic
    B. Superior vena cava, right atrium
32. True
33. True
34. A superior sagittal sinus
35. C internal occipital protuberance

Review Exercise B: Radiographic Anatomy of Thoracic and Abdominal Arteries and Veins, Portal System, Upper and Lower Arteries and Veins, and Lymphatic System

1. A. Aortic bulb
   B. Ascending aorta
   C. Aortic arch
   D. Descending aorta

2. A. Left circumflex
   B. Inverse aorta
   C. Pseudocoarctation
3. B (azygos vein)
4. 1. Celiac axis
   2. Superior mesenteric artery
   3. Right renal artery
   4. Left renal artery
   5. Inferior mesenteric artery
5. A. Common hepatic artery
   B. Splenic artery
   C. Left gastric artery
   D. Left common iliac artery
   E. Left external iliac artery
   F. Left internal iliac artery
6. B (T12)
7. L4
8. A. Left external iliac vein
   B. Left internal iliac vein
   C. Inferior mesenteric vein
   D. Splenic vein
   E. (Inferior vena cava)
   F. Hepatic vein
   G. Portal vein
   H. Right renal vein
   I. Superior mesenteric vein
   J. Right common iliac vein
9. A. Superior mesenteric vein
   B. Splenic vein
   C. (Hepatic portal vein)
   D. Hepatic veins
   E. Inferior vena cava
10. A. Brachiocephalic
    B. Subclavian
    C. Axillary
    D. Brachial
    E. Radial
    F. Ulnar
11. A. Superficial palmar arch vein
    B. Deep palmar arch vein
    C. Median cubital
    D. Brachial
    E. Superior vena cava
    F. Subclavian
    G. Cephalic
12. Median cubital
13. A. External iliac artery
    B. Common femoral
    C. Deep femoral
    D. Femoral
    E. Popliteal
    F. Dorsalis pedis
14. A. Anterior tibial
    B. Popliteal
    C. Deep femoral
    D. External iliac
    E. Left common iliac
    F. Inferior vena cava
    G. Internal iliac
    H. Femoral
    I. Great saphenous

15. Great saphenous vein
16. Thoracic duct
17. A. Fight diseases by producing lymphocytes and microphages
    B. Return proteins and other substances to the blood
    C. Filter lymph in the lymph nodes
    D. Transfer fats from the intestine to the blood
18. Lymphography
19. Lymphangiography
20. True
21. False (are commonly used)

Review Exercise C: Equipment and Supplies and Cerebral Angiographic Procedures

1. False (does require)
2. True
3. False (only 180°)
4. True
5. True
6. B. Respiratory therapist
7. Seldinger technique
8. A. Insertion of needle
   B. Placement of needle in lumen of vessel
   C. Insertion of guide wire
   D. Removal of needle
   E. Threading of catheter to area of interest
   F. Removal of guide wire
9. A. Cutdown
   B. Translumbar approach
10. C. Hypertension
11. A. Femoral artery
12. True

13. To maintain temperature of contrast media at body temperature
14. Oxygen and suction
15. True
16. False. (older film method resulted was not superior and was more time consuming)
17. A. Pixel-shifting or remasking
    B. Magnified or zooming
    C. Quantitative analysis of image to measure size or distances
18. False (does not require contrast media)
19. True
20. A. Vascular stenosis including arterial occlusions
    B. Aneurysms
    C. Arteriovenous malformations
    D. Trauma
    E. Neoplastic disease
21. Lateral
22. A. Internal carotid arteries
    B. Common carotid arteries
    C. External carotid arteries
    D. Vertebral arteries

Review Exercise D: Radiographic Procedures and Positioning for Thoracic, Angiocardiography, Abdominal, Peripheral, and Interventional Angiography

1. A. (Aneurysm)
   B. Congenital abnormalities
   C. Vessel stenosis
   D. Embolus
   E. Trauma
2. Pulmonary embolus

3. D. Femoral artery
4. A. Femoral vein
5. D. 30 to 50 ml
6. C. 45
7. A. Coronary arteries
8. Pigtail catheter
9. C. 15 to 30 frames per second
10. A. Ejection fraction
11. A. Aneurysm
    B. Congenital abnormality
    C. GI bleed
    D. Stenosis/occlusion
    E. Trauma
12. Femoral
13. A. Renal arteries
    B. Celiac artery
    C. Superior and inferior mesenteric arteries
14. Venacavagraphy
15. True
16. D. Left subclavian artery
17. True
18. A. Advanced pulmonary disease
19. C. Oil-based
20. A. Helps to identify lymph vessels
21. 1. A, 2. A, 3. B, 4. B, 5. A, 6. A, 7. B, 8. B, 9. A, 10. B, 11. B, 12. A
22. Vasopressin (Pitressin)
23. Basket catheter or loop snare
24. Balloon catheter
25. Thrombolysis
26. D (unresectable malignant disease)
27. False (70% to 80%)
28. True
29. False (primarily for treatment of disease)
30. False (performed primarily in angiographic suite)

SELF-TEST

Directions: This self-test should be taken only after completing all of the readings, review exercises, and laboratory activities for a particular section.   The purpose of this test is not only to provide a good learning exercise but also to serve as a good indicator of what your final evaluation grade will be. It is strongly suggested that if you do not get at least a 90% to 95% grade on this self-test, you should review those areas in which you missed questions before going to your instructor for the final evaluation exam for this chapter. (There are 73 questions or blanks—each is worth 1.4 points.)

1. The two arteries that deliver blood to the heart muscle are:

    A. Right and left pulmonary veins   C. Right and left pulmonary arteries

    B. Right and left brachiocephalic arteries   D. Right and left coronary arteries

2. Which of the following arteries does not originate from the arch of the aorta?

    A. Brachiocephalic   C. Left common carotid

    B. Left subclavian   D. Right common carotid

3. Each common carotid artery bifurcates into the internal and external arteries at the level of:

    A. Lower margin of thyroid cartilage   C. Upper margin of thyroid cartilage

    B. C6 vertebra   D. C2 vertebra

4. Which vessels carry oxygenated blood from the lungs back to the heart?

    A. Pulmonary veins   C. Coronary arteries

    B. Pulmonary arteries   D. Aorta

5. The _____ artery arises from the brachiocephalic artery rather than the aortic arch.

    A. Right vertebral   C. Right common carotid

    B. Left vertebral   D. Left common carotid

6. The external carotid does not supply blood to the:

    A. Anterior portion of brain   C. Anterior neck

    B. Facial area   D. Greater part of the scalp and meninges

7. Two branches of each internal carotid artery, which are well visualized with an internal carotid arteriogram, are the:

    A. Posterior and middle cerebral arteries   C. Right and left vertebral arteries

    B. Anterior and middle cerebral arteries   D. Facial and maxillary arteries

8. The two vertebral arteries enter the cranium through the foramen magnum and unite to form the:

    A. Brachiocephalic artery   C. Circle of Willis

    B. Vertebrobasilar artery   D. Basilar artery

9. The basilar artery rests upon the clivus of the _____ bone.

    A. Ethmoid   B. Parietal   C. Temporal   D. Sphenoid

10. Which of the following veins does not drain blood from the head, face, and neck regions?

    A. Right and left internal jugular veins   C. Internal and external cerebral veins

    B. Right and left vertebral veins   D. Right and left external jugular veins

11. The superior and inferior sagittal sinuses join certain other sinuses such as the transverse sinus at the base of the

    brain to become the _____ .

    A. External jugular vein   C. Subclavian vein

    B. Internal jugular vein   D. Vertebral vein

12. Which vein receives blood from the intercostal, esophageal, and phrenic veins?

    A. Superior vena cava   C. Azygos vein

    B. Inferior vena cava   D. Brachiocephalic veins

13. Match the following abdominal arteries with the labeled parts on Fig. 21-15.

    _____ 1. Inferior mesenteric

    _____ 2. Superior mesenteric

    _____ 3. Left renal

    _____ 4. Right renal

    _____ 5. Common hepatic

    _____ 6. Celiac (trunk) axis

    _____ 7. Left common iliac

    _____ 8. Left internal iliac

    _____ 9. Left external iliac

    _____ 10. Left gastric

    _____ 11. Abdominal aorta

    _____ 12. Splenic

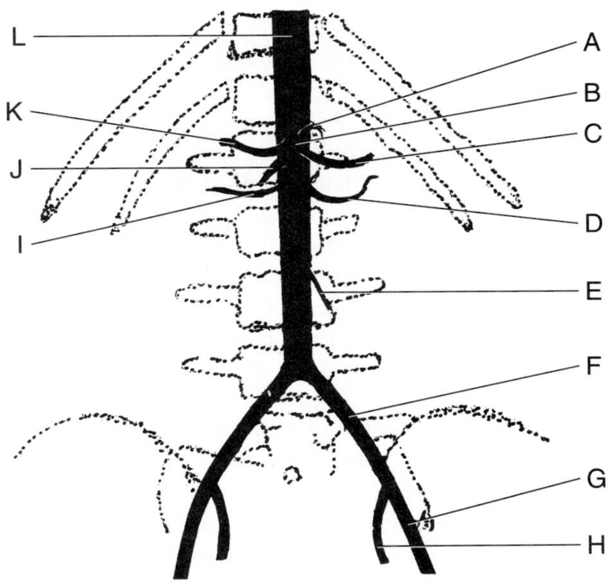

Fig. 21-15 Abdominal arteries.

14. True/False: The right subclavian artery arises directly from the aortic arch.

15. True/False: The cephalic vein is most commonly used for venipuncture.

16. True/False: The great saphenous vein is the longest vein in the body.

17. True/False: The thoracic duct is the largest lymph vessel in the body.

18. Which one of the following functions is *not* performed by the lymphatic system?

    A. Produce lymphocytes and microphages   C. Filter the lymph

    B. Synthesize simple carbohydrates   D. Return proteins and other substances to the blood

19. Solid food should be withheld for approximately _____ hours before an angiographic procedure.

   A. 1   C. 8

   B. 4   D. 24

20. Match the correct term best describing each of the following definitions:

   _____ 1. Also known as *red blood cells*

   _____ 2. Component of blood that helps repair tears in blood vessel walls and promotes blood clotting

   _____ 3. Carries deoxygenated blood from the right ventricle of the heart to the lungs

   _____ 4. Heart valve found between the left atrium and left ventricle

   _____ 5. Heart valve found between the right atrium and right ventricle

   _____ 6. The vessels that provide blood to the heart muscle

   _____ 7. The artery that bifurcates to form the right common carotid and right subclavian artery

   _____ 8. The artery that primarily supplies blood to the anterior neck, scalp, and meninges

   _____ 9. The artery that bifurcates into the anterior and middle cerebral artery

   _____ 10. The aspect of the sphenoid bone upon which the basilar artery rests

   _____ 11. The membranous portion of the dura mater containing the superior sagittal sinus

   _____ 12. The artery that forms the left gastric, hepatic, and splenic arteries

   _____ 13. The vein created by the splenic and superior mesenteric veins

   _____ 14. The vessel that carries oxygenated blood from the lungs to the left atrium of the heart

   _____ 15. A radiographic study of the lymph vessels

   A. Brachiocephlaic artery

   B. Pulmonary veins

   C. Celiac artery

   D. Coronary arteries

   E. Superior vena cava

   F. Portal vein

   G. Falx cerebri

   H. Lymphangiogram

   I. Inferior mesenteric artery

   J. Coronary sinus

   K. External carotid artery

   L. Tricuspid valve

   M. Clivus

   N. Mitral (bicuspid) valve

   O. Erythrocytes

   P. Pulmonary artery

   Q. Platelets

   R. Internal carotid artery

21. Injection flow rate in angiography is not affected by:

    A. Viscosity of contrast media   C. Body temperature

    B. Length and diameter of catheter   D. Injection pressure

22. Which one of the following imaging modalities will best demonstrate absence or presence of blood flow within a vessel?

    A. Computed tomography angiography   C. Magnetic resonance imaging

    B. Color duplex ultrasound   D. CO_2 angiography

23. True/False: Contrast media must be used during magnetic resonance angiography.

24. True/False: CO_2 angiography requires the use of a special injector.

25. Which of the following is not a pathologic indicator for cerebral angiography?

    A. Vascular lesions   C. Coarctation

    B. Aneurysm   D. Arteriovenous malformation

26. The imaging sequence during cerebral angiography, to include all phases of circulation, will typically require:

    A. 1 to 3 seconds   C. 8 to 10 seconds

    B. 4 to 6 seconds   D. 12 to 15 seconds

27. Pulmonary arteriography is usually performed to diagnose:

    A. Heart valve disease   C. Arteriovenous malformation

    B. Pulmonary emboli   D. Coarctation of the aorta

28. The most common vascular approach during pulmonary arteriography is the:

    A. Femoral vein   C. Superior vena cava

    B. Femoral artery   D. Axillary artery

29. Which one of the following positions will prevent superimposition of the proximal aorta during a thoracic aortogram?

    A. 45° RPO   C. AP

    B. 45° LPO   D. Lateral

30. During angiocardiography, the catheter is advanced from the aorta into the:

    A. Superior vena cava   C. Left ventricle

    B. Right ventricle   D. Brachiocephalic artery

31. The imaging rate during angiocardiography is between:

    A. 1 to 3 frames per second   C. 10 to 12 frames per second

    B. 4 to 8 frames per second   D. 15 to 30 frames per second

32. Which of the following would not be a common pathologic indicator for abdominal angiography?

    A. Aneurysm   C. Trauma

    B. Stenosis or occlusions of aorta   D. Malabsorption syndrome

33. The average amount of contrast media injected during a venacavagram is:

    A. 6 to 8 ml   C. 30 to 40 ml

    B. 10 to 15 ml   D. 50 to 70 ml

34. True/False: For peripheral angiography, imaging is commonly unilateral for both upper and lower limb exams.

35. True/False: Venograms of the extremity are rarely performed today because of the increased sensitivity of ultrasound.

36. Why is a blue dye injected during a lymphogram?

    A. Helps to visualize the lymph vessels   C. Helps to identify the veins of the limb

    B. Anesthetizes the vessels   D. Reduces spasm of the lymph vessels

37. True/False: Images are often taken 24 hours following injection during a lymphogram.

38. True/False: The most common contrast agent used during lymphography is water-soluble, non-ionic.

39. The most common pathologic indication for chemo-embolization is to treat:

    A. Brain aneurysm   C. AV malformation

    B. Stenosed vessels   D. Hepatic malignancies

40. Match the following descriptions to the correct term or interventional procedure.

    _____ 1. Infusion of therapeutic drugs   A. Embolization

    _____ 2. Device to extract urethral stones   B. Nephrostomy

    _____ 3. Procedure to dissolve blood clots   C. Infusion therapy

    _____ 4. Technique to restrict uncontrolled hemorrhage   D. Basket or loop snare catheter

    _____ 5. Technique to decompress obstructed bile duct   E. Percutaneous gastrostomy

    _____ 6. Direct puncture and catheterization of the renal pelvis   F. Thrombolysis

    _____ 7. Placement of an extended feeding tube into the stomach   G. Percutaneous biliary drainage

41. True/False: A vena cava filter is placed superior to the renal veins to prevent renal vein thrombosis.

42. True/False: The TIPS procedure involves placement of an intrahepatic stent.

CHAPTER 22

Computed Tomography

This chapter presents the general principles of computed tomography (CT) and the various equipment systems in use today. A study of soft tissue anatomy of the central nervous system (CNS) as viewed in axial sections is included. An introduction into the purpose, pathologic indications, and procedure of cranial, thoracic, abdominal, and pelvic computed tomography is also covered in this chapter. Selected sectional images of these three regions are presented.

CHAPTER OBJECTIVES

After you have completed **all** the activities of this chapter, you will be able to:

_____ 1. List three advantages of computed tomography over conventional radiography.

_____ 2. Identify the generational changes and advances in computed tomography systems.

_____ 3. List the major components of a computed tomographic system.

_____ 4. Explain the basic operating principles of computed tomography imaging to include x-ray transmission, data acquisition, image reconstruction, window width, window level, and slice thickness.

_____ 5. Identify the variables or image parameters controlled by the computed tomography technologist.

_____ 6. Calculate the pitch ratio for a helical CT scan using different variables.

_____ 7. List the two general divisions of the central nervous system (CNS).

_____ 8. Identify the specialized cells (neurons) of the nervous system and describe their specific parts and functions.

_____ 9. List the specific membranes or coverings of the CNS and identify the meningeal spaces or potential spaces associated with them.

_____ 10. List the three primary divisions of the brain.

_____ 11. List the four major cavities of the ventricular system and identify specific structures and passageways of the ventricular system.

_____ 12. Identify select gray and white matter structures in the brain.

_____ 13. Describe the concept of the "blood-brain barrier."

_____ 14. List the twelve cranial nerves.

_____ 15. List the common pathologic indicators for cranial, thoracic, abdominal, and pelvic computed tomography studies.

_____ 16. Identify specific structures of the brain, thorax, abdomen, and pelvis on axial drawings and CT images.

_____ 17. Identify the imaging parameters for cranial, thoracic, abdominal, and pelvic computed tomography studies.

Learning Exercises

Complete the following review exercises after reading the associated pages in the textbook as indicated by each exercise. Answers to each review exercise are given at the end of the review exercises.

REVIEW EXERCISE A: Basic Principles of Computed Tomography (see textbook pp. 700-704)

1. List the three advantages of CT over conventional radiography:

   A. _____

   B. _____

   C. _____

2. Match the following characteristics with the correct generation of CT scanner:

   _____ 1. Fan-shaped beam with 30 or more detectors   A. First-generation

   _____ 2. 1 to 2 detector system   B. Second-generation

   _____ 3. 8 times faster than a 1 second, single-slice scanner   C. Third-generation

   _____ 4. First scanner to rotate a full 360° around patient   D. Fourth-generation

   _____ 5. Capable of helical-type volume scanning (multiple answers)   E. Multi-slice CT

   _____ 6. Capable of 1-second or less scan times (multiple answers)

   _____ 7. Contains a bank of up to 960 detectors

   _____ 8. Scan times of 4 1/2 minutes per slice

   _____ 9. Up to 4800 detectors on a fixed ring

   _____ 10. Helical or continuous volume scanning (CVS) (multiple answers)

   _____ 11. The first type with fixed detectors rather than detectors rotating with x-ray tube

   _____ 12. Capable of acquiring 4 slices simultaneously

   _____ 13. First scanner with larger aperture, which permitted full body scanning

3. True/False: Noninvasive studies of the cardiovascular system are possible with multi-slice CT.

4. True/False: Helical CT scanners are limited to one 360° rotation per slice in the same direction.

5. Which of the following is *not* an advantage of multi-slice CT scanners?

   A. Fast imaging speed   C. Minimizes patient motion

   B. Acquires large number of slices rapidly D. Low-cost system to maintain

6. The actual thickness of tomographic slices with CT systems is:

    A. 1 to 3 or 4 centimeters   C. 1/4 to 1 or more centimeters

    B. 0.5 or more millimeters   D. 10 to 40 or more millimeters

7. The actual thickness of a tomographic slice is controlled by:

    A. Detectors   C. Effective focal spot

    B. Filament of x-ray tube   D. Source collimator

8. Define the term *voxel.* _____

9. What do the detectors measure in a CT system? _____

10. A voxel is a _____ dimensional image of the tissue while a pixel represents only _____ dimensions.

11. The depth of the voxels is determined by:

    A. Slice thickness   C. Actual scan time

    B. Speed of computer   D. Size of the pixel

12. Air would have a _____ (higher or lower) differential absorption as compared to soft tissue.

13. The purpose of the detector collimator is to:

    A. Reduce patient dose

    B. Minimize amount of scatter radiation that strikes detector

    C. Only allow high attenuation values to reach the detector

    D. Minimize patient motion artifact

14. List the two primary components of a computed tomographic system:

    A. _____   B. _____

15. Which aspect of the CT system houses the x-ray tube and detector array? _____

16. What is another term for image storage? _____

17. The central opening in the CT support structure where the patient is scanned is called the: _____.

18. CT numbers is a numerical scale that represents tissue _____

19. List the correct CT number range for the following tissue types:

    A. Cortical bone   _____

    B. White brain matter   _____

    C. Blood   _____

    D. Fat   _____

    E. Lung tissue   _____

    F. Air   _____

20. Which medium serves as the baseline for CT numbers? _____

21. Window width (WW) controls:

    A. Image density   C. Slice thickness

    B. Image contrast   D. Total number of slices

22. Window level (WL) controls:

    A. Image density   C. Slice thickness

    B. Image control   D. Total number of slices

23. Match the appearance of the following tissue types as seen on a CT image:

    _____ A. Bone   1. White

    _____ B. Gray brain matter   2. Gray

    _____ C. CSF   3. Black

    _____ D. Positive contrast media

24. Pitch is defined as _____ .

25. Calculate the pitch ratio using following parameters: Couch movement at a rate of 20 mm per second with a slice

    collimation of 10 mm. _____

26. The pitch ratio calculated in question 25 is an example of:

    A. Undersampling   C. Perfect pitch

    B. Oversampling   D. Intermittent pitch

27. Which of the following parameters would produce a 0.5:1.0 pitch ratio?

    A. 10 mm couch movement and 10 mm slice thickness

    B. 15 mm couch movement and 10 mm slice thickness

    C. 10 mm couch movement and 20 mm slice thickness

    D. 30 mm couch movement and 10 mm slice thickness

REVIEW EXERCISE B: Radiographic Anatomy of the Central Nervous System (see textbook pp. 705-713)

1. The central nervous system can be divided into two main divisions:

    A. _____

    B. _____

2. A. The solid spinal cord terminates at the level of the lower border of which vertebra? _____

   B. This tapered terminal area of the spinal cord is called the _____ .

3. A. The specialized cells of the nervous system that conduct electrical impulses are called _____ .

   B. The parts of these cells that receive the electrical impulse and conduct them toward the cell body are called

    _____ .

4. Three membranes or layers of coverings called *meninges* enclose both the brain and the spinal cord. Certain important spaces or potential spaces are associated with these meninges. List these three meninges and three associated spaces as follows:

MENINGES   *SPACES*

Skull or cranium

A. _____   D. _____
   (Outer "hard" or "tough" layer)   (Space or potential space)

B. _____   E. _____
   (Spider-like avascular membrane)   (Narrow space containing thin layer of fluid)

C. _____   F. _____
   (Inner "tender" layer)   (Wider space filled with cerebral spinal fluid)

5. The outer "hard" or "tough" membrane described above has an inner and outer layer tightly fused except for certain

   larger spaces between folds or creases of the brain and the skull, which provide for large venous blood channels

   called _____

6. The large cerebrum is divided into right and left hemispheres. Each hemisphere of the cerebrum is further divided into five lobes, with four of the lobes lying under the cranial bone of the same name. List these five lobes:

A. _____   D. _____

B. _____   E. _____

C. _____

7. The brain (encephalon) can be divided into three general divisions: the (1) forebrain, (2) midbrain, and (3) hindbrain. The forebrain and hindbrain are both divided into three divisions. List the three divisions of the forebrain and the hindbrain as labeled on Fig. 22-1. (Secondary terms for these divisions as found in the textbook are included in brackets.)

1. Forebrain   A. _____
   (Prosencephalon)   (Telencephalon) -Largest division

   (Diencephalon) { B. _____

                      C. _____

2. Midbrain
   (Mesencephalon)

3. Hindbrain   D. _____

   (Rhombencephalon) E. _____

                      F. _____

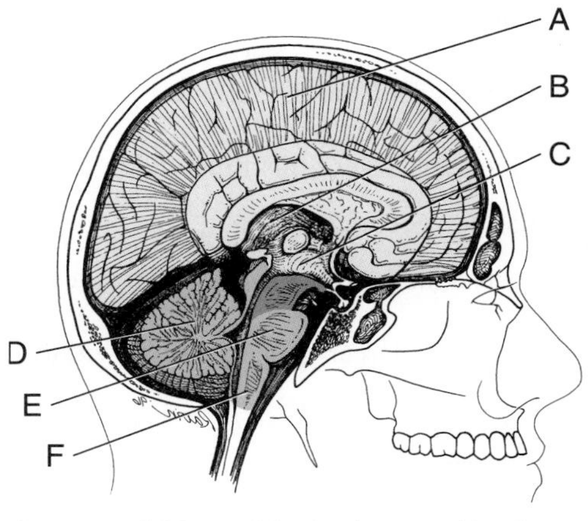

Fig. 22-1 Divisions of the forebrain and hindbrain, midsagittal view.

8. Identify the three lobes of the right cerebral hemisphere as labeled *A-C* in Fig. 22-2. The deep fissure separating the two cerebral hemispheres is labeled D. (Note: there is a fold of dura mater, called the *falx cerebri,* that extends deep within this fissure, separating the two hemispheres that is visualized on CT scans.)

A. _____ lobe

B. _____ lobe

C. _____ lobe

D. _____ fissure

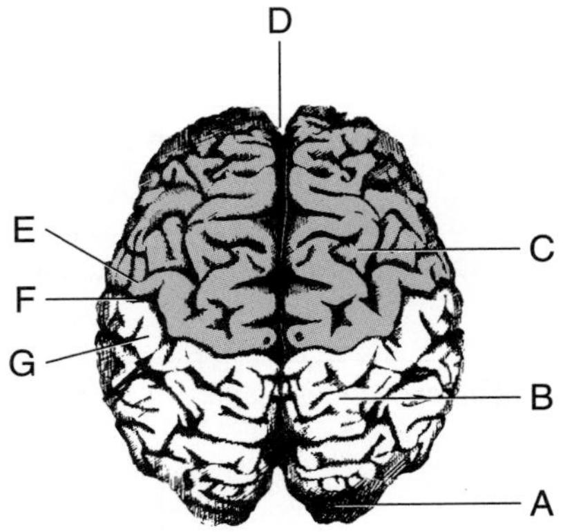

Fig. 22-2 Structures of the cerebral hemispheres.

9. The surface of each cerebral hemisphere contains numerous grooves and convolutions or raised areas. Identify labeled parts *E-G* in Fig. 22-2. Two of these raised areas, *E* and *G,* have specific names and are frequently demonstrated and identified on cranial CT scans. Part *F* is a shallow groove with a specific name.

E. _____

F. _____

G. _____

10. What is the name of the arched mass of white matter that connects the two cerebral hemispheres?

A. Falx cerebri   C. Central sulcus

B. Anterior central gyrus   D. Corpus callosum

11. What is the name of the large groove that separates the cerebral hemispheres?

A. Anterior central gyrus   C. Central sulcus

B. Longitudinal fissure   D. Posterior central gyrus

12. The fluid manufactured and stored in the ventricular system is called (A) _____ , abbreviated as (B) _____ . This fluid completely surrounds the brain and spinal cord by filling the space called the (C) _____ space. A blockage within this system may result in excessive accumulation of this fluid within the ventricles, creating a condition known as (D) _____ .

13. The cerebrospinal fluid-filled subarachnoid space and ventricular system are important in computed tomography because these areas can be differentiated from tissue structures by their density differences.

A. The larger spaces or areas within the subarachnoid space are called _____ .

B. The largest of these is the _____ , located just posterior and inferior to the fourth ventricle.

14. The central midline portion of the brain connecting the midbrain, pons, and medulla to the spinal cord is called the

_____ .

15. The optic chiasma, the site where some of the optic nerves cross to the opposite side, is located in the:

    A. _____ , a division of the forebrain.

    B. An important gland, which is located just inferior to this division of the forebrain is the

    _____ .

16. A second important midline structure gland is the (A) _____ , which is located just superior

    to the (B) _____ , a division of the hindbrain.

17. The central nervous system (CNS) can be divided by appearance into white matter and gray matter, which can be differentiated by CT. The difference in appearance between these two results from their makeup. Describe this difference by indicating what each consists of:

    A. White matter _____

    B. Gray matter _____

18. In general, the outer cerebral cortex is (A) _____ matter, while the more centrally located

    brain tissue is (B) _____ matter.

19. List the three structures associated with the hypothalamus:

    A. _____   B. _____   C. _____

20. List the three aspects of the brain stem:

    A. _____   B. _____   C. _____

21. Which aspect of the brain serves as an interpretation center for sensory impulses?
    A. Midbrain   C. Thalamus
    B. Pituitary gland   D. Hypothalamus

22. Which aspect of the brain coordinates important motor functions such as coordination, posture, and balance?
    A. Pons   C. Midbrain
    B. Cerebellum   D. Cerebrum

23. Which aspect of the brain controls important body activities related to homeostasis?
    A. Pons   C. Thalamus
    B. Cerebellum   D. Hypothalamus

24. Which aspect or structure of the brain controls a wide range of body functions including growth and reproductive functions?
    A. Pineal gland   C. Thalamus
    B. Pituitary gland   D. Hypothalamus

25. List the four cerebral nuclei or basal ganglia:

    A. _____   C. _____

    B. _____   D. _____

26. Ventricles: There are four cavities in the ventricular system. These are labeled in Fig. 22-3 and demonstrate the four ventricles in relationship to other brain structures. Two of the ventricles are located within the right and left cerebral hemispheres (A); the remaining two are midline structures (B and C).

    The larger two ventricles (A) have four significant parts labeled (1), (2), (3), and (6) in Fig. 22-4. The small duct-like structure (4) provides communication between ventricles, and (5) indicates a connection between the third and fourth ventricles. An important gland (8) is also shown. Number 7 represents an important communication with the subarachnoid space on each side of the fourth ventricle.

    Identify the ventricles and their parts as labeled on these two drawings.

    Fig. 22-3

    A.   Right and left _____ ventricles

    B.   _____ ventricle

    C.   _____ ventricle

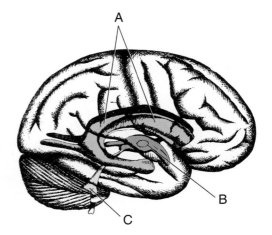

Fig. 22-3 Cavities in the ventricular system.

    Fig. 22-4

    1.   _____ (occipital)

    2.   _____

    3.   _____ (frontal)

    4.   _____ (foramen)

    5.   _____

    6.   _____ (temporal)

    7.   _____

    8.   _____ (gland)

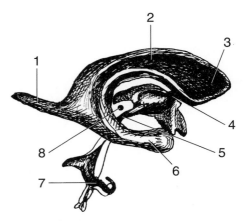

Fig. 22-4 Anatomy of the ventricles.

27. There are 12 pairs of cranial nerves, most of which originate from the brainstem and travel to various parts of the brain, controlling both sensory and motor functions. List these 12 pairs of cranial nerves:

    A.   _____   E.   _____   I.   _____

    B.   _____   F.   _____   J.   _____

    C.   _____   G.   _____   K.   _____

    D.   _____   H.   _____   L.   _____

REVIEW EXERCISE C: Cranial Computed Tomography and Sectional Anatomy of the Brain (see textbook pp. 714-716)

1. Which one of the following is not a common pathologic indicator for cranial computed tomography?

   A. Brain atrophy   C. Intracranial hemorrhage

   B. Multiple sclerosis   D. Aneurysm

2.   Approximately _____ to _____% of all cranial CTs require contrast media.

3.   True/False: Oxygen deprivation of 2 minutes will lead to permanent brain cell injury.

4.   True/False: Contrast media are able to pass through the blood-brain barrier in the normal individual.

5.   True/False: Contrast media are necessary for cranial CT for visualizing neoplasms.

6.   Which one of the following substances will not pass through the blood-brain barrier?

   A.   Proteins   C.   Oxygen

   B.   Glucose   D.   Select ions found in the blood

7.   Trauma to the skull may lead to a collection of blood accumulating under the dura mater called: _____

8.   With routine cranial CT positioning, the neck is flexed to create a _____ angle of the IOML vertical and parallel to the x-ray beam.

   A.   10°   C.   25°

   B.   20°   D.   30°

9.   On the average, it takes _____ to _____ axial scans to cover the entire brain.

10.   The most important aspect of positioning the head for cranial CT is to ensure there is no

   _____ and no _____ of the head.

11.   Identify the labeled parts on this axial section through the region of the mid-ventricular level (Figs. 22-5 and 22-6)

   A.   _____   E.   _____

   B.   _____   F.   _____

   C.   _____   G.   _____

   D.   _____

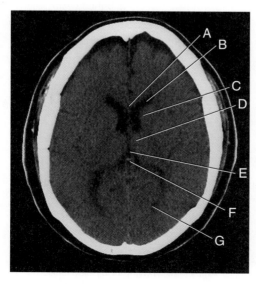

Fig. 22-5 Structure identification on an axial CT scan at mid-ventricular level.

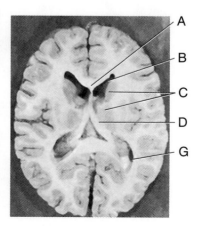

Fig. 22-6 Brain tissue specimen, mid-ventricular level.

12. Identify the labeled parts on this axial section through the level of the middle third ventricle (Figs. 22-7 and 22-8):

   A. _____

   B. _____

   C. _____

   D. _____

   E. _____

13. Axial section at the level of the mid orbits (Figs. 22-9 and 22-10):

   A. _____

   B. _____

   C. _____

   D. _____

   E. _____

   F. _____

   G. _____

   H. _____

   I. _____

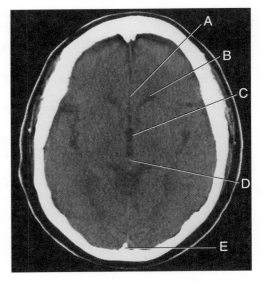

Fig. 22-7 Structure identification on an axial CT scan at mid-third ventricle level.

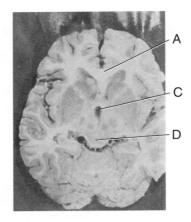

Fig. 22-8 Brain tissue specimen, mid-third ventricle level.

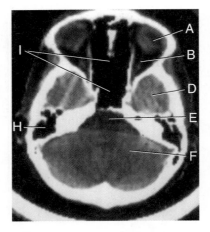

Fig. 22-9 Structure identification on an axial CT scan at the level of the mid orbits.

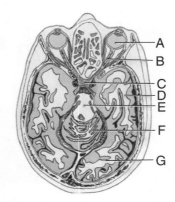

Fig. 22-10 Drawing of tissue in the axial section at the orbital plane level.

REVIEW EXERCISE D: Thoracic Computed Tomography Anatomy, Positioning, and Procedures (see textbook pp. 718-719)

Sectional Anatomy of the Thorax Identify the anatomy on these axial sections of the thorax at 10 mm-slice thickness obtained after bolus injections of contrast media. The patient's right is to your left as with conventional radiography.

1. Axial section through upper thorax at level of approximately T3 (Fig. 22-11). Parts *A, B, D,* and *E* represent veins and arteries of the lower neck and upper thorax just superior to the arch of the aorta. Parts *F* and *G* are well-known portions of the upper digestive tract and respiratory system that you should be able to identify by their relative locations

   A. _____ vein

   B. _____ artery

   C. _____

   D. _____ artery

   E. _____ artery

   F. _____

   G. _____

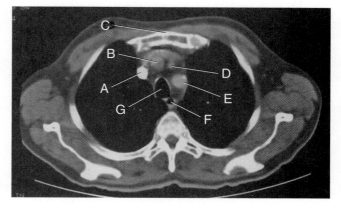

Fig. 22-11 Axial section through upper thorax at level of about T3.

2. Which one of the following structures is considered to be most posterior (as seen in Fig. 22-11)?

   A. Esophagus   C. Left brachiocephalic vein

   B. Trachea   D. Left common carotid artery

3. Axial section through level of carina (Fig. 22-12). Identify labeled structures *A-H,* which represent major vessels and bony structures of the chest.

   A. _____

   B. _____

   C. _____

   D. _____

   E. _____

   F. _____

   G. _____

   H. _____

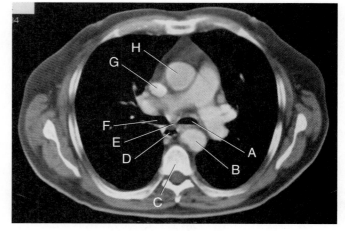

Fig. 22-12 Axial section through level of carina.

4. Which one of the following structures is located most anterior (as seen in Fig. 22-12)?

   A. Superior vena cava   C. Descending aorta

   B. Carina   D. Ascending aorta

5. Axial section through four chambers of the heart (Fig. 22-13). Identify labeled structures *A-H*, which represent the four chambers of the heart and other thoracic vessels and structures seen at this level.

   A. _____

   B. _____

   C. _____

   D. _____

   E. _____

   F. _____

   G. _____

   H. _____

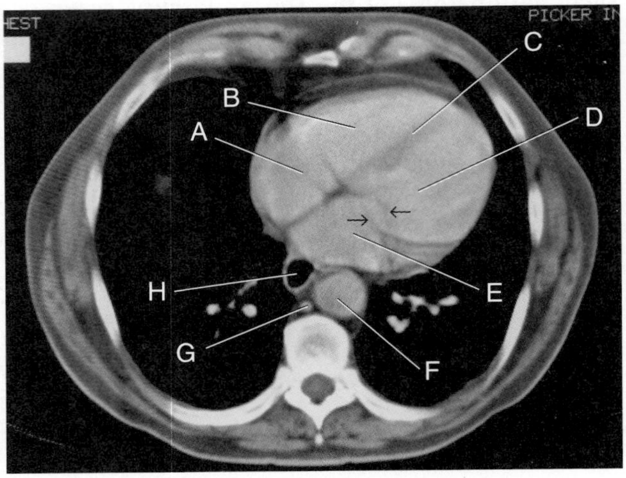

Fig. 22-13 Axial section through four chambers of the heart.

6. How can you determine whether structure *H* is the esophagus or the trachea?

   _____

7. The valve between heart chambers D and E is the _____ valve (see arrows).

8. Which chamber of the heart is located closest to the spine? _____

Positioning and Procedures for Thoracic CT:

9. Describe the projection of the chest taken as a localizing radiograph or pilot scan for CT of the chest.

   _____

10. What is the most common slice thickness for a CT study of the chest? _____

11. If a small pulmonary lesion is suspected, slice thickness will often be reduced to _____ .

12. Which of the following are not pathologic indicators for thoracic CT?

    A. Hilar lesions   E. Pericardial diseases

    B. Aneurysms   F. Evaluation of pulmonary nodules

    C. Abscess of thorax   G. All of the above are common indicators

    D. Cardiac disease

13. A mass seen on a thoracic CT study reveals a mass in the lungs. The attenuation of this mass is slightly above water (O). Which one of the following pathologic indicators would be most likely?

    A. Solid pulmonary nodule   C. Bronchogenic cyst

    B. Lung carcinoma   D. Pulmonary calcification

14. **Situation:** A patient with a clinical history of carcinoma of the lung comes to the radiology department for a CT of the thorax. Which one of the following scan ranges would be performed for this patient?

    A. From apex of lung to diaphragm   C. From apex of lung to left colic flexure

    B. From apex of lung to liver   D. From apex of lung to adrenal glands

15. Helical CT scanning uses a _____ breathing technique during CT of the thorax.

16. Describe the patient position for a routine CT examination of the thorax: _____

17. What is the name of the region located between the ascending aorta and the pulmonary artery? _____

_____ .

REVIEW EXERCISE E: Abdominal and Pelvic Computed Tomography Anatomy, Positioning, and Procedures (see textbook pp. 720-724)

The following CT images are 10 mm slice thickness. An intravenous contrast medium was given to enhance vascular structures as well as oral contrast for the GI tract.

1. Axial section through level of the pancreatic tail (Fig. 22-14). Identify labeled structures *A-K*, which represent major vessels and soft-tissue structures of the abdomen:

   A. _____

   B. _____

   C. _____

   D. _____

   E. _____

   F. _____

   G. _____

   H. _____

   I. _____

   J. _____

   K. _____

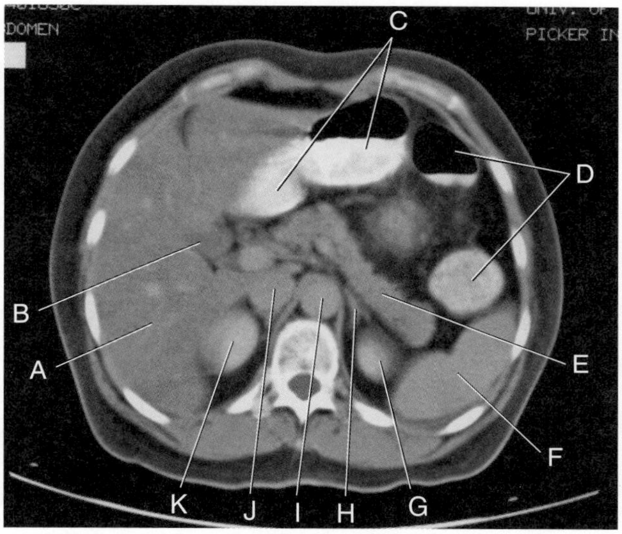

Fig. 22-14 Axial section through level of pancreatic tail.

Questions 2 and 3 relate to structures seen in Fig. 22-14.

2. Which two parts of the stomach are indicated by the two lead lines for label C? (Circle two of the four choices.)

   A. Pylorus   C. Fundus

   B. Body   D. Cardiac antrum

3. The adrenal glands often appear as an inverted _____ shape seen in sectional images of the abdomen.

4. Axial section through level of the second portion of duodenum (Fig. 22-15). Identify labeled structures *A-J,* which represent major vessels and soft-tissue structures of the abdomen:

A. _____

B. _____

C. _____

D. _____

E. _____

F. _____

G. _____

H. _____

I. _____

J. _____

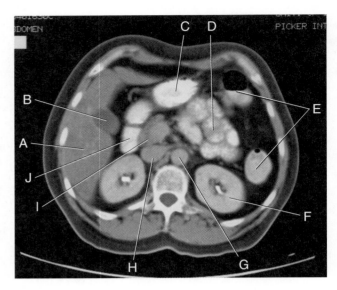

Fig. 22-15 Axial section through level of second portion of duodenum.

5. How can the second portion of the duodenum be distinguished from a tumor in the head of the pancreas as shown in Fig. 22-15?

_____

6. Axial section through level 2 cm caudad to the renal pelvis (Fig. 22-16). Identify labeled structures *A-I,* which represent major vessels and segments of both the large and small bowel, kidneys, and ureters.

A. _____

B. _____

C. _____

D. _____

E. _____

F. _____

G. _____

H. _____

I. _____

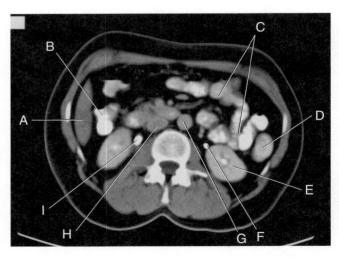

Fig. 22-16 Axial section through level 2 cm caudad to renal pelvis.

7. How can it be determined that the section in Fig. 22-16 is at a level just caudad to renal pelvis? (Hint: Look at the relationship of the kidneys and ureters.)

_____

8. How can it be determined which is the ascending colon and which is the descending colon on this section (Fig. 22-16)?

_____

9. Axial section through level of the ilium and the rectum (Fig. 22-17). Identify labeled structures *A-G*, which represent major vessels, soft tissues, and bony structures of the pelvis:

A. _____

B. _____

C. _____

D. _____

E. _____

F. _____

G. _____

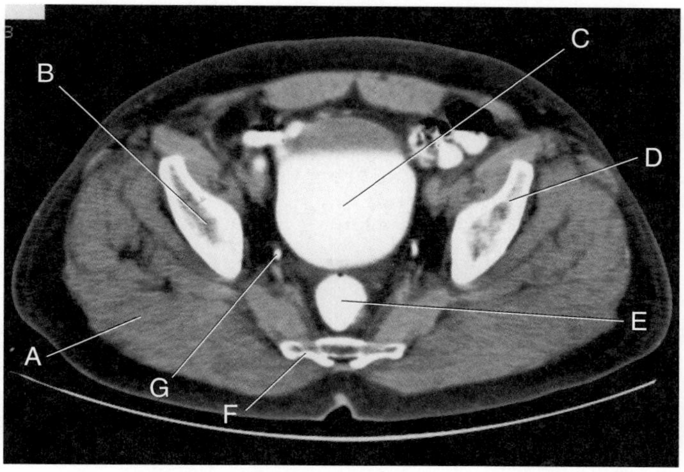

Fig. 22-17 Axial section through level of ilium and rectum.

Positioning and Procedures for Abdominal and Pelvic CT

10. True/False: The number of ERCP procedures performed has been greatly reduced due to the effectiveness of CT examinations of the abdomen.

11. True/False: Pregnancy is not a contraindication for CT of the abdomen.

12. True/False: CT has replaced (for the most part) lymphangiography in detecting lymph-node malignancies.

13. Pelvic CT is an excellent imaging modality for diagnosing occult disease. Occult disease is defined as:

_____

14. For most routine CT studies of the abdomen or pelvis, a slice thickness of _____ mm is often employed.

    A. 10 to 15   C. 5 to 8

    B. 20   D. 25 to 30

15. During a helical CT of the abdomen, a 15-mm couch movement per second with a slice collimation of 10 mm is used. Calculate the pitch ratio for this study.

_____

16. **Situation:** A patient with a clinical history of pancreatic cancer comes to CT for a study of the abdomen. What slice thickness should be used for this study at the level of the pancreas?

    A. 5 to 8 mm   C. 10 mm

    B. 2 to 3 mm   D. 1 to 1.5 mm

17. A. What percent of concentration of barium sulfate should be used for CT procedures of the abdomen and pelvis?

_____

    B. How does this compare with regular "thin" barium as used in conventional upper GI studies as described in

    Chapter 14? _____

18. Why is such a low concentration of barium used for CT studies?

_____

19. Describe the appearance of beam-hardening artifacts.

_____

20. When should the patient be given oral contrast media before a CT study of the small bowel?

   A. Night before the exam   C. Immediately before the exam

   B. 1 hour before the exam   D. 24 hours before the exam

21. What is the purpose of the insertion of a tampon for CT scans of the female pelvis and lower abdomen?

_____

22. If the upper abdomen is the area of interest, scanning generally begins at the level of the

(A) _____ , and continues inferiorly to the level of the (B) _____ .

23. If the pelvis is the area of interest, scanning begins at the level of the (A) _____ , and con-

tinues to the (B) _____ .

24. To prevent respiratory and peristaltic artifacts on CT scans of the abdomen, maximum exposure times of

_____ are needed.

25. A. What breathing instructions, if any, are required to obtain high-quality serial CT scans of the abdomen with

      non-spiral scanning? _____

    B. What are breathing requirements for volume (spiral) type scanning of the abdomen?

_____

Laboratory Exercises (see textbook pp. 714-724)

Part A of this learning activity needs to be carried out in a special procedures room equipped for whole-body CT. A supervising technologist or instructor should be present for this activity. Part B can be carried out in a classroom or any room where illuminators and other CT viewing facilities are available.

LABORATORY EXERCISE A: Positioning

Complete the following and place a check by each when completed.

_____ 1. Review the equipment in the room, noting the location of patient support equipment such as oxygen, suction, the IV pole, and the emergency cart.

_____ 2. Role play using another student as the patient. Prepare the patient by explaining the procedure, the breathing instructions they will be given, the sounds they will experience, and what they will see and experience as they are placed into the gantry aperture for the examination.

_____ 3. Place your patient on the table (couch) in a supine position with the arms above the head. Raise the patient and table to the correct height and slowly move into the gantry aperture until the x-ray beam trajectory coincides with the starting scan position for the part being examined. Using the intercom device, talk to the patient from the control console. Finally, remove your patient when the procedure is completed.

_____ 4. Review the controls and monitors at the operator console. Have someone demonstrate the image parameters and the other variables controlled by the technologist and explain how whole body scanning is different from cranial CT scanning.

LABORATORY EXERCISE B: Anatomy Review Using CT Scans

Use CT scans of the thorax (chest), abdomen, and pelvis as provided by your instructor. These may be "hard copies" as recorded on paper or film or they may be from disks or magnetic tape as displayed on monitors. They should include normal and abnormal sections displaying obvious pathology.

Locate and identify each of the organs and structures as labeled and identified on similar scans in the workbook and the textbook. (Pay particular attention to those parts you identified on similar scans in your workbook in the preceding Review Exercises A and B.)

_____ 1. Axial sections of the chest

_____ 2. Axial sections of the abdomen

_____ 3. Axial sections of the pelvis

Answers to Review Exercises

Review Exercise A: Basic Principles of Computed Tomography

1. A. Anatomy is presented in a series of slices that provides a more complete survey of a specific tissue.
   B. Better contrast resolution between various types of soft tissue.
   C. Ability to manipulate and adjust image after scanning is completed.
2. 1. B, 2. A, 3. E, 4. C, 5. C and D, 6. C, D and E, 7. C, 8. A, 9. D, 10. C and D 11. D, 12. E 13. C
3. True
4. False (multiple rotations possible)
5. D. Low cost system to maintain
6. B 0.5 mm or more
7. D source collimator
8. Volume element
9. Attenuation of radiation by a given tissue
10. Three, two
11. A. Slice thickness
12. Lower
13. B. Minimize amount of scatter radiation striking the detector
14. A. Scan unit
    B. Operator control console
15. Gantry
16. Image archiving
17. Aperture
18. Attenuation
19. A. Cortical bone: + 1000
    B. White brain matter: + 45
    C. Blood: + 20
    D. Fat: − 100
    E. Lung tissue: − 200
    F. Air: − 1000
20. Water
21. B. Image contrast
22. A. Image density
23. A. Bone - 1. white
    B. Gray brain matter - 2. gray
    C. CSF - 3. black
    D. Positive contrast media - 1. white
24. The ratio reflecting the relationship between patient couch movement and x-ray beam collimation or slice thickness
25. 2: 1 pitch
26. A. Undersampling
27. C. 10 mm couch movement and 20 mm slice thickness

Review Exercise B: Radiographic Anatomy of the Central Nervous System

1. A. Brain (encephalon)
   B. Spinal cord (medulla spinalis)
2. A. L1
   B. Conus medullaris
3. A. Neurons
   B. Dendrites
4. A. Dura mater
   B. Arachnoid
   C. Pia mater
   D. Epidural space
   E. Subdural space
   F. Subarachnoid space
5. Venous sinuses
6. A. Frontal lobe
   B. Parietal lobe
   C. Occipital lobe
   D. Temporal lobe
   E. Insula or central lobe
7. A. Cerebrum
   B. Thalamus
   C. Hypothalamus
   D. Cerebellum
   E. Pons
   F. Medulla (medulla oblongata)
8. A. Occipital lobe
   B. Parietal lobe
   C. Frontal lobe
   D. Longitudinal fissure
9. E. Anterior (precentral) central gyrus
   F. Central sulcus
   G. Posterior (post central) central gyrus
10. D corpus callosum
11. B longitudinal fissure
12. A. Cerebrospinal fluid
    B. CSF
    C. Subarachnoid
    D. Hydrocephalus
13. A. Cisterns
    B. Cistern cerebellomedullaris (Cisterna magna)
14. Brain stem
15. A. Hypothalamus
    B. Pituitary (hypophysis) gland
16. A. Pineal gland
    B. Cerebellum
17. A. Tracts of myelinated axons of nerve cells
    B. Primarily dendrites and cell bodies
18. A. Gray
    B. White
19. A. Infundibulum
    B. Posterior pituitary gland
    C. Optic chiasma
20. A. Midbrain
    B. Pons
    C. Medulla
21. C Thalamus
22. B Cerebellum
23. D Hypothalamus
24. B Pituitary gland
25. A. Caudate nucleus
    B. Lentiform nucleus
    C. Claustrum
    D. Amygdaloid nucleus
26. A. Right and left lateral ventricles
    B. Third ventricle
    C. Fourth ventricle
    1. Posterior horn
    2. Body
    3. Anterior horn
    4. Interventricular foramen
    5. Cerebral aqueduct
    6. Inferior horn
    7. Lateral recess
    8. Pineal gland
27. A. Olfactory
    B. Optic
    C. Oculomotor
    D. Trochlear
    E. Trigeminal
    F. Abducens
    G. Facial
    H. Acoustic
    I. Glossopharyngeal
    J. Vagus
    K. Spinal accessory
    L. Hypoglossal

Review Exercise C: Cranial Computed Tomography and Sectional Anatomy of the Brain

1. B. Multiple sclerosis
2. 50% to 90%
3. False. (4 minutes)
4. False (are not able to pass through)
5. True
6. A. proteins
7. Subdural hematoma
8. C. 25°
9. Six to ten
10. Rotation and no tilt
11. A. Anterior corpus callosum-genu
    B. Anterior horn of left lateral ventricle
    C. Region of caudate nuclei
    D. Region of thalamus
    E. Third ventricle
    F. Pineal gland or body
    G. Posterior horn of left lateral ventricle
12. A. Anterior corpus callosum-genu
    B. Anterior horn of left lateral ventricle (CT only)
    C. Third ventricle
    D. Region of pineal gland
    E. Internal occipital protuberance (CT only)
13. A. Orbital bulb or eyeball
    B. Left optic nerve
    C. Optic chiasma (drawing only)
    D. Temporal lobe of cerebrum

E. Pons
F. Cerebellum
G. Occipital lobe (drawing only)
H. Mastoid air cells (CT only)
I. Sphenoid and ethmoid sinuses-CT only

Review Exercise D: Thoracic Computed Tomography Anatomy, Positioning, and Procedures

1. A. Right brachiocephalic vein
   B. Brachiocephalic artery
   C. Sternum (manubrium)
   D. Left common carotid artery
   E. Left subclavian artery
   F. Esophagus
   G. Trachea
2. A esophagus
3. A. Left main stem bronchus
   B. Descending aorta
   C. T5 vertebra
   D. Esophagus
   E. Carina
   F. Right main stem bronchus
   G. Superior vena cava
   H. Ascending aorta
4. D ascending aorta
5. A. Right atrium
   B. Right ventricle
   C. Interventricular septum
   D. Left ventricle
   E. Left atrium
   F. Descending aorta
   G. Azygos vein
   H. Esophagus
6. This level (through the four chambers of the heart) is below or inferior to the carina, so *H* couldn't be the trachea.
7. Mitral
8. Left atrium
9. PA, tube and detectors stationary; patient and couch are moved at intervals through the aperture.
10. 10 mm
11. Scale 3 to 5 mm
12. G all are common indications
13. C. Bronchogenic cyst

14. D. From apex of lung to adrenal glands
15. Breath hold or single breath
16. Supine position with arms above head
17. Aortopulmonary window

Review Exercise E: Abdominal and Pelvic Computed Tomography Anatomy, Positioning, and Procedures

1. A. Right lobe of the liver (posterior segment)
   B. Gallbladder
   C. Stomach
   D. Colon
   E. Tail of pancreas
   F. Spleen
   G. Upper lobe of left kidney
   H. Left adrenal gland
   I. Aorta
   J. Inferior vena cava
   K. Upper lobe of right kidney
2. A and B (pylorus and body)
3. "V"
4. A. Right lobe of liver
   B. Gallbladder
   C. Stomach
   D. Jejunum
   E. Colon
   F. Left kidney
   G. Abdominal aorta
   H. Inferior vena cava
   I. Head of pancreas
   J. Second portion of duodenum
5. Give the patient oral contrast media to opacify the duodenum
6. A. Lower portion of right lobe of liver
   B. Ascending colon
   C. Jejunum
   D. Descending colon
   E. Left kidney
   F. Left ureter
   G. Abdominal aorta
   H. Inferior vena cava
   I. Right ureter

7. The ureters are seen in cross-section totally separate from the kidneys. (Above the renal pelvis ureters would not be visible, and at level of the renal pelvis ureters and kidneys would appear connected.)
8. Ascending would be on patient's right (side of liver) and descending would be on left.
9. A. Gluteus maximus muscle
   B. Right ilium
   C. Urinary bladder
   D. Left ilium
   E. Rectum
   F. Sacrum
   G. Right ureter
10. True
11. False (is a contraindication). Although the radiologist may still order CT if no other imaging modality will produce the needed diagnosis.
12. True
13. A hidden or concealed disease difficult to diagnose
14. A. 10 to 15
15. 1.5:1.0
16. A. 5 to 8 mm
17. A. 1% to 3%
    B. Much thinner, thin barium is about a 50% concentration for conventional upper GI studies
18. Higher concentrations of barium sulfate will produce beam-hardening artifacts.
19. Linear streaks arising from the high density structures
20. B. 1 hour before exam
21. To aid in localization of the vagina by entrapment of air
22. (A) Xiphoid process
    (B) Iliac crest
23. (A) Iliac crest
    (B) Symphysis pubis
24. 1 to 3 seconds
25. A. Ask patient to suspend respiration at same phase of respiration for all exposures for consistency
    B. With volume or spiral scanning a single breath hold of 20 to 30 seconds is needed.

SELF-TEST

This self-test should be taken only after completing all of the readings, review exercises, and laboratory activities for a particular section. The purpose of this test is not only to provide a good learning exercise but also to serve as a good indicator of what your final evaluation grade will be. It is strongly suggested that if you do not get at least a 90% to 95% grade on this self-test, you should review those areas in which you missed questions before going to your instructor for the final evaluation exam for this chapter. (There are 87 questions or blanks—each is worth 1.2 points.)

1. Which generation of CT scanner used a pencil-thin x-ray beam and a single detector?

    A. First-generation
    C. Third-generation

    B. Second-generation
    D. Fourth-generation

2. Which generation of CT scanner allows helical or continuous volume-type scanning (may be more than one correct answer)?

    A. First-generation
    C. Third-generation

    B. Second-generation
    D. Fourth-generation

3. Which devices in the helical CT scanners allow continual tube rotation in the same direction?

    _____

4. CT can detect tissue density (contrast) differences as low as:

    A. 1%
    C. 10%

    B. 5%
    D. 20%

5. Which device controls slice thickness in a CT image? _____

6. What must be done to the numerical data to create the actual CT image or picture?

    _____

7. The two major components of the scan unit are:

    A. _____
    B. _____

8. Each tiny picture element in the display matrix is called a (an) _____ .

9. Which of the following parameters *cannot* be varied by appropriate manipulation at the operator console?

    A. kVp
    D. Vertical adjustment of table height

    B. Scan time
    E. Thickness of slice

    C. Pitch selections

10. Contrast media will not ordinarily cross the _____ .

11. Which one of the following pathologic indications does *not* apply to cranial CT?

    A. Brain neoplasm
    D. Trauma

    B. Brain atrophy
    E. All of the above apply

    C. Multiple sclerosis

12. Considering the blood-brain phenomenon, which of the following would require the use of contrast media? (There may be more than one correct answer.)

    A. Hydrocephalus   D. Epidural hematoma

    B. Possible neoplasia   E. Brain tumor

    C. Subdural hematoma

13. In what year did the first successful clinical demonstration of computed tomography (CT) take place?

    A. 1895   B. 1966   C. 1972   D. 1981

14. A. The parts of the neuron that conduct impulses toward the cell body are called _____.

    B. The part that conducts impulses away from the cell body is the _____.

15. Three protective membranes that cover or enclose the entire central nervous system are called

_____

16. The three membranes from question 2 are called (starting externally):

    A. _____   B. _____   C. _____

17. The various layers of the membranes just discussed have specific spaces of various sizes between these layers. Each has a specific name. Identify these various membrane layers and their associated spaces on Fig. 22-18.

    Membranes and associated spaces:

    A. _____

    B. _____

    C. _____

    D. _____

    E. _____

    F. _____

    G. _____

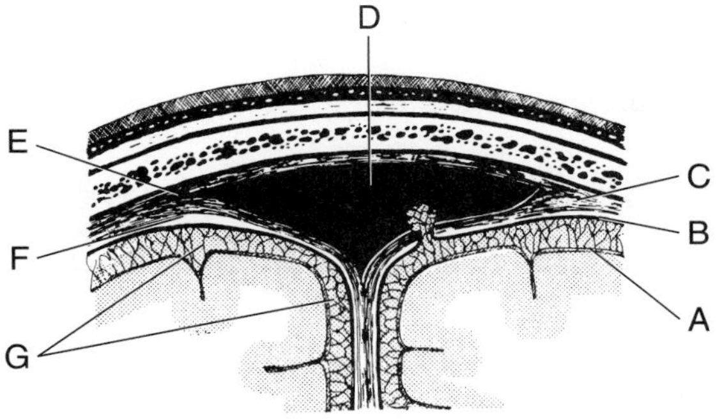

Fig. 22-18 Meninges and meningeal spaces.

18. Which of the spaces in Question 17 is normally filled with cerebrospinal fluid? _____

19. Match the following areas and divisions of the brain.

    _____ 1. Pons   A. Forebrain

    _____ 2. Cerebellum   B. Midbrain

    _____ 3. Cerebrum   C. Hindbrain

    _____ 4. Thalamus

    _____ 5. Medulla

20. The largest division of the brain is the _____.

21. The right and left cerebral hemispheres are separated by a deep fissure called the _____.

22. The fibrous band of white tissue deep within this fissure connecting the right and left hemispheres is called the

    _____.

23. What is the name of the tissue found within the fissure mentioned in question 22? _____

24. Which of the following ventricles are located within the cerebral hemispheres

    A. Lateral ventricles   C. Third ventricle

    B. Fourth ventricle   D. Cisterna magna

25. The diamond-shaped fourth ventricle connects inferiorly with a wide portion of subarachnoid space called the:

    A. Interventricular foramen   C. Cisterna cerebellomedullaris

    B. Lateral recesses   D. Cisterna pontis

26. Identify the ventricles, their parts, and their associated structures as labeled on both the lateral and top-view drawings (Figs. 22-19 and 22-20).

    Ventricles:

    A. _____

    B. _____

    C. _____

    Connecting ducts:

    a. _____

    b. _____

    c. _____

    Parts of lateral ventricles:

    1. _____

    2. _____

    3. _____

    4. _____

    Associated structure: (only in Fig. 22-19)

    5. _____

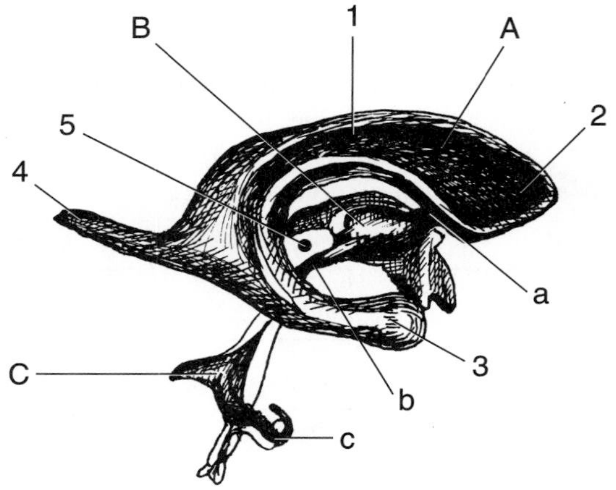

Fig. 22-19 Ventricles, lateral view.

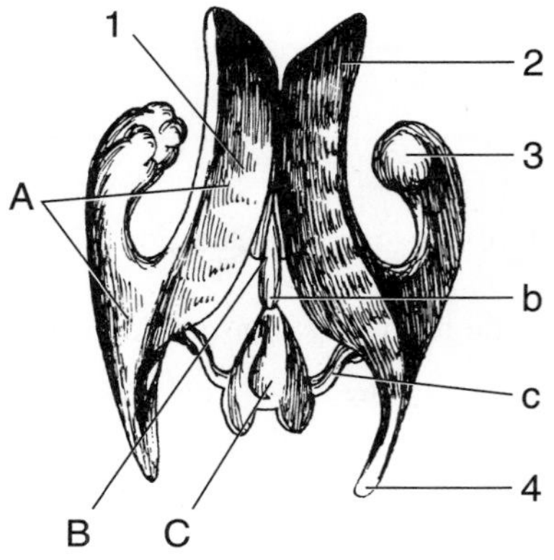

Fig. 22-20 Ventricles, superior view.

27. The condition known as _____ results from abnormal accumulation of cerebrospinal fluid

    within the _____.

28. Enlarged regions of the subarachnoid space are called _____.

29. Identify the four lobes of the cerebrum as labeled on

Fig. 22-21.

A. _____

B. _____

C. _____

D. _____

E. The fifth lobe, which is more centrally located and not
    shown on this drawing, is called the

_____.

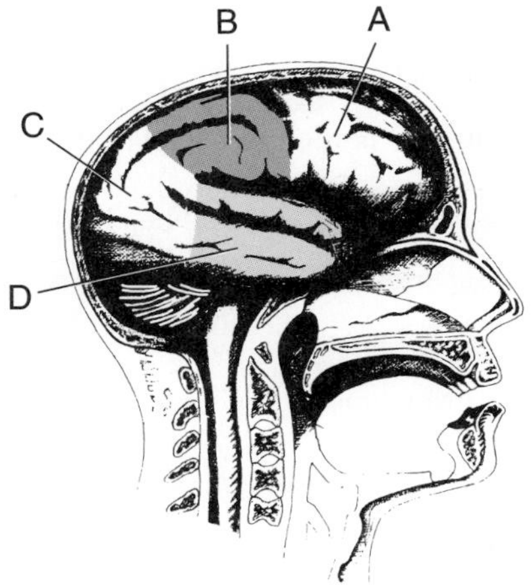

Fig. 22-21 Four lobes of the cerebrum.

30. Identify each of the following terms as either gray matter or white matter:

_____ 1. Cerebral cortex   A. Gray matter

_____ 2. Axons (fibrous parts of neuron)   B. White matter

_____ 3. Corpus callosum

_____ 4. Thalamus

_____ 5. Centrum semiovale

_____ 6. Cerebral nuclei

Questions 31 through 35 refer to anatomy as seen on the axial CT brain sections *(see textbook pp.715- 716)*

31. Select the structure that would *not* lie in the same axial section as the others (section through the orbital plane):

A. Temporal lobe   C. Longitudinal fissure

B. Cerebellum   D. Optic nerve

32. Select the structure that would not lie in the same axial section as the others (section through mid third ventricle):

A. Pons   D. Genu

B. Parietal lobe of cerebrum   E. Anterior horn of lateral ventricle

C. Internal occipital protuberance

33. Select the structure that would *not* lie in the same axial section as the others (section through mid ventricular level):

A. Frontal bone   D. Mid brain

B. Third ventricle   E. Caudate nucleus

C. Genu

Questions 34 through 37 refer to anatomy as seen on axial thoracic CT sections *(see textbook pp. 718 - 719)*

34. The brachiocephalic artery would be best demonstrated on an axial section at the level of the:

A. Sternal notch   C. Body portion of manubrium

B. Inferior portion of manubrium   D. Carina

35. The right internal jugular vein would only be clearly seen on axial sections at the level of the:

    A. Sternal notch   C. Carina

    B. Inferior portion of manubrium   D. Base of the heart

36. The ascending aorta would be clearly seen on axial sections at the level of the:

    A. Superior portion of manubrium   D. Carina

    B. Sternal notch   E. All of the above

    C. Aortopulmonary window

37. The right hemidiaphragm only would generally be seen on axial sections at the level of the:

    A. Base of the heart   D. Aortopulmonary window

    B. 2 cm below the base of the heart E. None of the above

    C. Carina

38. The space between the ascending and descending aorta is called _____.

39. Which one of the following structures is considered to be most anterior at the level of the carina?

    A. Ascending aorta   D. Left main stem bronchus

    B. Descending aorta   E. Azygos vein

    C. Carina

40. Which chamber of the heart is considered to be most posterior at the level of the base of the heart?

    A. Right atrium   C. Left atrium

    B. Right ventricle   D. Left ventricle

41. Which of the following is not a pathologic indication for CT of the thorax?

    A. Evaluation of pulmonary nodules   C. Hilar lesions

    B. Aneurysms   D. Mitral valve prolapse

42. A _____ slice thickness is commonly used for routine scans of the thorax.

    A. 10 mm   B. 5 mm   C. 2 mm   D. 10 cm

Questions 43 through 47 refer to anatomy as seen on the axial abdomen and pelvic CT sections *(see textbook pp. 722-724)*

43. The uncinate process refers to:

    A. A section of the liver located posteriorly and inferiorly

    B. A hooklike process of the spleen as seen lying next to the duodenum

    C. A process of the gallbladder seen only in the appropriate axial section

    D. The hooklike extension of the head of the pancreas

44. The right lobe of the liver is demonstrated on axial sections at the same level(s) of the:

    A. Pancreatic tail   C. Uncinate process of pancreas

    B. Mid portion of the kidneys   D. All of the above

45. The gallbladder is visualized on the same axial level as the:

    A. Renal pelves of kidneys   C. Right lobe of the liver

    B. Uncinate process of the pancreas D. All of the above

46. The prostate gland is best visualized at the same axial section level as the:

    A. Ischial rami   C. Urinary bladder

    B. Acetabular roof   D. Symphysis pubis

47. Which one of the following structures is considered to be most anterior (at the level of the femoral heads)?

    A. Rectum   C. Urinary bladder

    B. Seminal vesicles   D. Coccyx

48. A common couch incrementation for abdominal scanning is:

    A. 10 cm   B. 10 mm   C. 1 cm   D. 5 mm

49. Beam hardening artifacts for CT of the abdomen are most likely to occur when:

    A. Patient has metallic parts such as a hip prosthesis

    B. High concentration of a large bolus of barium is present with a low concentration of water

    C. Low concentration of barium (too diluted with water) is present

    D. Peristalsis occurs in GI tract

50. The first slice for an upper abdomen CT scan is commonly taken at the level of:

    A. First lumbar vertebrae   C. Xiphoid process

    B. Inferior rib margin   D. Iliac crest

51. True/False: The use of CT has greatly reduced the ERCP as a common standard diagnostic procedure for evaluating the biliary ducts.

52. True/False: The use of water-soluble contrast agents rather than barium sulfate suspensions for GI tract radiography is desirable because they tend to slow peristaltic action.

53. True/False: Because of the relatively short exposure times, patients are not required to hold their breath during CT exposures of the abdomen.

54. True/False: The use of both oral and/or rectal contrast media is essential for CT abdominal and pelvic exams.

55. True/False: Contrast media are injected intravenously in a similar manner to excretory urography to visualize structures within the mediastinum for thoracic CT.

Additional Imaging Procedures

This chapter discusses additional imaging procedures less common in most radiology departments. Arthrograms, sialograms, myelograms, and conventional tomograms are being replaced with other new imaging modalities such as computerized tomography (CT) or magnetic resonance imaging (MRI). However, in some departments, these procedures are still being performed in sufficient numbers that technologists need to be familiar with them so that they can perform them when requested.

The anatomy for these procedures has been studied in previous chapters; this chapter therefore covers only the procedures themselves and the related positioning. The exception to this is the anatomy of the female reproductive organs as described in the section on hysterosalpingography.

CHAPTER OBJECTIVES

After you have completed **all** the activities of this chapter, you will be able to:

ARTHROGRAPHY

_____ 1. Identify the purpose, indications, patient preparation, equipment, general procedure, and the positioning routines related to knee arthrography.

_____ 2. Identify the purpose, indications, patient preparation, equipment, general procedure, and the positioning and filming sequence related to shoulder arthrography.

HYSTEROSALPINOGRAPHY

_____ 1. Identify specific aspects of the female reproductive system.

_____ 2. Identify the purpose, indications, patient preparation, equipment, general procedure, and the positioning routines related to hysterosalpingography.

ORTHOROENTGENOGRAPHY

_____ 1. Define _orthoroentgenography_ and the purpose of this procedure.

_____ 2. Identify the specific positioning and procedure for lower and upper limb orthoroentgenography.

MYELOGRAPHY

_____ 1. Identify the purpose, indications, contraindications, equipment, and general procedure related to myelography.

_____ 2. Identify positioning routines performed for lumbar, thoracic, and cervical myelography.

SIALOGRAPHY

_____ 1. Identify major aspects of the salivary glands

_____ 2. Identify the purpose, indications, patient preparation, equipment, general procedure, and the positioning routines related to sialography.

BONE DENSITOMETRY

_____ 1. Define and list the risk factors for osteoporosis.

_____ 2. Identify the types of bone densitometry methods available, and the advantages and disadvantages for each method.

_____ 3. Identify the purpose, indications, patient preparation, equipment, general procedure, and the positioning routines related to bone densitometry.

CONVENTIONAL TOMOGRAPHY

_____ 1. Define the specific terms associated with conventional tomography.

_____ 2. Identify the five basic types of trajectories for tube movement in conventional tomography.

_____ 3. Identify the controls and variables that are common features on conventional tomographic units.

_____ 4. Define the difference between a variable and a fixed fulcrum.

_____ 5. Identify the four controlling factors related to tomographic blur.

_____ 6. Describe briefly the two variations of conventional tomography, including autotomography (breathing technique) and pantomography (Panorex).

_____ 7. Demonstrate the principles and controlling factors of conventional tomography in laboratory exercises.

Learning Exercises

Complete the following review exercises after reading the associated pages in the textbook as indicated by each exercise. Answers to each review exercise are given at the end of the review exercises.

REVIEW EXERCISE A: Arthrography (see textbook pp. 726-730)

1. What classifications of joints are studied with arthrography? _____

2. Other than conventional radiography of synovial joints (e.g., arthrography), what other imaging procedure is preferred by physicians for studying synovial joints? _____

3. List the three common forms of knee injury that require arthrography:

    A. _____

    B. _____

    C. _____

4. Give an example of nontraumatic pathology of the knee joint indicating arthrography. _____

5. What are the contraindications for arthrography of any joint? _____

6. True/False: An arthrogram must be approached as a sterile procedure; proper skin prep and sterility must be maintained.

7. True/False: Once the contrast medium is introduced into the knee joint, the knee must _not_ be flexed or exercised.

8. A. For a knee arthrogram, a _____ cc syringe is used with a _____ gauge needle to draw up _____ cc of positive contrast medial for injection.

    B. If dual contrast media is used, a _____ cc syringe is used to inject the negative contrast media.

9. List the two types of contrast media used for a knee arthrogram:

    A. _____

    B. _____

10. List the two projections for conventional "overhead" projections used for knee arthrography?

    A. _____

    B. _____

11. A. How much is the limb rotated between fluoroscopic spot films of the knee joint? _____

    B. How many exposures of each meniscus are generally taken with this method? _____

12. A. How many exposures are taken of each meniscus during horizontal beam arthrography of the knee?

        _____

    B. How many degrees of rotation of the leg between exposures? _____

13. What four aspects of shoulder anatomy are demonstrated with shoulder arthrography?

    A. _____   C. _____

    B. _____   D. _____

14. What is the general name for the conjoined tendons of the four major shoulder muscles? _____

15. What type of needle is commonly used for shoulder arthrograms? _____

16. A. For a single contrast study of the shoulder, how much positive contrast medium is commonly used?

        _____

    B. For a dual contrast study, _____ cc of positive contrast media and _____ cc of negative medium is used (e.g., room air).

17. List the five or six projections frequently taken during a shoulder arthrogram:

    A. _____   D. _____

    B. _____   E. _____

    C. _____   or F. _____

REVIEW EXERCISE B: Hysterosalpingography (see textbook pp. 731-733)

1. The hysterosalpingogram is a radiographic study of the _____ and _____ .

2. The uterus is situated between the _____ posteriorly and the

    _____ anteriorly.

3. List the four divisions of the uterus:

    A. _____

    B. _____

    C. _____

    D. _____

4. The largest division of the uterus is the _____ .

5. The distal aspect of the uterus extending to the vagina is the _____

6. List the three layers of tissue that form the uterus (from the innermost to the outermost layer):

    A. _____

    B. _____

    C. _____

7. Which of the following terms is not an aspect of the uterine tube?

    A. Cornu   C. Isthmus

    B. Ampulla   D. Infundibulum

8. True/False: Fertilization of the ovum occurs in the uterine tube.

9. True/False: The distal portion of the uterine tube opens into the peritoneal cavity.

10. Which of the following terms is used to describe the "degree of openness" of the uterine tube?

    A. Stenosis   C. Atresia

    B. Patency   D. Gauge

11. The most common indication for the hysterosalpingogram (HSG) is:

    _____

12. In addition to the answer for question 11, what are two additional pathologic indications for HSG?

    A. _____

    B. _____

13. List the three common types of lesions that can be demonstrated during a hysterosalpingogram:

    A. _____

    B. _____

    C. _____

14. The contrast medium preferred by most radiologists for a hysterosalpingogram is:

    A. Water-soluble, iodinated   C. Oxygen

    B. Oil-based, iodinated   D. Nitrogen

15. What device may be needed to aid the insertion and fixation of the cannula or catheter during the hysterosalpin-

    gogram? _____

16. To help facilitate the flow of contrast media into the uterine cavity, which position is the patient placed into follow-

    ing the injection of contrast media? _____

17. In addition to the supine position, what two other positions may be imaged to adequately visualize pertinent
    anatomy for an HSG?:

    A. _____

    B. _____

18. Where is the CR centered for overhead projections taken during a HSG using a 24 × 30 (10 × 12 in.) image receptor?

    A. At level of ASIS   C. Iliac crest

    B. Symphysis pubis   D. 2 in. (5 cm) superior to symphysis pubis

REVIEW EXERCISE C: Myelography (see textbook pp. 734-738)

1. Myelography is a radiographic study of the:

    A. _____

    B. _____

2. List the four common lesions or abnormalities (indications) demonstrated during myelography:

    A. _____   C. _____

    B. _____   D. _____

3. Of the four indications just mentioned, which is the most common for myelography?_____.

4. True/False: Myelography of the cervical and thoracic spine regions is most common.

5. List the four common contraindications for myelography:

    A. _____   C. _____

    B. _____   D. _____

6. What type of radiographic table must be used for myelography? _____

7. To reduce patient anxiety, a sedative is usually administered _____ hour(s) before the procedure.

8. Into what space is the contrast medium introduced with myelography? _____

9. List the two common puncture sites for contrast media injection during myelography:

    A. _____

    B. _____

10. Which one of the puncture sites from question 9 is preferred? _____

11. What is the patient's general body position(s) for the following punctures?

    A. Lumbar _____

    B. Cervical _____

12. Why is a large positioning block placed under the abdomen for a lumbar puncture in the prone position?

    _____

13. Which type of contrast medium is commonly used for myelography? _____

14. The contrast medium in question 13 will provide good radiopacity up to _____ after injection.

    A. 20 minutes   C. 1 hour

    B. 30 minutes   D. 8 hours

15. What dosage range of contrast medium is ideal for myelography?

    A. 8 to 10 cc   C. 6 to 17 cc

    B. 20 to 30 cc   D. Approximately 1 ml

16. Indicate the correct sequence of events for a myelogram by listing the following in order (1 through 8):

    _____ A. Introduce needle into subarachnoid space

    _____ B. Collect CSF and send to laboratory

    _____ C. Take conventional radiographic images

    _____ D. Explain the procedure to the patient

    _____ E. Introduce the contrast medium

    _____ F. Have patient sign informed consent form

    _____ G. Take fluoroscopic spot images

    _____ H. Prepare patient's skin for puncture

17. Which position is performed to demonstrate the region of C7 to T4 during a cervical myelogram?

    _____

18. Why should the patient's head and neck remain hyperextended during cervical myelography?

    _____

19. True/False: Generally, AP supine, PA prone, or horizontal beam lateral projections are not taken during thoracic spine myelography.

20. Complete the following for suggested basic routine projections (following fluoroscopy and spot-filming) for the different levels of the spine:

		PROJECTION/POSITION	*LEVEL OF CR*

1. Cervical region   A. _____

                               B. _____

2. Thoracic region   A. _____

                               B. _____

                               C. _____

3. Lumbar region   A. _____

21. True/False: Myelography is largely being replaced by MRI and CT.

REVIEW EXERCISE D: Sialography (see textbook pp. 739-741)

1. List the three pairs of salivary glands:

    A. _____

    B. _____

    C. _____

2. Which is the largest of the salivary glands? _____

3. Which is the smallest of the salivary glands? _____

4. List the two terms for the duct that carries saliva from the parotid gland to the oral cavity:

    A. _____

    B. _____

5. Which one of the following is not a correct term for the duct leading from the submandibular gland to the oral cavity?

    A. Wharton's duct   C. Submandibular duct

    B. Submaxillary duct   D. Bartholin's duct

6. The 12 small ducts leading form the sublingual glands to the oral cavity is/are called:

    A. Wharton's duct   C. Stenson's duct

    B. Duct of Rivinus   D. Accessory salivary ducts

7. What is the term for the center, vertical fold membrane located under the tongue? _____

8. Identify the salivary glands and associated structures labeled on Fig. 23-1:

    A. _____

    B. _____

    C. _____

    D. _____

    E. _____

    F. _____

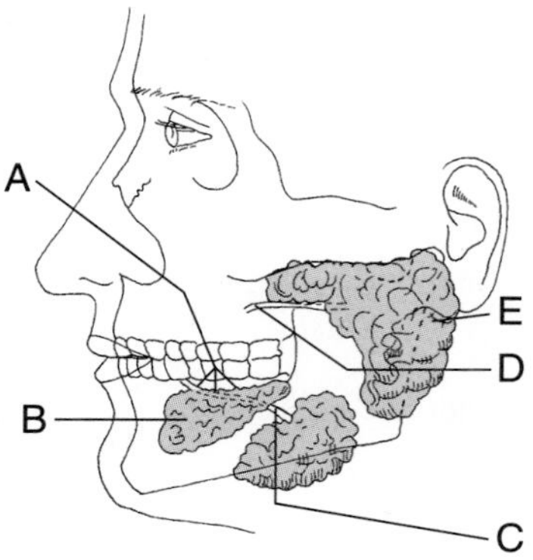

Fig. 23-1 Salivary glands and associated structures.

9. List the three most common pathologic indications that can lead to an obstruction of the salivary ductal system:

    A. _____

    B. _____

    C. _____

10. Sialectasia is:

    A. Dilation of the salivary duct   C. Inflammation of the salivary gland

    B. Stricture of the salivary duct   D. Inability to produce saliva

11. Why is the patient given a lemon slice to suck at the onset of the sialogram?

    _____

12. List the two devices used to cannulate a salivary duct once the duct is located.

    A. _____

    B. _____

13. If conventional tomography is used during a sialogram, _____ (oil-based or water-soluble) contrast media should be used.

14. If calculi in one of the salivary ducts are suspected, _____ contrast media should be used (oil-based or water-soluble).

15. On the average, how much contrast medium is injected to fill a salivary duct? _____

16. Which one of the following imaging modalities is not used during a sialogram?

    A. Conventional radiography   C. CT

    B. Sonography   D. Digital fluoroscopy

17. Which one of the following imaging positions is not performed during a sialogram?

    A. Superoinferior projection   C. AP/PA projection

    B. Lateral position   D. Lateral oblique position

REVIEW EXERCISE E: Orthoroentgenography (see textbook pp. 742-744)

1. Why is orthoroentgenography more commonly used in long bone measurements rather than CT?

   _____

2. What is the literal definition or meaning of the term *orthoroentgenogram*?

   _____

3. Why should separate projections be taken of limb joints rather than including the entire extremity on a single projection?

   _____

4. When performing an orthoroentgenographic procedure, what device needs to be placed on top of the table next to

   the affected limb? _____

5. What is the name of the surgical procedure that shortens a limb by fusing the epiphyses? _____

6. Which three joints are included on one image receptor for a long bone study of the lower limb?

   _____

7. True/False: Both right and left lower limbs can be placed on the same radiograph for a long bone study.

8. True/False: For a bilateral study, all three joints of both lower limbs can be placed on the same 35 × 43 cm (14 × 17 inch) IR.

9. If both lower limbs are radiographed together on one image receptor, why should two rulers be used with one under each limb rather than placing one midway between the two limbs?

   _____

10. True/False: For a long bone study of the upper limb, all three projections must be taken with the Bucky grid.

11. True/False: The wrist is examined in the pronated position (PA) for a long bone study of the upper limb.

12. True/False: The proximal humerus must be rotated internally for the shoulder projection taken during upper limb orthoroentgenography.

REVIEW EXERCISE F: Bone Densitometry (see textbook pp. 745-748)

1. Each year in the United States, approximately _____ million people have, or are at risk of developing, osteoporosis.

2. For osteoporosis to be visible radiographically, a loss of ____% to ____% of the trabecular bone must occur.

3. Cells responsible for new bone formation are called _____ , and cells that help to break

   down old bone are _____ .

4. The purpose of bone densitometry is to _____ .

5. Central or axial analysis includes bone density measurements of the:

   A. _____

   B. _____

6. Peripheral site analysis includes bone density measurements of the fingers, wrist, _____ ,

   _____ , or _____ .

7. True/False: Osteoporosis leads to an increased risk of fractures

8. True/False: Loss of magnesium and phosphorus from the bony cortex is the primary cause of osteoporosis

9. True/False: Osteoporosis affects primarily pre-menopausal women.

10. True/False: Hormone therapy may retard the effects of osteoporosis

11. Place a check by each of the following that are **not** risk factors for osteoporosis as listed in the texbook:

    _____ A. Family history of osteoporosis

    _____ B. Excessive physical activity

    _____ C. Low sodium and niacin intake

    _____ D. Smoking

    _____ E. Low body weight

    _____ F. Alcohol consumption

    _____ G. High fat diet

    _____ H. Low calcium intake

    _____ I. Height greater than 6 feet (180 cm)

    _____ J. Previous fractures

12. True/False: Severe scoliosis or kyphosis may result in less accurate results for bone densitometry procedures.

13. True/False: Bone densitometry needs to be scheduled at least 1 week following an iodinated contrast media or radionuclide procedure.

14. List the three most common types of bone densitometry equipment, methods, and techniques in current use:

    A. _____

    B. _____

    C. _____

15. Which one of the following bone densitometry techniques and equipment methods uses a dual-energy, fan-beam x-ray source?

    A. Radioabsorptiometry (RA)   C. (Dual-energy x-ray absorptiometry (DXA)

    B. Dual-energy photon absorptiometry D. Quantitative computed (DPA) tomography (QCT)

16. Z-score obtained with the DXA system compares the patient to:

    A. Young, healthy individual with peak bone mass
    C. Patient with moderate osteoporosis

    B. Patient with severe osteoporosis
    D. Average individual of the same age and gender

17. True/False: Patient dose with the DXA system ranges between 1 to 30 microSieverts.

18. Quantitative computed tomography (QCT) provides bone mineral density measurements of

    _____ and _____ bone.

19. The anatomical site most commonly evaluated with quantitative ultrasound (QUS) is _____.

20. True/False: DXA of the hip requires the lower limb to be rotated 15 to 20° internally.

21. The "T" score compares the patient's bone density to: _____.

22. Which of the following is the method of choice for evaluating both trabecular and cortical bone?

    A. Quantitative computed tomography (QCT)

    B. Dual-energy x-ray absorptiometry (DXA)

    C. Quantitative ultrasound (QUS)

    D. Dual-energy photon absorptiometry

23. Which of the methods from question 22 provides a true three-dimensional or volumetric analysis?

    _____

REVIEW EXERCISE G: Conventional Tomography (see textbook pp. 749-754)

1. Define each of the following terms. (Give short, concise answers.)

    A. Tomograph _____

    B. Fulcrum _____

    C. Fulcrum level _____

    D. Objective (focal) plane _____

    E. Sectional thickness _____

    F. Exposure angle _____

    G. Tube movement (shift) _____

    H. Amplitude _____

    I. Tube trajectory _____

    J. Blur _____

    K. Blur margin _____

2. Identify the correct term for the five tube movement
   trajectories in Fig. 23-2:

   A. _____

   B. _____

   C. _____

   D. _____

   E. _____

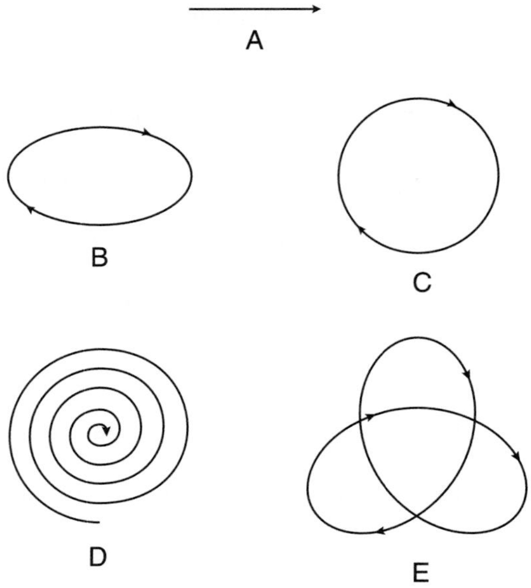

3. Which of the tube trajectories from the previous question are
   multidirectional? Which are unidirectional? (indicate by letter)

   1. Multidirectional _____

   2. Unidirectional _____

Fig. 23-2 Tube movement trajectories.

4. Which two of these tube trajectories are considered the most complex?

   _____

5. List the five common adjustments or settings found on the tomographic control panel:

   A. _____

   B. _____

   C. _____

   D. _____

   E. _____

6. True/False: Objects closer to the objective plane will experience maximum blurring.

7. True/False: The fixed-type fulcrum (rather than the variable type) is most commonly used with multidirectional specialized tomographic equipment.

8. Which one of the methods from the previous question (fixed or variable type) will alter the fulcrum by moving the

   patient and tabletop up or down? _____

9. Briefly describe the tomographic blurring principle. (Why, or how, does blurring of some objects occur while others remain in sharp focus?)

   _____

   _____

10. Describe the method of determining focal level settings and centering when beginning a tomographic procedure:

   _____

   _____

11. List the four factors that determine the amount of blurring:

A. _____

B. _____

C. _____

D. _____

12. True/False: As the exposure angle decreases, slice thickness also decreases (becomes thinner).

13. True/False: As the distance from the image receptor increases, object blurring will increase.

14. To explain how variations in tube trajectories or movement patterns influence the amount of blurring, complete the following (study the various tube trajectories of Fig. 23-2 as you answer these questions):

A. Maximum blurring occurs when objects are _____ (parallel or perpendicular) to the direction of tube movement.

B. A circular movement pattern will create _____ (more or less) blurring than an elliptical pattern.

C. The elliptical pattern has more objects nearer _____ (parallel or perpendicular) to the line of tube travel than the circular pattern.

D. Maximum blurring occurs with spiral and hypocycloidal tube patterns because they include a

_____ dimension as part of their movement.

15. Multidirectional tube trajectories are needed for visualizing small anatomical structures of _____ or less.

16. Which type of tomographic equipment demonstrates the following satisfactorily:

_____ 1. Lung tumor   A. Linear tomogram only

_____ 2. Nephrotomogram   B. Multidirectional or multitiered capabilities

_____ 3. Sella turcica

_____ 4. TMJs

_____ 5. Middle ear structures

_____ 6. Biliary ducts (ERCP)

17. True/False: The human eye accepts a certain degree of blurring as normal, making the actual amount of blurring somewhat subjective.

18. A tomographic principle in which the anatomical structure moves but the image receptor/tube remain stationary is

called _____. (Hint: It is used in certain lateral spine and sternum projections to blur out

overlying structures)

19. What is the most common application for pantotomography? _____

20. What device minimizes penumbra blurring during a pantotomographic procedure? _____

Laboratory Exercises

The following exercises are for two procedures for which supplies and equipment are most commonly available to students.

EXERCISE A. ORTHOROENTGENOGRAPHY-LONG BONE MEASUREMENT (see textbook pp. 742-744)

1. Using an upper and lower limb radiographic phantom (if available), produce long bone measurement radiographs of the following:

_____ Unilateral lower limb (AP projection of hip, knee, and ankle on one image receptor with a correctly placed Bell-Thompson ruler)

_____ Bilateral lower limbs (AP projections of hips, knees, and ankles on one image receptor with correctly placed Bell-Thompson rulers)

_____ Unilateral upper limb (AP projections of shoulder, elbow, and wrist on one image receptor with correctly placed ruler)

EXERCISE B. CONVENTIONAL TOMOGRAPHY (see textbook pp. 749-754)

This part of the learning exercise needs to be carried out in an energized radiographic room equipped with at least a linear type tomographic unit. The use of multidirectional and/or multitiered tomographic units is optional. Check the following steps when they are completed:

_____ **Step 1** **Equipment setup:** Set up the necessary tomographic equipment, including the adjustable fulcrum level attachment connected to the tube and to the Bucky.   Ensure that the Bucky tray locks are released (as well as the tube angle and tube distance locks), allowing the tube and Bucky tray to move freely.

_____ **Step 2** **Preparation of "phantom" for experiments:** Design a series of experiments to demonstrate the tomographic blurring principle and the effect of the four controlling and influencing factors on blurring.
Commercial tomographic phantoms are available with various lead numbers or other metallic devices placed at specific levels within the phantom.   If these are not readily available, one can easily be made with paper clips in combination with a wire mesh or other flat metallic objects placed in horizontal layers in three different books, or in three different layers within the same book. The shape or the configuration of the metallic objects can be varied in each layer so that the various levels can be differentiated on the radiograph.

_____ **Step 3** **Determine exposure factors:** Determine approximate exposure factors to visualize the metallic objects as placed in the books and stacked on the x-ray table.   Start with an approximate upper limb exposure technique. Make a test exposure. Set the factors on the control panel of the tomographic unit as needed.

OPTIONAL EXPERIMENTS TO DEMONSTRATE TOMOGRAPHIC PRINCIPLES AND VARIABLES:

Using your knowledge and understanding of tomographic blurring principles as studied in this chapter, design and carry out exercises as needed to demonstrate the following:

Experiment A: Orientation of Body Part to Tube Travel Demonstrate that those objects parallel to the direction of tube movement create "streaks" and are not as effectively blurred as when they are perpendicular to the tube movement.   This can be readily shown by changing the longitudinal direction of the metallic objects (e.g., paper clips) so the levels above and below the focal plane will be at some angle or completely perpendicular to the direction of the tube travel. This should demonstrate increased blurring of the objects above and below the focal plane.

Experiment B: Influencing and Controlling Factors for Tomographic Blurring Design experiments to demonstrate how each of the following four factors or variables influence or control the amount of blurring. On these types of experiments, remember to change only one factor at a time, keeping all other factors constant.

_____ **Factor 1** **Object-focal plane distance**

Demonstrate that those objects farther from the focal plane have greater movement on the image receptor and therefore increased blurring as compared with those closer to the focal plane.

This can be done by first taking tomographs with the objects above and below those in the focal plane. Compare these with tomographs taken when the objects above and below are placed at increased distances from the focal plane. You should be able to demonstrate markedly increased blurring on the second set of tomographs.

_____ **Factor 2 Exposure angle**

By changing the exposure angle, demonstrate that an increase in exposure angle with greater tube travel will increase the blurring, resulting in a thinner focal plane. Likewise, a decrease in exposure angle with less tube travel will decrease the movement of the objects above and below the focal plane, creating less blurring and a thicker section remaining in focus.

Remember that the amplitude or speed of tube movement must also increase as the exposure angle is increased so that the exposure continues throughout the full arc of tube travel.

_____ **Factor 3 Object-image receptor (IR) distance**

Demonstrate that as the distance of the objects from the IR is increased, greater blurring will occur.

Sponge blocks can be placed between objects (e.g., books or phantom) and the table to increase the object-IR distance. (This will demonstrate why the upside or side away from the IR on a tomogram of a lateral TMJ or of a lateral of inner ear structures should be examined rather than the downside.)

Optional

_____ **Factor 4 Tube trajectory** (if equipment is available)

This can be done only if equipment is available that has multidirectional and/or multitiered trajectory possibilities.

By changing to a circular or elliptical movement, demonstrate that increased blurring and a thinner focal plane can be achieved as compared with only linear tube movement.

Demonstrate that maximum blurring occurs with the multidirectional, multitiered (spiral and hypocycloidal) trajectories, even when the distance between the objects above and below the focal plane is very small. This should demonstrate that blurring of objects even as close as 1 mm to the focal plane can be achieved.

Answers to Review Exercises

Review Exercise A: Arthrography
1. Synovial joints
2. Magnetic resonance imaging (MRI)
3. A. Tears of the joint capsule
   B. Tears of the menisci
   C. Tears of ligaments
4. Baker's cyst
5. Allergic reactions to iodine-based contrast media, or to local anesthetics
6. True
7. False (needs to be flexed to distribute contrast media)
8. A. 10, 20, 5
   B. 50
9. A. Positive or radiopaque media such as iodinated, water-soluble contrast agent
   B. Negative or radiolucent contrast agents such as room air, oxygen, or carbon dioxide
10. A. AP
    B. Lateral
11. A. 20°
    B. 9
12. A. 6 (six views per meniscus)
    B. 30°
13. A. Joint capsule
    B. Rotator cuff
    C. Long tendon of biceps muscle
    D. Articular cartilage
14. Rotator cuff
15. 2½ to 3½ in. spinal needle
16. A. 10 to 12 cc
    B. 3 to 4, 10 to 12
17. A. AP scout
    B. AP internal rotation
    C. AP external rotation
    D. Glenoid fossa (Grashey) projection
    E. Transaxillary (inferosuperior axial) projection
    F. Bicipital (intertubercular) groove projection

Review Exercise B: Hysterosalpingography
1. Uterus
   Uterine tubes
2. Rectosigmoid colon
   Urinary bladder
3. A. Fundus
   B. Corpus (body)
   C. Isthmus
   D. Cervix
4. Corpus or body
5. Cervix
6. A. Endometrium
   B. Myometrium
   C. Serosa
7. A. Cornu
8. True
9. True
10. B. Patency
11. Assessment of female infertility
12. A. Demonstrate intrauterine pathology
    B. Evaluation of the uterine tubes following tubal ligation in reconstructive surgery
13. A. Endometrial polyps
    B. Uterine fibroids
    C. Intrauterine adhesions
14. A. Water-soluble, iodinated
15. Tenaculum
16. Slight Trendelenburg
17. A. LPO
    B. RPO
18. D. 2 in. (5 cm) superior to symphysis pubis

Review Exercise C: Myelography
1. A. Spinal cord
   B. Nerve root branches
2. A. Herniated nucleus pulposus (HNP)
   B. Cancerous or benign tumors
   C. Cysts
   D. Possible bone fragments
3. Herniated nucleus pulposus (HNP)
4. False (most common are cervical and lumbar regions)
5. A. Blood in the cerebrospinal fluid
   B. Arachnoiditis
   C. Increased intracranial pressure
   D. Recent lumbar puncture (within 2 weeks)
6. 90/15° tilting table
7. One (1)
8. Into the subarachnoid space (of spinal canal)
9. A. Lumbar (L3-4)
   B. Cervical (C1-2)
10. Lumbar (L3-4)
11. A. Prone or left lateral
    B. Erect or prone
12. For spinal flexion to widen the interspinous spaces to facilitate needle placement
13. Nonionic water-soluble iodine based
14. C. 1 hour
15. C. 6 to 17 cc
16. A. 4, B. 5, C. 8, D. 1, E. 6, F. 2, G. 7, H. 3
17. Swimmer's lateral using a horizontal x-ray beam
18. To keep the contrast media from entering the cranial subarachnoid space
19. True (right and left lateral decubitus positions are taken)
20. 1. A. Horizontal beam lateral (prone), C5
      B. Horizontal beam lateral (swimmers), C7
    2. A. R lateral decubitus (AP or PA), T7
      B. L lateral decubitus (AP or PA), T7
      C. R or L lateral, vertical beam, T7
    3. A. Semi-erect horizontal beam lateral (prone), L3
20. True

Review Exercise D: Sialography
1. A. Parotid glands
   B. Submandibular glands
   C. Sublingual glands
2. Parotid gland
3. Sublingual glands
4. A. Parotid duct
   B. Stensen's duct
5. D. Bartholin's duct
6. B. Ducts of Rivinus
7. Frenulum
8. A. Ducts of Rivinus (Bartholin's ducts)
   B. Sublingual gland
   C. Submandibular duct (Wharton's duct)
   D. Submandibular gland (submaxillary gland)
   E. Parotid duct (Stenson's duct)
   F. Parotid gland
9. A. Calculi
   B. Strictures
   C. Tumors
10. A. Dilation of the salivary duct
11. To cause the patient to express saliva and help locate the opening of a particular duct
12. A. Butterfly needle
    B. Sialography catheter
13. Oil-based
14. Water-soluble
15. 1 to 2 ml
16. B. Sonography
17. A. Superoinferior projection

Review Exercise E: Orthoroetgenography
1. CT is more costly and requires specialized equipment.
2. A straight or right angle radiograph
3. To prevent elongation of the limb due to the divergence of the x-ray beam
4. A special metallic (Bell-Thompson) ruler to measure bone length from one joint to another
5. Epiphysiodeses
6. Hip, knee, and ankle

7. True
8. True
9. A single center-placed ruler makes it difficult or impossible to shield the gonads without obscuring the upper part of the ruler.
10. True
11. False (PA would cross radius and ulna)
12. False (The proximal humerus is rotated into an external rotation position)

13. Review Exercise F: Bone Densitometry

1. 28
2. 30% to 50%
3. Osteoblasts, osteoclasts
4. Evaluate bone mineral density
5. A. Lumbar spine
   B. Proximal femur
6. Forearm, heel, or lower leg
7. True
8. False (loss of calcium and collagen)
9. False (post-menopausal)
10. True
11. B, C, G, I
12. True
13. True
14. A. Dual-energy x-ray absorptiometry (DXA)
   B. Quantitative computed tomography (QCT)
   C. Quantitative ultrasound (QUS)
15. C. Dual-energy x-ray absorptiometry (DXA)
16. D. Average individual of the same age and gender
17. True
18. Trabecular, cortical
19. Os calcis (heel)
20. True

21. An average healthy individual with peak bone mass
22. A. Quantitative computed tomography (QCT)
23. A. QCT

Review Exercise G: Conventional Tomography

1. A. The radiograph produced during a tomographic procedure
   B. The pivot point of the connecting rod between tube and film holder
   C. The distance from table top to fulcrum
   D. The plane or section of the object that is clear and in focus
   E. The thickness of the objective plane
   F. The angle resulting from the x-ray tube beam movement
   G. The distance the tube travels
   H. The speed the tube travels in inches per second or cm per second
   I. The geometric configuration or pattern of tube travel
   J. The area of distortion of objects outside the objective plane
   K. The outer edges of the blurred object
2. A. Linear
   B. Elliptical
   C. Circular
   D. Spiral
   E. Hypocycloidal
3. 1. B, C, D, E
2. A
4. D (spiral) and E (hypocycloidal)
5. A. Tube travel speed
   B. Objective plane

C. Direction or type of tube trajectory (for units that are multidirectional)
   D. Tube center
   E. Fulcrum level
6. False (objects away from objective plane have greatest blurring)
7. True
8. Fixed fulcrum type
9. Objects farther from the fulcrum level or objective plane will be blurred by the movement of the tube and film. Objects closer to this fulcrum level and those that are parallel to tube travel will remain almost stationary and experience little or no blurring.
10. Two 90° conventional radiographs are generally taken to determine depth and centering of the object of interest
11. A. Distance the object is from the objective plane
    B. Exposure angle
    C. Distance the object is from the film
    D. Tube trajectory
12. False (increases)
13. True
14. A. Perpendicular
    B. More
    C. Parallel
    D. Vertical or multitiered
15. 1 mm
16. 1. A, 2. A, 3. B, 4. B, 5. B, 6. A
17. True
18. Autotomography or breathing technique
19. Mandible studies
20. Slit beam restrictor or diaphragm

SELF-TEST

My Score = _____%

This self-test should be taken only after completing **all** the readings, review exercises, and laboratory activities for a particular section. The purpose of this test is not only to provide a good learning exercise but also to serve as a good indicator of what your final evaluation grade will be. It is strongly suggested that if you do not get at least a 90% to 95% grade on this self-test, you should review those areas in which you missed questions **before** going to your instructor for the final evaluation exam for this chapter. (There are 83 questions or blanks—each is worth 1.2 points.)

1. The formal term for a radiographic long bone measurement study is _____ .

2. True/False: To properly measure the length of a long bone, the entire lower limb should be included on a single projection.

3. True/False: Epiphysiodeses is an operation to lengthen bone by widening the epiphyseal plate.

4. True/False: Movement of the body part between exposures will compromise the long bone study.

5. True/False: If a long bone study of both lower limbs is ordered, the use of two metal rulers is recommended with both limbs exposed at the same time on the same image receptor.

6. What is the proper name for the special metal ruler used for long bone measurement? _____

7. What size of image receptor and how may exposures are recommended for a long bone study of the upper limbs for

   an adult? _____

8. List the two synovial-type joints most commonly examined with an arthrogram.

   A. _____   B. _____

9. List the two contraindications for an arthrogram:

   A. _____   B. _____

10. An indication of a possible "Baker's cyst" would suggest the need for an arthrogram procedure for the

    _____ .

11. List the two types and the amounts of contrast media commonly used for a knee arthrogram:

	TYPE	*AMOUNT*
A.	_____	_____
B.	_____	_____

12. What size needle is used to introduce the contrast media during a knee arthrogram? _____

13. What is the purpose of flexing the knee gently after the contrast media has been injected for an arthrogram procedure?

    _____

14. What size image receptor is recommended for horizontal beam arthrogram projections?

    _____

15. How many exposures are made, and how much is the leg rotated, between each exposure for horizontal beam knee arthrograms?

   A. Number of exposures: _____

   B. Degrees of rotation between exposures: _____

16. The term *rotator cuff* refers to what structures of the shoulder? _____

17. List the overhead projections that may be requested for a shoulder arthrogram:

   Scout

   A. _____

   Post Injection

   B. _____

   C. _____

   D. _____

   E. _____

   F. _____

18. List the three common lesions or conditions diagnosed through a myelogram:

   A. _____   C. _____

   B. _____

19. List the four common contraindications for a myelogram:

   A. _____   C. _____

   B. _____   D. _____

20. The most common clinical indication for a myelogram is:

   A. Benign tumors   C. HNP

   B. Spinal cysts   D. Bony injury to the spine

21. Which position will move the contrast media column from the lumbar to the cervical region during a myelogram?

   A. Fowler's   C. Trendelenburg

   B. Left lateral decubitus   D. Prone

22. What is the most common spinal puncture site for a lumbar myelogram?

   A. L3-4   C. L4-5

   B. L1-2   D. L5 -S1

24. A cervical puncture is indicated for an upper spinal region myelogram if:

   A. The patient has severe lordosis   C. The patient has HNP of the L4-5 level

   B. The patient has mild scoliosis   D. The patient has complete blockage at T-spine level

25. The absorption of the water-soluble contrast media into the vascular system of the body begins approximately _____ minutes after injection and is totally undetectable radiographically after _____ hours.

26. Which position is performed during a cervical myelogram to demonstrate the C7-T1 region?

    _____

27. Another term for tomography is _____.

28. Match the following tomographic terms with the correct definition:

    _____ 1. Objective plane   A. The area of distortion

    _____ 2. Exposure angle   B. The speed of tube travel

    _____ 3. Tomograph   C. Radiograph produced by a tomographic unit

    _____ 4. Blur   D. The plane where the object is clear

    _____ 5. Fulcrum   E. The pivot point between tube and image receptor

    _____ 6. Amplitude   F. The factor that determines slice thickness

29. Match the following tube trajectories: (Fig. 23-3)

    _____ 1. Spiral

    _____ 2. Elliptical

    _____ 3. Circular

    _____ 4. Hypocycloidal

    _____ 5. Linear

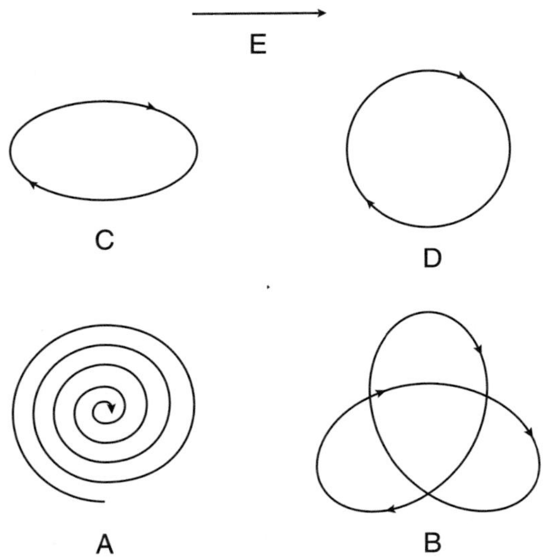

Fig. 23-3 Tube movement trajectories.

30. List the two methods of adjusting the fulcrum level:

    A. _____   B. _____

31. True/False: Maximum blurring of an object will be achieved when it is perpendicular to tube travel.

32. True/False: The primary factor affecting the sectional thickness as controlled by the operator is the type of tube trajectory.

33. True/False: Increased blurring occurs when the object is farther from the image receptor.

34. True/False: In pantomography, the image receptor and tube move with the patient stationary similar to conventional tomography.

35. True/False: Amplitude does not influence or control the amount of blurring.

36. Which one of the following exposure times would be suitable for breathing technique (autotomography)?

    A. 2 to 3 seconds　　　C. ½ second

    B. 1 second　　　　　　D. 10 milliseconds

37. List the four divisions of the uterus:

    A. _____

    B. _____

    C. _____

    D. _____

38. Which of the following is *not* a tissue layer of the uterus?

    A. Osseometrium　　　C. Endometrium

    B. Myometrium　　　　D. Serosa

39. True/False: The uterine tubes are connected directly to the ovaries.

40. List the two contraindications for a hysterosalpingogram:

    A. _____

    B. _____

41. True/False: Oil-based contrast medium is preferred for the majority of hysterosalpingograms.

42. True/False: Hysterosalpingography can be a therapeutic tool in correcting certain obstructions in the uterine tube.

43. Match the following salivary ducts to the correct salivary gland:

    _____ A. Parotid gland　　　　　　1. Ducts of Rivinus

    _____ B. Submandibular gland　　　2. Stenson's duct

    _____ C. Sublingual gland　　　　　3. Wharton's duct

44. Sialography is contraindicated for:

    A. Possible obstruction of the salivary duct　　　　　C. Salivary duct fistula

    B. Severe inflammation of the salivary gland or duct　　　D. Calculi lodged in salivary duct

45. What type of contrast media should be used for the majority of sialograms? _____

46. Which of the following is *not* a risk factor for osteoporosis:

    A. Excessive physical activity　　　C. Low body weight

    B. Alcohol consumption　　　　　　D. Low calcium intake

47. Newer dual-energy x-ray absorptiometry (DXA) uses:

    A. Fan-beam x-ray source　　　C. Pencil-thin x-ray source

    B. Positron-emission source　　D. Super voltage x-ray source

48. A T-score obtained with the DXA system compares the patient to a(n):

    A. Average patient of the same age and gender   C. Patient with moderate osteoporosis

    B. Healthy individual with peak bone mass   D. Patient with severe osteoporosis

49. The two negatives with quantitative computed tomography (QCT) are:

    A. _____

    B. _____

50. The area that is most commonly scanned with quantitative ultrasound (QUS) is the _____ .

CHAPTER 24

Additional Diagnostic and Therapeutic Modalities

This chapter introduces select alternative diagnostic and therapeutic imaging modalities, including nuclear medicine, radiation oncology, diagnostic ultrasound, and resonance imaging. The information and review exercises contained in Chapter 24 are intended to introduce students to basic concepts related to each of these modalities. Basic definitions, physical principles, clinical applications, and technologist responsibilities will be covered.

A more extensive presentation is provided in the magnetic resonance imaging (MRI) section, which introduces MRI terminology and the basics of MRI physics and instrumentation. The important clinical aspects related to personnel and patient safety are discussed. An introduction to the imaging parameters that affect the quality of the images and clinical applications of MRI is included. Although portions of the chapter may appear complex and will require careful study, the authors have provided a thorough introduction to understanding this exciting and rapidly developing field.

CHAPTER OBJECTIVES

After you have completed **all** the activities of this chapter, you will be able to:

———— 1. Identify basic operating principles related to nuclear medicine imaging.

———— 2. List the purpose, radionuclide used, and pathologic indications demonstrated with select nuclear medicine procedures.

———— 3. List specific responsibilities for members of the nuclear medicine team.

———— 4. Distinguish between internal and external types of radiation therapy.

———— 5. Identify the energy level, characteristics, and advantages of the major types of radiation therapy units.

———— 6. List the specific responsibilities of radiation oncology team members.

———— 7. Identify basic operating principles related to ultrasound.

———— 8. List the characteristics, advantages, and disadvantages of specific types of ultrasound systems.

———— 7. List the purpose, transducer used, and pathologic indications demonstrated with select ultrasound procedures.

———— 8. Explain how MRI produces an image.

———— 9. Compare the process of MRI image production with that of other imaging modalities.

———— 10. Explain how a signal is generated and received from body tissues.

———— 11. Explain how contrast is produced in the MR image.

———— 12. Identify specific MRI system components.

———— 13. Identify basic MRI safety considerations.

———— 14. Identify information to be included when preparing a patient for an MRI exam.

———— 15. Identify the type of contrast agent used in MRI.

———— 16. Identify the different types of RF coils.

———— 17. State the appearance of specific tissue types on both T1- and T2-weighted images.

———— 18. Define the terms and pathologic indications related to MRI.

Learning Exercises

Complete the following review exercises after reading the associated pages in the textbook as indicated by each exercise. Answers to each review exercise are given at the end of the review exercises.

REVIEW EXERCISE A: Nuclear Medicine (see textbook pp. 756-757)

1. Nuclear medicine uses radioactive materials called _____ in the study and treatment of various medical conditions.

2. Radioactive materials that are introduced into the body and concentrate in specific organs are called

   _____

3. How are the materials identified in question 2 introduced into the body?

   A. Inhalation   C. Injection

   B. Orally   D. All of the above

4. One of the most common radioactive materials used in nuclear medicine procedures is:

   A. Sulfur colloid   C. Technetium 99m

   B. Iodine 131   D. Thallium

5. The term *SPECT* is an abbreviation for _____.

6. The SPECT camera provides a _____ -dimensional view of the anatomy.

7. A study of the skeletal system using radioactive materials is called: _____ .

8. A common genitourinary nuclear medicine study is performed for:

   A. Kidney transplants   C. Pyelonephritis

   B. Renal cyst   D. All of the above

9. Nuclear medicine is considered the ideal modality for diagnosing _____ of the gastrointestinal tract.

   A. Peptic ulcers   C. Gastroesophageal reflux

   B. Meckel's diverticulum   D. Colitis

10. Which one of the following radiopharmaceutical is used during myocardial perfusion studies?

    A. Technetium 99m   C. Iodine 131

    B. Thallium   D. Neo Tect

11. Which one of the following radiopharmaceuticals is used to determine if a pulmonary lesion is benign or malignant?

    A. Technetium 99m   C. Iodine 131

    B. Thallium   D. Neo Tect

12. Match the following responsibilities to the correct nuclear medicine team member:

    ——— A. Properly disposes contaminated materials   1. Nuclear medicine technologist

    ——— B. Calibrates nuclear medicine imaging equipment   2. Nuclear medicine physician

    ——— C. Performs statistical analysis of study data   3. Medical nuclear physicist

    ——— D. Administers radionuclide to patient

    ——— E. Interprets procedure

    ——— F. Often serves as department radiation safety officer

    ——— G. Licensed to acquire and use radioactive materials

    ——— H. Prepares radioactive materials

    ——— I. Digitally processes the images

REVIEW EXERCISE B: Radiation Oncology (see textbook p. 758)

1. Cancer is second only to ————————————— as the leading cause of death in the United States and Canada.

2. Identify the two types of radiation therapy treatment:

    A. —————————————————

    B. —————————————————

3. Prostate cancer is a common candidate for which of the two types of radiation therapy treatment from question 2?

    ————————————————————————————————————

4. List the three sources of external beam radiation:

    A. —————————————————

    B. —————————————————

    C. —————————————————

5. Cobalt-60 units emit gamma rays at the intensity of ——— MeV.

    A. 1.25   C. 10.4

    B. 5.25   D. 15.25

6. What is the source of the high energy x-rays produced with a linear accelerator therapy unit?

    A. Cobalt-60   C. Uranium 235

    B. High-speed neutrons striking an anode   D. High-speed electrons striking an anode

7. Which of the following is most effective for the treatment of shallow or superficial cancerous tissue?

    A. Cobalt-60   C. High voltage x-ray type unit

    B. Linear accelerator   D. Internal, brachytherapy type

8.   Linear accelerators produce energy levels between _____ and _____ MeV.

   A.   1 to 2   C.   4 to 30

   B.   3 to 5   D.   30 to 50

9.   What is the purpose of radiation therapy simulation?

   _____

10.   Match the following responsibilities to the correct radiation oncology team member:

   _____ A.   Outlines plan to deliver the desired dosage   1.   Radiation therapist

   _____ B.   Administers radiation treatments   2.   Radiation oncologist

   _____ C.   May use fluoroscopy to determine treatment fields   3.   Medical dosimetrist

   _____ D.   Calibrates equipment   4.   Medical health physicist

   _____ E.   Prescribes treatment plan

   _____ F.   Advises oncologists on dosage calculations

   _____ G.   Maintains treatment records

REVIEW EXERCISE C: Ultrasound (see textbook pp 759-762)

1.   List three additional terms for ultrasound:

   A.   _____

   B.   _____

   C.   _____

2.   Medical ultrasound uses high frequency sound waves in the range between _____ to _____ MHz .

3.   True/False: Ultrasound is an ideal imaging modality for diagnosing an ileus.

4.   True/False: Ultrasound is often used to locate a bone cyst in the femur.

5.   True/False: Research studies conclude that there are no adverse biologic effects associated with the use of medical ultrasound.

6.   True/False: The first A-mode ultrasound unit was built in Germany in the late 1950s.

7.   Which generation of ultrasound unit introduced two-dimensional gray scale?

   A.   A-mode   C.   Real time dynamic

   B.   B-mode   D.   Doppler

8.   Which type of ultrasound unit is used to examine the structure and behavior of flowing blood?

   A.   A-mode   C.   Real time dynamic

   B.   B-mode   D.   Doppler

9. What major improvement is offered by the new high-definition digital ultrasound systems?

    A. Smaller size unit   C. Increase in dynamic range

    B. Can alter between A-mode and B-mode   D. Introduction of gray scale

10. What is the fundamental purpose or function of the transducer?

    _____

11. What type of material comprises the functional aspect of the transducer, which creates the high-frequency sound waves?

    A. Tungsten alloy   C. Silver/chromium alloy

    B. Ceramic   D. Ferrous alloy

12. What physical principle is applied when the transducer produces a sound wave?

    A. Piezoelectric effect   C. Thermionic emission

    B. Modulation transfer   D. Larmor effect

13. Match the correct frequency transducer to the following procedures and/or situations:

    _____ A. For an average or small abdomen   1. 3.5 MHz

    _____ B. For a larger abdomen   2. 5.0 to 7.0 MHz

    _____ C. For a study of a superficial structure   3. 17 MHz

14. True/False: A transducer serves as both a transmitter and receiver of echoes.

15. True/False: A sonographer must provide initial interpretation of the ultrasound images.

16. Ultrasound is the "gold standard" for studies of the following structures except the:

    A. Liver   C. Gallbladder

    B. Stomach   D. Uterus

17. What is the name of the ultrasound procedure in which amniotic fluid is withdrawn from the uterus for genetic analysis?

    _____

18. Ultrasound is very effective in evaluating the fetus before birth for early indications of:

    A. Heart defects   C. Spina bifida

    B. Hydrocephaly   D. All of the above

19. What is the advantage of using ultrasound for studies of the musculoskeletal system over MRI?

    A. Less expensive   C. Provides a functional study of joint movement

    B. Noninvasive   D. All of the above

20. Match the following sonographic terms to the correct definition:

_____ A. An image that possesses both width and height

1. Anechoic

_____ B. Alteration in frequency or wavelength reflected by moving objects

2. Backscatter

_____ C. Acoustic energy that travels through a medium

3. Doppler effect

_____ D. An anatomical object that does not produce any echoes

4. Echogenic

_____ E. Ultrasound images that demonstrate dynamic motion

5. Hyperechoic

_____ F. An anatomical object that produces more echoes than normal

6. Hypoechoic

_____ G. Acoustic energy reflected from a structure that interferes with the expected path of the acoustic wave

7. Real time imaging

_____ H. An anatomical structure that possesses echo-producing structures

8. Two-dimensional image

_____ I. An aspect of acoustic energy reflected back toward the source or origin

9. Wave

_____ J. An anatomical object that produces fewer echoes than normal

10. Reflection

REVIEW EXERCISE D: Physical Principles of MRI (see textbook pp. 763-768)

1. MRI uses _____ and _____ to obtain a mathematically reconstructed image.

2. The MRI image represents differences in the tissues of the patient in the number of _____ and the rate at which they recover from radiofrequency stimulation.

3. To compare the energy of x-rays and MRI radio waves and the relative effect on irradiated tissue, complete the following:

	WAVELENGTH	FREQUENCY	ENERGY
1. Typical x-rays	A. 10^{-9} cm	B. 10^{19} cycles/sec.	C. 60,000 electron volts
2. MRI radio waves	A. _____	B. _____	C. _____

4. A. Which nucleus is most suitable for MR? _____

   B. Why? _____

5. Which component of the nucleus is affected by radio waves and static magnetic fields?

   _____

6. A typical cubic centimeter of the human body may contain approximately how many _____ hydrogen atoms?

   A. 1000   C. 10^{10}

   B. 10,000   D. 10^{20}

7. Define and briefly describe the term *precession*. (Compare this with some well-known phenomenon.)

   _____

8. The rate of precession of a proton in a magnetic field _____ (increases or decreases) as the strength of the magnetic field increases.

9. Precession occurs due to _____ acting on a spinning nuclei.

10. The angle of precession of protons can be altered by the introduction of _____.

11. How does an increase in the length of applicaton time of the radio wave affect the angle of precession?

    _____

12. Timing of the radio wave to the rate of the precessing nuclei is an example of the concept of

    _____ .

13. The signal that is received by the antenna or the receiving coil comes from which part of the atoms in the body tissues?

    _____

14. The nucleus emits _____ waves because it is a tiny magnet that is also

    _____ .

15. Relaxation of the nuclei as soon as the radiofrequency pulse is turned off can be divided into two categories:

    _____ and _____ .

16. T1 relaxation is known as _____ or *spin-lattice relaxation.* (Hint: Transverse or longitudinal)

17. T2 relaxation is known as _____ or spin-spin relaxation.   (Hint: Transverse or longitudinal)

18. The quantity of hydrogen nuclei per given volume of tissue is referred to as the _____ ,

    which is a _____ (major or minor) contributor to the appearance of the MR image.

19. Describe the main purpose of the gradient magnetic fields (the magnetic field strengths through only specific regions or slices of body tissue).

    _____

20. What are three primary factors that determine the signal strength and therefore the brightness of an image?

    _____

    _____

    _____

REVIEW EXERCISE E: Equipment Components (see textbook pp.769-772)

1. List the five main components of the MRI system.

    A. _____   D. _____

    B. _____   E. _____

    C. _____

2. The two units of measurement pertaining to magnetic fields are _____ and _____.

3. List the three types of MRI magnet systems and their approximate field strengths.   (The earth's magnetic field strength is provided as a comparison.)

Type of Magnet	*Field Strength*	
Earth _____	.00005_____	Tesla
A. _____	_____	Tesla
B. _____	_____	Tesla
C. _____	_____	Tesla

4. MRI systems generally include gradient coils in _____ directions.

5. What is the major advantage of the new 3.0 Tesla ultra-fast MRI imaging systems?

   _____

6. What is the major advantage of the flared or short bore design MRI imaging systems?

   _____

7. The radiofrequency coils act as _____ to both produce and detect the radio waves, which are referred to as the MRI "signal."

8. A. A circumferential whole-volume coil is one which _____.

   B. Two examples of this type of coil are the _____ and _____.

9. An example of a surface coil is the _____.

10. The display or workstation allows the technologist to control the operation of the system and view the images. List at least three variables that can be controlled or set at this workstation.

   A. _____

   B. _____

   C. _____

Summary of MRI Imaging Process and System Components Used

Following is a five-step summary of the entire MR imaging process. It identifies the component used and the results of each step:

STEP	COMPONENT	RESULT
1. Apply static magnetic field	_____	Nuclei align and precess
2. Select slice by applying gradient magnetic field (variation of magnetic field strength over patient)	_____	Nuclei precess at a particular frequency
3. Apply RF pulses	_____	Nuclei in the slice area precess in phase at a greater angle
4. Receive RF signal	RF receiving coil or antenna	_____
5. Convert signal to image	_____	Reconstructed image is displayed

Fig. 24-1 Summary of MRI process and system components used.

11.   Complete the omitted parts by filling in the blanks of the steps, components, and results as listed in the following summary of MRI imaging process and system components used (Fig. 24-1).

REVIEW EXERCISE F: Clinical Applications, Safety Considerations, and Appearance of Anatomy (see textbook pp. 773-777)

1.   Complete the following list of MRI safety concerns.

   A.   _____

   B.   _____

   C.   _____

   D.   Local heating of tissues and metallic objects

   E.   Electrical interference with normal functions of nerve cells and muscle fibers.

2.   The danger of projectiles becomes _____ (greater/lesser) as ferromagnetic objects are

   moved toward the scanner because the field strength is _____ (directly/inversely) propor-

   tional to the cube of the distance from the bore of the magnet.

3.   In a code blue situation, the patient is removed from the scan room due to the danger of _____ .

4.   Pacemakers are not allowed inside the _____ gauss line.

5.   As a general rule, O_2 tanks, IV pumps, and wheelchairs are not allowed inside the _____ gauss line.

6.   Magnetic tapes, credit cards, and cochlear implants are not allowed inside the _____ gauss line.

7. Identify the most important contraindication to MRI involving torquing of metallic objects.

   _____

8. The unit for measuring local heating of tissues is: _____ (Hint: Initials are SAR)

   _____

9. MRI has the ability to show anatomy in _____, _____, and

   _____ planes.

10. MRI has excellent _____, which allows visualization of soft tissue structures.

11. Diagnosis of diseases such as those involving the CNS can be made with MRI by comparing the signals produced

    in _____ tissues with those produced in _____ tissues (normal or

    abnormal).

12. List three types of histories that should be obtained from patients before an MRI exam.

    A. _____   C. _____

    B. _____

13. Name the IV contrast agent commonly used in MRI: _____.

14. Describe how this contrast agent affects T1 and T2 relaxation rates: _____

    _____

15. The average amount of contrast media given during an MRI examination is _____ ml/kg; the injection rate should

    not exceed _____ ml/min.

16. List eight absolute contraindications to patient MRI scanning.

    A. _____

    B. _____

    C. _____

    D. _____

    E. _____

    F. _____

    G. _____

    H. _____

17. Match the following pulse sequence description with the correct designation.

    _____ 1. Pulse sequences using a combination of short TR and short TE   A. T1 relaxation

    _____ 2. Pulse sequences using a combination of long TR and long TE   B. T2 relaxation

18. List the T1- and T2-weighted appearances for the following tissues: dark, bright, light gray, or dark gray

		T1	T2
A.	Cortical bone	Dark	Dark
B.	Red bone marrow	____	____
C.	Fat	____	____
D.	White brain matter	____	____
E.	CSF	____	____
F.	Muscle	____	____
G.	Vessels	____	____

19. True/False: Flowing blood is not visualized with a conventional spin-echo pulse sequence.

20. True/False: Tissues filled with air do not produce a T1 or T2 signal and therefore appear as bright.

REVIEW EXERCISE G: MRI Examinations (see textbook: pp. 778-781)

1. Complete the list of six structures or tissue types best demonstrated by MRI of the brain.

    A. Gray matter   D. _____

    B. _____   E. Basal ganglia

    C. _____   F. Brain stem

2. Complete the list of six possible pathologies demonstrated by MRI of the brain.

    A. _____   E. Hemorrhagic disorders

    B. _____   F. CVA

    C. _____

    D. _____

3. MRI of the brain is considered superior to the CT in visualizing the following three regions of the body or tissue types.

    A. _____

    B. _____

    C. _____

4. Which of the following technical factors may be used in spine imaging?

    A. T1-weighted sequence   C. Cardiac gating

    B. T2-weighted sequence   D. All of the above

5. Complete the list of seven structures best demonstrated by MRI of the spine.

    A. _____   E. Facet joint spaces

    B. _____   F. Basivertebral vein

    C. _____   G. Ligamentus flavum

    D. _____

6. List two major advantages of MR over CT imaging of the spine.

    A. _____

    B. _____

7. True/False: CT is superior to MRI for evaluation of spinal trauma.

8. Complete the list of structures best demonstrated by MRI of the limb or joints.

    A. _____   C. _____   E. Blood vessels

    B. _____   D. _____   F. Marrow

                                                        G. Fat

9. Complete the list of structures (organs) best demonstrated by MRI of the abdomen and pelvis.

    A. _____   E. _____

    B. _____   F. Kidneys

    C. _____   G. Vessels

    D. _____   H. Reproductive organs

10. True/False: Sonography and CT are the modalities of choice for demonstrating renal cysts.

11. True/False: Transrectal coils may be used to demonstrate prostate and other reproductive organs.

12.   Match the following terms with the correct definition (refer to textbook [pp. 782-783] for questions 12 and 13):

_____   1.   MR technique to minimize motion artifacts   A.   T2

_____   2.   False features on an image caused by patient instability or   B.   Tesla
               equipment deficiencies

_____   3.   Slow gyration of an axis of a spinning body caused by an   C.   Signal averaging
               application of torque

_____   4.   Method of improving SNR by averaging several FIDs or spin   D.   Acoustic neuroma
               echos

_____   5.   Spin lattice or longitudinal relaxation time   E.   Fringe field

_____   6.   SI unit of magnetic field intensity   F.   Schwannoma

_____   7.   Stray magnetic field that exists outside the imager   G.   Artifacts

_____   8.   A new growth of the white substance of the nerve sheath   H.   Gating

_____   9.   A tumor growing from nerve cells affecting the sense of hearing   I.   Precession

_____ 10.   Spin-spin or transverse relaxation time   J.   T1

13.   Match the following terms with the correct definition:

_____   1.   Measure of the geometric relationship between the RF coil and the body. A.   Contrast resolution

_____   2.   Atmospheric gases such as nitrogen and helium used for cooling   B.   Chordoma

_____   3.   Reappearance of an NMR signal after the FID has disappeared   C.   Turbulence

_____   4.   Amount of rotation of the net magnetization vector produced by an RF   D.   Spin echo
               pulse.

_____   5.   Force that causes or tends to cause a body to rotate   E.   Filling factor

_____   6.   Repetition time   F.   Meningioma

_____   7.   In flowing fluid, velocity component that fluctuates randomly   G.   Cryogen

_____   8.   A malignant tumor arising form the embryonic remains of the notocord   H.   Torque

_____   9.   A hard, slow growing vascular tumor   I.   TR

_____ 10.   Ability of an imaging process to distinguish adjacent soft tissue structures   J.   Flip angle
               from one another

Answers to Review Exercises

Review Exercise A: Nuclear Medicine

1. Radiopharmaceuticals
2. Tracers
3. D. All of the above
4. C. Technetium 99m
5. Single photon emission computed tomography
6. Three
7. Bone scintigraphy
8. A. Kidney transplants
9. B. Meckel's diverticulum
10. B. Thallium
11. D. Neo Tect
12. A. 1
    B. 3
    C. 1
    D. 1
    E. 2
    F. 3
    G. 2
    H. 3
    I. 1

Review Exercise B: Radiation Oncology

1. Heart-related diseases
2. A. Internal, brachytherapy
    B. External beam, teletherapy
3. Internal, brachytherapy
4. A. X-ray units
    B. Cobalt-60 gamma rays units
    C. Linear accelerator or betatron units
5. A. 1.25
6. D. High-speed electrons striking an anode
7. B. Linear accelerator
8. C. 4 to 30
9. Determine the area and volume of tissue to be treated
10. A. 3
    B. 1
    C. 1
    D. 4
    E. 2
    F. 4
    G. 1

Review Exercise C: Ultrasound

1. A. Sonography
    B. Ultrasonography
    C. Echosonography
2. 1 to 17
3. False (is not ideal for ileus)
4. False (not used for bone cyst)
5. True
6. False (in the early 1950s)
7. B. B-mode
8. D. Doppler

9. C. Increase in dynamic range
10. Converts electrical energy to ultrasonic energy
11. B. Ceramic
12. A. Piezoelectric effect
13. A. 2
    B. 1
    C. 3
14. True
15. True
16. B. Stomach
17. Amniocentesis
18. D. All of the above
19. D. All of the above
20. A. 8
    B. 3
    C. 9
    D. 1
    E. 7
    F. 5
    G. 10
    H. 4
    I. 2
    J. 6

Review Exercise D: Physical Principles of MRI

1. Magnetic fields and radio waves
2. Nuclei
3. 2. A. 10^3 to 10^{-2} meters
    B. 10^5 to 10^{10} hertz
    C. 10^{-7} electron volts
4. A. Hydrogen (single proton nucleus)
    B. The large amount of hydrogen present in any organism.
5. Proton
6. A. 1000
7. Is similar to the wobble of a slowly spinning top
8. Increases
9. An outside force (the magnetic field)
10. Radio waves
11. Increase in time increases the angle of precession
12. Resonance
13. Nucleus, or proton
14. Radio, precessing or rotating
15. T1 relaxation and T2 relaxation
16. Longitudinal
17. Transverse
18. Spin density, minor
19. So that the returning signal can be located (because only the precessing nuclei within these regions or slice transmit signals).
20. A. Spin density
    B. T1 relaxation rate
    C. T2 relaxation rate

Review Exercise E: Equipment Components

1. A. Magnet
    B. Gradient coils
    C. Radiofrequency coils
    D. Electronic support system
    E. Computer and display
2. Tesla and Gauss
3. A. Resistive, 0.3
    B. Permanent, 0.3
    C. Superconducting, 2.0 to 3.0
4. Three (3)
5. Improved signal-to-noise ratio for brain mapping and real-time brain acquisitions
6. Helps to alleviate claustrophobia
7. Antennas
8. A. Encircles the part being imaged
    B. Any two of the following: body coil, limb (extremity) coil, head coil, or volume neck coil
9. Shoulder coil or planar coil
10. Any three of the following:
    A. Select pulse sequences
    B. Adjust parameters such as signal averages and pulse repetition time (TR)
    C. Initiate scan, or alter brightness and contrast of image
11. 1. Magnet
    2. Gradient coils
    3. RF sending coil or antenna
    4. Electric signal is received from nuclei and sent to computer
    5. Computer

Review Exercise F: Clinical Application, Safety Considerations, and Appearance of Anatomy

1. A. Potential hazards of projectiles
    B. Electrical interference with implants
    C. Torquing of metallic objects
2. Greater, directly
3. Metallic objects used in blue code situations becoming projectiles
4. 5
5. 50
6. 10
7. Presence of intracranial aneurysm clips
8. Specific absorption ratio
9. Transverse, sagittal, and coronal
10. Contrast resolution
11. Normal, abnormal
12. A. Surgical history
    B. Occupational history
    C. Accidental history
13. Gd - DTPA (Gadolinium - DTPA)
14. Shortens T1 and T2 relaxation rates

15. 0.2, 10
16. A. Cardiac pacemakers
    B. Electronic implant
    C. Aneurysm clip in the brain
    D. Inner ear surgery
    E. Metallic fragments in the body
    F. Metal in and/or removed from the eye
    G. Eye prostheses
    H. Pregnancy
17. 1. A. (T1 relaxation)
    2. B. (T2 relaxation)
18.

	T1	T2
B. Red bone marrow	Light gray	Dark gray
C. Fat	Bright	Dark
D. White brain matter	Light gray	Dark gray
E. CSF	Dark	Bright
F. Muscle	Dark gray	Dark gray
G. Vessels	Dark	Dark

19. True
20. False (appears black)

Review Exercise G: MRI Examinations

1. B. White matter
   C. Nerve tissue
   D. Ventricles
2. A. White matter disease (multiple sclerosis or demyelinating disease)
   B. Ischemic disorders
   C. Neoplasm
   D. Infectious diseases (such as AIDS and herpes)
3. A. Posterior fossa
   B. Brainstem
   C. Detecting small changes in tissue water content
4. D. All of the above
5. A. Spinal cord
   B. Nerve tissue
   C. Intervertebral disks
   D. Bone marrow
6. A. MR does not require the use of intrathecal (within a sheath) contrast media
   B. It covers a large area of the spine in a single sagittal view
7. True
8. A. Fat and Muscle
   B. Ligaments
   C. Tendons
   D. Nerves
9. A. Liver
   B. Pancreas
   C. Spleen
   D. Adrenals
   E. Gallbladder
10. True
11. True
12. 1. H, 2. G, 3. I, 4. C, 5. J,
    6. B, 7. E, 8. F, 9. D, 10. A
13. 1. E, 2. G, 3. D, 4. J, 5. H,
    6. I, 7. C, 8. B, 9. F, 10. A

SELF-TEST

This self-test should be taken only after completing all of the readings, review exercises, and laboratory activities for a particular section. The purpose of this test is not only to provide a good learning exercise but also to serve as a good indicator of what your final evaluation grade will be. It is strongly suggested that if you do not get at least a 90% to 95% grade on this self-test, you should review those areas where you missed questions before going to your instructor for the final evaluation exam for this chapter. (There are 75 questions or blanks—each is worth 1.3 points.)

1. One of the most common radionuclides used in nuclear medicine is:

   A. Thallium
   B. Techetium 99m
   C. Cardiolyte
   D. Sulfur colloid

2. What type of imaging device used in nuclear medicine provides a three-dimensional image of anatomical structures?

   A. SPECT camera
   B. B-mode unit
   C. Linear accelerator
   D. Real-time scanner

3. An abnormal region detected during a nuclear medicine skeletal scan is described as a/an:

   A. Signal void
   B. Hot spot
   C. Acoustic shadow
   D. Region of high attenuation

4. Which one of the following is a common pathologic indicator for a nuclear medicine gastrointestinal study?

   A. Duodenal ulcer
   B. Bezoar
   C. Meckel's diverticulum
   D. Ileus

5. If a treadmill is not available for a nuclear medicine cardiac study, the patient is given:

   A. Glucagon
   B. Valium
   C. Lasix
   D. Vasodilator

6. True/False: The perfusion phase of a nuclear medicine lung ventilation/perfusion study is performed **before** the ventilation phase.

7. Which one of the following duties is *not* a typical responsibility of the nuclear medicine technologist?

   A. Calibrate instrumentation
   B. Process images
   C. Administer radionuclides
   D. Decontaminate area due to spills

8. Which one of the following is *not* an example of a teletherapy unit?

   A. Linear accelerator
   B. Neutron accelerator
   C. X-ray units
   D. Cobalt-60 unit

9. Linear accelerators deliver energy levels to target tissues between:

   A. 50 to 100 kVp
   B. 1.25 to 5.0 MeV
   C. 100 to 300 kVp
   D. 4 to 30 MeV

10. True/False: The patient is often skin-tattooed during radiation therapy simulations.

11. Which one of the following is *not* a responsibility of the radiation therapist?

    A. Uses fluoroscopy for treatment planning   C. Prescribes the treatment

    B. Interacts directly with patient   D. Maintains therapy records

12. Which of the following is *not* an alternative term for medical ultrasound?

    A. Echosonography   C. Piezosonography

    B. Sonography   D. Ultrasonography

13. Medical ultrasound operates at a frequency range between:

    A. 1 to 5 KHz   C. 1 to 17 KHz

    B. 25 to 50 KHz   D. 1 to 17 MHz

14. Which generation of ultrasound equipment first introduced gray scale imaging?

    A. A-mode   C. Real time dynamic

    B. B-mode   D. Doppler

15. An ultrasound transducer converts _____ energy to ultrasonic energy.

    A. Electrical   C. Light

    B. Heat   D. Magnetic

16. Which one of the following transducers would be used on a large abdomen?

    A. 3.5 MHz   C. 10 MHz

    B. 5.0 to 7.0 MHz   D. 17 MHz

17. True/False: A higher frequency transducer will increase penetration through the anatomy but will produce lower image resolution.

18. True/False: A normal gallbladder is an example of a *hyperechoic* structure.

19. True/False: Breast ultrasound is used primarily to distinguish between solid and cystic masses.

20. With color-flow Doppler, blood flowing away from the transducer is:

    A. Red   C. Blue

    B. Gray   D. Black

21. The MR image represents differences in the number of:

    A. X-rays attenuated   C. Frequencies of nuclei

    B. Nuclei and the rate of their recovery   D. Radio waves

22. MRI technique makes use of:

    A. X-rays   C. Sound waves

    B. Radio waves   D. Visible light

23. The nuclei in the body used to receive and re-emit radio waves are:

    A. Hydrogen   C. Oxygen

    B. Carbon   D. Phosphorus

24. The nuclei that receive and re-emit radio waves are under the influence of:

   A. Gravitational force
   C. X-ray energy
   B. The sun and the planets
   D. A static magnetic field

25. Which of the following properties results in a nucleus becoming a small magnet?

   A. An even number of neutrons and protons
   C. An even number of electrons
   B. An odd number of neutrons or protons
   D. The presence of a magnet

26. Precession occurs because spinning magnetic nuclei:

   A. Oscillate in the presence of other atoms
   C. Are acted on by a static magnetic field
   B. Regress under the face of a magnet
   D. Ionize atoms

27. A precessing nucleus causes _____ to occur in a nearby loop of wire.

   A. An alternating current
   C. A direct current
   B. A dipole
   D. Magnetic regression

28. Precession can be altered by the application of:

   A. X-rays
   C. Microwaves
   B. Radio frequency waves
   D. Visible light

29. Resonance occurs when radio waves are:

   A. Of the same frequency as the precessing nuclei
   C. At the same rate as T2 relaxation
   B. At the same rate as T1 relaxation
   D. Received by an antenna

30. The angle of precession of the nuclei is altered because the:

   A. Nuclei must be vertical
   C. Electrostatic properties of the nuclei dominate
   B. The magnetic force dominates
   D. MR signal is strongest when nuclei are horizontal

31. Emitted waves from the nuclei are _____ and sent to the computer.

   A. Evaluated
   C. In resonance
   B. Received by an antenna
   D. Precessing

32. The _____ among T1, T2, and spin density of tissues produces image contrast.

   A. Similarities
   C. Differences
   B. Phase
   D. Frequency

33. In T2 relaxation, the spins:

   A. Are vertical in orientation
   C. Are reduced in density
   B. Move to the north
   D. Become out of phase with one another

34. In T1 relaxation, the spins:

   A. Are relaxing to a vertical orientation
   C. Are reduced in density
   B. Stay in a horizontal position
   D. Become out of phase with one another

35. Spin density refers to the _____ of hydrogen nuclei.

   A. Quality
   C. Phase D
   B. Quantity
   D. Wavelength

36. The signal strength and thus the brightness of points in the image is primarily determined by:

   A. Differences in T1 and T2 relaxation rates of tissues
   C. The longitudinal component of nuclei

   B. Differences in spin density of tissues
   D. Exposure of the nuclei to the static magnetic field

37. Gradient magnetic fields are useful because:

   A. The strength is consistent along the patient

   B. The strength determines the frequency of the MR signal

   C. They allow the location of the signal to be moved

   D. The precessional rate of the nuclei must be constant

38. Gradient magnetic fields allow:

   A. Slice selection and locating the signal
   C. Slice selection and spin echo

   B. Locating the signal and relaxation of nuclei
   D. Spin echo and relaxation of nuclei

39. TR can be defined as:

   A. Time reversal
   C. Timing range

   B. Repetition time
   D. Time of resonance

40. TE can be defined as:

   A. Echo phase
   C. Temporary echo

   B. Time net
   D. Echo time

41. TR and TE have a profound influence upon:

   A. Image noise deletion
   C. Signal averaging

   B. Image contrast
   D. Image density

42. One Tesla equals:

   A. 10,000 times the earth's magnetic field
   C. 10 Gauss

   B. 0.00005 Gauss
   D. 10,000 Gauss

43. Superconducting magnet systems produce magnetic field strengths of up to:

   A. 2.0 or 3.0 Tesla
   C. 0.3 Tesla

   B. 1.0 Tesla
   D. 0.1 Tesla

44. Which one of the following diagrams (Fig. 24-2) is correctly labeled according to the x, y, and z gradient coils (A, B, or C)? _____

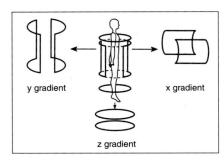
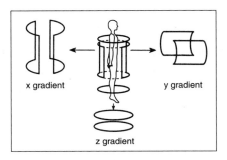
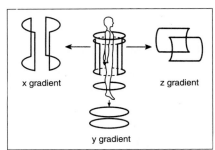

A   **B**   **C**

Fig. 24-2 Labeling of gradient coils.

45. Typical permanent magnet systems produce magnetic field strengths of up to:

    A. 2.0 Tesla   C. 0.3 Tesla

    B. 1.0 Tesla   D. 0.1 Tesla

46. Superconducting magnets require _____ to allow the low temperatures necessary for the property of superconductivity.

    A. Cryogens   C. Alternating electrical current

    B. Liquid hydrogen   D. Friction

47. The RF coils act as:

    A. The antennas to produce and receive radio waves   C. A shield from extraneous RF pulses

    B. A means of producing a gradient magnetic field   D. A superconducting magnet

48. Coils that are smaller than the body coil and that do not surround the anatomy are generally referred to as:

    A. Circumferential coils   C. Surface coils

    B. Whole-volume coils   D. Head coils

49. Which one of the following is not a similarity between MRI and CT?

    A. The outward appearance of the unit   C. The use of ionizing radiation

    B. The use of a computer to analyze information   D. Images viewed as a slice of tissue

50. Primary safety concerns for the technologist, patient, and medical personnel are due to:

    A. Fringe field strengths less than 1 Gauss

    B. Gravitational pull on metallic objects

    C. Magnetic fields and heat production

    D. Interaction of magnetic fields with metallic objects and tissues

51. Projectiles are a concern due to:

    A. Force of metallic objects being pulled to the magnet   C. Nerve cell function

    B. Fringe fields less than 10 Gauss   D. Local heating of tissues and metallic objects

52. Pacemakers are not allowed inside the:

    A. 5 Gauss line   C. 1.0 Gauss line

    B. 2.5 Gauss line   D. 0.5 Gauss line

53. IV pumps, wheelchairs, and O_2 tanks are not allowed inside the:

    A. 150 Gauss line   C. 5 Gauss line

    B. 50 Gauss line   D. 1 Gauss line

54. The most important contraindication in regard to torquing of metallic objects is:

    A. Intraabdominal surgical staples   C. Intracranial aneurysm clips

    B. Shrapnel   D. Hip prosthesis

55. Local heating of tissues (referred to as *SAR* or *specific absorption ratio*) is measured in:

    A. W/kg   C. RF frequency

    B. C°   D. F°

56. The contrast agent commonly used for MR examinations is:

    A. Iodine 131   C. Gadolinium oxysulfide

    B. Lanthanum oxybromide   D. Gadolinium-diethylene triamine pentaacetic acid

57. Contrast agents are generally used with:

    A. T1-weighted pulse sequences   C. Spin-density weighted pulse sequences

    B. T2-weighted pulse sequences   D. All of the above

58. Which of the following is considered a circumferential whole volume coil:

    A. Shoulder coil   C. Head coil

    B. C-spine coil   D. Planar coil

59. The three sets of gradient coils are typically:

    A. Visible on the external surface of the magnet

    B.   Situated in two different directions

    C. Located within the bore of the magnet or gantry

    D. All of the above

60. Surface coils improve:

    A. SNR   C. Safety

    B. Anatomical magnification   D. Heat dissipation

61. Proton (spin) density images use a pulse sequence that has a combination of:

    A. Long TR, short TE   C. Short TR, long TE

    B. Long TR, long TE   D. Short TR, short TE

62. T1-weighted images use a pulse sequence that has a combination of:

    A. Long TR, short TE   C. Short TR, long TE

    B. Long TR, long TE   D. Short TR, short TE

63. T2-weighted images use a pulse sequence that has a combination of:

    A. Long TR, short TE   C. Short TR, long TE

    B. Long TR, long TE   D. Short TR, short TE

64. On T1-weighted images, CSF will be:

    A. Dark   C. Same as white matter

    B. Bright   D. Same as gray matter

65. On T2-weighted images, CSF will be:

    A. Dark   C. Same as white matter

    B. Bright   D. Same as gray matter

66. MRI of the brain allows visualization of:

    A. White matter disease   C. Small calcifications

    B. Acute blood   D. Fractures

67. MRI of the brain includes the use of a standard head coil and:

    A. Prone position   C. Sedation

    B. Cardiac gating   D. T1- and T2-weighted pulse sequences

68. Which of the following is not best evaluated by MRI of the spine:

    A. Bone marrow changes   C. Disk herniation

    B. Cord abnormalities   D. Scoliosis

69. MRI of the lumbar spine requires the patient to be positioned:

    A. Feet first, prone   C. Head first, prone

    B. Feet first, supine   D. Head first, supine

70. MRI of the joints or limbs demonstrates all of the following except:

    A. Ligaments   C. Muscle

    B. Tendons   D. Skin

71. During MRI of the joints, the patient must lie so that the anatomy of interest is:

    A. Centered to the coil, coil then moved to magnet center   C. Prone and centered to the magnet

    B. Supine and centered to the magnet   D. None of the above

72. The patient is positioned for abdominopelvic MRI by placing the patient:

    A. Prone, head first   C. Prone, feet first

    B. Supine, feet first   D. Supine, head first

73. The largest drawback for MRI of the abdomen is:

    A. Motion artifacts   C. Coil selection

    B. Metallic implants   D. Sequence times

74. A RF pulse sequence for MRI in which the net magnetization is inverted is called:

    A. Inversion recovery   C. Flip angle

    B. Spin-echo   D. Saturation recovery

75. A mathematical procedure to separate frequency components of a signal from its amplitudes is called:

    A. Gradient moment nulling   C. Fourier transformation

    B. Signal averaging   D. Free induction decay

SELF-TEST ANSWERS

Chapter 14 Upper Gastrointestinal System

1. C. Production of hormones
2. C. Pineal
3. Barium swallow
4. Mumps
5. A. Mastication
6. B. Epiglottis
7. D. T11
8. A. Trachea
9. Peristalsis
10. Stomach
11. D. Incisura angularis
12. A. Fundus
13. False (in the stomach)
14. False (the greater curvature)
15. Fundus
16. Head of pancreas and C-loop of duodenum
17. 1. E, 2. F, 3. I, 4. H, 5. C, 6. A, 7 D, 8. G, 9. B
18. A. Distal esophagus
    B. Region of esophagogastric junction
    C. Fundus
    D. Greater curvature
    E. Body
    F. Pyloric antrum
    E. Pyloric canal
    H. Pyloric orifice (sphincter)
    I. Descending portion of duodenum
    J. Duodenal bulb
    K. Lesser curvature
19. A. Prone
    B. Air in fundus
20. Lateral
21. A. Supine
    B. Barium-filled fundus (air in pylorus)
22. A. Posterior
    B. Air in pylorus indicated semi-supine position
    C. (p. 440) RAO
    D. Air in fundus indicated a semi-prone position and duodenal bulb and C-loop in profile indicated an RAO and not an LAO.
23. Chyme
24. A. Vitamins
25. C. Rhythmic segmentation
26. Hyposthenic or asthenic, L3-4
27. Hypersthenic, T11-12
28. Barium sulfate
29. Carbon dioxide
30. A. Three or four parts of barium to one part of water
    B. One part barium to one part water

31. When there is a possibility that the contrast media may spill into the peritoneum (such as pre-surgery or a perforated bowel)
32. Output
33. C. 1000 to 6000 times
34. True
35. Lower
36. B. 0.50
37. A. Zenker's diverticulum
38. B. Nuclear medicine
39. D. Trapped vegetable fiber in the stomach
40. To detect signs of esophageal reflux (also see question 49 and answer)
41. 35 to 40°
42. The RAO visualizes the esophagus between the heart and vertebra better than an LAO.
43. Majority of esophagus is superimposed over the spine and thus is not well visualized
44. Shredded cotton or marshmallows
45. Right lateral
46. Reduce patient oblique to less than 40 degrees for asthenic patient.
47. Supine position for an AP projection
48. To rule-out esophageal varices (a condition of dilation of the veins, which in advanced stages may lead to internal bleeding)
49. The Valsalva maneuver, to rule out esophageal reflux (a condition wherein gastric contents return back through the gastric orifice into the esophagus causing irritation of esophageal lining).
50. An ulcer

Chapter 15 Lower Gastrointestinal System

1. A. 15 to 18 ft (4.5 to 5.5 m)
2. C. Ileum
3. D. Suspensory ligament of the duodenum
4. A. Ileum
5. C. Jejunum
6. A. Cecum
   B. Rectum
7. Veniform appendix
8. True
9. False (these are in large intestine)
10. Left
11. A. Jejunum
    B. Ileum
    C. Region of ileocecal valve
    D. Duodenum
    E. Pyloric portion of stomach
    F. Left colic (splenic) flexure

G. Descending colon
H. Sigmoid colon
I. Rectum
J. Cecum
K. Ascending colon
L. Right colic (hepatic)flexure
M. Transverse colon
12. C. Transverse colon
13. B. Large intestine
14. B. Rhythmic segmentation
15. 1. F, 2. D, 3. I, 4. L, 5. B, 6. G, 7. J, 8. C, 9. A, 10. E, 11. M, 12. K, 13. H
16. 1. D, 2. G, 3. E, 4. H, 5. A, 6. C, 7. B, 8. F
17. A. Barium enema
18. False
19. Hold breath on expiration
20. Produces compression of the abdomen that leads to separation of the loops of small intestine
21. 8 hours
22. Cathartic
23. Rectal retention enema tip
24. Glucagon
25. Lidocaine
26. D. Prolapse of rectum
27. B. Anorectal angle
28. True
29. RAO
30. Two hours
31. D. Anatrast
32. C. Center chamber only
33. 35 to 45 degrees
34. 2 inches (5 cm)
35. Defecography
36. LPO
37. Right lateral decubitus will drain excess barium from the descending colon allowing for detection of small polyp
38. Evacuative proctography
39. False
40. False
41. True
42. D. 2000 to 3000 mrad
43. A. Right. Iliac crest
    B. Left. 1 to 2 inches (2.5 to 5 cm) above the iliac crest

Chapter 16 Gallbladder and Biliary Ducts

1. A. Anterior inferior
2. C. Inferior
4. Falciform ligament
5. To break down or emulsify fats
6. Common hepatic duct
7. 30 to 40 cc
8. Hydrolysis

9. Cholecystokinin (CCK)
10. Common bile duct
11. 1. H, 2. F, 3. G, 4. A, 5. I, 6. B, 7. D, 8. E, 9. C
12. Supine, because the body and fundus of the gallbladder are anterior and the neck and cystic duct posterior
13. A. Fundus
   B. Body
   C. Neck
   D. Cystic duct
   E. Duodenum
   F. Common bile duct
   G. Common hepatic duct
   H. Right hepatic duct
   I. Left hepatic duct
14. 1. H, 2. I, 3. A, 4. B, 5. C, 6. F, 7. E, 8. G, 9. D
15. True
16. True
17. 1. C, 2. D, 3. E, 4. G, 5. B, 6. A, 7. F
18. At least 8 hours
19. 10 to 12 hours before the procedure
20. 70 to 76 kVp
21. Allow for better drainage of the gallbladder and free superimposition of biliary ducts and gallbladder from spine
22. 5 to 10 minutes
23. False (the patient needs to be NPO only 4 hours before the ultrasound procedure)
24. True
25. Through a small catheter placed into the remnant portion of the cystic duct after the gallbladder has been surgically removed
26. 6 to 8 cc
27. The grid must be turned crosswise to prevent grid cutoff.
28. A much smaller incision is required with the laparoscopic technique.
29. To detect postoperatively in the radiology department any residual stones in the biliary ducts that may have gone undetected during the cholecystectomy
30. B. Obstructive jaundice
31. D. Skinny needle
32. A. R, B. S, C. R
33. True
34. True
35. True
36. False
37. True
38. Center chamber
39. Operative cholangiogram is "immediate," performed during surgery, and the T-tube cholangiogram is "delayed," or done in radiology following surgery.

40. Increase the obliquity of the LAO position
41. Because of the more anterior location of the gallbladder
42. Either the erect, PA, or a right lateral decubitus positions will stratify or "layer" any possible stones in the gallbladder.
43. RPO
44. Keep the patient NPO for 4 hours then perform an ultrasound study of the gallbladder.
45. D. PTC

Chapter 17 Urinary System

1. A. Retroperitoneal
2. C. Posterolateral
3. Anterior
4. 30 degree
5. A. Uteropelvic junction
   B. Near brim of pelvis
   C. Ureterovesical (UV) junction
6. 2 inches, 5 cm
7. Uremia
8. D. 1.5 liter
9. D. Inferior vena cava
10. Renal pyramids
11. Renal pelvis
12. Nephron
13. True
14. False (99% is reabsorbed)
15. Trigone
16. A. Urinary bladder
   B. Ureter
   C. Ureteropelvic junction
   D. Renal pelvis
   E. Major calyces
   F. Minor calyces
17. Retrograde pyelogram (Note catheter in right ureter)
18. When the benefit of the procedure outweighs the risks of the radiation exposure
19. Ionic and nonionic
20. 1. I, 2. N, 3. I, 4. I, 5. I, 6. N, 7. I, 8. N, 9. I, 10. N
21. B. 0.6 to 1.5 mg/dl
22. A. 48 hours
23. C. Diabetes mellitus
24. A. Observe and reassure patient
25. B. Mild reaction
26. B. Mild reaction
27. D. Severe reaction
28. C. Moderate reaction
29. C. Axillary vein
30. 20 to 45 degrees
31. Anuria or anuresis
32. Lithotripsy
33. D. Vesicourethral reflux
34. A. Renal obstruction
35. A. Ectopic kidney
36. True
37. True
38. B. Ureteric calculi
39. 20 minutes following injection

40. Nephrogram or nephrotomography; immediately after completion of injection
41. Retrograde urethrogram on a male patient
42. Left posterior oblique (LPO)
43. False (higher for female)
44. False (primarily the ureter)
45. Angle the CR more caudally to project the symphysis pubis inferior to the bladder.

Chapter 18 Mammography

1. Mammography Quality Standards Act, 1994
2. Only VA facilities
3. 40
4. 8
5. Inframammary crease
6. Upper, outer quadrant (UOQ)
7. 11 o'clock
8. Pectoralis major muscle
9. Lactation or production of milk
10. Cooper's ligaments
11. Adipose (fatty)
12. Trabeculae
13. Base
14. A. Fibro-glandular
15. B. Fibro-fatty
16. C. Fatty
17. A. Fibro-fatty
18. A. Glandular tissue
   B. Nipple
   C. Adipose (fatty) tissue
   D. Pectoral muscle
   E. Mediolateral oblique (MLO)
   F. Axillary
19. Molybdenum
20. Apex
21. True (only not for implants)
22. True
23. False (grid is used due to the large amount of scatter and secondary)
24. 0.1 mm
25. 2x the original size of the object
26. B. 200 to 300 mrad (130 to 150 per projection)
27. Sonography (ultrasound)
28. Magnetic resonance imaging (MRI)
29. True
30. False (patient dose reduced by minimizing repeats)
31. True
32. A. Sulphur colloid
33. Noninvasive and invasive
34. D. XCCL
35. MLO
36. A. Craniocaudal (CC)
   B. Mediolateral oblique (MLO)
37. Mediolateral oblique projection
38. 25 to 28 kVp
39. Laterally exaggerated craniocaudal (XCCL) projection
40. LMO

41. Over
42. A. Eklund
    B. Implant displaced (ID)
43. Axillary tail view (AT); sometimes called the *Cleopatra view*
44. Axillary side
45. Have patient hold the breast back with her opposite hand
46. MLO (mediolateral oblique)
47. XXCL (laterally exaggerated cranio-caudad)
48. Inframammary crease at its upper limits
49. B. Mediolateral oblique
50. C. Use manual exposure factors

Chapter 19 Trauma and Mobile Radiography

1. A. Spiral fracture
   B. Compound fracture
   C. Comminuted fracture
   D. Greenstick fracture
   E. Colles' fracture
   F. Impacted fracture
   G. Compression fracture
   H. Stellate fracture
   I. Pott's fracture
2. A. Dislocation or luxation
   B. Subluxation
3. Spine (although, it can occur in the elbow as well)
4. B. lack of apposition
5. A. valgus angulation
6. 1. E, 2. I, 3. D, 4. H, 5. A, 6. B, 7. C, 8. G, 9. F
7. True
8. True
9. D AP shoulder
10. B 6:1 to 8:1
11. A. Grid frequency
    B. Grid ratio
12. True
13. Battery-operated, battery driven
14. Standard power source
15. False (mobile fluoroscopy units)
16. True
17. False (PA is recommended due to less exposure to operator and less OID)
18. True
19. Roadmapping
20. Reducing patient dose
21. A. Time
    B. Distance
    C. Shielding
22. Distance
23. A. less than 10 mR/hr
24. 4 mR (30 ÷ 60 × 8 = 4)
25. False (greater on tube side)
26. False (by a factor of four)
27. A right lateral decubitus
28. 3 to 4 in (7 to 10 cm) below the jugular notch

29. 15 to 20° mediolateral angle and horizontal beam lateral projections
30. C left lateral decubitus
31. Two
32. Parallel to the interepicondylar plane
33. A horizontal beam lateromedial projection
34. 25 to 30°, or until the CR can be projected parallel to the scapular blade (wing)
35. 10° posteriorly from perpendicular to the plantar surface of the foot
36. Perform a cross-angle CR projection of the ankle, with CR 15 to 20° lateromedial from the long axis of the foot
37. C affected leg is rotated 10 to 20° internally if possible
38. A 35 to 40° cephalad AP axial projection
39. C double angle oblique with IR perpendicular to CR
40. A. it reduces distortion
    B. the long OID produces an air gap effect, which improves image quality without the use of a grid thus allowing a double CR angle (which would cause grid cutoff if a grid were used)
41. B trauma, horizontal beam lateral
42. A. Crosswise
    B. 2 in. (5 cm) superior to EAM
43. C. Lateral
44. A. AP or PA and lateral wrist
45. D. Epiphyseal

Chapter 20 Pediatric Radiography

1. B. 2 years
2. D. Describe the . . .
3. D. Do none of the abovex
4. D. Hold-em Tiger
5. C. Pigg-O-Stat
6. A. Proper immobilization
   B. Short exposure times
   C. Accurate technique charts
7. Is she pregnant?
8. C. Pigg-O-Stat
9. D. 3-D ultrasound
10. B. Functional MRI
11. A. 4, B. 9, C. 7, D. 2, E. 13, F. 3, G. 12, H. 11, I. 1, J. 6, K. 10, L. 8, M. 5
12. A. (+), B. (+), C. (−), D. (+), E. (−), F. (+), G. (−)
13. C. Extend arms upward
14. 55 to 65 kVp
15. True
16. True
17. Kite method
18. Between the umbilicus and just above the pubis

19. 1. D, 2. E, 3. EP, 4. D, 5. E and EP
20. 1. B, 2. B, 3. E, 4. A, 5. E, 6. D, 7. A, 8. B, 9. D, 10. A, 11. E, 12. A, 13. A
21. D. 30°
22. B. Midway between glabella and inion
23. A. 4 hours
24. Diminish the risk of aspiration from vomiting
25 C. Appendicitis
26. A. Level of iliac crest
    B. 1 in. (2.5 cm) above umbilicus
27. Mammillary (nipple) level
28. 6 to 12 ounces
29. Manually, very slowly, using a 60 ml syringe and a #10 French flexible silicone catheter
30. No bowel prep is required
31. When the bladder is full and when voiding
32. One
33. A. Vesicoureteral reflux
    B. Before
34. False (shielding should be used in all positions using tape when necessary)
35. True

Chapter 21 Angiography and Interventional Procedures

1. D. Right and left coronary arteries
2. D. Right common carotid
3. C. Upper margin of thyroid cartilage
4. A. Pulmonary veins
5. C. Right common carotid
6. A. Anterior portion of brain
7. B. Anterior and middle cerebral arteries
8. D. Basilar artery
9. D. Sphenoid
10. C. Internal and external cerebral veins
11. B. Internal jugular vein
12. C. Azygos vein
13. 1. E, 2. J, 3. D, 4. I, 5. K, 6. B, 7. F, 8. H, 9. G, 10. A, 11. L, 12. C
14. False (from brachiocephalic)
15. False (median cubital vein)
16. True
17. True
18. B. Synthesize simple carbohydrates
19. C. 8
20. 1. O, 2. Q, 3. P, 4. N, 5. L, 6. D, 7 A, 8. K, 9. R, 10. M, 11. G, 12. C, 13. F, 14. B, 15. H
21. C. Body temperature
22. B. Color duplex ultrasound
23. False (Does not need to be used)
24. True

25. C. Coarctation
26. C. 8 to 10 seconds
27. B. Pulmonary emboli
28. A. Femoral vein
29. A. 45 RPO
30. C. Left ventricle
31. D. 15 to 30 frames per second
32. D. Malabsorption syndrome
33. C. 30 to 40 ml
34. False (unilateral for upper limb but bilateral for lower limb)
35. True
36. A. Helps to visualize the lymph vessels
37. True
38. False (oil-based is used. Water-soluble is too quickly absorbed)
39. D. Hepatic malignancies
40. 1. C, 2. D, 3. F, 4. A, 5. G, 6. B, 7. E
41. False (placed inferior to renal veins)
42. True

Chapter 22 Computed Tomography

1. A. First generation
2. C and D, third and fourth generation
3. Slip rings
4. A. 1%
5. Source collimator
6. Assign various shades of gray to the numerical values
7. A. Scan unit
   B. Operator control console
8. Pixel
9. D. Vertical adjustment of table height
10. Blood-brain barrier
11. C. Multiple sclerosis
12. B and E Possible neoplasia and brain tumor
13. C. 1972
14. A. Dendrites
    B. Axon
15. Meninges
16. A. Dura mater
    B. Arachnoid
    C. Pia mater
17. A. Pia mater
    B. Arachnoid mater
    C. Dura mater
    D. Venous sinus
    E. Epidural space
    F. Subdural space
    G. Subarachnoid spaces
18. Subarachnoid space
19. 1. C, 2. C, 3. A, 4. A, 5. C
20. Cerebrum
21. Longitudinal fissure
22. Corpus callosum
23. Falx cerebri

24. A. Lateral ventricles
25. C. Cisterna cerebellomedullaris
26. A. Lateral
    B. Third
    C. Fourth
    a. Interventricular foramen
    b. Cerebral aqueduct
    c. Lateral recess
    1. Body
    2. Anterior horn
    3. Inferior (temporal) horn
    4. Posterior horn
    5. Pineal gland
27. Hydrocephalus, ventricles
28. Cisterns
29. A. Frontal
    B. Parietal
    C. Occipital
    D. Temporal
    E. Insula or central lobe
30. 1. A, 2. B, 3. B, 4. B, 5. B, 6. A
31. C. Longitudinal fissure
32. A. Pons
33. D. Mid brain
34. B. Inferior portion of manubrium
35. A. Sternal notch
36. C. Aortopulmonary window
37. A. Base of heart
38. Aortopulmonary window
39. A. Ascending aorta
40. C. Left atrium
41. D. Mitral valve prolapse
42. A. 10 mm
43. D. The hooklike extension of the head of the pancreas
44. D. All of the above
45. D. All of the above
46. D. Symphysis pubis
47. C. Urinary bladder
48. B. 10 mm
49. B. High concentration of a large bolus of barium is present with a low concentration of water
50. C. Xiphoid process
51. True
52. False (They speed up peristaltic action)
53. False (Need to hold breath)
54. True
55. True

Chapter 23 Additional Imaging Procedures

1. Orthoroentgenography
2. False (Ends of bone must be on separate projections)
3. False (Is a premature fusion of the epiphysis to shorten a bone)
4. True
5. True
6. Bell-Thompson ruler

7. 24 x 39 cm (10 x 12 in.) or 30 x 35 cm (11 x 14 in.) with three exposures placed on the same IR
8. A. Knee
   B. Shoulder
9. A. Sensitivity to iodine
   B. Sensitivity to local anesthetics
10. Knee
11. A. Iodinated water soluble, 5 cc
    B. Room air, 80 to 100 cc
12. 20 gauge
13. To provide a thin, even coating of positive contrast media over the soft tissues of the knee joint
14. 18 x 43 cm (7 x 17 in.)
15. A. 6, B. 30°
16. The conjoined tendons of the four major shoulder muscles
17. A. AP internal and external rotation shoulder scout
    B. AP internal rotation
    C. AP external rotation
    D. Glenoid fossa projection (Grashey)
    E. Transaxillary (inferosuperior axial) projection
    F. Bicipital (intertubercular) groove projection
18. A. Herniated nucleus pulposus (HNP)
    B. Cancerous or benign tumors
    C. Cysts
19. A. Blood in the cerebrospinal fluid
    B. Arachnoiditis
    C. Increased intracranial pressure
    D. Recent lumbar puncture (2 weeks)
20. C HNP
21. C Trendelenburg
22. A L3-4
24. D blockage at T-spine level
25. 30, 24
26. Horizontal beam swimmer's lateral
27. Body section radiography
28. 1. D, 2. F, 3. C, 4. A, 5. E, 6. B
29. 1. A, 2. C, 3. D, 4. B, 5. E
30. A. Variable fulcrum
    B. Fixed fulcrum
31. True
32. False (is the exposure angle)
33. True
34. True
35. True
36. A 2 to 3 seconds
37. A. Fundus
    B. Corpus or body
    C. Isthmus
    D. Cervix
38. A. Osseometrium
39. False (connect to the uterus at the corna)

40. A. Acute pelvic inflammatory disease
    B. Active uterine bleeding
41. False (water-soluble is preferred)
42. True
43. A. 2
    B: 3
    C: 1
44. B. Severe inflammation of the salivary gland or duct
45. Water-soluble contrast media
46. A. Excessive physical activity
47. A. Fan-beam x-ray source
48. B. Healthy individual with peak bone mass
49. A. Higher patient dose
    B. More expensive as compared to other bone densitometry systems
50. Os calcis or calcaneus

Chapter 24 Additional Diagnostic and Therapeutic Modalities

1. B. Techetium 99m
2. A. SPECT camera
3. B. Hot spot
4. C. Meckel's diverticulum
5. D. Vasodilator
6. False (during the ventilation phase)
7. A. Calibrate instrumentation
8. B. Neutron accelerator
9. D. 4 to 30 MeV
10. True
11. C. Prescribes the treatment
12. C. Piezosonography
13. D. 1 to 17 MHz
14. B. B-mode
15. A. Electrical

16. A. 3.5 MHz
17. False (higher resolution)
18. False (gall bladder is anechonic)
19. True
20. C. Blue
21. B. Nuclei and the rate of their recovery
22. B. Radio waves
23. A. Hydrogen
24. D. A static magnetic field
25. B. An odd number of neutrons or protons
26. C. Are aced on by a static magnetic
27. A. An alternating current
28. B. Radio frequency waves
29. A. Of the same frequency as the precessing nuclei
30. D. MR signal is strongest when nuclei are horizontal
31. B. Received by an antenna
32. C. Differences
33. D. Become out of phase with one another
34. A. Are relaxing to a vertical orientation
35. B. Quantity
36. A. Differences in T1 and T2 relaxation rates of tissues nuclei
37. B. The strength determines the frequency of the MR signal
38. A. Slice selection and locating the signal
39. B. Repetition time
40. D. Echo time
41. B. Image contrast
42. D. 10,000 Gauss
43. A. 2.0 or 3.0 Tesla
44. B.

45. C. 0.3 tesla
46. A. Cryogens
47. A. The antennas to produce and receive radio waves
48. C. Surface coils
49. C. The use of ionizing radiation
50. D. Interaction of magnetic fields with metallic objects and tissues
51. A. Force of metallic objects being pulled to the magnet
52. A. 5 Gauss line
53. B. 50 Gauss line
54. C. Intracranial aneurysm clips
55. A. W/kg
56. D. Gadolinium-diethylene triamine pentaacetic acid
57. A. T1-weighted pulse sequences
58. C. Head coil
59. C. Located in bore of magnet
60. A. SNR
61. A. Long TR, short TE
62. D. Short TR, short TE
63. B. Long TR, long TE
64. A. Dark
65. B. Bright
66. A. White matter disease
67. D. T1- and T2-weighted pulse sequences
68. D. Scoliosis
69. B. Feet-first, supine
70. D. Skin
71. A. Centered to the coil, coil then moved to magnet center
72. B. Supine, feet first
73. A. Motion artifacts
74. A. Inversion recovery
75. C. Fourier transformation

The Human Comedy

PARISIAN LIFE

VOLUME IX

PEARSON CUSTOM LIBRARY

MGT 150: Principles of Management

Custom for York College of Pennsylvania
Stephen P. Robbins & Mary Coulter

PEARSON

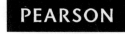

ISBN 10: 1-269-80934-2
ISBN 13: 978-1-269-80934-4

PEARSON

Table of Contents

Managers in the Workplace

From Chapter 1 of *Management*, Thirteenth Edition. Stephen P. Robbins and Mary Coulter. Copyright © 2016 by Pearson Education, Inc. All rights reserved.

It's Your Career

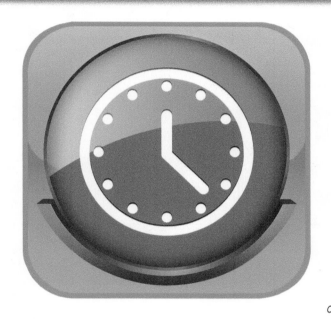

Source: valentint/Fotolia

A key to success in management and in your career is having *good time management skills.*

The ABC's of Managing Your Time

Are you BUSY? Do you always seem to have a lot to do and never seem to get it done, or done on time, or are things done at the last minute under a lot of pressure and stress? If you're like most people, the answer to these questions is YES! Well, maybe in a management textbook we need to do something about that by focusing on one aspect of management that can be tremendously useful to you...TIME MANAGEMENT! Time is a unique resource and one of your most valuable resources. First, if it's wasted, it can never be replaced. People talk about saving time, but time can never actually be saved. Second, unlike resources such as money or talent, which are distributed unequally in the world, time is an equal-opportunity resource. Each one of us gets exactly the same amount of time: 10,080 minutes a week. But as you have undoubtedly observed, some people are a lot more efficient in using their allotment. Commit to improving your ability to manage those 10,080 minutes so you can be more efficient and effective—in your career and in your personal life! Here are some suggestions to help you better use your time:

1. ***Make and keep a list of all your current, upcoming, and routine goals.*** *Know what needs to be done daily, weekly, and monthly.*
2. ***Rank your goals according to importance.*** *Not all goals are of equal importance. Given the limitations on your time, you want to make sure you give highest priority to the most important goals.*
3. ***List the activities/tasks necessary to achieve your goals.*** *What specific actions do you need to take to achieve your goals?*
4. ***Divide these activities/tasks into categories using an A, B, and C classification.*** *The As are important and urgent. Bs are either important or urgent, but not both. Cs are routine—not important nor urgent, but still need to be done.*

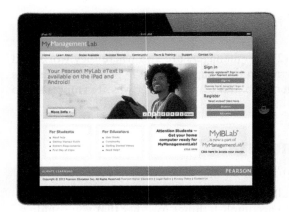

MyManagementLab®

⭐ **Improve Your Grade!**

When you see this icon, visit **www.mymanagementlab.com** for activities that are applied, personalized, and offer immediate feedback.

Learning Objectives

● **SKILL OUTCOMES**

1 **Explain** *why managers are important to organizations.*

2 **Tell** *who managers are and where they work.*

  ● **Know how to** manage your time.

3 **Describe** *the functions, roles, and skills of managers.*

  ● **Develop your skill** at being politically aware.

4 **Describe** *the factors that are reshaping and redefining the manager's job.*

5 **Explain** *the value of studying management.*

---

5. Schedule your activities/tasks according to the priorities you've set. *Prepare a daily plan. Every morning, or at the end of the previous workday, make a list of the five or so most important things you want to do for the day. Then set priorities for the activities listed on the basis of importance and urgency.*

6. Plan your to-do list each day so that it includes a mixture of A, B, and C activities/ tasks. *And it's best to spread the three types of tasks throughout your day so you're not lumping together all*

your demanding tasks. Also, be realistic about what you can achieve in a given time period.

7. Realize that priorities may change as your day or week proceeds. *New information may change a task's importance or urgency. As you get new information, reassess your list of priorities and respond accordingly.*

8. Remember that your goal is to manage getting your work done as efficiently and effectively as you can. *It's not to become an expert at creating to-do lists. Find what works best for you and use it!*

Like many students, you've probably had a job (or two) at some time or another while working on your degree. And your work experiences, regardless of where you've worked, are likely to have been influenced by the skills and abilities of your manager. What are today's successful managers like and what skills do they need in dealing with the problems and challenges of managing in the twenty-first century? This text is about the important work that managers do. The reality facing today's managers—and that might include you in the near future—is that the world is changing. In workplaces of all types—offices, stores, labs, restaurants, factories, and the like—managers deal with changing expectations and new ways of managing employees and organizing work. In this text, we introduce you to managers and management by looking

at (1) why managers are important, (2) who managers are and where they work, and (3) what managers do. Finally, we wrap up the chapter by (4) looking at the factors reshaping and redefining the manager's job and (5) discussing why it's important to study management.

WHY are managers important?

L01 What can a great boss do?

- Inspire you professionally and personally
- Energize you and your coworkers to accomplish things together that you couldn't get done by yourself
- Provide coaching and guidance with problems
- Provide you feedback on how you're doing
- Help you to improve your performance
- Keep you informed of organizational changes
- Change your life[1]

If you've worked with a manager like this, consider yourself lucky. Such a manager can make going to work a lot more enjoyable and productive. However, even managers who don't live up to such lofty ideals and expectations are important to organizations. Why? Let's look at three reasons.

The first reason why managers are important is because *organizations need their managerial skills and abilities* more than ever in uncertain, complex, and chaotic times. As organizations deal with today's challenges—changing workforce dynamics, the worldwide economic climate, changing technology, ever-increasing globalization, and so forth—managers play an important role in identifying critical issues and crafting responses. For example, at LVMH, the world's luxury-goods leader, you'd expect to find a team of exceptionally talented and creative innovators like Karl Lagerfeld, Carol Lim, Marc Jacobs, and Phoebe Philo. In the luxury-goods business, creative design and prestigious brands are vital. But it takes more than that to be successful. In this competitive industry, it takes more than creative design...there has to be a focus on commercial potential. That's why, behind the scenes, you'd also find a team of managers who scrutinize ideas and focus on the question: *Is this marketable?* These managers realize what is critical to success. The opposite "types" have worked together and created a successful business.[2]

Another reason why managers are important to organizations is because *they're critical to getting things done.* For instance, AT&T has some 6,750 general managers who manage the work of thousands of frontline employees.[3] These managers deal with all kinds of issues as the company's myriad tasks are carried out. They create and coordinate the workplace environment and work systems so that others can perform those tasks. Or, if work isn't getting done or isn't getting done as it should be, they're the ones who find out why and get things back on track. And these managers are key players in leading the company into the future.

Finally, *managers do matter* to organizations! How do we know that? The Gallup Organization, which has polled millions of employees and tens of thousands of managers, has found that the single most important variable in employee productivity and loyalty isn't pay or benefits or workplace environment—it's the quality of the relationship between employees and their direct supervisors.[4] In addition, global consulting firm Towers Watson found that the way a company manages and engages its people can significantly affect its financial performance.[5] That's scary considering another study by Towers Watson that found only 42 percent of respondents think their leaders inspire and engage them.[6] In yet another study by different researchers, 44 percent of the respondents said their supervisors strongly increased engagement.[7] However, in this same study, 41 percent of respondents also said their supervisors strongly decreased engagement. And, a different study of organizational performance found that managerial ability was important in creating organizational value.[8] So, as

you can see, managers can and do have an impact—positive and negative. What can we conclude from such reports? Managers are important—and they *do* matter!

WHO are managers and where
LO2 **do they work?**

Managers may not be who or what you might expect! Managers can range in age from 18 to 80+. They run large corporations, medium-sized businesses, and entrepreneurial start-ups. They're also found in government departments, hospitals, not-for-profit agencies, museums, schools, and even nontraditional organizations such as political campaigns and music tours. Managers can also be found doing managerial work in every country on the globe. In addition, some managers are top-level managers while others are first-line managers. And today, managers are just as likely to be women as they are men; however, the number of women in top-level manager positions remains low—only 45 women were CEOs of Fortune 1000 corporations in 2013.[9] But no matter where managers are found or what gender they are, managers have exciting and challenging jobs!

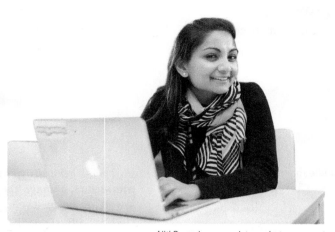

Ajiti Banga is an associate product manager at Pocket Gems, a firm in San Francisco that makes and publishes mobile games such as Pet Tap Hotel and Paradise Cove. Collaborating with multiple teams of engineers and designers, Banga manages games from initial concept through development to product launch.
Source: REUTERS/Stephen Lam

Who Is a Manager?

It used to be fairly simple to define who managers were: They were the organizational members who told others what to do and how to do it. It was easy to differentiate *managers* from *nonmanagerial employees*. Now, it isn't quite that simple. In many organizations, the changing nature of work has blurred the distinction between managers and nonmanagerial employees. Many traditional nonmanagerial jobs now include managerial activities.[10] For example, at General Cable Corporation's facility in Moose Jaw, Saskatchewan, Canada, managerial responsibilities are shared by managers and team members. Most of the employees at Moose Jaw are cross-trained and multiskilled. Within a single shift, an employee can be a team leader, equipment operator, maintenance technician, quality inspector, or improvement planner.[11] Or consider an organization like Morning Star Company, the world's largest tomato processor, where no employees are called managers—just 400 full-time employees who do what needs to be done and who together "manage" issues such as job responsibilities, compensation decisions, and budget decisions.[12] Sounds crazy, doesn't it? But it works—for this organization. (See Case Application #1 at the end of the chapter to see how another business—Zappos—has gone bossless!)

So, how *do* we define who managers are? A **manager** is someone who coordinates and oversees the work of other people so organizational goals can be accomplished. A manager's job is not about *personal* achievement—it's about helping *others* do their work. That may mean coordinating the work of a departmental group, or it might mean supervising a single person. It could involve coordinating the work activities of a team with people from different departments or even people outside the organization such as temporary employees or individuals who work for the organization's suppliers. Keep in mind that managers may also have work duties not related to coordinating and overseeing others' work. For example, an insurance claims supervisor might process claims in addition to coordinating the work activities of other claims clerks.

How can managers be classified in organizations? In traditionally structured organizations (often pictured as a pyramid because more employees are at lower organizational levels than at upper organizational levels), managers can be classified as first-line, middle, or top. (See Exhibit 1.) At the lowest level of management, **first-line (or frontline) managers** manage the work of nonmanagerial employees who typically are involved with producing the organization's products or servicing the organization's customers. These managers often have titles such as *supervisors* or even

manager
Someone who coordinates and oversees the work of other people so organizational goals can be accomplished

first-line (frontline) managers
Managers at the lowest level of management who manage the work of nonmanagerial employees

Exhibit 1
Levels of Management

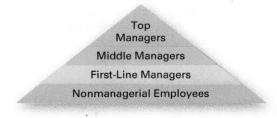

Top Managers
Middle Managers
First-Line Managers
Nonmanagerial Employees

middle managers
Managers between the lowest level and top levels of the organization who manage the work of first-line managers

top managers
Managers at or near the upper levels of the organization structure who are responsible for making organization-wide decisions and establishing the goals and plans that affect the entire organization

shift managers, district managers, department managers, or *office managers.* **Middle managers** manage the work of first-line managers and can be found between the lowest and top levels of the organization. They may have titles such as *regional manager, project leader, store manager,* or *division manager.* At the upper levels of the organization are the **top managers,** who are responsible for making organization-wide decisions and establishing the plans and goals that affect the entire organization. These individuals typically have titles such as *executive vice president, president, managing director, chief operating officer,* or *chief executive officer.*

Not all organizations are structured to get work done using a traditional pyramidal form, however. Some organizations, for example, are more loosely configured, with work done by ever-changing teams of employees who move from one project to another as work demands arise. Although it's not as easy to tell who the managers are in these organizations, we do know that someone must fulfill that role—that is, someone must coordinate and oversee the work of others, even if that "someone" changes as work tasks or projects change or that "someone" doesn't necessarily have the title of manager.

Where Do Managers Work?

organization
A deliberate arrangement of people to accomplish some specific purpose

It's obvious that managers work in organizations. But what is an **organization**? It's a deliberate arrangement of people to accomplish some specific purpose. Your college or university is an organization; so are fraternities and sororities, government departments, churches, Google, your neighborhood grocery store, the United Way, the St. Louis Cardinals baseball team, and the Mayo Clinic. All are considered organizations and have three common characteristics. (See Exhibit 2.)

First, an organization has a distinct purpose typically expressed through goals the organization hopes to accomplish. Second, each organization is composed of people. It takes people to perform the work that's necessary for the organization to achieve its goals. Third, all organizations develop a deliberate structure within which members do their work. That structure may be open and flexible, with no specific job duties or strict adherence to explicit job arrangements. For instance, most big projects at Google (at any one time, hundreds of projects are in process simultaneously) are tackled by small, focused employee teams that set up in an instant and complete work just as quickly.[15] Or the structure may be more traditional—like that of Procter & Gamble or General Electric or any large corporation—with clearly defined rules, regulations, job descriptions, and some members identified as "bosses" who have authority over other members.

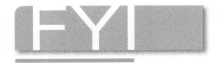

- Frontline managers directly supervise some 80 percent of the total workforce.[13]
- 10.8 million middle managers were in the U.S. workforce in 2012.[14]

Exhibit 2
Characteristics of Organizations

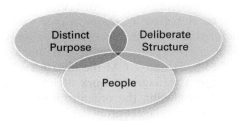

Distinct Purpose   Deliberate Structure

People

FUTURE VISION | Is It Still Managing When What You're Managing Are Robots?

While this text presents a fairly accurate description of today's workplace, you're going to spend most of your worklife in the future. What will that worklife look like? How will it be different from today? The workplace of tomorrow is likely to include workers that are faster, smarter, more responsible—and who just happen to be robots.[16] Are you at all surprised by this statement? Although robots have been used in factory and industrial settings for a long time, it's becoming more common to find robots in the office, and it's bringing about new ways of looking at how work is done and at what and how managers manage. So what *would* the manager's job be like managing robots? And even more intriguing is how these "workers" might affect how human coworkers interact with them.

As machines have become smarter, researchers have been looking at human-machine interaction and how people interact with the smart devices that are now such an integral part of our professional and personal lives. One conclusion is that people find it easy to bond with a robot, even one that doesn't look or sound anything like a real person. In a workplace setting, if a robot moves around in a "purposeful way," people tend to view it, in some ways, as a coworker. People name their robots and can even describe the robot's moods and tendencies. As telepresence robots become more common, the humanness becomes even more evident. For example, when Erwin Deininger, the electrical engineer at Reimers Electra Steam, a small company in Clear Brook, Virginia, moved to the Dominican Republic when his wife's job transferred her there, he was able to still be "present" at the company via his VGo robot. Now "robot" Deininger moves easily around the office and the shop floor, allowing the "real" Deininger to do his job just as if he were there in person. The company's president, satisfied with how the robot solution has worked out, has been surprised at how he acts around it, feeling at times that he's interacting with Deininger himself.

There's no doubt that robot technology will continue to be incorporated into organizational settings. The manager's job will become even more exciting and challenging as humans and machines work together to accomplish an organization's goals.

If your professor has chosen to assign this, go to **www.mymanagementlab.com** *to discuss the following questions.*

⭐ **TALK ABOUT IT 1:** What's your response to the title of this box: *Is* it still managing when what you're managing are robots? Discuss.

⭐ **TALK ABOUT IT 2:** If you had to "manage" people and robots, how do you think your job as manager might be different than what the chapter describes?

Many of today's organizations are structured more like Google, with flexible work arrangements, employee work teams, open communication systems, and supplier alliances. In these organizations, work is defined in terms of tasks to be done. And workdays have no time boundaries since work can be—and is—done anywhere, anytime. However, no matter what type of approach an organization uses, some deliberate structure is needed so work can get done, with managers overseeing and coordinating that work.

WHAT do managers do?

L03 Simply speaking, management is what managers do. But that simple statement doesn't tell us much, does it? Let's look first at what management is before discussing more specifically what managers do.

Management involves coordinating and overseeing the work activities of others so their activities are completed efficiently and effectively. We already know that coordinating and overseeing the work of others is what distinguishes a managerial position from a nonmanagerial one. However, this doesn't mean that managers or their employees can do what they want anytime, anywhere, or in any way. Instead, management involves ensuring that work activities are completed efficiently and effectively by the people responsible for doing them, or at least that's what managers should be doing.

management
Coordinating and overseeing the work activities of others so their activities are completed efficiently and effectively

Exhibit 3
Efficiency and Effectiveness
in Management

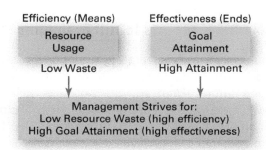

efficiency
Doing things right, or getting the most
output from the least amount of inputs

Efficiency refers to getting the most output from the least amount of inputs or resources. Managers deal with scarce resources—including people, money, and equipment—and want to use those resources efficiently. Efficiency is often referred to as "doing things right," that is, not wasting resources. For instance, at the HON Company plant in Cedartown, Georgia, where employees make and assemble office furniture, efficient manufacturing techniques were implemented by cutting inventory levels, decreasing the amount of time to manufacture products, and lowering product reject rates. These efficient work practices paid off, as the plant reduced costs by more than $7 million in one year.[17]

effectiveness
Doing the right things, or doing those
work activities that will result in achieving
goals

It's not enough, however, just to be efficient. Management is also concerned with employee effectiveness. **Effectiveness** is often described as "doing the right things," that is, doing those work activities that will result in achieving goals. For instance, at the HON factory, goals included meeting customers' rigorous demands, executing world-class manufacturing strategies, and making employees' jobs easier and safer. Through various employee work initiatives, these goals were pursued *and* achieved. Whereas efficiency is concerned with the *means* of getting things done, effectiveness is concerned with the *ends*, or attainment of organizational goals (see Exhibit 3). In successful organizations, high efficiency and high effectiveness typically go hand in hand. Poor management (which leads to poor performance) usually involves being inefficient and ineffective or being effective but inefficient.

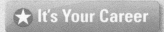 **It's Your Career**

Time Management—If your instructor is using MyManagementLab, log onto **www.mymanagementlab.com** and test your *time management knowledge*. **Be sure to refer back to the chapter opener!**

Now let's take a more detailed look at what managers do. Describing what managers do isn't easy. Just as no two organizations are alike, no two managers' jobs are alike. In spite of this, management researchers have developed three approaches to describe what managers do: functions, roles, and skills.

Management Functions

According to the functions approach, managers perform certain activities or functions as they efficiently and effectively coordinate the work of others. What are these functions? Henri Fayol, a French businessman in the early part of the twentieth century, suggested that all managers perform five functions: planning, organizing, commanding, coordinating, and controlling.[18] Today, we use four functions to describe a manager's work: planning, organizing, leading, and controlling (see Exhibit 4). Let's briefly look at each.

Planning	Organizing	Leading	Controlling	
Setting goals, establishing strategies, and developing plans to coordinate activities	Determining what needs to be done, how it will be done, and who is to do it	Motivating, leading, and any other actions involved in dealing with people	Monitoring activities to ensure that they are accomplished as planned	**Lead to** → Achieving the organization's stated purposes

Exhibit 4
Four Functions of Management

If you have no particular destination in mind, then any road will do. However, if you have someplace in particular you want to go, you've got to plan the best way to get there. Because organizations exist to achieve some particular purpose, someone must define that purpose and the means for its achievement. Managers are that someone. As managers engage in **planning**, they set goals, establish strategies for achieving those goals, and develop plans to integrate and coordinate activities.

Managers are also responsible for arranging and structuring work that employees do to accomplish the organization's goals. We call this function **organizing**. When managers organize, they determine what tasks are to be done, who is to do them, how the tasks are to be grouped, who reports to whom, and where decisions are to be made.

Every organization has people, and a manager's job is to work with and through people to accomplish goals. This is the **leading** function. When managers motivate subordinates, help resolve work group conflicts, influence individuals or teams as they work, select the most effective communication channel, or deal in any way with employee behavior issues, they're leading.

The final management function is **controlling**. After goals and plans are set (planning), tasks and structural arrangements are put in place (organizing), and people are hired, trained, and motivated (leading), there has to be an evaluation of whether things are going as planned. To ensure goals are met and work is done as it should be, managers monitor and evaluate performance. Actual performance is compared with the set goals. If those goals aren't achieved, it's the manager's job to get work back on track. This process of monitoring, comparing, and correcting is the controlling function.

Just how well does the functions approach describe what managers do? Do managers always plan, organize, lead, and then control? Not necessarily. What a manager does may not always happen in this sequence. However, regardless of the order in which these functions are performed, managers do plan, organize, lead, and control as they manage.

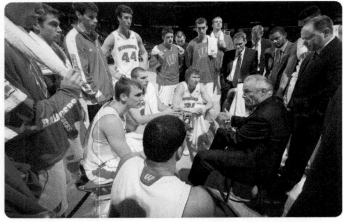

Leading is an important function that Bo Ryan performs as head basketball coach for UW-Madison. He manages effectively by directing and coordinating the work activities of his coaching staff and team of athletes and by motivating them to achieve the goals and objectives of the university's basketball program.
Source: David Stluka /AP Images

planning
Management function that involves setting goals, establishing strategies for achieving those goals, and developing plans to integrate and coordinate activities

organizing
Management function that involves arranging and structuring work to accomplish the organization's goals

leading
Management function that involves working with and through people to accomplish organizational goals

If your professor has assigned this, go to **www.mymanagementlab.com** to complete the **Simulation: *What Is Management?*** and see how well you can apply the ideas of planning, organizing, leading, and controlling.

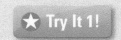
⭐ Try It 1!

Although the functions approach is a popular way to describe what managers do, some have argued that it isn't relevant.[19] So let's look at another perspective.

controlling
Management function that involves monitoring, comparing, and correcting work performance

let's get REAL

The Scenario:

Micah, one of your best employees, was just promoted to a managerial position. You invited him to lunch to celebrate and to see what was on his mind about his new position. Waiting for your food to arrive, you asked him if he had any concerns or questions about being a manager. Looking straight at you, Micah said, "How is being a manager going to be different? What will I do as a manager?"

How would you respond?

Being a manager means that you have a greater responsibility to consider, and keep in mind big-picture organizational goals and how your work and that of your staff contributes to those goals. As a manager you also have a responsibility to think about development opportunities for any team members who may now report to you. How will you help to put them on a path toward growth and success?

Maribel Lara
Director,
Account Management

Mintzberg's Managerial Roles and a Contemporary Model of Managing

Henry Mintzberg, a well-known management researcher, studied actual managers at work. In his first comprehensive study, Mintzberg concluded that what managers do can best be described by looking at the managerial roles they engage in at work.[20] The term **managerial roles** refers to specific actions or behaviors expected of and exhibited by a manager. (Think of the different roles you play—student, employee, student organization member, volunteer, sibling, and so forth—and the different things you're expected to do in these roles.) When describing what managers do from a roles perspective, we're not looking at a specific person per se, but at the expectations and responsibilities associated with the person in that role—the role of a manager.[21] As shown in Exhibit 5, these 10 roles are grouped around interpersonal relationships, the transfer of information, and decision making.

The **interpersonal roles** involve people (subordinates and persons outside the organization) and other ceremonial and symbolic duties. The three interpersonal roles include figurehead, leader, and liaison. The **informational roles** involve collecting, receiving, and disseminating information. The three informational roles include monitor, disseminator, and spokesperson. Finally, the **decisional roles** entail making decisions or choices and include entrepreneur, disturbance handler, resource allocator, and negotiator. As managers perform these roles, Mintzberg proposed that their activities included both reflection (thinking) and action (doing).[22]

A number of follow-up studies have tested the validity of Mintzberg's role categories, and the evidence generally supports the idea that managers—regardless of the type of organization or level in the organization—perform similar roles.[23] However, the emphasis that managers give to the various roles seems to change with organizational level.[24] At higher levels of the organization, the roles of disseminator, figurehead, negotiator, liaison, and spokesperson are more important; while the leader role (as Mintzberg defined it) is more important for lower-level managers than it is for either middle or top-level managers.

managerial roles
Specific actions or behaviors expected of and exhibited by a manager

interpersonal roles
Managerial roles that involve people and other duties that are ceremonial and symbolic in nature

informational roles
Managerial roles that involve collecting, receiving, and disseminating information

decisional roles
Managerial roles that revolve around making choices

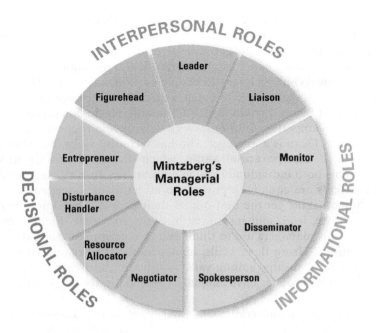

Exhibit 5
Mintzberg's Managerial Roles

Source: Based on Mintzberg, H., *The Nature of Managerial Work* (New York: Prentice Hall, 1983).

So which approach is better, managerial functions or Mintzberg's propositions? Although each does a good job of depicting what managers do, the functions approach still seems to be the generally accepted way of describing the manager's job. "The classical functions provide clear and discrete methods of classifying the thousands of activities managers carry out and the techniques they use in terms of the functions they perform for the achievement of goals."[25] However, Mintzberg's role approach and additional model of managing do offer us other insights into managers' work.

Management Skills

UPS is a company that understands the importance of management skills.[26] The company's new on-road supervisors are immersed in a new manager orientation where they learn people and time management skills. The company started an intensive eight-day offsite skills training program for first-line managers as a way to improve its operations. What have supervisors learned from the skills training? Some things they mentioned learning were how to communicate more effectively and important information about safety compliance and labor practices.

What types of skills do managers need? Robert L. Katz proposed that managers need three critical skills in managing: technical, human, and conceptual.[27] (Exhibit 6 shows the relationships of these skills to managerial levels.) **Technical skills** are the job-specific knowledge and techniques needed to proficiently perform work tasks. These skills tend to be more important for first-line managers

technical skills
Job-specific knowledge and techniques needed to proficiently perform work tasks

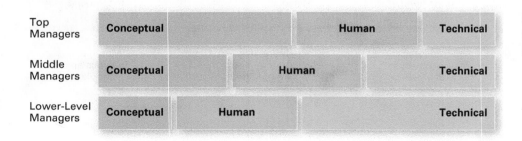

Top Managers	Conceptual	Human	Technical
Middle Managers	Conceptual	Human	Technical
Lower-Level Managers	Conceptual	Human	Technical

Exhibit 6
Skills Needed at Different Managerial Levels

because they typically manage employees who use tools and techniques to produce the organization's products or service the organization's customers. Often, employees with excellent technical skills get promoted to first-line manager. For example, Dean White, a production supervisor at Springfield Remanufacturing, started as a parts cleaner. Now, White manages 25 people in six departments. He noted that at first it was difficult to get people to listen, especially his former peers. "I learned I had to gain respect before I could lead," White said. He credits mentors—other supervisors whose examples he followed—with helping him become the type of manager he is today.[28] Dean is a manager who has technical skills, but also recognizes the importance of **interpersonal skills**, which involve the ability to work well with other people both individually and in a group. Because all managers deal with people, these skills are equally important to all levels of management. Managers with good human skills get the best out of their people. They know how to communicate, motivate, lead, and inspire enthusiasm and trust. Finally, **conceptual skills** are the skills managers use to think and to conceptualize about abstract and complex situations. Using these skills, managers see the organization as a whole, understand the relationships among various subunits, and visualize how the organization fits into its broader environment. These skills are most important to top managers.

Other important managerial skills that have been identified are listed in Exhibit 7. In today's demanding and dynamic workplace, employees who want to be valuable assets must constantly upgrade their skills, and developing management skills can be particularly beneficial.

interpersonal skills
The ability to work well with other people individually and in a group

conceptual skills
The ability to think and to conceptualize about abstract and complex situations

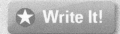 **Write It!** If your professor has assigned this, go to **mymanagementlab.com** and complete the **Writing Assignment** *MGMT 1: Management Skills*.

Exhibit 7
Important Managerial Skills

Source: Based on *Workforce Online*; J. R. Ryan, *Bloomberg BusinessWeek Online*; In-Sue Oh and C. M. Berry; and R. S. Rubin and E. C. Dierdorff.

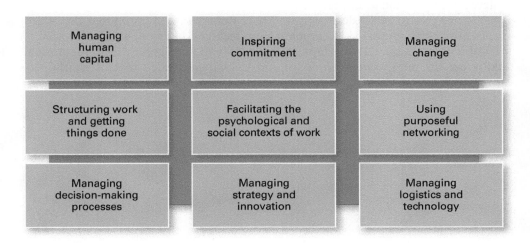

Managing human capital

Inspiring commitment

Managing change

Structuring work and getting things done

Facilitating the psychological and social contexts of work

Using purposeful networking

Managing decision-making processes

Managing strategy and innovation

Managing logistics and technology

let's get REAL

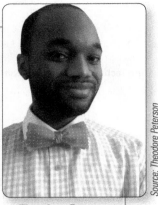

Theodore Peterson
Lead Mentor/
Behavioral Assistant

The Scenario:

Recently, one of your employees, Ryan, was moved from team member to team leader. Walking down the hallway, you overhear this conversation, "I don't understand what's up with Ryan these days. Just Tuesday, he went out with us for a while after work, laughing and joking like always. Then today he calls me in to tell me I need to put more effort in on the Langley project and to stop wasting time. One minute he wants to be my friend, and the next he acts all boss-like. I never thought he'd turn on us like that when he got promoted to team leader."

What advice would you give Ryan?

I would remind Ryan that he is in a different position now, and that he has to set an example. One of the things about being a leader is you cannot ask someone to do something that you're not willing to do yourself or haven't done. The second thing I would tell Ryan is that he has to begin to set boundaries; a lot of people don't understand the difference between business and friendship. At the end of the day, Ryan is the lead and will be held responsible first; which is why he was placed in the position in the first place. Pay attention and be careful about what you say and do around others outside of work.

HOW is the manager's job changing?

LO4 Welcome to the new world of managing! Using game-like software that can meticulously track worker productivity, some workplaces are turning to "games" to hire, monitor, motivate, and manage employees.[29] For instance, Marriott Hotels uses a mobile app with job candidates to assess virtually how they perform hotel service tasks. SAP uses games to educate its employees on sustainability, and Unilever uses them for training purposes. This so-called "gamification" is a relatively new approach being explored by organizations looking for ways to engage employees and add value to the workplace.

In today's world, managers are dealing with global economic and political uncertainties, changing workplaces, ethical issues, security threats, and changing technology. For example, Dave Maney, the top manager of Headwaters MB, a Denver-based investment bank, had to fashion a new plan during the recession. When the company's board of directors gave senior management complete freedom to ensure the company's survival, they made a bold move. All but seven key employees were laid off. Although this doesn't sound very responsible or resourceful, it invited those laid-off employees to form independent member firms. Now, Headwaters steers investment transactions to those firms, while keeping a small percentage for itself. The new organizational arrangement drastically reduced fixed costs and also gave managers more time to do the all-important job of marketing. As Maney said, "It was a good strategy for us and positioned us for the future."[30] It's likely that more managers *will* have to manage

Exhibit 8
Changes Facing Managers

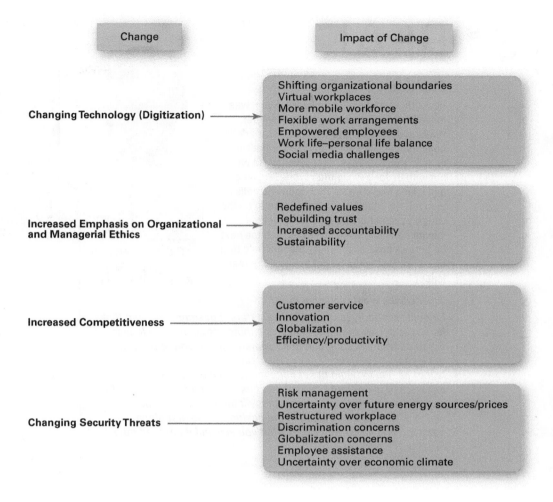

Change	Impact of Change
Changing Technology (Digitization)	Shifting organizational boundaries Virtual workplaces More mobile workforce Flexible work arrangements Empowered employees Work life–personal life balance Social media challenges
Increased Emphasis on Organizational and Managerial Ethics	Redefined values Rebuilding trust Increased accountability Sustainability
Increased Competitiveness	Customer service Innovation Globalization Efficiency/productivity
Changing Security Threats	Risk management Uncertainty over future energy sources/prices Restructured workplace Discrimination concerns Globalization concerns Employee assistance Uncertainty over economic climate

under such demanding circumstances, and the fact is that *how* managers manage is changing. Exhibit 8 shows some of the most important changes facing managers. Throughout the rest of this text, we'll discuss these and other changes and how they affect the way managers plan, organize, lead, and control. We want to highlight four of these changes: the increasing importance of customers, social media, innovation, and sustainability.

Importance of Customers to the Manager's Job

John Chambers, CEO of Cisco Systems, likes to listen to voice mails forwarded to him from dissatisfied customers because he wants to hear firsthand the emotions and frustrations they're experiencing. He can't get that type of insight by reading an e-mail.[31] This manager understands the importance of customers. You need customers. Without them, most organizations would cease to exist. Yet, focusing on the customer has long been thought to be the responsibility of marketing types. "Let the marketers worry about the customers" is how many managers felt. We're discovering, however, that employee attitudes and behaviors play a big role in customer satisfaction. For instance, passengers of Qantas Airways were asked to rate their "essential needs" in air travel. Almost every factor listed was one directly influenced by the actions of company employees—from prompt baggage delivery, to courteous and efficient cabin crews, to assistance with connections, to quick and friendly check-ins.[32]

Today, the majority of employees in developed countries work in service jobs. For instance, almost 80 percent of the U.S. labor force is employed in service industries. In Australia, 69 percent work in service industries, and in Canada, 70 percent do. In the United Kingdom, Germany, and Japan, the percentages are 78, 69, and 73, respectively. Even in developing countries such as Colombia, Dominican Republic, Vietnam, and Bangladesh, we find 68 percent, 63 percent, 31 percent, and 54 percent of the labor force employed in service jobs.[33] Examples of service jobs include technical support representatives, food servers or fast-food counter workers, sales clerks, custodians and housekeepers, teachers, nurses, computer repair technicians, front-desk clerks, consultants, purchasing agents, credit representatives, financial planners, and bank tellers. The odds are pretty good that when you graduate, you'll go to work for a company that's in a service industry, not in manufacturing or agriculture.

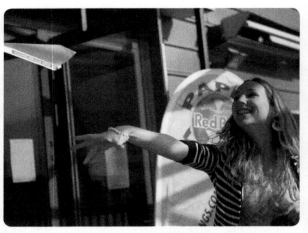

Red Bull, the Austrian-based energy-drink firm, launched its own global media company that integrates innovative social media strategies into each of its marketing events. Through its network of more than 35 million followers, Red Bull creates a strong bond with its young target audience, such as the woman shown here competing in a worldwide paper airplane contest.
Source: Maurin Bisig/ZUMA Press/Newscom

Managers are recognizing that delivering consistent, high-quality customer service is essential for survival and success in today's competitive environment and that employees are an important part of that equation.[34] The implication is clear: managers must create a customer-responsive organization where employees are friendly and courteous, accessible, knowledgeable, prompt in responding to customer needs, and willing to do what's necessary to please the customer.[35] Before we leave the topic of customer service management, we want to share one more story that illustrates why it's important for today's managers (all managers, not just those in marketing) to understand what it takes to serve customers. During a broadcasted Stanley Cup playoff game, Comcast subscribers suddenly found themselves staring at a blank screen. Many of those customers got on Twitter to find out why. And it was there, not on a phone system, that they discovered a lightning strike in Atlanta had caused the power outage and that transmission would be restored as quickly as possible. Managers at Comcast understood how to exploit popular communications technology, and the company's smart use of Twitter accentuates the importance of social media tools in communicating with customers.[36]

If your professor has assigned this, go to **www.mymanagementlab.com** to watch a video titled *Zane's Cycles: The Management Environment* and to respond to questions.

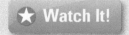

★ Watch It!

Importance of Social Media to the Manager's Job

You probably can't imagine a time when employees did their work without smart devices, e-mail, or Internet access. Yet, some 20 years ago, as these tools were becoming more common in workplaces, managers struggled with the challenges of providing guidelines for using the Internet and e-mail in their organizations. Today, the new frontier is **social media**, forms of electronic communication through which users create online communities to share ideas, information, personal messages, and other content. And employees don't just use these on their personal time, but also for work purposes. That's why managers need to understand and manage the power and peril of social media. For instance, at grocery chain SuperValu, managers realized that keeping 135,000-plus employees connected and engaged was imperative to continued success.[37] They decided to adopt an internal social media tool to foster

social media
Forms of electronic communication through which users create online communities to share ideas, information, personal messages, and other content

LEADER *making a* DIFFERENCE

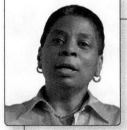

Source: Jemal Countess/Getty Images Entertainment/Gettyimages.com

Ursula Burns *is the first African American woman to lead a company the size of Xerox.[38] Appointed to the CEO position in 2009, Burns is known for her courage to "tell the truth in ugly times." Having grown up in the projects on the Lower East Side of New York, Burns understands what it takes to get through those uncertainties. With her aptitude for math, Burns went on to earn a mechanical engineering degree from Polytechnic Institute of New York. After a summer engineering internship at Xerox, she was hooked. At Xerox, Burns was mentored by individuals who saw her potential. Throughout her more than 30-year career at Xerox, Burns had a reputation for being bold. As a mechanical engineer, she got noticed because she wasn't afraid to speak up bluntly in a culture that's known more for being polite, courteous, and discreet than for being outspoken. Although Burns is still radically honest and direct, she has become more of a listener, calling herself a "listener-in-chief."* What can you learn from this leader making a difference?

cooperation and collaboration among the 10 distinct store brands operating in 44 states. And they're not alone. More and more businesses are turning to social media not just as a way to connect with customers, but also as a way to manage their human resources and tap into their innovation and talent. That's the potential power of social media. But the potential peril is in how it's used. When the social media platform becomes a way for boastful employees to brag about their accomplishments, for managers to publish one-way messages to employees, or for employees to argue or gripe about something or someone they don't like at work, then it's lost its usefulness. To avoid this, managers need to remember that social media is a tool that needs to be managed to be beneficial. At SuperValu, about 9,000 store managers and assistant managers use the social media system. Although sources say it's too early to draw any conclusions, it appears that managers who actively make use of the system are having better store sales revenues than those who don't.

Importance of Innovation to the Manager's Job

Success in business today demands innovation. Innovation means exploring new territory, taking risks, and doing things differently. And innovation isn't just for high-tech or other technologically sophisticated organizations. Innovative efforts can be found in all types of organizations. For instance, the manager of the Best Buy store in Manchester, Connecticut, clearly understood the importance of being innovative, a task made particularly challenging because the average Best Buy store is often staffed by young adults in their first or second jobs who aren't always committed long term to a retail career. Yet, the increasingly sophisticated products carried by the store required a high level of employee training. The store manager tackled this challenge by getting employees to suggest new ideas. One idea—a "team close," in which employees scheduled to work at the store's closing time closed the store together and walked out together as a team—had a remarkable impact on employee attitudes and commitment.[39] Innovation is critical throughout all levels and parts of an organization.

Importance of Sustainability to the Manager's Job

It's the world's largest retailer with over $469 billion in annual sales, 2.2 million employees, and 10,100 stores. Yes, we're talking about Walmart. And Walmart is probably the last company that you'd think about in a section describing sustainability. However, Walmart announced at the beginning of this decade that it would "cut some 20 million metric tons of greenhouse gas emissions from its supply chain by the end of 2015—the equivalent of removing more than 3.8 million cars from the road for a year."[40] The company recently announced that it now reuses or recycles more than 80 percent of the waste produced in its domestic stores and in other U.S. operations.[41] This corporate action affirms that sustainability and green management have become mainstream issues for managers.

What's emerging in the twenty-first century is the concept of managing in a sustainable way, which has had the effect of widening corporate responsibility not only to managing in an efficient and effective way, but also to responding strategically to a wide range of environmental and societal challenges.[42] Although "sustainability" means different things to different people, the World Business Council for Sustainable Development describes a situation where all earth's inhabitants can live well with adequate resources.[43] From a business perspective, **sustainability** has been described as a company's ability to achieve its business goals and increase long-term shareholder value by integrating economic, environmental, and social opportunities into its business strategies.[44] Sustainability issues are now moving up the agenda of business leaders and the boards of thousands of companies. Like the managers at Walmart are discovering, running an organization in a more sustainable way will mean that managers have to make informed business decisions based on thorough communication with various stakeholders; understanding their requirements; and starting to factor economic, environmental, and social aspects into how they pursue their business goals.

sustainability
A company's ability to achieve its business goals and increase long-term shareholder value by integrating economic, environmental, and social opportunities into its business strategies

WHY study management?

L05 You may be wondering why you need to study management. If you're majoring in accounting or marketing or any field other than management, you may not understand how studying management is going to help your career. We can explain the value of studying management by looking at three things: the universality of management, the reality of work, and the rewards and challenges of being a manager.

The Universality of Management

Just how universal is the need for management in organizations? We can say with absolute certainty that management is needed in all types and sizes of organizations, at all organizational levels and in all organizational work areas, and in all organizations, no matter where they're located. This is known as the **universality of management**. (See Exhibit 9.) In all these organizations, managers must plan, organize, lead, and control. However, that's not to say that management is done the same way. What a supervisor in an applications testing group at Twitter does versus what the CEO of Twitter does is a matter of degree and emphasis, not function. Because both are managers, both will plan, organize, lead, and control. How much and how they do so will differ, however.

universality of management
The reality that management is needed in all types and sizes of organizations, at all organizational levels, in all organizational areas, and in organizations no matter where located

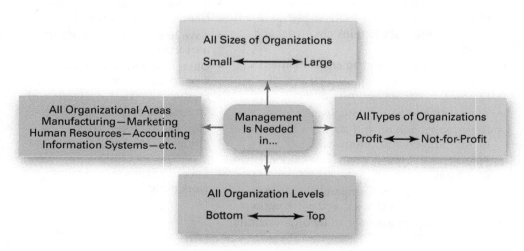

Exhibit 9
Universal Need for Management

Management is universally needed in all organizations, so we want to find ways to improve the way organizations are managed. Why? Because we interact with organizations every single day. Organizations that are well managed—and we'll share many examples of these throughout the text—develop a loyal customer base, grow, and prosper, even during challenging times. Those that are poorly managed find themselves losing customers and revenues. By studying management, you'll be able to recognize poor management and work to get it corrected. In addition, you'll be able to recognize and support good management, whether it's in an organization with which you're simply interacting or whether it's in an organization in which you're employed.

★ **Try It 2!**   If your professor has assigned this, go to **www.mymanagementlab.com** to complete the *Simulation: Managing Your Career* and get a feel for your career goals.

The Reality of Work

Another reason for studying management is the reality that for most of you, once you graduate from college and begin your career, you will either manage or be managed. For those who plan to be managers, an understanding of management forms the foundation upon which to build your management knowledge and skills. For those of you who don't see yourself managing, you're still likely to have to work with managers. Also, assuming that you'll have to work for a living and recognizing that you're very likely to work in an organization, you'll probably have some managerial responsibilities even if you're not a manager. Our experience tells us that you can gain a great deal of insight into the way your boss (and fellow employees) behave and how organizations function by studying management. Our point is that you don't have to aspire to be a manager to gain something valuable from a course in management.

Rewards and Challenges of Being a Manager

We can't leave our discussion here without looking at the rewards and challenges of being a manager. (See Exhibit 10.) What *does* it mean to be a manager in today's workplace?

Exhibit 10
Rewards and Challenges of Being a Manager

Rewards	Challenges
• Create a work environment in which organizational members can work to the best of their ability	• Do hard work
• Have opportunities to think creatively and use imagination	• May have duties that are more clerical than managerial
• Help others find meaning and fulfillment in work	• Have to deal with a variety of personalities
• Support, coach, and nurture others	• Often have to make do with limited resources
• Work with a variety of people	• Motivate workers in chaotic and uncertain situations
• Receive recognition and status in organization and community	• Blend knowledge, skills, ambitions, and experiences of a diverse work group
• Play a role in influencing organizational outcomes	• Success depends on others' work performance
• Receive appropriate compensation in the form of salaries, bonuses, and stock options	
• Good managers are needed by organizations	

First, there are many challenges. It can be a tough and often thankless job. In addition, a portion of a manager's job (especially at lower organizational levels) may entail duties that are often more clerical (compiling and filing reports, dealing with bureaucratic procedures, or doing paperwork) than managerial.[45] Managers also spend significant amounts of time in meetings and dealing with interruptions, which can be time consuming and sometimes unproductive.[46] Managers often have to deal with a variety of personalities and have to make do with limited resources. It can be a challenge to motivate workers in the face of uncertainty and chaos, as this recession has illustrated time and time again. And managers may find it difficult to successfully blend the knowledge, skills, ambitions, and experiences of a diverse work group. Finally, as a manager, you're not in full control of your destiny. Your success typically is dependent on others' work performance.

Despite these challenges, being a manager *can* be rewarding. You're responsible for creating a work environment in which organizational members can do their work to the best of their ability and thus help the organization achieve its goals. You help others find meaning and fulfillment in their work. You get to support, coach, and nurture others and help them make good decisions. In addition, as a manager, you often have the opportunity to think creatively and use your imagination. You'll get to meet and work with a variety of people—both inside and outside the organization. Other rewards may include receiving recognition and status in your organization and in the community, playing a role in influencing organizational outcomes, and receiving attractive compensation in the form of salaries, bonuses, and stock options. Finally, as we said earlier in the chapter, organizations need good managers. It's through the combined efforts of motivated and passionate people working together that organizations accomplish their goals. As a manager, you can be assured that your efforts, skills, and abilities are needed.

PREPARING FOR: Exams/Quizzes

CHAPTER SUMMARY by Learning Objectives

LO1   EXPLAIN **why managers are important to organizations.**

Managers are important to organizations for three reasons. First, organizations need their managerial skills and abilities in uncertain, complex, and chaotic times. Second, managers are critical to getting things done in organizations. Finally, managers contribute to employee productivity and loyalty; the way employees are managed can affect the organization's financial performance, and managerial ability has been shown to be important in creating organizational value.

LO2   TELL **who managers are and where they work.**

Managers coordinate and oversee the work of other people so that organizational goals can be accomplished. Nonmanagerial employees work directly on a job or task and have no one reporting to them. In traditionally structured organizations, managers can be first-line, middle, or top. In other more loosely configured organizations, the managers may not be as readily identifiable, although someone must fulfill that role.

Managers work in an organization, which is a deliberate arrangement of people to accomplish some specific purpose. Organizations have three characteristics: they have a distinctive purpose, they are composed of people, and they have a deliberate structure. Many of today's organizations are structured to be more open, flexible, and responsive to changes.

LO3 | DESCRIBE **the functions, roles, and skills of managers.**

Broadly speaking, management is what managers do and involves coordinating and overseeing the efficient and effective completion of others' work activities. Efficiency means doing things right; effectiveness means doing the right things.

The four functions of management include planning (defining goals, establishing strategies, and developing plans), organizing (arranging and structuring work), leading (working with and through people), and controlling (monitoring, comparing, and correcting work performance).

Mintzberg's managerial roles include interpersonal, which involve people and other ceremonial/symbolic duties (figurehead, leader, and liaison); informational, which involve collecting, receiving, and disseminating information (monitor, disseminator, and spokesperson); and decisional, which involve making choices (entrepreneur, disturbance handler, resource allocator, and negotiator).

Katz's managerial skills include technical (job-specific knowledge and techniques), interpersonal (ability to work well with people), and conceptual (ability to think and express ideas). Technical skills are most important for lower-level managers, while conceptual skills are most important for top managers. Interpersonal skills are equally important for all managers. Some other managerial skills identified include managing human capital, inspiring commitment, managing change, using purposeful networking, and so forth.

LO4 | DESCRIBE **the factors that are reshaping and redefining the manager's job.**

The changes impacting managers' jobs include global economic and political uncertainties, changing workplaces, ethical issues, security threats, and changing technology. Managers must be concerned with customer service because employee attitudes and behaviors play a big role in customer satisfaction. Managers must be concerned with social media because these forms of communication are becoming important and valuable tools in managing. Managers must also be concerned with innovation because it is important for organizations to be competitive. And finally, managers must be concerned with sustainability as business goals are developed.

LO5 | EXPLAIN **the value of studying management.**

It's important to study management for three reasons: (1) the universality of management, which refers to the fact that managers are needed in all types and sizes of organizations, at all organizational levels and work areas, and in all global locations; (2) the reality of work—that is, you will either manage or be managed; and (3) the awareness of the significant rewards (such as creating work environments to help people work to the best of their ability, supporting and encouraging others, helping others find meaning and fulfillment in work, etc.) and challenges (having to work hard, sometimes having more clerical than managerial duties, interacting with a variety of personalities, etc.) in being a manager.

MyManagementLab

Go to **mymanagementlab.com** to complete the problems marked with this icon ⭐.

✪ REVIEW AND DISCUSSION QUESTIONS

1. How do managers differ from nonmanagerial employees?

2. Is your course instructor a manager? Discuss in terms of managerial functions, managerial roles, and skills.

3. "The manager's most basic responsibility is to focus people toward performance of work activities to achieve desired outcomes." Why do you agree or disagree with this statement?

4. Explain why the universality-of-management concept still holds true or doesn't hold true in today's world.

5. Is business management a profession? After doing some external research, why is management a profession or why is it not?

6. Does the way contemporary organizations are structured appeal to you? Why or why not?

7. In today's environment, explain which is more important to organizations—efficiency or effectiveness.

8. "Management is undoubtedly one of humankind's most important inventions." Explain why you do or do not agree with this statement.

MyManagementLab

If your professor has assigned these, go to **mymanagementlab.com** for Auto-graded writing questions as well as the following Assisted-graded writing questions:

9. Is there one best "style" of management? Why or why not?

10. Researchers at Harvard Business School found that the most important managerial behaviors involve two fundamental things: enabling people to move forward in their work and treating them decently as human beings. What do you think of these two managerial behaviors? What are the implications for someone, like yourself, who is studying management?

PREPARING FOR: My Career

✪ PERSONAL INVENTORY ASSESSMENTS 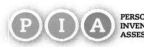 PERSONAL INVENTORY ASSESSMENT

Time Management Assessment

Take a look at how well *you* manage time. This PIA will help you determine how skillfully you do that.

✪ ETHICS DILEMMA

• 26 percent of new managers feel they are unprepared to transition into management roles • 58 percent of new managers don't receive any training to help them make the transition • 50 percent of first-time managers fail in that transition.[47] Moving to a management position isn't easy as these statistics indicate.

11. Explain why an organization does or does not have an ethical responsibility to assist its new managers in their new positions.

12. What could organizations do to make the transition into a management role easier?

SKILL EXERCISE Developing Your Political Skill

About the Skill
Research has shown that people differ in their political skills.[48] Those who are politically skilled are more effective in their use of influence tactics. Political skill also appears to be more effective when the stakes are high. Finally, politically skilled individuals are able to exert their influence without others detecting it, which is important in being effective so that you're not labeled political. A person's political skill is determined by his or her networking ability, interpersonal influence, social astuteness, and apparent sincerity.

Steps in Practicing the Skill

- *Develop your networking ability*. A good network can be a powerful tool. You can begin building a network by getting to know important people in your work area and the organization and then developing relationships with individuals in positions of power. Volunteer for committees or offer your help on projects that will be noticed by those in positions of power. Attend important organizational functions so that you can be seen as a team player and someone who's interested in the organization's success. Start a rolodex file of individuals that you meet, even if for a brief moment. Then, when you need advice on work, use your connections and network with others throughout the organization.

- *Work on gaining interpersonal influence*. People will listen to you when they're comfortable and feel at ease around you. Work on your communication skills so that you can communicate easily and effectively with others. Work on developing good rapport with people in all areas and at all levels of your organization. Be open, friendly, and willing to pitch in. The amount of interpersonal influence you have will be affected by how well people like you.

- *Develop your social astuteness*. Some people have an innate ability to understand people and sense what they're thinking. If you don't have that ability, you'll have to work at developing your social astuteness by doing things such as saying the right things at the right time, paying close attention to people's facial expressions, and trying to determine whether others have hidden agendas.

- *Be sincere*. Sincerity is important to getting people to want to associate with you. Be genuine in what you say and do. And show a genuine interest in others and their situations.

Practicing the Skill
Select each of the components of political skill and spend one week working on it. Write a brief set of notes describing your experiences—good and bad. Were you able to begin developing a network of people throughout the organization or did you work at developing your social astuteness, maybe by starting to recognize and interpret people's facial expressions and the meaning behind those expressions? What could you have done differently to be more politically skilled? Once you begin to recognize what's involved with political skills, you should find yourself becoming more connected and politically adept.

WORKING TOGETHER Team Exercise

By this time in your life, all of you have had to work with individuals in managerial positions (or maybe *you* were the manager), either through work experiences or through other organizational experiences (social, hobby/interest, religious, and so forth). What do you think makes some managers better than others? Do certain characteristics distinguish good managers? Form small groups with 3–4 other class members. Discuss your experiences with managers—good and bad. Draw up a list of the characteristics of those individuals you felt were good managers. For each item, indicate which management function and which management skill you think it falls under. As a group, be prepared to share your list with the class and to explain your choice of management function and skill.

LEARNING TO BE A MANAGER

- Use the most current *Occupational Outlook Handbook* (U.S. Department of Labor, Bureau of Labor Statistics) to research three different categories of managers. For each, prepare a bulleted list that describes the following: the nature of the work, training and other qualifications needed, earnings, and job outlook and projections data.

- Get in the habit of reading at least one current business periodical (*Wall Street Journal, Bloomberg BusinessWeek, Fortune, Fast Company, Forbes*, etc.). Keep a file with interesting information you find about managers or managing.

- Using current business periodicals, find three examples of managers you would describe as *Master Managers*. Write

a paper describing these individuals as managers and why you feel they deserve this title.

- Interview two different managers and ask them the following questions: What are the best and worst parts about being a manager? What's the best management advice you ever received? Type up the questions and their answers to turn in to your professor.

- Accountants and other professionals have certification programs to verify their skills, knowledge, and professionalism. What about managers? Two certification programs for managers include the Certified Manager (Institute of Certified Professional Managers) and the

Certified Business Manager (Association of Professional in Business Management). Research each of these programs. Prepare a bulleted list of what each involves.

- If you're involved in student organizations, volunteer for leadership roles or for projects where you can practice planning, organizing, leading, and controlling different projects and activities. You can also gain valuable managerial experience by taking a leadership role in class team projects.

- In your own words, write down three things you learned in this text about being a good manager. Keep a copy of this for future reference.

CASE APPLICATION 1 Who Needs a Boss?

"Holacracy."[49] That's the word of the day at Zappos, the Nevada-based online shoe and apparel retailer. During a four-hour, year-end employee meeting in 2013, CEO Tony Hsieh announced that he was eliminating the company's traditional managerial and structural hierarchy to implement a holacracy. What is a holacracy, you ask? In a nutshell, it's an organizational system with no job titles, no managers, and no top-down hierarchy with upper, middle, or lower levels where decisions can get hung up. The idea behind this new type of arrangement is to focus on the work that needs to be done and not on some hierarchical structure where great ideas and suggestions can get lost in the channels of reporting. The holacracy concept was dreamed up by Brian Robertson, the founder of a Pennsylvania software startup. Its name comes from the Greek word *holos,* a single, autonomous, self-sufficient unit that's also dependent on a larger unit.[50] A simple explanation of Robertson's vision of a holacracy is: workers as partners, job descriptions as roles, and partners organized into circles.[51]

At Zappos, work (and the 1,500 employees who do it) will be organized around self-governing employee circles—around 400 of these circles when the reorganization is complete sometime in December 2014. (It might help you grasp this idea by thinking of these employee circles as types of overlapping employee "groups" but with more fluid membership and individual roles/responsibilities.) In these circles, employees can take on any number of roles, and the expectation is that each employee will help out wherever he or she can. Without titles or a hierarchy, anyone can initiate a project and implement innovative ideas. The hope is that circle members will pool ideas and watch out for each other. The goal is radical transparency and to get more people to take charge. Yet, trusting individuals who probably know the details of the job better than any "manager" to work conscientiously, creatively, and efficiently is good as long as there is a way to keep standards high. The last thing Zappos wants is for a "slacker" mentality to take hold.

Hsieh has always approached leading his business in unique and radical ways. He strongly believes in the power of the individual and has created a highly successful organization (which is now part of Amazon) that's known for its zany culture where corporate values are matched with personal values, and where "weirdness and humility" are celebrated.[52] However, as the company moves away from the traditional work model to this new system, it may face some challenges. Both Zappos and Robertson caution that while a holacracy might eliminate the traditional manager's job, there is still structure and accountability. Poor performers will be obvious because they

won't have enough "roles" to fill their time, or a circle charged with monitoring the company's culture may decide they're not a good fit. Also, just because there are no "traditional" managers doesn't mean that leaders won't emerge. But it will be important to watch for dominant personalities emerging as authority figures, which could potentially cause other employees to be resentful or to rebel. Zappos says that it will not be leaderless. Some individuals will have a bigger role and scope of purpose, but leadership is also distributed and expected in each role. "Everybody is expected to lead and be an entrepreneur in their own roles, and holacracy empowers them to do so."[53] Also, there will be some structure arrangement where "the broadest circles can to some extent tell sub-groups what they're accountable for doing."[54] But accountability, rather than flowing only up, will flow throughout the organization in different paths. Other challenges they're still trying to figure out include who has the ultimate authority to hire, fire, and decide pay. The hope is that eventually the authority for each of these roles will be done within the holacratic framework as well. So, if no one has a title and there are no bosses, is Tony Hsieh still the CEO? So far, he hasn't publicly commented about how his own role is impacted.

⭐ **DISCUSSION QUESTIONS**

13. What is a holacracy?

14. What benefits do you see to an organization where there are no job titles, no managers, and no hierarchy?

15. What challenges does a holacratic approach have?

16. Discuss why you would or would not like to work in an organization like this.

CASE APPLICATION **2** Building a Better Boss

Google doesn't do anything halfway. So when it decided to "build a better boss," it did what it does best...look at data.[55] Using data from performance reviews, feedback surveys, and supporting papers turned in for individuals being nominated for top-manager awards, Google tried to find what a great boss is and does. The project, dubbed Project Oxygen, examined some 100 variables and ultimately identified eight characteristics or habits of Google's most effective managers. Here are the "big eight":

- Provide an unambiguous vision of the future;
- Help individuals to reach their long-term work goals;
- Express interest in employees' well-being;
- Insure you have the necessary technical abilities to support employee efforts;
- Display effective communication skills, especially listening;
- Provide coaching support when needed;
- Focus on being productive and on end results; and
- Avoid over-managing; let your team be responsible.

At first glance, you're probably thinking that these eight attributes seem pretty simplistic and obvious, and you may be wondering why Google spent all this time and effort to uncover these. Even Google's vice president for people operations, Laszlo Bock, said, "My first reaction was, that's it?" Another writer described it as "reading like a whiteboard gag from an episode of *The Office*." But, as the old saying goes, there *was* more to this list than meets the eye.

When Bock and his team began looking closer and rank ordering the eight items by importance, Project Oxygen got interesting—a lot more interesting! And

to understand this, you have to understand something about Google's approach to management since its founding in 1999. Plain and simple, managers were encouraged to "leave people alone. Let the engineers do their stuff. If they become stuck, they'll ask their bosses, whose deep technical expertise propelled them to management in the first place." It's not hard to see what Google wanted its managers to be—outstanding technical specialists. Mr. Bock explains, "In the Google context, we'd always believed that to be a manager, particularly on the engineering side, you need to be as deep or deeper a technical expert than the people who work for you." However, Project Oxygen revealed that technical expertise was ranked number eight (very last) on the list. So, here's the complete list from most important to least important, along with what each characteristic entails:

- *Provide coaching support when needed* (provide specific feedback and have regular one-on-one meetings with employees; offer solutions tailored to each employee's strengths)
- *Avoid over-managing; let your team be responsible* (give employees space to tackle problems themselves, but be available to offer advice)
- *Express interest in employees' well-being* (make new team members feel welcome and get to know your employees as people)
- *Focus on being productive and on end results* (focus on helping the team achieve its goals by prioritizing work and getting rid of obstacles)
- *Display good communication skills, especially listening* (learn to listen and to share information; encourage open dialogue and pay attention to the team's concerns)
- *Help individuals to reach their long-term work goals* (notice employees' efforts so they can see how their hard work is furthering their careers; appreciate employees' efforts and make that appreciation known)
- *Provide an unambiguous vision of the future* (lead the team but keep everyone involved in developing and working towards the team's vision)
- *Insure you have the necessary technical abilities to support employee efforts* (understand the challenges facing the team and be able to help team members solve problems)

Now, managers at Google aren't just encouraged to be great managers, they know what being a great manager involves. And the company is doing its part as well. Using the list, Google started training managers, as well as providing individual coaching and performance review sessions. You can say that Project Oxygen breathed new life into Google's managers. Bock says the company's efforts paid off quickly. "We were able to have a statistically significant improvement in manager quality for 75 percent of our worst-performing managers."

⭐ DISCUSSION QUESTIONS

17. Describe the findings of Project Oxygen using the functions approach, Mintzberg's roles approach, and the skills approach.

18. Are you surprised at what Google found out about "building a better boss?" Explain your answer.

19. What's the difference between encouraging managers to be great managers and knowing what being a great manager involves?

20. What could other companies learn from Google's experiences?

21. Would you want to work for a company like Google? Why or why not?

ENDNOTES

1. J. Welch and S. Welch, "An Employee Bill of Rights," *Bloomberg BusinessWeek*, March 16, 2009, p. 72.

2. R. Goffee and G. Jones, "Creating the Best Workplace on Earth," *Harvard Business Review,* May 2013.

3. R. Feintzeig, "Building Middle-Manager Morale," *Wall Street Journal,* August 8, 2013, pp. B1+.

4. R. Beck and J. Harter, "Why Great Managers Are So Rare," *Gallup Business Journal* [businessjournal.gallup.com], March 25, 2014; E. Frauenheim, "Managers Don't Matter," *Workforce Management Online*, April 2010; and K. A. Tucker and V. Allman, "Don't Be a Cat-and-Mouse Manager," The Gallup Organization [www.brain.gallup.com], September 9, 2004.

5. "Work USA 2008/2009 Report: Driving Business Results through Continuous Engagement," Watson Wyatt Worldwide, Washington, DC.

6. "The New Employment Deal: How Far, How Fast and How Enduring? Insights from the 2010 Global Workforce Study," Towers Watson, Washington, DC.

7. R. R. Hastings, "Study: Supervisors Drive Employee Engagement," *HR Magazine*, August 2011, p. 22.

8. T. R. Holcomb, R. M. Holmes, Jr., and B. L. Connelly, "Making the Most of What You Have: Managerial Ability as a Source of Resource Value Creation," *Strategic Management Journal*, May 2009, pp. 457–485.

9. http://www.catalyst.org/knowledge/women-ceos-fortune-1000, January 1, 2014.

10. D. J. Campbell, "The Proactive Employee: Managing Workplace Initiative," *Academy of Management Executive*, August 2000, pp. 52–66.

11. J. S. McClenahen, "Prairie Home Champion," *Industry Week*, October 2005, pp. 45–47.

12. "Interaction: First, Let's Fire All the Managers," *Harvard Business Review*, March 2012, pp. 20–21; and G. Hamel, "First, Let's Fire All the Managers," *Harvard Business Review*, December 2011, pp. 48–60.

13. F. Hassan, "The Frontline Advantage," *Harvard Business Review,* May 2011, p. 109.

14. L. Weber and L. A. Santiago, "By The Numbers," *Wall Street Journal,* August 6, 2013, p. B4.

15. Q. Hardy, "Google Thinks Small," *Forbes*, November 14, 2005, pp. 198–202.

16. Future Vision box based on M. Saltsman, "The Employee of the Month Has a Battery," *Wall Street Journal*, January 30, 2014, p. A13; L. Weber, "Robots Need Supervisors Too," *Wall Street Journal,* August 8, 2013, p. B5; S. Grobart, "Robot Workers: Coexistence Is Possible," *Bloomberg BusinessWeek Online,* December 13, 2012; and D. Bennett, "I'll Have My Robots Talk to Your Robots," *Bloomberg BusinessWeek* (February 21–27, 2011), pp. 52–62.

17. P. Panchak, "Sustaining Lean," *Industry Week*, October 2005, pp. 48–50.

18. H. Fayol, *Industrial and General Administration* (Paris: Dunod, 1916).

19. For a comprehensive review of this question, see C. P. Hales, "What Do Managers Do? A Critical Review of the Evidence," *Journal of Management*, January 1986, pp. 88–115.

20. J. T. Straub, "Put on Your Manager's Hat," *USA Today Online* [www.usatoday.com], October 29, 2002; and H. Mintzberg, *The Nature of Managerial Work* (New York: Harper & Row, 1973).

21. E. C. Dierdorff, R. S. Rubin, and F. P. Morgeson, "The Milieu of Managerial Work: An Integrative Framework Linking Work Context to Role Requirements," *Journal of Applied Psychology*, June 2009, pp. 972–988.

22. H. Mintzberg and J. Gosling, "Educating Managers Beyond Borders," *Academy of Management Learning and Education*, September 2002, pp. 64–76.

23. See, for example, M. J. Martinko and W. L. Gardner, "Structured Observation of Managerial Work: A Replication and Synthesis," *Journal of Management Studies*, May 1990, pp. 330–357; A. I. Kraut, P. R. Pedigo, D. D. McKenna, and M. D. Dunnette, "The Role of the Manager: What's Really Important in Different Management Jobs," *Academy of Management Executive*, November 1989, pp. 286–293; and

C. M. Pavett and A. W. Lau, "Managerial Work: The Influence of Hierarchical Level and Functional Specialty," *Academy of Management Journal*, March 1983, pp. 170–77.

24. Pavett and Lau, "Managerial Work."

25. S. J. Carroll and D. J. Gillen, "Are the Classical Management Functions Useful in Describing Managerial Work?" *Academy of Management Review*, January 1987, p. 48.

26. K. Tyler, "Train Your Front Line," *HR Magazine,* December 2013, pp. 43–45.

27. See, for example, J. G. Harris, D. W. DeLong, and A. Donnellon, "Do You Have What It Takes to Be an E-Manager?" *Strategy and Leadership*, August 2001, pp. 10–14; C. Fletcher and C. Baldry, "A Study of Individual Differences and Self-Awareness in the Context of Multi-Source Feedback," *Journal of Occupational and Organizational Psychology*, September 2000, pp. 303–319; and R. L. Katz, "Skills of an Effective Administrator," *Harvard Business Review*, September/October 1974, pp. 90–102.

28. K. Fivecoat-Campbell, "Up the Corporate Ladder," *Springfield, Missouri, Business Journal*, March 12–18, 2012, pp. 9+.

29. P. Shergill, "Winning the Talent Game: How Gamification Is Impacting Business and HR," www.wired.com/insights/, January 29, 2014; T. Harbert, "Giving Gamification A Go," *Computerworld*, January 13, 2014, pp. 12–17; and F. Manjoo, "The 'Gamification' of the Office," *Wall Street Journal*, January 13, 2014, pp. B1+.

30. C. Ansberry, "Firms Map Routes to Recovery," *Wall Street Journal*, March 2, 2010, pp. B1+.

31. F. F. Reichheld, "Lead for Loyalty," *Harvard Business Review*, July/August 2001, Vol. 79(7) p. 76.

32. Cited in E. Naumann and D. W. Jackson, Jr., "One More Time: How Do You Satisfy Customers?" *Business Horizons*, May/June 1999, p. 73.

33. Data from *The World Factbook 2014*, https://www.cia.gov/library/publications/the-world-factbook/geos/ch.html.

34. C. B. Blocker, D. J. Flint, M. B. Myers, and S. F. Slater, "Proactive Customer Orientation and Its Role for Creating Customer Value in Global Markets," *Journal of the Academy of Marketing Science*, April 2011, pp. 216–233; D. Dougherty and A. Murthy, "What Service Customers Really Want," *Harvard Business Review*, September 2009, p. 22; and K. A. Eddleston, D. L. Kidder, and B. E. Litzky, "Who's the Boss? Contending With Competing Expectations From Customers and Management," *Academy of Management Executive*, November 2002, pp. 85–95.

35. See, for instance, D. Meinert, "Aim to Serve," *HR Magazine*, December 2011, p. 18; D. M. Mayer, M. G. Ehrhart, and B. Schneider, "Service Attribute Boundary Conditions of the Service Climate-Customer Satisfaction Link," *Academy of Management Journal*, October 2009, pp. 1034–1050; M. Groth, T. Hennig-Thurau, and G. Walsh, "Customer Reactions to Emotional Labor: The Roles of Employee Acting Strategies and Customer Detection Accuracy," *Academy of Management Journal*, October 2009, pp. 958–974; J. W. Grizzle, A. R. Zablah, T. J. Brown, J. C. Mowen, and J. M. Lee, "Employee Customer Orientation in Context: How the Environment Moderates the Influence of Customer Orientation on Performance Outcomes," *Journal of Applied Psychology*, September 2009, pp. 1227–1242; B. A. Gutek, M. Groth, and B. Cherry, "Achieving Service Success Through Relationships and Enhanced Encounters," *Academy of Management Executive*, November 2002, pp. 132–144; Eddleston, Kidder, and Litzky, "Who's the Boss? Contending With Competing Expectations From Customers and Management"; S. D. Pugh, J. Dietz, J. W. Wiley, and S. M. Brooks, "Driving Service Effectiveness Through Employee-Customer Linkages," *Academy of Management Executive*, November 2002, pp. 73–84; S. D. Pugh, "Service With a Smile: Emotional Contagion in the Service Encounter," *Academy of Management Journal*, October 2001, pp. 1018–1027; W. C. Tsai, "Determinants and Consequences of Employee Displayed Positive Emotions," *Journal of Management*, vol. 27, no. 4, 2001, pp. 497–512; Naumann and Jackson, Jr., "One More Time: How Do You Satisfy Customers?"; and M. D. Hartline and O. C. Ferrell, "The Management of Customer-Contact Service Employees: An Empirical Investigation," *Journal of Marketing*, October 1996, pp. 52–70.

36. J. Swartz, "Twitter Helps Customer Service," *USA Today*, November 18, 2009, p. 3B; and J. Swartz, "Businesses Get Cheap Help from a Little Birdie," *USA Today*, June 26, 2009, p. 1B.

37. D. Ferris, "Social Studies: How to Use Social Media to Build a Better Organization," *Workforce Online*, February 12, 2012.

38. Leader Making a Difference box based on C. Hymowitz, "Ursula Burns," *Bloomberg BusinessWeek*, August 12–25, 2013, pp. 56–58; "What Do CEOs Admire?" *Fortune*, March 19, 2012, p. 143; N. Kolakowski, "Ursula Burns: Focused on the Core," *eWeek*, February 13, 2012, pp. 10–13; E. McGert, "Fresh Copy," *Fast Company*, December 2011/January 2012, pp. 132–138; and D. Mattioli, "Xerox Chief Looks Beyond Photocopiers Toward Services," *Wall Street Journal*, June 13, 2011, p. B9.

39. R. Wagner, "One Store, One Team at Best Buy," *Gallup Brain* [http://brain.gallup.com/content/], August 12, 2004.

40. S. Clifford, "Unexpected Ally Helps Wal-Mart Cut Waste," *New York Times Online*, April 13, 2012; and S. Rosenbloom, "Wal-Mart Unveils Plan to Make Supply Chain Greener," *New York Times Online*, February 25, 2010.

41. S. Clifford, "Unexpected Ally Helps Wal-Mart Cut Waste," *New York Times Online*, April 13, 2012.

42. KPMG Global Sustainability Services, *Sustainability Insights*, October 2007.

43. *Vision 2050* Report, Overview, www.wbcsd.org/vision2050.aspx.

44. *Symposium on Sustainability—Profiles in Leadership*, New York, October 2001.

45. R. E. Silverman, "Where's the Boss? Trapped in a Meeting," *Wall Street Journal*, February 14, 2012, pp. B1+; and J. Sandberg, "Down over Moving Up: Some New Bosses Find They Hate Their Jobs," *Wall Street Journal*, July 27, 2005, p. B1.

46. Silverman, "Where's the Boss? Trapped in a Meeting."

47. M. S. Plakhotnik and T. S. Rocco, "A Succession Plan for First-Time Managers," *T&D*, December 2011, pp. 42–45; P. Brotherton, "New Managers Feeling Lost at Sea," *T&D*, June 2011, p. 25; and "How Do We Help a New Manager Manage?" *Workforce Management Online*, June 16, 2011.

48. S. Y. Todd, K. J. Harris, R. B. Harris, and A. R. Wheeler, "Career Success Implications of Political Skill," *Journal of Social Psychology*, June 2009, pp. 179–204; G. R. Ferris, D. C. Treadway, P. L. Perrewé, R. L. Brouer, C. Douglas, and S. Lux, "Political Skill in Organizations," *Journal of Management*, June 2007, pp. 290–329; K. J. Harris, K. M. Kacmar, S. Zivnuska, and J. D. Shaw, "The Impact of Political Skill on Impression Management Effectiveness," *Journal of Applied Psychology*, January 2007, pp. 278–285; and G. R. Ferris, D. C. Treadway, R. W. Kolodinsky, W. A. Hochwarter, C. J. Kacmar, C. Douglas, and D. D. Frink, "Development and Validation of the Political Skill Inventory," *Journal of Management*, February 2005, pp. 126–152.

49. E. Kampf, "Can You Really Manage Engagement Without Managers?" *Gallup Business Journal* [businessjournal.gallup.com], April 24, 2014; "Holacracy," *T&D*, March 2014, p. 17; S. Helgesen, "An Extreme Take on Restructuring: No Job Titles, No Managers, No Politics," *Strategy + Business*, www.strategy-business.com, February 11, 2014; R. Trikha, "Zappos Says Bye to Managers—What if You Had No Boss?" www.cybercoders.com/insights/, January 7, 2014; G. Anders, "No More Bosses for Zappos (A Cautionary Tale)," jobs.aol.com/articles/, January 7, 2014; M. Wohlsen, "The Next Big Thing You Missed: Companies That Work Better Without Bosses," www.wired.com/business/, January 7, 2014; C. Sweeney and J. Gosfield, "No Managers Required: How Zappos Ditched the Old Corporate Structure for Something New," www.fastcompany.com, January 6, 2014; J. McGregor, "Zappos Says Goodbye to Bosses," www.washingtonpost.com/blogs/on-leadership/, January 3, 2014; J. Edwards, "Zappos Is Getting Rid of All Job Titles and Managers, But Some Bosses Will Still Decide Who Gets Paid What," www.businessinsider.com/, January 2, 2014; A. Groth, "Zappos is Going Holacratic: No Job Titles, No Managers, No Hierarchy," qz.com/, December 30, 2013; R. E. Silverman, "Managers? Who Needs Those?" *Wall Street Journal*, August 7, 2013, pp. B1+; M. Shaer, "The Boss Stops Here," nymag.com/news/features/, June 16, 2013; S. Wagreich, "A Billion Dollar Company With *No* Bosses? Yes, It Exists," www.inc.com/, March 14, 2013; R. E. Silverman, "Who's the Boss? There Isn't One," *Wall Street Journal*, June 20, 2012, pp. B1+; G. Hamel, "First, Let's Fire All the Managers;" and J. Badal, "Can a Company Be Run as a Democracy?" *Wall Street Journal*, April 23, 2007, p. B1.

50. C. Sweeney and J. Gosfield, "No Managers Required: How Zappos Ditched the Old Corporate Structure for Something New."

51. C. Sweeney and J. Gosfield, "No Managers Required: How Zappos Ditched the Old Corporate Structure for Something New."

52. D. Richards, "At Zappos, Culture Pays," www.strategy-business.com/article, August 24, 2010.

53. A. Groth, "Zappos is Going Holacratic: No Job Titles, No Managers, No Hierarchy," qz.com, December 30, 2013.

54. G. Anders, "No More Bosses for Zappos (A Cautionary Tale)," jobs.aol.com/articles, January 7, 2014.

55. D. A. Garvin, "How Google Sold Its Engineers on Management," *Harvard Business Review*, December 2013, pp. 74–82; R. D'Aprix, "A Simple Effective Formula for Leadership," *Strategic Communication Management*, May 2011, p. 14; R. Jaish, "Pieces of Eight," *e-learning age*, May 2011, p. 6; M. L. Stallard, "Google's Project Oxygen: A Case-Study in Connection Culture," www.humanresourcesiq.com, March 25, 2011; J. Aquino, "8 Traits of Stellar Managers, Defined by Googlers," www.businessinsider.com, March 15, 2011; and A. Bryant, "Google's Quest to Build a Better Boss," *New York Times Online*, March 12, 2011.

Management History *Module*

Management History *Module*

Henry Ford once said, "History is more or less bunk." Well, he was wrong! History is important because it can put current activities in perspective. In this module, we're going to take a trip back in time to see how the field of study called management has evolved. What you're going to see is that today's managers still use many elements of the historical approaches to management. Focus on the following learning objectives as you read and study this module.

Learning Objectives

1 **Describe** some early management examples.
2 **Explain** the various theories in the classical approach.
3 **Discuss** the development and uses of the behavioral approach.
4 **Describe** the quantitative approach.
5 **Explain** the various theories in the contemporary approach.

3000 BC – 1776	1911 – 1947	Late 1700s – 1950s	1940s – 1950s	1960s – present
Early Management	Classical Approach	Behavioral Approach	Quantitative Approach	Contemporary Approaches

EARLY Management

MH1

Management has been practiced a long time. Organized endeavors directed by people responsible for planning, organizing, leading, and controlling activities have existed for thousands of years. Let's look at some of the most interesting examples.

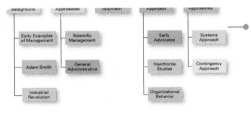

Source: Stephen Studd/Getty Images

The Egyptian pyramids and the Great Wall of China are proof that projects of tremendous scope, employing tens of thousands of people, were completed in ancient times.[1] It took more than 100,000 workers some 20 years to construct a single pyramid. Who told each worker what to do? Who ensured there would be enough stones at the site to keep workers busy? The answer is *managers*. Someone had to plan what was to be done, organize people and materials to do it, make sure those workers got the work done, and impose some controls to ensure that everything was done as planned.

Another example of early management can be found in the city of Venice, which was a major economic and trade center in the 1400s. The Venetians developed an early form of business enterprise and engaged in many activities common to today's organizations. For instance, at the arsenal of Venice, warships were floated along the canals, and at each stop, materials and riggings were added to the ship.[2] Sounds a lot like a car "floating" along an assembly line, doesn't it? In addition, the Venetians used warehouse and inventory systems to keep track of materials, human resource management functions to manage the labor force (including wine breaks), and an accounting system to keep track of revenues and costs.

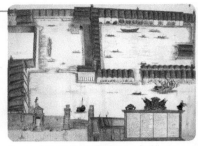

Source: Antonio Natale/Bridgeman Art Library

In 1776, Adam Smith published *The Wealth of Nations*, in which he argued the economic advantages that organizations and society would gain from the **division of labor** (or **job specialization**)—that is, breaking down jobs into narrow and repetitive tasks. Using the pin industry as an example, Smith claimed that 10 individuals, each doing a specialized task, could produce about 48,000 pins a day among them. However, if each person worked alone performing each task separately, it would be quite an accomplishment to produce even 10 pins a day! Smith concluded that division of labor increased productivity by increasing each worker's skill and dexterity, saving time lost in changing tasks and creating labor-saving inventions and machinery. Job specialization continues to be popular. For example, think of the specialized tasks performed by members of a hospital surgery team, meal preparation tasks done by workers in restaurant kitchens, or positions played by players on a football team.

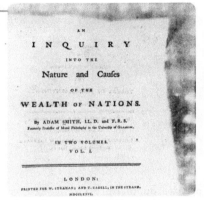

Source: Fotosearch/Stringer/Getty Images

Starting in the late eighteenth century when machine power was substituted for human power, a point in history known as the **industrial revolution**, it became more economical to manufacture goods in factories rather than at home. These large, efficient factories needed someone to forecast demand, ensure that enough material was on hand to make products, assign tasks to people, direct daily activities, and so forth. That "someone" was a manager. These managers would need formal theories to guide them in running these large organizations. It wasn't until the early 1900s, however, that the first steps toward developing such theories were taken.

In this module, we'll look at four major approaches to management theory: classical, behavioral, quantitative, and contemporary. (See Exhibit 1.) Keep in

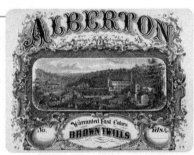

Source: Transcendental Graphics/Getty Images

Exhibit 1
Major Approaches to Management

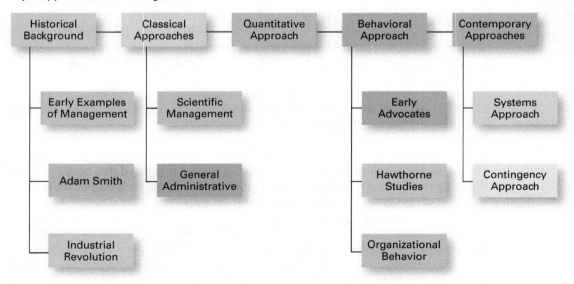

division of labor (job specialization)
The breakdown of jobs into narrow and repetitive tasks

industrial revolution
A period during the late eighteenth century when machine power was substituted for human power, making it more economical to manufacture goods in factories than at home

mind that each approach is concerned with trying to explain management from the perspective of what was important at that time in history and the backgrounds and interests of the researchers. Each of the four approaches contributes to our overall understanding of management, but each is also a limited view of what it is and how to best practice it.

3000 BC – 1776	1911 – 1947	Late 1700s – 1950s	1940s – 1950s	1960s – present
Early Management	Classical Approach	Behavioral Approach	Quantitative Approach	Contemporary Approaches

CLASSICAL Approach

MH2

classical approach
First studies of management, which emphasized rationality and making organizations and workers as efficient as possible

Although we've seen how management has been used in organized efforts since early history, the formal study of management didn't begin until early in the twentieth century. These first studies of management, often called the **classical approach**, emphasized rationality and making organizations and workers as efficient as possible. Two major theories comprise the classical approach: scientific management and general administrative theory. The two most important contributors to scientific management theory were Frederick W. Taylor and the husband-wife team of Frank and Lillian Gilbreth. The two most important contributors to general administrative theory were Henri Fayol and Max Weber. Let's take a look at each of these important figures in management history.

Scientific Management

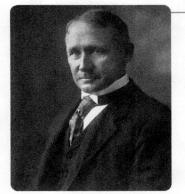

Source: Jacques Boyer/The Image Works

scientific management
An approach that involves using the scientific method to find the "one best way" for a job to be done

If you had to pinpoint when modern management theory was born, 1911 might be a good choice. That was when Frederick Winslow Taylor's *Principles of Scientific Management* was published. Its contents were widely embraced by managers around the world. Taylor's book described the theory of **scientific management**: the use of scientific methods to define the "one best way" for a job to be done.

Taylor worked at the Midvale and Bethlehem Steel Companies in Pennsylvania. As a mechanical engineer with a Quaker and Puritan background, he was continually appalled by workers' inefficiencies. Employees used vastly different techniques to do the same job. They often "took it easy" on the job, and Taylor believed that worker output was only about one-third of what was possible. Virtually no work standards existed, and workers were placed in jobs with little or no concern for matching their abilities and aptitudes with the tasks they were required to do. Taylor set out to remedy that by applying the scientific method to shop-floor jobs. He spent more than two decades passionately pursuing the "one best way" for such jobs to be done.

Taylor's experiences at Midvale led him to define clear guidelines for improving production efficiency. He argued that these four principles of management (see Exhibit 2) would result in prosperity for both workers and managers.[3] How did these scientific principles really work? Let's look at an example.

Probably the best known example of Taylor's scientific management efforts was the pig iron experiment. Workers loaded "pigs" of iron (each weighing 92 lbs.) onto rail cars. Their daily average output was 12.5 tons. However, Taylor believed that by scientifically analyzing the job to determine the "one best way" to load pig iron, output could be increased to 47 or 48 tons per day. After scientifically applying different combinations of procedures, techniques, and tools, Taylor succeeded in getting that level of productivity. How? By putting the right person on the job with the correct tools and equipment, having the worker follow his instructions exactly, and motivating the worker with an economic incentive of a significantly higher daily wage. Using similar approaches for other jobs, Taylor was able to define the "one best way" for doing each job. Overall, Taylor

1. Develop a science for each element of an individual's work to replace the old rule-of-thumb method.
2. Scientifically select and then train, teach, and develop the worker.
3. Heartily cooperate with the workers to ensure that all work is done in accordance with the principles of the science that has been developed.
4. Divide work and responsibility almost equally between management and workers. Management does all work for which it is better suited than the workers.

Source: Taylor, Frederick Winslow, Principles of Scientific Management (New York: Harper, 1911).

Exhibit 2
Taylor's Scientific Management Principles

achieved consistent productivity improvements in the range of 200 percent or more. Based on his groundbreaking studies of manual work using scientific principles, Taylor became known as the "father" of scientific management. His ideas spread in the United States and to other countries and inspired others to study and develop methods of scientific management. His most prominent followers were Frank and Lillian Gilbreth.

A construction contractor by trade, Frank Gilbreth gave up that career to study scientific management after hearing Taylor speak at a professional meeting. Frank and his wife Lillian, a psychologist, studied work to eliminate inefficient hand-and-body motions. The Gilbreths also experimented with the design and use of the proper tools and equipment for optimizing work performance.[4] Also, as parents of 12 children, the Gilbreths ran their household using scientific management principles and techniques. In fact, two of their children wrote a book, *Cheaper by the Dozen*, which described life with the two masters of efficiency.

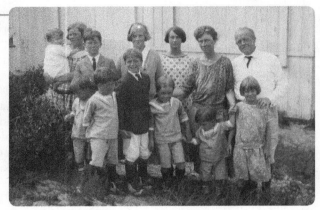

Source: Bettmann/Corbis

Frank is probably best known for his bricklaying experiments. By carefully analyzing the bricklayer's job, he reduced the number of motions in laying exterior brick from 18 to about 5, and in laying interior brick from 18 to 2. Using Gilbreth's techniques, a bricklayer was more productive and less fatigued at the end of the day.

The Gilbreths invented a device called a microchronometer that recorded a worker's hand-and-body motions and the amount of time spent doing each motion. Wasted motions missed by the naked eye could be identified and eliminated. The Gilbreths also devised a classification scheme to label 17 basic hand motions (such as search, grasp, hold), which they called **therbligs** (Gilbreth spelled backward with the *th* transposed). This scheme gave the Gilbreths a more precise way of analyzing a worker's exact hand movements.

therbligs
A classification scheme for labeling basic hand motions

general administrative theory
An approach to management that focuses on describing what managers do and what constitutes good management practice

HOW TODAY'S MANAGERS USE SCIENTIFIC MANAGEMENT Many of the guidelines and techniques Taylor and the Gilbreths devised for improving production efficiency are still used in organizations today. When managers analyze the basic work tasks that must be performed, use time-and-motion study to eliminate wasted motions, hire the best-qualified workers for a job, or design incentive systems based on output, they're using the principles of scientific management.

General Administrative Theory

General administrative theory focused more on what managers do and what constituted good management practice. Henri Fayol first identified five functions that managers perform: planning, organizing, commanding, coordinating, and controlling.[5]

Fayol wrote during the same time period as Taylor. While Taylor was concerned with first-line managers and the scientific method, Fayol's attention was directed at the activities of *all* managers. He wrote from his personal experience as the managing director of a large French coal-mining firm.

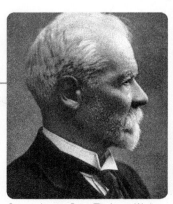

Source: Jacques Boyer/The Image Works

Fayol described the practice of management as something distinct from accounting, finance, production, distribution, and other typical business functions. His belief that management was an activity common to all business endeavors, government, and even the home led him to develop 14 **principles of management**—fundamental rules of management that could be applied to all organizational situations and taught in schools. These principles are shown in Exhibit 3.

Max Weber (pronounced VAY-ber) was a German sociologist who studied organizations.[6] Writing in the early 1900s, he developed a theory of authority structures and relations based on an ideal type of organization he called a **bureaucracy**—a form of organization characterized by division of labor, a clearly defined hierarchy, detailed rules and regulations, and impersonal relationships. (See Exhibit 4.) Weber recognized that this "ideal bureaucracy" didn't exist in reality. Instead, he intended it as a basis for theorizing about how work could be done in large groups. His theory became the structural design for many of today's large organizations.

Bureaucracy, as described by Weber, is a lot like scientific management in its ideology. Both emphasized rationality, predictability, impersonality, technical competence, and authoritarianism. Although Weber's ideas were less practical than Taylor's, the fact that his "ideal type" still describes many contemporary organizations attests to their importance.

HOW TODAY'S MANAGERS USE GENERAL ADMINISTRATIVE THEORY Several of our current management ideas and practices can be directly traced to the contributions of general administrative theory. For instance, the functional view of the manager's job can be attributed to Fayol. In addition, his 14 principles serve as a frame of reference from which many current management concepts—such as managerial authority, centralized decision making, reporting to only one boss, and so forth—have evolved.

principles of management
Fundamental rules of management that could be applied in all organizational situations and taught in schools

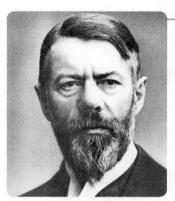

Source: Hulton Archive/Getty Images

bureaucracy
A form of organization characterized by division of labor, a clearly defined hierarchy, detailed rules and regulations, and impersonal relationships

Exhibit 3
Fayol's Fourteen Principles of Management

1. **Division of work.** Specialization increases output by making employees more efficient.
2. **Authority.** Managers must be able to give orders, and authority gives them this right.
3. **Discipline.** Employees must obey and respect the rules that govern the organization.
4. **Unity of command.** Every employee should receive orders from only one superior.
5. **Unity of direction.** The organization should have a single plan of action to guide managers and workers.
6. **Subordination of individual interests to the general interest.** The interests of any one employee or group of employees should not take precedence over the interests of the organization as a whole.
7. **Remuneration.** Workers must be paid a fair wage for their services.
8. **Centralization.** This term refers to the degree to which subordinates are involved in decision making.
9. **Scalar chain.** The line of authority from top management to the lowest ranks is the scalar chain.
10. **Order.** People and materials should be in the right place at the right time.
11. **Equity.** Managers should be kind and fair to their subordinates.
12. **Stability of tenure of personnel.** Management should provide orderly personnel planning and ensure that replacements are available to fill vacancies.
13. **Initiative.** Employees allowed to originate and carry out plans will exert high levels of effort.
14. **Esprit de corps.** Promoting team spirit will build harmony and unity within the organization.

Source: Based on Henri Fayol's 1916 Principles of Management, "Administration Industrielle et Générale," translated by C. Storrs, General and Industrial Management (London: Sir Isaac Pitman & Sons, London, 1949).

Exhibit 4
Characteristics of Weber's Bureaucracy

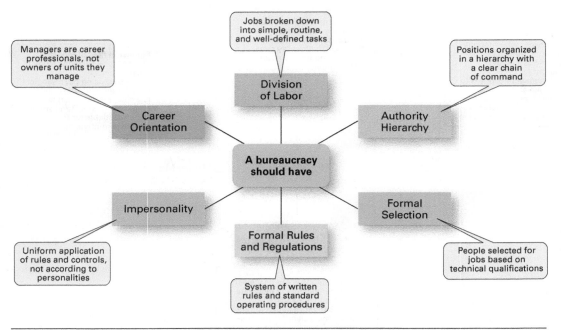

Source: Based on *Essays in Sociology* by Max Weber, translated, edited, and introduction by H. H. Gerth and C. Wright Mills (New York: Oxford University Press, 1946).

Weber's bureaucracy was an attempt to formulate an ideal prototype for organizations. Although many characteristics of Weber's bureaucracy are still evident in large organizations, his model isn't as popular today as it was in the twentieth century. Many managers feel that a bureaucratic structure hinders individual employees' creativity and limits an organization's ability to respond quickly to an increasingly dynamic environment. However, even in flexible organizations of creative professionals—such as Google, Samsung, General Electric, or Cisco Systems—bureaucratic mechanisms are necessary to ensure that resources are used efficiently and effectively.

3000 BC – 1776	1911 – 1947	Late 1700s – 1950s	1940s – 1950s	1960s – present
Early Management	Classical Approach	Behavioral Approach	Quantitative Approach	Contemporary Approaches

BEHAVIORAL Approach

As we know, managers get things done by working with people. This explains why some writers have chosen to look at management by focusing on the organization's people. The field of study that researches the actions (behavior) of people at work is called **organizational behavior (OB)**. Much of what managers do today when managing people—motivating, leading, building trust, working with a team, managing conflict, and so forth—has come out of OB research.

Although a number of individuals in the early twentieth century recognized the importance of people to an organization's success, four stand out as early advocates of the OB approach: Robert Owen, Hugo Munsterberg, Mary Parker Follett, and Chester Barnard. Their contributions were varied and distinct, yet all believed that people were the most important asset of the organization and should be managed accordingly. Their ideas provided the foundation for such management practices as employee selection procedures, motivation programs, and work teams. Exhibit 5 summarizes each individual's most important ideas.

organizational behavior (OB)
The study of the actions of people at work

Exhibit MH-5
Early OB Advocates

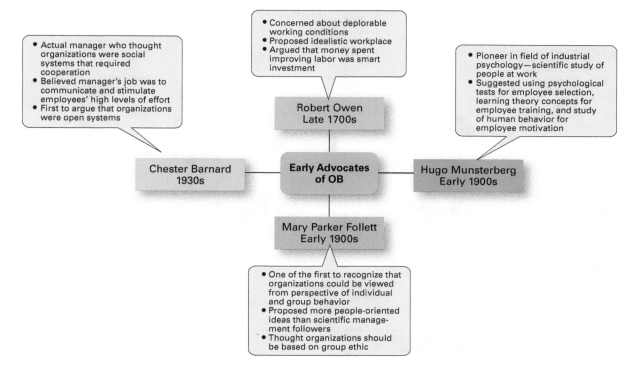

- Actual manager who thought organizations were social systems that required cooperation
- Believed manager's job was to communicate and stimulate employees' high levels of effort
- First to argue that organizations were open systems

- Concerned about deplorable working conditions
- Proposed idealistic workplace
- Argued that money spent improving labor was smart investment

- Pioneer in field of industrial psychology—scientific study of people at work
- Suggested using psychological tests for employee selection, learning theory concepts for employee training, and study of human behavior for employee motivation

Robert Owen
Late 1700s

Chester Barnard
1930s

Early Advocates of OB

Hugo Munsterberg
Early 1900s

Mary Parker Follett
Early 1900s

- One of the first to recognize that organizations could be viewed from perspective of individual and group behavior
- Proposed more people-oriented ideas than scientific management followers
- Thought organizations should be based on group ethic

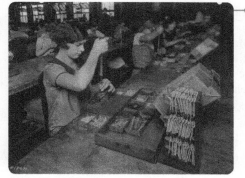

Source: Morton College

Hawthorne Studies
A series of studies during the 1920s and 1930s that provided new insights into individual and group behavior

Without question, the most important contribution to the OB field came out of the **Hawthorne Studies**, a series of studies conducted at the Western Electric Company Works in Cicero, Illinois. These studies, which started in 1924, were initially designed by Western Electric industrial engineers as a scientific management experiment. They wanted to examine the effect of various lighting levels on worker productivity. Like any good scientific experiment, control and experimental groups were set up, with the experimental group exposed to various lighting intensities, and the control group working under a constant intensity. If you were the industrial engineers in charge of this experiment, what would you have expected to happen? It's logical to think that individual output in the experimental group would be directly related to the intensity of the light. However, they found that as the level of light was increased in the experimental group, output for both groups increased. Then, much to the surprise of the engineers, as the light level was decreased in the experimental group, productivity continued to increase in both groups. In fact, a productivity decrease was observed in the experimental group *only* when the level of light was reduced to that of a moonlit night. What would explain these unexpected results? The engineers weren't sure, but concluded that lighting intensity was not directly related to group productivity and that something else must have contributed to the results. They weren't able to pinpoint what that "something else" was, though.

In 1927, the Western Electric engineers asked Harvard professor Elton Mayo and his associates to join the study as consultants. Thus began a relationship that would last through 1932 and encompass numerous experiments in the redesign of jobs, changes in workday and workweek length, introduction of rest periods, and individual versus group wage plans.[7] For example, one experiment was designed to evaluate the effect of a group piecework incentive pay system on group productivity. The results indicated that the incentive plan had less effect on a worker's output than

group pressure, acceptance, and security. The researchers concluded that social norms or group standards were the key determinants of individual work behavior.

Scholars generally agree that the Hawthorne Studies had a game-changing impact on management beliefs about the role of people in organizations. Mayo concluded that people's behavior and attitudes are closely related, that group factors significantly affect individual behavior, that group standards establish individual worker output, and that money is less a factor in determining output than group standards, group attitudes, and security. These conclusions led to a new emphasis on the human behavior factor in the management of organizations.

Although critics attacked the research procedures, analyses of findings, and conclusions, it's of little importance from a historical perspective whether the Hawthorne Studies were academically sound or their conclusions justified.[8] What *is* important is that they stimulated an interest in human behavior in organizations.

HOW TODAY'S MANAGERS USE THE BEHAVIORAL APPROACH The behavioral approach has largely shaped how today's organizations are managed. From the way managers design jobs to the way they work with employee teams to the way they communicate, we see elements of the behavioral approach. Much of what the early OB advocates proposed and the conclusions from the Hawthorne studies have provided the foundation for our current theories of motivation, leadership, group behavior and development, and numerous other behavioral approaches.

3000 BC – 1776	1911 – 1947	Late 1700s – 1950s	1940s – 1950s	1960s – present
Early Management	Classical Approach	Behavioral Approach	Quantitative Approach	Contemporary Approaches

QUANTITATIVE Approach

Although passengers bumping into each other when trying to find their seats on an airplane can be a mild annoyance for them, it's a bigger problem for airlines because lines get backed up, slowing down how quickly the plane can get back in the air. Based on research in space-time geometry, one airline innovated a unique boarding process called "reverse pyramid" that has saved at least two minutes in boarding time.[9] This is an example of the **quantitative approach**, which is the use of quantitative techniques to improve decision making. This approach also is known as *management science*.

quantitative approach
The use of quantitative techniques to improve decision making

The quantitative approach evolved from mathematical and statistical solutions developed for military problems during World War II. After the war was over, many of these techniques used for military problems were applied to businesses. For example, one group of military officers, nicknamed the Whiz Kids, joined Ford Motor Company in the mid-1940s and immediately began using statistical methods and quantitative models to improve decision making.

What exactly does the quantitative approach do? It involves applying statistics, optimization models, information models, computer simulations, and other quantitative techniques to management activities. Linear programming, for instance, is a technique that managers use to improve resource allocation decisions. Work scheduling can be more efficient as a result of critical-path scheduling analysis. The economic order quantity model helps managers determine optimum inventory levels. Each of these is an example of quantitative techniques being applied to improve managerial decision making. Another area where quantitative techniques are used frequently is in total quality management.

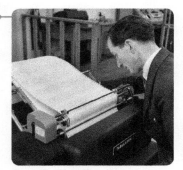

Source: Bert Hardy/Getty Images

Exhibit 6
What Is Quality Management?

1. **Intense focus on the customer.** The customer includes outsiders who buy the organization's products or services and internal customers who interact with and serve others in the organization.

2. **Concern for continual improvement.** Quality management is a commitment to never being satisfied. "Very good" is not good enough. Quality can always be improved.

3. **Process focused.** Quality management focuses on work processes as the quality of goods and services is continually improved.

4. **Improvement in the quality of everything the organization does.** This relates to the final product, how the organization handles deliveries, how rapidly it responds to complaints, how politely the phones are answered, and the like.

5. **Accurate measurement.** Quality management uses statistical techniques to measure every critical variable in the organization's operations. These are compared against standards to identify problems, trace them to their roots, and eliminate their causes.

6. **Empowerment of employees.** Quality management involves the people on the line in the improvement process. Teams are widely used in quality management programs as empowerment vehicles for finding and solving problems.

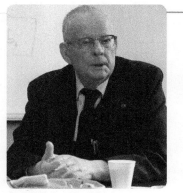

Source: AP Photo/David Stluka

total quality management (TQM)
A philosophy of management that is driven by continuous improvement and responsiveness to customer needs and expectations

A quality revolution swept through both the business and public sectors in the 1980s and 1990s.[10] It was inspired by a small group of quality experts, the most famous being W. Edwards Deming (pictured at right) and Joseph M. Juran. The ideas and techniques they advocated in the 1950s had few supporters in the United States but were enthusiastically embraced by Japanese organizations. As Japanese manufacturers began beating U.S. competitors in quality comparisons, however, Western managers soon took a more serious look at Deming's and Juran's ideas, which became the basis for today's quality management programs.

Total quality management, or **TQM**, is a management philosophy devoted to continual improvement and responding to customer needs and expectations. (See Exhibit 6.) The term *customer* includes anyone who interacts with the organization's product or services, internally or externally. It encompasses employees and suppliers, as well as the people who purchase the organization's goods or services. *Continual improvement* isn't possible without accurate measurements, which require statistical techniques that measure every critical variable in the organization's work processes. These measurements are compared against standards to identify and correct problems.

HOW TODAY'S MANAGERS USE THE QUANTITATIVE APPROACH No one likes long lines, especially residents of New York City. If they see a long checkout line, they often go somewhere else. However, at Whole Foods' first gourmet supermarkets in Manhattan, customers found something different—that is, the longer the line, the shorter the wait. When ready to check out, customers are guided into serpentine single lines that feed into numerous checkout lanes. Whole Foods, widely known for its organic food selections, can charge premium prices, which allow it the luxury of staffing all those checkout lanes. And customers are finding that their wait times are shorter than expected.[11] The science of keeping lines moving is known as queue management. And for Whole Foods, this quantitative technique has translated into strong sales at its Manhattan stores.

The quantitative approach contributes directly to management decision making in the areas of planning and control. For instance, when managers make budgeting, queuing, scheduling, quality control, and similar decisions, they typically rely on quantitative techniques. Specialized software has made the use of these techniques less intimidating for managers, although many still feel anxious about using them.

3000 BC - 1776	1911 - 1947	Late 1700s - 1950s	1940s - 1950s	1960s - present
Early Management	Classical Approach	Behavioral Approach	Quantitative Approach	Contemporary Approaches

CONTEMPORARY Approaches

MH5

As we've seen, many elements of the earlier approaches to management theory continue to influence how managers manage. Most of these earlier approaches focused on managers' concerns *inside* the organization. Starting in the 1960s, management researchers began to look at what was happening in the external environment *outside* the boundaries of the organization. Two contemporary management perspectives—systems and contingency—are part of this approach. Systems theory is a basic theory in the physical sciences, but had never been applied to organized human efforts. In 1938, Chester Barnard, a telephone company executive, first wrote in his book, *The Functions of an Executive,* that an organization functioned as a cooperative system. However, it wasn't until the 1960s that management researchers began to look more carefully at systems theory and how it related to organizations.

A **system** is a set of interrelated and interdependent parts arranged in a manner that produces a unified whole. The two basic types of systems are closed and open. **Closed systems** are not influenced by and do not interact with their environment. In contrast, **open systems** are influenced by and do interact with their environment. Today, when we describe organizations as systems, we mean open systems. Exhibit 7 shows a diagram of an organization from an open systems perspective. As you can see, an organization takes in inputs (resources) from the environment and transforms or processes these resources into outputs that are distributed into the environment. The organization is "open" to and interacts with its environment.

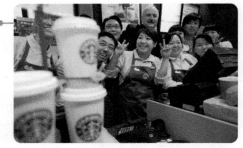
Source: Frederic J. Brown/AFP/Getty Images/Newscom

How does the systems approach contribute to our understanding of management? Researchers envisioned an organization as made up of "interdependent factors, including individuals, groups, attitudes, motives, formal structure, interactions, goals, status, and authority."[12] What this means is that as managers coordinate work activities in the various parts of the organization, they ensure that all these parts are working together so the organization's goals can be achieved. For example, the systems approach recognizes that, no matter how efficient the production department, the marketing department must anticipate changes in customer tastes and work with the product development department in creating products customers want—or the organization's overall performance will suffer.

system
A set of interrelated and interdependent parts arranged in a manner that produces a unified whole

closed systems
Systems that are not influenced by and do not interact with their environment

open systems
Systems that interact with their environment

Exhibit 7
Organization as an Open System

Inputs	Transformation Process	Outputs
Raw Materials Human Resources Capital Technology Information	Employees' Work Activities Management Activities Technology and Operations Methods	Products and Services Financial Results Information Human Results

Environment — Organization — Feedback — Environment

In addition, the systems approach implies that decisions and actions in one organizational area will affect other areas. For example, if the purchasing department doesn't acquire the right quantity and quality of inputs, the production department won't be able to do its job.

Finally, the systems approach recognizes that organizations are not self-contained. They rely on their environment for essential inputs and as outlets to absorb their outputs. No organization can survive for long if it ignores government regulations, supplier relations, or the varied external constituencies on which it depends.

How relevant is the systems approach to management? Quite relevant. Consider, for example, a shift manager at a Starbucks restaurant who must coordinate the work of employees filling customer orders at the front counter and the drive-through windows, direct the delivery and unloading of food supplies, and address any customer concerns that come up. This manager "manages" all parts of the "system" so that the restaurant meets its daily sales goals.

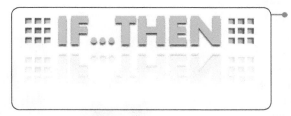

contingency approach
A management approach that recognizes organizations as different, which means they face different situations (contingencies) and require different ways of managing

The early management theorists came up with management principles they generally assumed to be universally applicable. Later research found exceptions to many of these principles. For example, division of labor is valuable and widely used, but jobs can become *too* specialized. Bureaucracy is desirable in many situations, but in other circumstances, other structural designs are *more* effective. Management is not (and cannot be) based on simplistic principles to be applied in all situations. Different and changing situations require managers to use different approaches and techniques. The **contingency approach** (sometimes called the *situational approach*) says that organizations are different, face different situations (contingencies), and require different ways of managing.

A good way to describe contingency is "if, then." *If* this is the way my situation is, *then* this is the best way for me to manage in this situation. It's intuitively logical because organizations and even units within the same organization differ—in size, goals, work activities, and the like. It would be surprising to find universally applicable management rules that would work in *all* situations. But, of course, it's one thing to say that the way to manage "depends on the situation" and another to say what the situation is. Management researchers continue working to identify these situational variables. Exhibit 8 describes four popular contingency variables. Although the list is by no means comprehensive—more than 100 different variables have been identified—it represents those most widely used and gives you an idea of what we mean by

Exhibit 8
Popular Contingency Variables

Organization Size. As size increases, so do the problems of coordination. For instance, the type of organization structure appropriate for an organization of 50,000 employees is likely to be inefficient for an organization of 50 employees.

Routineness of Task Technology. To achieve its purpose, an organization uses technology. Routine technologies require organizational structures, leadership styles, and control systems that differ from those required by customized or nonroutine technologies.

Environmental Uncertainty. The degree of uncertainty caused by environmental changes influences the management process. What works best in a stable and predictable environment may be totally inappropriate in a rapidly changing and unpredictable environment.

Individual Differences. Individuals differ in terms of their desire for growth, autonomy, tolerance of ambiguity, and expectations. These and other individual differences are particularly important when managers select motivation techniques, leadership styles, and job designs.

the term *contingency variable*. The primary value of the contingency approach is that it stresses there are no simplistic or universal rules for managers to follow.

So what do managers face today when managing? Although the dawn of the information age is said to have begun with Samuel Morse's telegraph in 1837, dramatic changes in information technology that occurred in the latter part of the twentieth century and continue through today directly affect the manager's job. Managers now may manage employees who are working from home or working halfway around the world. An organization's computing resources used to be mainframe computers locked away in temperature-controlled rooms and only accessed by the experts. Now, practically everyone in an organization is connected—wired or wireless—with devices no larger than the palm of the hand. Just like the impact of the industrial revolution in the 1700s on the emergence of management, the information age has brought dramatic changes that continue to influence the way organizations are managed.

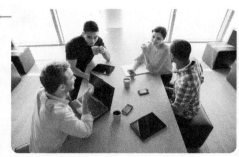
Source: Image Source/Getty Images

PREPARING FOR: Exams/Quizzes

CHAPTER SUMMARY by Learning Objectives

MH1 | DESCRIBE **some early management examples.**
Studying history is important because it helps us see the origins of today's management practices and recognize what has and has not worked. We can see early examples of management practice in the construction of the Egyptian pyramids and in the arsenal of Venice. One important historical event was the publication of Adam Smith's *Wealth of Nations*, in which he argued the benefits of division of labor (job specialization). Another was the industrial revolution, where it became more economical to manufacture in factories than at home. Managers were needed to manage these factories, and these managers needed formal management theories to guide them.

MH2 | EXPLAIN **the various theories in the classical approach.**
Frederick W. Taylor, known as the "father" of scientific management, studied manual work using scientific principles—that is, guidelines for improving production efficiency—to find the one best way to do those jobs. The Gilbreths' primary contribution was finding efficient hand-and-body motions and designing proper tools and equipment for optimizing work performance. Fayol believed the functions of management were common to all business endeavors but also were distinct from other business functions. He developed 14 principles of management from which many current management concepts have evolved. Weber described an ideal type of organization he called a bureaucracy—characteristics that many of today's large organizations still have. Today's managers use the concepts of scientific management when they analyze basic work tasks to be performed, use time-and-motion study to eliminate wasted motions, hire the best qualified workers for a job, and design incentive systems based on output. They use general administrative theory when they perform the functions of management and structure their organizations so that resources are used efficiently and effectively.

MH3 DISCUSS **the development and uses of the behavioral approach.**

The early OB advocates (Robert Owen, Hugo Munsterberg, Mary Parker Follett, and Chester Barnard) contributed various ideas, but all believed that people were the most important asset of the organization and should be managed accordingly. The Hawthorne Studies dramatically affected management beliefs about the role of people in organizations, leading to a new emphasis on the human behavior factor in managing. The behavioral approach has largely shaped how today's organizations are managed. Many current theories of motivation, leadership, group behavior and development, and other behavioral issues can be traced to the early OB advocates and the conclusions from the Hawthorne Studies.

MH4 DESCRIBE **the quantitative approach.**

The quantitative approach involves applications of statistics, optimization models, information models, and computer simulations to management activities. Today's managers use the quantitative approach, especially when making decisions, as they plan and control work activities such as allocating resources, improving quality, scheduling work, or determining optimum inventory levels. Total quality management—a management philosophy devoted to continual improvement and responding to customer needs and expectations—also makes use of quantitative methods to meet its goals.

MH5 EXPLAIN **the various theories in the contemporary approach.**

The systems approach says that an organization takes in inputs (resources) from the environment and transforms or processes these resources into outputs that are distributed into the environment. This approach provides a framework to help managers understand how all the interdependent units work together to achieve the organization's goals and that decisions and actions taken in one organizational area will affect others. In this way, managers can recognize that organizations are not self-contained, but instead rely on their environment for essential inputs and as outlets to absorb their outputs.

The contingency approach says that organizations are different, face different situations, and require different ways of managing. It helps us understand management because it stresses there are no simplistic or universal rules for managers to follow. Instead, managers must look at their situation and determine that *if* this is the way my situation is, *then* this is the best way for me to manage.

MyManagementLab

Go to **mymanagementlab.com** to complete the problems marked with this icon ✪.

✪ REVIEW AND DISCUSSION QUESTIONS

1. Explain why studying management history is important.

2. What early evidence of management practice can you describe?

3. Describe the important contributions made by the classical theorists.

4. What did the early advocates of OB contribute to our understanding of management?

5. Why were the Hawthorne Studies so critical to management history?

6. What kind of workplace would Henri Fayol create? How about Mary Parker Follett? How about Frederick W. Taylor?

7. Explain what the quantitative approach has contributed to the field of management.

8. Describe total quality management.

9. How do systems theory and the contingency approach make managers better at what they do?

10. How do societal trends influence the practice of management? What are the implications for someone studying management?

PREPARING FOR: My Career

MY TURN TO BE A MANAGER

- Choose two nonmanagement classes you are currently enrolled in or have taken previously. Describe three ideas and concepts from those subject areas that might help you be a better manager.

- Read at least one current business article from any popular business periodical each week for four weeks. Describe what each of the four articles is about and how each relates to any (or all) of the four approaches to management.

- Choose an organization with which you are familiar and describe the job specialization used there. Is it efficient and effective? Why or why not? How could it be improved?

- Can scientific management principles help you be more efficient? Choose a task you do regularly (such as laundry, fixing dinner, grocery shopping, studying for exams, etc.). Analyze it by writing down the steps involved in completing that task. See if any activities could be combined or eliminated. Find the "one best way" to do this task! And the next time you have to do the task, try the scientifically managed way! See if you become more efficient (keeping in mind that changing habits isn't easy to do).

- How do business organizations survive for 100+ years? Obviously, they've seen a lot of historical events come and go. Choose one of these companies and research their history: Coca-Cola, Procter & Gamble, Avon, or General Electric. How has it changed over the years?

From your research on this company, what did you learn that could help you be a better manager?

- Find the current top three best-selling management books. Read a review of the book or the book covers (or even the book!). Write a short paragraph describing what each book is about. Also, write about which of the historical management approaches you think the book fits into and how you think it fits into that approach.

- Pick one historical event from this century and do some research on it. Write a paper describing the impact this event might be having or has had on how workplaces are managed.

- Come on, admit it, you multitask, don't you? And if not, you probably know people who do. Multitasking is also common in the workplace. But does it make employees more efficient and effective? Pretend you're the manager in charge of a loan-processing department. Describe how you would research this issue using each of the following management approaches or theories: scientific management, general administrative theory, quantitative approach, behavioral approach, systems theory, and contingency theory.

- In your own words, write down three things you learned in this module about being a good manager. Keep a copy of this for future reference.

ENDNOTES

1. C. S. George, Jr., *The History of Management Thought,* 2d ed. (Upper Saddle River, NJ: Prentice Hall, 1972), p. 4.
2. Ibid., pp. 35–41.
3. F. W. Taylor, *Principles of Scientific Management* (New York: Harper, 1911), p. 44. For other information on Taylor, see S. Wagner-Tsukamoto, "An Institutional Economic Reconstruction of Scientific Management: On the Lost Theoretical Logic of Taylorism," *Academy of Management Review,* January 2007, pp. 105–117; R. Kanigel, *The One Best Way: Frederick Winslow Taylor and the Enigma of Efficiency* (New York: Viking, 1997); and M. Banta, *Taylored Lives: Narrative Productions in the Age of Taylor, Veblen, and Ford* (Chicago: University of Chicago Press, 1993).
4. See for example, F. B. Gilbreth, *Motion Study* (New York: Van Nostrand, 1911); and F. B. Gilbreth and L. M. Gilbreth, *Fatigue Study* (New York: Sturgis and Walton, 1916).
5. H. Fayol, *Industrial and General Administration* (Paris: Dunod, 1916).
6. M. Weber, *The Theory of Social and Economic Organizations,* ed. T. Parsons, trans. A. M. Henderson and T. Parsons (New York: Free Press, 1947); and M. Lounsbury and E. J. Carberry, "From King to Court Jester? Weber's Fall from Grace in Organizational Theory," *Organization Studies,* vol. 26, no. 4, 2005, pp. 501–525.
7. E. Mayo, *The Human Problems of an Industrial Civilization* (New York: Macmillan, 1933); and F. J. Roethlisberger and W. J. Dickson, *Management and the Worker* (Cambridge, MA: Harvard University Press, 1939).
8. See, for example, G. W. Yunker, "An Explanation of Positive and Negative Hawthorne Effects: Evidence from the Relay Assembly Test Room and Bank Wiring Observation Room Studies," paper presented at Academy of Management Annual Meeting, August 1993, Atlanta, Georgia; S. R. Jones, "Was There a Hawthorne Effect?" *American Sociological Review,* November 1992, pp. 451–468; and S. R. G. Jones, "Worker Interdependence and Output: The Hawthorne Studies Reevaluated," *American Sociological Review,* April 1990, pp. 176–190; J. A. Sonnenfeld, "Shedding Light on the Hawthorne Studies," *Journal of Occupational Behavior,* April 1985, pp. 111–130; B. Rice, "The Hawthorne Defect: Persistence of a Flawed Theory," *Psychology Today,* February 1982, pp. 70–74; R. H. Franke and J. Kaul, "The Hawthorne Experiments: First Statistical

Interpretations," *American Sociological Review*, October 1978, pp. 623–643; and A. Carey, "The Hawthorne Studies: A Radical Criticism," *American Sociological Review*, June 1967, pp. 403–416.

9. N. Zamiska, "Plane Geometry: Scientists Help Speed Boarding of Aircraft," *Wall Street Journal*, November 2, 2005, p. A1+.

10. See, for example, J. Jusko, "Tried and True," *IW*, December 6, 1999, pp. 78–84; T. A. Stewart, "A Conversation with Joseph Juran," *Fortune*, January 11, 1999, pp. 168–170; J. R. Hackman and R. Wageman, "Total Quality Management: Empirical, Conceptual, and Practical Issues," *Administrative Science Quarterly*, June 1995, pp. 309–342; T. C. Powell, "Total Quality Management as Competitive Advantage: A Review and Empirical Study," *Strategic Management Journal*, January 1995, pp. 15–37; R. K. Reger, L. T. Gustafson, S. M. Demarie, and J. V. Mullane, "Reframing the Organization: Why Implementing Total Quality Is Easier Said Than Done," *Academy of Management Review*, July 1994, pp. 565–584; C. A. Reeves and D. A. Bednar, "Defining Quality: Alternatives and Implications," *Academy of Management Review*, July 1994, pp. 419–445; J. W. Dean, Jr. and D. E. Bowen, "Management Theory and Total Quality: Improving Research and Practice through Theory Development," *Academy of Management Review*, July 1994, pp. 392–418; B. Krone, "Total Quality Management: An American Odyssey," *The Bureaucrat*, Fall 1990, pp. 35–38; and A. Gabor, *The Man Who Discovered Quality* (New York: Random House, 1990).

11. M. Barbaro, "A Long Line for a Shorter Wait at the Supermarket," *New York Times Online*, June 23, 2007.

12. S. Haines, "Become a Strategic Thinker," *Training,* October/November 2009, p. 64; and K. B. DeGreene, *Sociotechnical Systems: Factors in Analysis, Design, and Management* (Upper Saddle River, NJ: Prentice Hall, 1973), p. 13.

Making Decisions

From Chapter 2 of *Management*, Thirteenth Edition. Stephen P. Robbins and Mary Coulter. Copyright © 2016 by Pearson Education, Inc. All rights reserved.

Making Decisions

Source: Zudy and Kysa/Shutterstock

A key to success in management and in your career is knowing *how to be an effective decision maker.*

Be a Better Decision Maker

Decisions are an essential part of your life... personally and professionally. When you make a decision, you're making a judgment or choice between two or more alternatives: Do I sign up for this professor or this other one? What's better for my résumé—study abroad for a semester or do a summer internship or get involved with student organizations? What do I want for lunch— tacos, pizza, salad? Or do I even have time to eat before I go to class?

Each and every day is a series of decisions— from minor to significant, and everything in between. That's kind of a daunting thought, isn't it! Obviously, you want to make the best decisions you can... especially when it comes to those significant decisions. And, when you're finally out of school and working, making good decisions at your job also will be important and may even influence your performance evaluations and future career prospects. However, making the right decision every single time is practically impossible. (Yes, we've all made decisions we've regretted.) Good decision making is a skill, and like any skill, it can be learned and improved. So, how can you improve your decision-making skills? Here's an overview of what you need to know (each numbered item will be further described and explained in the chapter):

1. **Know, understand, and use the decision-making process.** *Yes, there is a "method" to making decisions that takes you from identifying problems to evaluating the effectiveness of your decision. It works. Know it. Understand it. Use it.*

2. **Know when and how to use rational or intuitive decision making or both.** *Different types of problems and different types of conditions will influence how you approach making a decision.*

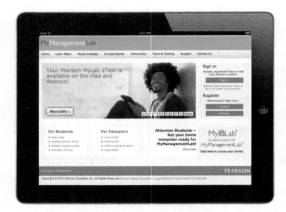

MyManagementLab®

⭐ **Improve Your Grade!**

When you see this icon, visit
www.mymanagementlab.com for activities that are
applied, personalized, and offer immediate feedback.

Learning Objectives

● **SKILL OUTCOMES**

1 **Describe** *the eight steps in the decision-making process.*

● **Develop your skill** at being creative.

2 **Explain** *the four ways managers make decisions.*

3 **Classify** *decisions and decision-making conditions.*

4 **Describe** *different decision-making styles and discuss how biases affect decision making.*

● **Know how to** recognize when you're using decision-making errors and biases and what
to do about it.

5 **Identify** *effective decision-making techniques.*

---

3. *Know your decision-making style.* *Not
everyone approaches decision making the same
way. Some people's style is more "fact" oriented
and blunt, ready to take action; others tend to be
more introspective and cautious. It doesn't mean
one style is better than another. But you do need
to recognize how you're most comfortable when
making a decision—and how others around you
make decisions. (This can be especially useful
when working on team projects, when other
team members may approach decision making
differently than you do!)*

**4. *Know, recognize, and understand the
biases and errors that may influence your decision
making.*** *Yes, biases and errors can creep into your
decision making. You may think you're making good
decisions and may not even recognize you're doing
these things. Yet, these errors and biases are likely
undermining your ability to make good judgments and
good choices. Beware! Be aware!*

Decision making is the essence of management. It's what managers do (or try to
avoid). And all managers would like to make good decisions because they're judged
on the outcomes of those decisions. In this text, we examine the concept of decision
making and how managers make decisions.

THE Decision-Making Process

L01 It was the type of day that airline managers dread. A record-setting bliz-
zard moving up the East Coast—covering roads, railroads, and airport
runways with as much as 27 inches of snow. One of the major airlines that would

have to deal with the storm, American Airlines, has over 78,000 employees who make flights possible and four who cancel those flights, if needed. Working out of the Fort Worth, Texas, control center, these employees, who deal with all kinds of situations, know that snowstorms are relatively simple because they can be forecasted in advance fairly easily and airline crews can quickly deploy equipment and procedures to deal with ice and snow. But still, even this doesn't mean that the decisions they have to make are easy, especially when those decisions affect hundreds of flights and thousands of passengers![1] Although most decisions managers make don't involve blizzards (or other weather-related uncertainties), you can see that decisions—choices, judgments—play an important role in what an organization has to do or is able to do.

Managers at all levels and in all areas of organizations make **decisions**. That is, they make choices. For instance, top-level managers make decisions about their organization's goals, where to locate manufacturing facilities, or what new markets to move into. Middle- and lower-level managers make decisions about production schedules, product quality problems, pay raises, and employee discipline. Our focus in this text is on how *managers* make decisions, but making decisions isn't something that just managers do. All organizational members make decisions that affect their jobs and the organization they work for.

Although decision making is typically described as choosing among alternatives, there's more to it than that! Why? Because decision making is (and should be) a process, not just a simple act of choosing among alternatives.[2] Even for something as straightforward as deciding where to go for lunch, you do more than just choose burgers or pizza or hot dogs. Granted, you may not spend a lot of time contemplating your lunch decision, but you still go through the process when making that decision. Exhibit 1 shows the eight steps in the decision-making process. This process is as relevant to personal decisions as it is to corporate decisions. Let's use an example—a manager deciding what laptop computers to purchase—to illustrate the steps in the process.

decision
A choice among two or more alternatives

Step 1: Identify a Problem

Your team is dysfunctional, your customers are leaving, or your plans are no longer relevant.[3] Every decision starts with a **problem**, a discrepancy between an existing and a desired condition.[4] Let's work through an example. Amanda is a sales manager whose reps need new laptops because their old ones are outdated and inadequate for doing their job. To make it simple, assume it's not economical to add memory to the old computers and it's the company's policy to purchase, not lease. Now we have a problem—a disparity between the sales reps' current computers (existing condition) and their need to have more efficient ones (desired condition). Amanda has a decision to make.

How do managers identify problems? In the real world, most problems don't come with neon signs flashing "problem." When her reps started complaining about their computers, it was pretty clear to Amanda that something needed to be done, but few problems are that obvious. Managers also have to be cautious not to confuse problems with symptoms of the problem. Is a 5 percent drop in sales a problem? Or are declining sales merely a symptom of the real problem, such as poor-quality products, high prices, or bad advertising? Also, keep in mind that problem identification is subjective. What one manager considers a problem might not be considered a problem by another manager. In addition, a manager who resolves the wrong problem perfectly is likely to perform just as poorly as the manager who doesn't even recognize a problem and does nothing. As you can see, effectively identifying problems is important, but not easy.[5]

problem
An obstacle that makes it difficult to achieve a desired goal or purpose

Step 2: Identify Decision Criteria

Once a manager has identified a problem, he or she must identify the **decision criteria** important or relevant to resolving the problem. Every decision maker has criteria guiding his or her decisions even if they're not explicitly stated. In our example, Amanda

decision criteria
Criteria that define what's important or relevant to resolving a problem

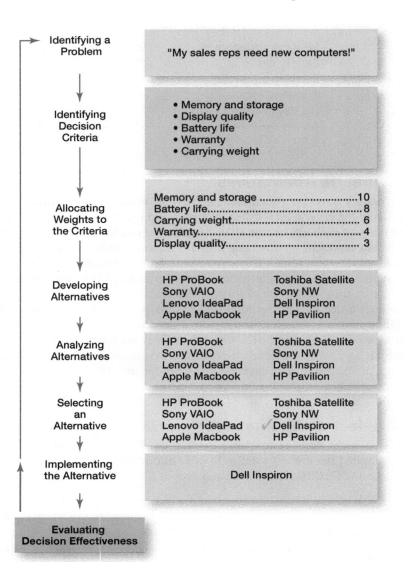

Exhibit 1
Decision-Making Process

Identifying a Problem — "My sales reps need new computers!"

Identifying Decision Criteria
- Memory and storage
- Display quality
- Battery life
- Warranty
- Carrying weight

Allocating Weights to the Criteria
Memory and storage 10
Battery life...8
Carrying weight.. 6
Warranty... 4
Display quality.. 3

Developing Alternatives
HP ProBook	Toshiba Satellite
Sony VAIO	Sony NW
Lenovo IdeaPad	Dell Inspiron
Apple Macbook	HP Pavilion

Analyzing Alternatives
HP ProBook	Toshiba Satellite
Sony VAIO	Sony NW
Lenovo IdeaPad	Dell Inspiron
Apple Macbook	HP Pavilion

Selecting an Alternative
HP ProBook	Toshiba Satellite
Sony VAIO	Sony NW
Lenovo IdeaPad	✓ Dell Inspiron
Apple Macbook	HP Pavilion

Implementing the Alternative — Dell Inspiron

Evaluating Decision Effectiveness

decides after careful consideration that memory and storage capabilities, display quality, battery life, warranty, and carrying weight are the relevant criteria in her decision.

Step 3: Allocate Weights to the Criteria

If the relevant criteria aren't equally important, the decision maker must weight the items in order to give them the correct priority in the decision. How? A simple way is to give the most important criterion a weight of 10 and then assign weights to the rest using that standard. Of course, you could use any number as the highest weight. The weighted criteria for our example are shown in Exhibit 2.

Step 4: Develop Alternatives

The fourth step in the decision-making process requires the decision maker to list viable alternatives that could resolve the problem. In this step, a decision maker needs to be creative, and the alternatives are only listed—not evaluated just yet. Our sales manager, Amanda, identifies eight laptops as possible choices. (See Exhibit 3.)

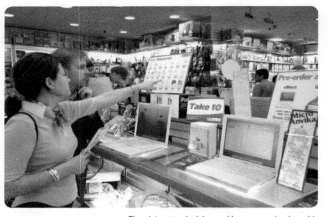

The eight-step decision-making process begins with identifying a problem and ends with evaluating the result of the decision. After identifying the need to buy new laptop computers for her sales reps, the manager must identify relevant criteria such as price, display quality, and memory that will help guide her final decision.
Source: Alex Segre/Alamy

Exhibit 2
Important Decision Criteria

Memory and storage	10
Battery life	8
Carrying weight	6
Warranty	4
Display quality	3

Step 5: Analyze Alternatives

Once alternatives have been identified, a decision maker must evaluate each one. How? By using the criteria established in Step 2. Exhibit 3 shows the assessed values that Amanda gave each alternative after doing some research on them. Keep in mind that these data represent an assessment of the eight alternatives using the decision criteria, but *not* the weighting. When you multiply each alternative by the assigned weight, you get the weighted alternatives as shown in Exhibit 4. The total score for each alternative, then, is the sum of its weighted criteria.

Sometimes a decision maker might be able to skip this step. If one alternative scores highest on every criterion, you wouldn't need to consider the weights because that alternative would already be the top choice. Or if the weights were all equal, you could evaluate an alternative merely by summing up the assessed values for each one. (Look again at Exhibit 3.) For example, the score for the HP ProBook would be 36, and the score for the Sony NW would be 35.

Step 6: Select an Alternative

The sixth step in the decision-making process is choosing the best alternative or the one that generated the highest total in Step 5. In our example (Exhibit 4), Amanda would choose the Dell Inspiron because it scored higher than all other alternatives (249 total).

Step 7: Implement the Alternative

In Step 7 in the decision-making process, you put the decision into action by conveying it to those affected and getting their commitment to it. We know that if the people who must implement a decision participate in the process, they're more likely to support it than if you just tell them what to do. Another thing managers may need to do during implementation is reassess the environment for any changes, especially if it's a long-term decision. Are the criteria, alternatives, and choices still the best ones, or has the environment changed in such a way that we need to reevaluate?

Exhibit 3
Possible Alternatives

	Memory and Storage	Battery Life	Carrying Weight	Warranty	Display Quality
HP ProBook	10	3	10	8	5
Sony VAIO	8	7	7	8	7
Lenovo IdeaPad	8	5	7	10	10
Apple Macbook	8	7	7	8	7
Toshiba Satellite	7	8	7	8	7
Sony NW	8	3	6	10	8
Dell Inspiron	10	7	8	6	7
HP Pavilion	4	10	4	8	10

	Memory and Storage	Battery Life	Carrying Weight	Warranty	Display Quality	Total
HP ProBook	100	24	60	32	15	231
Sony VAIO	80	56	42	32	21	231
Lenovo IdeaPad	80	40	42	40	30	232
Apple Macbook	80	56	42	32	21	231
Toshiba Satellite	70	64	42	32	21	229
Sony NW	80	24	36	40	24	204
Dell Inspiron	100	56	48	24	21	249
HP Pavilion	40	80	24	32	30	206

Exhibit 4
Evaluation of Alternatives

Step 8: Evaluate Decision Effectiveness

The last step in the decision-making process involves evaluating the outcome or result of the decision to see whether the problem was resolved. If the evaluation shows that the problem still exists, then the manager needs to assess what went wrong. Was the problem incorrectly defined? Were errors made when evaluating alternatives? Was the right alternative selected but poorly implemented? The answers might lead you to redo an earlier step or might even require starting the whole process over.

MANAGERS Making Decisions

LO2 Although everyone in an organization makes decisions, decision making is particularly important to managers. As Exhibit 5 shows, it's part of all four managerial functions. That's why managers—when they plan, organize, lead, and control—are called *decision makers*.

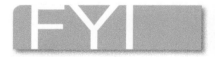

• Decision making is the essence of management.[6]

Exhibit 5
Decisions Managers May Make

Planning
- What are the organization's long-term objectives?
- What strategies will best achieve those objectives?
- What should the organization's short-term objectives be?
- How difficult should individual goals be?

Organizing
- How many employees should I have report directly to me?
- How much centralization should there be in an organization?
- How should jobs be designed?
- When should the organization implement a different structure?

Leading
- How do I handle employees that appear to be unmotivated?
- What is the most effective leadership style in a given situation?
- How will a specific change affect worker productivity?
- When is the right time to stimulate conflict?

Controlling
- What activities in the organization need to be controlled?
- How should those activities be controlled?
- When is a performance deviation significant?
- What type of management information system should the organization have?

The fact that almost everything a manager does involves making decisions doesn't mean that decisions are always time-consuming, complex, or evident to an outside observer. Most decision making is routine. For instance, every day of the year you make a decision about what to eat for dinner. It's no big deal. You've made the decision thousands of times before. It's a pretty simple decision and can usually be handled quickly. It's the type of decision you almost forget *is* a decision. And managers also make dozens of these routine decisions every day, for example, which employee will work what shift next week, what information should be included in a report, or how to resolve a customer's complaint. Keep in mind that even though a decision seems easy or has been faced by a manager a number of times before, it still is a decision. Let's look at four perspectives on how managers make decisions.

Making Decisions: Rationality

rational decision making
Describes choices that are logical and consistent and maximize value

We assume that managers will use **rational decision making**; that is, they'll make logical and consistent choices to maximize value.[7] After all, managers have all sorts of tools and techniques to help them be rational decision makers. What does it mean to be a "rational" decision maker?

ASSUMPTIONS OF RATIONALITY   A rational decision maker would be fully objective and logical. The problem faced would be clear and unambiguous, and the decision maker would have a clear and specific goal and know all possible alternatives and consequences. Finally, making decisions rationally would consistently lead to selecting the alternative that maximizes the likelihood of achieving that goal. These assumptions apply to any decision—personal or managerial. However, for managerial decision making, we need to add one additional assumption—decisions are made in the best interests of the organization. These assumptions of rationality aren't very realistic and managers don't always act rationally, but the next concept can help explain how most decisions get made in organizations.

Making Decisions: Bounded Rationality

Despite the unrealistic assumptions, managers are *expected* to be rational when making decisions.[8] They understand that "good" decision makers are supposed to do certain things and exhibit good decision-making behaviors as they identify problems, consider alternatives, gather information, and act decisively but prudently. When they do so, they show others that they're competent and that their decisions are the result of intelligent deliberation. However, a more realistic approach to describing how managers make decisions is the concept of **bounded rationality**, which says that managers make decisions rationally, but are limited (bounded) by their ability to process information.[9] Because they can't possibly analyze all information on all alternatives, managers **satisfice**, rather than maximize. That is, they accept solutions that are "good enough." They're being rational within the limits (bounds) of their ability to process information. Let's look at an example.

bounded rationality
Decision making that's rational, but limited (bounded) by an individual's ability to process information

satisfice
Accept solutions that are "good enough"

Suppose you're a finance major and upon graduation you want a job, preferably as a personal financial planner with a minimum salary of $45,000 and within 100 miles of your hometown. You accept a job offer as a business credit analyst—not exactly a personal financial planner but still in the finance field—at a bank 50 miles from home at a starting salary of $42,500. If you had done a more comprehensive job search, you would have discovered a job in personal financial planning at a trust company only 25 miles from your hometown and starting at a salary of $45,000. You weren't a perfectly rational decision maker because you didn't maximize your decision by searching all possible alternatives and then choosing the best. But because the first job offer was satisfactory (or "good enough"), you behaved in a bounded-rationality manner by accepting it.

Most decisions that managers make don't fit the assumptions of perfect rationality, so they satisfice. However, keep in mind that their decision making is also likely

influenced by the organization's culture, internal politics, power considerations, and by a phenomenon called **escalation of commitment**, an increased commitment to a previous decision despite evidence that it may have been wrong.[10] The *Challenger* space shuttle disaster is often used as an example of escalation of commitment. Decision makers chose to launch the shuttle that day even though the decision was questioned by several individuals who believed it was a bad one. Why would decision makers escalate commitment to a bad decision? Because they don't want to admit that their initial decision may have been flawed. Rather than search for new alternatives, they simply increase their commitment to the original solution.

escalation of commitment
An increased commitment to a previous decision despite evidence it may have been wrong

Making Decisions: The Role of Intuition

When managers at stapler-maker Swingline saw the company's market share declining, they used a logical scientific approach to address the issue. For three years, they exhaustively researched stapler users before deciding what new products to develop. However, at Accentra, Inc., founder Todd Moses used a more intuitive decision approach to come up with his line of unique PaperPro staplers.[11]

Like Todd Moses, managers often use their intuition to help their decision making. What is **intuitive decision making**? It's making decisions on the basis of experience, feelings, and accumulated judgment. Researchers studying managers' use of intuitive decision making have identified five different aspects of intuition, which are described in Exhibit 6.[12] How common is intuitive decision making? One survey found that almost half of the executives surveyed "used intuition more often than formal analysis to run their companies."[13]

Intuitive decision making can complement both rational and bounded rational decision making.[14] First of all, a manager who has had experience with a similar type of problem or situation often can act quickly with what appears to be limited information because of that past experience. In addition, a recent study found that individuals who experienced intense feelings and emotions when making decisions actually

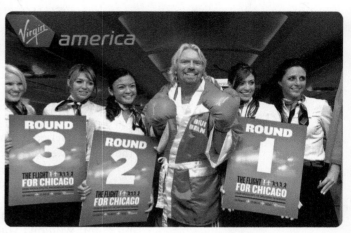

Virgin Group founder Richard Branson relied on his guiding principle of "Trust your instincts" when deciding to enter the airline business. Facing tough competition, Branson used his intuition to launch his new venture and promoted it by dressing up as a prize fighter determined to knock out his competitors. *Source: ZUMA Wire Service/Alamy*

intuitive decision making
Making decisions on the basis of experience, feelings, and accumulated judgment

Exhibit 6
What Is Intuition?

Managers make decisions based on their past experiences

Managers make decisions based on ethical values or culture

Managers make decisions based on feelings or emotions

Experience-based decisions

Values or ethics-based decisions

Affect-initiated decisions

Intuition

Subconscious mental processing

Cognitive-based decisions

Managers use data from subconscious mind to help them make decisions

Managers make decisions based on skills, knowledge, and training

Source: Based on L. A. Burke and M. K. Miller, "Taking the Mystery Out of Intuitive Decision Making," *Academy of Management Executive,* October 1999, pp. 91–99.

achieved higher decision-making performance, especially when they understood their feelings as they were making decisions. The old belief that managers should ignore emotions when making decisions may not be the best advice.[15]

★ **Watch It 1!**   If your professor has assigned this, go to **www.mymanagementlab.com** to watch a video titled *CH2MHill - Decision Making* and to respond to questions.

Making Decisions: The Role of Evidence-Based Management

evidence-based management (EBMgt)
The systematic use of the best available evidence to improve management practice

Sales associates at the cosmetics counter at department store Bon-Ton Stores Inc. had the highest turnover of any store sales group. Using a data-driven decision approach, managers devised a more precise pre-employment assessment test. Now, not only do they have lower turnover, they actually have better hires.[16]

Suppose you were exhibiting some strange, puzzling physical symptoms. In order to make the best decisions about proper diagnosis and treatment, wouldn't you want your doctor to base her decisions on the best available evidence? Now suppose you're a manager faced with putting together an employee recognition program. Wouldn't you want those decisions also to be based on the best available evidence? "Any decision-making process is likely to be enhanced through the use of relevant and reliable evidence, whether it's buying someone a birthday present or wondering which new washing machine to buy."[17] That's the premise behind **evidence-based management (EBMgt)**, the "systematic use of the best available evidence to improve management practice."[18]

EBMgt is quite relevant to managerial decision making. The four essential elements of EBMgt are: (1) the decision maker's expertise and judgment; (2) external evidence that's been evaluated by the decision maker; (3) opinions, preferences, and

---

let's get REAL

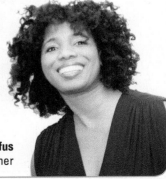

The Scenario:

Juan Hernandez is a successful business owner. His landscaping business is growing, and a few months ago he decided to bring in somebody to manage his office operations since he had little time to keep on top of that activity. However, this individual can't seem to make a decision without agonizing over and over and on and on about it.

What could Juan do to help this person become a better decision maker?

Juan could give his office assistant a more complete picture of the tasks at hand for the day/week/month as well as timelines for each. It would force his decision to be made within a certain timeframe as well as give him a bigger-picture view of the workload. It would make him realize that there are many more tasks to accomplish.

Prudence Rufus
Business Owner/Photographer

Source: Prudence Rufus

values of those who have a stake in the decision; and (4) relevant organizational (internal) factors such as context, circumstances, and organizational members. The strength or influence of each of these elements on a decision will vary with each decision. Sometimes, the decision maker's intuition (judgment) might be given greater emphasis in the decision; other times it might be the opinions of stakeholders; and at other times, it might be ethical considerations (organizational context). The key for managers is to recognize and understand the mindful, conscious choice as to which elements are most important and should be emphasized in making a decision.

TYPES of Decisions and Decision-Making Conditions

LO3 Restaurant managers in Portland make routine decisions weekly about purchasing food supplies and scheduling employee work shifts. It's something they've done numerous times. But now they're facing a different kind of decision—one they've never encountered: how to adapt to a new law requiring that nutritional information be posted.

Types of Decisions

Such situations aren't all that unusual. Managers in all kinds of organizations face different types of problems and decisions as they do their jobs. Depending on the nature of the problem, a manager can use one of two different types of decisions.

STRUCTURED PROBLEMS AND PROGRAMMED DECISIONS Some problems are straightforward. The decision maker's goal is clear, the problem is familiar, and information about the problem is easily defined and complete. Examples might include when a customer returns a purchase to a store, when a supplier is late with an important delivery, a news team's response to a fast-breaking event, or a college's handling of a student wanting to drop a class. Such situations are called **structured problems** because they're straightforward, familiar, and easily defined. For instance, a server spills a drink on a customer's coat. The customer is upset and the manager needs to do something. Because it's not an unusual occurrence, there's probably some standardized routine for handling it. For example, the manager offers to have the coat cleaned at the restaurant's expense. This is what we call a **programmed decision**, a repetitive decision that can be handled by a routine approach. Because the problem is structured, the manager doesn't have to go to the trouble and expense of going through an involved decision process. The "develop-the-alternatives" stage of the decision-making process either doesn't exist or is given little attention. Why? Because once the structured problem is defined, the solution is usually self-evident or at least reduced to a few alternatives that are familiar and have proved successful in the past. The spilled drink on the customer's coat doesn't require the restaurant manager to identify and weight decision criteria or to develop a long list of possible solutions. Instead, the manager relies on one of three types of programmed decisions: procedure, rule, or policy.

A **procedure** is a series of sequential steps a manager uses to respond to a structured problem. The only difficulty is identifying the problem. Once it's clear, so is the procedure. For instance, a purchasing manager receives a request from a warehouse manager for 15 tablets for the inventory clerks. The purchasing manager knows how to make this decision by following the established purchasing procedure.

A **rule** is an explicit statement that tells a manager what can or cannot be done. Rules are frequently used because they're simple to follow and ensure consistency. For example, rules about lateness and absenteeism permit supervisors to make disciplinary decisions rapidly and fairly.

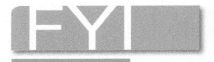

structured problems
Straightforward, familiar, and easily defined problems

programmed decision
A repetitive decision that can be handled by a routine approach

procedure
A series of sequential steps used to respond to a well-structured problem

rule
An explicit statement that tells managers what can or cannot be done

policy
A guideline for making decisions

The third type of programmed decisions is a **policy**, a guideline for making a decision. In contrast to a rule, a policy establishes general parameters for the decision maker rather than specifically stating what should or should not be done. Policies typically contain an ambiguous term that leaves interpretation up to the decision maker. Here are some sample policy statements:

- The customer always comes first and should always be *satisfied.*
- We promote from within, *whenever possible.*
- Employee wages shall be *competitive* within community standards.

Notice that the terms *satisfied, whenever possible,* and *competitive* require interpretation. For instance, the policy of paying competitive wages doesn't tell a company's human resources manager the exact amount he or she should pay, but it does guide them in making the decision.

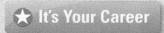 **It's Your Career**

Decision Making, Part 1—If your instructor is using MyManagementLab, log onto **mymanagementlab.com** and test your *decision-making knowledge.* **Be sure to refer back to the chapter opener!**

unstructured problems
Problems that are new or unusual and for which information is ambiguous or incomplete

nonprogrammed decisions
Unique and nonrecurring decisions that require a custom-made solution

UNSTRUCTURED PROBLEMS AND NONPROGRAMMED DECISIONS Not all the problems managers face can be solved using programmed decisions. Many organizational situations involve **unstructured problems**, new or unusual problems for which information is ambiguous or incomplete. Whether to build a new manufacturing facility in China is an example of an unstructured problem. So, too, is the problem facing restaurant managers in Portland who must decide how to modify their businesses to comply with the new law. When problems are unstructured, managers must rely on nonprogrammed decision making in order to develop unique solutions. **Nonprogrammed decisions** are unique and nonrecurring and involve custom-made solutions.

Exhibit 7 describes the differences between programmed and nonprogrammed decisions. Lower-level managers mostly rely on programmed decisions (procedures, rules, and policies) because they confront familiar and repetitive problems. As managers move up the organizational hierarchy, the problems they confront become more unstructured. Why? Because lower-level managers handle the routine decisions and let upper-level managers deal with the unusual or difficult decisions. Also, upper-level managers delegate routine decisions to their subordinates so they can deal with more difficult issues.[20] Thus, few managerial decisions in the real world are either fully programmed or nonprogrammed. Most fall somewhere in between.

Exhibit 7
Programmed Versus
Nonprogrammed Decisions

Characteristic	Programmed Decisions	Nonprogrammed Decisions
Type of problem	Structured	Unstructured
Managerial level	Lower levels	Upper levels
Frequency	Repetitive, routine	New, unusual
Information	Readily available	Ambiguous or incomplete
Goals	Clear, specific	Vague
Time frame for solution	Short	Relatively long
Solution relies on...	Procedures, rules, policies	Judgment and creativity

If your professor has assigned this, go to **www.mymanagementlab.com** to complete the Writing Assignment MGMT 8: Decision Making.

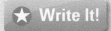 ★ Write It!

Decision-Making Conditions

When making decisions, managers may face three different conditions: certainty, risk, and uncertainty. Let's look at the characteristics of each.

CERTAINTY   The ideal situation for making decisions is one of **certainty**, a situation where a manager can make accurate decisions because the outcome of every alternative is known. For example, when Wyoming's state treasurer decides where to deposit excess state funds, he knows exactly the interest rate offered by each bank and the amount that will be earned on the funds. He is certain about the outcomes of each alternative. As you might expect, most managerial decisions aren't like this.

RISK   A far more common situation is one of **risk**, conditions in which the decision maker is able to estimate the likelihood of certain outcomes. Under risk, managers have historical data from past personal experiences or secondary information that lets them assign probabilities to different alternatives. Let's do an example.

Suppose you manage a Colorado ski resort, and you're thinking about adding another lift. Obviously, your decision will be influenced by the additional revenue that the new lift would generate, which depends on snowfall. You have fairly reliable weather data from the last 10 years on snowfall levels in your area—three years of

certainty
A situation in which a manager can make accurate decisions because all outcomes are known

risk
A situation in which the decision maker is able to estimate the likelihood of certain outcomes

---

FUTURE VISION | **Who Makes the Decisions, Person or Machine?**

Do you have an e-book reader? About 50 percent of the U.S. population does. You'd be surprised at what digital-book publishers and retailers now know about you. The major players in e-book publishing—Amazon, Apple, and Google—can easily track readers' moves and actions. For instance, this passage from *Catching Fire*, the second book of the Hunger Games series, was the most highlighted among Kindle readers: "Because sometimes things happen to people and they're not equipped to deal with them" (Collins, Suzanne, *Catching Fire*, the Second Book from the Hunger Games, © Suzanne Collins, New York: Scholastic Press, 2009, pp. 31–32). Subscription services Scribd and Oyster know that sci-fi readers prefer beer over wine and that romance readers are more likely to read in the early hours of the morning. And according to Nook data, science-fiction, romance, and crime-fiction fans often read more books more quickly than readers of literary fiction.[21]

The possibilities of technology as a tool for managerial decision making are endless and fascinating! Artificial intelligence software soon will be available to approach problems the way the human brain does—by trying to recognize patterns that underlie a complex set of data. Like people, this software will "learn" to pick out subtle patterns. In so doing, it will be able to perform a number of decision-making tasks.

Just as today's computers allow you to access information quickly from sources such as spreadsheets or search engines, most of the routine decisions that employees now make on the job are likely to be delegated to a software program in the future. For instance, much of the diagnostic work now done by doctors will be done by software. Patients will describe their symptoms to a computer in a medical kiosk, possibly at their neighborhood drugstore; from answers the patient provides, the computer will render a decision. Similarly, many hiring decisions will be made by software programmed to simulate the successful decision processes used by recruiters and managers. Welcome to the future of decision making!

*If your professor has chosen to assign this, go to **www.mymanagementlab.com** to discuss the following questions.*

⭐ **TALK ABOUT IT 1:** What steps of the decision-making process will technology be most useful for? Explain.

⭐ **TALK ABOUT IT 2:** How can technology be a "tool" for managerial decision making?

Exhibit 8
Expected Value

Event	Expected Revenues	×	Probability	=	Expected Value of Each Alternative
Heavy snowfall	$850,000		0.3		$255,000
Normal snowfall	725,000		0.5		362,500
Light snowfall	350,000		0.2		70,000
					$687,500

heavy snowfall, five years of normal snowfall, and two years of light snow. And you have good information on the amount of revenues generated during each level of snow. You can use this information to help you make your decision by calculating expected value—the expected return from each possible outcome—by multiplying expected revenues by snowfall probabilities. The result is the average revenue you can expect over time if the given probabilities hold. As Exhibit 8 shows, the expected revenue from adding a new ski lift is $687,500. Of course, whether that's enough to justify a decision to build depends on the costs involved in generating that revenue.

UNCERTAINTY What happens if you face a decision where you're not certain about the outcomes and can't even make reasonable probability estimates? We call this condition **uncertainty**. Managers face decision-making situations of uncertainty. Under these conditions, the choice of alternatives is influenced by the limited amount of available information and by the psychological orientation of the decision maker. An optimistic manager will follow a *maximax* choice (maximizing the maximum possible payoff); a pessimist will follow a *maximin* choice (maximizing the minimum possible payoff); and a manager who desires to minimize his maximum "regret" will opt for a *minimax* choice. Let's look at these different choice approaches using an example.

A marketing manager at Visa has determined four possible strategies (S_1, S_2, S_3, and S_4) for promoting the Visa card throughout the West Coast region of the United States. The marketing manager also knows that major competitor MasterCard has three competitive actions (CA_1, CA_2, and CA_3) it's using to promote its card in the same region. For this example, we'll assume that the Visa manager had no previous knowledge that would allow her to determine probabilities of success of any of the four strategies. She formulates the matrix shown in Exhibit 9 to show the various Visa strategies and the resulting profit, depending on the competitive action used by MasterCard.

In this example, if our Visa manager is an optimist, she'll choose strategy 4 (S_4) because that could produce the largest possible gain: $28 million. Note that this choice maximizes the maximum possible gain (maximax choice).

If our manager is a pessimist, she'll assume that only the worst can occur. The worst outcome for each strategy is as follows: S_1 = $11 million; S_2 = $9 million; S_3 = $15 million; S_4 = $14 million. These are the most pessimistic outcomes from each strategy.

uncertainty
A situation in which a decision maker has neither certainty nor reasonable probability estimates available

Exhibit 9
Payoff Matrix

Visa Marketing Strategy (in millions of dollars)	MasterCard's Competitive Action		
	CA$_1$	CA$_2$	CA$_3$
S$_1$	13	14	11
S$_2$	9	15	18
S$_3$	24	21	15
S$_4$	18	14	28

Exhibit 10
Regret Matrix

Visa Marketing Strategy (in millions of dollars)	MasterCard's Competitive Action		
	CA₁	CA₂	CA₃
S₁	11	7	17
S₂	15	6	10
S₃	0	0	13
S₄	6	7	0

Following the *maximin* choice, she would maximize the minimum payoff; in other words, she'd select S_3 ($15 million is the largest of the minimum payoffs).

In the third approach, managers recognize that once a decision is made, it will not necessarily result in the most profitable payoff. There may be a "regret" of profits given up—*regret* referring to the amount of money that could have been made had a different strategy been used. Managers calculate regret by subtracting all possible payoffs in each category from the maximum possible payoff for each given event, in this case for each competitive action. For our Visa manager, the highest payoff—given that MasterCard engages in CA_1, CA_2, or CA_3—is $24 million, $21 million, or $28 million, respectively (the highest number in each column). Subtracting the payoffs in Exhibit 9 from those figures produces the results shown in Exhibit 10.

The maximum regrets are $S_1 = $17 million, $S_2 = $15 million, $S_3 = $13 million, and $S_4 = $7 million. The *minimax* choice minimizes the maximum regret, so our Visa manager would choose S_4. By making this choice, she'll never have a regret of profits given up of more than $7 million. This result contrasts, for example, with a regret of $15 million had she chosen S_2 and MasterCard had taken CA_1.

Although managers try to quantify a decision when possible by using payoff and regret matrices, uncertainty often forces them to rely more on intuition, creativity, hunches, and "gut feel."

LEADER *making a* DIFFERENCE

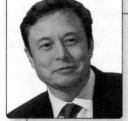

Source: Kristoffer Tripplaar/Sipa USA (Sipa via AP Images)

He's not your typical CEO. In fact, some might call him a little crazy, except for the fact that his track record at turning crazy ideas into profitable ventures is pretty good. We're talking about Elon Musk.[22] In 2002, he sold his second Internet startup, PayPal, to eBay for $1.5 billion. (His first company, a Web software firm, was acquired by Compaq.) Currently, Musk is CEO of Space Exploration Technologies (SpaceX) and Tesla Motors, and chairman and largest shareholder of SolarCity, an energy technology company. SpaceX, which builds rockets for companies and countries to put satellites in space, was the first private company to deliver cargo to the International Space Station. It's reigniting interest in space exploration. Tesla Motors is the world's most prominent maker of electric cars and is proving that electric cars can be green, sexy, and profitable. SolarCity is now the leading provider of domestic solar panels in the United States. Each of these ventures has transformed (or is transforming) an industry: PayPal—Internet payments; Tesla—automobiles; SpaceX—aeronautics; and SolarCity—energy. As a decision maker, Musk deals mostly with unstructured problems in risky conditions. However, like other business innovators, Musk is comfortable with that and in pursuing what many might consider "crazy" idea territory. His genius has been compared to that of the late Steve Jobs. And Fortune magazine named him the 2013 Businessperson of the Year. What can you learn from this leader making a difference?

DECISION-MAKING Styles

LO4 William D. Perez's tenure as Nike's CEO lasted a short and turbulent 13 months. Analysts attributed his abrupt dismissal to a difference in decision-making approaches between him and Nike cofounder Phil Knight. Perez tended to rely more on data and facts when making decisions, whereas Knight highly valued, and had always used, his judgment and feelings to make decisions.[23] As this example clearly shows, managers have different styles when it comes to making decisions.

Linear–Nonlinear Thinking Style Profile

Suppose you're a new manager. How will you make decisions? Recent research done with four distinct groups of people says the way a person approaches decision making is likely affected by his or her thinking style.[24] Your thinking style reflects two things: (1) the source of information you tend to use (external data and facts OR internal sources such as feelings and intuition), and (2) whether you process that information in a linear way (rational, logical, analytical) OR a nonlinear way (intuitive, creative, insightful). These four dimensions are collapsed into two styles. The first, **linear thinking style**, is characterized by a person's preference for using external data and facts and processing this information through rational, logical thinking to guide decisions and actions. The second, **nonlinear thinking style**, is characterized by a preference for internal sources of information (feelings and intuition) and processing this information with internal insights, feelings, and hunches to guide decisions and actions. Look back at the earlier Nike example and you'll see both styles described.

Managers need to recognize that their employees may use different decision-making styles. Some employees may take their time weighing alternatives and relying on how they feel about it, while others rely on external data before logically making a decision. These differences don't make one person's approach better than the other. It just means their decision-making styles are different.

linear thinking style
Decision style characterized by a person's preference for using external data and facts and processing this information through rational, logical thinking

nonlinear thinking style
Decision style characterized by a person's preference for internal sources of information and processing this information with internal insights, feelings, and hunches

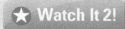 **Watch It 2!**

If your professor has assigned this, go to **www.mymanagementlab.com** to watch a video titled *Rudi's Bakery - Decision Making* and to respond to questions.

Decision-Making Biases and Errors

When managers make decisions, they not only use their own particular style, they may use "rules of thumb," or **heuristics**, to simplify their decision making. Rules of thumb can be useful because they help make sense of complex, uncertain, and ambiguous information.[25] Even though managers may use rules of thumb, that doesn't mean those rules are reliable. Why? Because they may lead to errors and biases in processing and evaluating information. Exhibit 11 identifies 12 common decision errors of managers and biases they may have. Let's look at each.[26]

When decision makers tend to think they know more than they do or hold unrealistically positive views of themselves and their performance, they're exhibiting the *overconfidence bias*. The *immediate gratification bias* describes decision makers who tend to want immediate rewards and to avoid immediate costs. For these individuals, decision choices that provide quick payoffs are more appealing than those with payoffs in the future. The *anchoring effect* describes how decision makers fixate on initial information as a starting point and then, once set, fail to adequately adjust for subsequent information. First impressions, ideas, prices, and estimates carry unwarranted weight relative to information received later. When decision makers selectively organize and interpret events based on their biased perceptions, they're using the *selective perception bias*. This influences the information they pay attention to, the problems they identify, and the alternatives they develop. Decision makers who seek out information that reaffirms their past choices and discounts information that contradicts past judgments exhibit the *confirmation bias*. These people tend to accept at face value information that confirms their preconceived views and are critical and skeptical of information that challenges these views. The *framing bias* is when decision makers select and highlight certain aspects of a situation while excluding others. By drawing attention to specific aspects of a situation and highlighting them, while at the same time downplaying or omitting other

heuristics
Rules of thumb that managers use to simplify decision making

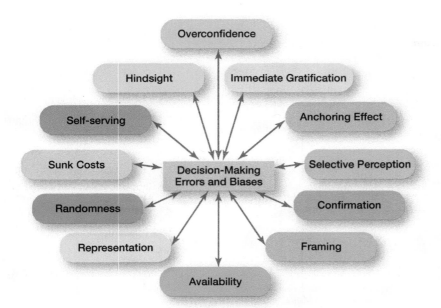

Exhibit 11
Common Decision-Making Biases

aspects, they distort what they see and create incorrect reference points. The *availability bias* happens when decision makers tend to remember events that are the most recent and vivid in their memory. The result? It distorts their ability to recall events in an objective manner and results in distorted judgments and probability estimates. When decision makers assess the likelihood of an event based on how closely it resembles other events or sets of events, that's the *representation bias.* Managers exhibiting this bias draw analogies and see identical situations where they don't exist. The *randomness bias* describes the actions of decision makers who try to create meaning out of random events. They do this because most decision makers have difficulty dealing with chance even though random events happen to everyone, and there's nothing that can be done to predict them. The *sunk costs error* occurs when decision makers forget that current choices can't correct the past. They incorrectly fixate on past expenditures of time, money, or effort in assessing choices rather than on future consequences. Instead of ignoring sunk costs, they can't forget them. Decision makers who are quick to take credit for their successes and to blame failure on outside factors are exhibiting the *self-serving bias.* Finally, the *hindsight bias* is the tendency for decision makers to falsely believe that they would have accurately predicted the outcome of an event once that outcome is actually known.

Managers avoid the negative effects of these decision errors and biases by being aware of them and then not using them! Beyond that, managers also should pay attention to "how" they make decisions and try to identify the heuristics they typically use and critically evaluate the appropriateness of those heuristics. Finally, managers might want to ask trusted individuals to help them identify weaknesses in their decision-making style and try to improve on those weaknesses.

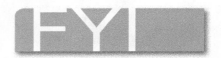

- When managers reduced the effects of bias in their decision making, their organizations' performance returns were 7 percent higher.[27]

Decision Making, Part 2—If your instructor is using MyManagementLab, log onto **mymanagementlab.com** and test your *decision-making knowledge.* **Be sure to refer back to the chapter opener!**

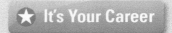

Exhibit 12
Overview of Managerial Decision Making

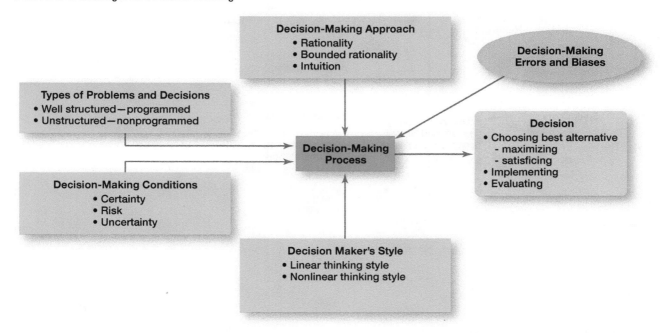

Decision-Making Approach
- Rationality
- Bounded rationality
- Intuition

Decision-Making Errors and Biases

Types of Problems and Decisions
- Well structured—programmed
- Unstructured—nonprogrammed

Decision-Making Process

Decision
- Choosing best alternative
  - maximizing
  - satisficing
- Implementing
- Evaluating

Decision-Making Conditions
- Certainty
- Risk
- Uncertainty

Decision Maker's Style
- Linear thinking style
- Nonlinear thinking style

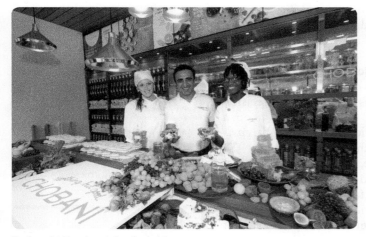

Nonlinear thinking characterizes the decision-making style of Hamdi Ulukaya, founder of the Chobani yogurt brand. Shown here with employees at his first-of-its-kind Mediterranean yogurt bar in New York City, Ulukaya introduced his Greek-style yogurt in the United States without having any knowledge about how to launch a new business.
Source: Diane Bondareff/Invision for Chobani/AP Images

Overview of Managerial Decision Making

Exhibit 12 provides an overview of managerial decision making. Because it's in their best interests, managers *want* to make good decisions—that is, choose the "best" alternative, implement it, and determine whether it takes care of the problem, which is the reason the decision was needed in the first place. Their decision-making process is affected by four factors: the decision-making approach, the type of problem, decision-making conditions, and their decision-making style. In addition, certain decision-making errors and biases may impact the process. Each factor plays a role in determining how the manager makes a decision. So whether a decision involves addressing an employee's habitual tardiness, resolving a product quality problem, or determining whether to enter a new market, it has been shaped by a number of factors.

EFFECTIVE Decision Making in Today's World

LO5 Per Carlsson, a product development manager at IKEA, "spends his days creating Volvo-style kitchens at Yugo prices." His job is to take the "problems" identified by the company's product-strategy council (a group of globe-trotting senior managers that monitors consumer trends and establishes product priorities) and turn them into furniture that customers around the world want to buy. One "problem" identified by the council: the kitchen has replaced the living room as the social and entertaining center in the home. Customers are looking for kitchens that convey comfort and cleanliness while still allowing them to pursue their gourmet aspirations. Carlsson must take this information and make things happen. There are a lot of decisions to make—programmed and nonprogrammed—and the fact that IKEA is

a global company makes it even more challenging. Comfort in Asia means small, cozy appliances and spaces, while North American customers want oversized glassware and giant refrigerators. His ability to make good decisions quickly has significant implications for IKEA's success.[28]

Today's business world revolves around making decisions, often risky ones, usually with incomplete or inadequate information, and under intense time pressure. Making good business decisions in today's rapid-paced and messy world isn't easy. Things happen too fast. Customers come and go in the click of a mouse or the swipe of a screen. Market landscapes can shift dramatically overnight along several dimensions. Competitors can enter a market and exit it just as quickly as they entered. Thriving and prospering under such conditions means managerial decision making must adapt to these realities. Most managers make one decision after another; and as if that weren't challenging enough, more is at stake than ever before. Bad decisions can cost millions. What do managers need to do to make effective decisions in today's fast-moving world? First, let's look at some suggested guidelines. Then, we'll discuss an interesting new line of thinking that has implications for making effective decisions—especially for business types—called design thinking.

If your professor has assigned this, go to **www.mymanagementlab.com** to complete the Simulation: *Decision Making* and see how well you can apply the ideas behind the decision-making process.

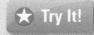

Guidelines for Effective Decision Making

Decision making is serious business. Your abilities and track record as an effective decision maker will determine how your organizational work performance is evaluated and whether you'll be promoted to higher and higher positions of responsibility. Here are some additional guidelines to help you be a better decision maker.

- *Understand cultural differences.* Managers everywhere want to make good decisions. However, is there only one "best" way worldwide to make decisions? Or does the "best way depend on the values, beliefs, attitudes, and behavioral patterns of the people involved?"[29]
- *Create standards for good decision making.* Good decisions are forward-looking, use available information, consider all available and viable options, and do not create conflicts of interest.[30]
- *Know when it's time to call it quits.* When it's evident that a decision isn't working, don't be afraid to pull the plug. For instance, the CEO of L.L.Bean pulled the plug on building a new customer call center in Waterville, Maine—"literally stopping the bulldozers in their tracks"—after T-Mobile said it was building its own call center right next door. He was afraid that the city would not have enough qualified workers for both companies and so decided to build 55 miles away in Bangor.[31] He knew when it was time to call it quits. However, as we said earlier, many decision makers block or distort negative information because they don't want to believe their decision was bad. They become so attached to a decision that they refuse to recognize when it's time to move on. In today's dynamic environment, this type of thinking simply won't work.
- *Use an effective decision-making process.* Experts say an effective decision-making process has these six characteristics: (1) it focuses on what's important; (2) it's logical and consistent; (3) it acknowledges both subjective and objective thinking and blends analytical with intuitive thinking; (4) it requires only as much information and analysis as is necessary to resolve a particular dilemma; (5) it encourages and guides the gathering of relevant information and informed opinion; and (6) it's straightforward, reliable, easy to use, and flexible."[32]

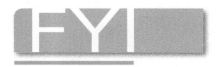

• 77 percent of managers say the number of decisions they make during a typical day has increased.[34]

design thinking
Approaching management problems as designers approach design problems

• *Develop your ability to think clearly* so you can make better choices at work and in your life.[33] Making good decisions doesn't come naturally. You have to work at it. Read and study about decision making. Keep a journal of decisions in which you evaluate your decision making successes and failures by looking at the process you used and the outcomes you got.

Design Thinking and Decision Making

The way managers approach decision making—using a rational and analytical mindset in identifying problems, coming up with alternatives, evaluating alternatives, and choosing one of those alternatives—may not be the best, and is certainly not the only, choice in today's environment. That's where design thinking comes in. **Design thinking** has been described as "approaching management problems as designers approach design problems."[35] More organizations are beginning to recognize how design thinking can benefit them.[36] For instance, Apple has long been celebrated for its design thinking. The company's lead designer, Jonathan "Jony" Ive (who was behind some of Apple's most successful products, including the iPod and iPhone and was just knighted in the United Kingdom for services to design and enterprise) had this to say about Apple's design approach: "We try to develop products that seem somehow inevitable—that leave you with the sense that that's the only possible solution that makes sense."[37]

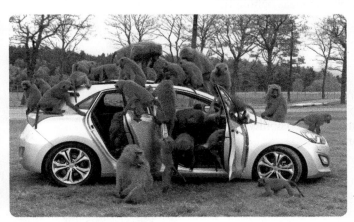

Korean carmaker Hyundai decided to take the design thinking approach in testing the durability and quality of its i30 hatchback family car by letting a group of forty safari park baboons examine it for ten hours. Hyundai hopes that the lessons learned from the excessive wear-and-tear test of the car's parts and interior can be applied to the research and development of future cars.
Source: REX Features/AP Imagres

While many managers don't deal specifically with product or process design decisions, they still make decisions about work issues that arise, and design thinking can help them be better decision makers. What can the design thinking approach teach managers about making better decisions? Well, it begins with the first step of identifying problems. Design thinking says that managers should look at problem identification collaboratively and integratively, with the goal of gaining a deep understanding of the situation. They should look not only at the rational aspects, but also at the emotional elements. Then invariably, of course, design thinking would influence how managers identify and evaluate alternatives. "A traditional manager (educated in a business school, of course) would take the options that have been presented and analyze them based on deductive reasoning and then select the one with the highest net present value. However, using design thinking, a manager would say, "What is something completely new that would be lovely if it existed but doesn't now?"[38] Design thinking means opening up your perspective and gaining insights by using observation and inquiry skills and not relying simply on rational analysis. We're not saying that rational analysis isn't needed; we are saying that there's more needed in making effective decisions, especially in today's world. Just a heads up: Design thinking also has broad implications for managers in other areas.

Big Data and Decision Making

• Amazon.com, Earth's biggest online retailer, earns billions of dollars of revenue each year—estimated at one-third of sales—from its "personalization technologies" such as product recommendations and computer-generated e-mails.[39]
• At AutoZone, decision makers are using new software that gleans information from a variety of databases and allows its 5,000-plus local stores to target deals and hopefully reduce the chance that customers will walk away without making a purchase. AutoZone's chief information officer says, "We think this is the direction of the future."[40]

- It's not just businesses that are exploiting big data. A team of San Francisco researchers was able to predict the magnitude of a disease outbreak halfway around the world by analyzing phone patterns from mobile phone usage.[41]

Yes, there's a ton of information out there—100 petabytes here in the decade of the 2010s, according to experts. (In bytes, that translates to 1 plus 17 zeroes, in case you were wondering!)[42] And businesses—and other organizations—are finally figuring out how to use it. So what is **big data**? It's the vast amount of quantifiable information that can be analyzed by highly sophisticated data processing. One IT expert described big data with "3V's: high volume, high velocity, and/or high variety information assets."[43]

What does big data have to do with decision making? A lot, as you can imagine. With this type of data at hand, decision makers have very powerful tools to help them make decisions. However, experts caution that collecting and analyzing data for data's sake is wasted effort. Goals are needed when collecting and using this type of information. As one individual said, "Big data is a descendant of Taylor's 'scientific management' of more than a century ago."[44] While Taylor used a stopwatch to time and monitor a worker's every movement, big data is using math modeling, predictive algorithms, and artificial intelligence software to measure and monitor people and machines like never before. But managers need to really examine and evaluate how big data might contribute to their decision making before jumping in with both feet. Why? Because big data, no matter how comprehensive or well analyzed, needs to be tempered by good judgment.

big data
The vast amount of quantifiable information that can be analyzed by highly sophisticated data processing

PREPARING FOR: Exams/Quizzes

CHAPTER SUMMARY by Learning Objectives

LO1 DESCRIBE the eight steps in the decision-making process.

A decision is a choice. The decision-making process consists of eight steps: (1) identify problem; (2) identify decision criteria; (3) weight the criteria; (4) develop alternatives; (5) analyze alternatives; (6) select alternative; (7) implement alternative; and (8) evaluate decision effectiveness.

LO2 EXPLAIN the four ways managers make decisions.

The assumptions of rationality are as follows: the problem is clear and unambiguous; a single, well-defined goal is to be achieved; all alternatives and consequences are known; and the final choice will maximize the payoff. Bounded rationality says that managers make rational decisions but are bounded (limited) by their ability to process information. Satisficing happens when decision makers accept solutions that are good enough. With escalation of commitment, managers increase commitment to a decision even when they have evidence it may have been a wrong decision. Intuitive decision making means making decisions on the basis of experience, feelings, and accumulated judgment. Using evidence-based management, a manager makes decisions based on the best available evidence.

LO3 CLASSIFY decisions and decision-making conditions.

Programmed decisions are repetitive decisions that can be handled by a routine approach and are used when the problem being resolved is straightforward, familiar, and easily defined (structured). Nonprogrammed decisions are unique decisions that require

a custom-made solution and are used when the problems are new or unusual (unstructured) and for which information is ambiguous or incomplete. Certainty is a situation in which a manager can make accurate decisions because all outcomes are known. Risk is a situation in which a manager can estimate the likelihood of certain outcomes. Uncertainty is a situation in which a manager is not certain about the outcomes and can't even make reasonable probability estimates. When decision makers face uncertainty, their psychological orientation will determine whether they follow a maximax choice (maximizing the maximum possible payoff); a maximin choice (maximizing the minimum possible payoff); or a minimax choice (minimizing the maximum regret—amount of money that could have been made if a different decision had been made).

LO4 DESCRIBE **different decision-making styles and discuss how biases affect decision making.**

A person's thinking style reflects two things: the source of information you tend to use (external or internal) and how you process that information (linear or nonlinear). These four dimensions were collapsed into two styles. The linear thinking style is characterized by a person's preference for using external data and processing this information through rational, logical thinking. The nonlinear thinking style is characterized by a preference for internal sources of information and processing this information with internal insights, feelings, and hunches. The 12 common decision-making errors and biases include overconfidence, immediate gratification, anchoring, selective perception, confirmation, framing, availability, representation, randomness, sunk costs, self-serving bias, and hindsight. The managerial decision-making model helps explain how the decision-making process is used to choose the best alternative(s), either through maximizing or satisficing and then implementing and evaluating the alternative. It also helps explain what factors affect the decision-making process, including the decision-making approach (rationality, bounded rationality, intuition), the types of problems and decisions (well structured and programmed or unstructured and non-programmed), the decision-making conditions (certainty, risk, uncertainty), and the decision maker's style (linear or nonlinear).

LO5 IDENTIFY **effective decision-making techniques.**

Managers can make effective decisions by understanding cultural differences in decision making, creating standards for good decision making, knowing when it's time to call it quits, using an effective decision-making process, and developing their ability to think clearly. An effective decision-making process (1) focuses on what's important; (2) is logical and consistent; (3) acknowledges both subjective and objective thinking and blends both analytical and intuitive approaches; (4) requires only "enough" information as is necessary to resolve a problem; (5) encourages and guides gathering relevant information and informed opinions; and (6) is straightforward, reliable, easy to use, and flexible.

Design thinking is "approaching management problems as designers approach design problems." It can be useful when identifying problems and when identifying and evaluating alternatives. Using big data, decision makers have power tools to help them make decisions. However, no matter how comprehensive or well analyzed the big data, it needs to be tempered by good judgment.

MyManagementLab

Go to **mymanagementlab.com** to complete the problems marked with this icon ⭐.

⭐ REVIEW AND DISCUSSION QUESTIONS

1. Why is decision making often described as the essence of a manager's job?

2. Describe the eight steps in the decision-making process.

3. Compare and contrast the four ways managers make decisions.

4. Explain the two types of problems and decisions. Contrast the three decision-making conditions.

5. Would you call yourself a linear or nonlinear thinker? What are the decision-making implications of these labels? What are the implications for choosing where you want to work?

6. "As managers use computers and software tools more often, they'll be able to make more rational decisions." Do you agree or disagree with this statement? Why?

7. How can managers blend the guidelines for making effective decisions in today's world with the rationality and bounded rationality models of decision making, or can they? Explain.

8. Is there a difference between wrong decisions and bad decisions? Why do good managers sometimes make wrong decisions? Bad decisions? How can managers improve their decision-making skills?

MyManagementLab

If your professor has assigned these, go to **www.mymanagementlab.com** for Auto-graded writing questions as well as the following Assisted-graded writing questions:

9. How might an organization's culture influence the way managers make decisions?

10. All of us bring biases to the decisions we make. What would be the drawbacks of having biases? Could there be any advantages to having biases? Explain. What are the implications for managerial decision making?

PREPARING FOR: My Career

⭐ PERSONAL INVENTORY ASSESSMENTS 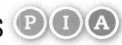 PERSONAL INVENTORY ASSESSMENT

Solving Problems Analytically and Creatively

Making decisions is all about solving problems. Do this PIA and find out about your level of creativity and innovation in problem solving.

⭐ ETHICS DILEMMA

A baggage handler at Reno-Tahoe International Airport refused to load a dangerously thin hunting dog with bloody paws and body covered with sores onto a flight home to its owner.[45] Transportation Safety Authority (TSA) officers couldn't even get the dog to stand up to be X-rayed, and everyone who saw it—ticket counter personnel, the TSA employees, and even the airport police officers—was concerned about the dog's condition. The baggage handler was afraid that the dog wouldn't survive the flight, so she refused to load it onto the plane. Her supervisor told her that the animal's paperwork was in order and its condition "wasn't her concern" and to load the dog. When she

refused, she was fired. Eventually, the dog was taken away by animal control officers and nursed back to health before being sent to its owner in Texas. And some days later, the fired baggage handler was offered her job back with missed pay. The baggage handler's employer called the incident "regrettable" and said it would be used as a "teachable moment for the company."

11. Was the decision by the supervisor to fire the baggage handler appropriate? Explain both "why" and "why not."

12. If you were a manager, how would you use this incident to "teach" employees about ethics and decision making?

SKILLS EXERCISE   Developing Your Creativity Skill

About the Skill

Creativity is a frame of mind. You need to open your mind to new ideas. Every individual has the ability to be creative, but many people simply don't try to develop that ability. In contemporary organizations, such people may have difficulty achieving success. Dynamic environments and managerial chaos require that managers look for new and innovative ways to attain their goals as well as those of the organization.[46]

Steps in Practicing the Skill

- *Think of yourself as creative*. Although it's a simple suggestion, research shows that if you think you can't be creative, you won't be. Believing in yourself is the first step in becoming more creative.

- *Pay attention to your intuition*. Every individual's subconscious mind works well. Sometimes answers come to you when least expected. For example, when you are about to go to sleep, your relaxed mind sometimes whispers a solution to a problem you're facing. Listen to that voice. In fact, most creative people keep a notepad near their bed and write down those great ideas when they occur. That way, they don't forget them.

- *Move away from your comfort zone*. Every individual has a comfort zone in which certainty exists. But creativity and the known often do not mix. To be creative, you need to move away from the status quo and focus your mind on something new.

- *Engage in activities that put you outside your comfort zone.* You not only must think differently; you need to do things differently and thus challenge yourself. Learning to play a musical instrument or learning a foreign language, for example, opens your mind to a new challenge.

- *Seek a change of scenery*. People are often creatures of habit. Creative people force themselves out of their habits by changing their scenery, which may mean going into a quiet and serene area where you can be alone with your thoughts.

- *Find several right answers*. In the discussion of bounded rationality, we said that people seek solutions that are good enough. Being creative means continuing to look for other solutions even when you think you have solved the problem. A better, more creative solution just might be found.

- *Play your own devil's advocate*. Challenging yourself to defend your solutions helps you to develop confidence in your creative efforts. Second-guessing yourself may also help you find more creative solutions.

- *Believe in finding a workable solution.* Like believing in yourself, you also need to believe in your ideas. If you don't think you can find a solution, you probably won't.

- *Brainstorm with others*. Being creative is not a solitary activity. Bouncing ideas off others creates a synergistic effect.

- *Turn creative ideas into action.* Coming up with ideas is only half the process. Once the ideas are generated, they must be implemented. Keeping great ideas in your mind or on paper that no one will read does little to expand your creative abilities.

Practicing the Skill

How many words can you make using the letters in the word *brainstorm*? There are at least 95.

WORKING TOGETHER   Team Exercise

Being effective in decision making is something that managers obviously want. What's involved with being a good decision maker? Form groups of three to four students. Discuss your experiences making decisions—for example, buying a car or some other purchase, choosing classes and professors, making summer or spring break plans, and so forth. Each of you should share times when you felt you made good decisions. Analyze what happened during that decision-making process that contributed to it being a good decision. Then, consider some decisions that you felt were bad. What happened to make them bad? What common characteristics, if any, did you identify among the good decisions? The bad decisions? Come up with a bulleted list of practical suggestions for making good decisions. As a group, be prepared to share your list with the class.

MY TURN TO BE A MANAGER

- For one week, pay close attention to the decisions you make and how you make them. Write a description of five of those decisions using the steps in the decision-making process as your guide. Also, describe whether you relied on external or internal sources of information to help you make the decision and whether you think you were more linear or nonlinear in how you processed that information.

- When you feel you haven't made a good decision, assess how you could have made a better decision.

- Find two examples of a procedure, a rule, and a policy. Bring a description of these examples to class and be prepared to share them.

- Write a procedure, a rule, and a policy for your instructor to use in your class. Be sure that each one is clear and understandable. And be sure to explain how it fits the characteristics of a procedure, a rule, or a policy.

- Find three examples of managerial decisions described in any of the popular business periodicals (*Wall Street*

Journal, BusinessWeek, Fortune, etc.). Write a paper describing each decision and any other information, such as what led to the decision, what happened as a result of the decision, etc. What did you learn about decision making from these examples?

- Interview two managers and ask them for suggestions on what it takes to be a good decision maker. Write down their suggestions and be prepared to present them in class.

- Do a Web search on the phrase "101 dumbest moments in business." Get the most current version of this end-of-year list. Pick three of the examples and describe what happened. What's your reaction to the examples? How could the managers have made better decisions?

- In your own words, write down three things you learned in this text about being a good manager. Keep a copy of this for future reference.

CASE APPLICATION 1 Tasting Success

The Coca-Cola Company (Coke) is in a league by itself.[47] As the world's largest and number one nonalcoholic beverage company, Coke makes or licenses more than 3,500 drinks in more than 200 countries. Coke has built 15 billion-dollar brands and also claims four of the top five soft-drink brands (Coke, Diet Coke, Fanta, and Sprite). Although it fell to the number-three spot in 2013, each year since 2001, global brand consulting firm Interbrand, in conjunction with *Bloomberg BusinessWeek,* has identified Coke as the number-one best global brand. Coke's executives and managers are focusing on ambitious, long-term growth for the company—doubling Coke's business by 2020. A big part of achieving this goal is building up its Simply Orange juice business into a powerful global juice brand. Decision making is playing a crucial role as managers try to beat rival PepsiCo, which has a 40 percent market share in the not-from-concentrate juice category compared to Coke's 28 percent share. And those managers aren't leaving anything to chance in this hot—umm, cold—pursuit!

You'd think that making orange juice (OJ) would be relatively simple—pick, squeeze, pour. While that would probably be the case in your own kitchen, in Coke's case, that glass of 100 percent OJ is possible only through "satellite imagery, complicated data algorithms, and even a juice pipeline." The purchasing director for Coke's massive Florida juice packaging facility says, "Mother Nature doesn't like to be standardized." Yet, standardization is what it takes for Coke to make this work profitably. And producing a juice beverage is far more complicated than bottling soda.

Using what it calls its "Black Book model," Coke wants to ensure that customers have consistently fresh, tasty OJ 12 months a year despite a peak growing season that's only three months long. To help in this, Coke is relying on a "revenue analytic consultant." He says, "Orange juice is definitely one of the most complex applications of business analytics." To consistently deliver an optimal blend given the challenges of nature requires some 1 quintillion (that's 1 followed by 18 zeroes) decisions.

There's no secret formula to Black Book, it's simply an algorithm. It includes detailed data about the more than 600 different flavors that make up an orange and about customer preferences. This data is correlated to a profile of each batch of raw juice. The algorithm then determines how to blend batches to match a certain taste and consistency. At the juice bottling plant, "blend technicians carry out Black Book instructions prior to bottling." The weekly OJ recipe they use is "tweaked" constantly. Black Book also includes data on external factors such as weather patterns, crop yields, and other cost pressures. This is useful for Coke's decision makers as they ensure they'll have enough supplies for at least 15 months. One Coke executive says, "If we have a hurricane or freeze, we can quickly replan the business in 5 or 10 minutes just because we've mathematically modeled it."

⭐ DISCUSSION QUESTIONS

13. Which decisions in this story could be considered unstructured problems? Structured problems?

14. How does the Black Book help Coke's managers and other employees in decision making?

15. What does Coke's big data have to do with its goals?

16. Do some research on revenue analytics. What is it? How can it help managers make better decisions?

CASE APPLICATION 2 The Business of Baseball

Baseball has long been called "America's national pastime" (although according to a Harris Interactive survey, the NFL has been, hands down, the favorite sport of Americans).[48] Now, the game of baseball can probably be better described as America's number crunchers. Take, for instance, Sandy Alderson, the general manager of the New York Mets. He explained the team's decision to let batting champion and free agent shortstop Jose Reyes go to the Miami Marlins. "I'm happy with the analysis we used and the strategy we pursued." As he made this announcement, three members of his baseball operations staff stood by with their laptops open and ready to provide any needed data. A baseball writer has described the sport's move to data analysis this way, "Don't overlook the increasing value of facts, figures, and other data ... and the people who interpret them."

As the 2011 film *Moneyball* (based on an earlier book by the same name) emphasizes, statistics—the "right" statistics—are crucial aspects of effective decision making in the sport of baseball. The central premise of *Moneyball* was that the collected wisdom of baseball insiders (players, managers, coaches, scouts, and the front office) had pretty much been flawed almost from the onset of the game. Commonly-used statistics—such as stolen bases, runs batted in, and batting averages—that were typically used to evaluate players' abilities and performances were inadequate and poor gauges of potential. Rigorous statistical analysis showed that on-base percentages and slugging percentages were better indicators of a player's offensive potential. The goal of all this number crunching? To make better decisions. Team managers want to allocate their limited payroll in the best way possible to help the team be a winner.

The move to more systematic data usage can also be seen in college baseball. At this level, coaches have long used their faces (touching their ears, noses, and chins at a "dizzying speed") to communicate pitch selection to the catcher. Now, however,

hundreds of college teams at all levels have abandoned these body signals and are using a system in which the coach yells out a series of numbers. "The catcher decodes the sequence by looking at a chart tucked into a wristband—the kind football quarterbacks have worn since 1965—and then relays the information to the pitcher the way he always has." Coaches say this approach is not only faster and more efficient, it's not decipherable by "dugout spies" wanting to steal the signs. Since the method allows for many combinations that can mean many different pitches, the same number sequence won't be used for the rest of the game—and maybe not even for the rest of the season.

⭐ DISCUSSION QUESTIONS

17. In a general sense, what kinds of decisions are made in baseball? Would you characterize these decisions as structured or unstructured problems? Explain. What type(s) of decision-making condition would you consider this to be? Explain.

18. Is it appropriate for baseball managers to use only quantitative, objective criteria in evaluating their players? What do you think? Why?

19. Do some research on Sabermetrics. What is it? What does it have to do with decision making?

20. Describe how baseball front office executives and college coaches could use each of the following to make better decisions: (a) rationality, (b) bounded rationality, (c) intuition, and (d) evidence-based management.

21. Can there be too much information in managing the business of baseball? Discuss.

ENDNOTES

1. M. Trottman, "Choices in Stormy Weather," *Wall Street Journal,* February 14, 2006, pp. B1+.
2. S. Minter, "The Season of Snap Judgments," *Industry Week,* May 2010, p. 6; and D. A. Garvin and M. A. Roberto, "What You Don't Know About Making Decisions," *Harvard Business Review,* September 2001, pp. 108–116.
3. "A Bold Alternative to the Worst 'Best' Practices," *BusinessWeek Online* [www.businessweek.com], September 15, 2009.
4. W. Pounds, "The Process of Problem Finding," *Industrial Management Review,* Fall 1969, pp. 1–19.
5. R. J. Volkema, "Problem Formulation: Its Portrayal in the Texts," *Organizational Behavior Teaching Review,* 11, No. 3 (1986–1987), pp. 113–126.
6. T. A. Stewart, "Did You Ever Have to Make Up Your Mind?" *Harvard Business Review,* January 2006, p. 12; and E. Pooley, "Editor's Desk," *Fortune,* June 27, 2005, p. 16.
7. See A. Langley, "In Search of Rationality: The Purposes Behind the Use of Formal Analysis in Organizations," *Administrative Science Quarterly,* December 1989, pp. 598–631; and H. A. Simon, "Rationality in Psychology and Economics," *Journal of Business,* October 1986, pp. 209–224.
8. J. G. March, "Decision-Making Perspective: Decisions in Organizations and Theories of Choice," in A. H. Van de Ven and W. F. Joyce (eds.), *Perspectives on Organization Design and Behavior* (New York: Wiley-Interscience, 1981), pp. 232–233.
9. See P. Hemp, "Death by Information Overload," *Harvard Business Review,* September 2009, pp. 82–89; D. Heath and C. Heath, "The Gripping Statistic," *Fast Company,* September 2009, pp. 59–60; D. R. A. Skidd, "Revisiting Bounded Rationality," *Journal of Management Inquiry,* December 1992, pp. 343–347; B. E. Kaufman, "A New Theory of Satisficing," *Journal of Behavioral Economics,* Spring 1990, pp. 35–51; and N. M. Agnew and J. L. Brown, "Bounded Rationality: Fallible Decisions in Unbounded Decision Space," *Behavioral Science,* July 1986, pp. 148–161.
10. See, for example, G. McNamara, H. Moon, and P. Bromiley, "Banking on Commitment: Intended and Unintended Consequences of an Organization's Attempt to Attenuate Escalation of Commitment," *Academy of Management Journal,* April 2002, pp. 443–452; V. S. Rao and A. Monk, "The Effects of Individual Differences and Anonymity on Commitment to Decisions," *Journal of Social Psychology,* August 1999, pp. 496–515; C. F. Camerer and R. A. Weber, "The Econometrics and Behavioral Economics of Escalation of Commitment: A Re-examination of Staw's Theory," *Journal of Economic Behavior and Organization,* May 1999, pp. 59–82; D. R. Bobocel and J. P. Meyer, "Escalating Commitment to a Failing Course of Action: Separating the Roles of Choice and Justification," *Journal of Applied Psychology,* June 1994, pp. 360–363; and B. M. Staw, "The Escalation of Commitment to a Course of Action," *Academy of Management Review,* October 1981, pp. 577–587.
11. W. Cole, "The Stapler Wars," *Time Inside Business,* April 2005, p. A5.
12. See E. Dane and M. G. Pratt, "Exploring Intuition and Its Role in Managerial Decision Making," *Academy of Management Review,* January 2007, pp. 33–54; M. H. Bazerman and D. Chugh, "Decisions Without Blinders," *Harvard Business Review,* January 2006, pp. 88–97; C. C. Miller and R. D. Ireland, "Intuition in Strategic Decision Making: Friend or Foe in the Fast-Paced 21st Century," *Academy of Management Executive,* February 2005, pp. 19–30; E. Sadler-Smith and E. Shefy, "The Intuitive Executive: Understanding and Applying 'Gut Feel' in Decision Making," *Academy of Management Executive,* November 2004, pp. 76–91; and L. A. Burke and M. K. Miller, "Taking the Mystery Out of Intuitive Decision Making," *Academy of Management Executive,* October 1999, pp. 91–99.

13. C. C. Miller and R. D. Ireland, "Intuition in Strategic Decision Making: Friend or Foe," p. 20.

14. E. Sadler-Smith and E. Shefy, "Developing Intuitive Awareness in Management Education," *Academy of Management Learning & Education,* June 2007, pp. 186–205.

15. M. G. Seo and L. Feldman Barrett, "Being Emotional During Decision Making—Good or Bad? An Empirical Investigation," *Academy of Management Journal,* August 2007, pp. 923–940.

16. B. Roberts, "Hire Intelligence," *HR Magazine,* May 2011, p. 63.

17. R. B. Briner, D. Denyer, and D. M. Rousseau, "Evidence-Based Management: Concept Cleanup Time?" *Academy of Management Perspective,* November 2009, p. 22.

18. J. Pfeffer and R. Sutton, "Trust the Evidence, Not Your Instincts," *New York Times Online,* September 3, 2011; and T. Reay, W. Berta, and M. K. Kohn, "What's the Evidence on Evidence-Based Management?" *Academy of Management Perspectives,* November 2009, p. 5.

19. "Hurry Up and Decide," *Bloomberg BusinessWeek,* May 14, 2001, p. 16.

20. K. R. Brousseau, M. J. Driver, G. Hourihan, and R. Larsson, "The Seasoned Executive's Decision-Making Style," *Harvard Business Review,* February 2006, pp. 111–121.

21. Future Vision box based on S. Jayson, "They're Studying You," *USA Today,* March 11, 2014, p. 6B; A. Chen, "You Are What You e-Read," *Wall Street Journal,* February 19, 2014, pp. D1+; A. Alter, "Your E-Book Is Reading You," *Wall Street Journal,* June 29, 2012, pp. D1+; R. Kurzweil, "Man or Machine?" *Wall Street Journal,* June 29, 2012, p. C12; D. Jones and A. Shaw, "Slowing Momentum: Why BPM Isn't Keeping Pace with Its Potential," *BPM Magazine,* February 2006, pp. 4–12; B. Violino, "IT Directions," *CFO,* January 2006, pp. 68–72; D. Weinberger, "Sorting Data to Suit Yourself," *Harvard Business Review,* March 2005, pp. 16–18; and C. Winkler, "Getting a Grip on Performance," *CFO-IT,* Winter 2004, pp. 38–48.

22. Leader Making a Difference box based on J. Weisenthal, "Here's Why Elon Musk Built Tesla Even Though He Thought It Was Probably Going to Fail," www.businessinsider.com, March 30, 2014; M. Adamo and C. Leahey, "The List: 2013's Top People in Business," *Fortune,* December 9, 2013, pp. 90–91; A. Vandermey, "Businessperson of the Year," *Fortune,* December 9, 2013, pp. 98–108; T. Hessman, "The World According to Elon Musk," *Industry Week,* October 2013, pp. 12–17; and A. Vance, "Electric Company," *Bloomberg BusinessWeek,* July 22, 2013, pp. 48–52.

23. S. Holmes, "Inside the Coup at Nike," *BusinessWeek,* February 6, 2006, pp. 34–37; and M. Barbaro, "Slightly Testy Nike Divorce Came Down to Data vs. Feel," *New York Times Online* [www.nytimes.com], January 28, 2006.

24. C. M. Vance, K. S. Groves, Y. Paik, and H. Kindler, "Understanding and Measuring Linear–Nonlinear Thinking Style for Enhanced Management Education and Professional Practice," *Academy of Management Learning & Education,* June 2007, pp. 167–185.

25. E. Teach, "Avoiding Decision Traps," *CFO,* June 2004, pp. 97–99; and D. Kahneman and A. Tversky, "Judgment Under Uncertainty: Heuristics and Biases," *Science* 185 (1974), pp. 1124–1131.

26. Information for this section taken from D. Kahneman, D. Lovallo, and O. Sibony, "Before You Make That Decision . . ." *Harvard Business Review,* June 2011, pp. 50–60; and S. P. Robbins, *Decide & Conquer* (Upper Saddle River, NJ: Financial Times/Prentice Hall), 2004.

27. D. Kahneman, D. Lovallo, and O. Siboney, "Before You Make That Big Decision," *Harvard Business Review,* June 2011, pp. 50–60.

28. L. Margonelli, "How IKEA Designs Its Sexy Price Tags," *Business 2.0,* October 2002, p. 108.

29. P. C. Chu, E. E. Spires, and T. Sueyoshi, "Cross-Cultural Differences in Choice Behavior and Use of Decision Aids: A Comparison of Japan and the United States," *Organizational Behavior & Human Decision Processes,* vol. 77, no. 2 (1999), pp. 147–170.

30. D. Ariely, "Good Decisions. Bad Outcomes," *Harvard Business Review,* December 2010, p. 40.

31. S. Thurm, "Seldom-Used Executive Power: Reconsidering," *Wall Street Journal,* February 6, 2006, p. B3.

32. J. S. Hammond, R. L. Keeney, and H. Raiffa, *Smart Choices: A Practical Guide to Making Better Decisions* (Boston, MA: Harvard Business School Press, 1999), p. 4.

33. R. Dobelli, *The Art of Thinking Clearly* (New York: HarperCollins), 2013; and *Decisive: How to Make Better Choices in Life and Work* (New York: Random House/Crown Business), 2013.

34. J. MacIntyre, "Bosses and Bureaucracy," *Springfield Business Journal,* August 1–7, 2005, p. 29.

35. D. Dunne and R. Martin, "Design Thinking and How It Will Change Management Education: An Interview and Discussion," *Academy of Management Learning & Education,* December 2006, p. 512.

36. M. Korn and R. E. Silverman, "Forget B-School, D-School Is Hot," *Wall Street Journal,* June 7, 2012, pp. B1+; R. Martin and J. Euchner, "Design Thinking," *Research Technology Management,* May/June 2012, pp. 10–14; T. Larsen and T. Fisher, "Design Thinking: A Solution to Fracture-Critical Systems," *DMI News & Views,* May 2012, p. 31; T. Berno, "Design Thinking versus Creative Intelligence," *DMI News & Views,* May 2012, p. 28; J. Liedtka and Tim Ogilvie, "Helping Business Managers Discover Their Appetite for Design Thinking," *Design Management Review,* Issue 1, 2012, pp. 6–13; and T. Brown, "Strategy By Design," *Fast Company,* June 2005, pp. 52–54.

37. C. Guglielmo, "Apple Loop: The Week in Review," *Forbes.com,* May 25, 2012, p. 2.

38. D. Dunne and R. Martin, "Design Thinking and How It Will Change Management Education: An Interview and Discussion," p. 514.

39. K. Cukier and V. Mayer-Schönberger, "The Financial Bonanza of Big Data," *Wall Street Journal,* March 8, 2013, p. A15.

40. R. King and S. Rosenbush, "Big Data Broadens Its Range," *Wall Street Journal,* March 14, 2013, p. B5.

41. "Big Data, Big Impact: New Possibilities for International Development," World Economic Forum, weforum.org, 2012.

42. M. Kassel, "From a Molehill To a Mountain," *Wall Street Journal,* March 11, 2013, p. R1.

43. D. Laney, "The Importance of 'Big Data': A Definition," www.gartner.com/it-glossary/big-data/, March 22, 2013.

44. S. Lohr, "Sure, Big Data Is Great. But So Is Intuition," *New York Times Online,* December 29, 2012.

45. Based on A. Newcomb, "Fired Baggage Handler Offered Job Back," abcnews.go.com, December 7, 2011; The Associated Press, "Worker Won't Load Injured Dog, Loses Job," *Springfield News-Leader,* December 6, 2011, p. 3A; and "Baggage Handler Fired After Refusing to Load Dog on Plane," www.foxnews.com, December 5, 2011.

46. Developing Your Creative Skill exercise based on S. P. Robbins, *Essentials of Organizational Behavior,* 8th ed. (Upper Saddle River, NJ: Prentice Hall, 2004); C. W. Wang and R. Y. Horng, "The Effects of Creative Problem Solving Training on Creativity, Cognitive Type, and R & D Performance," *R&D Management* (January 2002), pp. 35–46; S. Caudron, "Creativity 101," *Workforce* (March 2002), pp. 20, 24; and T. M. Amabile, "Motivating Creativity in Organizations," *California Management Review* (Fall 1997), pp. 42–52.

47. D. D. Stanford, "Coke Has a Secret Formula For Orange Juice, Too," *Bloomberg Businessweek,* February 4–10, 2013, pp. 19–20; P. Sellers, "The New Coke," *Fortune,* May 21, 2012, pp. 138–144; and Adi Ignatious, "Shaking Things Up at Coca-Cola," *Harvard Business Review,* October 2011, pp. 94–99.

48. J. Green, "John Henry and the Making of a Red Sox Baseball Dynasty," www.BloombergBusinessweek.com, April 24, 2014; S. Amick, "Analytics Take Game by Storm," *USA Today,* March 4, 2014, p. 7C; P. White, "More Managers Embrace Analytics," *USA Today,* February 11, 2014, p. 1C+; J. Swartz, "Batting Cleanup for Giants: Technology," *USA Today,* April 1, 2013, p. 3B; T. Caporale and T.C. Collier, "Scouts versus Stats: The Impact of Moneyball on the Major League Baseball Draft," *Applied Economics,* vol. 45, Issue 15, 2013, pp. 1983–1990; B. Cohen, "College Baseball Showing Signs of a Revolution," *Wall Street Journal,* June 22, 2012, p. D10; T. Van Riper and C. Semmimi, "The New Moneyball," *Forbes,* April 9, 2012, pp. 70–76; D. K. Berman, "So, What's Your Algorithm?" *Wall Street Journal,* January 4, 2012, pp. B1+; P. White, "The Suits Behind the Uniforms," *USA Today,* December 7, 2011, pp. 1C+; K. L. Papps, A. Bryson, and R. Gomez, "Heterogeneous Worker Ability and Team-Based Production: Evidence from Major League Baseball, 1920–2009," *Labour Economics,* June 2011, pp. 310–319; Michael Lewis, *Moneyball,* (New York: W. W. Norton & Co., 2011); and B. Curtis, "Debating America's Pastime(s)," *New York Times Online,* January 2, 2009.

Management Practice: Part 1

Management Practice

A Manager's Dilemma

Selina Lo loves her job as the manager of a toy store in San Francisco. She loves the chaos and the excitement of kids as they wander around the store searching for their favorite toys. Teddy bears pulled off the shelves and toy trucks left on the floor are part and parcel of managing a toy store. Yet, her biggest challenge, which is a problem faced by many retailers, is employee turnover. Many of her employees leave after just a few months on the job because of hectic schedules and long work hours. Selina is always looking for new ways to keep her employees committed to their jobs. She also takes care of customers' requests and complaints and tries to address them satisfactorily. This is what Selina's life as a manager is like. However, retailers are finding that people with Selina's skills and enthusiasm for store management are few and far between. Managing a retail store is not the career that most college graduates aspire to. Attracting and keeping talented managers continues to be a challenge for all kinds of retailers.

Suppose you're a recruiter for a large retail chain and want to get college graduates to consider store management as a career option. Using what you learned, how would you do that?

Global Sense

Who holds more managerial positions worldwide: women or men? Statistics tell an interesting story. In the United States, women held 50 percent of all managerial positions, but only 4.8 percent of the Fortune 500 CEO spots. In the United Kingdom, only 1.8 percent of the FTSE 500 companies' top positions are held by women. In Germany, women hold 35.6 percent of all management positions, but only 3 percent of women are executive board members. Asian countries have a much higher percentage of women in CEO positions. In Thailand, 30 percent of female managers hold the title of CEO, as do 18 percent in Taiwan. In China, 19 percent of the female workforce are CEOs. Even in Japan, 8 percent of senior managers are women. A census of Australia's top 200 companies listed on the Australian Stock Exchange showed that 11 percent of company executive managers were women. Finally, in Arab countries, the percentage of women in management positions is less than 10 percent.

As you can see, companies across the globe have a large gender gap in leadership. Men far outnumber women in senior business leadership positions. These circumstances exist despite efforts and campaigns to improve equality in the workplace. One company—Deutsche Telekom—is tackling the problem head-on. It says it intends to "more than double the number of women who are managers within five years." In addition, it plans to increase the number of women in senior and middle management to 30 percent by the end of 2015. One action the company is taking is to improve and increase the recruiting of female university graduates. The company's goal: at least 30 percent of the places in executive development programs held by women. Other steps taken by the company revolve around the work environment and work-family issues. Deutsche's chief executive René Obermann said, "Taking on more women in management positions is not about the enforcement of misconstrued egalitarianism. Having a greater number of women at the top will quite simply enable us to operate better."

Discuss the following questions in light of what you learned:

- *What issues might Deutsche Telekom face in recruiting female university graduates?*
- *How could it address those issues?*
- *What issues might it face in introducing changes in work-family programs, and how could it address those issues?*
- *What do you think of Obermann's statement that having a greater number of women at the top will enable the company to operate better?*
- *What could other organizations around the globe learn from Deutsche Telekom?*

Sources: "Women CEOs of the Fortune 1000," [www.catalyst.org/knowledge/women-ceos-fortune-1000], May 9, 2014; J. Nerenberg, "Nearly 20 percent of Female Chinese Managers Are CEOs," [www.fastcompany.com], March 8, 2011; S. Doughty, "Cracking the Glass Ceiling: Female Staff Have the Same Chance as Men of Reaching the Top, Figures Reveal," [www.dailymail.co.uk], March 4, 2011; G. Toegel, "Disappointing Statistics, Positive Outlook," Forbes.com, February 18, 2011; E. Butler, "Wanted: Female Bosses for Germany," [www.bbc.co.uk], February 10, 2011; S. P. Robbins, M. Coulter, Y. Sidani, and D. Jamali, Management: Arab World Edition (London: Pearson Education Limited, 2011), p. 5; "Proportion of Executive Managers and Board Directors of ASX 200 Companies Who Are Women," Australian Bureau of Statistics [www.abs.gov.au], September 15, 2010; Stevens and J. Espinoza, "Deutsche Telekom Sets Women-Manager Quota," Wall Street Journal Online, March 22, 2010; J. Blaue, "Deutsche Telekom Launches Quota for Top Women Managers," www.german-info.com/business_shownews; and N. Clark, "Goal at Deutsche Telekom: More Women as Managers," New York Times Online, March 15, 2010.

Continuing Case

Starbucks—Introduction

Community. Connection. Caring. Committed. Coffee. Five Cs that describe the essence of Starbucks Corporation—what it stands for and what it wants to be as a business. With more than 19,000 stores in 62 countries, Starbucks is the world's number one specialty coffee retailer. The company also owns Seattle's Best Coffee, Teavana, Tazo, Starbucks VIA, Starbucks Refreshers, Evolution Fresh, La

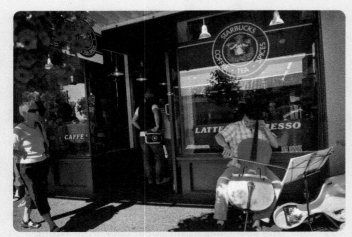

Beginning in 1971 as a coffee shop in Seattle's Pike's Place Market, Starbucks has grown to become the world's top specialty coffee retailer with shops in more than 62 countries and an expanded product line including merchandise, beverages and fresh food, global consumer products, and a Starbucks card and consumer rewards program. Starbucks first store, shown here today, retains its original look with signs and other items bearing the company's first logo.
Source: Martin Zlimek/ZUMApress/Alamy

Boulange, and Verismo brands. It's a company that truly epitomizes the challenges facing managers in today's globally competitive environment. To help you better understand these challenges, we're going to take an in-depth look at Starbucks through these continuing cases. Each of these six continuing cases will look at Starbucks from the perspective of the material presented. Although each case "stands alone," you'll be able to see the progression of the management process as you work through each one.

The Beginning

"We aren't in the coffee business, serving people. We're in the people business, serving coffee." That's the philosophy of Howard Schultz, chairman and chief global strategist of Starbucks. It's a philosophy that has shaped—and continues to shape—the company.

The first Starbucks, which opened in Seattle's famous Pike Place Market in 1971, was founded by Gordon Bowker, Jerry Baldwin, and Zev Siegl. The company was named for the coffee-loving first mate in the book *Moby Dick,* which also influenced the design of Starbucks' distinctive two-tailed siren logo. Schultz, a successful New York City businessperson, first walked into Starbucks in 1981 as a sales representative for a Swedish kitchenware manufacturer. He was hooked immediately. He knew that he wanted to work for this company, but it took almost a year before he could persuade the owners to hire him. After all, he *was* from New York and he hadn't grown up with the values of the company. The owners thought Schultz's style and high energy would clash with the existing culture. But Schultz was quite persuasive and was able to allay the owners' fears. They asked him to join the company as director of retail operations and

marketing, which he enthusiastically did. Schultz's passion for the coffee business was obvious. Although some of the company's employees resented the fact that he was an "outsider," Schultz had found his niche and he had lots of ideas for the company. As he says, "I wanted to make a positive impact."

About a year after joining the company, while on a business trip to Milan, Schultz walked into an espresso bar and right away knew that this concept could be successful in the United States. He said, "There was nothing like this in America. It was an extension of people's front porch. It was an emotional experience. I believed intuitively we could do it. I felt it in my bones." Schultz recognized that although Starbucks treated coffee as produce, something to be bagged and sent home with the groceries, the Italian coffee bars were more like an experience—a warm, community experience. That's what Schultz wanted to recreate in the United States. However, Starbucks' owners weren't really interested in making Starbucks big and didn't really want to give the idea a try. So Schultz left the company in 1985 to start his own small chain of espresso bars in Seattle and Vancouver called *Il Giornale*. Two years later when Starbucks' owners finally wanted to sell, Schultz raised $3.8 million from local investors to buy them out. That small investment has made him a very wealthy person indeed!

Company Facts

Starbucks' main product is coffee—more than 30 blends and single-origin coffees. In addition to fresh-brewed coffee, here's a sampling of other products the company also offers:

- **Handcrafted beverages:** Hot and iced espresso beverages, coffee and noncoffee blended beverages, Tazo® teas, and smoothies
- **Merchandise:** Home espresso machines, coffee brewers and grinders, premium chocolates, coffee mugs and coffee accessories, compact discs, and other assorted items
- **Fresh food:** Baked pastries, sandwiches, salads, hot breakfast items, and yogurt parfaits
- **Global consumer products:** Starbucks Frappuccino® coffee drinks, Starbucks Iced Coffee drinks, Starbucks Liqueurs, and a line of super-premium ice creams
- **Starbucks card and My Starbucks Rewards® program:** A reloadable stored-value card and a consumer rewards program
- **Brand portfolio:** Starbucks Entertainment, Ethos™ Water, Seattle's Best Coffee, and Tazo® Tea

At the end of 2013, the company had more than 200,000 full- and part-time partners (employees) around the world. Howard Schultz is the chairman, president, and CEO of Starbucks. Some of the other "interesting" executive positions include chief operating officer; global chief marketing officer; chief creative officer; executive vice president of partner resources and chief community officer; executive

vice president, global supply chain; executive vice president, global coffee; learning business partner; and international partner resource coordinator.

Decisions, Decisions

One thing you may not realize is that after running the show for 15 years at Starbucks, Howard Schultz, at age 46, stepped out of the CEO job in 2000 (he remained as chairman of the company) because he was "a bit bored." By stepping down as CEO—which he had planned to do, had prepared for, and had no intention of returning to—essentially he was saying that he agreed to trust the decisions of others. At first the company thrived, but then the perils of rapid mass-market expansion began to set in and customer traffic began to fall for the first time ever. As he watched what was happening, there were times when he felt the decisions being made were not good ones. Schultz couldn't shake his gut feeling that Starbucks had lost its way. In fact, in a memo dubbed the "espresso shot heard round the world," he wrote to his top managers explaining in detail how the company's unprecedented growth had led to many minor compromises that when added up led to a "watering down of the Starbucks experience." Among his complaints: sterile "cookie cutter" store layouts, automatic espresso machines that robbed the "barista theater" of roasting and brewing a cup of coffee, and flavor-locked packaging that didn't allow customers to inhale and savor that distinctive coffee aroma. Starbucks had lost its "cool" factor, and Schultz's criticism of the state of the company's stores was blunt and bold. There was no longer a focus on coffee but only on making the cash register ring. Within a year of the memo (and eight years after he left the CEO gig), Schultz was back in charge and working to restore the Starbucks experience. His goals were to fix the troubled stores, to reawaken the emotional attachment with customers, and to make long-term changes like reorganizing the company and revamping the supply chain. The first thing he did, however, was to apologize to the staff for the decisions that had brought the company to this point. In fact, his intention to restore quality control led him to a decision to close all (at that time) 7,100 U.S. stores for one evening to retrain 135,000 baristas on the coffee experience...what it meant, what it was. It was a bold decision, and one that many "experts" felt would be a public relations and financial disaster. But Schultz felt doing so was absolutely necessary to revive and reenergize Starbucks. Another controversial decision was to hold a leadership conference with all store managers (some 8,000 of them) and 2,000 other partners—all at one time and all in one location. Why? To energize and galvanize these employees around what Starbucks stands for and what needed to be done for the company to survive and prosper. Schultz was unsure about how Wall Street would react to the cost, which was around $30 million total (airfare, meals, hotels, etc.), but again he didn't care because he felt doing so was absolutely necessary and critical. And

rather than gathering together in Seattle, where Starbucks is headquartered, Schultz chose New Orleans as the site for the conference. Here was a city still recovering from Hurricane Katrina, which had totally devastated it five years earlier in 2005. Talk about a logistical nightmare—and it was. But, the decision was a symbolic choice. New Orleans was in the process of rebuilding itself and succeeding, and Starbucks was in the process of rebuilding itself and could succeed, too. While there, Starbucks partners volunteered some 50,000 hours of time, reinforcing to Schultz and to all the managers that despite all the problems, Starbucks had not lost its values. Other decisions, like closing 800 stores and laying off 4,000 partners, were more difficult. Since that transition time, Schultz has made lots of decisions. Starbucks has again come back even stronger in what it stands for, achieving in 2013 record financial results, and it is on track to continue those record results.

So we're beginning to see how Starbucks epitomizes the five Cs—community, connection, caring, committed, and coffee. In this *Continuing Case* in the Management Practice sections, you'll discover more about Starbucks' unique and successful ways of managing. As you work on these remaining continuing cases, keep in mind that there may be information included in this introduction you might want to review.

Discussion Questions

1. What management skills do you think would be most important for Howard Schultz to have? Why? What skills do you think would be most important for a Starbucks store manager to have? Why?
2. How might the following management theories/approaches be useful to Starbucks: scientific management, organizational behavior, quantitative approach, systems approach?
3. Choose three of the current trends and issues facing managers and explain how Starbucks might be impacted. What might be the implications for first-line managers? Middle managers? Top managers?
4. Give examples of how Howard Schultz might perform the interpersonal roles, the informational roles, and the decisional roles.
5. Look at Howard Schultz's philosophy of Starbucks. How will this affect the way the company is managed?
6. Go to the company's Web site [www.starbucks.com], and find the list of senior officers. Pick one of those positions and describe what you think that job might involve. Try to envision what types of planning, organizing, leading, and controlling this person would have to do.
7. Look up the company's mission and guiding principles at the company's Web site. What do you think of the mission and guiding principles?

Describe how these would influence how a barista at a local Starbucks store does his or her job. Describe how these would influence how one of the company's top executives does his or her job.

8. Starbucks has some pretty specific goals it wants to achieve. Given this, do you think managers would be more likely to make rational decisions, bounded rationality decisions, or intuitive decisions? Explain.

9. Give examples of decisions that Starbucks managers might made under conditions of certainty. Under conditions of risk. Under conditions of uncertainty.

10. What kind of decision maker does Howard Schultz appear to be? Explain your answer.

11. How might biases and errors affect the decision making done by Starbucks executives? By Starbucks store managers? By Starbucks partners?

12. How might design thinking be important to a company like Starbucks? Do you see any indication that Starbucks uses design thinking? Explain.

Notes for the Continuing Case

Information from company Web site, www.starbucks.com, including 2013 Annual Report; H. Schultz (with J. Gordon), *Onward: How Starbucks Fought for Its Life without Losing Its Soul* (New York: Rodale, 2011); J. Cummings, "Legislative Grind," *Wall Street Journal*, April 12, 2005, pp. A1+; A. Serwer and K. Bonamici, "Hot Starbucks to Go," *Fortune*, January 26, 2004, pp. 60–74; R. Gulati, Sarah Huffman, and G. Neilson, "The Barista Principle," *Strategy and Business*, Third Quarter 2002, pp. 58–69; B. Horovitz, "Starbucks Nation," *USA Today*, May 29–21, 2006, pp. A1+; and H. Schultz and D. Jones Yang, *Pour Your Heart into It: How Starbucks Built a Company One Cup at a Time* (New York: Hyperion, 1997).

Managing the External Environment and the Organization's Culture

From Chapter 3 of *Management*, Thirteenth Edition. Stephen P. Robbins and Mary Coulter. Copyright © 2016 by Pearson Education, Inc. All rights reserved.

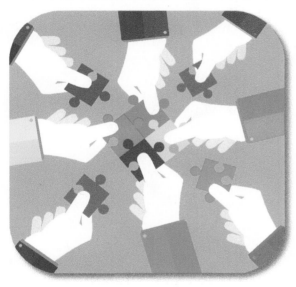

Managing the External Environment and the Organization's Culture

Source: Robuart/Shutterstock.

A key to success in management and in your career is knowing how to "read" an organization's culture so you can find one in which you'll be happy.

Reading an Organization's Culture: Find One Where You'll Be Happy

Wouldn't it be nice to one day find a job you enjoy in an organization you're excited to go to every day (or at least most days!)? Although other factors influence job choice, an organization's culture can be an important indicator of "fit." Organizational cultures differ and so do individuals. Being able to "read" an organization's culture should help you find one that's right for you. By matching your personal preferences to an organization's culture, you are more likely to find satisfaction in your work, are less likely to leave, and have a greater probability of getting positive performance evaluations. Here's a list of things you can do to "read" culture:

*1. **Do background work.** Check out the company's Web site. What impression do you get from it? Are corporate values listed? Mission statement? Look for current news items about the company, especially for evidence of high turnover or recent management shake-ups. Look for clues in stories told in annual reports and other organizational literature. Get the names of former employees if you can and talk with them. You might also talk with members of professional trade associations to which the organization's employees belong.*

*2. **Observe the physical surroundings and corporate symbols.** Pay attention to logos, signs, posters, pictures, photos, style of dress, length of hair, degree of openness between offices, and office furnishings and arrangements. Where do employees park? What does the physical condition of the building and offices look like? What does the office layout look like? What activities are encouraged or discouraged by the physical layout? What do these things say about what the organization values? Could you see yourself working there—and enjoying it?*

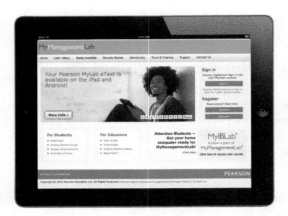

MyManagementLab®

⭐ **Improve Your Grade!**

When you see this icon, visit
www.mymanagementlab.com for activities that are
applied, personalized, and offer immediate feedback.

Learning Objectives

● SKILL OUTCOMES

1 Contrast *the actions of managers according to the omnipotent and symbolic views.*

2 Describe *the constraints and challenges facing managers in today's external environment.*

   ● **Develop your skill** at scanning the environment so you can anticipate and interpret changes taking place.

3 Discuss *the characteristics and importance of organizational culture.*

   ● **Know how** to read and assess an organization's culture.

4 Describe *current issues in organizational culture.*

---

3. How would you characterize the people you meet? *Are they formal? Casual? Serious? Jovial? Open? Restrained in providing information? What stories are repeated? Are jokes/anecdotes used in conversation? How are employees addressed? What do job titles say about the organization? Does the organization's hierarchy appear to be strict or loose? What do these things say about what the organization values?*

4. Look at the organization's HR manual (if you can). *Are there formal rules and regulations? How detailed are they? What do they cover? Could you see yourself working within these parameters?*

5. Ask questions of the people you meet. *For instance: What's the background of current senior managers? Were they promoted from within or hired from the outside? What does the organization do to get new employees up and running? How is job success defined/determined? What rituals are important, and what events get commemorated? Why? Can you describe a decision that didn't work out well, and what the consequences were for that decision maker? Could you describe a crisis or critical event that occurred recently in the organization and how top management responded? What do these things say about what the organization values?*

When you apply for a job, much about the organization's culture is right there for you to see. Know the clues to look for and decide if it's for you!

In this text, we're going to look at culture and other important aspects of management's context. We'll examine the challenges in the external environment and discuss the characteristics of organizational culture. But before we address these topics, we first need to look at two perspectives on how much impact managers actually have on an organization's success or failure.

THE MANAGER: Omnipotent or Symbolic?

LO1 A slumping stock price and continued criticism by many Wall Street analysts about brand performance led to a top management shake-up at PepsiCo. Two top managers in the company's PepsiCo Americas Beverages unit were affected. One was reassigned to a position with lesser responsibility and the other "retired."[1] Such a move shuffling managers is not all that uncommon in the corporate world, but why?

How much difference *does* a manager make in how an organization performs? The dominant view in management theory and society in general is that managers are directly responsible for an organization's success or failure. We call this perspective the **omnipotent view of management**. In contrast, others have argued that much of an organization's success or failure is due to external forces outside managers' control. This perspective is called the **symbolic view of management**. Let's look at each perspective to try and clarify just how much credit or blame managers should get for their organization's performance.

omnipotent view of management
The view that managers are directly responsible for an organization's success or failure

symbolic view of management
The view that much of an organization's success or failure is due to external forces outside managers' control

The Omnipotent View

Managers are extremely important to organizations. Differences in an organization's performance are assumed to be due to the decisions and actions of its managers. Good managers anticipate change, exploit opportunities, correct poor performance, and lead their organizations. When profits are up, managers take the credit and are rewarded with bonuses, stock options, and the like. When profits are down, top managers are often fired in the belief that "new blood" will bring improved results. In the omnipotent view, someone has to be held accountable when organizations perform poorly regardless of the reasons, and that "someone" is the manager. Of course, when things go well, managers also get the credit—even if they had little to do with achieving the positive outcomes.

This view of managers as omnipotent is consistent with the stereotypical picture of the take-charge business executive who overcomes any obstacle in seeing that the organization achieves its goals. And this view isn't limited to business organizations. It also explains turnover among college and professional sports coaches, who are considered the "managers" of their teams. Coaches who lose more games than they win are usually fired and replaced by new coaches who are expected to correct the poor performance.

The Symbolic View

In the 1990s, Cisco Systems was the picture of success. Growing rapidly, it was widely praised by analysts for its "brilliant strategy, masterful management of acquisitions and superb customer focus."[2] However, as Cisco's performance declined during the early part of the twenty-first century, analysts said its strategy was flawed, its acquisition approach was haphazard, and its customer service was poor. Was declining performance due to the managers' decisions and actions, or was it due to external circumstances beyond their control? The symbolic view would suggest the latter.

The symbolic view says that a manager's ability to affect performance outcomes is influenced and constrained by external factors.[3] According to this view, it's unreasonable to expect managers to significantly affect an organization's performance. Instead, performance is influenced by factors over which managers have little control, such as the economy, customers, governmental policies, competitors' actions, industry conditions, and decisions made by previous managers.

This view is labeled "symbolic" because it's based on the belief that managers symbolize control and influence.[4] How? By developing plans, making decisions, and engaging in other managerial activities to make sense out of random, confusing, and ambiguous situations. However, the actual part that managers play in organizational success or failure is limited according to this view.

Exhibit 1
Constraints on Managerial Discretion

Organizational Environment	Managerial Discretion	Organizational Culture

In reality, managers are neither all-powerful nor helpless. But their decisions and actions are constrained. As you can see in Exhibit 1, external constraints come from the organization's environment and internal constraints come from the organization's culture.

THE EXTERNAL ENVIRONMENT:
Constraints and Challenges

LO2 Digital technology has disrupted all types of industries—from financial services and retail to entertainment and automotive. Choosing to embrace these changes, BMW borrowed a page from Apple's playbook and decided to replace its old way of doing things at dealerships.[5] Rather than the standard rows of cars, banners, and showroom cubicles, they're bringing in "product geniuses" to help shoppers better understand and to demonstrate the complex technology now in cars. Other car manufacturers are doing similar things. For instance, General Motors is working with its dealerships to install "connection centers" in showrooms. Anyone who doubts the impact the external environment has on managing just needs to look at what's happened in the automotive industry and many other industries during the last few years.

The term **external environment** refers to factors and forces outside the organization that affect its performance. As shown in Exhibit 2, it includes several different components. The economic component encompasses factors such as interest rates, inflation, changes in disposable income, stock market fluctuations, and business cycle stages. The demographic component is concerned with trends in population characteristics such as age, race, gender, education level, geographic location, income, and family composition. The political/legal component looks at federal, state, and local laws as well as global laws and laws of other countries. It also includes a country's political conditions and stability. The sociocultural component is concerned with societal and cultural factors such as values, attitudes, trends, traditions, lifestyles, beliefs, tastes, and patterns of behavior. The technological component is concerned with scientific or industrial innovations. The global component encompasses those issues associated with globalization and a world economy. Although all these components pose potential constraints on managers' decisions and actions, we're going to take a closer look at two of them—the economic and demographic—by looking at how changes taking place in those components constrain managers and organizations. Then, we'll wrap up this section by examining environmental uncertainty and stakeholder relationships.

external environment
Those factors and forces outside the organization that affect its performance

The Economic Environment

Like many global businesses, Nestlé is facing increased commodity costs.[6] The maker of products from Crunch chocolate bars to Nescafé coffee to Purina pet food spends more than $30 billion a year on raw materials. To get a better feel for what that number

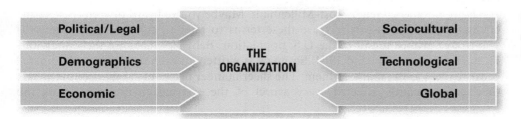

Political/Legal		Sociocultural
Demographics	THE ORGANIZATION	Technological
Economic		Global

Exhibit 2
Components of External Environment

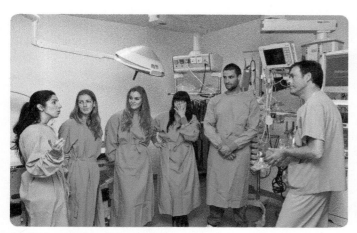

Jens Schriewe (right), head of nursing services at a hospital in Germany, talks with young Spanish nurses he hired to join his clinical staff. To keep Germany's economy improving in the aftermath of the global economic crisis, managers like Jens who face a shortage of skilled workers look for job seekers from Spain and other nations where unemployment remains high.
Source: Daniel Karmann/EPA/Newscom

reflects, think about this: annually, the company purchases about 10 percent of the world's coffee crop, 12 million metric tons of milk, and more than 300,000 tons of cocoa.

Commodity (raw materials) costs are just one of the many volatile economic factors facing organizations. Managers need to be aware of the economic context so they can make the best decisions for their organizations.

THE GLOBAL ECONOMY AND THE ECONOMIC CONTEXT The lingering global economic challenges—once described as the "Great Recession" by some analysts—began with turmoil in home mortgage markets in the United States, as many homeowners found themselves unable to make their mortgage payments.[7] The problems soon affected businesses as credit markets collapsed. All of a sudden, credit was no longer readily available to fund business activities. And due to our globally connected world, it didn't take long for economic troubles in the United States to spread to other countries. The slow, fragile recovery of global economies has continued to be a constraint on organizational decisions and actions. Christine Lagarde, the Managing Director of the International Monetary Fund said that while the global economy appears to be strengthening, global growth is still sluggish.[8] In addition, the World Economic Forum identified two significant risks facing business leaders and policy makers over the next decade: "severe income disparity and chronic fiscal imbalances."[9] Let's take a quick look at the first of these risks, economic inequality, since it reflects that it's not just the economic numbers, but also societal attitudes that can constrain managers.

ECONOMIC INEQUALITY AND THE ECONOMIC CONTEXT A Harris Interactive Poll found that only 10 percent of adults think economic inequality is "not a problem at all." Most survey respondents believed it is either a major problem (57 percent) or a minor problem (23 percent).[10] Why has this issue become so sensitive? After all, those who worked hard and were rewarded because of their hard work or innovativeness have long been admired. And yes, an income gap has always existed. In the United States, that gap between the rich and the rest has been much wider than in other developed nations for decades and was accepted as part of our country's values and way of doing things. However, our acceptance of an ever-increasing income gap may be diminishing.[11] As economic growth has languished and sputtered, and as people's belief that anyone could grab hold of an opportunity and have a decent shot at prosperity has wavered, social discontent over growing income gaps has increased. The bottom line is that business leaders need to recognize how societal attitudes in the economic context also may create constraints as they make decisions and manage their businesses.[12]

The Demographic Environment

Demography is destiny. Have you ever heard this phrase? What it means is that the size and characteristics of a country's population can have a significant effect on what it's able to achieve and on virtually every aspect of life including politics, economics, and culture. This should make it obvious why it's important to examine demographics. Age is a particularly important demographic since the workplace often has different age groups all working together.

Baby Boomers. Gen Y. Post-Millennials. Maybe you've heard or seen these terms before. Population researchers use these terms to refer to three of the more well-known age groups found in the U.S. population. Baby Boomers are those individuals born between 1946 and 1964. So much is written and reported about "boomers" because there are so many of them. The sheer number of people in that cohort means they've significantly affected every aspect of the external environment (from the

educational system to entertainment/lifestyle choices to the Social Security system and so forth) as they've cycled through the various life stages.

Gen Y (or the "Millennials") is typically considered to encompass those individuals born between 1978 and 1994. As the children of the Baby Boomers, this age group is also large in number and making its imprint on external environmental conditions as well. From technology to clothing styles to work attitudes, Gen Y is making its imprint on workplaces.

Then, we have the Post-Millennials—the youngest identified age group—basically teens and middle-schoolers.[13] This group has also been called the iGeneration, primarily because they've grown up with technology that customizes everything to the individual. Population experts say it's too early to tell whether elementary school-aged children and younger are part of this demographic group or whether the world they live in will be so different that they'll comprise a different demographic cohort.[14] Although this youngest group has not officially been "named," some are referring to them as the "touch-screen generation."[15]

Demographic age cohorts are important to our study of management because, as we said earlier, large numbers of people at certain stages in the life cycle can constrain decisions and actions taken by businesses, governments, educational institutions, and other organizations. Demographics not only looks at current statistics, but also looks to the future. For instance, recent analysis of birth rates shows that more than 80 percent of babies born worldwide are from Africa and Asia.[16] And here's an interesting fact: India has one of the world's youngest populations with more males under the age

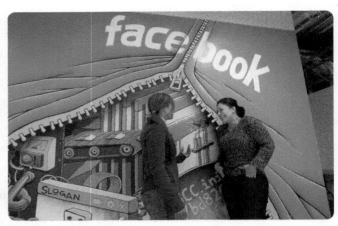

Gen Y is an important demographic at Facebook, where most employees are under 40. The company values the passion and pioneering spirit of its young employees who embrace the challenges of building groundbreaking technology and of working in a fast-paced environment with considerable change and ambiguity.
Source: Paul Sakuma/AP Images

FUTURE VISION | Tomorrow's Workforce: More Diverse Than Ever

Two of the largest changes happening in the makeup of the workforce in the United States are significant increases in Hispanic and senior-citizen participation.

Hispanic-Americans continue to be the fastest-growing segment of the U.S. population. They currently make up 17 percent of the population, although that number is forecasted to increase to 20 percent by 2025. In the southern part of the United States, the percentages will be higher. In cities such as Los Angeles, Phoenix, Tucson, El Paso, and Miami, more than a third of the population will be Hispanic. These general population percentages should translate equivalently to the labor force. The likelihood that you'll have a coworker whose first language is Spanish will be quite high.

You can also expect to see a graying of the workforce. By 2025, most employees will be working beyond normal retirement ages. People are living longer and enjoying good health well into their 70s. Those who enjoy being actively engaged in a job won't want to give that up. On the other hand, there also will be those senior citizens who can't afford to retire and have to continue working to avoid financial strains. In fact, we saw this happening in the most recent recession.

Individuals who would like to have stepped away from their 8-to-5 jobs were happy to have a job and held onto that job. Now, envision that workplace where you'll also likely be working with many older (age 65+) coworkers. However, when those individuals *do* decide to retire, it could leave many organizations scrambling as these individuals take their institutional knowledge, communication skills, and professionalism gained from years of work experience with them.

Again, these two demographic changes foretell a workplace in which, as a manager or as coworkers, you're going to be interacting and working with others who may not think or act or do things the way you would.

If your professor has chosen to assign this, go to ***www.mymanagementlab.com*** *to discuss the following questions.*

⭐ **TALK ABOUT IT 1:** Why is it important for managers to be aware of demographic changes?

⭐ **TALK ABOUT IT 2:** What can managers do to stay on top of demographic changes?

of 5 than the entire population of France. And by 2050, it's predicted that China will have more people age 65 and older than the rest of the world combined.[17] Consider the impact of such population trends on future organizations and managers.

How the External Environment Affects Managers

Knowing *what* the various components of the external environment are and examining certain aspects of that environment are important to managers. However, understanding *how* the environment affects managers is equally as important. We're going to look at three ways the environment constrains and challenges managers—first, through its impact on jobs and employment; next, through the environmental uncertainty that is present; and finally, through the various stakeholder relationships that exist between an organization and its external constituencies.

JOBS AND EMPLOYMENT   As any or all external environmental conditions (economic, demographic, technological, globalization, etc.) change, one of the most powerful constraints managers face is the impact of such changes on jobs and employment—both in poor conditions and in good conditions. The power of this constraint was painfully obvious during the last global recession as millions of jobs were eliminated and unemployment rates rose to levels not seen in many years. Businesses have been slow to reinstate jobs, creating continued hardships for those individuals looking for work.[18] Many college grads have struggled to find jobs or ended up taking jobs that don't require a college degree.[19] Other countries face the same issues. Although such readjustments aren't bad in and of themselves, they do create challenges for managers who must balance work demands and having enough of the right types of people with the right skills to do the organization's work.

Not only do changes in external conditions affect the types of jobs that are available, they affect how those jobs are created and managed. For instance, many employers use flexible work arrangements to meet work output demand.[20] For instance, work

let's get REAL

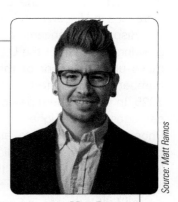

Source: Matt Ramos

Matt Ramos
Director of Marketing

The Scenario:

Kerri and Ralf co-own a full-line, full-service insurance agency. Their customers cover a wide range of ages from young professionals to families to retired seniors. They're considering using social media, especially Facebook and Twitter, for most communications with their customers. Before investing time, money, and other resources in this venture, they want to make sure the investment will benefit their business, especially given their broad customer base. Is the timing right?

What advice about external environmental trends would you give Kerri and Ralf?

The timing is right to get the basics down. But should you invest a lot of money and resources into it? Not quite. Only 8% of consumers think companies are delivering superior customer service on social media. Invest time while collecting customer feedback. Always test, if customer feedback is positive, that's a great sign to begin investing more resources into this new and unproven idea.

tasks may be done by freelancers hired to work on an as-needed basis, or by temporary workers who work full-time but are not permanent employees, or by individuals who share jobs. Keep in mind that such responses have come about because of the constraints from the external environment. As a manager, you'll need to recognize how these work arrangements affect the way you plan, organize, lead, and control. This whole issue of flexible work arrangements has become so prevalent and part of how work is done in organizations.

ASSESSING ENVIRONMENTAL UNCERTAINTY Another constraint posed by external environments is the amount of uncertainty found in that environment, which can affect organizational outcomes. **Environmental uncertainty** refers to the degree of change and complexity in an organization's environment. The matrix in Exhibit 3 shows these two aspects.

The first dimension of uncertainty is the degree of change. If the components in an organization's environment change frequently, it's a *dynamic* environment. If change is minimal, it's a *stable* one. A stable environment might be one with no new competitors, few technological breakthroughs by current competitors, little activity by pressure groups to influence the organization, and so forth. For instance, Zippo Manufacturing, best known for its Zippo lighters, faces a relatively stable environment, with few competitors and little technological change. The main external concern for the company is probably the declining numbers of tobacco smokers, although the company's lighters have other uses, and global markets remain attractive. In contrast, the recorded music industry faces a dynamic (highly uncertain and unpredictable) environment. Digital formats and music-downloading sites turned the industry upside down and brought high levels of uncertainty.

If change is predictable, is that considered dynamic? No. Think of department stores that typically make one-quarter to one-third of their sales in November and December. The drop-off from December to January is significant. But because the change is predictable, the environment isn't considered dynamic. When we talk about degree of change, we mean change that's unpredictable. If change can be accurately anticipated, it's not an uncertainty for managers.

The other dimension of uncertainty describes the degree of **environmental complexity**, which looks at the number of components in an organization's environment and the extent of the knowledge that the organization has about those components. An organization with fewer competitors, customers, suppliers, government agencies, and so forth faces a less complex and uncertain environment. Organizations deal with environmental complexity in various ways. For example, Hasbro Toy Company simplified its environment by acquiring many of its competitors.

environmental uncertainty
The degree of change and complexity in an organization's environment

environmental complexity
The number of components in an organization's environment and the extent of the organization's knowledge about those components

Exhibit 3
Environmental Uncertainty Matrix

		Degree of Change	
		Stable	**Dynamic**
Degree of Complexity	**Simple**	**Cell 1** Stable and predictable environment Few components in environment Components are somewhat similar and remain basically the same Minimal need for sophisticated knowledge of components	**Cell 2** Dynamic and unpredictable environment Few components in environment Components are somewhat similar but are continually changing Minimal need for sophisticated knowledge of components
	Complex	**Cell 3** Stable and predictable environment Many components in environment Components are not similar to one another and remain basically the same High need for sophisticated knowledge of components	**Cell 4** Dynamic and unpredictable environment Many components in environment Components are not similar to one another and are continually changing High need for sophisticated knowledge of components

LEADER making a DIFFERENCE

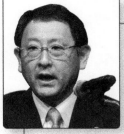
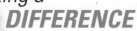

Source: Ahn Young-joon/AP Images

Akio Toyoda's first three years on the job were quite interesting, to put it mildly! Akio, the grandson of Toyota's founder, became the company's president in 2009, which was also the year the company had its first operating loss in 70 years.[21] In 2010, Toyota's excellent reputation for quality was damaged by a global recall fiasco. Then, on March 11, 2011, the devastating earthquake and tsunami and consequent nuclear crisis in Japan disrupted the company's global supply chain, forcing Toyota to slash production worldwide. What a set of challenges for this new leader! However, Akio was not deterred. Instead, he looked at what he could do to bring Toyota through the crises to once again be the leader in the global car market. One thing he did was "dramatically change the way the company is managed." Most Japanese companies use a "bottom-up" management approach, which slows down decision making as ideas make their way through the organization for approval. Akio's management style is to "be fast" and to "be flexible." Such an approach was particularly crucial during the difficult aftermath of the earthquake and tsunami. Akio "took the unusual step of instructing the general managers of departments such as body engineering and powertrain to restore production and not waste time reporting upward." As Akio steers the company toward sustainable growth, he recognizes the importance of Toyota's different stakeholders including shareholders, employees, and customers. Five years after being named Toyota's CEO, Akio was named one of the best CEOs of 2013. What can you learn from this leader making a difference?

Complexity is also measured in terms of the knowledge an organization needs about its environment. For instance, managers at Pinterest must know a great deal about their Internet service provider's operations if they want to ensure their Web site is available, reliable, and secure for their customers. On the other hand, managers of college bookstores have a minimal need for sophisticated knowledge about their suppliers.

How does the concept of environmental uncertainty influence managers? Looking again at Exhibit 3, each of the four cells represents different combinations of degree of complexity and degree of change. Cell 1 (stable and simple environment) represents the lowest level of environmental uncertainty and cell 4 (dynamic and complex environment) the highest. Not surprisingly, managers have the greatest influence on organizational outcomes in cell 1 and the least in cell 4. Because uncertainty poses a threat to an organization's effectiveness, managers try to minimize it. Given a choice, managers would prefer to operate in the least uncertain environments. However, they rarely control that choice. In addition, the nature of the external environment today is that most industries are facing more dynamic change, making their environments more uncertain.

MANAGING STAKEHOLDER RELATIONSHIPS What makes MTV a popular cable channel for young adults year after year? One factor is its success in building relationships with its various stakeholders: viewers, celebrities and reality stars, advertisers, affiliate TV stations, public service groups, and others. The nature of stakeholder relationships is another way in which the environment influences managers. The more obvious and secure these relationships, the more influence managers will have over organizational outcomes.

stakeholders
Any constituencies in the organization's environment that are affected by an organization's decisions and actions

Stakeholders are any constituencies in the organization's environment affected by an organization's decisions and actions. These groups have a stake in or are significantly influenced by what the organization does. In turn, these groups can influence the organization. For example, think of the groups that might be affected by the decisions and actions of Starbucks—coffee bean farmers, employees, specialty coffee competitors, local communities, and so forth. Some of these stakeholders also, in turn, may influence decisions and actions of Starbucks' managers. The idea that organizations have stakeholders is now widely accepted by both management academics and practicing managers.[22]

Exhibit 4 identifies some of an organization's most common stakeholders. Note that these stakeholders include internal and external groups. Why? Because both can affect what an organization does and how it operates.

Why should managers even care about managing stakeholder relationships?[23] For one thing, it can lead to desirable organizational outcomes such as improved predictability of environmental changes, more successful innovations, greater degree of trust among stakeholders, and greater organizational flexibility to reduce the

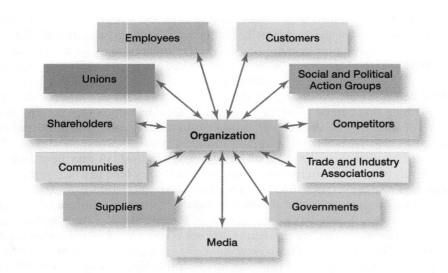

Exhibit 4
Organizational Stakeholders

impact of change. But does it affect organizational performance? The answer is yes! Management researchers who have looked at this issue are finding that managers of high-performing companies tend to consider the interests of all major stakeholder groups as they make decisions.[24]

Another reason for managing external stakeholder relationships is that it's the "right" thing to do. Because an organization depends on these external groups as sources of inputs (resources) and as outlets for outputs (goods and services), managers need to consider their interests as they make decisions.

ORGANIZATIONAL CULTURE: Constraints and Challenges

LO3   Each of us has a unique personality—traits and characteristics that influence the way we act and interact with others. When we describe someone as warm, open, relaxed, shy, or aggressive, we're describing personality traits. An organization, too, has a personality, which we call its *culture*. And that culture influences the way employees act and interact with others. An organization's culture can make employees feel included, empowered, and supported or it can have the opposite effect. Because culture can be powerful, it's important for managers to pay attention to it.

What Is Organizational Culture?

W. L. Gore & Associates, a company known for its innovative and high-quality fabrics used in outdoor wear and other products, understands the importance of organizational culture. Since its founding in 1958, Gore has used employee teams in a flexible, nonhierarchical organizational arrangement to develop its innovative products. Associates (employees) at Gore are committed to four basic principles articulated by company founder Bill Gore: (1) fairness to one another and everyone you come in contact with; (2) freedom to encourage, help, and allow other associates to grow in knowledge, skill, and scope of responsibility; (3) the ability to make your own commitments and keep them; and (4) consulting other associates before taking actions that could affect the company's reputation. After a visit to the company, one analyst reported that an associate told him, "If you tell anybody what to do here, they'll never work for you again." That's the type of independent, people-oriented culture Bill Gore wanted. And it works well for the company—it's earned a position on *Fortune's* annual list of "100 Best Companies to Work For" every year since the list began in 1998, one of only three companies to achieve that distinction.[26]

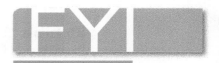

- 84 percent of managers believe culture is critical to business success.
- 35 percent think their company's culture is effectively managed.[25]

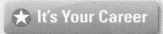

organizational culture
The shared values, principles, traditions, and ways of doing things that influence the way organizational members act and that distinguish the organization from other organizations

Organizational culture has been described as the shared values, principles, traditions, and ways of doing things that influence the way organizational members act and that distinguish the organization from other organizations. In most organizations, these shared values and practices have evolved over time and determine, to a large extent, how "things are done around here."[27]

Our definition of culture implies three things. First, culture is a *perception*. It's not something that can be physically touched or seen, but employees perceive it on the basis of what they experience within the organization. Second, organizational culture is *descriptive*. It's concerned with how members perceive the culture and describe it, not with whether they like it. Finally, even though individuals may have different backgrounds or work at different organizational levels, they tend to describe the organization's culture in similar terms. That's the *shared* aspect of culture.

Research suggests seven dimensions that seem to capture the essence of an organization's culture.[28] These dimensions (shown in Exhibit 5) range from low to high, meaning it's not very typical of the culture (low) or is very typical of the culture (high). Describing an organization using these seven dimensions gives a composite picture of the organization's culture. In many organizations, one cultural dimension often is emphasized more than the others and essentially shapes the organization's personality and the way organizational members work. For instance, at Sony Corporation, the focus is product innovation (innovation and risk taking). The company "lives and breathes" new product development and employees' work behaviors support that goal. In contrast, Southwest Airlines has made its employees a central part of its culture (people orientation). Exhibit 6 describes how the dimensions can create significantly different cultures.

★ It's Your Career

Organizational Culture—If your instructor is using MyManagementLab, log onto **mymanagementlab.com** and test your *organizational culture knowledge*. **Be sure to refer back to the chapter opener!**

Exhibit 5
Dimensions of Organizational Culture

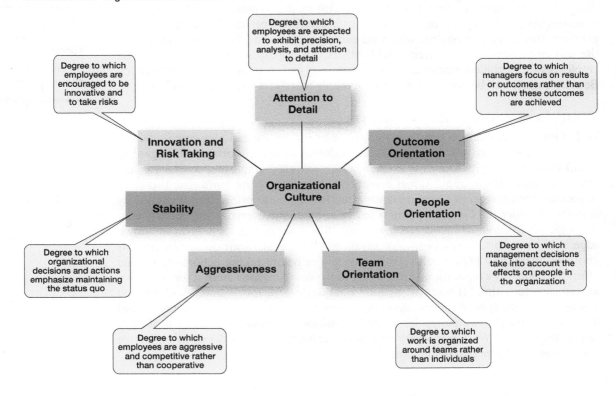

Organization A

 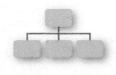

Exhibit 6
Contrasting Organizational
Cultures

This organization is a manufacturing firm. Managers are expected to fully document all decisions, and "good managers" are those who can provide detailed data to support their recommendations. Creative decisions that incur significant change or risk are not encouraged. Because managers of failed projects are openly criticized and penalized, managers try not to implement ideas that deviate much from the status quo. One lower-level manager quoted an often-used phrase in the company: "If it ain't broke, don't fix it."

Employees are required to follow extensive rules and regulations in this firm. Managers supervise employees closely to ensure there are no deviations. Management is concerned with high productivity, regardless of the impact on employee morale or turnover.

Work activities are designed around individuals. There are distinct departments and lines of authority, and employees are expected to minimize formal contact with other employees outside their functional area or line of command. Performance evaluations and rewards emphasize individual effort, although seniority tends to be the primary factor in the determination of pay raises and promotions.

Organization B

 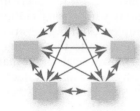 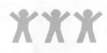

This organization is also a manufacturing firm. Here, however, management encourages and rewards risk taking and change. Decisions based on intuition are valued as much as those that are well rationalized. Management prides itself on its history of experimenting with new technologies and its success in regularly introducing innovative products. Managers or employees who have a good idea are encouraged to "run with it," and failures are treated as "learning experiences." The company prides itself on being market driven and rapidly responsive to the changing needs of its customers.

There are few rules and regulations for employees to follow, and supervision is loose because management believes its employees are hardworking and trustworthy. Management is concerned with high productivity but believes this comes through treating its people right. The company is proud of its reputation as a good place to work.

Job activities are designed around work teams, and team members are encouraged to interact with people across functions and authority levels. Employees talk positively about the competition between teams. Individuals and teams have goals, and bonuses are based on achievement of outcomes. Employees are given considerable autonomy in choosing the means by which the goals are attained.

Exhibit 7
Strong Versus Weak Cultures

Strong Cultures	Weak Cultures
Values widely shared	Values limited to a few people—usually top management
Culture conveys consistent messages about what's important	Culture sends contradictory messages about what's important
Most employees can tell stories about company history or heroes	Employees have little knowledge of company history or heroes
Employees strongly identify with culture	Employees have little identification with culture
Strong connection between shared values and behaviors	Little connection between shared values and behaviors

Strong Cultures

strong cultures
Organizational cultures in which the key values are intensely held and widely shared

All organizations have cultures, but not all cultures equally influence employees' behaviors and actions. **Strong cultures**—those in which the key values are deeply held and widely shared—have a greater influence on employees than weaker cultures. (Exhibit 7 contrasts strong and weak cultures.) The more employees accept the organization's key values and the greater their commitment to those values, the stronger the culture. Most organizations have moderate to strong cultures, that is, there is relatively high agreement on what's important, what defines "good" employee behavior, what it takes to get ahead, and so forth. The stronger a culture becomes, the more it affects the way managers plan, organize, lead, and control.[29]

Why is having a strong culture important? For one thing, in organizations with strong cultures, employees are more loyal than employees in organizations with weak cultures.[30] Research also suggests that strong cultures are associated with high organizational performance.[31] And it's easy to understand why. After all, if values are clear and widely accepted, employees know what they're supposed to do and what's expected of them, so they can act quickly to take care of problems. However, the drawback is that a strong culture also might prevent employees from trying new approaches, especially when conditions change rapidly.[32]

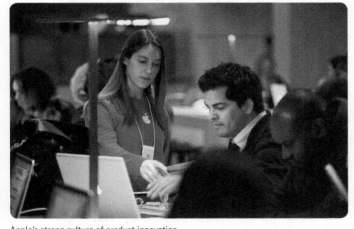

Apple's strong culture of product innovation and customer-responsive service reflects the core values of its visionary cofounder Steve Jobs. Jobs instilled these core values in all employees, from top executives to sales associates, such as the Genius Bar employee shown here training a customer at the Apple Store in Manhattan.
Source: Rex Features/AP Images

Where Culture Comes From and How It Continues

Exhibit 8 illustrates how an organization's culture is established and maintained. The original source of the culture usually reflects the vision of the founders. For instance, as we described earlier, W. L. Gore's culture reflects the values of founder Bill Gore. Company founders are not constrained by previous customs or approaches and

Exhibit 8
Establishing and Maintaining Culture

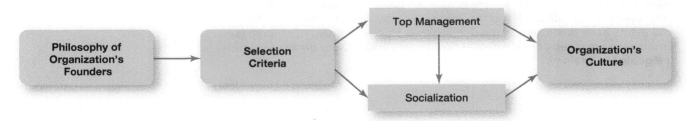

can establish the early culture by articulating a vision of what they want the organization to be. Also, the small size of most new organizations makes it easier to instill that vision with all organizational members.

Once the culture is in place, however, certain organizational practices help maintain it. For instance, during the employee selection process, managers typically judge job candidates not only on the job requirements, but also on how well they might fit into the organization. At the same time, job candidates find out information about the organization and determine whether they are comfortable with what they see.

The actions of top managers also have a major impact on the organization's culture. For instance, at CarMax, CEO Tom Folliard was a key member of the team that developed and launched CarMax. As one of the original developers of the company's unique and strong culture, Folliard is very focused on listening. He visits numerous stores every year, connecting with associates and answering questions and soliciting feedback. Does it work? You bet! CarMax has grown to be the nation's largest retailer of used vehicles by keeping associates happy, leading to happy customers.[33] The company has been on *Fortune*'s 100 Best Companies to Work For list since 2006. Through what they say and how they behave, top managers establish norms that filter down through the organization and can have a positive effect on employees' behaviors. For instance, former IBM CEO Sam Palmisano wanted employees to value teamwork so he chose to take several million dollars from his yearly bonus and give it to his top executives based on their teamwork. He said, "If you say you're about a team, you have to be a team. You've got to walk the talk, right?"[34] However, as we've seen in numerous corporate ethics scandals, the actions of top managers also can lead to undesirable outcomes.

let's get REAL

The Scenario:

Paulo, the manager of a Web communications agency, is discovering that hiring employees can be frustrating. His last three hires are having trouble fitting in with the other 12 employees. For instance, one of the individuals—who's actually been there for six months now—doesn't want to jump in and help out the other team members when a deadline is fast approaching. And this same person doesn't say anything in team meetings and lets everyone else make decisions. And then there's the way they dress. "I don't expect them to 'suit up' or wear ties, but ripped cargo shorts and tattered flip-flops are a little too casual. Why don't these people 'get it'?"

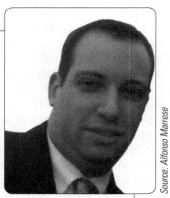

Source: Alfonso Marrese

Alfonso Marrese
Retail Executive

What advice about organizational culture would you give Paulo?

During the interview process Human Resources needs to explain the company's brand values and how the company works as a team to meet goals. Depending on what level or position the candidate is being hired for, maybe a second interview with a senior manager would help to see if the candidate will fit in with the group. During the interview process, dress code, policies and procedures should be explained to the candidate. During the first week or two on the job, the manager should be giving the new hire feedback on how he/she is doing. If there are any issues, they need to be addressed.

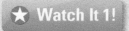

Watch It 1! If your professor has assigned this, go to **www.mymanagementlab.com** to watch a video titled *Rudi's Bakery: Organizational Culture* and to respond to questions.

socialization
The process that helps employees adapt to the organization's culture

Finally, organizations help employees adapt to the culture through **socialization**, a process that helps new employees learn the organization's way of doing things. For instance, new employees at Starbucks stores go through 24 hours of intensive training that helps turn them into brewing consultants (baristas). They learn company philosophy, company jargon, and even how to assist customers with decisions about beans, grind, and espresso machines. One benefit of socialization is that employees understand the culture and are enthusiastic and knowledgeable with customers.[35] Another benefit is that it minimizes the chance that new employees who are unfamiliar with the organization's culture might disrupt current beliefs and customs.

How Employees Learn Culture

Employees "learn" an organization's culture in a number of ways. The most common are stories, rituals, material symbols, and language.

STORIES Organizational "stories" typically contain a narrative of significant events or people, including such things as the organization's founders, rule breaking, reactions to past mistakes, and so forth.[36] Managers at Southwest Airlines tell stories celebrating employees who perform heroically for customers.[37] Such stories help convey what's important and provide examples that people can learn from. At 3M Company, the product innovation stories are legendary. There's the story about the 3M scientist who spilled chemicals on her tennis shoe and came up with Scotchgard. Then, there's the story about Art Fry, a 3M researcher who wanted a better way to mark the pages of his church hymnal and invented the Post-It Note. These stories reflect what made 3M great and what it will take to continue that success.[38] To help employees learn the culture, organizational stories anchor the present in the past, provide explanations and legitimacy for current practices, exemplify what is important to the organization, and provide compelling pictures of an organization's goals.[39]

RITUALS In the early days of Facebook, founder Mark Zuckerberg had an artist paint a mural at company headquarters showing children taking over the world with laptops. Also, he would end employee meetings by pumping his fist in the air and leading employees in a chant of "domination." Although the cheering ritual was intended to be something simply fun, other company executives suggested he drop it because it made him seem silly, and they feared that competitors might cite it as evidence of monopolistic goals.[40] That's the power that rituals can have in shaping what employees believe is important. Corporate rituals are repetitive sequences of activities that express and reinforce the important values and goals of the organization. One of the best-known corporate rituals is Mary Kay Cosmetics' annual awards ceremony for its sales representatives. The company spends more than $50 million annually on rewards and prize incentives. Looking like a cross between a circus and a Miss America pageant, the ceremony takes place in a large auditorium, on a stage in front of a large, cheering audience, with all the participants dressed in glamorous evening clothes. Salespeople are rewarded for sales goal achievements with an array of expensive gifts, including big-screen televisions, diamond rings, trips, and pink Cadillacs. This "show" acts as a motivator by publicly acknowledging outstanding sales performance. In addition, the ritual aspect reinforces late founder Mary Kay's determination and optimism, which enabled her to overcome personal hardships, start her own company, and achieve material success. It conveys to her salespeople that reaching their sales goals is important and through hard work and encouragement, they too can achieve success. The contagious enthusiasm and excitement of Mary Kay sales representatives make it obvious that this annual "ritual" plays a

significant role in establishing desired levels of motivation and behavioral expectations, which is, after all, what management hopes an organization's culture does. But rituals don't have to be this elaborate. For instance, at Minneapolis-based Salo LLC, employees ring an office gong when a deal is signed.[41]

MATERIAL ARTIFACTS AND SYMBOLS When you walk into different businesses, do you get a "feel" for what type of work environment it is—formal, casual, fun, serious, and so forth? These reactions demonstrate the power of material symbols or artifacts in creating an organization's personality.[42] The layout of an organization's facilities, how employees dress, the types of automobiles provided to top executives, and the availability of corporate aircraft are examples of material symbols. Others include the size of offices, the elegance of furnishings, executive "perks" (extra benefits provided to managers such as health club memberships, use of company-owned facilities, and so forth), employee fitness centers or on-site dining facilities, and reserved parking spaces for certain employees. At WorldNow, a business that helps local media companies develop new online distribution channels and revenue streams, an important material symbol is an old dented drill that the founders purchased for $2 at a thrift store. The drill symbolizes the company's culture of "drilling down to solve problems." When an employee is presented with the drill in recognition of outstanding work, he or she is expected to personalize the drill in some way and devise a new rule for caring for it. One employee installed a Bart Simpson trigger; another made the drill wireless by adding an antenna. The company's "icon" carries on the culture even as the organization evolves and changes.[43]

Material symbols convey to employees who is important and the kinds of behavior (for example, risk taking, conservative, authoritarian, participative, individualistic, and so forth) that are expected and appropriate.

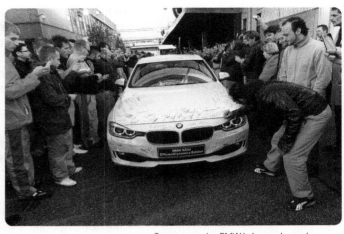

German carmaker BMW helps employees learn about its culture by telling the "story of 1959"—the year when BMW almost went bankrupt. To keep the company afloat, managers asked employees to help them implement a turnaround plan. The employees shown here signing a new car model they produced signifies the powerful role they continue to play in BMW's success.
Source: Andreas Gebert/EPA/Newscom

If your professor has assigned this, go to **www.mymanagementlab.com** to watch a video titled *CH2MHill: Organizational Culture* and to respond to questions.

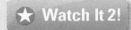

LANGUAGE Many organizations and units within organizations use language as a way to identify and unite members of a culture. By learning this language, members attest to their acceptance of the culture and their willingness to help preserve it. For instance, at Cranium, a Seattle board game company, "chiff" is used to remind employees of the need to be incessantly innovative in everything they do. "Chiff" stands for "clever, high-quality, innovative, friendly, fun."[44] At Build-A-Bear Workshop stores, employees are encouraged to use a sales technique called "Strive for Five," in which they work to sell each customer five items. The simple rhyming slogan is a powerful tool to drive sales.[45]

Over time, organizations often develop unique terms to describe equipment, key personnel, suppliers, customers, processes, or products related to its business. New employees are frequently overwhelmed with acronyms and jargon that, after a short period of time, become a natural part of their language. Once learned, this language acts as a common denominator that bonds members.

How Culture Affects Managers

Houston-based Apache Corp. has become one of the best performers in the independent oil drilling business because it has fashioned a culture that values risk taking and quick decision making. Potential hires are judged on how much initiative they've shown in getting projects done at other companies. And company employees

are handsomely rewarded if they meet profit and production goals.[46] Because an organization's culture constrains what they can and cannot do and how they manage, it's particularly relevant to managers. Such constraints are rarely explicit. They're not written down. It's unlikely they'll even be spoken. But they're there, and all managers quickly learn what to do and not do in their organization. For instance, you won't find the following values written down, but each comes from a real organization.

- Look busy, even if you're not.
- If you take risks and fail around here, you'll pay dearly for it.
- Before you make a decision, run it by your boss so that he or she is never surprised.
- We make our product only as good as the competition forces us to.
- What made us successful in the past will make us successful in the future.
- If you want to get to the top here, you have to be a team player.

The link between values such as these and managerial behavior is fairly straightforward. Take, for example, a so-called "ready-aim-fire" culture. In such an organization, managers will study and analyze proposed projects endlessly before committing to them. However, in a "ready-*fire*-aim" culture, managers take action and then analyze what has been done. Or, say an organization's culture supports the belief that profits can be increased by cost cutting and that the company's best interests are served by achieving slow but steady increases in quarterly earnings. Managers are unlikely to pursue programs that are innovative, risky, long term, or expansionary. In an organization whose culture conveys a basic distrust of employees, managers are more likely to use an authoritarian leadership style than a democratic one. Why? The culture establishes for managers appropriate and expected behavior. For example, Banco Santander, whose headquarters are located 20 kilometers from downtown Madrid, has been described as a "risk-control freak." The company's managers adhered to "banking's stodgiest virtues—conservatism and patience." However, it's those values that triggered the company's growth from the sixth largest bank in Spain to the leading bank in the euro zone.[47]

As shown in Exhibit 9, a manager's decisions are influenced by the culture in which he or she operates. An organization's culture, especially a strong one, influences and constrains the way managers plan, organize, lead, and control.

Exhibit 9
Types of Managerial Decisions Affected by Culture

Planning
Culture
- The degree of risk that plans should contain
- Whether plans should be developed by individuals or teams
- The degree of environmental scanning in which management will engage

Organizing
Culture
- How much autonomy should be designed into employees' jobs
- Whether tasks should be done by individuals or in teams
- The degree to which department managers interact with each other

Leading
Culture
- The degree to which managers are concerned with increasing employee job satisfaction
- What leadership styles are appropriate
- Whether all disagreements— even constructive ones— should be eliminated

Controlling
Culture
- Whether to impose external controls or to allow employees to control their own actions
- What criteria should be emphasized in employee performance evaluations
- What repercussions will occur from exceeding one's budget

CURRENT Issues in Organizational Culture

L04   Nordstrom, the specialty retail chain, is renowned for its attention to customers. Nike's innovations in athletic shoe and apparel technology are legendary. Tom's of Maine is known for its commitment to doing things ethically and spiritually. How have these organizations achieved such reputations? Their organizational cultures have played a crucial role. Let's look at three current cultural issues: creating an innovative culture, creating a customer-responsive culture, and nurturing workplace spirituality.

Creating an Innovative Culture

You may not recognize IDEO's name, but you've probably used a number of its products. As a product design firm, it takes the ideas that corporations bring it and turns those ideas into reality. Some of its creations range from the first commercial mouse (for Apple) to the first stand-up toothpaste tube (for Procter & Gamble), to the handheld personal organizer (for Palm), to the Contour USB glucose meter (for Bayer AG). It's critical that IDEO's culture support creativity and innovation.[48] And you might actually own and use products from another well-known innovative organization—Apple.[49] From its founding in 1976 to today, Apple has been on the forefront of product design and development. They've brought us Mac, iPod, iTunes, iPhone, and the iPad, which has changed the way you read and interact with materials such as this text. Although both these companies are in industries where innovation is critical to success, the fact is that any successful organization needs a culture that supports innovation. How important is culture to innovation? In a recent survey of senior executives, over half said that the most important driver of innovation for companies was a supportive corporate culture.[50]

What does an innovative culture look like? According to Swedish researcher Goran Ekvall, it would be characterized by the following:

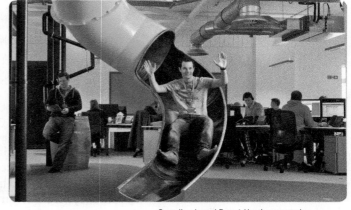

Canadian-based Peer 1 Hosting created a culture that supports creativity and innovation. At its European headquarters, the youthful staff of the global Web infrastructure and cloud hosting provider interact in a casual and playful environment of trust and openness, personal and professional challenge, debate, and risk taking.
Source: Solent News/Rex Features/AP Images

- **Challenge and involvement**—Are employees involved in, motivated by, and committed to the long-term goals and success of the organization?
- **Freedom**—Can employees independently define their work, exercise discretion, and take initiative in their day-to-day activities?
- **Trust and openness**—Are employees supportive and respectful of each other?
- **Idea time**—Do individuals have time to elaborate on new ideas before taking action?
- **Playfulness/humor**—Is the workplace spontaneous and fun?
- **Conflict resolution**—Do individuals make decisions and resolve issues based on the good of the organization versus personal interest?
- **Debates**—Are employees allowed to express opinions and put forth ideas for consideration and review?
- **Risk taking**—Do managers tolerate uncertainty and ambiguity, and are employees rewarded for taking risks?[51]

Creating a Customer-Responsive Culture

Harrah's Entertainment, the world's largest gaming company, is fanatical about customer service—and for good reason. Company research showed that customers satisfied with the service they received at a Harrah's casino increased their gaming expenditures by 10 percent, and those extremely satisfied increased their gaming expenditures by 24 percent.

Exhibit 10

Creating a Customer-Responsive Culture

Characteristics of Customer-Responsive Culture	Suggestions for Managers
Type of employee	Hire people with personalities and attitudes consistent with customer service: friendly, attentive, enthusiastic, patient, good listening skills
Type of job environment	Design jobs so employees have as much control as possible to satisfy customers, without rigid rules and procedures
Empowerment	Give service-contact employees the discretion to make day-to-day decisions on job-related activities
Role clarity	Reduce uncertainty about what service-contact employees can and cannot do by continual training on product knowledge, listening, and other behavioral skills
Consistent desire to satisfy and delight customers	Clarify organization's commitment to doing whatever it takes, even if it's outside an employee's normal job requirements

When customer service translates into these types of results, of course managers would want to create a customer-responsive culture![52]

What does a customer-responsive culture look like?[53] Exhibit 10 describes five characteristics of customer-responsive cultures and offers suggestions as to what managers can do to create that type of culture.

 Try It!

If your professor has assigned this, go to **www.mymanagementlab.com** to complete the Simulation: *Organizational Culture* and see how well you can apply the ideas of organizational culture.

Spirituality and Organizational Culture

workplace spirituality

A culture where organizational values promote a sense of purpose through meaningful work that takes place in the context of community

What do Southwest Airlines, Men's Wearhouse, Chick-fil-A, Ford, Xerox, Tyson Foods, and Hewlett-Packard have in common? They're among a growing number of organizations that have embraced workplace spirituality. What is **workplace spirituality**? It's a culture in which organizational values promote a sense of purpose through meaningful work taking place in the context of community.[54] Organizations with a spiritual culture recognize that people have a mind and a spirit, seek to find meaning and purpose in their work, and desire to connect with other human beings and be part of a community. And such desires aren't limited to workplaces, as a recent study showed that college students also are searching for meaning and purpose in life.[55]

Workplace spirituality seems to be important now for a number of reasons. Employees are looking for ways to cope with the stresses and pressures of a turbulent pace of life. Contemporary lifestyles—single-parent families, geographic mobility, temporary jobs, economic uncertainty, technologies that create distance between people—underscore the lack of community that many people feel. As humans, we crave involvement and connection. In addition, as baby boomers navigate mid-life issues, they're looking for something meaningful, something beyond the job. Others

wish to integrate their personal life values with their professional lives. For others, formalized religion hasn't worked, and they continue to look for anchors to replace a lack of faith and to fill a growing sense of emptiness. What type of culture can do all these things? What differentiates spiritual organizations from their nonspiritual counterparts? Research shows that spiritual organizations tend to have five cultural characteristics.[56]

1. *Strong sense of purpose.* Spiritual organizations build their cultures around a meaningful purpose. While profits are important, they're not the primary values of the organization. For instance, Timberland's slogan is "Boots, Brand, Belief," which embodies the company's intent to use its "resources, energy, and profits as a publicly traded footwear-and-apparel company to combat social ills, help the environment, and improve conditions for laborers around the globe...and to create a more productive, efficient, loyal, and committed employee base."[57]

2. *Focus on individual development.* Spiritual organizations recognize the worth and value of individuals. They aren't just providing jobs; they seek to create cultures in which employees can continually grow and learn.

3. *Trust and openness.* Spiritual organizations are characterized by mutual trust, honesty, and openness. Managers aren't afraid to admit mistakes. And they tend to be extremely up-front with employees, customers, and suppliers.

4. *Employee empowerment.* Managers trust employees to make thoughtful and conscientious decisions. For instance, at Southwest Airlines, employees—including flight attendants, baggage handlers, gate agents, and customer service representatives—are encouraged to take whatever action they deem necessary to meet customer needs or help fellow workers, even if it means going against company policies.

5. *Tolerance of employee expression.* The final characteristic that differentiates spiritually based organizations is that they don't stifle employee emotions. They allow people to be themselves—to express their moods and feelings without guilt or fear of reprimand.

Using a different approach, a recent study suggests that the concept of spirituality in the workplace can best be captured by three factors: interconnection with a higher power, interconnection with human beings, and interconnection with nature and all living things.[58]

Critics of the spirituality movement have focused on two issues: legitimacy (Do organizations have the right to impose spiritual values on their employees?) and economics (Are spirituality and profits compatible?).

An emphasis on spirituality clearly has the potential to make some employees uneasy. Critics might argue that secular institutions, especially businesses, have no business imposing spiritual values on employees. This criticism is probably valid when spirituality is defined as bringing religion into the workplace.[59] However, it's less valid when the goal is helping employees find meaning in their work. If concerns about today's lifestyles and pressures truly characterize a growing number of workers, then maybe it is time for organizations to help employees find meaning and purpose in their work and to use the workplace to create a sense of community.

The issue of whether spirituality and profits are compatible is certainly important. Limited evidence suggests that the two may be compatible. One study found that companies that introduced spiritually based techniques improved productivity and significantly reduced turnover.[60] Another found that organizations that provided their employees with opportunities for spiritual development outperformed those that didn't.[61] Others reported that spirituality in organizations was positively related to creativity, ethics, employee satisfaction, job involvement, team performance, and organizational commitment.[62]

PREPARING FOR: Exams/Quizzes

CHAPTER SUMMARY by Learning Objectives

LO1 CONTRAST **the actions of managers according to the omnipotent and symbolic views.**

According to the omnipotent view, managers are directly responsible for an organization's success or failure. The symbolic view argues that much of an organization's success or failure is due to external forces outside managers' control. The two constraints on manager's discretion are the organization's culture (internal) and the environment (external). Managers aren't totally constrained by these two factors since they can and do influence their culture and environment.

LO2 DESCRIBE **the constraints and challenges facing managers in today's external environment.**

The external environment includes those factors and forces outside the organization that affect its performance. The main components include economic, demographic, political/legal, sociocultural, technological, and global. Managers face constraints and challenges from these components because of the impact they have on jobs and employment, environmental uncertainty, and stakeholder relationships.

LO3 DISCUSS **the characteristics and importance of organizational culture.**

The seven dimensions of culture are attention to detail, outcome orientation, people orientation, team orientation, aggressiveness, stability, and innovation and risk taking. In organizations with strong cultures, employees are more loyal and performance tends to be higher. The stronger a culture becomes, the more it affects the way managers plan, organize, lead, and control. The original source of a culture reflects the vision of organizational founders. A culture is maintained by employee selection practices, the actions of top managers, and socialization processes. Also, culture is transmitted to employees through stories, rituals, material symbols, and language. These elements help employees "learn" what values and behaviors are important as well as who exemplifies those values. The culture affects how managers plan, organize, lead, and control.

LO4 DESCRIBE **current issues in organizational culture.**

The characteristics of an innovative culture are challenge and involvement, freedom, trust and openness, idea time, playfulness/humor, conflict resolution, debates, and risk taking. A customer-responsive culture has five characteristics: outgoing and friendly employees; jobs with few rigid rules, procedures, and regulations; empowerment; clear roles and expectations; and employees who are conscientious in their desire to please the customer. Workplace spirituality is important because employees are looking for a counterbalance to the stresses and pressures of a turbulent pace of life. Aging baby boomers and other workers are looking for something meaningful in their lives, an involvement and connection that they often don't find in contemporary lifestyles, and to meet the needs that organized religion is not meeting for some of them. Spiritual organizations tend to have five characteristics: strong sense of purpose, focus on individual development, trust and openness, employee empowerment, and toleration of employee expression.

MyManagementLab

Go to **mymanagementlab.com** to complete the problems marked with this icon ⭐.

⭐ REVIEW AND DISCUSSION QUESTIONS

1. Describe the two perspectives on how much impact managers have on an organization's success or failure.

2. "Businesses are built on relationships." What do you think this statement means? What are the implications for managing the external environment?

3. Refer to Exhibit 6. How would a first-line manager's job differ in these two organizations? How about a top-level manager's job?

4. Classrooms have cultures. Describe your classroom culture using the seven dimensions of organizational culture. Does the culture constrain your instructor? How? Does it constrain you as a student? How?

5. Can culture be a liability to an organization? Explain.

6. Discuss the impact of a strong culture on organizations and managers.

7. Using Exhibit 8, explain how a culture is formed and maintained.

8. Explain why workplace spirituality seems to be an important concern.

MyManagementLab

If your professor has assigned these, go to **mymanagementlab.com** for Auto-graded writing questions as well as the following Assisted-graded writing questions:

9. Why is it important for managers to understand the external environmental components?

10. Describe an effective culture for (a) a relatively stable environment and (b) a dynamic environment. Explain your choices.

PREPARING FOR: My Career

⭐ PERSONAL INVENTORY ASSESSMENTS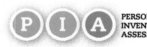

What's My Comfort with Change?

As you saw in this text, change is a big part of the external environment and an organization's culture. This PIA will assess how comfortable you are with change.

⭐ ETHICS DILEMMA

In many ways, technology has made all of us more productive. However, ethical issues do arise in how and when technology is used. Take the sports arena. All kinds of technologically advanced sports equipment (swimsuits, golf clubs, ski suits, etc.) have been developed that can sometimes give competitors/players an edge over their opponents.[63] We saw it in swim meets at the Summer Olympics and on the ski slopes and ice rinks at the Winter Olympics.

11. What do you think? Is this an ethical use of technology?

12. What if your school (or country) was competing for a championship and couldn't afford to outfit athletes in such equipment and it affected your ability to compete? Would that make a difference?

13. What ethical guidelines might you suggest for such situations?

SKILLS EXERCISE Developing Your Environmental Scanning Skill

About the Skill
Anticipating and interpreting changes that take place in the environment is an important skill managers need. Information that comes from scanning the environment can be used in making decisions and taking actions. And managers at all levels of an organization need to know how to scan the environment for important information and trends.

Steps in Practicing the Skill
You can be more effective at scanning the environment if you use the following suggestions:[64]

- *Decide which type of environmental information is important to your work.* Perhaps you need to know changes in customers' needs and desires, or perhaps you need to know what your competitors are doing. Once you know the type of information you'd like to have, you can look at the best ways to get that information.

- *Regularly read and monitor pertinent information.* There is no scarcity of information to scan, but what you need to do is read pertinent information sources. How do you know information sources are pertinent? They're pertinent if they provide you with the information you identified as important.

- *Incorporate the information you get from your environmental scanning into your decisions and actions.* Unless you use the information you're getting, you're wasting your time getting it. Also, the more you use information from your environmental scanning, the more likely it is that you'll want to continue to invest time and other resources into gathering it. You'll see that

this information is important to your ability to manage effectively and efficiently.

- *Regularly review your environmental scanning activities.* If you're spending too much time getting information you can't use, or if you're not using the pertinent information you've gathered, you need to make some adjustments.

- *Encourage your subordinates to be alert to information that is important.* Your employees can be your "eyes and ears" as well. Emphasize to them the importance of gathering and sharing information that may affect your work unit's performance.

Practicing the Skill
The following suggestions are activities you can do to practice and reinforce the behaviors associated with scanning the environment.

14. Select an organization with which you're familiar either as an employee or perhaps as a frequent customer. Assume you're the top manager in this organization. What types of information from environmental scanning do you think would be important to you? Where would you find this information? Now assume you're a first-level manager in this organization. Would the types of information you'd get from environmental scanning change? Explain.

15. Assume you're a regional manager for a large bookstore chain. Using the Internet, what types of environmental and competitive information were you able to identify? For each source, what information did you find that might help you do your job better?

WORKING TOGETHER Team Exercise

Although all organizations face environmental constraints, the components in their external environments differ. Get into a small group with three to four other class members and choose one organization from two different industries. Describe the external components for each organization.

How are your descriptions different for the two organizations? How are they similar? Now, using the same two organizations, see if you can identify the important stakeholders for these organizations. As a group, be prepared to share your information with the class and to explain your choices.

LEARNING TO BE A MANAGER

- Find two current examples in any popular business periodicals of the omnipotent and symbolic views of management. Write a paper describing what you found and how the two examples you found represent these views of management.

- Choose an organization with which you're familiar or one you would like to know more about. Create a table identifying potential stakeholders of this organization. Then, indicate what particular interests or concerns these stakeholders might have.

- If you belong to a student organization, evaluate its culture by answering the following: How would you describe the culture? How do new members learn the culture? How is the culture maintained? If you don't belong to a student organization, talk to another student who does and evaluate it using the same questions.

- Find one example of a company that represents each of the current issues in organizational culture. Describe what the company is doing that reflects its commitment to this culture.

- In your own words, write down three things you learned in this text about being a good manager. Keep a copy of this for future reference.

CASE APPLICATION 1 Going to Extremes

Number-one best e-retailer. For those of you who have shopped on Zappos.com, that number one ranking probably isn't a surprise.[65] For those of you who haven't shopped on Zappos.com, it wouldn't take long for you to see why Zappos deserves that accolade. And it's more than the fact that Zappos has a great selection of products, super-fast shipping, and free returns. The real secret to its success is its people, who make the Zappos shopping experience truly unique and outstanding. The company, which began selling shoes and other products online in 1999, has put "extraordinary effort into building a desirable organizational culture, which has provided a sure path to business success." As part of its culture, Zappos espouses 10 corporate values. At the top of that list is "Deliver WOW through service." And do they ever deliver the WOW! Even through the recent economic challenges, Zappos has continued to thrive—a sure sign its emphasis on organizational culture is paying off.

Zappos is not only the number-one e-retailer but also one of the 100 best companies to work for. Okay. So what is it *really* that makes Zappos' culture so great? Let's take a closer look.

Zappos began selling shoes and other products online in 1999. Four years later, it was profitable, and it reached more than $1 billion in sales by 2009. Also in 2009, Zappos was named Customer Service Champ by *BusinessWeek* and was given an A+ rating by the Better Business Bureau. Also that year, Amazon (yeah, that Amazon) purchased Zappos for 10 million Amazon shares, worth almost $928 million at the time. Zappos' employees divided up $40 million in cash and restricted stock and were assured that Zappos management would remain in place.

The person who was determined to "build a culture that applauds such things as weirdness and humility" was Tony Hsieh (pronounced *Shay*), who became CEO of Zappos in 2000. And Tony is the epitome of weirdness and humility. For instance, on April Fools' Day 2010, he issued a press release announcing that "Zappos was suing Walt Disney Company in a class action suit claiming that Disney was misleading the public by saying that Disneyland is 'the happiest place on earth' because clearly," Hsieh argued, "Zappos is."

Before joining Zappos, Hsieh had been cofounder of the Internet advertising network LinkExchange and had seen firsthand the "dysfunction that can arise from building a company in which technical skill is all that matters." He was determined to do it differently at Zappos. Hsieh first invited Zappos' 300 employees to list the core values the culture should be based on. That process led to the 10 values that continue to drive the organization, which now employs about 1,400 people.

Another thing that distinguishes Zappos culture is the recognition that organizational culture is more than a list of written values. The culture has to be "lived." And Zappos does this by maintaining a "complex web of human interactions."

At Zappos, social media is used liberally to link employees with one another and with the company's customers. For instance, one recent tweet said, "Hey. Did anyone bring a hairdryer to the office today?" This kind of camaraderie can maintain and sustain employee commitment to the company.

Also at Zappos, the company's "pulse" or "health" of the culture is surveyed monthly. In these happiness surveys, employees answer such "unlikely questions as whether they believe that the company has a higher purpose than profits, whether their own role has meaning, whether they feel in control of their career path, whether they consider their co-workers to be like family and friends, and whether they are happy in their jobs." Survey results are broken down by department, and opportunities for "development" are identified and acted on. For example, when one month's survey showed that a particular department had "veered off course and felt isolated from the rest of the organization," actions were taken to show employees how integral their work was to the rest of the company.

Oh, and one other thing about Zappos. Every year, to celebrate its accomplishments, it publishes a *Culture Book,* a testimonial to the power of its culture. "Zappos has a belief that the right culture with the right values will always produce the best organizational performance, and this belief trumps everything else."

⭐ DISCUSSION QUESTIONS

16. Find a list of all 10 of Zappos' corporate values. Pick two of the values and explain how you think those values would influence the way employees do their work.

17. Using this list of corporate values and Exhibit 5, describe Zappos' organizational culture. In which areas would you say that Zappos' culture is very high (or typical)? Explain.

18. How did Zappos' corporate culture begin? How is Zappos' corporate culture maintained?

19. The right culture with the right values will always produce the best organizational performance. Do you agree or disagree with this statement? Why?

20. What could other companies learn from Tony Hsieh and Zappos' experiences?

CASE APPLICATION 2 Not Sold Out

Competitors in the movie theater industry had hoped that they were through the challenges they'd faced during the economic downturn.[66] After ticket sales revenue in 2011 fell 4 percent from the previous year, revenue in 2012 was up 6.1 percent. However, in 2013, revenues were up again, but just barely—not even by 1 percent. The numbers of people going to see a movie continue to stall. So, the industry has tried to pump up revenue with high-profile movies, higher ticket prices, and premium amenities.

The number of movie screens in the United States totals a little more than 39,000. Together, the four largest movie theater chains in the United States have a little over 19,200 screens—and a lot of seats to fill. The largest, Regal Entertainment Group (based in Knoxville, Tennessee), has more than 7,300 screens. AMC Entertainment (based in Kansas City, Missouri) has almost 5,000 screens. The other two major competitors are Cinemark (based in Plano, Texas—about 4,400 screens) and Carmike Cinemas (based in Columbus, Georgia—almost 2,500 screens). The challenge for

these companies is getting people to watch movies on all those screens, a decision that encompasses many factors.

One important factor, according to industry analysts, is the uncertainty over how people want their movies delivered, which is largely a trade-off between convenience and quality (or what the experts call fidelity experience). Will consumers choose convenience over quality and use mobile devices such as iPads? Will they trade some quality for convenience and watch at home on surround-sound, flat-screen, high-definition home theater systems? Or will they go to a movie theater with wide screens, high-quality sound systems, and the social experience of being with other moviegoers and enjoy the highest-fidelity experience—even with the inconveniences? Movie theater managers believe that mobile devices aren't much of a threat, even though they may be convenient. On the other hand, home theater systems may be more of a threat as they've become extremely affordable and have "acceptable" quality. Although not likely to replace any of these higher-quality offerings, drive-in theaters, analysts note, are experiencing a resurgence, especially in geographic locations where they can be open year-round. The movie theater chains are also battling IMAX Corporation for customers as movie screens get bigger and bigger. Over the last five years, the number of these oversized screens built by the five largest theater companies has grown to the point where it almost equals the number of IMAX locations. The movie theater chains have invested in these formats because it can add several extra dollars to the ticket price, resulting in increased revenues.

Another factor managers need to wrestle with is the impression consumers have of the movie-going experience. A consumer lifestyle poll showed that the major dislike about going to the movies was the cost, a drawback cited by 36 percent of the respondents. Other factors noted included the noise, uncomfortable seats, the inconvenience, the crowds, and too many previews/commercials before the movie.

A final question facing the movie theater industry *and* the major film studios is how to be proactive in avoiding the problems that the recorded music industry faced with the illegal downloading of songs. The amount of entertainment streamed online (which includes both music and video) continues to experience double-digit growth. The biggest threat so far has been YouTube, which has become a powerful force in the media world with owner Google's backing. But now Amazon and Netflix are flexing their movie muscles as well. To counter that threat, industry executives have asked for filtering mechanisms to keep unlawful material off these sites and to develop some type of licensing arrangements whereby the industry has some protection over its copyrighted film content.

⭐ DISCUSSION QUESTIONS

21. Using Exhibit 2, what external components might be most important for managers in movie theater chains to know about? Why?

22. According to the case, what external trends do managers at the movie theater chains have to deal with?

23. How do you think these trends might constrain decisions made by managers at the movie theater chains?

24. What stakeholders do you think might be most important to movie theater chains? What interests might these stakeholders have?

ENDNOTES

1. "Industry & People," *Food Engineering,* November 2011, p. 16; and M. Esterl, "PepsiCo Shakes Up Management," *Wall Street Journal,* September 15, 2011, p. B3.

2. P. Rozenzweig, "The Halo Effect and Other Managerial Delusions," *The McKinsey Quarterly Online Journal,* no. 1, March 9, 2007.

3. For insights into the symbolic view, see "Why CEO Churn Is Healthy," *BusinessWeek*, November 13, 2000, p. 230; S. M. Puffer and J. B. Weintrop, "Corporate Performance and CEO Turnover: The Role of Performance Expectations," *Administrative Science Quarterly*, March 1991, pp. 1–19; C. R. Schwenk, "Illusions of Management Control? Effects of Self-Serving Attributions on Resource Commitments and Confidence in Management," *Human Relations*, April 1990, pp. 333–347; J. R. Meindl and S. B. Ehrlich, "The Romance of Leadership and the Evaluation of Organizational Performance," *Academy of Management Journal*, March 1987, pp. 91–109; J. A. Byrne, "The Limits of Power," *BusinessWeek*, October 23, 1987, pp. 33–35; D. C. Hambrick and S. Finkelstein, "Managerial Discretion: A Bridge Between Polar Views of Organizational Outcomes," in L. L. Cummings and B. M. Staw (eds.), *Research in Organizational Behavior*, vol. 9 (Greenwich, CT: JAI Press, 1987), pp. 369–406; and J. Pfeffer, "Management as Symbolic Action: The Creation and Maintenance of Organizational Paradigms," in L. L. Cummings and B. M. Staw (eds.), *Research in Organizational Behavior*, vol. 3 (Greenwich, CT: JAI Press, 1981), pp. 1–52.

4. T. M. Hout, "Are Managers Obsolete?" *Harvard Business Review*, March–April 1999, pp. 161–168; and Pfeffer, "Management as Symbolic Action."

5. C. Rogers and J. B. White, "BMW Tosses Salesmen for 'Geniuses,'" *Wall Street Journal,* February 20, 2014, p. B1+; M. Campbell, "BMW Advancing 'Product Geniuses' Plans as Apple's Retail Model Extends into Automotive," appleinsider.com, February 19, 2014; "BMW Geniuses to Help Shoppers Understand Technology," www.autotrader.com, February 19, 2014; and K. Kerwin, "BMW Asks, Does It Take a Genius to Sell a Car?" www.forbes.com, January 13, 2014.

6. R. Roberson, "Are High Commodity Prices Here to Stay?" *Southeast Farm Press,* October 5, 2011, pp. 18–20; A. Hanacek, "Deli Processing: Cost Crunch," *National Provisioner*, October 2011, pp. 111–114; and T. Mulier, "Nestlé's Recipe for Juggling Volatile Commodity Costs," *Bloomberg BusinessWeek,* March 21–27, 2011, pp. 29–30.

7. A. R. Sorkin, "What Might Have Been, and the Fall of Lehman," *New York Times Online,* September 9, 2013; and D. H. Henderson, "When the Rain Came Down: A Masterful Account of How the Housing Crisis and Credit Crunch Nearly Brought Down the Economy," *Wall Street Journal,* January 19–20, 2013, p. C5.

8. P. Davidson, "Global Growth Appears Stunted, IMF Chief Says," *USA Today,* April 3, 2014, p. 2B.

9. E. Pfanner, "Economic Troubles Cited as the Top Risks in 2012," *New York Times Online,* January 11, 2012; and E. Pfanner, "Divining the Business and Political Risks of 2012," *New York Times Online,* January 11, 2012.

10. C. Hausman, "Americans See Inequality as a Major Problem," Ethics Newsline [www.globalethics.org/newsline], April 9, 2012.

11. E. Porter, "Inequality Undermines Democracy," *New York Times Online,* March 20, 2012.

12. D. M. Owens, "Why Care About Income Disparity: An Interview with Timothy Noah," *HRMagazine,* March 2013, p. 53; J. Cox, "Occupy Wall Street: They're Back, But Does Anyone Care?" CNBC.com, April 30, 2012; L. Visconti, "Ask the White Guy: Why Are Disparities in Income Distribution Increasing?" DiversityInc.com, April 10, 2012; P. Meyer, "Income Inequality *Does* Matter," *USA Today,* March 28, 2012, p. 9A; E. Porter, "Inequality Undermines Democracy," *New York Times Online,* March 20, 2012; T. Cowen, "Whatever Happened to Discipline and Hard Work?" *New York Times Online,* November 12, 2011; and A. Davidson, "It's Not Just About the Millionaires," *New York Times Online,* November 9, 2011.

13. S. Jayson, "iGeneration Has No Off Switch," *USA Today,* February 10, 2010, pp. 1D+; and L. Rosen, *Rewired: Understanding the iGeneration and the Way They Learn* (New York: Palgrave-McMillan, 2010).

14. B. Horovitz, "Generation Whatchamacallit," *USA Today,* May 4, 2012, p. 1B+.

15. H. Rosin, "The Touch-Screen Generation," *The Atlantic,* April 2013, pp. 56-65.

16. S. Cardwell, "Where Do Babies Come From?" *Newsweek,* October 19, 2009, p. 56.

17. Y. Hori, J-P. Lehmann, T. Ma Kam Wah, and V. Wang, "Facing Up to the Demographic Dilemma," *Strategy & Business Online,* Spring 2010; and E. E. Gordon, "Job Meltdown or Talent Crunch?" *Training,* January 2010, p. 10.

18. S. Jayson, "Recession Has Broad Effects for Ages 18–34," *USA Today,* February 9, 2012, p. 4D; and M. Rich, "For Jobless, Little Hope of Restoring Better Days," *New York Times Online,* December 1, 2011.

19. R. Singh, "Generation U: Too Many Underemployed College Grads," www.ere.net, July 19, 2013.

20. S. G. Hauser, "Independent Contractors Helping to Shape the New World of Work," Workforce.com, February 3, 2012; H. G. Jackson, "Flexible Workplaces: A Business Imperative," *HRMagazine,* October 2011, p. 10; I. Speitzer, "Contingent Staffing," Workforce.com, October 4, 2011; M. Steen, "More Employers Take on Temps, but Planning Is Paramount," Workforce.com, May 2011; P. Davidson, "More Temp Workers Are Getting Hired," *USA Today,* March 8, 2010, p. 1B; S. Reddy, "Wary Companies Rely on Temporary Workers," *Wall Street Journal,* March 6/7, 2010, p. A4; P. Davidson, "Cuts in Hours Versus Cuts in Jobs," *USA Today,* February 25, 2010, p. 1B; and S. A. Hewlett, L. Sherbin, and K. Sumberg, "How Gen Y and Boomers Will Reshape Your Agenda," *Harvard Business Review,* July–August, 2009, pp. 71–76.

21. Leader Making a Difference box based on J. Reingold, "Sydney Finkelstein's Best and Worst CEOs of 2013," fortune.com, December 13, 2013; A. Taylor III, "Akio Toyoda: Toyota's Comeback Kid," *Fortune,* February 27, 2012, pp. 72–79; J. E. Vascellaro and others, "Twelve Global Executives to Watch in 2012," *Wall Street Journal,* December 29, 2011, pp. B1+; "Steeled by 3 Years of Crises, Toyoda Steers Toward Growth," *Automotive News,* November 14, 2011, p. 18; W. Boccard, M. Francis, B. Powell, and R. Arora, "The Changing Face of Asian Business," *Fortune,* May 2, 2011, pp. 81+; "A New-Model Toyoda Is at Ease in Media Spotlight," *Automotive News,* March 14, 2011, p. 22; and K. Mitra, "Still Apologizing," *Business Today,* January 23, 2011, p. 125.

22. J. P. Walsh, "Book Review Essay: Taking Stock of Stakeholder Management," *Academy of Management Review*, April 2005, pp. 426–438; R. E. Freeman, A. C. Wicks, and B. Parmar, "Stakeholder Theory and 'The Corporate Objective Revisited,'" *Organization Science*, June 2004, pp. 364–369; T. Donaldson and L. E. Preston, "The Stakeholder Theory of the Corporation: Concepts, Evidence, and Implications," *Academy of Management Review*, January 1995, pp. 65–91; and R. E. Freeman, *Strategic Management: A Stakeholder Approach* (Boston: Pitman/Ballinger, 1984).

23. J. S. Harrison and C. H. St. John, "Managing and Partnering With External Stakeholders," *Academy of Management Executive*, May 1996, pp. 46–60.

24. S. L. Berman, R. A. Phillips, and A. C. Wicks, "Resource Dependence, Managerial Discretion, and Stakeholder Performance," *Academy of Management Proceedings* Best Conference Paper, August 2005; A. J. Hillman and G. D. Keim, "Shareholder Value, Stakeholder Management, and Social Issues: What's the Bottom Line?" *Strategic Management Journal*, March 2001, pp. 125–139; J. S. Harrison and R. E. Freeman, "Stakeholders, Social Responsibility, and Performance: Empirical Evidence and Theoretical Perspectives," *Academy of Management Journal*, July 1999, pp. 479–487; and J. Kotter and J. Heskett, *Corporate Culture and Performance* (New York: The Free Press, 1992).

25. Booz & Company, "Culture and Change: Why Culture Matters and How It Makes Change Stick," www.strategy-business.com, January 9, 2014.

26. M. Moskowitz, R. Levering, C. Bessette, C. Dunn, C. Fairchild, and B. Southward, "The 100 Best Companies to Work For," *Fortune,* February 3, 2014, pp. 108–115; M. Moskowitz, R. Levering, O. Akhtar, E. Fry, C. Leahey, and A. Vandermey, "The 100 Best Companies to Work For," *Fortune,* February 4, 2013, pp. 85–96; M. Moskowitz, R.

Levering, C. Tkaczyk, C. Keating, A. Konrad, A. Vandermey, and C. Kapelke, "The 100 Best Companies to Work For," *Fortune,* February 6, 2012, pp. 117+; M. Moskowitz, R. Levering, and C. Tkaczyk, "The List," *Fortune,* February 8, 2010, pp. 75–88; E. Ruth, "Gore-Tex Maker Decides It's Time to Demand Some Attention," The Wilmington, DE, *News Journal, USA Today,* October 24, 2007, p. 5B; and A. Deutschman, "The Fabric of Creativity," *Fast Company,* December 2004, pp. 54–62.

27. K. Shadur and M. A. Kienzle, "The Relationship Between Organizational Climate and Employee Perceptions of Involvement," *Group & Organization Management,* December 1999, pp. 479–503; M. J. Hatch, "The Dynamics of Organizational Culture," *Academy of Management Review,* October 1993, pp. 657–693; D. R. Denison, "What Is the Difference between Organizational Culture and Organizational Climate? A Native's Point of View on a Decade of Paradigm Wars," paper presented at Academy of Management Annual Meeting, 1993, Atlanta, GA; and L. Smircich, "Concepts of Culture and Organizational Analysis," *Administrative Science Quarterly,* September 1983, p. 339.

28. J. A. Chatman and K. A. Jehn, "Assessing the Relationship between Industry Characteristics and Organizational Culture: How Different Can You Be?" *Academy of Management Journal,* June 1994, pp. 522–553; and C. A. O'Reilly III, J. Chatman, and D. F. Caldwell, "People and Organizational Culture: A Profile Comparison Approach to Assessing Person-Organization Fit," *Academy of Management Journal,* September 1991, pp. 487–516.

29. Y. Berson, S. Oreg, and T. Dvir, "CEO Values, Organizational Culture, and Firm Outcomes," *Journal of Organizational Behavior,* July 2008, pp. 615–633; and E. H. Schien, *Organizational Culture and Leadership* (San Francisco: Jossey-Bass, 1985), pp. 314–315.

30. A. E. M. Va Vianen, "Person-Organization Fit: The Match Between Newcomers' and Recruiters' Preferences for Organizational Cultures," *Personnel Psychology,* Spring 2000, pp. 113–149; K. Shadur and M. A. Kienzle, *Group & Organization Management;* P. Lok and J. Crawford, "The Relationship Between Commitment and Organizational Culture, Subculture, and Leadership Style," *Leadership & Organization Development Journal,* vol. 20, no. 6/7, 1999, pp. 365–374; C. Vandenberghe, "Organizational Culture, Person-Culture Fit, and Turnover: A Replication in the Health Care Industry," *Journal of Organizational Behavior,* March 1999, pp. 175–184; and C. Orphen, "The Effect of Organizational Cultural Norms on the Relationships between Personnel Practices and Employee Commitment," *Journal of Psychology,* September 1993, pp. 577–579.

31. See, for example, J. B. Sorensen, "The Strength of Corporate Culture and the Reliability of Firm Performance," *Administrative Science Quarterly,* 2002, vol. 47, no. 1, pp. 70–91; R. Goffee and G. Jones, "What Holds the Modern Company Together?" *Harvard Business Review,* November–December 1996, pp. 133–148; Collins and Porras, "Building Your Company's Vision," *Harvard Business Review,* September–October 1996, pp. 65–77; J. C. Collins and J. I. Porras, *Built to Last* (New York: HarperBusiness, 1994); G. G. Gordon and N. DiTomaso, "Predicting Corporate Performance from Organizational Culture," *Journal of Management Studies,* November 1992, pp. 793–798; J. P. Kotter and J. L. Heskett, *Corporate Culture and Performance* (New York: Free Press, 1992), pp. 15–27; and D. R. Denison, *Corporate Culture and Organizational Effectiveness* (New York: Wiley, 1990).

32. Sorensen, pp. 70–91; and L. B. Rosenfeld, J. M. Richman, and S. K. May, "Information Adequacy, Job Satisfaction, and Organizational Culture in a Dispersed-Network Organization," *Journal of Applied Communication Research,* vol. 32, 2004, pp. 28–54.

33. "What They Do - What Makes CarMax Great - What Employees Say - Great Perks," us.greatrated.com/carmax, February 2014; and "Great Workplaces: How CarMax Cares," *Fortune,* April 8, 2013, p. 21.

34. S. E. Ante, "The New Blue," *BusinessWeek,* March 17, 2003, p. 82.

35. C. C. Miller, "Now at Starbucks: A Rebound," *New York Times Online,* January 21, 2010; J. Jargon, "Latest Starbucks Buzzword: 'Lean' Japanese Techniques," *Wall Street Journal,* August 4, 2009, pp. A1+; P. Kafka, "Bean Counter," *Forbes,* February 28, 2005, pp. 78–80; A. Overholt, "Listening to Starbucks," *Fast Company,* July 2004, pp. 50–56; and B. Filipczak, "Trained by Starbucks," *Training,* June 1995, pp. 73–79.

36. P. Guber, "The Four Truths of the Storyteller," *Harvard Business Review,* December 2007, pp. 53–59; S. Denning, "Telling Tales," *Harvard Business Review,* May 2004, pp. 122–129; T. Terez, "The Business of Storytelling," *Workforce,* May 2002, pp. 22–24; J. Forman, "When Stories Create an Organization's Future," *Strategy & Business,* Second Quarter 1999, pp. 6–9; C. H. Deutsch, "The Parables of Corporate Culture," *New York Times,* October 13, 1991, p. F25; and D. M. Boje, "The Storytelling Organization: A Study of Story Performance in an Office-Supply Firm," *Administrative Science Quarterly,* March 1991, pp. 106–126.

37. G. Colvin, "Value Driven," *Fortune,* November 23, 2009, p. 24.

38. J. Useem, "Jim McNerney Thinks He Can Turn 3M From a Good Company Into a Great One—With a Little Help From His Former Employer, General Electric," *Fortune,* August 12, 2002, pp. 127–132.

39. Denning, 2004; and A. M. Pettigrew, "On Studying Organizational Cultures," *Administrative Science Quarterly,* December 1979, p. 576.

40. J. E. Vascellaro, "Facebook CEO in No Rush to 'Friend' Wall Street," *Wall Street Journal,* March 4, 2010, p. A1+.

41. S. Shellenbarger, "Believers in the 'Project Beard' and Other Office Rituals," *Wall Street Journal,* June 26, 2013, pp. D1+.

42. E. H. Schein, "Organizational Culture," *American Psychologist,* February 1990, pp. 109–119.

43. M. Zagorski, "Here's the Drill," *Fast Company,* February 2001, p. 58.

44. "Slogans That Work," Forbes.com Special, January 7, 2008, p. 99.

45. P. Keegan, "Best Companies to Work For: Maxine Clark and Kip Tindell Exchange Jobs," *Fortune,* February 8, 2010, pp. 68–72.

46. C. Palmeri, "The Fastest Drill in the West," *BusinessWeek,* October 24, 2005, pp. 86–88.

47. J. Levine, "Dare to Be Boring," *Time,* February 1, 2010, pp. Global Business 1–2.

48. J. Guthrie, "David Kelley of IDEO Raises Level of Design," SFGate.com, October 23, 2011; C. T. Greer, "Innovation 101," WSJ.com, October 17, 2011; "The World's 50 Most Innovative Companies," *Fast Company,* March 2010, p. 90; L. Tischler, "A Designer Takes On His Biggest Challenge," *Fast Company,* February 2009, pp. 78+; T. Kelley and J. Littman, *The Ten Faces of Innovation: IDEO's Strategies for Defeating the Devil's Advocate and Driving Creativity Throughout Your Organization* (New York: Currency, 2005); C. Fredman, "The IDEO Difference," *Hemispheres,* August 2002, pp. 52–57; and T. Kelley and J. Littman, *The Art of Innovation* (New York: Currency, 2001).

49. D. Lyons, "Think Really Different," *Newsweek,* April 5, 2010, pp. 46–51; and R. Brands, "Innovation Made Incarnate," *Bloomberg BusinessWeek Online,* January 11, 2010.

50. J. Yang and R. W. Ahrens, "Culture Spurs Innovation," *USA Today,* February 25, 2008, p. 1B.

51. J. Cable, "Building an Innovative Culture," *Industry Week,* March 2010, pp. 32–37; M. Hawkins, "Create a Climate of Creativity," *Training,* January 2010, p. 12; and L. Simpson, "Fostering Creativity," *Training,* December 2001, p. 56.

52. M. Millstein, "Customer Relationships Make Playing the Odds Easy," *Chain Store Age,* December 2007, p. 22A; and L. Gary, "Simplify and Execute: Words to Live By in Times of Turbulence," *Harvard Management Update,* January 2003, p. 12.

53. Based on J. McGregor, "Customer Service Champs," *BusinessWeek,* March 3, 2008, pp. 37–57; B. Schneider, M. G. Ehrhart, D. M. Mayer, J. L. Saltz, and K. Niles-Jolly, "Understanding Organization-Customer Links in Service Settings," *Academy of Management Journal,* December 2006, pp. 1017–1032; B. A. Gutek, M. Groth, and B. Cherry, "Achieving Service Success Through Relationships and Enhanced Encounters," *Academy of Management Executive,* November 2002, pp. 132–144; K. A. Eddleston, D. L. Kidder, and B. E. Litzky, "Who's the Boss? Contending With Competing Expectations From Customers and Management," *Academy of Management Executive,* November 2002, pp. 85–95; S. D. Pugh, J. Dietz, J. W. Wiley, and S. M. Brooks, "Driving Service Effectiveness Through Employee-Customer Linkages," *Academy of Management Executive,* November 2002, pp. 73–84; L. A. Bettencourt, K. P. Gwinner, and M. L. Mueter, "A Comparison of Attitude, Personality, and Knowledge Predictors of Service-Oriented Organizational Citizenship Behaviors," *Journal of Applied Psychology,* February 2001, pp. 29–41; M. D. Hartline, J. G. Maxham III, and D. O. McKee, "Corridors of Influence in the Dissemination of Customer-

Oriented Strategy to Customer Contact Service Employees," *Journal of Marketing*, April 2000, pp. 35–50; L. Lengnick-Hall and C. A. Lengnick-Hall, "Expanding Customer Orientation in the HR Function," *Human Resource Management*, Fall 1999, pp. 201–214; M. D. Hartline and O. C. Ferrell, "The Management of Customer-Contact Service Employees: An Empirical Investigation," *Journal of Marketing*, October 1996, pp. 52–70; and M. J. Bitner, B. H. Booms, and L. A. Mohr, "Critical Service Encounters: The Employee's Viewpoint," *Journal of Marketing*, October 1994, pp. 95–106.

54. R. A. Giacalone and C. L. Jurkiewicz (eds.), *Handbook of Workplace Spirituality and Organizational Performance* (New York: M. E. Sharp, 2003).

55. M. B. Marklein, "Study: College Students Seeking Meaning of Life," *USA Today*, *Springfield News-Leader*, December 22, 2007, p. 6C.

56. This section is based on L. Lambert III, "God Goes to the Office," *USA Today*, February 8, 2010, p. 7A; B. S. Pawar, "Workplace Spirituality Facilitation: A Comprehensive Model," *Journal of Business Ethics*, December 2009, pp. 375–386; "Faith and Spirituality in the Workplace," *Walton Business Perspective*, Fall 2009, p. 22; B. S. Pawar, "Some of the Recent Organizational Behavior Concepts as Precursors to Workplace Spirituality," *Journal of Business Ethics*, August 2009, pp. 245–261; L. Lambert III, *Spirituality Inc: Religion in the American Workplace*, (New York: New York University Press, 2009); A. Gross-Schaefer, "Reaching for the Stars: Effective Tools for the Creation of a More Spiritual Workplace," *Employee Relations Law Journal*, Summer 2009, pp. 25–42; D. Grant, "What Should a Science of Workplace Spirituality Study? The Case for a Relational Approach," *Academy of Management Proceedings* Best Paper, August 2005; C. D. Pielstick, "Teaching Spirituality Synchronicity in a Business Leadership Class," *Journal of Management Education*, February 2005, pp. 153–168; H. Ashar and M. Lane-Maher, "Success and Spirituality in the New Business Paradigm," *Journal of Management Inquiry*, June 2004, pp. 249–260; G. A. Gull and J. Doh, "The 'Transmutation' of the Organization: Toward a More Spiritual Workplace," *Journal of Management Inquiry*, June 2004, pp. 128–139; K. C. Cash and G. R. Gray, "A Framework for Accommodating Religion and Spirituality in the Workplace," *Academy of Management Executive*, August 2000, pp. 124–133; F. Wagner-Marsh and J. Conley, "The Fourth Wave: The Spiritually-Based Firm," *Journal of Organizational Change Management*, vol. 12, no. 3, 1999, pp. 292–302; E. H. Burack, "Spirituality in the Workplace," *Journal of Organizational Change Management*, vol. 12, no. 3, 1999, pp. 280–291; J. Milliman, J. Ferguson, D. Trickett, and B. Condemi, "Spirit and Community at Southwest Airlines: An Investigation of a Spiritual Values-Based Model," *Journal of Organizational Change Management*, vol. 12, no. 3, 1999, pp. 221–233; and I. A. Mitroff and E. A. Denton, *A Spiritual Audit of Corporate America: A Hard Look at Spirituality, Religion, and Values in the Workplace* (San Francisco: Jossey-Bass, 1999).

57. J. Reingold, "Walking the Walk," *Fast Company*, November 2005, p. 82.

58. C. H. Liu and P. J. Robertson, "Spirituality in the Workplace: Theory and Measurement," *Journal of Management Inquiry*, March 2011, pp. 35–50.

59. M. Lips-Wiersma, K. L. Dean, and C. J. Fornaciari, "Theorizing the Dark Side of the Workplace Spirituality Movement," *Journal of Management Inquiry*, December 2009, pp. 288–300; P. Paul, "A Holier Holiday Season," *American Demographics*, December 2001, pp. 41–45; and M. Conlin, "Religion in the Workplace: The Growing Presence of Spirituality in Corporate America," *Business Week*, November 1, 1999, pp. 151–158.

60. Cited in M. Conlin, "Religion in the Workplace," p. 153.

61. C. P. Neck and J. F. Milliman, "Thought Self-Leadership: Finding Spiritual Fulfilment in Organizational Life," *Journal of Managerial Psychology*, vol. 9, no. 8, 1994, p. 9.

62. J. Marques, "Toward Greater Consciousness in the 21st-Century Workplace: How Buddhist Practices Fit In," *Journal of Business Ethics*, March 2010, pp. 211–225; L. Kim, "Improving the Workplace with Spirituality," *Journal for Quality and Participation*, October 2009, pp. 32–35; M. Stevenson, "Toward a Greater Understanding of Spirit at Work: A Model of Spirit at Work and Outcomes," *Academy of Management Proceedings Online*, August 2009; P. D. Corner, "Workplace Spirituality and Business Ethics: Insights from an Eastern Spiritual Tradition," *Journal of Business Ethics*, March 2009, pp. 377–389; M.

L. Lynn, M. J. Naughton, and S. VanderVeen, "Faith at Work Scale (FWS): Justification, Development, and Validation of a Measure of Judaeo-Christian Religion in the Workplace," *Journal of Business Ethics*, March 2009, pp. 227–243; R. W. Kolodinsky, R. A. Giacalone, and C. L. Jurkiewicz, "Workplace Values and Outcomes: Exploring Personal, Organizational, and Interactive Workplace Spirituality," *Journal of Business Ethics*, August 2008, pp. 465–480; and J. Millman, A. Czaplewski, and J. Ferguson, "An Exploratory Empirical Assessment of the Relationship Between Spirituality and Employee Work Attitudes," paper presented at Academy of Management, Washington, DC, August 2001.

63. M. V. Copeland, "Can the Ski Suit Make the Man (and Woman)?" *Fortune Online*, February 16, 2010; C. Hausman, "New and Old Technologies Keep Officials, Ethicists, Debating Questions of Fairness," *Global Ethics Newsline Online*, February 8, 2010; and S. Sataline, "Some Aging Competitors Call High-Tech Swimsuits Dirty Pool," *Wall Street Journal*, November 3, 2009, p. A1.

64. Based on C. K. Prahalad, "Best Practices Get You Only So Far," *Harvard Business Review*, April 2010, p. 32; J. R. Oreja-Rodriguez and V. Yanes-Estévez, "Environmental Scanning: Dynamism with Rack and Stack Rasch Model," *Management Decision*, vol. 48, no. 2, 2010, pp. 260–276; C. Heavey, Z. Simsek, F. Roche, and A. Kelly, "Decision Comprehensiveness and Corporate Entrepreneurship: The Moderating Role of Managerial Uncertainty Preferences and Environmental Dynamism," *Journal of Management Studies*, December 2009, pp. 1289–1314; R. Subramanian, N. Fernandes, and E. Harper, "Environmental Scanning in U.S. Companies: Their Nature and Their Relationship to Performance," *Management International Review*, July 1993, pp. 271–286; E. H. Burack and N. J. Mathys, "Environmental Scanning Improves Strategic Planning," *Personnel Administrator*, 1989, pp. 82–87; and L. M. Fuld, *Monitoring the Competition* (New York: Wiley, 1988).

65. M. Moskowitz, R. Levering, C. Tkaczyk, C. Keating, A. Konrad, A. Vandermey, and C. Kapelke, "The 100 Best Companies to Work For," *Fortune*, February 6, 2012, pp. 117+; K. Gurchiek, "Delivering HR at Zappos," *HRMagazine*, June 2011, pp. 44–45; V. Nayar, "Employee Happiness: Zappos vs. HCL," Businessweek.com, January 5, 2011; D. Richards, "At Zappos, Culture Pays," *Strategy+Business Online*, August 2010; T. Hseih, "Zappos's CEO on Going to Extremes for Customers," *Harvard Business Review*, July–August 2010, pp. 41–45; A. Perschel, "Work-Life Flow: How Individuals, Zappos, and Other Innovative Companies Achieve High Engagement," *Global Business & Organizational Excellence*, July 2010, pp. 17–30; T. Hseih, "Why I Sold Zappos," *Inc.*, June 2010, pp. 100–104; T. Hseih, "Happy Feet," *Newsweek*, June 21, 2010, p. 10; M. Betts, "Zappos Earns No. 1 Ranking for E-retailing," *Computerworld*, June 7, 2010, p. 4; S. Elliott, "Tireless Employees Get Their Tribute, Even if It's in Felt and Polyester," *New York Times Online*, March 4, 2010; C. Palmeri, "Now for Sale, Zappos Culture," *Bloomberg BusinessWeek*, January 11, 2010, p. 57; E. Frauenheim, "Can Zappos Culture Survive the Amazon Jungle?"; and Zappos, *Culture Book*. *Workforce Management Online*, September 14, 2009.

66. "Yearly Box Office," boxofficemojo.com/yearly/, March 7, 2014; "Can the Movie Theater Be Saved," *Fast Company*, December 2013/January 2014, pp. 69–72; E. Schwartzel, "Movie-Theater Chains Take on IMAX," *Wall Street Journal*, December 13, 2013, p. B6; A. Sharma, "Hollywood Feels Netflix's Influence," *Wall Street Journal*, July 8, 2013, pp. B1+; C. Bialik, "Studios Struggle for Focus on Film Pirates' Booty," *Wall Street Journal*, April 6–7, 2013, p. A2; M. Rosenbaum, "Box Office Bust: Movie Attendance Hits 16-Year Low," ABCNews.com, December 28, 2011; M. Cieply, "Charging a Premium for Movies, At a Cost," *New York Times Online*, July 31, 2011; B. Barnes and M. Cieply, "Graying Audience Returns to Movies," *New York Times Online*, February 25, 2011; L. A. E. Schuker, "Double Feature: Dinner and a Movie," *Wall Street Journal*, January 5, 2011, pp. D1+; J. O'Donnell, "Going to the Movies At Home," *USA Today*, January 5, 2011, p. 3B; M. DeCuir, "Some Food and Alcohol with Your Flick? Cinemas Hope So," *USA Today*, March 27, 2008, p. 3A; B. Barnes, "At Cineplexes, Sports, Opera, Maybe a Movie," *New York Times Online*, March 23, 2008; D. Stuckey and K. Gelles, "Entertainment Sold Online," *USA Today*, February 26, 2008; and J. Carroll, "Americans Dislike the Cost of Going to the Movies," *Gallup News Service*, December 22, 2006.

Managing Social Responsibility and Ethics

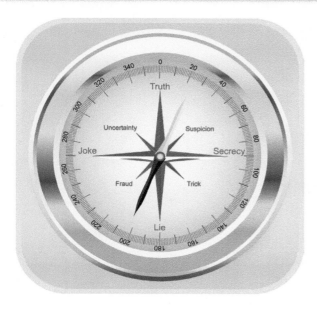

Source: Cattallina/Shutterstock.

A key to success in management and in your career is knowing how to make good decisions about ethical dilemmas.

How to Be Ethical When No One Else Seems to Be

You make choices every day: Your boss asks you to do something questionable; you see a colleague doing something that violates a company rule or policy; you think about calling in sick because it's a beautiful day, and boy oh boy do you need a day off; you need to make copies of some personal documents and the company copier isn't monitored by anyone; you need to get some bills paid online and your boss is in meetings all day. Choices, choices, choices. What do you do?

When an ethical dilemma occurs at work— the place where you spend the vast majority of your week and the source of your income that pays your bills and provides benefits—it can be challenging to decide what to do. In addition to the chapter suggestions (see Exhibit 8), here are some ideas that might help nudge you to be ethical when no one else seems to be:

*1. **Make sure you have all the information you need to make a decision.** Sometimes, ethical "dilemmas" at work turn out to be nothing more than rumors or speculation about worst-case-scenarios. "You can only do the right thing when you're not looking at things all wrong."[1] Get the facts, but use your discretion, patience, and common sense. Seek out advice from someone you trust and who you think is knowledgeable and wise.*

*2. **Recognize that we don't always act the way we think we're going to act when faced with an ethical dilemma.**[2] Most of us would say that we know we should be fair, be respectful, be trustworthy, be responsible, treat others as we want to be treated, etc. We have a set*

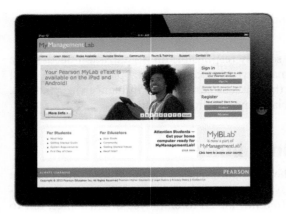

MyManagementLab®

⭐ **Improve Your Grade!**

When you see this icon, visit
www.mymanagementlab.com for activities that are
applied, personalized, and offer immediate feedback.

Learning Objectives

● SKILL OUTCOMES

1 ***Discuss*** *what it means to be socially responsible and what factors influence that decision.*

2 ***Explain*** *green management and how organizations can go green.*

3 ***Discuss*** *the factors that lead to ethical and unethical behavior.*

   ● **Develop your skill at** creating trust in work groups.

4 ***Describe*** *management's role in encouraging ethical behavior.*

   ● **Know how** to make good decisions about ethical dilemmas.

5 ***Discuss*** *current social responsibility and ethics issues.*

---

of values we want—and strive—to live by. What happens, though, is that when faced with an ethical dilemma, our "I" self rationalizes by saying: I don't want to lose my job, I don't want to be punished, I don't want to look foolish, etc. And so when something happens that we know is ethically questionable or even wrong, we "know" we should speak up or make it right. But we can't quite figure out how to do that, and then we explain it away by saying that it's okay that we acted the way we did. So, be aware of the way you "fool" yourself. Don't ignore or downplay ethical dilemmas.

    3.   **TEST yourself.** *When faced with an ethical dilemma, use these "tests:"[3]*

   ● *The Golden Rule Test: Would I want people to do this to me?*

   ● *The Truth Test: Does this action represent the whole truth and nothing but the truth?*

   ● *The Stench Test: Does this action "stink" when I contemplate doing it?*

   ● *The What-If-Everybody-Did-This Test: Would I want everyone to do this? Would I want to live in that kind of world?*

   ● *The Family Test: How would my parents/ spouse/significant other/children feel if they found out I did this?*

   ● *The Conscience Test: Does this action go against my conscience? Will I feel guilty afterwards?*

   ● *The Consequences Test: Might this action have bad consequences? Might I regret doing this?*

   ● *The Front Page/Social Media Test: How would I feel if this action was reported on the front page of my hometown newspaper or splashed across social media outlets for all to see?*

Deciding when and how ethical and socially responsible an organization needs to be raises complicated issues managers may have to address as they plan, organize, lead, and control. As managers manage, these issues can and do influence their actions. Let's see what we can learn about social responsibility and ethics.

WHAT Is Social Responsibility?

LO1 Organizations profess their commitment to sustainability and package their products in non-recyclable materials. Companies have large pay inequities; however, the difference is often not linked to employee performance, but to entitlement and "custom." Large global corporations lower their costs by outsourcing to countries where human rights are not a high priority and justify it by saying they're bringing in jobs and helping to strengthen the local economies. Businesses facing a difficult economic environment offer employees reduced hours and early retirement packages. Are these companies being socially responsible? Managers regularly face decisions that have a dimension of social responsibility in areas such as employee relations, philanthropy, pricing, resource conservation, product quality and safety, and doing business in countries that devalue human rights. What does it mean to be socially responsible?

From Obligations to Responsiveness to Responsibility

The concept of *social responsibility* has been described in different ways. For instance, it's been called "profit making only," "going beyond profit making," "any discretionary corporate activity intended to further social welfare," and "improving social or environmental conditions."[4] We can understand it better if we first compare it to two similar concepts: social obligation and social responsiveness.[5] **Social obligation** is when a firm engages in social actions because of its obligation to meet certain economic and legal responsibilities. The organization does what it's obligated to do and nothing more. This idea reflects the **classical view** of social responsibility, which says that management's only social responsibility is to maximize profits. The most outspoken advocate of this approach is economist and Nobel laureate Milton Friedman. He argued that managers' primary responsibility is to operate the business in the best interests of the stockholders, whose primary concerns are financial.[6] He also argued that when managers decide to spend the organization's resources for "social good," they add to the costs of doing business, which have to be passed on to consumers through higher prices or absorbed by stockholders through smaller dividends. Friedman doesn't say that organizations shouldn't be socially responsible, but his interpretation of social responsibility is to maximize profits for stockholders—a view still held by some today. An advisory firm that works with major corporations says, "Companies would achieve more social good by simply focusing on the bottom line rather than social responsibility programs."[7]

The other two concepts—social responsiveness and social responsibility—reflect the **socioeconomic view**, which says that managers' social responsibilities go beyond making profits to include protecting and improving society's welfare. This view is based on the belief that corporations are *not* independent entities responsible only to stockholders, but have an obligation to the larger society. Organizations around the world have embraced this view, as shown by a survey of global executives in which 84 percent said that companies must balance obligations to shareholders with obligations to the public good.[8] But how do these two concepts differ?

Social responsiveness is when a company engages in social actions in response to some popular social need. Managers are guided by social norms and values and make practical, market-oriented decisions about their actions.[9] For instance, Ford Motor Company became the first automaker to endorse a federal ban on sending text messages while driving. A company spokesperson explained that research has found that activities, such as text messaging, distract a drivers' eyes from watching

social obligation
When a firm engages in social actions because of its obligation to meet certain economic and legal responsibilities

classical view
The view that management's only social responsibility is to maximize profits

socioeconomic view
The view that management's social responsibility goes beyond making profits to include protecting and improving society's welfare

social responsiveness
When a firm engages in social actions in response to some popular social need

the road and traffic and contribute to an increased risk of getting in an accident.[10] By supporting this ban, company managers "responded" to what they felt was an important social need. After Japan's massive earthquake and tsunami, many tech companies responded with resources and support. For instance, social networking giant Facebook set up a Japan earthquake page for users to find information about disaster relief. After the devastating Haiti earthquake, many companies responded to the immense needs in that region. For instance, UPS has a company-wide policy that urges employees to volunteer during natural disasters and other crises. In support of this policy, UPS maintains a 20-person logistics emergency team in Asia, Europe, and the Americas that's trained in humanitarian relief.[11]

A socially *responsible* organization views things differently. It goes beyond what it's obligated to do or chooses to do because of some popular social need and does what it can to help improve society because it's the right thing to do. We define **social responsibility** as a business's intention, beyond its legal and economic obligations, to do the right things and act in ways that are good for society.[12] Our definition assumes that a business obeys the law and cares for its stockholders, but adds an ethical imperative to do those things that make society better and not to do those that make it worse. A socially responsible organization does what is right because it feels it has an ethical responsibility to do so. For example, according to our definition, Abt Electronics in Glenview, Illinois, would be described as socially responsible. As one of the largest single-store electronics retailers in the United States, Abt responded to soaring energy costs and environmental concerns by shutting off lights more frequently and reducing air conditioning and heating. However, an Abt family member said, "These actions weren't just about costs, but about doing the right thing. We don't do everything just because of money."[13]

So, how should we view an organization's social actions? A U.S. business that meets federal pollution control standards or that doesn't discriminate against employees over the age of 40 in job promotion decisions is meeting its social obligation because laws mandate these actions. However, when it provides on-site child-care facilities for employees or packages products using recycled paper, it's being socially responsive. Why? Working parents and environmentalists have voiced these social concerns and demanded such actions.

For many businesses, their social actions are better viewed as socially responsive, rather than socially responsible (at least according to our definition). However, such actions are still good for society. For example, Chick-fil-A announced that by 2019, it would no longer sell products containing meat from poultry raised with antibiotics. And CVS Caremark Corporation announced that it would stop selling all tobacco products by October of 2014.[14] These types of actions are in response to societal concerns.

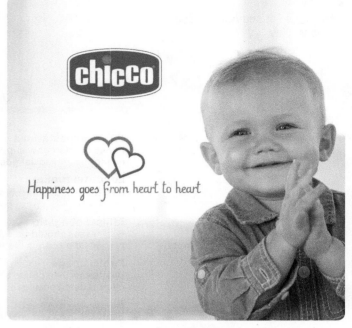

Artsana, the Italian maker of Chicco baby care products, invests in social responsibility initiatives that help children in need both in Italy and in the poorest regions of the world. Chicco's global "Happiness Goes from Heart to Heart" project is aimed at treating childhood heart disease and supports the brand's mission of "making children happy and giving them something to smile about."
Source: PRNewsFoto/Chicco USA/AP Images

social responsibility
A business's intention, beyond its legal and economic obligations, to do the right things and act in ways that are good for society

If your professor has assigned this, go to **www.mymanagementlab.com** to watch a video titled: *Honest Tea: Corporate Social Responsibility* and to respond to questions.

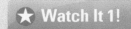

Should Organizations Be Socially Involved?

Other than meeting their social obligations (which they *must* do), should organizations be socially involved? One way to look at this question is by examining arguments for and against social involvement. Several points are outlined in Exhibit 1.[15]

Exhibit 1
Arguments For and Against Social
Responsibility

FOR

Public expectations
Public opinion now supports businesses pursuing economic and social goals.

Long-run profits
Socially responsible companies tend to have more secure long-run profits.

Ethical obligation
Businesses should be socially responsible because responsible actions are the right thing to do.

Public image
Businesses can create a favorable public image by pursuing social goals.

Better environment
Business involvement can help solve difficult social problems.

Discouragement of further governmental regulation
By becoming socially responsible, businesses can expect less government regulation.

Balance of responsibility and power
Businesses have a lot of power and an equally large amount of responsibility is needed to balance against that power.

Stockholder interests
Social responsibility will improve a business's stock price in the long run.

Possession of resources
Businesses have the resources to support public and charitable projects that need assistance.

Superiority of prevention over cures
Businesses should address social problems before they become serious and costly to correct.

AGAINST

Violation of profit maximization
Business is being socially responsible only when it pursues its economic interests.

Dilution of purpose
Pursuing social goals dilutes business's primary purpose—economic productivity.

Costs
Many socially responsible actions do not cover their costs and someone must pay those costs.

Too much power
Businesses have a lot of power already; if they pursue social goals, they will have even more.

Lack of skills
Business leaders lack the necessary skills to address social issues.

Lack of accountability
There are no direct lines of accountability for social actions.

Numerous studies have examined whether social involvement affects a company's economic performance.[16] Although most found a small positive relationship, no generalizable conclusions can be made, because these studies have shown that relationship is affected by various contextual factors such as firm size, industry, economic conditions, and regulatory environment.[17] Another concern was causation. If a study showed that social involvement and economic performance were positively related, this correlation didn't necessarily mean that social involvement *caused* higher economic performance—it could simply mean that high profits afforded companies the "luxury" of being socially involved.[18] Such methodological concerns can't be taken lightly. In fact, one study found that if the flawed empirical analyses in these studies were "corrected," social responsibility had a neutral impact on a company's financial performance.[19] Another found that participating in social issues not related to

the organization's primary stakeholders was negatively associated with shareholder value.[20] A re-analysis of several studies concluded that managers can afford to be (and should be) socially responsible.[21]

Another way to view social involvement and economic performance is by looking at socially responsible investing (SRI) funds, which provide a way for individual investors to support socially responsible companies. (You can find a list of SRI funds at www.socialfunds.com.) Typically, these funds use some type of **social screening**; that is, they apply social and environmental criteria to investment decisions. For instance, SRI funds usually will not invest in companies involved in liquor, gambling, tobacco, nuclear power, weapons, price fixing, fraud, or in companies that have poor product safety, employee relations, and environmental track records. The number of socially screened mutual funds has grown from 55 to 146, and assets in these funds have grown to more than $3.7 trillion—an amount that equals the combined GDPs of Brazil and Canada.[22] But more important than the total amount invested in these funds is that the Social Investment Forum reports that the performance of most SRI funds is comparable to that of non-SRI funds.[23]

So, what can we conclude about social involvement and economic performance? It appears that a company's social actions *don't hurt* its economic performance. Given political and societal pressures to be socially involved, managers probably need to take social issues and goals into consideration as they plan, organize, lead, and control.

social screening
Applying social criteria (screens) to investment decisions

If your professor has assigned this, go to **www.mymanagementlab.com** to watch a video titled: *CH2MHill: Ethics and Social Responsibility* and to respond to questions.

★ **Watch It 2!**

GREEN Management and Sustainability

LO2   Nike Inc. launched an app called Making, which allows its design engineers to see the environmental effects of their material choices on water, energy and waste, and chemistry.[24] Coca-Cola, the world's largest soft drink company, has worked to make 100 percent of its new vending machines and coolers hydrofluorocarbon-free (HFC-free) by 2015. This initiative alone will have the same effect on global carbon emissions as taking 11 million cars off the road for a single year.[25] The Fairmont Hotel chain generated a lot of buzz over its decision to set up rooftop beehives to try and help strengthen the population of honeybees, which have been mysteriously abandoning their hives and dying off by the millions worldwide. This Colony Collapse Disorder could have potentially disastrous consequences since one-third of the food we eat comes from plants that depend on bee pollination. At Toronto's Fairmont Royal York, six hives are home to some 360,000 bees that forage in and around the city *and* produce a supply of award-winning honey.[26] Did you know that planning a driving route with more right-hand turns than left can save you money? UPS does. That's just one of many stats the global logistics leader can quote about how research-based changes in its delivery route design contribute to the sustainability of the planet.[27] Being green is in!

Until the late 1960s, few people (and organizations) paid attention to the environmental consequences of their decisions and actions. Although some groups were concerned with conserving natural resources, about the only reference to saving the environment was the ubiquitous printed request "Please Don't Litter." However, a number of environmental disasters brought a new spirit of environmentalism to individuals, groups, and organizations. Increasingly, managers have begun to consider the impact of their organization on the natural environment, which we call **green management**. What do managers need to know about going green?

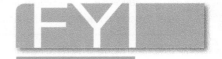

- 75 percent of workplaces have at least one green technology practice.[28]

green management
Managers consider the impact of their organization on the natural environment

How Organizations Go Green

Managers and organizations can do many things to protect and preserve the natural environment.[29] Some do no more than what is required by law; that is, they fulfill their social obligation. However, others have radically changed their products and production processes. For instance, Fiji Water uses renewable energy sources, preserves forests, and conserves water. Carpet-maker Mohawk Industries uses recycled plastic containers to produce fiber used in its carpets. Google and Intel initiated an effort to get computer makers and customers to adopt technologies that reduce energy consumption. Paris-based TOTAL, SA, one of the world's largest integrated oil companies, is going green by implementing tough new rules on oil tanker safety and working with groups such as Global Witness and Greenpeace. UPS, the world's largest package delivery company, has done several things—from retrofitting its aircraft with advanced technology and fuel-efficient engines to developing a computer network that efficiently dispatches its fleet of brown trucks to using alternative fuel to run those trucks. Although interesting, these examples don't tell us much about how organizations go green. One model uses the terms *shades of green* to describe the different environmental approaches that organizations may take.[30] (See Exhibit 2.)

The first approach, the *legal (or light green) approach,* is simply doing what is required legally. In this approach, which illustrates social obligation, organizations exhibit little environmental sensitivity. They obey laws, rules, and regulations without legal challenge and that's the extent of their being green.

As an organization becomes more sensitive to environmental issues, it may adopt the *market approach* and respond to environmental preferences of customers. Whatever customers demand in terms of environmentally friendly products will be what the organization provides. For example, DuPont developed a new type of herbicide that helped farmers around the world reduce their annual use of chemicals by more than 45 million pounds. By developing this product, the company was responding to the demands of its customers (farmers) who wanted to minimize the use of chemicals on their crops. This is a good example of social responsiveness, as is the next approach.

LEADER *making a* DIFFERENCE

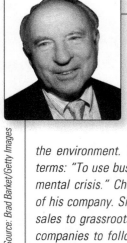

Source: Brad Barket/Getty Images

Yvon Chouinard *is a self-taught blacksmith who, in 1957, started crafting mountain climbing pitons he and other climbing enthusiasts used as anchors on risky climbs.[31] His hardware became so popular that he would go on to found the outdoor-clothing company Patagonia. As his company grew, Chouinard realized that everything his company did had an effect—mostly negative—on the environment. Today, he defines the company's mission in eco-driven terms: "To use business to inspire and implement solutions to the environmental crisis." Chouinard has put environmental activism at the forefront of his company. Since 1985, Patagonia has donated 1 percent of its annual sales to grassroots environmental groups and has gotten more than 1,300 companies to follow its lead as part of its "1% for the Planet" group. He recognizes that "every product, no matter how much thought goes into it, has a destructive impact on Earth." But nonetheless, he keeps doing what he does because "it's the right thing to do."* What can you learn from this leader making a difference?

Exhibit 2
Green Approaches

Source: Based on R. E. Freeman, J. Pierce, and R. Dodd, *Shades of Green: Business Ethics and the Environment* (New York: Oxford University Press, 1995).

High → Activist Approach (Dark Green)

Stakeholder Approach

Market Approach

Low Legal Approach (Light Green)

Environmental Sensitivity

In the *stakeholder approach*, an organization works to meet the environmental demands of multiple stakeholders such as employees, suppliers, or community. For instance, Hewlett-Packard has several corporate environmental programs in place for its supply chain (suppliers), product design and product recycling (customers and society), and work operations (employees and community).

Finally, if an organization pursues an *activist (or dark green) approach*, it looks for ways to protect the earth's natural resources. The activist approach reflects the highest degree of environmental sensitivity and illustrates social responsibility. For example, Belgian company Ecover produces ecological cleaning products in a near-zero-emissions factory. This factory (the world's first ecological one) is an engineering marvel with a huge grass roof that keeps things cool in summer and warm in winter and a water treatment system that runs on wind and solar energy. The company chose to build this facility because of its deep commitment to the environment.

Evaluating Green Management Actions

As businesses become "greener," they often release detailed reports on their environmental performance. Almost 6,000 companies around the globe voluntarily report their efforts in promoting environmental sustainability using the guidelines developed by the Global Reporting Initiative (GRI). These reports, which can be found on the GRI Web site (www.globalreporting.org), describe the numerous green actions of these organizations.

Another way organizations show their commitment to being green is through pursuing standards developed by the nongovernmental International Organization for Standardization (ISO). Although ISO has developed more than 18,000 international standards, it's probably best known for its ISO 9000 (quality management) and ISO 14000 (environmental management) standards. Organizations that want to become ISO 14000 compliant must develop a total management system for meeting

let's get REAL

The Scenario:

Like many students, Sonjia Kresnik has to work part-time, mostly on the weekends, while taking classes at the local university. She likes her job as team leader for a popular restaurant in downtown Portland and has worked there for three years. She's also always had a strong interest in green issues and would like to see her weekend crew be more involved in sustainable practices. How can she get her employees involved in "greening" their workplace?

What do you suggest Sonjia do?

Sonjia should get her employees involved by providing incentives for their accomplishments toward being "green." A simple way to get people to cooperate is to make things fun, perhaps making it a competition, or providing prizes when they reach certain goals. They can get a gift card or something that will make them want to work harder at being more "green." Even a group effort can be rewarding, if you set team goals. I've found that the incentive techniques motivate people to try harder.

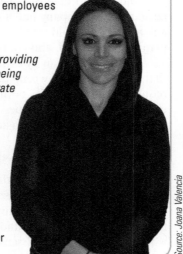

Joana Valencia
Senior Project Manager

Source: Joana Valencia

environmental challenges. In other words, it must minimize the effects of its activities on the environment and continually improve its environmental performance. If an organization can meet these standards, it can state that it's ISO 14000 compliant—an accomplishment achieved by organizations in over 155 countries.

One final way to evaluate a company's green actions is to use the Global 100 list of the most sustainable corporations in the world (www.global100.org).[32] To be named to this list—announced each year at the renowned World Economic Forum in Davos, Switzerland—a company has displayed a superior ability to effectively manage environmental and social factors. In 2014, the United States led the list with 18 Global 100 companies. Canada followed with 13 spots, and the United Kingdom and France tied for third with 8 spots each. Emerging markets Brazil and China accounted for 3 spots on the index. Some companies on the 2014 list included Novo Nordisk A/S (Denmark), Cisco Systems Inc. (United States), The Sage Group PLC (United Kingdom), and Natura Cosmeticos SA (Brazil).

MANAGERS and Ethical Behavior

LO3 One hundred fifty years. That was the maximum prison sentence handed to financier Bernard Madoff, who stole billions of dollars from his clients, by a U.S. district judge who called his crimes "evil." In Britain, which has been characterized by some critics as a "nanny state because of its purported high level of social control and surveillance," a controversy arose over the monitoring of garbage cans. Many local governments have installed monitoring chips in municipally distributed trash cans. These chips match cans with owners and can be used to track the weight of the bins, leading some critics to fear that the country is moving to a pay-as-you-go system, which they believe will discriminate against large families. A government report says that Iceland, hit hard by both the global economic meltdown and a pesky volcano, was "victimized by politicians, bankers, and regulators who engaged in acts of extreme negligence."[33] When you hear about such behaviors—especially after the high-profile financial misconduct at Enron, WorldCom, Lehman Brothers, and other organizations—you might conclude that businesses aren't ethical. Although that's not the case, managers—at all levels, in all areas, in all sizes, and in all kinds of organizations—do face ethical issues and dilemmas. For instance, is it ethical for a sales representative to bribe a purchasing agent as an inducement to buy? Would it make a difference if the bribe came out of the sales rep's commission? Is it ethical for someone to use a company car for private use? How about using company e-mail for personal correspondence or using the company phone to make personal phone calls? What if you managed an employee who worked all weekend on an emergency situation and you told him to take off two days sometime later and mark it down as "sick days" because your company had a clear policy that overtime would not be compensated for any reason?[34] Would that be okay? How will you handle such situations? As managers plan, organize, lead, and control, they must consider ethical dimensions.

What do we mean by **ethics**? We're defining it as the principles, values, and beliefs that define right and wrong decisions and behavior.[35] Many decisions managers make require them to consider both the process and who's affected by the result.[36] To better understand the ethical issues involved in such decisions, let's look at the factors that determine whether a person acts ethically or unethically.

ethics
Principles, values, and beliefs that define what is right and wrong behavior

Factors That Determine Ethical and Unethical Behavior

Whether someone behaves ethically or unethically when faced with an ethical dilemma is influenced by several things: his or her stage of moral development and other moderating variables, including individual characteristics, the organization's structural design, the organization's culture, and the intensity of the ethical issue. (See Exhibit 3.) People who lack a strong moral sense are much less likely to do the wrong things if they're constrained by rules, policies, job descriptions, or strong cultural norms that disapprove

Exhibit 3

Factors That Determine Ethical and Unethical Behavior

Individual Characteristics | Issue Intensity

Ethical Dilemma → Stage of Moral Development → Moderators → Ethical/Unethical Behavior

Structural Variables | Organizational Culture

of such behaviors. Conversely, intensely moral individuals can be corrupted by an organizational structure and culture that permits or encourages unethical practices. Let's look more closely at these factors.

STAGE OF MORAL DEVELOPMENT   Research divides moral development into three levels, each having two stages.[37] At each successive stage, an individual's moral judgment becomes less dependent on outside influences and more internalized.

At the first level, the *preconventional* level, a person's choice between right and wrong is based on personal consequences from outside sources, such as physical punishment, reward, or exchange of favors. At the second level, the *conventional* level, ethical decisions rely on maintaining expected standards and living up to the expectations of others. At the *principled* level, individuals define moral values apart from the authority of the groups to which they belong or society in general. The three levels and six stages are described in Exhibit 4.

What can we conclude about moral development?[38] First, people proceed through the six stages sequentially. Second, there is no guarantee of continued moral development. Third, the majority of adults are at stage four: They're limited to obeying the rules and will be inclined to behave ethically, although for different reasons. A manager at stage three is likely to make decisions based on peer approval; a manager at stage four will try to be a "good corporate citizen" by making decisions that respect the organization's rules and procedures; and a stage five manager is likely to challenge organizational practices that he or she believes to be wrong.

INDIVIDUAL CHARACTERISTICS   Two individual characteristics—values and personality—play a role in determining whether a person behaves ethically. Each person comes to an organization with a relatively entrenched set of personal **values,** which represent basic convictions about what is right and wrong. Our values develop from a young age based on what we see and hear from parents, teachers, friends, and others. Thus, employees in the same organization often possess very different values.[39] Although *values* and *stage of moral development* may seem similar, they're not. Values are broad and cover a wide range of issues; the stage of moral development is a measure of independence from outside influences.

values
Basic convictions about what is right and wrong

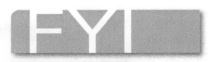

- An organization devoted to global ethics says that societies share five core moral values— honesty, respect, responsibility, fairness, and compassion.[40]

Level		Description of Stage
	Principled	6. Following self-chosen ethical principles even if they violate the law
		5. Valuing rights of others and upholding absolute values and rights regardless of the majority's opinion
	Conventional	4. Maintaining conventional order by fulfilling obligations to which you have agreed
		3. Living up to what is expected by people close to you
Preconventional		2. Following rules only when doing so is in your immediate interest
		1. Sticking to rules to avoid physical punishment

Exhibit 4

Stages of Moral Development

Source: L. Kohlberg, "Moral Stages and Moralization: The Cognitive-Development Approach," in T. Lickona (ed.), *Moral Development and Behavior: Theory, Research, and Social Issues* (New York: Holt, Rinehart & Winston, 1976), pp. 34–35.

ego strength
A personality measure of the strength of a person's convictions

locus of control
A personality attribute that measures the degree to which people believe they control their own fate

Two personality variables have been found to influence an individual's actions according to his or her beliefs about what is right or wrong: ego strength and locus of control. **Ego strength** measures the strength of a person's convictions. People with high ego strength are likely to resist impulses to act unethically and instead follow their convictions. That is, individuals high in ego strength are more likely to do what they think is right and be more consistent in their moral judgments and actions than those with low ego strength.

Locus of control is the degree to which people believe they control their own fate. People with an *internal* locus of control believe they control their own destinies. They're more likely to take responsibility for consequences and rely on their own internal standards of right and wrong to guide their behavior. They're also more likely to be consistent in their moral judgments and actions. People with an *external* locus of control believe what happens to them is due to luck or chance. They're less likely to take personal responsibility for the consequences of their behavior and more likely to rely on external forces.[41]

STRUCTURAL VARIABLES   An organization's structural design can influence whether employees behave ethically. Those structures that minimize ambiguity and uncertainty with formal rules and regulations and those that continuously remind employees of what is ethical are more likely to encourage ethical behavior. Other structural variables that influence ethical choices include goals, performance appraisal systems, and reward allocation procedures.

Although many organizations use goals to guide and motivate employees, those goals can create some unexpected problems. One study found that people who don't reach set goals are more likely to engage in unethical behavior, even if they do or don't have economic incentives to do so. The researchers concluded that "goal setting can lead to unethical behavior."[42] Examples of such behaviors abound—from companies shipping unfinished products just to reach sales goals or "managing earnings" to meet financial analysts' expectations, to schools excluding certain groups of students when reporting standardized test scores to make their "pass" rate look better.[43]

An organization's performance appraisal system also can influence ethical behavior. Some systems focus exclusively on outcomes, while others evaluate means as well as ends. When employees are evaluated only on outcomes, they may be pressured to do whatever is necessary to look good on the outcomes and not be concerned with how they got those results. Research suggests that "success may serve to excuse unethical behaviors."[44] The danger of such thinking is that if managers are more lenient in correcting unethical behaviors of successful employees, other employees will model their behavior on what they see.

Closely related to the organization's appraisal system is how rewards are allocated. The more that rewards or punishment depend on specific goal outcomes, the more employees are pressured to do whatever they must to reach those goals—perhaps to the point of compromising their ethical standards. Experts say that "It's a good idea to look at what you're encouraging employees to do. A sales goal of $147 an hour led auto mechanics at Sears to 'repair' things that weren't broken."[45]

ORGANIZATION'S CULTURE   As Exhibit 3 showed, the content and strength of an organization's culture also influence ethical behavior.[46] An organization's culture consists of the shared organizational values. These values reflect what the organization stands for and what it believes in as well as create an environment that influences employee behavior ethically or unethically. When it comes to ethical behavior, a culture most likely to encourage high ethical standards is one that's high in risk tolerance, control, and conflict tolerance. Employees in such a culture are encouraged to be aggressive and innovative, are aware that unethical practices will be discovered, and feel free to openly challenge expectations they consider to be unrealistic or personally undesirable.

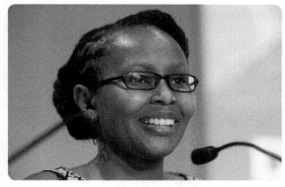

Juliana Rotich has high ego strength. A native of Kenya, she believes in the transformational power of technology to address social problems. Determined to speed up the digital revolution in Africa, Rotich and her team of innovators have developed open disaster-mapping software, formed a technology hub in Nairobi, and created a new Internet connectivity device to overcome problems of poor reception and power outages in Africa.
Source: Robert Schlesinger/Picture Alliance/Robert Schles/Newscom

Because shared values can be powerful influences, many organizations are using **values-based management**, in which the organization's values guide employees in the way they do their jobs. For instance, Timberland is an example of a company using values-based management. With a simple statement, "Make It Better," employees at Timberland know what's expected and valued; that is, they find ways to "make it better"—whether it's creating quality products for customers, performing community service activities, designing employee training programs, or figuring out ways to make the company's packaging more environmentally friendly. As it says on the company's Web site, "Everything we do at Timberland grows out of our relentless pursuit to find a way to make it better." At Corning, one of the core values guiding employee behavior is integrity. Employees are expected to work in ways that are honest, decent, and fair. Timberland and Corning aren't alone in their use of values-based management. A survey of global companies found that a large number (more than 89 percent) said they had a written corporate values statement.[47] This survey also found that most of the companies believed their values influenced relationships and reputation, the top-performing companies consciously connected values with the way employees did their work, and top managers were important to reinforcing the importance of the values throughout the organization.

Thus, an organization's managers do play an important role here. They're responsible for creating an environment that encourages employees to embrace the culture and the desired values as they do their jobs. In fact, *research shows that the behavior of managers is the **single most important influence** on an individual's decision to act ethically or unethically.*[48] People look to see what those in authority are doing and use that as a benchmark for acceptable practices and expectations.

values-based management
The organization's values guide employees in the way they do their jobs

FUTURE VISION | Building an Ethical Culture That Lasts

Let's start off with the bad news about the state of ethics in the U.S. workplace:

- 60 percent of misdeeds reported by workers involved someone with managerial authority.
- 24 percent of those observed misdeeds involved senior managers.
- In organizations with *weak* ethical cultures, 88 percent of workers reported seeing misconduct.[49]

Now, how about some better news:

- In organizations with *strong* ethical cultures, only 20 percent of workers reported seeing misconduct.[50]
- Companies on Ethisphere's World's Most Ethical Companies list had 20 percent greater profits and 6 percent better shareholder returns than other companies.[51]

Ethics *is* a part of an organization's culture. And it's becoming ever more critical for businesses to "do things around here" ethically. Society expects it. Customers demand it. And with the speed and spread of news globally—bad and good—you can't hide! So what are the critical aspects of an ethical culture? Certainly, it encompasses things like whether an organization's employees are trustworthy, reliable, fair, honest,

compassionate, and respectful in dealings with customers, peers, and other stakeholders. But it's also whether managers at all levels talk about ethics and model appropriate behavior. Is ethical behavior reinforced? However, the responsibility for doing things ethically isn't just on managers' backs. In ethical cultures, organizational colleagues support one another in making ethical decisions and in doing ethical work. It can be an infectious type of atmosphere in which good people do good and the organization where they work prospers by achieving those greater profits and better shareholder returns. A win-win in anyone's book! This vision of an ethical workplace isn't just for the future, but is also important for today.

If your professor has chosen to assign this, go to ***www.mymanagementlab.com*** *to discuss the following questions.*

⭐ **TALK ABOUT IT 1:** Why do you think organizations with *weak* ethical cultures have four times as many workers witnessing misconduct?

⭐ **TALK ABOUT IT 2:** "Society expects it (ethical practices). Customers demand it." Discuss why you agree or disagree with this.

Finally, a strong culture exerts more influence on employees than a weak one. If a culture is strong and supports high ethical standards, it has a powerful and positive influence on the decision to act ethically or unethically. For example, IBM has a strong culture that has long stressed ethical dealings with customers, employees, business partners, and communities.[52] To reinforce the importance of ethical behaviors, the company developed an explicitly detailed set of guidelines for business conduct and ethics. And the penalty for violating the guidelines: disciplinary actions, including dismissal. IBM's managers continually reinforce the importance of ethical behavior and reinforce the fact that a person's actions and decisions are important to the way the organization is viewed.

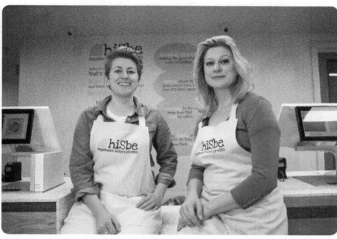

Sisters Amy and Ruth Anslow launched a new type of sustainable and affordable supermarket in Brighton, England, based on eight core values that guide employee behavior: go local, pick seasonal, protect nature, support ethical, think welfare, save fish, consider waste, and choose real. Called hiSbe (How It Should Be), the store puts people—rather than profits—first.
Source: David McHugh/AP Images

ISSUE INTENSITY A student who would never consider breaking into an instructor's office to steal an accounting exam doesn't think twice about asking a friend who took the same course from the same instructor last semester what questions were on an exam. Similarly, a manager might think nothing about taking home a few office supplies yet be highly concerned about the possible embezzlement of company funds. These examples illustrate the final factor that influences ethical behavior: the intensity of the ethical issue itself.[53]

As Exhibit 5 shows, six characteristics determine issue intensity or how important an ethical issue is to an individual: greatness of harm, consensus of wrong, probability of harm, immediacy of consequences, proximity to victim(s), and concentration of effect. These factors suggest that:

- the larger the number of people harmed
- the more agreement that the action is wrong
- the greater the likelihood that the action will cause harm
- the more immediately the consequences of the action will be felt
- the closer the person feels to the victim(s)
- the more concentrated the effect of the action on the victim(s)...

Exhibit 5
Issue Intensity

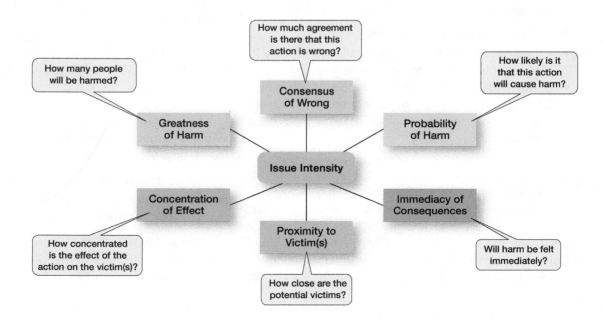

the greater the issue intensity or importance. When an ethical issue is important, employees are more likely to behave ethically.

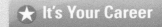

Ethics—If your instructor is using MyManagementLab, log onto **mymanagementlab.com** and test your *knowledge about being ethical.* **Be sure to refer back to the chapter opener!**

Ethics in an International Context

Are ethical standards universal? Although some common moral beliefs exist, social and cultural differences between countries are important factors that determine ethical and unethical behavior.[54]

Should Coca-Cola employees in Saudi Arabia adhere to U.S. ethical standards, or should they follow local standards of acceptable behavior? If Airbus (a European company) pays a "broker's fee" to an intermediary to get a major contract with a Middle Eastern airline, should Boeing be restricted from doing the same because such practices are considered improper in the United States? (Note: In the United Kingdom, the Law Commission, a governmental advisory body, has said that bribing officials in foreign countries should be a criminal offense. It said that claims of "it's local custom" should not be a reason for allowing it.[55]) British defense giant BAE, which has been the target of various bribery and corruption allegations, was ordered to "submit to the supervision of an ethics monitor and pay nearly $500 million to resolve the corruption allegations."[56]

In the case of payments to influence foreign officials or politicians, U.S. managers are guided by the Foreign Corrupt Practices Act (FCPA), which makes it illegal to knowingly corrupt a foreign official. However, even this law doesn't always reduce ethical dilemmas to black and white. In some countries, government bureaucrat salaries are low because custom dictates that they receive small payments from those they serve. Payoffs to these bureaucrats "grease the machinery" and ensure that things get done. The FCPA does not expressly prohibit small payoffs to foreign government employees whose duties are primarily administrative or clerical *when* such payoffs are an accepted part of doing business in that country. Any action other than this is illegal. In 2013 (latest numbers available), the U.S. Department of Justice brought seven FCPA enforcement actions, collecting approximately $420 million in fines.[57]

It's important for individual managers working in foreign cultures to recognize the social, cultural, and political-legal influences on what is appropriate and acceptable behavior.[58] And international businesses must clarify their ethical guidelines so that employees know what's expected of them while working in a foreign location, which adds another dimension to making ethical judgments.

Another guide to being ethical in international business is the United Nations Global Compact, which is an initiative created by the United Nations outlining principles for doing business globally in the areas of human rights, labor, the environment, and anti-corruption (see Exhibit 6). More than 10,000 participants and stakeholders from over 145 countries have committed to the UN Global Compact, making it the world's largest voluntary corporate citizenship initiative.[59] The goal of the UN Global Compact is a more sustainable and inclusive global economy. Organizations making this commitment do so because they believe that the world business community plays a significant role in improving economic and social conditions. In addition, the Organization for Economic Co-operation and Development (OECD) has made fighting bribery and corruption in international business a high priority. The centerpiece of its efforts is the Anti-Bribery Convention (or set of rules and guidelines), which was the first global instrument to combat corruption in cross-border business deals. To date, significant gains have been made in fighting corruption in the 40 countries that have ratified it.[60]

Exhibit 6

The Ten Principles of the United Nations Global Compact

The UN Global Compact asks companies to embrace, support, and enact, within their sphere of influence, a set of core values in the areas of human rights, labor standards, the environment, and anti-corruption:

Human Rights

Principle 1:	Business should support and respect the protection of internationally-proclaimed human rights within their sphere of influence; and
Principle 2:	Make sure they are not complicit in human rights abuses.

Labor Standards

Principle 3:	Business should uphold the freedom of association and the effective recognition of the right to collective bargaining;
Principle 4:	The elimination of all forms of forced and compulsory labor;
Principle 5:	The effective abolition of child labor; and
Principle 6:	The elimination of discrimination in respect to employment and occupation.

Environment

Principle 7:	Business should support a precautionary approach to environmental challenges;
Principle 8:	Undertake initiatives to promote greater environmental responsibility; and
Principle 9:	Encourage the development and diffusion of environmentally friendly technologies.

Anti-Corruption

Principle 10:	Business should work against corruption in all its forms, including extortion and bribery.

Source: Copyright © 2012 by United Nations Global Compact (www.unglobalcompact.org). Reprinted with permission.

ENCOURAGING Ethical Behavior

LO4 At a Senate hearing exploring the accusations that Wall Street firm Goldman Sachs deceived its clients during the housing-market meltdown, Arizona senator John McCain said, "I don't know if Goldman has done anything illegal, but there's no doubt their behavior was unethical."[61] You have to wonder what the firm's managers were thinking or doing while such ethically questionable decisions and actions were taking place.

Managers can do a number of things if they're serious about encouraging ethical behaviors—hire employees with high ethical standards, establish codes of ethics, lead by example, and so forth. By themselves, such actions won't have much of an impact. But if an organization has a comprehensive ethics program in place, it can potentially improve an organization's ethical climate. The key variable, however, is *potentially.* There are no guarantees that a well-designed ethics program will lead to the desired outcome. Sometimes corporate ethics programs are little more than public relations gestures that do little to influence managers and employees. For instance, Sears had a long history of encouraging ethical business practices through its corporate Office of Ethics and Business Practices. However, its ethics programs didn't stop managers from illegally trying to collect payments from bankrupt charge account holders or from routinely deceiving automotive service center customers into thinking they needed unnecessary repairs. Even Enron, often referred to as the "poster child" of corporate wrongdoing, outlined values in its final annual report that most would consider ethical—communication, respect, integrity, and excellence.

let's get REAL

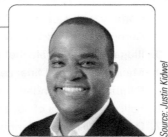

Justin Kidwell
Management Consultant

The Scenario

All through university, Finlay Roberts wasn't sure what he really wanted to do. But now he had found what he thought was a great job, one where he could enhance his leadership skills in a competitive environment with teams of employees who sold security systems over the phone. What he soon discovered, though, was that competing to meet sales goals often led to unethical actions.

After learning about ethics in pretty much every management class he took, Finlay wanted to show his employees that he was committed to an ethical workplace.

What advice would you give Finlay?

One of the cornerstones to professional success is to maintain and demonstrate strong ethics—often by exceeding the standards set by the organization. One potential path for Finlay is to remember that damaging the company's brand can risk destroying his career, but missing sales/performance targets will only impede his career. Over the long run, professionals with strong reputations will outlast those with questionable character.

Yet the way top managers behaved didn't reflect those values at all.[62] Let's look at some specific ways that managers can encourage ethical behavior and create a comprehensive ethics program.

Employee Selection

Wanting to reduce workers' compensation claims, Hospitality Management Corp. did pre-employment integrity testing at one hotel to see if the tests could "weed out applicants likely to be dishonest, take dangerous risks or engage in other undesirable behaviors." After six months, claims were down among new hires.[63]

The selection process (interviews, tests, background checks, and so forth) should be viewed as an opportunity to learn about an individual's level of moral development, personal values, ego strength, and locus of control.[64] However, a carefully designed selection process isn't foolproof and, even under the best circumstances, individuals with questionable standards of right and wrong may be hired. That means having other ethics controls in place.

Codes of Ethics and Decision Rules

George David, former CEO and chairman of Hartford, Connecticut-based United Technologies Corporation (UTC), believed in the power of a code of ethics. That's why UTC has always had one that was quite explicit and detailed. Employees know the company's behavioral expectations, especially when it comes to ethics. UBS AG, the Swiss bank, also has an explicit employee code crafted by the CEO that bans staff from helping clients cheat on their taxes.[65] However, not all organizations have such explicit ethical guidelines.

Uncertainty about what is and is not ethical can be a problem for employees. A **code of ethics**, a formal statement of an organization's values and the ethical rules it expects employees to follow, is a popular choice for reducing that ambiguity. Research shows that 97 percent of organizations with more than 10,000 employees have a

code of ethics
A formal statement of an organization's primary values and the ethical rules it expects its employees to follow

Exhibit 7
Codes of Ethics

Cluster 1. Be a Dependable Organizational Citizen

1. Comply with safety, health, and security regulations.
2. Demonstrate courtesy, respect, honesty, and fairness.
3. Illegal drugs and alcohol at work are prohibited.
4. Manage personal finances well.
5. Exhibit good attendance and punctuality.
6. Follow directives of supervisors.
7. Do not use abusive language.
8. Dress in business attire.
9. Firearms at work are prohibited.

Cluster 2. Do Not Do Anything Unlawful or Improper That Will Harm the Organization

1. Conduct business in compliance with all laws.
2. Payments for unlawful purposes are prohibited.
3. Bribes are prohibited.
4. Avoid outside activities that impair duties.
5. Maintain confidentiality of records.
6. Comply with all antitrust and trade regulations.
7. Comply with all accounting rules and controls.
8. Do not use company property for personal benefit.
9. Employees are personally accountable for company funds.
10. Do not propagate false or misleading information.
11. Make decisions without regard for personal gain.

Cluster 3. Be Good to Customers

1. Convey true claims in product advertisements.
2. Perform assigned duties to the best of your ability.
3. Provide products and services of the highest quality.

Source: F. R. David, "An Empirical Study of Codes of Business Ethics: A Strategic Perspective," paper presented at the 48th Annual Academy of Management Conference, Anaheim, California, August 1988. Used with permission of Fred David.

written code of ethics. Even in smaller organizations, nearly 93 percent have one.[66] And codes of ethics are becoming more popular globally. Research by the Institute for Global Ethics says that shared values such as honesty, fairness, respect, responsibility, and caring are pretty much universally embraced.[67] In addition, a survey of businesses in 22 countries found that 78 percent have formally stated ethics standards and codes of ethics; and more than 85 percent of *Fortune* Global 200 companies have a business code of ethics.[68]

What should a code of ethics look like? It should be specific enough to show employees the spirit in which they're supposed to do things yet loose enough to allow for freedom of judgment. A survey of companies' codes of ethics found their content tended to fall into three categories, as shown in Exhibit 7.[69]

Unfortunately, codes of ethics may not work as well as we think they should. A survey of employees in U.S. businesses found that 41 percent of those surveyed had observed ethical or legal violations in the previous 12 months, including such things as conflicts of interest, abusive or intimidating behavior, and lying to employees. And 37 percent of those employees didn't report observed misconduct.[70] Does this mean

Exhibit 8
A Process for Addressing Ethical Dilemmas

Step 1: What is the **ethical dilemma?**

Step 2: Who are the **affected stakeholders?**

Step 3: Which **personal, organizational,** and **external factors** are important in this decision?

Step 4: What are possible **alternatives?**

Step 5: What is my **decision** and how will I act on it?

that codes of ethics shouldn't be developed? No. However, in doing so, managers should use these suggestions:[71]

1. Organizational leaders should model appropriate behavior and reward those who act ethically.
2. All managers should continually reaffirm the importance of the ethics code and consistently discipline those who break it.
3. The organization's stakeholders (employees, customers, and so forth) should be considered as an ethics code is developed or improved.
4. Managers should communicate and reinforce the ethics code regularly.
5. Managers should use the five-step process (see Exhibit 8) to guide employees when faced with ethical dilemmas.

Leadership at the Top

In 2011, Tim Cook was named CEO of Apple Inc. Although it's an extremely successful company, Apple is viewed by some as the epitome of greedy capitalism with no concern for how its products are manufactured. Cook, who was named one of the 100 Most Influential People in Business Ethics by *Ethisphere*, has increased the company's focus on supply chain ethics and compliance issues. It was the first technology company to join the Fair Labor Association, which means that organization can now review the labor practices within the company's supply chain. In addition, at a recent annual stockholders' meeting with investors and journalists, Cook, who was challenged by a spokesperson from a conservative think tank to explain how the company's sustainability efforts were in the best interests of shareholders, bluntly and clearly said that Apple wasn't just about making a profit and that "We want to leave the world better than we found it."[72]

Doing business ethically requires a commitment from managers at all levels, but especially the top level. Why? Because they're the ones who uphold the shared values and set the cultural tone. They're role models in terms of both words and actions, though what they *do* is far more important than what they *say.* If top managers, for example, take company resources for their personal use, inflate their expense accounts, or give favored treatment to friends, they imply that such behavior is acceptable for all employees.

Top managers also set the tone by their reward and punishment practices. The choices of whom and what are rewarded with pay increases and promotions send a strong signal to employees. As we said earlier, when an employee is rewarded for achieving impressive results in an ethically questionable manner, it indicates to others that those ways are acceptable. When an employee does something unethical, managers must punish the offender and publicize the fact by making the outcome visible to everyone in the organization. This practice sends a message that doing wrong has a price and it's not in employees' best interests to act unethically!

Job Goals and Performance Appraisal

Employees in three Internal Revenue Service offices were found in the bathrooms flushing tax returns and other related documents down the toilets. When questioned, they openly admitted doing it, but offered an interesting explanation for their

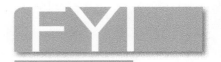

• 67 percent of companies include ethical conduct as a performance measure in employee evaluations.[73]

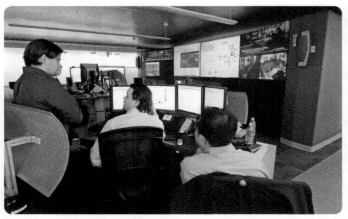

An innovative training video called "Ethics Idol" teaches Cisco Systems' employees how to deal with ethical problems at work. Featured on Cisco's intranet, the video presents ethical scenarios from Cisco's Code of Business Conduct that are evaluated by judges, asks employees questions related to which judge's answer they agree with, and then shows the official Cisco answer.
Source: AP Photo/Paul Sakuma

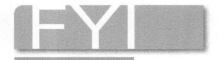

- 81 percent of companies provide ethics training.[75]

behavior. The employees' supervisors had been pressuring them to complete more work in less time. If the piles of tax returns weren't processed and moved off their desks more quickly, they were told their performance reviews and salary raises would be adversely affected. Frustrated by few resources and an overworked computer system, the employees decided to "flush away" the paperwork on their desks. Although these employees knew what they did was wrong, it illustrates how powerful unrealistic goals and performance appraisals can be.[74] Under the stress of unrealistic goals, otherwise ethical employees may feel they have no choice but to do whatever is necessary to meet those goals. Also, goal achievement is usually a key issue in performance appraisal. If performance appraisals focus only on economic goals, ends will begin to justify means. To encourage ethical behavior, both ends *and* means should be evaluated. For example, a manager's annual review of employees might include a point-by-point evaluation of how their decisions measured up against the company's code of ethics as well as how well goals were met.

Ethics Training

More organizations are setting up seminars, workshops, and similar ethics training programs to encourage ethical behavior. Such training programs aren't without controversy, as the primary concern is whether ethics can be taught. Critics stress that the effort is pointless because people establish their individual value systems when they're young. Proponents note, however, that several studies have shown that values can be learned after early childhood. In addition, they cite evidence that shows that teaching ethical problem solving can make an actual difference in ethical behaviors;[76] that training has increased individuals' level of moral development;[77] and that, if nothing else, ethics training increases awareness of ethical issues in business.[78]

How can ethics be taught? Let's look at an example involving global defense contractor Lockheed Martin, one of the pioneers in the case-based approach to ethics training.[79] Lockheed Martin's employees take annual ethics training courses delivered by their managers. The main focus of these short courses features department or job-specific issues. In each department, employee teams review and discuss the cases and then apply an "Ethics Meter" to "rate whether the real-life decisions were ethical, unethical, or somewhere in between." For example, one of the possible ratings on the Ethics Meter, "On Thin Ice," is explained as "bordering on unethical and should raise a red flag." After the teams have applied their ratings, managers lead discussions about the ratings and examine why the company's core ethics principles were or were not applied in the cases. In addition to its ethics training, Lockheed Martin has a widely used written code of ethics, an ethics helpline that employees can call for guidance on ethical issues, and ethics officers based in the company's various business units.

Independent Social Audits

The fear of being caught can be an important deterrent to unethical behavior. Independent social audits, which evaluate decisions and management practices in terms of the organization's code of ethics, increase that likelihood. Such audits can be regular evaluations or they can occur randomly with no prior announcement. An effective ethics program probably needs both. To maintain integrity, auditors should be responsible to the company's board of directors and present their findings directly to the board. This arrangement gives the auditors clout and lessens the opportunity for retaliation from those being audited. Because the Sarbanes-Oxley Act holds businesses to more rigorous standards of financial disclosure and corporate governance, more organizations are finding the idea of independent social audits appealing.

As the publisher of *Business Ethics* magazine stated, "The debate has shifted from *whether* to be ethical to *how* to be ethical."[80]

Protective Mechanisms

Employees who face ethical dilemmas need protective mechanisms so they can do what's right without fear of reprimand. An organization might designate ethical counselors for employees facing an ethics dilemma. These advisors also might advocate the ethically "right" alternatives. Other organizations have appointed ethics and compliance officers who design, direct, and modify the organization's ethics/compliance programs as needed.[81] In fact, many organizations have raised the visibility of their compliance officers, even to the point of being a direct report to the CEO.[82]

If your professor has assigned this, go to **www.mymanagementlab.com** to complete the Writing Assignment MGMT 4: Ethics.

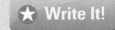 Write It!

SOCIAL Responsibility and Ethics
Issues in Today's World

LO5 Today's managers continue to face challenges in being socially responsible and ethical. Next, we examine three current issues: managing ethical lapses and social irresponsibility, social entrepreneurship, and promoting positive social change.

Managing Ethical Lapses and Social Irresponsibility

Even after public outrage over the Enron-era misdeeds, irresponsible and unethical practices by managers in all kinds of organizations haven't gone away, as you've observed with some of the questionable behaviors that took place at financial services firms such as Goldman Sachs and Lehman Brothers. But what's more alarming is what's going on "in the trenches," in offices, warehouses, and stores. One survey reported that among 5,000 employees: 45 percent admitted falling asleep at work; 22 percent said they spread a rumor about a coworker; 18 percent said they snooped after hours; and 2 percent said they took credit for someone else's work.[83] Some interesting recent research suggests that men are more likely to act unethically than women in situations where failure could harm their sense of masculinity.[84] The researchers suggest that the reason is that losing a "battle, particularly in contexts that are highly competitive and historically male oriented, presents a threat to masculine competency. To ensure victory, men will sacrifice moral standards if doing so means winning."

Unfortunately, it's not just at work that we see such behaviors; they're prevalent throughout society. Studies conducted by the Center for Academic Integrity showed that 26 percent of college and university business majors admitted to "serious cheating" on exams and 54 percent admitted to cheating on written assignments. But business students weren't the worst cheaters—that distinction belonged to journalism majors, of whom 27 percent said they had cheated.[85] And a survey by Students in Free Enterprise (SIFE) found that only 19 percent of students would report a classmate who cheated.[86] But even more frightening is what today's teenagers say is "acceptable." In a survey, 23 percent said they thought violence toward another person is acceptable on some level.[87] What do such statistics say about what managers may have to deal with in the future? It's not too far-fetched to say that organizations may have difficulty upholding high ethical standards when their future employees so readily accept unethical behavior.

What can managers do? Two actions seem particularly important: ethical leadership and protecting those who report wrongdoing.

9
Ethical Leader

- Be a good role model by being ethical and honest.
  - Tell the truth always.
  - Don't hide or manipulate information.
  - Be willing to admit your failures.
- Share your personal values by regularly communicating them to employees.
- Stress the organization's or team's important shared values.
- Use the reward system to hold everyone accountable to the values.

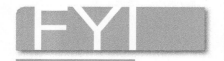

- The strongest predictor of ethical leadership behavior: empathy.[90]

whistle-blower
Individual who raises ethical concerns or issues to others

ETHICAL LEADERSHIP   Not long after Herb Baum took over as CEO of Dial Corporation, he got a call from Reuben Mark, the CEO of competitor Colgate-Palmolive, who told him he had a copy of Dial's strategic marketing plan that had come from a former Dial salesperson who recently had joined Colgate-Palmolive. Mark told Baum he had not looked at it, didn't intend to look at, and was returning it. In addition, he himself was going to deal appropriately with the new salesperson.[88] As this example illustrates, managers must provide ethical leadership. As we said earlier, what managers *do* has a strong influence on employees' decisions whether to behave ethically.[89] When managers cheat, lie, steal, manipulate, take advantage of situations or people, or treat others unfairly, what kind of signal are they sending to employees (or other stakeholders)? Probably not the one they want to send. Exhibit 9 gives some suggestions on how managers can provide ethical leadership.

PROTECTION OF EMPLOYEES WHO RAISE ETHICAL ISSUES   What would you do if you saw other employees doing something illegal, immoral, or unethical? Would you step forward? Many of us wouldn't because of the perceived risks. That's why it's important for managers to assure employees who raise ethical concerns or issues that they will face no personal or career risks. These individuals, often called **whistle-blowers,** can be a key part of any company's ethics program. For example, Sherron Watkins, who was a vice president at Enron, clearly outlined her concerns about the company's accounting practices in a letter to chairman Ken Lay. Her statement that, "I am incredibly nervous that we will implode in a wave of accounting scandals" couldn't have been more prophetic.[91] However, surveys show that most observers of wrongdoing don't report it and that's the attitude managers have to address.[92] Reasons employees give for not blowing the whistle include: fear it might damage someone's career, fear that it would make it harder to work with that individual, fear that he/she (the whistle-blower) wouldn't be taken seriously, fear of not having enough proof, thought someone else would report it, and fear of losing job or other retaliation.[93] So, how can employees be protected so they're willing to step up if they see unethical or illegal things occurring?

One way is to set up toll-free ethics hotlines. For instance, Dell has an ethics hotline that employees can call anonymously to report infractions that the company will then investigate.[94] In addition, managers need to create a culture where bad news can be heard and acted on before it's too late. Michael Josephson, founder of the Josephson Institute of Ethics (www.josephsoninstitute.org) said, "It is absolutely and unequivocally important to establish a culture where it is possible for employees to complain and protest and to get heard."[95] Even if some whistle-blowers have a personal agenda they're pursuing, it's important to take them seriously. Another way is to have in place a "procedurally just process," which means making sure the decision-making process is fair and that employees are treated respectfully about their concerns.[96] Finally, the federal legislation Sarbanes-Oxley offers some legal protection. Any manager who retaliates against an employee for reporting violations faces a stiff penalty: a 10-year jail sentence.[97] Unfortunately, despite this protection, hundreds of employees who have stepped forward and revealed wrongdoings at their companies have been fired or let go from their jobs.[98] At the present time, it's not a perfect solution, but it is a step in the right direction.

If your professor has assigned this, go to **www.mymanagementlab.com** to complete the Simulation: Management and Ethics and get a better understanding of the challenges of managing ethically in organizations.

Social Entrepreneurship

The world's social problems are many and viable solutions are few. But numerous people and organizations are trying to do something. For instance, Reed Paget, founder and CEO of British bottled water company Belu, made his company the world's first to become carbon-neutral. Its bottles are made from corn and can be composted into soil. Also, Belu's profits go toward projects that bring clean water to parts of the world that lack access to it. Paget has chosen to pursue a purpose as well as a profit.[99] He is an example of a **social entrepreneur**, an individual or organization who seeks out opportunities to improve society by using practical, innovative, and sustainable approaches.[100] "What business entrepreneurs are to the economy, social entrepreneurs are to social change."[101] Social entrepreneurs want to make the world a better place and have a driving passion to make that happen. For example, AgSquared aims to help small farmers, who make up 90 percent of the farms in the United States, keep better track of critical information such as basic accounting of seeds, soil data and weather mapping, and even best practices from the farm community.[102] Also, social entrepreneurs use creativity and ingenuity to solve problems. For instance, Seattle-based PATH (Program for Appropriate Technology in Health) is an international nonprofit organization that uses low-cost technology to provide needed health-care solutions for poor, developing countries. By collaborating with public groups and for-profit businesses, PATH has developed simple life-saving solutions such as clean birthing kits, credit-card sized lab test kits, and disposable vaccination syringes that can't be reused. PATH has pioneered innovative approaches to solving global medical problems.[103]

What can we learn from these social entrepreneurs? Although many organizations have committed to doing business ethically and responsibly, perhaps there is more they can do, as these social entrepreneurs show. Maybe, as in the case of PATH, it's simply a matter of business organizations collaborating with public groups or nonprofit organizations to address a social issue. Or maybe, as in the case of AgSquared, it's providing expertise where needed. Or it may involve nurturing individuals who passionately and unwaveringly believe they have an idea that could make the world a better place and simply need the organizational support to pursue it.

social entrepreneur
An individual or organization that seeks out opportunities to improve society by using practical, innovative, and sustainable approaches

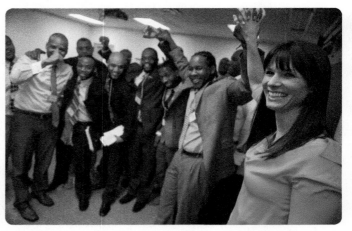

Social entrepreneur Catherine Rohr is the founder and CEO of Defy Ventures, an organization that provides men who have criminal histories with entrepreneurship training, intensive character development, and career opportunities to help them transform their lives and succeed as income earners, fathers, and role models in their communities.
Source: Ann Hermes/The Christian Science Monitor via Getty Images

Businesses Promoting Positive Social Change

Since 1946, Target has contributed 5 percent of its annual income to support community needs, an amount that adds up to more than $3 million a week. And it's not alone in those efforts. "Over the past two decades, a growing number of corporations, both within and beyond the United States, have been engaging in activities that promote positive social change."[104] Businesses can do this in a couple of ways: through corporate philanthropy and through employee volunteering efforts.

CORPORATE PHILANTHROPY Corporate philanthropy can be an effective way for companies to address societal problems.[105] For instance, the breast cancer "pink" campaign and the global AIDS Red campaign (started by Bono) are ways that companies support social causes.[106] Many organizations also donate money to various causes that employees and customers care about. In 2012 (latest numbers

available), the sum of corporate giving totaled over $20.3 billion in cash and products.[107] Other corporations have funded their own foundations to support various social issues. For example, Google's foundation—called DotOrg by its employees—has about $2 billion in assets that it uses to support five areas: developing systems to help predict and prevent disease pandemics, empowering the poor with information about public services, creating jobs by investing in small and midsized businesses in the developing world, accelerating the commercialization of plug-in cars, and making renewable energy cheaper than coal.[108]

EMPLOYEE VOLUNTEERING EFFORTS Employee volunteering is another popular way for businesses to be involved in promoting social change. For instance, Dow Corning sent a small team of employees to rural India helping women "examine stitchery and figure out prices for garments to be sold in local markets."[109] Molson-Coors' eleven-member executive team spent a full day at their annual team-building retreat building a house in Las Vegas with Habitat for Humanity. PricewaterhouseCoopers employees renovated an abandoned school in Newark, New Jersey. Every Wachovia employee is given six paid days off from work each year to volunteer in his or her community. Other businesses are encouraging their employees to volunteer in various ways. The Committee to Encourage Corporate Philanthropy says that more than 90 percent of its members had volunteer programs and almost half encouraged volunteerism by providing paid time off or by creating volunteer events.[110] Many businesses have found that such efforts not only benefit communities, but enhance employees' work efforts and motivation.

PREPARING FOR: Exams/Quizzes

CHAPTER SUMMARY by Learning Objective

LO1 DISCUSS **what it means to be socially responsible and what factors influence that decision.**

Social obligation, which reflects the classical view of social responsibility, is when a firm engages in social actions because of its obligation to meet certain economic and legal responsibilities. Social responsiveness is when a firm engages in social actions in response to some popular social need. Social responsibility is a business's intention, beyond its economic and legal obligations, to pursue long-term goals that are good for society. Both of these reflect the socioeconomic view of social responsibility. Determining whether organizations should be socially involved can be done by looking at arguments for and against it. Other ways are to assess the impact of social involvement on a company's economic performance and evaluate the performance of SRI funds versus non-SRI funds. We can conclude that a company's social responsibility doesn't appear to hurt its economic performance.

LO2 EXPLAIN **green management and how organizations can go green.**

Green management is when managers consider the impact of their organization on the natural environment. Organizations can "go green" in different ways. The light green approach is doing what is required legally, which is social obligation. Using the market approach, organizations respond to the environmental preferences of their customers. Using the stakeholder approach, organizations respond to the environmental demands of multiple stakeholders. Both the market and stakeholder approaches can be viewed as social responsiveness. With an activist or dark green approach, an organization looks for ways to respect and preserve the earth and its natural resources, which can be viewed as social responsibility.

Green actions can be evaluated by examining reports that companies compile about their environmental performance, by looking for compliance with global standards for environmental management (ISO 14000), and by using the Global 100 list of the most sustainable corporations in the world.

LO3 DISCUSS **the factors that lead to ethical and unethical behavior.**

Ethics refers to the principles, values, and beliefs that define right and wrong decisions and behavior. The factors that affect ethical and unethical behavior include an individual's level of moral development (preconventional, conventional, or principled), individual characteristics (values and personality variables—ego strength and locus of control), structural variables (structural design, use of goals, performance appraisal systems, and reward allocation procedures), organizational culture (shared values and cultural strength), and issue intensity (greatness of harm, consensus of wrong, probability of harm, immediacy of consequences, proximity to victims, and concentration of effect).

Since ethical standards aren't universal, managers should know what they can and cannot do legally as defined by the Foreign Corrupt Practices Act. It's also important to recognize any cultural differences and to clarify ethical guidelines for employees working in different global locations. Finally, managers should know about the principles of the Global Compact and the Anti-Bribery Convention.

LO4 DESCRIBE **management's role in encouraging ethical behavior.**

The behavior of managers is the single most important influence on an individual's decision to act ethically or unethically. Some specific ways managers can encourage

ethical behavior include paying attention to employee selection, having and using a code of ethics, recognizing the important ethical leadership role they play and how what they do is far more important than what they say, making sure that goals and the performance appraisal process don't reward goal achievement without taking into account how those goals were achieved, using ethics training and independent social audits, and establishing protective mechanisms.

LO5 DISCUSS **current social responsibility and ethics issues.**

Managers can manage ethical lapses and social irresponsibility by being strong ethical leaders and by protecting employees who raise ethical issues. The example set by managers has a strong influence on whether employees behave ethically. Ethical leaders also are honest, share their values, stress important shared values, and use the reward system appropriately. Managers can protect whistle-blowers (employees who raise ethical issues or concerns) by encouraging them to come forward, by setting up toll-free ethics hotlines, and by establishing a culture in which employees can complain and be heard without fear of reprisal. Social entrepreneurs play an important role in solving social problems by seeking out opportunities to improve society by using practical, innovative, and sustainable approaches. Social entrepreneurs want to make the world a better place and have a driving passion to make that happen. Businesses can promote positive social change through corporate philanthropy and employee volunteering efforts.

MyManagementLab

Go to **mymanagementlab.com** to complete the problems marked with this icon ⭐.

⭐ REVIEW AND DISCUSSION QUESTIONS

1. Differentiate between social obligation, social responsiveness, and social responsibility.

2. What does social responsibility mean to you personally? Do *you* think business organizations should be socially responsible? Explain.

3. What factors influence whether a person behaves ethically or unethically? Explain all relevant factors.

4. Do you think values-based management is just a "do-gooder" ploy? Explain your answer.

5. Internet file sharing programs are popular among college students. These programs work by allowing nonorganizational users to access any local network where desired files are located. Because these types of file sharing programs tend to clog bandwidth,

local users' ability to access and use a local network is reduced. What ethical and social responsibilities does a university have in this situation? To whom do they have a responsibility? What guidelines might you suggest for university decision makers?

6. What are some problems that could be associated with employee whistle-blowing for (a) the whistle-blower and (b) the organization?

7. Describe the characteristics and behaviors of someone you consider to be an ethical person. How could the types of decisions and actions this person engages in be encouraged in a workplace?

8. Explain the ethical and social responsibility issues facing managers today.

MyManagementLab

If your professor has assigned these, go to **mymanagementlab.com** for Auto-graded writing questions as well as the following Assisted-graded writing questions:

9. What is green management and how can organizations go green?

10. Discuss specific ways managers can encourage ethical behavior.

PREPARING FOR: My Career

⊕ PERSONAL INVENTORY ASSESSMENTS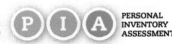

Ethical Leadership Assessment

Organizations need ethical leadership from all employees, but especially from managers. In this PIA, you'll see how much thought and effort goes into your being ethical in your workplace behavior.

⊕ ETHICS DILEMMA

70 percent of adults say that most students cheat at least once in school. • 42 percent of those same adults said they cheated on a test or exam while in school.[111]

Cheating. Is technology enabling more cheating on tests and exams? Students cheating (or trying to cheat) isn't new. It's an age-old battle in education. However, the battle has become much more sophisticated. From hacking to wirelessly transmitting questions outside the testing room to installing a keylogger (a small device that can be placed in the back of a computer to monitor keystrokes) on a teacher's computer—technology has enabled those bent on cheating more ways, and more sophisticated ways, to get it done.

11. Cheating scandals uncovered at Harvard, the Air Force Academy, New York City's Stuyvesant High School, Corona del Mar, and many others are often described as having a "culture of cheating."[112] Explain what you think this means. Could such a culture be changed? If so, how? If not, why not?

12. Do you think that those who use technology to cheat know that what they're doing is wrong and that it's damaging their education? Explain.

13. What might work best for controlling high-tech cheating—changing people's attitudes towards cheating or developing high-tech deterrents to make sure cheating can't take place? Explain.

SKILLS EXERCISE Developing Your Building Trust Skill

About the Skill

Trust plays an important role in the manager's relationships with his or her employees.[113] Given the importance of trust in setting a good ethical example for employees, today's managers should actively seek to develop it within their work group.

Steps in Practicing the Skill

- *Practice openness.* Mistrust comes as much from what people don't know as from what they do. Being open with employees leads to confidence and trust. Keep people informed. Make clear the criteria you use in making decisions. Explain the rationale for your decisions. Be forthright and candid about problems. Fully disclose all relevant information.

- *Be fair.* Before making decisions or taking actions, consider how others will perceive them in terms of objectivity and fairness. Give credit where credit is due. Be objective and impartial in performance appraisals. Pay attention to equity perceptions in distributing rewards.

- *Speak your feelings.* Managers who convey only hard facts come across as cold, distant, and unfeeling. When you share your feelings, others will see that you are real

and human. They will know you for who you are and their respect for you is likely to increase.

- *Tell the truth.* Being trustworthy means being credible. If honesty is critical to credibility, then you must be perceived as someone who tells the truth. Employees are more tolerant of hearing something "they don't want to hear" than of finding out that their manager lied to them.

- *Be consistent.* People want predictability. Mistrust comes from not knowing what to expect. Take the time to think about your values and beliefs, and let those values and beliefs consistently guide your decisions. When you know what's important to you, your actions will follow, and you will project a consistency that earns trust.

- *Fulfill your promises.* Trust requires that people believe that you are dependable. You need to ensure that you keep your word. Promises made must be promises kept.

- *Maintain confidences.* You trust those whom you believe to be discreet and those on whom you can rely. If people open up to you and make themselves vulnerable by telling you something in confidence, they need to feel assured you won't discuss it with others or betray that confidence.

If people perceive you as someone who leaks personal confidences or someone who can't be depended on, you've lost their trust.

- *Demonstrate competence.* Develop the admiration and respect of others by demonstrating technical and professional ability. Pay particular attention to developing and displaying your communication, negotiation, and other interpersonal skills.

Practicing the Skill

Read through the following scenario. Write a paper describing how you would handle the situation. Be sure to refer to the eight behaviors described previously for developing trust.

Scenario

Donna Romines is the shipping department manager at Tastefully Tempting, a gourmet candy company based in Phoenix. Orders for the company's candy come from around the world. Your six-member team processes these orders. Needless to say, the two months before Christmas are quite hectic. Everybody counts the days until December 24 when the phones finally stop ringing off the wall, at least for a couple of days. You and all of your team members breathe a sigh of relief as the last box of candy is sent on its way out the door.

When the company was first founded five years ago, after the holiday rush, the owners would shut down Tastefully Tempting for two weeks after Christmas. However, as the business has grown and moved into Internet sales, that practice has become too costly. There's too much business to be able to afford that luxury. And the rush for Valentine's Day orders start pouring in the week after Christmas. Although the two-week, post-holiday, company-wide shutdown has been phased out formally, some departments have found it difficult to get employees to gear up once again after the Christmas break. The employees who come to work after Christmas usually accomplish little. This year, though, things have got to change. You know that the cultural "tradition" won't be easy to overcome, but your shipping team needs to be ready to tackle the orders that have piled up. After all, Tastefully Tempting's customers want their orders filled promptly and correctly!

WORKING TOGETHER Team Exercise

In an effort to be (or at least appear to be) socially responsible, many organizations donate money to philanthropic and charitable causes. In addition, many organizations ask their employees to make individual donations to these causes. Suppose you're the manager of a work team, and you know that several of your employees can't afford to pledge money right now because of personal or financial problems. You've also been told by your supervisor that the CEO has been known to check the list of individual contributors to see who is and is not "supporting these very important causes." Working together in a small group of three or four, answer the following questions:

- How would you handle this situation?
- What ethical guidelines might you suggest for individual and organizational contributions in such a situation?
- Create a company policy statement that expresses your ethical guidelines.

MY TURN TO BE A MANAGER

- Find five different examples of organizational codes of ethics. Using Exhibit 7, describe what each contains. Compare and contrast the examples.

- Using the examples of codes of ethics you found, create what you feel would be an appropriate and effective organizational code of ethics. In addition, create your own *personal code of ethics* you can use as a guide to ethical dilemmas.

- Take advantage of volunteer opportunities. Be sure to include these on your résumé. If possible, try to do things in these volunteer positions that will improve your managerial skills in planning, organizing, leading, or controlling.

- Go to the Global Reporting Initiative Web site (www. globalreporting.org) and choose three businesses from the list that have filed reports. Look at those reports and describe/evaluate what's in them. In addition, identify the stakeholders that might be affected and how they might be affected by the company's actions.

- Make a list of what green management things your school is doing. If you're working, make a list of what green management things your employer is doing. Do some research on being green. Are there additional things your school or employer could be doing? Write a report to each describing any suggestions. (Look for ways you could use these suggestions to be more "green" in your personal life.)

- Over the course of two weeks, see what ethical "dilemmas" you observe. These could be ones you face personally or they could be ones that others (friends, colleagues, other students talking in the hallway or before class, and so forth) face. Write these dilemmas down

and think about what you might do if faced with that dilemma.

- Interview two different managers about how they encourage their employees to be ethical. Write down their comments and discuss how these ideas might help you be a better manager.

- If you have the opportunity, take a class on business or managerial ethics or on social responsibility—often called

business and society—or both. Not only will this look good on your résumé, it could help you personally grapple with some of the tough issues managers face in being ethical and responsible.

- In your own words, write down three things you learned in this text about being a good manager. Keep a copy of this for future reference.

CASE APPLICATION 1 A Better Tomorrow

It's an incredibly simple but potentially world-changing idea.[114] For each pair of shoes sold, a pair is donated to a child in need. That's the business model followed by TOMS Shoes. During a visit to Argentina in 2006 as a contestant on the CBS reality show *The Amazing Race,* Blake Mycoskie, founder of TOMS, "saw lots of kids with no shoes who were suffering from injuries to their feet." Just think what it would be like to be barefoot, not by choice, but from lack of availability and ability to own a pair. He was so moved by the experience that he wanted to do something. That something is what TOMS does now by blending charity with commerce. (The name TOMS is actually short for "Shoes for a better tomorrow," which eventually became "Tomorrow's Shoes," which then became "Toms.") And a better tomorrow is what Blake wanted to provide to shoeless children around the world. Those shoe donations have been central to the success of the TOMS brand, which is popular among tweens, teens, and twenty-somethings. And TOMS has helped provide more than 1 million shoes to kids in need in the United States and abroad since its founding. Hoping to build on this success, the company recently launched its second one-for-one product—an eyewear line whose sales will help provide improved vision to those in need.

⭐ DISCUSSION QUESTIONS

14. How can TOMS balance being socially responsible *and* being focused on profits?

15. Would you describe TOMS' approach as social obligation, social responsiveness, or social responsibility? Explain.

16. It's time to think like a manager. TOMS' one-for-one approach is a wonderful idea, but what would be involved with making it work?

17. Do you think consumers are drawn to products with a charitable connection? Why or why not?

Lessons from Lehman Brothers: Will We Ever Learn?

On September 15, 2008, financial services firm Lehman Brothers filed for bankruptcy with the U.S. Bankruptcy Court in the Southern District of New York.[115] That action—the largest Chapter 11 filing in financial history—started an escalating and spiraling "crisis of confidence" that destabilized world financial markets and set off the worst financial scenario since the Great Depression. The fall of this Wall Street icon is, unfortunately, not a new thing, as we've seen in the stories of Enron, WorldCom, and others. In a report released by bankruptcy court-appointed examiner Anton Valukas, Lehman executives and the firm's auditor, Ernst & Young, were lambasted for actions that led to the firm's collapse. Valukas said, "Lehman repeatedly exceeded its own internal risk limits and controls, and a wide range of bad calls by its management led to the bank's failure." Let's look behind the scenes at some of the issues.

One of the major problems at Lehman was its culture and reward structure. Excessive risk taking by employees was openly lauded and rewarded handsomely. Individuals making questionable deals were hailed and treated as "conquering heroes." On the other hand, anyone who questioned decisions was often ignored or overruled. For instance, Oliver Budde, who served as an associate general counsel at Lehman for nine years, was responsible for preparing the firm's public filings on executive compensation. Infuriated by what he felt was the firm's "intentional under-representation of how much top executives were paid," Budde argued with his bosses for years about that matter, to no avail. Then, one time he objected to a tax deal that an outside accounting firm had proposed to lower medical insurance costs saying, "My gut feeling was that this was just reshuffling some papers to get an expense off the balance sheet. It was not the right thing, and I told them." However, Budde's bosses disagreed and okayed the deal.

Another problem at Lehman was the firm's top leadership. Valukas's report was highly critical of Lehman's executives who "should have done more, done better." He pointed out that the executives made the company's problems worse by their conduct, which ranged from "serious but nonculpable errors of business judgment to actionable balance sheet manipulation." Valukas went on to say that "former chief executive Richard Fuld was at least grossly negligent in causing Lehman to file misleading periodic reports." These reports were part of an accounting device called "Repo 105." Lehman used this device to get some $50 billion of undesirable assets off its balance sheet at the end of the first and second quarters of 2008, instead of selling those assets at a loss. The examiner's report "included e-mails from Lehman's global financial controller confirming that the only purpose or motive for Repo 105 transactions was reduction in the balance sheet, adding that there was no substance to the transactions." Lehman's auditor was aware of the use of Repo 105 but did not challenge or question it. Sufficient evidence indicated that Fuld knew about the use of it as well; however, he signed off on quarterly reports that made no mention of it. Fuld's attorney claimed that Mr. Fuld had no knowledge of these transactions or how they were recorded on the books since he was not involved in structuring or negotiating them. A spokesperson from auditor Ernst & Young said that Lehman's bankruptcy was due to several unprecedented unfavorable and hostile events in the financial markets.

⭐ DISCUSSION QUESTIONS

18. Describe the situation at Lehman Brothers from an ethics perspective. What's your opinion of what happened here?

19. What was the culture at Lehman Brothers like? How did this culture contribute to the company's downfall?

20. What role did Lehman's executives play in the company's collapse? Were they being responsible and ethical? Discuss.

21. Could anything have been done differently at Lehman Brothers to prevent what happened? Explain.

22. After all the public uproar over Enron and then the passage of the Sarbanes-Oxley Act to protect shareholders, why do you think we still continue to see these types of situations? Is it unreasonable to expect that businesses can and should act ethically?

ENDNOTES

1. S. Welch, "The Uh-Oh Feeling: Sticky Situations at Work," www.oprah.com/money/, from the November 2007 issue of *O, the Oprah Magazine*.

2. A. Tugend, "In Life and Business, Learning to Be Ethical," *New York Times Online*, January 10, 2014.

3. A. Goodman, "The Dilemma: Addicted & Conflicted About Laughing at the Afflicted," www.globalethics.org/newsline, June 3, 2013; and T. Lickona, *Character Matters: How to Help Our Children Develop Good Judgment, Integrity, and Other Essential Virtues* (New York: Touchstone Publishing, 2004).

4. M. L. Barnett, "Stakeholder Influence Capacity and the Variability of Financial Returns to Corporate Social Responsibility," *Academy of Management Review*, July 2007, pp. 794–816; A. Mackey, T. B. Mackey, and J. B. Barney, "Corporate Social Responsibility and Firm Performance: Investor Preferences and Corporate Strategies," *Academy of Management Review*, July 2007, pp. 817–835; and A. B. Carroll, "A Three-Dimensional Conceptual Model of Corporate Performance," *Academy of Management Review*, October 1979, p. 499.

5. See K. Basu and G. Palazzo, "Corporate Social Performance: A Process Model of Sensemaking," *Academy of Management Review*, January 2008, pp. 122–136; and S. P. Sethi, "A Conceptual Framework for Environmental Analysis of Social Issues and Evaluation of Business Response Patterns," *Academy of Management Review*, January 1979, pp. 68–74.

6. M. Friedman, *Capitalism and Freedom* (Chicago: University of Chicago Press, 1962); and Friedman, "The Social Responsibility of Business Is to Increase Profits," *New York Times Magazine*, September 13, 1970, p. 33.

7. V. Vermaelen, "An Innovative Approach to Funding CSR Projects," *Harvard Business Review*, June 2011, p. 28; S. Strom, "To Be Good Citizens, Report Says Companies Should Just Focus on Bottom Line," *New York Times Online*, June 14, 2011; and A. Karnani, "The Case Against Social Responsibility," *Wall Street Journal*, August 23, 2010, pp. R1+.

8. S. Lohr, "First, Make Money. Also, Do Good," *New York Times Online*, August 13, 2011; and S. Liebs, "Do Companies Do Good Well?" *CFO*, July 2007, p. 16.

9. See, for example, D. J. Wood, "Corporate Social Performance Revisited," *Academy of Management Review*, October 1991, pp. 703–708; and S. L. Wartick and P. L. Cochran, "The Evolution of the Corporate Social Performance Model," *Academy of Management Review*, October 1985, p. 763.

10. N. Bunkley, "Ford Backs Ban on Text Messaging by Drivers," *New York Times Online*, September 11, 2009.

11. B. X. Chen, "Tech Companies Respond to Japan Quake With Resources, Support," wired.com, March 15, 2011; and J. O'Donnell, "UPS Workers Head to Haiti to Provide Help," *USA Today*, January 25, 2010, p. 4B.

12. See, for example, R. A. Buchholz, *Essentials of Public Policy for Management*, 2d ed. (Upper Saddle River, NJ: Prentice Hall, 1990).

13. I. Brat, "The Extra Step," *Wall Street Journal*, March 24, 2008, p. R12.

14. S. Strom, "Chick-fil-A Commits to Stop Sales of Poultry Raised with Antibiotics," *New York Times Online*, February 11, 2014; and "CVS to Become First Major U.S. Drugstore to Drop Cigarettes," foxnews.com, February 5, 2014.

15. This section is based on J. D. Margolis and J. P. Walsh, "Misery Loves Companies: Rethinking Social Initiatives by Business," *Administrative Science Quarterly*, vol. 48, no. 2, 2003, pp. 268–305; K. Davis and W. C. Frederick, *Business and Society: Management, Public Policy, Ethics*, 5th ed. (New York: McGraw-Hill, 1984), pp. 28–41; and R. J. Monsen Jr., "The Social Attitudes of Management," in J. M. McGuire (ed.), *Contemporary Management: Issues and Views* (Upper Saddle River, NJ: Prentice Hall, 1974), p. 616.

16. See, for instance, J. Surroca, J. A. Tribo, and S. Waddock, "Corporate Responsibility and Financial Performance: The Role of Intangible Resources," *Strategic Management Journal*, May 2010, pp. 463–490; R. Garcia-Castro, M. A. Ariño, and M. A. Canela, "Does Social Performance Really Lead to Financial Performance? Accounting for Endogeneity," *Journal of Business Ethics*, March 2010, pp. 107–126; J. Peloza, "The Challenge of Measuring Financial Impacts from Investments in Corporate Social Performance," *Journal of Management*, December 2009, pp. 1518–1541; J. D. Margolis and H. Anger Elfenbein, "Do Well by Doing Good? Don't Count on It," *Harvard Business Review*, January 2008, pp. 19–20; M. L. Barnett, "Stakeholder Influence Capacity and the Variability of Financial Returns to Corporate Social Responsibility," 2007; D. O. Neubaum and S. A. Zahra, "Institutional Ownership and Corporate Social Performance: The Moderating Effects of Investment Horizon, Activism, and Coordination," *Journal of Management*, February 2006, pp. 108–131; B. A. Waddock and S. B. Graves, "The Corporate Social Performance–Financial Performance Link," *Strategic Management Journal*, April 1997, pp. 303–319; J. B. McGuire, A. Sundgren, and T. Schneeweis, "Corporate Social Responsibility and Firm Financial Performance," *Academy of Management Journal*, December 1988, pp. 854–872; K. Aupperle, A. B. Carroll, and J. D. Hatfield, "An Empirical Examination of the Relationship Between Corporate Social Responsibility and Profitability," *Academy of Management Journal*, June 1985, pp. 446–463; and P. Cochran and R. A. Wood, "Corporate Social Responsibility and Financial Performance," *Academy of Management Journal*, March 1984, pp. 42–56.

17. Peloza, "The Challenge of Measuring Financial Impacts from Investments in Corporate Social Performance."

18. B. Seifert, S. A. Morris, and B. R. Bartkus, "Having, Giving, and Getting: Slack Resources, Corporate Philanthropy, and Firm Financial Performance," *Business & Society,* June 2004, pp. 135–161; and McGuire, Sundgren, and Schneeweis, "Corporate Social Responsibility and Firm Financial Performance."

19. A. McWilliams and D. Siegel, "Corporate Social Responsibility and Financial Performance: Correlation or Misspecification?" *Strategic Management Journal,* June 2000, pp. 603–609.

20. A. J. Hillman and G. D. Keim, "Shareholder Value, Stakeholder Management, and Social Issues: What's the Bottom Line?" *Strategic Management Journal,* vol. 22, 2001, pp. 125–139.

21. M. Orlitzky, F. L. Schmidt, and S. L. Rynes, "Corporate Social and Financial Performance," *Organization Studies,* vol. 24, no. 3, 2003, pp. 403–441.

22. "Growth of Sustainable and Responsible Investment," The Forum for Sustainable and Responsible Investment, www.ussif.org, March 29, 2014; R. Kapadia, "Blind Faith," *SmartMoney,* February 2011, pp. 72–76; and A. Hughey and P. Villareal, "Socially Responsible Investing," *National Center for Policy Analysis* [www.ncpa.org/pdfs/ba657.pdf], May 11, 2009.

23. Social Investment Forum, "Socially Responsible Mutual Fund Charts: Financial Performance," www.socialinvest.org/resources/performance.cfm, April 28, 2010.

24. "Sustainability: Just Do It," *Industry Week,* February 2014, pp. 22–23.

25. A. Salkever, "Why Are Coke Drinkers Smiling? Vending Machines to Be More Eco-Friendly," *Daily Finance Online* [www.dailyfinance.com], December 3, 2009.

26. "Hive Mentality," *Body + Soul,* December 2009, p. 26.

27. "The Total Package," *Bloomberg BusinessWeek,* March 19 March 25, 2012, p. 6.

28. J. Yang and P. Trap, "Applying Green Tech at Work," *USA Today,* May 13, 2013, p. 1B.

29. D. A. Lubin and D. C. Esty, "The Sustainability Imperative," *Harvard Business Review,* May 2010, pp. 42–50; J. Pfeffer, "Building Sustainable Organizations: The Human Factor," *Academy of Management Perspectives,* February 2010, pp. 34–45; R. Nidumolu, C. K. Prahalad, and M. R. Rangaswami, "Why Sustainability Is Now the Key Driver of Innovation," *Harvard Business Review,* September 2009, pp. 56–64; A. A. Marcus and A. R. Fremeth, "Green Management Matters Regardless," *Academy of Management Perspectives,* August 2009, pp. 17–27; D. S. Siegel, "Green Management Matters Only If It Yields More Green: An Economic/Strategic Perspective," *Academy of Management Perspectives,* August 2009, pp. 5–16; and A. White, "The Greening of the Balance Sheet," *Harvard Business Review,* March 2006, pp. 27–28.

30. The concept of shades of green can be found in R. E. Freeman, J. Pierce, and R. Dodd, *Shades of Green: Business Ethics and the Environment* (New York: Oxford University Press, 1995).

31. Leader Making a Difference box based on "Questions for Rick Ridgeway," *Fortune,* September 16, 2013, p. 25; C. Winter, "Patagonia's Latest Product: A Venture Fund," *Bloomberg BusinessWeek,* May 13–19, 2013, pp. 23–24; One Percent for the Planet, http://www.onepercentfortheplanet.org/en/, June 12, 2012; S. Stevenson, "Patagonia's Founder Is America's Most Unlikely Business Guru," *Wall Street Journal Magazine,* May 2012; "Responsible Company," *Wall Street Journal Online,* April 25, 2012; T. Henneman, "Patagonia Fills Payroll With People Who Are Passionate," *Workforce Management Online,* November 4, 2011; M. J. Ybarra, "Book Review: The Fun Hog Expedition Revisited," *Wall Street Journal,* February 19, 2010, p. W8; K. Garber, "Not in the Business of Hurting the Planet," *US News & World Report,* November 2009, p. 63; and T. Foster, "No Such Thing As Sustainability," *Fast Company,* July/August 2009, pp. 46–48.

32. The Global 100 list is a collaborative effort of Corporate Knights Inc. and Innovest Strategic Value Advisors. Information from Global 100 Web site [www.global100.org], January 22, 2014.

33. C. Hausman, "Financial News Focuses on Questions of Ethics," *Ethics Newsline* [www.globalethics.org/newsline], April 20, 2010; C. Hausman, "Privacy Issues Prominent in Week's Tech News," *Ethics Newsline* [www.globalethics.org/newsline], March 9, 2010; and H. Maurer and C. Lindblad, "Madoff Gets the Max," *Bloomberg BusinessWeek,* July 13 & 20, 2009, p. 6.

34. This last example is based on J. F. Viega, T. D. Golden, and K. Dechant, "Why Managers Bend Company Rules," *Academy of Management Executive,* May 2004, pp. 84–90.

35. K. Davis and W. C. Frederick, *Business and Society*, p. 76.

36. F. D. Sturdivant, *Business and Society: A Managerial Approach,* 3rd ed. (Homewood, IL: Richard D. Irwin, 1985), p. 128.

37. L. K. Treviño, G. R. Weaver, and S. J. Reynolds, "Behavioral Ethics in Organizations: A Review," *Journal of Management,* December 2006, pp. 951–990; T. Kelley, "To Do Right or Just to Be Legal," *New York Times,* February 8, 1998, p. BU12; J. W. Graham, "Leadership, Moral Development, and Citizenship Behavior," *Business Ethics Quarterly,* January 1995, pp. 43–54; L. Kohlberg, *Essays in Moral Development: The Psychology of Moral Development,* vol. 2 (New York: Harper & Row, 1984); and L. Kohlberg, *Essays in Moral Development: The Philosophy of Moral Development,* vol. 1 (New York: Harper & Row, 1981).

38. See, for example, J. Weber, "Managers' Moral Reasoning: Assessing Their Responses to Three Moral Dilemmas," *Human Relations,* July 1990, pp. 687–702.

39. W. C. Frederick and J. Weber, "The Value of Corporate Managers and Their Critics: An Empirical Description and Normative Implications," in W. C. Frederick and L. E. Preston (eds.) *Business Ethics: Research Issues and Empirical Studies* (Greenwich, CT: JAI Press, 1990), pp. 123–144; and J. H. Barnett and M. J. Karson, "Personal Values and Business Decisions: An Exploratory Investigation," *Journal of Business Ethics,* July 1987, pp. 371–382.

40. K. Strom-Gottfried, "A Personal Take on Global Ethics," *Ethics Newsline,* globalethics.org, March 25, 2013; and "Creating-Value Skeptics," *Ethics Newsline,* globalethics.org, August 13, 2012.

41. M. E. Baehr, J. W. Jones, and A. J. Nerad, "Psychological Correlates of Business Ethics Orientation in Executives," *Journal of Business and Psychology,* Spring 1993, pp. 291–308; and L. K. Treviño and S. A. Youngblood, "Bad Apples in Bad Barrels: A Causal Analysis of Ethical Decision-Making Behavior," *Journal of Applied Psychology,* August 1990, pp. 378–385.

42. M. E. Schweitzer, L. Ordonez, and B. Douma, "Goal Setting as a Motivator of Unethical Behavior," *Academy of Management Journal,* June 2004, pp. 422–432.

43. M. C. Jensen, "Corporate Budgeting is Broken—Let's Fix It," *Harvard Business Review,* June 2001, pp. 94–101.

44. R. L. Cardy and T. T. Selvarajan, "Assessing Ethical Behavior Revisited: The Impact of Outcomes on Judgment Bias," paper presented at the Annual Meeting of the Academy of Management, Toronto, 2000.

45. M. H. Bazerman and A. E. Tenbrunsel, "Ethical Breakdowns," *Harvard Business Review,* April 2011, pp. 58–65.

46. M. C. Gentile, "Keeping Your Colleagues Honest," *Harvard Business Review,* March 2010, pp. 114–117; J. R. Edwards and D. M. Cable, "The Value of Value Congruence," *Journal of Applied Psychology,* May 2009, pp. 654–677; G. Weaver, "Ethics and Employees: Making the Connection," *Academy of Management Executive,* May 2004, pp. 121–125; V. Anand, B. E. Ashforth, and M. Joshi, "Business as Usual: The Acceptance and Perpetuation of Corruption in Organizations," *Academy of Management Executive,* May 2004, pp. 39–53; J. Weber, L. B. Kurke, and D. W. Pentico, "Why Do Employees Steal?" *Business & Society,* September 2003, pp. 359–380; V. Arnold and J. C. Lampe, "Understanding the Factors Underlying Ethical Organizations: Enabling Continuous Ethical Improvement," *Journal of Applied Business Research,* Summer 1999, pp. 1–19.

47. P. Van Lee, L. Fabish, and N. McCaw, "The Value of Corporate Values," *Strategy & Business,* Summer 2005, pp. 52–65.

48. F. O. Walumba and J. Schaubroeck, "Leader Personality Traits and Employee Voice Behavior: Mediating Roles of Ethical Leadership and Work Group Psychological Safety," *Journal of Applied Psychology,* September 2009, pp. 1275–1286; G. Weaver, "Ethics and Employees: Making the Connection," May 2004; G. Weaver, L. K. Treviño, and P. L. Cochran, "Integrated and Decoupled Corporate Social Performance: Management Commitments, External Pressures, and Corporate Ethics Practices," *Academy of Management Journal,* October 1999, pp. 539–552; G. R. Weaver, L. K. Treviño, and P. L. Cochran, "Corporate Ethics Programs as Control Systems: Influences of Executive Commitment

and Environmental Factors," *Academy of Management Journal*, February 1999, pp. 41–57; R. B. Morgan, "Self- and Co-Worker Perceptions of Ethics and Their Relationships to Leadership and Salary," *Academy of Management Journal*, February 1993, pp. 200–214; and B. Z. Posner and W. H. Schmidt, "Values and the American Manager: An Update," *California Management Review*, Spring 1984, pp. 202–216.

49. National Business Ethics Survey of the U.S. Workforce, 2013, *Ethics Resource Center* [www.ethics.org], March, 2014.

50. Ibid.

51. S. Watkins, "Set Example, Train Employees to Build Ethical Culture," investors.com, February 28, 2013.

52. IBM Corporate Responsibility Report, 2007 [www.ibm.com]; and A. Schultz, "Integrating IBM," *CRO*, March/April 2007, pp. 16–21.

53. T. Barnett, "Dimensions of Moral Intensity and Ethical Decision Making: An Empirical Study," *Journal of Applied Social Psychology*, May 2001, pp. 1038–1057; and T. M. Jones, "Ethical Decision Making by Individuals in Organizations: An Issue-Contingent Model," *Academy of Management Review*, April 1991, pp. 366–395.

54. W. Bailey and A. Spicer, "When Does National Identity Matter? Convergence and Divergence in International Business Ethics," *Academy of Management Journal*, December 2007, pp. 1462–1480; and R. L. Sims, "Comparing Ethical Attitudes Across Cultures," *Cross Cultural Management: An International Journal*, vol. 13, no. 2, 2006, pp. 101–113.

55. BBC News Online, "Legal Review of Overseas Bribery," November 29, 2007.

56. C. Hausman, "British Defense Giant BAE Must Hire Ethics Monitor and Pay Huge Penalties Under Corruption Settlement," *Ethics Newsline* [www.globalethics.org], February 15, 2010.

57. "DOJ Enforcement of the FCPA—Year in Review," www.fcpaprofessor.com, January 8, 2014.

58. L. Paine, R. Deshpande, J. D. Margolis, and K. E. Bettcher, "Up to Code: Does Your Company's Conduct Meet World-Class Standards?" *Harvard Business Review*, December 2005, pp. 122–133; G. R. Simpson, "Global Heavyweights Vow 'Zero Tolerance' for Bribes," *Wall Street Journal*, January 27, 2005, pp. A2+; A. Spicer, T. W. Dunfee, and W. J. Bailey, "Does National Context Matter in Ethical Decision Making? An Empirical Test of Integrative Social Contracts Theory," *Academy of Management Journal*, August 2004, pp. 610–620; J. White and S. Taft, "Frameworks for Teaching and Learning Business Ethics Within the Global Context: Background of Ethical Theories," *Journal of Management Education*, August 2004, pp. 463–477; J. Guyon, "CEOs on Managing Globally," *Fortune*, July 26, 2004, p. 169; A. B. Carroll, "Managing Ethically with Global Stakeholders: A Present and Future Challenge," *Academy of Management Executive*, May 2004, pp. 114–120; and C. J. Robertson and W. F. Crittenden, "Mapping Moral Philosophies: Strategic Implications for Multinational Firms," *Strategic Management Journal*, April 2003, pp. 385–392.

59. United Nations Global Compact, http://www.unglobalcompact.org/ParticipantsAndStakeholders/index.html, March 31, 2014.

60. Organization for Economic Cooperation and Development, "About Bribery in International Business," www.oecd.org, April 30, 2010.

61. R. M. Kidder, "Can Disobedience Save Wall Street?" *Ethics Newsline* [www.globalethics.org], May 3, 2010.

62. Enron example taken from P. M. Lencioni, "Make Your Values Mean Something," *Harvard Business Review*, July 2002, p. 113; and Sears example taken from series of posters called "Sears Ethics and Business Practices: A Century of Tradition," in *Business Ethics*, May/June 1999, pp. 12–13; and B. J. Feder, "The Harder Side of Sears," *New York Times*, July 20, 1997, pp. BU1+.

63. B. Roberts, "Your Cheating Heart," *HR Magazine*, June 2011, pp. 55–60.

64. J. R. Edwards and D. M. Cable, "The Value of Value Congruence," *Journal of Applied Psychology*, May 2009, pp. 654–677; and Treviño and Youngblood, "Bad Apples in Bad Barrels," p. 384.

65. K. Bart, "UBS Lays Out Employee Ethics Code," *Wall Street Journal Online* [online.wsj.com], January 12, 2010; J. L. Lunsford, "Transformer in Transition," *Wall Street Journal*, May 17, 2007, pp. B1+; and J. S. McClenahen, "UTC's Master of Principle," *Industry Week*, January 2003, pp. 30–36.

66. M. Weinstein, "Survey Says: Ethics Training Works," *Training*, November 2005, p. 15.

67. J. E. Fleming, "Codes of Ethics for Global Corporations," *Academy of Management News*, June 2005, p. 4.

68. "Corporate Codes of Ethics Spread," *Ethics Newsline* [www.globalethics.org], October 12, 2009; "Global Ethics Codes Gain Importance as a Tool to Avoid Litigation and Fines," *Wall Street Journal*, August 19, 1999, p. A1; and J. Alexander, "On the Right Side," *World Business*, January/February 1997, pp. 38–41.

69. F. R. David, "An Empirical Study of Codes of Business Ethics: A Strategic Perspective," paper presented at the 48th Annual Academy of Management Conference; Anaheim, California, August 1988.

70. National Business Ethics Survey of the U.S. Workforce, 2013, *Ethics Resource Center* [www.ethics.org], March, 2014.

71. J. B. Singh, "Determinants of the Effectiveness of Corporate Codes of Ethics: An Empirical Study," *Journal of Business Ethics*, July 2011, pp. 385–395; P. M. Erwin, "Corporate Codes of Conduct: The Effects of Code Content and Quality on Ethical Performance," *Journal of Business Ethics*, April 2011, pp. 535–548; "Codes of Conduct," Center for Ethical Business Cultures [www.cebcglobal.org], February 15, 2006; L. Paine, R. Deshpande, J. D. Margolis, and K. E. Bettcher, "Up to Code: Does Your Company's Conduct Meet World-Class Standards"; and A. K. Reichert and M. S. Webb, "Corporate Support for Ethical and Environmental Policies: A Financial Management Perspective," *Journal of Business Ethics*, May 2000.

72. L-M. Eleftheriou-Smith, "Apple's Tim Cook: 'Business Isn't Just About Making Profit'"; and P. Elmer-Dewitt, "Apple's Tim Cook Picks a Fight with Climate Change Deniers," tech.fortune.com, March 1, 2014.

73. National Business Ethics Survey of the U.S. Workforce, 2013, *Ethics Resource Center* [www.ethics.org], March, 2014.

74. V. Wessler, "Integrity and Clogged Plumbing," *Straight to the Point*, newsletter of VisionPoint Corporation, Fall 2002, pp. 1–2.

75. National Business Ethics Survey of the U.S. Workforce, 2013, Ethics Resource Center [www.ethics.org/nbes], 2014.

76. T. A. Gavin, "Ethics Education," *Internal Auditor*, April 1989, pp. 54–57.

77. L. Myyry and K. Helkama, "The Role of Value Priorities and Professional Ethics Training in Moral Sensitivity," *Journal of Moral Education*, 2002, vol. 31, no. 1, pp. 35–50; W. Penn and B. D. Collier, "Current Research in Moral Development as a Decision Support System," *Journal of Business Ethics*, January 1985, pp. 131–136.

78. J. A. Byrne, "After Enron: The Ideal Corporation," *Business Week*, August 19, 2002, pp. 68–71; D. Rice and C. Dreilinger, "Rights and Wrongs of Ethics Training," *Training & Development Journal*, May 1990, pp. 103–109; and J. Weber, "Measuring the Impact of Teaching Ethics to Future Managers: A Review, Assessment, and Recommendations," *Journal of Business Ethics*, April 1990, pp. 182–190.

79. E. White, "What Would You Do? Ethics Courses Get Context," *Wall Street Journal*, June 12, 2006, p. B3; and D. Zielinski, "The Right Direction: Can Ethics Training Save Your Company?" *Training*, June 2005, pp. 27–32.

80. G. Farrell and J. O'Donnell, "Ethics Training as Taught by Ex-Cons: Crime Doesn't Pay," *USA Today*, November 16, 2005, p. 1B+.

81. J. Weber, "The New Ethics Enforcers," *Business Week*, February 13, 2006, pp. 76–77.

82. G. J. Millman and S. Rubenfeld, "For Corporate America, Risk is Big Business," *Wall Street Journal*, January 16, 2014, pp. B1+; and G. J. Millman and B. DiPietro, "For Compliance Chiefs, Who's the Boss?" *Wall Street Journal*, January 16, 2014, p. B7.

83. "Survey Reveals How Many Workers Commit Office Taboos," *Ethics Newsline* [www.globalethics.org], September 18, 2007.

84. C. Hausman, "Men Are Less Ethical than Women, Claims Researcher," *Ethics Newsline*, www.globaletehics.org/newsline, June 25, 2012; and C. May, "When Men Are Less Moral Than Women," ScientificAmerican.com, June 19, 2012.

85. H. Oh, "Biz Majors Get an F for Honesty," *Business Week*, February 6, 2006, p. 14.

86. "Students Aren't Squealers," *USA Today*, March 27, 2003, p. 1D; and J. Merritt, "You Mean Cheating Is Wrong?" *Business Week*, December 9, 2002, p. 8.

87. J. Hyatt, "Unethical Behavior: Largely Unreported in Offices and Justified by Teens," *The CRO Online*, February 13, 2008.

88. D. Lidsky, "Transparency: It's Not Just for Shrink Wrap Anymore," *Fast Company,* January 2005, p. 87.

89. S. S. Wiltermuth and F. J. Flynn, "Power, Moral Clarity, and Punishment in the Workplace," *Academy of Management Journal,* August 2013, pp. 1002–1023; M. Crossnan, D. Mazutis, G. Seijts, and J. Gandz, "Developing Leadership Character in Business Programs," *Academy of Management Learning and Education,* June 2013, pp. 285–305; D. M. Mayer, K. Aquino, R. L. Greenbaum, and M. Kuenze, "Who Displays Ethical Leadership, and Why Does It Matter? An Examination of Antecedents and Consequences of Ethical Leadership," *Academy of Management Journal,* February 2012, pp. 151–171; and F. O. Walumbwa, D. M. Mayer, P. Wang, H. Wang, K. Workman, and A. L. Christensen, "Linking Ethical Leadership to Employee Performance: The Roles of Leader-Member Exchange, Self-Efficacy, and Organizational Identification," *Organizational Behavior & Human Decision Processes,* July 2011, pp. 204–213.

90. C. Dowden, "Forget Ethics Training: Focus on Empathy," business.financialpost.com, June 21, 2013.

91. W. Zellner, "A Hero—and a Smoking-Gun Letter," *Business Week,* January 28, 2002, pp. 34–35.

92. National Business Ethics Survey, Ethics Resource Center (Arlington, VA), 2007.

93. R. Bell, "Blowing the Whistle, Blowing Your Career?" *Workforce,* December 2013, p. 12; and A. Fredin, "The Unexpected Cost of Staying Silent," *Strategic Finance,* April 2012, pp. 53–59.

94. S. Armour, "More Companies Urge Workers to Blow the Whistle," *USA Today,* December 16, 2002, p. 1B.

95. J. Wiscombe, "Don't Fear Whistleblowers," *Workforce,* July 2002, pp. 26–27.

96. "ERC Releases New Research: Reporting Improves with a Procedurally Just Process," Ethics Resource Center, www.ethics.org, May 30, 2013.

97. T. Reason, "Whistle Blowers: The Untouchables," *CFO,* March 2003, p. 18; and C. Lachnit, "Muting the Whistle-Blower?" *Workforce,* September 2002, p. 18.

98. J. Hyatt, "Corporate Whistleblowers Might Need a Monetary Nudge, Researchers Suggest," *CRO Newsletter Online,* April 11, 2007; J. O'Donnell, "Blowing the Whistle Can Lead to Harsh Aftermath, Despite Law," *USA Today,* August 1, 2005, p. 2B; and D. Solomon, "For Financial Whistle-Blowers, New Shield Is An Imperfect One," *Wall Street Journal,* October 4, 2004, pp. A1+.

99. A. Smith, "Bottled Up," *Time,* August 14, 2009, p. Global 6.

100. This definition based on P. Tracey and N. Phillips, "The Distinctive Challenge of Educating Social Entrepreneurs: A Postscript and Rejoinder to the Special Issue on Entrepreneurship Education," *Academy of Management Learning & Education,* June 2007, pp. 264–271; Schwab Foundation for Social Entrepreneurship [www.schwabfound.org], February 20, 2006; and J. G. Dees, J. Emerson, and P. Economy, *Strategic Tools for Social Entrepreneurs* (New York: John Wiley & Sons, Inc., 2002).

101. P. Margulies, "Linda Rottenberg's High-Impact Endeavor," *Strategy + Business Online,* Spring 2012; S. Moran, "Some Ways to Get Started as a Social Entrepreneur," *New York Times Online,* June 22, 2011; P. A. Dacin, M. T. Dacin, and M. Matear, "Social Entrepreneurship: Why We Don't Need a New Theory and How We Move Forward From Here," *Academy of Management Perspective,* August 2010, pp. 37–57; and D. Bornstein, *How to Change the World: Social Entrepreneurs and the Power of New Ideas* (New York: Oxford University Press, 2004), inside cover jacket.

102. A. Kamenetz, "Five Social Capitalists Who Will Change the World in 2010," *Fast Company Online* [www.fastcompany.com], February 1, 2010.

103. K. H. Hammonds, "Now the Good News," *Fast Company,* December 2007/January 2008, pp. 110–121; C. Dahle, "Filling the Void," *Fast Company,* January/February 2006, pp. 54–57; and PATH [www.path.org].

104. R. J. Bies, J. M. Bartunek, T. L. Fort, and M. N. Zald, "Corporations as Social Change Agents: Individual, Interpersonal, Institutional, and Environmental Dynamics," *Academy of Management Review,* July 2007, pp. 788–793.

105. "The State of Corporate Philanthropy: A McKinsey Global Survey," *The McKinsey Quarterly Online,* February 2008.

106. R. Nixon, The Associated Press, "Bottom Line for (Red)," *New York Times Online,* February 6, 2008; and G. Mulvihill, "Despite Cause, Not Everyone Tickled Pink by Campaign," *Springfield News-Leader,* October 15, 2007, p. 2E.

107. Giving in Numbers: 2013 Edition, Committee Encouraging Corporate Philanthropy, http://cecp.co/research.html.

108. K. J. Delaney, "Google: From 'Don't be Evil' to How to Do Good," *Wall Street Journal,* January 18, 2008, pp. B1+; H. Rubin, "Google Offers a Map for Its Philanthropy," *New York Times Online,* January 18, 2008; and K. Hafner, "Philanthropy Google's Way: Not the Usual," *New York Times Online,* September 14, 2006.

109. A. Tergesen, "Doing Good to Do Well," *Wall Street Journal,* January 9, 2012, p. B7.

110. Committee to Encourage Corporate Philanthropy [www.corporatephilanthropy.org], April 7, 2008; "Investing in Society," *Leaders,* July–September 2007, pp. 12+; M. C. White, "Doing Good on Company Time," *New York Times Online,* May 8, 2007; and M. Lowery, "How Volunteerism is Changing the Face of Philanthropy," *DiversityInc,* December 2006, pp. 45–47.

111. R. Huggins and P. Trap, "How Honest We Are About Cheating in School," *USA Today,* September 21, 2012, p. 1A.

112. J. Beck, "Who Cheats and Why?" *The Atlantic,* January/February 2014, p. 27; H. Fry, "Culture of Cheating at Corona del Mar High, Parents Warn," www.latimes.com, January 29, 2014; and C. McWhirter, "High-Tech Cheaters Pose Test," *Wall Street Journal,* June 11, 2013, p. A3.

113. Skills Exercise based on F. Bartolome, "Nobody Trusts the Boss Completely—Now What?" *Harvard Business Review,* March–April 1989, pp. 135–142; and J. K. Butler Jr., "Toward Understanding and Measuring Conditions of Trust: Evolution of a Condition of Trust Inventory," *Journal of Management,* September 1991, pp. 643–663.

114. "20 Odd Questions: Sole Man Blake Mycoskie," *Wall Street Journal,* January 2012, p. D8; "Your Childhood Saw It Coming," *Fast Company,* December 2011/January 2012, p. 25; C. Garton, "Consumers Are Drawn to Products With a Charitable Connection," *USA Today Online,* July 18, 2011; "Ten Companies With Social Responsibility at the Core," *Advertising Age,* April 19, 2010, p. 88; C. Binkley, "Charity Gives Shoe Brand Extra Shine," *Wall Street Journal,* April 1, 2010, p. D7; J. Shambora, "How I Got Started: Blake Mycoskie, Founder of TOMS Shoes," *Fortune,* March 22, 2010, p. 72; and "Making A Do-Gooder's Business Model Work," *BusinessWeek Online,* January 26, 2009.

115. J. Sterngold, "Who Cares About Another $200 Million?" *Bloomberg BusinessWeek,* May 3–9, 2010, pp. 56–59; L. Story and E. Dash, "Lehman Channeled Risks Through Alter Ego Firm," *New York Time Online,* April 12, 2010; P. M. Barrett, "Cold Case: Lessons From the Lehman Autopsy," *Bloomberg BusinessWeek,* April 5, 2010, pp. 20–22; A. Smith, "What's Left of Lehman: A Plan," *CNNMoney* [www.money.cnn.com], March 16, 2010; and G. Wong and A. Smith, "What Killed Lehman," *CNNMoney* [www.money.cnn.com], March 15, 2010.

Managing Change and Innovation

From Chapter 7 of *Management*, Thirteenth Edition. Stephen P. Robbins and Mary Coulter. Copyright © 2016 by Pearson Education, Inc. All rights reserved.

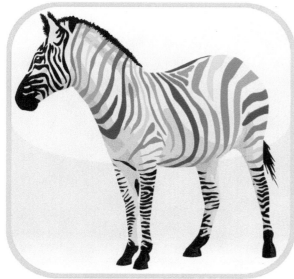

Managing Change and Innovation

It's Your Career

Source: spline_x/Shutterstock

A key to success in management and in your career is knowing *how to overcome your resistance to change and be change ready.*

Be Change Ready: Overcoming Resistance

Change takes us out of our comfort zone. And most of us don't like being out of our comfort zone. But to survive and thrive in your career, you're going to have to be change ready. As you'll see throughout this chapter, change is inevitable. So, the more easily you can adapt...the more successful, appreciated, and happy you'll be. Here are some suggestions for you to overcome your resistance to change:

*1.   **Evaluate your change readiness.** Some people flow with change easily and naturally. Others find it more difficult to deal with change. How would you rate your change readiness? Do you like change? Are you intimidated by change? Do you take steps to change or are you just daydreaming and talking big? Do you avoid decisions just so you don't have to change? Do you fear criticism, rejection, failure, success? You might be surprised to see "success" listed here along with criticism, rejection, and failure. But some people fear succeeding, especially if it means that they'll have to change. Think about it...if you're successful in your career, that likely will entail changes in job responsibilities, changes in the people you work with, and maybe even changes in geographical location. How okay are you with that?*

*2.   **Accept the idea of change.** Although change brings unknowns and uncertainties—even fears, suspicions, and doubts—change how you look at change. Don't be afraid of it. Yes, it can take you out of your comfort zone, but change isn't always such a bad thing. It's not your enemy, and it doesn't always bring unwelcomed events or outcomes. Accept the fact that change happens and make a mental note to work at being more comfortable with that. Getting comfortable with change may take some effort, but it's important to accept the idea of change.*

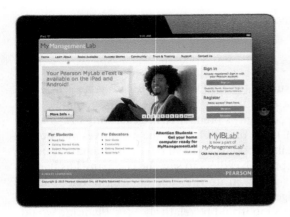

MyManagementLab®

⭐ Improve Your Grade!

When you see this icon, visit
www.mymanagementlab.com for activities that are
applied, personalized, and offer immediate feedback.

Learning Objectives

● SKILL OUTCOMES

1 *Compare* and contrast views on the change process.

2 *Classify* types of organizational change.

3 *Explain* how to manage resistance to change.

 ● **Know how** to be change ready by overcoming your resistance to change.

4 *Discuss* contemporary issues in managing change.

 ● **Develop your skill** in change management so you can serve as a catalyst for change.

5 *Describe* techniques for stimulating innovation.

---

3. Develop your flexibility. *Look for the opportunities and possibilities that change will bring. Shift from focusing on the "change" to focusing on the "new experiences." How can you benefit from this change? What challenges and constraints are there likely to be? Be confident about your ability to adapt and adjust. Be okay with making mistakes. Realize that these are ways to build on your experiences and to develop your flexibility.*

4. Prepare for change. *Learn as much as you can about impending changes. Understand the reason/rationale for changes. As we discuss* in the chapter, it's okay to raise concerns you may have about changes, but the goal should be to find the best solutions. By being prepared for change, you can then help others accept change. Have a positive attitude about change. Be the person who's a positive force in your workplace. Don't be the complainer. When things become chaotic and uncertain, be prepared to embrace change. When fear/resistance starts to build, remember that change implies progress. Progress implies moving forward. And moving forward implies you're change ready.

In today's world, big companies and small businesses, universities and colleges, state and city governments, and even the military are forced to be innovative. Although innovation has always been a part of the manager's job, it has become even more important in recent years. In this text, we'll describe why innovation is important and how managers can manage innovation. Because innovation is often closely tied to an organization's change efforts, let's start by looking at change and how managers manage change.

THE CHANGE Process

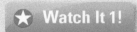 When John Lechleiter assumed the CEO's job at Eli Lilly, he sent each of his senior executives a clock ticking down the hours, minutes, and seconds until the day when one of the company's premier cash-generating drugs went off patent. It was a visual reminder of some major changes the executives had better be prepared for. By the end of 2016, Lilly stood to lose $10 billion in annual revenues as patents on three of its key drugs expired. Needless to say, the company has had to make some organizational changes as it picked up the pace of drug development.[1] Lilly's managers are doing what managers everywhere must do—implement change!

If it weren't for change, a manager's job would be relatively easy. Planning would be simple because tomorrow would be no different from today. The issue of effective organizational design would also be resolved because the environment would not be uncertain and there would be no need to redesign the structure. Similarly, decision making would be dramatically streamlined because the outcome of each alternative could be predicted with almost certain accuracy. But that's not the way it is. Change is an organizational reality.[2] Organizations face change because external and internal factors create the need for change (see Exhibit 1). When managers recognize that change is needed, then what? How do they respond?

★ **Watch It 1!** If your professor has assigned this, go to **www.mymanagementlab.com** to watch a video titled: *Rudi's Bakery: Organizational Change and Development* and to respond to questions.

Two Views of the Change Process

Two very different metaphors can be used to describe the change process.[3] One metaphor envisions the organization as a large ship crossing a calm sea. The ship's captain and crew know exactly where they're going because they've made the trip many times before. Change comes in the form of an occasional storm, a brief distraction in an otherwise calm and predictable trip. In the calm waters metaphor, change is seen as an occasional disruption in the normal flow of events. In the other metaphor, the organization is seen as a small raft navigating a raging river with uninterrupted white-water rapids. Aboard the raft are half a dozen people who have never worked together before, who are totally unfamiliar with the river, who are unsure of their eventual destination, and who, as if things weren't bad enough, are traveling at night. In the white-water rapids metaphor, change is normal and expected and managing it is a continual process. These two metaphors present very different approaches to understanding and responding to change. Let's take a closer look at each one.

Exhibit 1
External and Internal Forces for Change

External

- Changing consumer needs and wants
- New governmental laws
- Changing technology
- Economic changes

Internal

- New organizational strategy
- Change in composition of workforce
- New equipment
- Changing employee attitudes

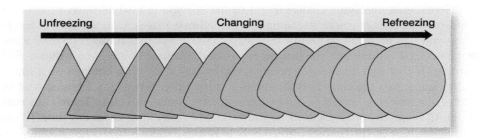

Exhibit 2
The Three-Step Change Process

THE CALM WATERS METAPHOR At one time, the calm waters metaphor was fairly descriptive of the situation managers faced. It's best understood by using Kurt Lewin's three-step change process.[4] (See Exhibit 2.)

According to Lewin, successful change can be planned and requires *unfreezing* the status quo, *changing* to a new state, and *refreezing* to make the change permanent. The status quo is considered equilibrium. To move away from this equilibrium, unfreezing is necessary. Unfreezing can be thought of as preparing for the needed change. It can be done by increasing the *driving forces,* which are forces pushing for change; by decreasing the *restraining forces*, which are forces that resist change; or by combining the two approaches.

Once unfreezing is done, the change itself can be implemented. However, merely introducing change doesn't ensure that it will take hold. The new situation needs to be *refrozen* so that it can be sustained over time. Unless this last step is done, there's a strong chance that employees will revert back to the old equilibrium state—that is, the old ways of doing things. The objective of refreezing, then, is to stabilize the new situation by reinforcing the new behaviors.

Lewin's three-step process treats change as a move away from the organization's current equilibrium state. It's a calm waters scenario where an occasional disruption (a "storm") means planning and implementing change to deal with the disruption. Once the disruption has been dealt with, however, things continue on under the new changed situation. This type of environment isn't what most managers face today.

WHITE-WATER RAPIDS METAPHOR DJ Patil, an expert in chaos theory, first made his name as a researcher of weather patterns at the University of Maryland. He says, "There are some times when you can predict weather well for the next 15 days. Other times, you can only really forecast a couple of days. Sometimes you can't predict the next two hours." The business climate is turning out to be a lot like that two-hour weather scenario. "The pace of change in our economy and our culture is accelerating and our visibility about the future is declining."[5]

As senior vice president and general manager of Connected Energy, a unit of Cisco, Laura Ipsen's company works on developing energy ecosystems for the smart-grid market. She describes her job as follows, "My job is like having to put together a 1,000-piece puzzle but I don't have the box top with the picture of what it looks like, and some of the pieces are missing."[6] Susan Whiting is chairman of Nielsen Media Research, the company best known for its television ratings, which are frequently used to determine how much advertisers pay for TV commercials. The media research business isn't what it used to be, however, as the Internet, video on demand, cell phones, iPods, digital video recorders, and other changing technologies have made data collection much more challenging. Whiting says, "If you look at a typical week I have, it's a combination of trying to lead a company in change in an industry in change."[7] These are pretty accurate descriptions of what change is like in our second change metaphor—white-water rapids. It's also consistent with a world that's increasingly dominated by information, ideas, and knowledge.[8]

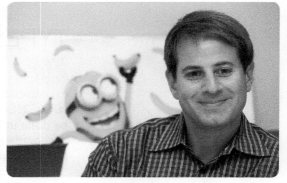

David Newman is the director of the new Target Technology Innovation Center in San Francisco. Target competes in a white-water rapids environment where major changes in technology and shopping behavior continue to reshape retailing. Newman and his team of innovators are studying evolving technologies and interactive devices to improve Target's performance and customers' shopping experiences online and in stores.
Source: Jeff Chiu/AP Images

Here's what managing change might be like for you in a white-water rapids environment: The college you're attending has the following rules: Courses vary in length. When you sign up, you don't know how long a course will run. It might go for 2 weeks or 15 weeks. Furthermore, the instructor can end a course at any time with no prior warning. If that isn't challenging enough, the length of the class changes each time it meets: Sometimes the class lasts 20 minutes; other times it runs for 3 hours. And the time of the next class meeting is set by the instructor during this class. There's one more thing: All exams are unannounced, so you have to be ready for a test at any time. To succeed in this type of environment, you'd have to respond quickly to changing conditions. Students who are overly structured or uncomfortable with change wouldn't succeed.

Increasingly, managers are realizing that their job is much like what a student would face in such a college. The stability and predictability of the calm waters metaphor don't exist. Disruptions in the status quo are not occasional and temporary, and they are not followed by a return to calm waters. Many managers never get out of the rapids. Like DJ Patil, Laura Ipsen, and Susan Whiting, they face constant change.

Is the white-water rapids metaphor an exaggeration? Probably not! Although you'd expect a chaotic and dynamic environment in high-tech industries, even organizations in non-high-tech industries are faced with constant change. Take the case of Swedish home appliance company Electrolux. You might think the home appliances industry couldn't be all that difficult—after all, most households need the products, which are fairly uncomplicated—but that impression would be wrong. Electrolux's chief executive Keith McLoughlin has had several challenges to confront.[9] First, there's the challenge of developing products that will appeal to a wide range of global customers. For instance, only 4 in 10 adults in the United Kingdom own a dishwasher. On the other hand, about 78 percent of U.S. homeowners have a dishwasher. Then, there's the challenge of cheaper alternatives flooding the market. Electrolux faces intense competition in the United States, and during the economic slowdown, the global appliance market tumbled on stubbornly weak demand. In addition, with a unionized labor force in Sweden, Electrolux faces expectations as far as how they treat their employees. McLoughlin recognizes that his company will have to continue to change if it's going to survive and prosper in the white-water rapids environment in which it operates.

Today, any organization that treats change as the occasional disturbance in an otherwise calm and stable world runs a great risk. Too much is changing too fast for an organization or its managers to be complacent. It's no longer business as usual. And managers must be ready to efficiently and effectively manage the changes facing their organization or their work area.

TYPES of Organizational Change

L02 Have you seen (or used) the 3M Co.'s Command picture-hanging hooks (which can actually be used to hang many different items)? They're an easy-to-use, relatively simple product consisting of plastic hooks and sticky foam strips. The manufacturing process, however, was far from simple. The work used to be done in four different states and take 100 days. However, a couple of years ago, the company's former CEO decided to start "untangling its hairballs" by streamlining complex and complicated production processes. Needless to say, a lot of changes had to take place. Today, those Command products are produced at a consolidated production "hub" in a third less time.[10] 3M Co. was up for the "hairball" challenge and focused its change efforts on its people and processes.

What Is Organizational Change?

Most managers, at one point or another, will have to change some things in their workplace. We classify these changes as **organizational change**, which is any alteration of people, structure, or technology. Organizational changes often need someone to act as a catalyst and assume the responsibility for managing the change

organizational change
Any alteration of people, structure, or technology in an organization

process—that is, a **change agent**. Change agents can be a manager within the organization, but could be a nonmanager—for example, a change specialist from the HR department or even an outside consultant.[11] For major changes, an organization often hires outside consultants to provide advice and assistance. Because they're from the outside, they have an objective perspective that insiders may lack. But outside consultants have a limited understanding of the organization's history, culture, operating procedures, and people. They're also more likely to initiate drastic change than insiders because they don't have to live with the repercussions after the change is implemented. In contrast, internal managers may be more thoughtful, but possibly overcautious, because they must live with the consequences of their decisions.

change agent
Someone who acts as a catalyst and assumes the responsibility for managing the change process

Types of Change

Managers face three main types of change: structure, technology, and people (see Exhibit 3). Changing *structure* includes any change in structural variables such as reporting relationships, coordination mechanisms, employee empowerment, or job redesign. Changing *technology* encompasses modifications in the way work is performed or the methods and equipment that are used. Changing *people* refers to changes in attitudes, expectations, perceptions, and behavior of individuals or groups.

CHANGING STRUCTURE   Jin Zhiguo, chairman of Tsingtao Brewery understands how important structural change can be. When the company shifted from a government-run company to a market-led company, many changes had to take place. He says, "Having worked for a state-owned enterprise, our people weren't used to competing for jobs or to being replaced for performance."[12] The change from a bureaucratic and risk-averse company to one that could compete in a global market required structural change.

Changes in the external environment or in organizational strategies often lead to changes in the organizational structure. Because an organization's structure is defined by how work gets done and who does it, managers can alter one or both of these *structural components*. For instance, departmental responsibilities could be combined, organizational levels eliminated, or the number of persons a manager supervises could be increased. More rules and procedures could be implemented to increase standardization. Or employees could be empowered to make decisions so decision making could be faster.

Another option would be to make major changes in the actual *structural design*. For instance, when Hewlett-Packard acquired Compaq Computer, product divisions were dropped, merged, or expanded. Structural design changes also might include, for instance, a shift from a functional to a product structure or the creation of a project

Structure	Structural components and structural design
Technology	Work processes, methods, and equipment
People	Attitudes, expectations, perceptions, and behavior—individual and group

Exhibit 3
Three Types of Change

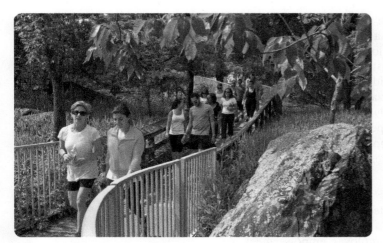

Hiking four round-trip miles together is a healthy team-building exercise managers of Wellness Corporate Solutions use as an organizational development method to bring about changes in employees that improve the quality of their interpersonal work relationships. Taking long walks together helps Wellness employees learn how other employees think and work.
Source: Chikwendiu/The Washington Post/Getty Images

organizational development (OD)
Change methods that focus on people and the nature and quality of interpersonal work relationships

structure design. Avery-Dennis Corporation, for example, revamped its structure to a new design that arranges work around teams.

CHANGING TECHNOLOGY Managers can also change the technology used to convert inputs into outputs. Most early management studies dealt with changing technology. For instance, scientific management techniques involved implementing changes that would increase production efficiency. Today, technological changes usually involve the introduction of new equipment, tools, or methods; automation; or computerization.

Competitive factors or new innovations within an industry often require managers to introduce *new equipment, tools,* or *operating methods.* For example, coal mining companies in New South Wales updated operational methods, installed more efficient coal handling equipment, and made changes in work practices to be more productive.

Automation is a technological change that replaces certain tasks done by people with tasks done by machines. Automation has been introduced in organizations such as the U.S. Postal Service, where automatic mail sorters are used, and in automobile assembly lines, where robots are programmed to do jobs that workers used to perform.

The most visible technological changes have come from *computerization.* Most organizations have sophisticated information systems. For instance, supermarkets and other retailers use scanners that provide instant inventory information and many are starting to accept mobile payments. Also, most offices are computerized. At BP p.l.c., for example, employees had to learn how to deal with the personal visibility and accountability brought about by an enterprise-wide information system. The integrative nature of this system meant that what any employee did on his or her computer automatically affected other computer systems on the internal network.[13] At the Benetton Group SpA, computers link its manufacturing plants outside Treviso, Italy, with the company's various sales outlets and a highly automated warehouse. Now, product information can be transmitted and shared instantaneously, a real plus in today's environment.[14]

CHANGING PEOPLE Changing people involves changing attitudes, expectations, perceptions, and behaviors—something that's not easy to do. **Organizational development (OD)** is the term used to describe change methods that focus on people and the nature and quality of interpersonal work relationships.[15] The most popular OD techniques are described in Exhibit 4. Each seeks to bring about changes in the organization's people and make them work together better. For example, executives at Scotiabank, one of Canada's Big Five banks, knew that the success of a new customer sales and service strategy depended on changing employee attitudes and behaviors. Managers used different OD techniques during the strategic change, including team building, survey feedback, and intergroup development. One indicator of how well these techniques worked in getting people to change was that every branch in Canada implemented the new strategy on or ahead of schedule.[16]

Much of what we know about OD practices has come from North American research. However, managers need to recognize that some techniques that work for U.S. organizations may not be appropriate for organizations or organizational divisions based in other countries.[17] For instance, a study of OD interventions showed that "multirater [survey] feedback as practiced in the United States is not embraced in Taiwan" because the cultural value of "saving face is simply more powerful than the value of receiving feedback from subordinates."[18] What's the lesson for managers? Before using the same OD techniques to implement

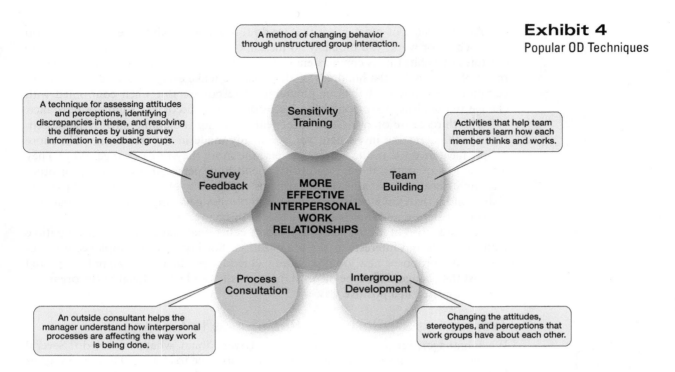

Exhibit 4
Popular OD Techniques

A method of changing behavior through unstructured group interaction.

A technique for assessing attitudes and perceptions, identifying discrepancies in these, and resolving the differences by using survey information in feedback groups.

Activities that help team members learn how each member thinks and works.

Sensitivity Training

Survey Feedback

MORE EFFECTIVE INTERPERSONAL WORK RELATIONSHIPS

Team Building

Process Consultation

Intergroup Development

An outside consultant helps the manager understand how interpersonal processes are affecting the way work is being done.

Changing the attitudes, stereotypes, and perceptions that work groups have about each other.

behavioral changes, especially across different countries, managers need to be sure they've taken into account cultural characteristics and whether the techniques "make sense for the local culture."

MANAGING Resistance to Change

LO3 We know it's better for us to eat healthy and to be active, yet few of us follow that advice. We resist making changes in our lifestyle. Volkswagen Sweden and ad agency DDB Stockholm did an experiment to see if they could get people to change their behavior and take the healthier option of using the stairs instead of riding an escalator.[19] How? They put a working piano keyboard on a stairway in a Stockholm subway station (you can see a video of it on YouTube) to see if commuters would use it. The experiment was a resounding success as stair traffic rose 66 percent. The lesson—people can change if you make the change appealing.

Change can be a threat to people in an organization. Organizations can build up inertia that motivates people to resist changing their status quo, even though change might be beneficial. Why do people resist change, and what can be done to minimize their resistance?

Why Do People Resist Change?

It's often said that most people hate any change that doesn't jingle in their pockets. This resistance to change is well documented.[20] Why *do* people resist change? The main reasons include uncertainty, habit, concern over personal loss, and the belief that the change is not in the organization's best interest.[21]

Change replaces the known with uncertainty. No matter how much you may dislike attending college, at least you know what's expected of you. When you leave college for the world of full-time employment, you'll trade the known for the unknown. Employees in organizations are faced with similar uncertainty. For example, when quality control methods based on statistical models are introduced into manufacturing plants, many quality control inspectors have to learn the new methods. Some may fear that they will be unable to do so and may develop a negative attitude toward the change or behave poorly if required to use them.

Another cause of resistance is that we do things out of habit. Every day when you go to school or work, you probably go the same way, if you're like most people. We're creatures of habit. Life is complex enough—we don't want to have to consider the full range of options for the hundreds of decisions we make every day. To cope with this complexity, we rely on habits or programmed responses. But when confronted with change, our tendency to respond in our accustomed ways becomes a source of resistance.

The third cause of resistance is the fear of losing something already possessed. Change threatens the investment you've already made in the status quo. The more people have invested in the current system, the more they resist change. Why? They fear the loss of status, money, authority, friendships, personal convenience, or other economic benefits they value. This fear helps explain why older workers tend to resist change more than younger workers. Older employees generally have more invested in the current system and thus have more to lose by changing.

A final cause of resistance is a person's belief that the change is incompatible with the goals and interests of the organization. For instance, an employee who believes that a proposed new job procedure will reduce product quality can be expected to resist the change. This type of resistance actually can be beneficial to the organization if expressed in a positive way.

Techniques for Reducing Resistance to Change

When managers see resistance to change as dysfunctional, what can they do? Several strategies have been suggested in dealing with resistance to change. These approaches include education and communication, participation, facilitation and support, negotiation, manipulation and co-optation, and coercion. These tactics are summarized here and described in Exhibit 5. Managers should view these techniques as tools and use the most appropriate one, depending on the type and source of the resistance.

let's get REAL

The Scenario:

After the National Transportation Safety Board recommended that states ban the use of cell phones while driving because of safety concerns, many companies are changing their policy on employee cell phone use. Jeff Turner, owner of an appliance repair service company in Toledo, Ohio, has told his employees that the company's new policy is "No cell phone use while driving." However, he's having a difficult time enforcing the policy.

What suggestions would you give Jeff about getting his employees to change their behavior?

I would suggest having a briefing with all employees and explaining to them why it is important to follow this policy, as it involves people's lives. Furthermore, I would enforce the policy by giving out formal warnings when anyone is reported using their phones while driving. If that has no impact, I would then suggest suspension without pay. I've found that sometimes people need to see consequences in order to cooperate and comply with policies.

Oscar Valencia
Manufacturing Manager

Source: Oscar Valencia

Technique	When Used	Advantage	Disadvantage
Education and communication	When resistance is due to misinformation	Clear up misunderstandings	May not work when mutual trust and credibility are lacking
Participation	When resisters have the expertise to make a contribution	Increase involvement and acceptance	Time-consuming; has potential for a poor solution
Facilitation and support	When resisters are fearful and anxiety ridden	Can facilitate needed adjustments	Expensive; no guarantee of success
Negotiation	When resistance comes from a powerful group	Can "buy" commitment	Potentially high cost; opens doors for others to apply pressure too
Manipulation and co-optation	When a powerful group's endorsement is needed	Inexpensive, easy way to gain support	Can backfire, causing change agent to lose credibility
Coercion	When a powerful group's endorsement is needed	Inexpensive, easy way to gain support	May be illegal; may undermine change agent's credibility

Exhibit 5
Techniques for Reducing Resistance to Change

Education and communication can help reduce resistance to change by helping employees see the logic of the change effort. This technique, of course, assumes that much of the resistance lies in misinformation or poor communication.

Participation involves bringing those individuals directly affected by the proposed change into the decision-making process. Their participation allows these individuals to express their feelings, increase the quality of the process, and increase employee commitment to the final decision.

Facilitation and support involve helping employees deal with the fear and anxiety associated with the change effort. This help may include employee counseling, therapy, new skills training, or a short paid leave of absence.

Negotiation involves exchanging something of value for an agreement to lessen the resistance to the change effort. This resistance technique may be quite useful when the resistance comes from a powerful source.

Manipulation and co-optation refer to covert attempts to influence others about the change. It may involve distorting facts to make the change appear more attractive.

Finally, *coercion* can be used to deal with resistance to change. Coercion involves the use of direct threats or force against the resisters.

Change Readiness—If your instructor is using MyManagementLab, log onto **mymanagementlab.com** and test your *change readiness knowledge*. **Be sure to refer back to the chapter opener!**

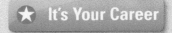

CONTEMPORARY Issues in Managing Change

L04 When CEO David Gray joined Daxko, a small software vendor based in Birmingham, Alabama, he wanted a more collegial workplace and he wanted to relieve employee stress. Now with a Wii console and a 52-inch plasma TV in the work/play lounge and an open-office layout, the company's "casual but

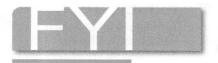
driven environment now resembles Silicon Valley more than the Deep South." One employee said, "It's pretty intense here. Expectations for what I need to accomplish are clearly set. And if I can play the Wii while doing it, that's even better."[22] Employee stress is one of the major critical concerns for managers today. In this section, we're going to discuss stress and two other critical concerns—changing organizational culture and making change happen successfully. Let's look first at changing culture.

Changing Organizational Culture

Korean Air CEO Cho Yang-Ho had a challenging change situation facing him. He wanted to transform his airline's image of an accident-prone airline from a developing country to that of a strong international competitor.[24] His main focus was on improving safety above all else, which meant making significant changes to the organization's culture. What made his task even more challenging was Korea's hierarchical culture that teaches Koreans to be deferential toward their elders and superiors. Cho says, "It (the hierarchical culture) exists in all Oriental culture." His approach to changing his company's culture involved implementing a "systems approach aimed at minimizing the personality-driven, top-down culture that is a legacy of Korean business managers who place emphasis on intuition and responding to orders." The cultural change must have worked. Korean Air is now the world's largest commercial cargo carrier, and it has earned a four-star rating (out of five possible stars) from a London aviation firm that rates airlines on quality.

The fact that an organization's culture is made up of relatively stable and permanent characteristics tends to make it very resistant to change.[25] A culture takes a long time to form, and once established it tends to become entrenched. Strong cultures are particularly resistant to change because employees have become so committed to them. For instance, it didn't take long for Lou Gerstner, who was CEO of IBM from 1993 to 2002, to discover the power of a strong culture. Gerstner, the first outsider to lead IBM, needed to overhaul the ailing, tradition-bound company if it was going to regain its role as the dominant player in the computer industry. However, accomplishing that feat in an organization that prided itself on its long-standing culture was Gerstner's biggest challenge. He said, "I came to see in my decade at IBM that culture isn't just one aspect of the game—it *is* the game."[26] Over time, if a certain culture becomes a handicap, a manager might be able to do little to change it, especially in the short run. Even under the most favorable conditions, cultural changes have to be viewed in years, not weeks or even months.

LEADER *making a* DIFFERENCE

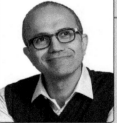

Source: Stuart Isett/Polaris/Newscom

When the news broke late summer 2013 that Microsoft's CEO (Steve Ballmer) was stepping down, the search for his replacement was on. Analysts said that whoever the replacement was, that individual would face the challenge of "rebooting Microsoft's corporate culture, in which charting the safe but profitable course...too often wins out over innovation...."[27] Satya Nadella is that person. Named CEO in February 2014, Nadella is a 22-year veteran of Microsoft. His new "slogan" is innovation, innovation, innovation. When asked what his plans are for the software giant, he answered with that one word, innovation. How does he plan to make innovation part of the culture? By "ruthlessly removing any obstacles that allow us to be innovative; every individual to innovate."[28] What can you learn from this leader making a difference?

UNDERSTANDING THE SITUATIONAL FACTORS What "favorable conditions" facilitate cultural change? One is that *a dramatic crisis occurs,* such as an unexpected financial setback, the loss of a major customer, or a dramatic technological innovation by a competitor. Such a shock can weaken the status quo and make people start thinking about the relevance of the current culture. Another condition may be that *leadership changes hands.* New top leadership can provide an alternative set of key values and may be perceived as more capable of responding to the crisis than the old leaders were. Another is that *the organization is young and small.* The younger the organization, the less entrenched its culture. It's easier for managers to communicate new

Exhibit 6
Changing Culture

- **Set the tone through management behavior;** top managers, particularly, need to be positive role models.

- Create **new stories, symbols, and rituals** to replace those currently in use.

- Select, promote, and support employees who **adopt** the new values.

- **Redesign socialization processes** to align with the new values.

- To encourage acceptance of the new values, **change the reward system.**

- Replace unwritten norms with **clearly specified expectations.**

- **Shake up current subcultures** through job transfers, job rotation, and/or terminations.

- Work to get consensus through **employee participation** and creating a **climate with a high level of trust.**

values in a small organization than in a large one. Finally, the *culture is weak.* Weak cultures are more receptive to change than strong ones.[29]

MAKING CHANGES IN CULTURE If conditions are right, how do managers change culture? No single action is likely to have the impact necessary to change something ingrained and highly valued. Managers need a strategy for managing cultural change, as described in Exhibit 6. These suggestions focus on specific actions that managers can take. Following them, however, is no guarantee that the cultural change efforts will succeed. Organizational members don't quickly let go of values that they understand and that have worked well for them in the past. Change, if it comes, will be slow. Also, managers must stay alert to protect against any return to old, familiar traditions.

Employee Stress

"Most weekdays at 5:30 p.m., after putting in eight hours as an insurance agent in Lawrenceville, Georgia, April Hamby scurries about 100 yards to the Kroger supermarket two doors away. She's not there to pick up some milk and bread, but instead to work an additional six hours as a cashier before driving home 35 miles and slipping into bed by 2 a.m. so she can get up at 7 a.m. and begin the grind anew."[30] And April's situation isn't all that unusual. In today's still-uncertain economic environment, many people found themselves working two or more jobs and battling stress.[31]

As a student, you've probably experienced stress—class projects, exams, even juggling a job and school. Then, there's the stress associated with getting a decent job after graduation. But even after you've landed that job, stress isn't likely to stop. For many employees, organizational change creates stress. An uncertain environment characterized by time pressures, increasing workloads, mergers, and restructuring has created a large number of employees who are overworked and stressed.[32] In fact, depending on which survey you look at, the number of employees experiencing job stress in the United States ranges anywhere from 40 percent to 80 percent.[33] However, workplace stress isn't just an American problem. Global studies indicate that some 50 percent of workers surveyed in 16 European countries reported that stress and job responsibility have risen significantly over a five-year period; 35 percent of Canadian workers surveyed said they are under high job stress; in Australia, cases of occupational stress jumped 21 percent in a one-year period; more than 57 percent of Japanese employees suffer from work-related stress; some 83 percent of call-center workers in India suffer from sleeping disorders; and a study of stress in China showed that managers are experiencing more stress.[34] Another interesting study found that stress was the leading cause of people quitting their jobs. Surprisingly, however, employers were clueless. They said that stress wasn't even among the top five reasons why people leave and instead wrongly believed that insufficient pay was the main reason.[35]

stress
The adverse reaction people have to excessive pressure placed on them from extraordinary demands, constraints, or opportunities

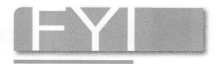

- 64 percent of employees describe their "typical" workday stress level as very/somewhat stressed.[38]

stressors
Factors that cause stress

role conflicts
Work expectations that are hard to satisfy

role overload
Having more work to accomplish than time permits

role ambiguity
When role expectations are not clearly understood

WHAT IS STRESS? **Stress** is the adverse reaction people have to excessive pressure placed on them from extraordinary demands, constraints, or opportunities.[36] Stress isn't always bad. Although it's often discussed in a negative context, stress can be positive, especially when it offers a potential gain. For instance, functional stress allows an athlete, stage performer, or employee to perform at his or her highest level at crucial times.

However, stress is more often associated with constraints and demands. A constraint prevents you from doing what you desire; demands refer to the loss of something desired. When you take a test at school or have your annual performance review at work, you feel stress because you confront opportunity, constraints, and demands. A good performance review may lead to a promotion, greater responsibilities, and a higher salary. But a poor review may keep you from getting the promotion. An extremely poor review might lead to your being fired.

One other thing to understand about stress is that just because the conditions are right for stress to surface doesn't always mean it will. Two conditions are necessary for *potential* stress to become *actual* stress.[37] First, there must be uncertainty over the outcome, and second, the outcome must be important.

WHAT CAUSES STRESS? Stress can be caused by personal factors and by job-related factors called **stressors**. Clearly, change of any kind—personal or job-related—has the potential to cause stress because it can involve demands, constraints, or opportunities. Organizations have no shortage of factors that can cause stress. Pressures to avoid errors or complete tasks in a limited time period, changes in the way reports are filed, a demanding supervisor, and unpleasant coworkers are a few examples. Let's look at five categories of organizational stressors: task demands, role demands, interpersonal demands, organization structure, and organizational leadership.

Task demands are factors related to an employee's job. They include the design of a person's job (autonomy, task variety, degree of automation), working conditions, and the physical work layout. Work quotas can put pressure on employees when their "outcomes" are perceived as excessive.[39] The more interdependence between an employee's tasks and the tasks of others, the greater the potential for stress. *Autonomy*, on the other hand, tends to lessen stress. Jobs in which temperatures, noise, or other working conditions are dangerous or undesirable can increase anxiety. So, too, can working in an overcrowded room or in a visible location where interruptions are constant.

Role demands relate to pressures placed on an employee as a function of the particular role he or she plays in the organization. **Role conflicts** create expectations that may be hard to reconcile or satisfy. **Role overload** is experienced when the employee is expected to do more than time permits. **Role ambiguity** is created when role expectations are not clearly understood and the employee is not sure what he or she is to do.

Interpersonal demands are pressures created by other employees. Lack of social support from colleagues and poor interpersonal relationships can cause considerable stress, especially among employees with a high social need.

Organization structure can increase stress. Excessive rules and an employee's lack of opportunity to participate in decisions that affect him or her are examples of structural variables that might be potential sources of stress.

Organizational leadership represents the supervisory style of the organization's managers. Some managers create a culture characterized by tension, fear, and anxiety. They establish unrealistic pressures to perform in the short run, impose excessively tight controls, and routinely fire employees who don't measure up. This style of leadership filters down through the organization and affects all employees.

Personal factors that can create stress include family issues, personal economic problems, and inherent personality characteristics. Because employees bring their personal problems to work with them, a full understanding of employee stress requires a manager to be understanding of these personal factors.[40] Evidence also indicates that employees' personalities have an effect on how susceptible they are to stress. The most commonly used labels for these personality traits are Type A and Type B.

let's get REAL

The Scenario:

Sondra Chan manages a team of 12 researchers at an organics-based cosmetics company. Like many companies during the past few years, she's asked her employees to take on greater responsibility since budgets are tight and no new hires have been brought onboard. Although she wants her team members to view these added responsibilities as furthering their own personal development, she also doesn't want to stretch them too far, causing out-of-control workplace stress and burnout.

What can Sondra do so her team doesn't get too stressed?

Sondra should meet with each team member to review the details of their new job responsibilities and how she will use a structured and supportive approach to incorporate these tasks into their daily routine. Be positive and encouraging, but firm and forward-thinking by focusing on the opportunities for personal and professional growth. Sondra should consistently touch base with each team member to gauge their progress and morale.

ToniAnn Petrella-Diaz
Retail Manager

Type A personality is characterized by chronic feelings of a sense of time urgency, an excessive competitive drive, and difficulty accepting and enjoying leisure time. The opposite of Type A is **Type B personality**. Type Bs don't suffer from time urgency or impatience. Until quite recently, it was believed that Type As were more likely to experience stress on and off the job. A closer analysis of the evidence, however, has produced new conclusions. Studies show that only the hostility and anger associated with Type A behavior are actually associated with the negative effects of stress. And Type Bs are just as susceptible to the same anxiety-producing elements. For managers, it is important to recognize that Type A employees are more likely to show symptoms of stress, even if organizational and personal stressors are low.

Type A personality
People who have a chronic sense of urgency and an excessive competitive drive

Type B personality
People who are relaxed and easygoing and accept change easily

WHAT ARE THE SYMPTOMS OF STRESS? We see stress in a number of ways. For instance, an employee who is experiencing high stress may become depressed, accident prone, or argumentative; may have difficulty making routine decisions; may be easily distracted, and so on. As Exhibit 7 shows, stress symptoms can be grouped under

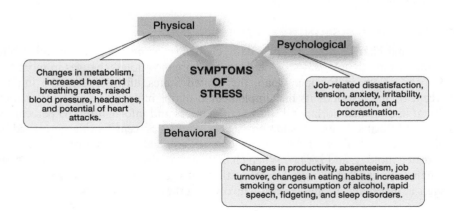

Exhibit 7
Symptoms of Stress

Physical: Changes in metabolism, increased heart and breathing rates, raised blood pressure, headaches, and potential of heart attacks.

Psychological: Job-related dissatisfaction, tension, anxiety, irritability, boredom, and procrastination.

SYMPTOMS OF STRESS

Behavioral: Changes in productivity, absenteeism, job turnover, changes in eating habits, increased smoking or consumption of alcohol, rapid speech, fidgeting, and sleep disorders.

three general categories: physical, psychological, and behavioral. All of these can significantly affect an employee's work.

In Japan, there's a stress phenomenon called *karoshi* (pronounced kah-roe-she), which is translated literally as "death from overwork." During the late 1980s, "several high-ranking Japanese executives still in their prime years suddenly died without any previous sign of illness."[41] As Japanese multinational companies expand operations to China, Korea, and Taiwan, it's feared that the karoshi culture may follow.

HOW CAN STRESS BE REDUCED? As mentioned earlier, not all stress is dysfunctional. Because stress can never be totally eliminated from a person's life, managers want to reduce the stress that leads to dysfunctional work behavior. How? Through controlling certain organizational factors to reduce job-related stress, and to a more limited extent, offering help for personal stress.

Things managers can do in terms of job-related factors begin with employee selection. Managers need to make sure an employee's abilities match the job requirements. When employees are in over their heads, their stress levels are typically high. A realistic job preview during the selection process can minimize stress by reducing ambiguity over job expectations. Improved organizational communications will keep ambiguity-induced stress to a minimum. Similarly, a performance planning program such as MBO (management by objectives) will clarify job responsibilities, provide clear performance goals, and reduce ambiguity through feedback. Job redesign is also a way to reduce stress. If stress can be traced to boredom or to work overload, jobs should be redesigned to increase challenge or to reduce the workload. Redesigns that increase opportunities for employees to participate in decisions and to gain social support also have been found to reduce stress.[42] For instance, at U.K. pharmaceutical maker GlaxoSmithKline, a team-resilience program in which employees can shift assignments, depending on people's workload and deadlines, has helped reduce work-related stress by 60 percent.[43]

Stress from an employee's personal life raises two problems. First, it's difficult for the manager to control directly. Second, ethical considerations include whether the manager has the right to intrude—even in the most subtle ways—in an employee's personal life. If a manager believes it's ethical and the employee is receptive, the manager might consider several approaches. Employee *counseling* can provide stress relief. Employees often want to talk to someone about their problems, and the organization—through its managers, in-house human resource counselors, or free or low-cost outside professional help—can meet that need. Companies such as Citicorp, AT&T, and Johnson & Johnson provide extensive counseling services for their employees. A *time management program* can help employees whose personal lives suffer from a lack of planning to sort out their priorities.[44] Still another approach is organizationally sponsored *wellness programs*. For example, Wellmark Blue Cross Blue Shield of Des Moines, Iowa, offers employees an onsite health and fitness facility that is open six days a week. Employees at Cianbro, a general contracting company located in the northeastern United States, are provided a wellness program tailored to the unique demands of the construction environment.[45]

Making Change Happen Successfully

Organizational change is an ongoing daily challenge facing managers in the United States and around the globe. In a global study of organizational changes in more than 2,000 organizations in Europe, Japan, the United States, and the United Kingdom, 82 percent of the respondents had implemented major information systems changes, 74 percent had created horizontal sharing of services and information, 65 percent had implemented flexible human resource practices, and 62 percent had decentralized operational decisions.[46] Each of these major changes entailed numerous other changes in structure, technology, and people. When changes are needed, who makes them happen? Who manages them? Although you may think it's just top-level managers, actually managers at *all* organizational levels are involved in the change process.

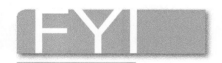

• Only 43 percent of change initiatives achieved the desired goal.[47]

Even with the involvement of all levels of managers, change efforts don't always work the way they should. In fact, a global study of organizational change concluded that "Hundreds of managers from scores of U.S. and European companies [are] satisfied with their operating prowess...[but] dissatisfied with their ability to implement change."[48] How can managers make change happen successfully? They can (1) make the organization change capable, (2) understand their own role in the process, and (3) give individual employees a role in the change process. Let's look at each of these suggestions.

In an industry where growth is slowing and competitors are becoming stronger, United Parcel Service (UPS) prospers. How? By embracing change! Managers spent a decade creating new worldwide logistics businesses because they anticipated slowing domestic shipping demand. They continue change efforts in order to exploit new opportunities.[49] UPS is what we call a change-capable organization. What does it take to be a change-capable organization? Exhibit 8 summarizes the characteristics.

The second component of making change happen successfully is for managers to recognize their own important role in the process. Managers can, and do, act as change agents. But their role in the change process includes more than being catalysts for change; they must also be change leaders. When organizational members resist change, it's the manager's responsibility to lead the change effort. But even when there's no resistance to the change, someone has to assume leadership. That someone is managers.

The final aspect of making change happen successfully revolves around getting all organizational members involved. Successful organizational change is not a one-person job. Individual employees are a powerful resource in identifying and addressing change issues. "If you develop a program for change and simply hand it to your people, saying, 'Here, implement this,' it's unlikely to work. But when people help to build something, they will support it and make it work."[50] Managers need to encourage employees to be change agents—to look for those day-to-day improvements and changes that individuals and teams can make. For instance, a study of organizational change found that 77 percent of changes at the work group level were reactions to a specific, current problem or to a suggestion from someone outside the work group; and 68 percent of those changes occurred in the course of employees' day-to-day work.[51]

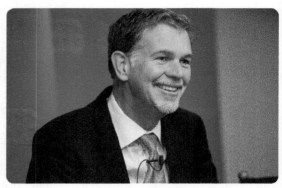

Netflix CEO Reed Hastings leads a change-capable organization. He cofounded Netflix as a DVD rental service, then added an Internet video streaming service, and now offers its own content such as *House of Cards.* Hastings makes change at Netflix happen successfully by innovating and adapting quickly to how people want to see movies and television programs.
Source: Kristoffer Tripplaar/Sipa USA/AP Images

Exhibit 8
Change-Capable Organizations

Sources: Based on S. Ante, "Change Is Good—So Get Used to It," *BusinessWeek,* June 22, 2009, pp. 69–70; and P. A. McLagan, "The Change-Capable Organization," *T&D,* January 2003, pp. 50–59.

- **_Link the present and the future._** Think of work as more than an extension of the past; think about future opportunities and issues and factor them into today's decisions.

- **_Make learning a way of life._** Change-friendly organizations excel at knowledge sharing and management.

- **_Actively support and encourage day-to-day improvements and changes._** Successful change can come from the small changes as well as the big ones.

- **_Ensure diverse teams._** Diversity ensures that things won't be done like they've always been done.

- **_Encourage mavericks._** Because their ideas and approaches are outside the mainstream, mavericks can help bring about radical change.

- **_Shelter breakthroughs._** Change-friendly organizations have found ways to protect those breakthrough ideas.

- **_Integrate technology._** Use technology to implement changes.

- **_Build and deepen trust._** People are more likely to support changes when the organization's culture is trusting and managers have credibility and integrity.

- **_Couple permanence with perpetual change._** Because change is the only constant, companies need to figure out how to protect their core strengths during times of change.

- **_Support an entrepreneurial mindset._** Many younger employees bring a more entrepreneurial mindset to organizations and can serve as catalysts for radical change.

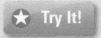

If your professor has assigned this, go to **www.mymanagementlab.com** to complete the Simulation: Change and get a better understanding of the challenges of managing change in organizations.

STIMULATING Innovation

LO5 "Innovation is the key to continued success." "We innovate today to secure the future."[52] These two quotes (the first by Ajay Banga, the CEO of MasterCard, and the second by Sophie Vandebroek, chief technology officer of Xerox Innovation Group) reflect how important innovation is to organizations. Success in business today demands innovation. In the dynamic, chaotic world of global competition, organizations must create new products and services and adopt state-of-the-art technology if they're going to compete successfully.[53]

What companies come to mind when you think of successful innovators? Maybe it's Apple with its iPad, iPhone, iPod, and wide array of computers. Maybe it's Google with its continually evolving Web platform. And Google is a good example of the new, faster pace of innovation. The company runs 50 to 200 online search experiments with users at any given time. In one instance, Google asked selected users how many search results they'd like to see on a single screen. The reply from the users was more, many more. So Google ran an experiment that tripled the number of search results per screen to 30. The result: traffic declined because "it took about a third of a second longer for search results to appear—a seemingly insignificant delay that nonetheless upset many of the users."[55] Google tried something new and quickly found out it wasn't something they wanted to pursue. Even Procter & Gamble, the global household and personal products giant, is doing the "vast majority of our concept testing online, which has created truly substantial savings in money and time," according to the company's global consumer and market knowledge officer.[56] What's the secret to the success of these and other innovator champions? What can other managers do to make their organizations more innovative? In the following sections, we'll try to answer those questions as we discuss the factors behind innovation.

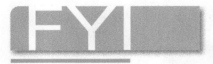

- Only 28 percent of organizations consider themselves innovative.[54]

Creativity Versus Innovation

The definition of innovation varies widely, depending on who you ask. For instance, the Merriam-Webster dictionary defines innovation as "the introduction of something new" and "a new idea, method, or device; novelty." The CEO of the company that makes Bubble Wrap says, "It means inventing a product that has never existed." To the CEO of Ocean Spray Cranberries, it means "turning an overlooked commodity, such as leftover cranberry skins into a consumer snack like Craisins."[57] We're going to define it by first looking at the concept of creativity. **Creativity** refers to the ability to combine ideas in a unique way or to make unusual associations between ideas.[58] A creative organization develops unique ways of working or novel solutions to problems. But creativity by itself isn't enough. The outcomes of the creative process need to be turned into useful products or work methods, which is defined as **innovation**. Thus, the innovative organization is characterized by its ability to generate new ideas that are implemented into new products, processes, and procedures designed to be useful—that is, to channel creativity into useful outcomes. When managers talk about changing an organization to make it more creative, they usually mean they want to stimulate and nurture innovation.

creativity
The ability to combine ideas in a unique way or to make unusual associations between ideas

innovation
Taking creative ideas and turning them into useful products or work methods

Stimulating and Nurturing Innovation

The systems model can help us understand how organizations become more innovative.[59] Getting the desired outputs (innovative products and work methods) involves transforming inputs. These inputs include

FUTURE VISION | Company-Mandated "Experiment" Time

When employees are busy doing their regular job tasks, how can innovation ever flourish? When job performance is evaluated by what you get done, how you get it done, and when you get it done, how can innovation ever happen? This has been the challenge facing organizations wanting to be more innovative. One solution has been to give employees mandated time to experiment with their own ideas on company-related projects.[60] For instance, Google has its "20% Time" initiative, which encourages employees to spend 20 percent of their time at work on projects not related to their job descriptions. Other companies—Facebook, Apple, LinkedIn, 3M, Hewlett-Packard, among others—have similar initiatives. Hmmmm...so having essentially one day a week to work on company-related ideas you have almost seems too good to be true. But, more importantly, does it really spark innovation? Well, it can. At Google, it led to the autocomplete system, Google News, GMail, and Adsense. However, such "company" initiatives do face tremendous obstacles, despite how good they sound on paper. One challenge is that today's employees face strict monitoring in terms of time and resources. Thus, there's a reluctance on their part to use this time since most employees have enough to do just keeping up with their regular tasks. And if bonuses/incentives are based on goals achieved, employees are smart about what to spend their time on.

Other challenges include what happens to the ideas that employees do have, unsupportive managers and coworkers who may view this as a "goof-around-for-free-day," and obstacles in the corporate bureaucracy. So, how can companies make it work? Here are some suggestions: top managers need to support the initiatives/projects and make that support known; managers need to support employees who have that personal passion and drive, that creative spark—clear a path for them to pursue their ideas; perhaps allow employees more of an incentive to innovate (rights to design, etc.); and last, but not least, don't institutionalize it. Creativity and innovation, by their very nature, involve risk and reward. Give creative individuals the space to try and to fail and to try and to fail as needed.

If your professor has chosen to assign this, go to **www.mymanagementlab.com** *to discuss the following questions.*

⭐ **TALK ABOUT IT 1:** What benefits do you see with such mandated experiment time for (a) organizations? (b) Individuals?

⭐ **TALK ABOUT IT 2:** What obstacles do these initiatives face and how can managers overcome those obstacles?

---

creative people and groups within the organization. But having creative people isn't enough. It takes the right environment to help transform those inputs into innovative products or work methods. This "right" environment—that is, an environment that stimulates innovation—includes three variables: the organization's structure, culture, and human resource practices. (See Exhibit 9.)

Structural Variables

An organization's structure can have a huge impact on innovativeness. Research into the effect of structural variables on innovation shows five things.[62] First, an organic-type structure positively influences innovation. Because this structure is low in formalization, centralization, and work specialization, it facilitates the flexibility and sharing of ideas that are critical to innovation. Second, the availability of plentiful resources provides a key building block for innovation. With an abundance of resources, managers can afford to purchase innovations, can afford the cost of instituting innovations, and can absorb failures. For example, at Smart Balance Inc., the heart-healthy food developer uses its resources efficiently by focusing on product development and outsourcing almost everything else, including manufacturing, product distribution, and sales. The company's CEO says this approach allows them to be "a pretty aggressive innovator" even during economic downturns.[63] Third, frequent communication between organizational units helps break down barriers to innovation.[64] Cross-functional teams, task forces, and other such organizational

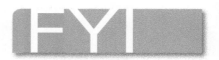

- 65 percent of companies innovate by integrating both the past and the future.[61]

Exhibit 9

Innovation Variables

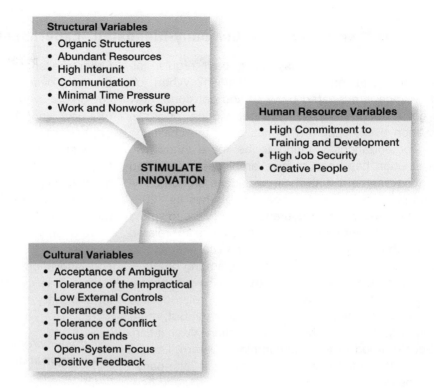

designs facilitate interaction across departmental lines and are widely used in innovative organizations. For instance, Pitney Bowes, the mail and documents company, uses an electronic meeting place called IdeaNet, where its employees can collaborate and provide comments and input on any idea they think will help create new sources of revenue, improve profitability, or add new value for customers. IdeaNet isn't just an electronic suggestion box or open forum; employees are presented with specific idea challenges. A recent one involved how to expand its mail service business into new segments. Hundreds of employees from multiple functions and business units weighed in with ideas, and eight promising ideas were generated.[65] Fourth, innovative organizations try to minimize extreme time pressures on creative activities despite the demands of white-water rapids environments. Although time pressures may spur people to work harder and may make them feel more creative, studies show that it actually causes them to be less creative.[66] Companies such as Google, 3M, and Hewlett-Packard actually urge staff researchers to spend a chunk of their workweek on self-initiated projects, even if those projects are outside the individual's work area of expertise.[67] Finally, studies have shown that an employee's creative performance was enhanced when an organization's structure explicitly supported creativity. Beneficial kinds of support included things like encouragement, open communication, readiness to listen, and useful feedback.[68]

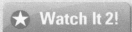 **Watch It 2!** If your professor has assigned this, go to **www.mymanagementlab.com** to watch a video titled: *CH2MHill: Innovation* and to respond to questions.

CULTURAL VARIABLES "Throw the bunny" is part of the lingo used by a product development team at toy company Mattel. It refers to a juggling lesson where team members learn to juggle two balls and a stuffed bunny. Most people easily learn to juggle two balls but can't let go of that third object. Creativity, like juggling, is learn-

ing to let go—that is, to "throw the bunny." And for Mattel, having a culture where people are encouraged to "throw the bunny" is important to its continued product innovations.[69]

Innovative organizations tend to have similar cultures.[70] They encourage experimentation, set creativity goals, reward both successes and failures, and celebrate mistakes. An innovative organization is likely to have the following characteristics.

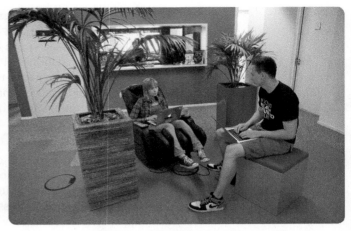

These Google Inc. employees working at the company's offices in Berlin, Germany, are encouraged to accept the inevitability of failure as part of the way to be innovative and successful. Google nurtures a culture of innovation that tolerates risks, encourages experimentation, and views mistakes as learning opportunities.
Source: Krisztian Bocsi/Bloomberg/Getty Images

- *Accept ambiguity.* Too much emphasis on objectivity and specificity constrains creativity.
- *Tolerate the impractical.* Individuals who offer impractical, even foolish, answers to what-if questions are not stifled. What at first seems impractical might lead to innovative solutions. Encourage entrepreneurial thinking.[71]
- *Keep external controls minimal.* Rules, regulations, policies, and similar organizational controls are kept to a minimum.
- *Tolerate risk.* Employees are encouraged to experiment without fear of consequences should they fail.[72] "Failure, and how companies deal with failure, is a very big part of innovation."[73] Treat mistakes as learning opportunities. You don't want your employees to fear putting forth new ideas. In an uncertain economic environment, it's especially important that employees don't feel they have to avoid innovation and initiative because it's unsafe for them to do so. A recent study found that one fear employees have is that their coworkers will think negatively of them if they try to come up with better ways of doing things. Another fear is that they'll "provoke anger among others who are comfortable with the status quo."[74] In an innovative culture, such fears are not an issue.
- *Tolerate conflict.* Diversity of opinions is encouraged. Harmony and agreement between individuals or units are *not* assumed to be evidence of high performance.
- *Focus on ends rather than means.* Goals are made clear, and individuals are encouraged to consider alternative routes toward meeting the goals. Focusing on ends suggests that several right answers might be possible for any given problem.[75]
- *Use an open-system focus.* Managers closely monitor the environment and respond to changes as they occur. For example, at Starbucks, product development depends on "inspiration field trips to view customers and trends." When Michelle Gass was the company's senior vice president of global strategy (she's now the president of Starbucks Europe, Middle East, and Africa), she "took her team to Paris, Düsseldorf, and London to visit local Starbucks and other restaurants to get a better sense of local cultures, behaviors, and fashions." She says, "You come back just full of different ideas and different ways to think about things than you would had you read about it in a magazine or e-mail."[76]
- *Provide positive feedback.* Managers provide positive feedback, encouragement, and support so employees feel that their creative ideas receive attention.
- *Exhibit empowering leadership.* Be a leader who lets organizational members know that the work they do is significant. Provide organizational members the opportunity to participate in decision making. Show them you're confident they can achieve high performance levels and outcomes. Being this type of leader will have a positive influence on creativity.[77]

HUMAN RESOURCE VARIABLES In this category, we find that innovative organizations actively promote the training and development of their members so their knowledge remains current; offer their employees high job security to reduce the fear of getting fired for making mistakes; and encourage individuals to become **idea champions**, actively and enthusiastically supporting new ideas, building support, overcoming resistance, and ensuring that innovations are implemented. Research finds that idea champions have common personality characteristics: extremely high

idea champion
Individual who actively and enthusiastically supports new ideas, builds support, overcomes resistance, and ensures that innovations are implemented

self-confidence, persistence, energy, and a tendency toward risk taking. They also display characteristics associated with dynamic leadership. They inspire and energize others with their vision of the potential of an innovation and through their strong personal conviction in their mission. They're also good at gaining the commitment of others to support their mission. In addition, idea champions have jobs that provide considerable decision-making discretion. This autonomy helps them introduce and implement innovations in organizations.[78]

Innovation and Design Thinking

Undoubtedly, a strong connection exists between design thinking and innovation. "Design thinking can do for innovation what TQM did for quality."[79] Just as TQM provides a process for improving quality throughout an organization, design thinking can provide a process for coming up with things that don't exist. When a business approaches innovation with a design-thinking mentality, the emphasis is on getting a deeper understanding of what customers need and want. It entails knowing customers as real people with real problems—not just as sales targets or demographic statistics. But it also entails being able to convert those customer insights into real and usable products. For instance, at Intuit, the company behind TurboTax software, founder Scott Cook felt "the company wasn't innovating fast enough."[80] So he decided to apply design thinking. He called the initiative "Design for Delight" and it involved customer field research to understand their "pain points"—that is, what most frustrated them as they worked in the office and at home. Then, Intuit staffers brainstormed (they nicknamed it "painstorm") a "variety of solutions to address the problems and experiment with customers to find the best ones." For example, one pain point uncovered by an Intuit team was how customers could take pictures of tax forms to reduce typing errors. Some younger customers, used to taking photos with their smartphones, were frustrated that they couldn't just complete their taxes on their mobiles. To address this, Intuit developed a mobile app called SnapTax, which the company says has been downloaded more than a million times since it was introduced in 2010. That's how design thinking works in innovation.

CHAPTER SUMMARY by Learning Objectives

LO1 COMPARE and contrast views on the change process.

The calm waters metaphor suggests that change is an occasional disruption in the normal flow of events and can be planned and managed as it happens. In the white-water rapids metaphor, change is ongoing and managing it is a continual process.

Lewin's three-step model says change can be managed by unfreezing the status quo (old behaviors), changing to a new state, and refreezing the new behaviors.

LO2 CLASSIFY types of organizational change.

Organizational change is any alteration of people, structure, or technology. Making changes often requires a change agent to act as a catalyst and guide the change process.

Changing structure involves any changes in structural components or structural design. Changing technology involves introducing new equipment, tools, or methods; automation; or computerization. Changing people involves changing attitudes, expectations, perceptions, and behaviors.

LO3 EXPLAIN how to manage resistance to change.

People resist change because of uncertainty, habit, concern over personal loss, and the belief that the change is not in the organization's best interest.

The techniques for reducing resistance to change include education and communication (educating employees about and communicating to them the need for the change), participation (allowing employees to participate in the change process), facilitation and support (giving employees the support they need to implement the change), negotiation (exchanging something of value to reduce resistance), manipulation and co-optation (using negative actions to influence), and coercion (using direct threats or force).

LO4 DISCUSS contemporary issues in managing change.

The shared values that comprise an organization's culture are relatively stable, which makes it difficult to change. Managers can do so by being positive role models; creating new stories, symbols, and rituals; selecting, promoting, and supporting employees who adopt the new values; redesigning socialization processes; changing the reward system, clearly specifying expectations; shaking up current subcultures; and getting employees to participate in change.

Stress is the adverse reaction people have to excessive pressure placed on them from extraordinary demands, constraints, or opportunities. To help employees deal with stress, managers can address job-related factors by making sure an employee's abilities match the job requirements, improve organizational communications, use a performance planning program, or redesign jobs. Addressing personal stress factors is trickier, but managers could offer employee counseling, time management programs, and wellness programs.

Making change happen successfully involves focusing on making the organization change capable, making sure managers understand their own role in the process, and giving individual employees a role in the process.

LO5 DESCRIBE techniques for stimulating innovation.

Creativity is the ability to combine ideas in a unique way or to make unusual associations between ideas. Innovation is turning the outcomes of the creative process into useful products or work methods.

Important structural variables include an organic-type structure, abundant resources, frequent communication between organizational units, minimal time pressure, and support. Important cultural variables include accepting ambiguity, tolerating the impractical, keeping external controls minimal, tolerating risk, tolerating conflict, focusing on ends not means, using an open-system focus, providing positive feedback, and being an empowering leader. Important human resource variables include high commitment to training and development, high job security, and encouraging individuals to be idea champions.

A close and strong connection exists between design thinking and innovation. It involves knowing customers as real people with real problems and converting those insights into usable and real products.

MyManagementLab

Go to **mymanagementlab.com** to complete the problems marked with this icon ⭐.

⭐ REVIEW AND DISCUSSION QUESTIONS

1. Contrast the calm waters and white-water rapids metaphors of change.

2. Explain Lewin's three-step model of the change process.

3. Describe how managers might change structure, technology, and people.

4. Can a low-level employee be a change agent? Explain your answer.

5. How are opportunities, constraints, and demands related to stress? Give an example of each.

6. Planned change is often thought to be the best approach to take in organizations. Can unplanned change ever be effective? Explain.

7. Organizations typically have limits to how much change they can absorb. As a manager, what signs would you look for that might suggest your organization has exceeded its capacity to change?

8. Innovation requires allowing people to make mistakes. However, being wrong too many times can be disastrous to your career. Do you agree? Why or why not? What are the implications for nurturing innovation?

MyManagementLab

If your professor has assigned these, go to **mymanagementlab.com** for Auto-graded writing questions as well as the following Assisted-graded writing questions:

9. Why do people resist change? How can resistance to change be reduced?

10. Describe the structural, cultural, and human resources variables that are necessary for innovation.

PREPARING FOR: My Career

⭐ PERSONAL INVENTORY ASSESSMENTS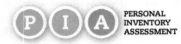

Are You a Type A Personality?

Do you think you're a Type A personality? Take this PIA and find out so you can better control the negative aspects of being a Type A!

⭐ ETHICS DILEMMA

Half of all Americans say they've taken on major new roles and duties at work since the recession ended, often without extra pay. One in five companies offers some form of stress management program.[81] Although employee assistance programs (EAPs) are available, many employees may choose not to participate. Why? Many employees are reluctant to ask for help, especially if a major source of that stress is job overload or job insecurity. After all, there's still a stigma associated with stress. Employees don't want to be perceived as being unable to handle the demands of their job. Although they may need stress management now more than ever, few employees want to admit they're stressed.

11. What can be done about this paradox of needing stress management assistance but being reluctant to admit it?

12. Do organizations even *have* an ethical responsibility to help employees deal with stress? Discuss.

SKILLS EXERCISE Developing Your Change Management Skill

About the Skill

Managers play an important role in organizational change. That is, they often serve as a catalyst for the change—a change agent. However, managers may find that change is resisted by employees. After all, change represents ambiguity and uncertainty, or it threatens the status quo. How can this resistance to change be effectively managed? Here are some suggestions.[82]

Steps in Practicing the Skill

- *Assess the climate for change.* One major factor in why some changes succeed while others fail is the readiness for change. Assessing the climate for change involves asking several questions. The more affirmative answers you get, the more likely it is that change efforts will succeed. Here are some guiding questions:

  a. Is the sponsor of the change high enough in the organization to have power to effectively deal with resistance?

  b. Is senior management supportive of the change and committed to it?

  c. Do senior managers convey the need for change, and is this feeling shared by others in the organization?

  d. Do managers have a clear vision of how the future will look after the change?

  e. Are objective measures in place to evaluate the change effort, and have reward systems been explicitly designed to reinforce them?

  f. Is the specific change effort consistent with other changes going on in the organization?

  g. Are managers willing to sacrifice their personal self-interests for the good of the organization as a whole?

  h. Do managers pride themselves on closely monitoring changes and actions by competitors?

  i. Are managers and employees rewarded for taking risks, being innovative, and looking for new and better solutions?

  j. Is the organizational structure flexible?

  k. Does communication flow both down and up in the organization?

  l. Has the organization successfully implemented changes in the past?

  m. Are employees satisfied with, and do they trust, management?

  n. Is a high degree of interaction and cooperation typical between organizational work units?

  o. Are decisions made quickly, and do they take into account a wide variety of suggestions?

- *Choose an appropriate approach for managing the resistance to change.* In this text, six strategies have been suggested for dealing with resistance to change—education and communication, participation, facilitation and support, negotiation, manipulation and co-optation, and coercion. Review Exhibit 5 for the advantages and disadvantages and when it is best to use each approach.

167

- *During the time the change is implemented and after the change is completed, communicate with employees regarding what support you may be able to provide.* Your employees need to know you are there to support them during change efforts. Be prepared to offer the assistance that may be necessary to help them enact the change.

Practicing the Skill

Read through the following scenario. Write down some notes about how you would handle the situation described. Be sure to refer to the three suggestions for managing resistance to change.

You're the nursing supervisor at a community hospital employing both emergency room and floor nurses. Each of these teams of nurses tends to work almost exclusively with others doing the same job. In your professional reading, you've come across the concept of cross-training nursing teams and giving them more varied responsibilities, which in turn has been shown to improve patient care while lowering costs. You call the two team leaders, Sue and Scott, into your office to discuss your plan to have the nursing teams move to this approach. To your surprise, they're both opposed to the idea. Sue says she and the other emergency room nurses feel they're needed in the ER, where they fill the most vital role in the hospital. They work special hours when needed, do whatever tasks are required, and often work in difficult and stressful circumstances. They think the floor nurses have relatively easy jobs for the pay they receive. Scott, leader of the floor nurses team, tells you that his group believes the ER nurses lack the special training and extra experience that the floor nurses bring to the hospital. The floor nurses claim they have the heaviest responsibilities and do the most exacting work. Because they have ongoing contact with the patients and their families, they believe they shouldn't be pulled away from vital floor duties to help ER nurses complete their tasks. Now—what would you do?

WORKING TOGETHER Team Exercise

Let's see how creative you can be! Form teams of 3–4 people. From the list below, choose one activity to complete (or your professor may assign you one).

- How could you recycle old keys? Come up with as many suggestions as you can. (The more the better!)

- Think about different uses for a golf tee. Be as creative as possible as you list your suggestions.
- List different ways that a brick can be used. See how many ideas you can come up with. Think beyond the obvious.

MY TURN TO BE A MANAGER

- Take responsibility for your own future career path. Don't depend on your employer to provide you with career development and training opportunities. Right now, sign up for things that will help you enhance your skills—workshops, seminars, continuing education courses, etc.

- Pay attention to how you handle change. Try to figure out why you resist certain changes and not others.

- Pay attention to how others around you handle change. When friends or family resist change, practice using different approaches to managing this resistance to change.

- When you find yourself experiencing dysfunctional stress, write down what's causing the stress, what stress symptoms you're exhibiting, and how you're dealing with the stress. Keep this information in a journal and evaluate how well your stress reducers are working and how you could handle stress better. Your goal is to get to a point where you recognize that you're stressed and can take positive actions to deal with the stress.

- Research information on how to be a more creative person. Write down suggestions in a bulleted-list format and be prepared to present your information in class.

- Is innovation more about (1) stopping something old, or (2) starting something new? Prepare arguments supporting or challenging each view.

- Choose two organizations you're familiar with and assess whether these organizations face a calm waters or white-water rapids environment. Write a short report describing these organizations and your assessment of the change environment each faces. Be sure to explain your choice of change environment.

- Choose an organization with which you're familiar (employer, student organization, family business, etc.). Describe its culture (shared values and beliefs). Select two of those values/beliefs and describe how you would go about changing them. Put this information in a report.

- In your own words, write down three things you learned in this text about being a good manager. Keep a copy of this for future reference.

CASE APPLICATION **1** In Search of the Next Big Thing

It all started with a simple plan to make a superior T-shirt. As special teams captain during the mid-1990s for the University of Maryland football team, Kevin Plank hated having to repeatedly change the cotton T-shirt he wore under his jersey as it became wet and heavy during the course of a game.[83] He knew there had to be a better alternative and set out to make it. After a year of fabric and product testing, Plank introduced the first Under Armour compression product—a synthetic shirt worn like a second skin under a uniform or jersey. And it was an immediate hit! The silky fabric was light and made athletes feel faster and fresher, giving them, according to Plank, an important psychological edge. Today, Under Armour continues to passionately strive to make all athletes better by relentlessly pursuing innovation and design. A telling sign of the company's philosophy is found over the door of its product design studios: "We have not yet built our defining product."

Today, Baltimore-based Under Armour (UA) is a $1.4 billion company. In 16 years, it has grown from a college start-up to a "formidable competitor of the Beaverton, Oregon behemoth" (better known as Nike, a $21 billion company). The company has nearly 3 percent of the fragmented U.S. sports apparel market and sells products from shirts, shorts, and cleats to underwear. In addition, more than 100 universities wear UA uniforms. The company's logo—an interlocking U and A—is becoming almost as recognizable as the Nike swoosh.

Starting out, Plank sold his shirts using the only advantage he had—his athletic connections. "Among his teams from high school, military school, and the University of Maryland, he knew at least 40 NFL players well enough to call and offer them the shirt." He was soon joined by another Maryland player, Kip Fulks, who played lacrosse. Fulks used the same "six-degrees strategy" in the lacrosse world. (Today, Fulks is the company's COO.) Believe it or not, the strategy worked. UA sales quickly gained momentum. However, selling products to teams and schools would take a business only so far. That's when Plank began to look at the mass market. In 2000, he made his first deal with a big-box store, Galyan's (which was eventually bought by Dick's Sporting Goods). Today, almost 30 percent of UA's sales come from Dick's and the Sports Authority. But they haven't forgotten where they started, either. The company has all-school deals with 10 Division 1 schools. "Although these deals don't bring in big bucks, they deliver brand visibility...."

Despite their marketing successes, innovation continues to be the name of the game at UA. How important is innovation to the company's heart and soul? Consider what you have to do to enter its new products lab. "Place your hands inside a state-of-the-art scanner that reads—and calculates—the exact pattern of the veins on the back. If it recognizes the pattern, which it does for only 20 out of 5,000 employees, you're in. If it doesn't, the vault-like door won't budge." In the unmarked lab at the company's headquarters campus in Baltimore, products being developed include a shirt that can monitor an athlete's heart rate, a running shoe designed like your back spine, and a sweatshirt that repels water almost as well as a duck's feathers. There's also work being done on a shirt that may help air-condition your body by reading your vital signs.

So what's next for Under Armour? With a motto that refers to protecting this house, innovation will continue to be important. Building a business beyond what it's known for—that is, what athletes wear next to their skin—is going to be challenging. However, Plank is "utterly determined to conquer that next layer, and the layer after that." He says, "There's not a product we can't build."

⭐ DISCUSSION QUESTIONS

13. What do you think of UA's approach to innovation? Would you expect to see this type of innovation in an athletic wear company? Explain.

14. What do you think UA's culture might be like in regards to innovation?

15. Could design thinking help UA improve its innovation efforts? Discuss.

16. What's your interpretation of the company's philosophy posted prominently over the door of its design studio? What does it say about innovation?

17. What could other companies learn from the way UA innovates?

CASE APPLICATION 2 Workplace Stress Can Kill

We know that too much stress can be bad for our health and well-being. That connection has proved itself painfully and tragically in two high-profile situations, at France Télécom and at China's Foxconn Technology Group.[84]

Between 2008 and 2011, more than 50 people at France Télécom committed suicide. The situation captured the attention of the worldwide media, the public, and the French government because many of the suicides and more than a dozen failed suicide attempts were attributed to work-related problems. Although France has a higher suicide rate than any other large Western country, this scenario is particularly troublesome. So much so, that the Paris prosecutor's office opened an investigation of the company over accusations of psychological harassment. The judicial inquiry began with a complaint by the union Solidares Unitaires Démocratiques against France Télécom's former chief executive and two members of his top management team. The complaint accused management of conducting a "pathogenic restructuring." Excerpts of the inspector's report, although not public, were published in the French media and described a situation in which the company used various forms of psychological pressure in an effort to eliminate 22,000 jobs. Company doctors alerted management about the possible psychological dangers of the stress that could accompany such drastic change. "The spate of suicides highlighted a quirk at the heart of French society: Even with robust labor protection, workers see themselves as profoundly insecure in the face of globalization, with many complaining about being pushed beyond their limits." A company lawyer denied that France Télécom had systematically pressured employees to leave.

Company executives realized they needed to take drastic measures to address the issue. One of the first changes was a new CEO, Stéphane Richard, who said his priority "would be to rebuild the morale of staff who have been through trauma, suffering and much worse." The company halted some workplace practices identified as particularly disruptive, like involuntary transfers, and began encouraging more supportive practices, including working from home. A company spokesperson says the company has completed two of six agreements with unions that cover a wide range of workplace issues such as mobility, work-life balance, and stress. Yet, France isn't the only country dealing with worker suicides.

Workplace conditions at China's Foxconn Technology Group—the world's largest maker of electronic components, which employs over a million workers—were strongly criticized after a series of suicides among young workers. In what was described as sweatshop conditions, employees often worked 76-hour weeks for low wages. Some workers said they had to stand so long, their legs swelled until they could

barely walk. Other complaints revolved around child labor and hazardous waste. One worker said, "The assembly line ran very fast and after just one morning we all had blisters and the skin on our hand was black. The factory was also really choked with dust and no one could bear it." In early 2012, Apple and Foxconn reached an agreement to improve conditions for the workers assembling iPhones and iPads. According to the agreement, Foxconn would hire thousands of new workers to reduce overtime work, improve safety protocols, and upgrade housing and other amenities. It's also reported that the company has launched a $224 million project to build one million robots in the next three years to use in its factories. This "empire of robots" will replace half a million Foxconn employees and move them "higher up the value chain."

⭐ DISCUSSION QUESTIONS

18. What is your reaction to the situations described in this case? What factors, both inside the companies and externally, appear to have contributed to this situation?

19. What appeared to be happening in the France Télécom's workplace? What stress symptoms might have alerted managers to a problem?

20. Should managers be free to make decisions that are in the best interests of the company without worrying about employee reactions? Discuss. What are the implications for managing change?

21. What are France Télécom's and Foxconn's executives doing to address the situation? Do you think it's enough? Are there other actions they might take? If so, describe those actions. If not, why not?

22. What could other companies and managers learn from this situation?

ENDNOTES

1. A. Weintraub and M. Tirrell, "Eli Lilly's Drug Assembly Line," *Bloomberg BusinessWeek,* March 8, 2010, pp. 56–57.

2. "Clear Direction in a Complex World: How Top Companies Create Clarity, Confidence and Community to Build Sustainable Performance," Towers Watson [www.towerswatson.com], 2011–2012; R. Soparnot, "The Concept of Organizational Change Capacity," *Journal of Organizational Change,* vol. 24, no. 1, 2011, pp. 640–661; A. H. Van de Ven and K. Sun, "Breakdowns in Implementing Models of Organization Change," *Academy of Management Perspectives,* August 2011, pp. 58–74; L. Dragoni, P. E. Tesluk, J. E. A. Russell, and I. S. Oh, "Understanding Managerial Development: Integrating Developmental Assignments, Learning Orientation, and Access to Developmental Opportunities in Predicting Managerial Competencies," *Academy of Management Journal,* August 2009, pp. 731–743; G. Nadler and W. J. Chandon, "Making Changes: The FIST Approach," *Journal of Management Inquiry,* September 2004, pp. 239–246; and C. R. Leana and B. Barry, "Stability and Change as Simultaneous Experiences in Organizational Life," *Academy of Management Review,* October 2000, pp. 753–759.

3. The idea for these metaphors came from J. E. Dutton, S. J. Ashford, R. M. O'Neill, and K. A. Lawrence, "Moves That Matter: Issue Selling and Organizational Change," *Academy of Management Journal,* August 2001, pp. 716–736; B. H. Kemelgor, S. D. Johnson, and S. Srinivasan, "Forces Driving Organizational Change: A Business School Perspective," *Journal of Education for Business,* January/February 2000, pp. 133–137; G. Colvin, "When It Comes to Turbulence, CEOs Could Learn a Lot from Sailors," *Fortune,* March 29, 1999, pp. 194–196; and P. B. Vaill, *Managing as a Performing Art: New Ideas for a World of Chaotic Change* (San Francisco: Jossey-Bass, 1989).

4. K. Lewin, *Field Theory in Social Science* (New York: Harper & Row, 1951).

5. R. Safian, "Generation Flux," *FastCompany.com,* February 2012, p. 62.

6. "Who's Next," *FastCompany.com,* December 2010/January 2011, p. 39.

7. D. Lieberman, "Nielsen Media Has Cool Head at the Top," *USA Today,* March 27, 2006, p. 3B.

8. S. A. Mohrman and E. E. Lawler III, "Generating Knowledge That Drives Change," *Academy of Management Perspectives,* February 2012, pp. 41–51; S. Ante, "Change Is Good—So Get Used to It," *BusinessWeek,* June 22, 2009, pp. 69–70; L. S. Lüscher and M. W. Lewis, "Organizational Change and Managerial Sensemaking: Working Through Paradox," *Academy of Management Journal,* April 2008, pp. 221–240; F. Buckley and K. Monks, "Responding to Managers' Learning Needs in an Edge-of-Chaos Environment: Insights from Ireland," *Journal of Management,* April 2008, pp. 146–163; and G. Hamel, "Take It Higher," *Fortune,* February 5, 2001, pp. 169–170.

9. "Electrolux Cops Top Design Honors," *This Week in Consumer Electronics,* June 4, 2012, p. 48; A. Wolf, "Electrolux Q1 Profits Up 23%," *This Week in Consumer Electronics,* May 7, 2012, p. 30; M. Boyle, "Persuading Brits to Give Up Their Dishrags," *Bloomberg BusinessWeek,* March 26, 2012, pp. 20–21; "Electrolux Earnings Down in 2011, Hopeful for 2012," *Appliance* Design.com, March 2012, pp. 7–8; "Electrolux Breaks Ground on Memphis Factory," *Kitchen & Bath Design News,* December 2011, p. 15; J. R. Hagerty and B. Tita, "Appliance Sales Tumble," *Wall Street Journal,* October 29, 2011, p. B1; and A. Sains and S. Reed, "Electrolux Cleans Up," *BusinessWeek,* February 27, 2006, pp. 42–43.

10. J. R. Hagerty, "3M Begins Untangling Its Hairballs," *Wall Street Journal,* May 17, 2012, p. B1+.

11. R. Lawrence, "Many Fish In A Global Development Pond," *Chief Learning Officer,* November 2011, pp. 26–31; K. Roose, "Outsiders' Ideas Help Bank of America Cut Jobs and Costs," *New York Times Online,* September 12, 2011; and "How HR Made A Difference," *PeopleManagement.co.uk,* February 2011, p. 31.

12. J. Zhiguo, "How I Did It: Tsingtao's Chairman on Jump-Starting a Sluggish Company," *Harvard Business Review,* April 2012, pp. 41–44.

13. J. Jesitus, "Change Management: Energy to the People," *Industry Week,* September 1, 1997, pp. 37, 40.

14. D. Lavin, "European Business Rushes to Automate," *Wall Street Journal*, July 23, 1997, p. A14.

15. See, for example, B. B. Bunker, B. T. Alban, and R. J. Lewicki, "Ideas in Currency and OD Practice," *The Journal of Applied Behavioral Science*, December 2004, pp. 403–422; L. E. Greiner and T. G. Cummings, "Wanted: OD More Alive Than Dead!" *Journal of Applied Behavioral Science*, December 2004, pp. 374–391; S. Hicks, "What Is Organization Development?" *Training & Development*, August 2000, p. 65; W. Nicolay, "Response to Farias and Johnson's Commentary," *Journal of Applied Behavioral Science*, September 2000, pp. 380–381; and G. Farias, "Organizational Development and Change Management," *Journal of Applied Behavioral Science*, September 2000, pp. 376–379.

16. T. White, "Supporting Change: How Communicators at Scotiabank Turned Ideas into Action," *Communication World*, April 2002, pp. 22–24.

17. M. Javidan, P. W. Dorfman, M. S. deLuque, and R. J. House, "In the Eye of the Beholder: Cross-Cultural Lessons in Leadership from Project GLOBE," *Academy of Management Perspective*, February 2006, pp. 67–90; and E. Fagenson-Eland, E. A. Ensher, and W. W. Burke, "Organization Development and Change Interventions: A Seven-Nation Comparison," *The Journal of Applied Behavioral Science*, December 2004, pp. 432–464.

18. E. Fagenson-Eland, Ensher, and Burke, "Organization Development and Change Interventions: A Seven-Nation Comparison," p. 461.

19. S. Shinn, "Stairway to Reinvention," *BizEd*, January/February 2010, p. 6; M. Scott, "A Stairway to Marketing Heaven," *BusinessWeek*, November 2, 2009, p. 17; and The Fun Theory [http://thefuntheory.com], November 10, 2009.

20. See, for example, J. D. Ford, L. W. Ford, and A. D'Amelio, "Resistance to Change: The Rest of the Story," *Academy of Management Review*, April 2008, pp. 362–377; A. Deutschman, "Making Change: Why Is It So Hard to Change Our Ways?" *Fast Company*, May 2005, pp. 52–62; S. B. Silverman, C. E. Pogson, and A. B. Cober, "When Employees at Work Don't Get It: A Model for Enhancing Individual Employee Change in Response to Performance Feedback," *Academy of Management Executive*, May 2005, pp. 135–147; C. E. Cunningham, C. A. Woodward, H. S. Shannon, J. MacIntosh, B. Lendrum, D. Rosenbloom, and J. Brown, "Readiness for Organizational Change: A Longitudinal Study of Workplace, Psychological and Behavioral Correlates," *Journal of Occupational and Organizational Psychology*, December 2002, pp. 377–392; M. A. Korsgaard, H. J. Sapienza, and D. M. Schweiger, "Beaten Before Begun: The Role of Procedural Justice in Planning Change," *Journal of Management*, 2002, vol. 28, no. 4, pp. 497–516; R. Kegan and L. L. Lahey, "The Real Reason People Won't Change," *Harvard Business Review*, November 2001, pp. 85–92; S. K. Piderit, "Rethinking Resistance and Recognizing Ambivalence: A Multidimensional View of Attitudes Toward an Organizational Change," *Academy of Management Review*, October 2000, pp. 783–794; C. R. Wanberg and J. T. Banas, "Predictors and Outcomes of Openness to Changes in a Reorganizing Workplace," *Journal of Applied Psychology*, February 2000, pp. 132–142; A. A. Armenakis and A. G. Bedeian, "Organizational Change: A Review of Theory and Research in the 1990s," *Journal of Management*, vol. 25, no. 3, 1999, pp. 293–315; and B. M. Staw, "Counterforces to Change," in P. S. Goodman and Associates (eds.), *Change in Organizations* (San Francisco: Jossey-Bass, 1982), pp. 87–121.

21. A. Reichers, J. P. Wanous, and J. T. Austin, "Understanding and Managing Cynicism about Organizational Change," *Academy of Management Executive*, February 1997, pp. 48–57; P. Strebel, "Why Do Employees Resist Change?" *Harvard Business Review*, May–June 1996, pp. 86–92; and J. P. Kotter and L. A. Schlesinger, "Choosing Strategies for Change," *Harvard Business Review*, March–April 1979, pp. 107–109.

22. A. Foege, "Wii at Work," *CNNMoney* [cnnmoney.com], June 5, 2009.

23. D. Aguirre and R. von Post, "Culture's Critical Role in Change Management," www.strategy-business.com, December 5, 2013.

24. R. Yu, "Korean Air Upgrades Service, Image," *USA Today*, August 24, 2009, pp. 1B+.

25. See P. Anthony, *Managing Culture* (Philadelphia: Open University Press, 1994); P. Bate, *Strategies for Cultural Change* (Boston: Butterworth-Heinemann, 1994); C. G. Smith and R. P. Vecchio, "Organizational Culture and Strategic Management: Issues in the Strategic Management of Change," *Journal of Managerial Issues*, Spring 1993, pp. 53–70; P. F. Drucker, "Don't Change Corporate Culture—Use It!" *Wall Street Journal*, March 28, 1991, p. A14; and T. H. Fitzgerald, "Can Change in Organizational Culture Really Be Managed?" *Organizational Dynamics*, Autumn 1988, pp. 5–15.

26. K. Maney, "Famously Gruff Gerstner Leaves IBM a Changed Man," *USA Today*, November 11, 2002, pp. 1B+; and Louis V. Gerstner, *Who Says Elephants Can't Dance: Inside IBM's Historic Turnaround* (New York: Harper Business, 2002).

27. S. Ovide, "Next CEO's Job: Fix Microsoft Culture," *Wall Street Journal*, August 26, 2013, pp. B1+.

28. N. Bilton, "With New Chief, Microsoft's New Mantra Is 'Innovation' Over and Over," *New York Times Online*, February 4, 2014.

29. See, for example, D. C. Hambrick and S. Finkelstein, "Managerial Discretion: A Bridge between Polar Views of Organizational Outcomes," in L. L. Cummings and B. M. Staw (eds.), *Research in Organizational Behavior*, vol. 9 (Greenwich, CT: JAI Press, 1987), p. 384; and R. H. Kilmann, M. J. Saxton, and R. Serpa (eds.), *Gaining Control of the Corporate Culture* (San Francisco: Jossey-Bass, 1985).

30. P. Davidson, "Moonlighting Becomes a Way of Life for Many," *USA Today*, June 24, 2009, p. 3B.

31. P. Korkki, "Driven to Worry, and to Procrastinate," *New York Times Online*, February 25, 2012; E. Frauenheim, "To the Limit," *Workforce Management Online*, December 16, 2011; A. Kadet, "Surviving the Superjob," *SmartMoney*, June 2011, pp. 75–79; L. J. Dugan, "Working Two Jobs and Still Underemployed," *Wall Street Journal*, December 1, 2009, p. A15; N. Parmar, "The New Balancing Act," *Smart Money*, October 2009, p. 59; and Davidson "Moonlighting Becomes a Way of Life for Many."

32. S. Ilgenfritz, "Are We Too Stressed to Reduce Our Stress?" *Wall Street Journal*, November 10, 2009, p. D2; C. Daniels, "The Last Taboo," *Fortune*, October 28, 2002, pp. 137–144; J. Laabs, "Time-Starved Workers Rebel," *Workforce*, October 2000, pp. 26–28; M. A. Verespej, "Stressed Out," *Industry Week*, February 21, 2000, pp. 30–34; and M. A. Cavanaugh, W. R. Boswell, M. V. Roehling, and J. W. Boudreau, "An Empirical Examination of Self-Reported Work Stress Among U.S. Managers," *Journal of Applied Psychology*, February 2000, pp. 65–74.

33. A report on job stress compiled by the American Institute of Stress [www.stress.org/job], 2002–2003.

34. M. Conlin, "Go-Go-Going to Pieces in China," *Business Week*, April 23, 2007, p. 88; V. P. Sudhashree, K. Rohith, and K. Shrinivas, "Issues and Concerns of Health Among Call Center Employees," *Indian Journal of Occupational Environmental Medicine*," vol. 9, no. 3, 2005, pp. 129–132; E. Muehlchen, "An Ounce of Prevention Goes a Long Way," Wilson Banwell [www.wilsonbanwell.com], January 2004; UnionSafe, "Stressed Employees Worked to Death" [unionsafe.labor.net.au/news], August 23, 2003; O. Siu, "Occupational Stressors and Well-Being Among Chinese Employees: The Role of Organizational Commitment," *Applied Psychology: An International Review*, October 2002, pp. 527–544; O. Siu, P. E. Spector, C. L. Cooper, L. Lu, and S. Yu, "Managerial Stress in Greater China: The Direct and Moderator Effects of Coping Strategies and Work Locus of Control," *Applied Psychology: An International Review*, October 2002, pp. 608–632; A. Oswald, "New Research Reveals Dramatic Rise in Stress Levels in Europe's Workplaces," University of Warwick [www.warwick.ac.uk/news/pr], 1999; and Y. Shimizu, S. Makino, and T. Takata, "Employee Stress Status During the Past Decade [1982–1992] Based on a Nation-Wide Survey Conducted by the Ministry of Labour in Japan," Japan Industrial Safety and Health Association, July 1997, pp. 441–450.

35. G. Kranz, "Job Stress Viewed Differently by Workers, Employers," *Workforce Management* [www.workforce.com], January 15, 2008.

36. Adapted from the UK National Work-Stress Network [www.workstress.net].

37. R. S. Schuler, "Definition and Conceptualization of Stress in Organizations," *Organizational Behavior and Human Performance*, April 1980, p. 191.

38. A. R. Carey and P. Trap, "Feeling Stressed at Work," *USA Today*, June 12, 2013, p. 1A.

39. J. B. Rodell and T. A. Judge, "Can 'Good' Stressors Spark 'Bad' Behaviors? The Mediating Role of Emotions in Links of Challenge and Hindrance Stressors with Citizenship and Counterproductive Behaviors," *Journal of Applied Psychology,* November 2009, pp. 1438–1451; and see, for example, "Stressed Out: Extreme Job Stress: Survivors' Tales," *Wall Street Journal,* January 17, 2001, p. B1.

40. See, for instance, S. Bates, "Expert: Don't Overlook Employee Burnout," *HR Magazine,* August 2003, p. 14.

41. "The Japanese Are Dying to Get to Work," www.tofugu.com, January 26, 2012; A. Kanai, "Karoshi (Work to Death) in Japan," *Journal of Business Ethics,* January 2009, Supplement 2, pp. 209–216; "Jobs for Life," *The Economist* [www.economist.com], December 19, 2007; and B. L. de Mente, "Karoshi: Death from Overwork," Asia Pacific Management Forum [www.apmforum.com], May 2002.

42. H. Benson, "Are You Working Too Hard?" *Harvard Business Review,* November 2005, pp. 53–58; B. Cryer, R. McCraty, and D. Childre, "Pull the Plug on Stress," *Harvard Business Review,* July 2003, pp. 102–107; C. Daniels, "The Last Taboo;" C. L. Cooper and S. Cartwright, "Healthy Mind, Healthy Organization—A Proactive Approach to Occupational Stress," *Human Relations,* April 1994, pp. 455–471; C. A. Heaney et al., "Industrial Relations, Worksite Stress Reduction and Employee Well-Being: A Participatory Action Research Investigation," *Journal of Organizational Behavior,* September 1993, pp. 495–510; C. D. Fisher, "Boredom at Work: A Neglected Concept," *Human Relations,* March 1993, pp. 395–417; and S. E. Jackson, "Participation in Decision Making as a Strategy for Reducing Job-Related Strain," *Journal of Applied Psychology,* February 1983, pp. 3–19.

43. C. Mamberto, "Companies Aim to Combat Job-Related Stress," *Wall Street Journal,* August 13, 2007, p. B6.

44. J. Goudreau, "Dispatches from the War on Stress," *BusinessWeek,* August 6, 2007, pp. 74–75.

45. Well Workplace 2008 Award Executive Summaries, Wellmark BlueCross BlueShield and Zimmer Holdings, Inc., available on Wellness Councils of America Web site [www.welcoa.org].

46. P. A. McLagan, "Change Leadership Today," *T&D,* November 2002, pp. 27–31.

47. D. Meinert, "Wings of Change," *HR Magazine,* November 2012, p. 32.

48. P. A. McLagan, "Change Leadership Today," *T&D,* November 2002, p. 29.

49. K. Kingsbury, "Road to Recovery," *Time,* March 18, 2010, pp. Global 14–16; and C. Haddad, "UPS: Can It Keep Delivering?" *BusinessWeek Online Extra* [www.businessweek.com], Spring 2003.

50. W. Pietersen, "The Mark Twain Dilemma: The Theory and Practice for Change Leadership," *Journal of Business Strategy,* September/October 2002, p. 35.

51. P. A. McLagan, "The Change-Capable Organization," *T&D,* January 2003, pp. 50–58.

52. A. Saha-Bubna and M. Jarzemsky, "MasterCard President Is Named CEO," *Wall Street Journal,* April 13, 2010, p. C3; and S. Vandebook, "Quotable," *IndustryWeek,* April 2010, p. 18.

53. R. M. Kanter, "Think Outside the Building," *Harvard Business Review,* March 2010, p. 34; T. Brown, "Change By Design," *BusinessWeek,* October 5, 2009, pp. 54–56; J. E. Perry-Smith and C. E. Shalley, "The Social Side of Creativity: A Static and Dynamic Social Network Perspective," *Academy of Management Review,* January 2003, pp. 89–106; and P. K. Jagersma, "Innovate or Die: It's Not Easy, But It Is Possible to Enhance Your Organization's Ability to Innovate," *Journal of Business Strategy,* January–February 2003, pp. 25–28.

54. S. Castellano, "Guidelines to Innovation," *T&D,* September 2013, p. 20.

55. E. Brynjolfsson and M. Schrage, "The New Faster Face of Innovation," *Wall Street Journal,* August 17, 2009, p. R3.

56. Ibid.

57. L. Kwoh, "You Call That Innovation?" *Wall Street Journal,* May 23, 2012, pp. B1+.

58. These definitions are based on E. Miron-Spektor, M. Erez, and E. Naveh, "The Effect of Conformist and Attentive-to-Detail Members on Team Innovation: Reconciling the Innovation Paradox," *Academy of Management Journal,* August 2011, pp. 740–760; and T. M. Amabile, *Creativity in Context* (Boulder, CO: Westview Press, 1996).

59. U. R. Hülsheger, N. Anderson, and J. F. Salgado, "Team-Level Predictors of Innovation at Work: A Comprehensive Meta-Analysis Spanning Three Decades of Research," *Journal of Applied Psychology,* September 2009, pp. 1128–1145; R. W. Woodman, J. E. Sawyer, and R. W. Griffin, "Toward a Theory of Organizational Creativity," *Academy of Management Review,* April 1993, pp. 293–321.

60. Future Vision box based on R. Tate, "Google Couldn't Kill 20 Percent Time Even If It Wanted To," wired.com, August 21, 2013; C. Mims, "Google Engineers Insist 20% Time Is Not Dead—It's Just Turned Into 120% Time," qz.com, August 16, 2013; R. Neimi, "Inside the Moonshot Factory," *Bloomberg BusinessWeek,* May 22, 2013, pp. 56–61; and A. Foege, "The Trouble With Tinkering Time," *Wall Street Journal,* January 19/20, 2013, p. C3.

61. "SmartPulse," smartbrief.com, June 19, 2013.

62. G. Hirst, D. Van Knippenberg, C. H. Chen, and C. A. Sacramento, "How Does Bureaucracy Impact Individual Creativity? A Cross-Level Investigation of Team Contextual Influences on Goal Orientation-Creativity Relationships," *Academy of Management Journal,* June 2011, pp. 624–641; L. Sagiv, S. Arieli, J. Goldenberg, and A. Goldschmidt, "Structure and Freedom in Creativity: The Interplay Between Externally Imposed Structure and Personal Cognitive Style," *Journal of Organizational Behavior,* November 2010, pp. 1086–1100; J. van denEnde and G. Kijkuit, "Nurturing Good Ideas," *Harvard Business Review,* April 2009, p. 24; T. M. Egan, "Factors Influencing Individual Creativity in the Workplace: An Examination of Quantitative Empirical Research," *Advances in Developing Human Resources,* May 2005, pp. 160–181; N. Madjar, G. R. Oldham, and M. G. Pratt, "There's No Place Like Home? The Contributions of Work and Nonwork Creativity Support to Employees' Creative Performance," *Academy of Management Journal,* August 2002, pp. 757–767; T. M. Amabile, C. N. Hadley, and S. J. Kramer, "Creativity Under the Gun," *Harvard Business Review,* August 2002, pp. 52–61; J. B. Sorensen and T. E. Stuart, "Aging, Obsolescence, and Organizational Innovation," *Administrative Science Quarterly,* March 2000, pp. 81–112; G. R. Oldham and A. Cummings, "Employee Creativity: Personal and Contextual Factors at Work," *Academy of Management Journal,* June 1996, pp. 607–634; and F. Damanpour, "Organizational Innovation: A Meta-Analysis of Effects of Determinants and Moderators," *Academy of Management Journal,* September 1991, pp. 555–590.

63. J. S. Lublin, "Smart Balance Keeps Tight Focus on Creativity," *Wall Street Journal,* June 8, 2009, p. B4.

64. P. R. Monge, M. D. Cozzens, and N. S. Contractor, "Communication and Motivational Predictors of the Dynamics of Organizational Innovations," *Organization Science,* May 1992, pp. 250–274.

65. D. Dobson, "Integrated Innovation at Pitney Bowes," *Strategy+Business* [www.strategy-business.com], October 26, 2009.

66. T. M. Amabile, C. N. Hadley, and S. J. Kramer, "Creativity Under the Gun."

67. T. Jana, "Dusting Off a Big Idea in Hard Times," *BusinessWeek,* June 22, 2009, pp. 44–46.

68. N. Madjar, G. R. Oldham, and M. G. Pratt, "There's No Place Like Home? The Contributions of Work and Nonwork Creativity Support to Employees' Creative Performance."

69. C. Salter, "Mattel Learns to 'Throw the Bunny,'" *Fast Company,* November 2002, p. 22.

70. See, for instance, K. E. M. De Stobbeleir, S. J. Ashford, and D. Buyens, "Self-Regulation of Creativity at Work: The Role of Feedback-Seeking Behavior in Creative Performance," *Academy of Management Journal,* August 2011, pp. 811–831; J. Cable, "Building an Innovation Culture," *Industry Week,* March 2010, pp. 32–37; M. Hawkins, "Create a Climate of Creativity," *Training,* January 2010, p. 12; D. C. Wyld, "Keys to Innovation: The Right Measures and the Right Culture?" *Academy of Management Perspective,* May 2009, pp. 96–98; J. E. Perry-Smith, "Social Yet Creative: The Role of Social Relationships in Facilitating Individual Creativity," *Academy of Management Journal,* February 2006, pp. 85–101; C. E. Shalley, J. Zhou, and G. R. Oldham, "The Effects of Personal and Contextual Characteristics on Creativity: Where Should We Go from Here?" *Journal of Management,* vol. 30, no. 6, 2004, pp. 933–958; J. E. Perry-Smith and C. E. Shalley, "The Social Side of Creativity: A Static and Dynamic Social Network Perspective;" J. M. George and J. Zhou, "When Openness to Experience and

Conscientiousness are Related to Creative Behavior: An Interactional Approach," *Journal of Applied Psychology,* June 2001, pp. 513–524; J. Zhou, "Feedback Valence, Feedback Style, Task Autonomy, and Achievement Orientation: Interactive Effects on Creative Behavior," *Journal of Applied Psychology,* 1998, vol. 83, pp. 261–276; T. M. Amabile, R. Conti, H. Coon, J. Lazenby, and M. Herron, "Assessing the Work Environment for Creativity," *Academy of Management Journal,* October 1996, pp. 1154–1184; S. G. Scott and R. A. Bruce, "Determinants of Innovative People: A Path Model of Individual Innovation in the Workplace," *Academy of Management Journal,* June 1994, pp. 580–607; R. Moss Kanter, "When a Thousand Flowers Bloom: Structural, Collective, and Social Conditions for Innovation in Organization," in B. M. Staw and L. L. Cummings (eds.), *Research in Organizational Behavior,* vol. 10 (Greenwich, CT: JAI Press, 1988), pp. 169–211; and Amabile, *Creativity in Context.*

71. L. A. Schlesinger, C. F. Kiefer, and P. B. Brown, "New Project? Don't Analyze—Act," *Harvard Business Review,* March 2012, pp. 154–158.

72. T. L. Stanley, "Creating a No-Blame Culture," *Supervision,* October 2011, pp. 3–6; S. Shellenbarger, "Better Ideas Through Failure," *Wall Street Journal,* October 27, 2011, pp. D1+; and R. W. Goldfarb, "When Fear Stifles Initiative," *New York Times Online,* May 14, 2011.

73. S. Shellenbarger, "Better Ideas Through Failure."

74. F. Yuan and R. W. Woodman, "Innovative Behavior in the Workplace: The Role of Performance and Image Outcome Expectations," *Academy of Management Journal,* April 2010, pp. 323–342.

75. K. E. M. De Stobbeleir, S. J. Ashford, and D. Buyens, "Self-Regulation of Creativity at Work: The Role of Feedback-Seeking Behavior in Creative Performance."

76. J. McGregor, "The World's Most Innovative Companies," *Business-Week,* April 24, 2006, p. 70.

77. X. Zhang and K. M. Bartol, "Linking Empowering Leadership and Employee Creativity: The Influence of Psychological Empowerment, Intrinsic Motivation, and Creative Process Engagement," *Academy of Management Journal,* February 2010, pp. 107–128.

78. J. H. Dyer, H. B. Gregersen, and C. M. Christensen, "The Innovator's DNA," *Harvard Business Review,* December 2009, pp. 60–67; J. Gong, J-C Huang, and J-L. Farh, "Employee Learning Orientation, Transformational Leadership, and Employee Creativity: The Mediating Role of Employee Creative Self-Efficacy," *Academy of Management Journal,* August 2009, pp. 765–778; B. Buxton, "Innovation Calls for I-Shaped People," *BusinessWeek Online* [www.businessweek.com], July 13, 2009; J. Ramos, "Producing Change That Lasts," *Across the Board,* March 1994, pp. 29–33; T. Stjernberg and A. Philips, "Organizational Innovations in a Long-Term Perspective: Legitimacy and Souls-of-Fire as Critical Factors of Change and Viability," *Human Relations,* October 1993, pp. 1193–2023; and J. M. Howell and C. A. Higgins, "Champions of Change," *Business Quarterly,* Spring 1990, pp. 31–32.

79. J. Liedtka and T. Ogilvie, *Designing for Growth: A Design Thinking Tool Kit for Managers,* (New York: Columbia Business School Press, 2011).

80. R. E. Silverman, "Companies Change Their Way of Thinking," *Wall Street Journal,* June 7, 2012, p. B8; and R. L. Martin, "The Innovation Catalysts," *Harvard Business Review,* June 2011, pp. 82–87.

81. Ethics Dilemma based on T. Roth and J. Harter, "Unhealthy, Stressed Employees Are Hurting Your Business," *Gallup Business Journal Online,* May 22, 2012; R. Vesely, "EAPs Modernize, But Employees Are Slow to Catch On," *Workforce Management Online,* February 20, 2012; A. Kadet, "Surviving the Superjob;" P. F. Weisberg, "Wellness Programs: Legal Requirements and Risks," *Workforce Management Online* [www.workforce.com], March 2010; S. S. Wang, "Workplace Mental-Health Services Expand," *Wall Street Journal,* December 15, 2009, p. D8; and D. Cole, "The Big Chill," *US News & World Report,* December 6, 2004, pp. EE2–EE5.

82. Developing Your Skill box based on J. P. Kotter and L. A. Schlesinger, "Choosing Strategies for Change," *Harvard Business Review,* March–April 1979, pp. 106–114; and T. A. Stewart, "Rate Your Readiness to Change," *Fortune,* February 7, 1994, pp. 106–110.

83. B. Horovitz, "In Search of Next Big Thing," *USA Today,* July 9, 2012, pp. 1B+; Press Release, "Under Armour Reports Fourth Quarter Net Revenues Growth of 34% and Fourth Quarter EPS Growth of 40%," [investor.underarmour.com], January 26, 2012; D. Roberts, "Under Armour Gets Serious," *Fortune,* November 7, 2011, pp. 153–162; E. Olson, "Under Armour Applies Its Muscle to Shoes," *New York Times Online,* August 8, 2011; M. Townsend, "Under Armour's Daring Half-Court Shot," *Bloomberg BusinessWeek,* November 1–November 7, 2010, pp. 24–25; and E. Olson, "Under Armour Wants to Dress Athletic Young Women," *New York Times Online,* August 31, 2010.

84. J. Clare, "Foxconn Says Another Worker Committed Suicide," Reuters, [www.businessinsider.com], June 14, 2012; M. Moore, "Mass Suicide Protest at Apple Manufacturer Foxconn Factory," [www.telegraph.co.uk], January 11, 2012; C. Campbell, "Foxconn's Robot Empire," *Macleans,* November 21, 2011, p. 41; T. Culpan, Z. Lifei, B. Einhorn, "How to Beat the High Cost of Happy Workers," *Bloomberg Business-Week,* May 9, 2011, pp. 39–40; A. Chrisafis, "France Télécom Worker Kills Himself in Office Car Park," [www.guardian.co.uk], April 26, 2011; M. Saltmarsh, "France Télécom Suicides Prompt an Investigation," *New York Times Online,* April 9, 2010; C. Stievenard, "France's Approach to Workplace Bullying," *Workforce Management Online* [www.workforce.com], March 2010; R. Bender and M. Colchester, "Morale Is Priority for France Télécom," *Wall Street Journal,* February 4, 2010, p. B2; The Associated Press, "Executive Quits After Suicides at France Télécom," *New York Times Online,* October 6, 2009; and D. Jolly and M. Saltmarsh, "Suicides in France Put Focus on Workplace," *New York Times Online,* September 30, 2009.

Management Practice: Part 2

Management Practice

A Manager's Dilemma

One of the biggest fears of a food service company manager has to be the hepatitis A virus, a highly contagious virus transmitted by sharing food, utensils, cigarettes, or drug paraphernalia with an infected person. Food service workers aren't any more susceptible to the illness than anyone else, but an infected employee can easily spread the virus by handling food, especially cold foods. The virus, which is rarely fatal, can cause flulike illness for several weeks. There is no cure for hepatitis A, but a vaccine can prevent it. Jim Brady, manager of a restaurant, is facing a serious dilemma. He recently learned one of his cooks could have exposed as many as 350 people to hepatitis A during a five-day period when he was at work. The cook was thought to have contracted the virus through an infant living in his apartment complex. Because children usually show no symptoms of the disease, they can easily pass it on to adults. Jim has a decision to make. Should he go public with the information, or should he only report it to the local health department as required by law?

Using what you've learned, what would you do in this situation?

Global Sense

A vice president for engineering at a major chip manufacturer who found one of his projects running more than a month late felt that perhaps the company's Indian engineers "didn't understand the sense of urgency" in getting the project completed. In the Scottish highlands, the general manager of O'Bryant's Kitchens is quite satisfied with his non-Scottish employees—cooks who are German, Swedish, and Slovak, and waitresses who are mostly Polish. Other highland hotels and restaurants also have a large number of Eastern European staff. Despite the obvious language barriers, these Scottish employers are finding ways to help their foreign employees adapt and be successful. When the manager of a telecommunications company's developer forum gave a presentation to a Finnish audience and asked for feedback, he was told, "That was good." Based on his interpretation of that phrase, he assumed it must have been just an okay presentation—nothing spectacular. However, since Finns tend to be generally much quieter and more reserved than Americans, that response actually meant, "That was great, off the scale." And the owner of a Chicago-based manufacturing company, who now has two factories in Suzhou, China, is dealing with the challenges that many companies moving to China face: understanding the way their Chinese employees view work and nurturing Chinese managerial talent.

It's not easy being a successful global manager, especially when it comes to dealing with cultural differences. Those cultural differences have been described as an "iceberg," of which we only see the top 15 percent, mainly food, appearance, and language. Although these elements can be complicated, it's the other 85 percent of the "iceberg" that's not apparent initially that managers need to be especially concerned about. What does that include? Workplace issues such as communication styles, priorities, role expectations, work tempo, negotiation styles, nonverbal communication, attitudes toward planning, and so forth. Understanding these issues requires developing a global mindset and skill set. Many organizations are relying on cultural awareness training to help them do just that.

Discuss the following questions in light of what you learned:

- *What global attitude do you think would most encourage, support, and promote cultural awareness? Explain.*
- *Would legal-political and economic differences play a role as companies design appropriate cultural awareness training for employees? Explain.*
- *Is diversity management related to cultural awareness? Discuss.*
- *Pick one of the countries mentioned above and do some cultural research on it. What did you find out about the culture of that country? How might this information affect the way a manager in that country plans, organizes, leads, and controls?*
- *What advice might you give to a manager who has little experience globally?*

Sources: P. Korkki, "More Courses Get You Ready to Face the World," New York Times Online, February 29, 2012; N. Bloom, C. Genakos, R. Sadun, and J. Van Reenen, "Management Practices Across Firms and Countries," Academy of Management Perspectives, February 2012, pp. 12–33; E. Spitznagel, "Impress Your Chinese Boss," Bloomberg BusinessWeek, January 9–15, 2012, pp. 80–81; R. S. Vassolo, J. O. De Castro, and L. R. Gomez-Meija, "Managing in Latin America: Common Issues and A Research Agenda," Academy of Management Perspectives, November 2011, pp. 22–37; P. Thorby, "Great Expectations: Mastering Cultural Sensitivity in Business and HR," [www.workforce.com], August 17, 2011; K. Tyler, "Global Ease," HR Magazine, May 2011, pp. 41–48; J. S. Lublin, "Cultural Flexibility In Demand," Wall Street Journal, April 11, 2011, pp. B1+; and S. Russwurm, L. Hernandez, S. Chambers, and K. Chung, "Developing Your Global Know-How," Harvard Business Review, March 2011, pp. 70–75.

Continuing Case

Starbucks—Basics of Managing in Today's Workplace

As managers manage in today's workplace, they must be aware of some specific integrative issues that can affect the way they plan, organize, lead, and control. The

characteristics and nature of these integrative issues will influence what managers and other employees do and how they do it. And more importantly, it will affect how efficiently and effectively managers do their job of coordinating and overseeing the work of other people so that goals—organizational and work-level or work-unit—can be accomplished. What are these integrative managerial issues, and how does Starbucks accommodate and respond to them as they manage in today's workplace? In this part of the Continuing Case, we're going to look at Starbucks' external environment/organizational culture, global business, diversity, and social responsibility/ethical challenges.

Starbucks—Defining the Terrain: Culture and Environment

As managers manage, they must be aware of the terrain or broad environment within which they plan, organize, lead, and control. The characteristics and nature of this "terrain" will influence what managers and other employees do and how they do it. And more importantly, it will affect how efficiently and effectively managers do their job of coordinating and overseeing the work of other people so that goals—organizational and work-level or work-unit—can be accomplished. What does Starbucks' terrain look like, and how is the company adapting to that terrain?

An organization's culture is a mix of written and unwritten values, beliefs, and codes of behavior that influence the way work gets done and the way people behave in organizations. And the distinct flavor of Starbucks' culture can be traced to the original founders' philosophies and Howard Schultz's unique beliefs about how a company should be run. The three friends (Jerry Baldwin, Gordon Bowker, and Zev Siegl) who founded Starbucks in 1971 as a store in Seattle's historic Pike Place Market district did so for one reason: They loved coffee and tea and wanted Seattle to have access to the best. They had no intention of building a business empire. Their business philosophy, although never written down, was simple: "Every company must stand for something; don't just give customers what they ask for or what they think they want; and assume that your customers are intelligent and seekers of knowledge." The original Starbucks was a company passionately committed to world-class coffee and dedicated to educating its customers, one-on-one, about what great coffee can be. It was these qualities that ignited Howard Schultz's passion for the coffee business and inspired him to envision what Starbucks could become. Schultz continues to have that passion for his business—he is the visionary and soul behind Starbucks. He visits at least 30 to 40 stores a week, talking to partners (employees) and to customers. His ideas for running a business have been called "unconventional," but Schultz doesn't care. He says, "We can be extremely profitable and competitive, with a highly regarded brand, and also be respected for treating our people well." One member of the company's board of directors says about him, "Howard is consumed

with his vision of Starbucks. That means showing the good that a corporation can do for its workers, shareholders, and customers."

The company's mission and guiding principles (which you can find at www.starbucks.com) are meant to guide the decisions and actions of company partners from top to bottom. They also have significantly influenced the organization's culture. Starbucks' culture emphasizes keeping employees motivated and content. One thing that's been important to Howard Schultz from day one is the relationship he has with his employees. He treasures those relationships and feels they're critically important to the way the company develops its relationships with its customers and the way it is viewed by the public. He says, "We know that our people are the heart and soul of our success." Starbucks' 200,000-plus employees worldwide serve millions of customers each week. That's a lot of opportunities to either satisfy or disappoint the customer. The experiences customers have in the stores ultimately affect the company's relationships with its customers. That's why Starbucks has created a unique relationship with its employees. Starbucks provides all employees who work more than 20 hours a week health care benefits and stock options. Schultz says, "The most important thing I ever did was give our partners (employees) bean stock (options to buy the company's stock). That's what sets us apart and gives us a higher-quality employee, an employee that cares more." And Starbucks does care about its employees. For instance, when three Starbucks employees were murdered in a botched robbery attempt in Washington, D.C., Schultz immediately flew there to handle the situation. In addition, he decided that all future profits from that store would go to organizations working for victims' rights and violence prevention. Another example of the company's concern: recently, Starbucks announced that it was committed to hiring 10,000 veterans and military spouses over the next five years.

As a global company with revenues of $14.9 billion, Starbucks' executives recognize they must be aware of the impact the environment has on their decisions and actions. Starbucks began lobbying legislators in Washington, D.C., on issues including lowering trade barriers, health care costs, and tax breaks. It's something that Schultz didn't really want to do, but he recognized that such efforts could be important to the company's future.

Global Challenges

You could say that Starbucks has been a global business from day one. While on a business trip in 1983 to Milan, Howard Schultz (who worked in marketing for Starbucks' original founders and is now the company's CEO) experienced firsthand Italy's coffee culture and had an epiphany about how such an approach might work back home in the United States. Now, almost 40 years later, Starbucks stores are found in 62 countries (as of 2014), including stores from China and Australia to the Netherlands and Switzerland,

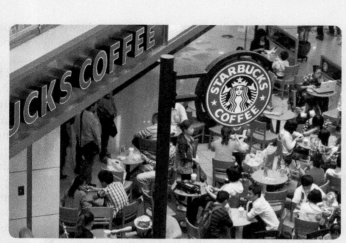

These customers are enjoying "the Starbucks experience" at a coffee shop in Guangzhou, China. Starbucks sees an enormous potential for growth in China, where 140 cities have a population exceeding one million people. While expanding in China and other global markets, Starbucks managers must take into account the cultural, economic, legal, and political aspects of different markets as they plan, organize, lead, and control.
Source: Imaginechina/Associated Press

among others. Doing business globally can be challenging. Since much of the company's future growth prospects are global, the company has targeted some markets for additional global expansion, including China, Brazil, and Vietnam. Schultz is clear about the fact that his company sees China as the number one growth opportunity for Starbucks. During a visit in late 2011, a government official informed him that 140 cities in China now have a population exceeding one million people. That's a lot of potential coffee drinkers buying cups of Starbucks coffee and other Starbucks products! But in China and all of its global markets, Starbucks must be cognizant of the economic, legal-political, and cultural aspects that characterize those markets. For instance, in Europe—the "birthplace of café and coffeehouse culture"—Starbucks is struggling, even after a decade of doing business there. Take France, where Starbucks has been since 2004 and has 63 stores. It has never made a profit. Of course, part of that could be attributed to the debt crisis and sluggish economy. And rents and labor costs are notoriously high. Yet, the biggest challenge for Starbucks may be trying to appeal to the vast array of European tastes. The company's chief of Starbucks operations for Europe, the Middle East, and Africa decided to take an "anthropological tour" to get a better feel for the varying wants and needs of coffee lovers in Europe. Although it was initially thought that the well-established coffeehouse culture in places like Paris or Vienna might be what customers wanted, what was discovered instead was that customers wanted the "Starbucks experience." But even that means different things in different markets. For instance, the British drink take-away (to-go) coffee, so Starbucks is planning for hundreds of drive-through locations there. In the rest of Europe, Starbucks plans to put many new sites in airports and railway stations on the continent. Although the growth potential seems

real, cultural challenges still remain, not only in Europe but in Starbucks' other markets as well. The company is recognizing that not every customer wants a "watered-down Starbucks" experience. So, as Starbucks continues its global expansion, it's attempting to be respectful of the cultural differences, most especially in that important market, China.

Managing Diversity and Inclusion

Not only does Starbucks attempt to be respectful of global cultural differences, it is committed to being an organization that embraces and values diversity in how it does business. The company-wide diversity strategy encompasses four areas: customers, suppliers, partners (employees), and communities. Starbucks attempts to make the Starbucks Experience accessible to all customers and to respond to each customer's unique preferences and needs. Starbucks' supplier diversity program works to provide opportunities for developing a business relationship to women- and minority-owned suppliers. As far as its partners, the company is committed to a workplace that values and respects people from diverse backgrounds. The most current company diversity statistics available show that 33 percent of employees are minorities and 64 percent are women. And Starbucks aims to enable its partners to do their best work and to be successful in the Starbucks environment. The company does support partner networks. Some of the current ones include Starbucks Access Alliance, a forum for partners with disabilities; Starbucks Armed Forces Support Network, which supports veterans and those currently in the armed forces and their families; and the Starbucks Black Partner Network, which strengthens relationships and connections among partners of African descent. Finally, Starbucks supports diversity in its local neighborhoods and global communities through programs and investments that deepen its ties in those areas. Although Starbucks is committed to practicing and valuing diversity, by no means is it perfect. For instance, an Americans with Disabilities Act case was filed against a specific Starbucks store by a job applicant who had short height because of the condition of dwarfism. The store management refused to hire her for a barista job even though she claimed she could do the job using a step stool. And they did not even offer to try this accommodation. Starbucks quickly settled the case and agreed to provide training to managers on proper ADA procedures. The company's response earned praise from the Equal Employment Opportunity Commission for its prompt resolution of the issue.

Social Responsibility and Ethics

Doing good coffee is important to Starbucks, but so is doing good. Starbucks takes its social responsibility and ethical commitments seriously. In 2001, the company began issuing an annual corporate social responsibility report, which

addresses the company's decisions and actions in relation to its products, society, the environment, and the workplace. These reports aren't simply a way for Starbucks to brag about its socially responsible actions, but are intended to stress the importance of doing business in a responsible way and to hold employees and managers accountable for their actions.

Starbucks focuses its corporate responsibility efforts on three main areas: ethical sourcing (buying), environmental stewardship, and community involvement. Starbucks approaches ethical sourcing from the perspective of helping the farmers and suppliers who grow and produce their products use responsible growing methods and helping them be successful, thus promoting long-term sustainability of the supply of quality coffee. It's a win-win situation. The farmers have a better (and more secure) future and Starbucks is helping create a long-term supply of a commodity they depend on. Environmental stewardship has been one of the more challenging undertakings for Starbucks, especially when you think about the number of disposable containers generated by the more than three billion customers served annually. And front-of-the-store waste is only half the battle. Behind-the-counter waste is also generated in the form of cardboard boxes, milk jugs, syrup bottles, and, not surprisingly, coffee grounds. Even with recycling bins provided, one wrong item in a recycle bin can make the whole thing unrecyclable to a hauler. Despite this, the company has made significant strides in recycling. In a 2010 test program, 100,000 paper coffee cups were made into new ones. The company's goal by 2015 was to recycle all four-billion-plus cups sold annually. An ambitious goal, for sure. And it wasn't able to meet that goal, as customer recycling is available at only 39 percent of its company-operated stores. However, the company has made progress possible only through a cooperative effort with other companies in the materials value chain (even competitors) to find recycling solutions that work. Starbucks is totally committed to being a good environmental steward. Finally, Starbucks has always strived to be a good neighbor by providing a place for people to come together and by committing to supporting financially and in other ways the communities where its stores are located. Partners (and customers, for that matter) are encouraged to get involved in volunteering in their communities. In addition, the Starbucks Foundation, which started in 1997 with funding for literacy programs in the United States and Canada, now makes grants to a wide variety of community projects and service programs.

Starbucks is also very serious about doing business ethically. In fact, it was named to the 2014 list of World's Most Ethical Companies, as it has been for the last eight years. From the executive level to the store level, individuals are expected and empowered to protect Starbucks' reputation through how they conduct business and how they treat others. And individuals are guided by the *Standards of Business Conduct,* a resource created for employees in doing business ethically, with integrity and honesty. These business conduct standards cover the workplace environment, business practices, intellectual property and proprietary information, and community involvement. A flow-chart model included in the standards document is used to illustrate an ethical decision-making framework for partners. Despite the thorough information in the standards, if partners face a situation where they're unsure how to respond or where they want to voice concerns, they're encouraged to seek out guidance from their manager, their partner resources representative, or even the corporate office of business ethics and compliance. The company also strongly states that it does not tolerate any retaliation against or victimization of any partner who raises concerns or questions.

Innovation, Innovation

Starbucks has always thought "outside the box." From the beginning, it took the concept of the corner coffee shop and totally revamped the coffee experience. And the company has always had the ability to roll out new products relatively quickly. The company's R&D (research and development) teams are responsible for innovating food and beverage products and new equipment. In 2011, the company spent nearly $15 million on technical R&D, product testing, and product and process improvements in all areas of the business. That was a 67 percent increase over 2010 expenditures and a 114 percent increase over 2009 expenditures. R&D expenditures are no longer reported in the Annual Report. (Here is a link to an interesting discussion of Starbucks' innovative efforts: [http://www.innovationmanagementcenter.com/wordpress/wp-content/uploads/2013/11/Starbucks-Paper-on-Controlled-Innovation.pdf].)

A glimpse of Starbucks' innovation process can be seen in how it approaches the all-important Christmas season, since "Starbucks has Christmas down to a science." It takes many months of meetings and tastings before rolling out the flavors and aromas. For the 2011 season, the process started in October 2010, when customers had the opportunity to fill out in-store and online surveys used to gauge their "mindset." In mid-December 2010, Schultz—who has final approval on all new products and themes—reviewed the 2011 theme. And things better be "Christmas-perfect." In March 2011, the 2011 theme (Let's Merry) was approved. By mid-March, the "core holiday team" started to meet weekly. On June 1, production cranked up on the company's seasonal red cups (which were introduced in 1997 and remain very popular). By the end of June, the holiday team has assembled a mock-up of a Starbucks café for Schultz to review and approve. By mid-August, all of the in-store signs, menu boards, and window decals are on their way to the printer. All of these pieces come together for the full holiday rollout on November 15, 2011. It's important to get everything right for this season. Want proof?

The company had revenues of almost $3 billion during the holiday quarter. That's a lot of Christmas cheer!

The company's product innovation process must be doing something right, as many of its Christmas products have been popular for years. For instance, the company's Christmas Blend debuted in 1985. The Gingerbread Latte was a Christmas 2000 innovation. The Caramel Brulée Latte came out during the 2009 holiday season. During the Christmas 2011 season, customers got their first taste of the Skinny Peppermint Mocha—a nod to the trend of healthier, but still tasty, products—and the line of petite desserts, which were introduced to commemorate the company's 40th birthday. But obviously, given Starbucks' outcomes, it's not only the Christmas products that have been successful. One of Starbucks' creations was a line of light-roasted coffee beans and brews. And the popularity of energy drinks led the company to create a line of "natural" energy drinks called Refreshers. The new fruity, carbonated drink that's high in antioxidants will get its energy boost from unroasted green coffee extract. Schultz told shareholders that the company is continuing to create lots of Starbucks products that "live outside of our stores." Starbucks Refreshers are sold at 160,000 grocery stores and made-to-order versions are sold in Starbucks stores.

Starbucks doesn't always get new products through in-house development. There are times when it "buys" the product. For instance, it purchased Evolution Fresh Inc. in late 2011. Evolution Fresh™ juice is available in more than 8,000 locations. Starbucks also plans on opening juice bars that will sell the juice products as well as health foods.

Discussion Questions

1. Do you think Howard Schultz views his role more from the omnipotent or from the symbolic perspective? Explain.
2. What has made Starbucks' culture what it is? How is that culture maintained?
3. Does Starbucks encourage a customer responsive culture? An ethical culture? Explain.
4. Describe some of the specific and general environmental components that are likely to impact Starbucks.
5. How would you classify the uncertainty of the environment in which Starbucks operates? Explain.
6. What stakeholders do you think Starbucks might be most concerned with? Why? What issue(s) might each of these stakeholders want Starbucks to address?
7. Why do you think Howard Schultz is uncomfortable with the idea of legislative lobbying? Do you think his discomfort is appropriate? Why or why not?
8. What types of global economic and legal-political issues might Starbucks face as it does business globally?
9. You're responsible for developing a global cultural awareness program for Starbucks' executives who are leading the company's international expansion efforts. Describe what you think will be important for these executives to know.
10. Using information from the case and information you pull from Starbucks' Web site, what global attitude do you think Starbucks exhibits? Defend your choice.
11. Pick one of the countries mentioned as an important target for Starbucks. Make a bulleted list of economic, political-legal, and cultural characteristics of this country.
12. What workforce challenges might Starbucks face in global markets in regard to its partners?
13. How does Starbucks manage diversity? What is Starbucks doing to manage diversity in each of the four areas: customers, suppliers, partners, and communities?
14. With more than 149,000 partners worldwide, what challenges would Starbucks face in making sure its diversity values are practiced and adhered to?
15. Starbucks defines diversity on its Web site in the form of an equation:

$$\text{Diversity} = \text{Inclusion} + \text{Equity} + \text{Accessibility.}$$

Explain what you think this means. What do you think of this definition of diversity?
16. What other workplace diversity initiatives (besides employee resource groups) might be appropriate for an organization like Starbucks?
17. Go to the company's Web site [www.starbucks.com] and find the latest corporate social responsibility report. Choose one of the key areas in the report (or your professor may assign one of these areas). Describe and evaluate what the company has done in this key area.
18. What do you think of Starbucks' goal to recycle all four billion cups sold annually by 2015? What challenges did it face in meeting that goal?
19. Why is the concept of "empowering" employees important in doing business ethically?
20. Again, go to the company's Web site. Find the *Standards of Business Conduct* document. First, what's your impression of this document? Then, choose one topic from one of the main areas covered. Describe what advice is provided to partners.

21. What do you think the company's use of the term *partners* instead of employees implies? What's your reaction to this? Do you think it matters what companies call their employees? (For instance, Walmart calls its employees *associates*.) Why or why not?

22. Howard Schultz is adamant about providing the best "Starbucks experience" to each and every customer. As a store manager, how would you keep your employees from experiencing high levels of stress when lines are out the door and customers want their Starbucks now?

23. Would you classify Starbucks' environment as more calm waters or white-water rapids? Explain. How does the company manage change in this type of environment?

24. Describe Starbucks' innovation environment.

25. Review the company's mission and guiding principles (at www.starbucks.com). Explain how these might affect the following: managing its external environment and its organizational culture, global efforts, diversity efforts, social responsibility and ethics issues, and change and innovation issues.

Notes for the Continuing Case

Information from Starbucks Corporation 2013 Annual Report, www.investor.starbucks.com, May, 2014; "2014 World's Most Ethical Companies," www.ethispere.com/worlds-most-ethical/wme-honorees/, May 2014; A. Minter, "Why Starbucks Won't Recycle Your Cup," www.bloombergview.com, April 7, 2014; "Starbucks Corporation Business Ethics and Compliance: Standards of Business Conduct," www.assets.starbucks.com, August 6, 2012; Starbucks News Release, "Starbucks Reports Record Third Quarter Results," www.investor.starbucks.com, July 26, 2012; L. Alderman, "In Europe, Starbucks Adjusts to a Café Culture," *New York Times Online,* March 30, 2012; V. Varma and B. Packard, "Starbucks Global Responsibility Report Year in Review: Fiscal 2011," www.starbucks.com, March 16, 2012; B. Gregg, "Is Professor's 'Hi, Sweetie' Comment Sexual Harassment?" www.diversityinc.com, March 12, 2012; S. Faris, "Grounds Zero," *Bloomberg BusinessWeek Online,* February 9, 2012; "Howard Schultz, on Getting a Second Shot," *Inc.,* April 2011, pp. 52–54; "A Shout Out to Starbucks," *Wholeliving.com,* April 2011, p. 111; and "Starbucks Quest for Healthy Growth: An Interview with Howard Schultz," *McKinsey Quarterly,* Issue 2, 2011, pp. 34–43.

Planning Work Activities

From Chapter 8 of *Management*, Thirteenth Edition. Stephen P. Robbins and Mary Coulter. Copyright © 2016 by Pearson Education, Inc. All rights reserved.

Planning Work Activities

It's Your Career

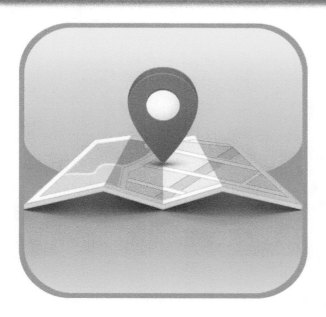

Source: Davooda/Shutterstock

A key to success in management and in your career is knowing *how to set goals, professionally and personally.*

You Gotta Have Goals

It's been said that if you don't know where you're going, any road will get you there. It has also been said that the shortest distance between two points is a straight line. These two sayings emphasize the importance of goals. Organizations want people who can get things done. And goal setting is an essential component of long-term career success. Successful athletes, businesspeople, and achievers in all fields use goals (a) to focus their efforts, (b) as short-term motivation, and (c) to build self-confidence as goals are successfully completed. You need to do the same thing. So how can you be better at setting goals? Here are some suggestions:

*1.   **Identify what you'd like to do or achieve in important life areas** such as career, financial, education, family, physical, public service/community involvement, and so forth. Focus on your most important broad goals. Try to identify where or what you'd like to be in 5 years, 10 years, 20 years. What is your dream? Your vision? If you're having trouble doing that, try thinking about what you don't want (I don't want to be working for someone else), and then turn that around to find your goal (I'd like to start my own business).*

*2.   **Make your goals actionable.** Although having broad, visionary goals is important, you need to set smaller goals with more specific, achievable actions. You can do this by:*

- *WRITING YOUR GOALS DOWN. Something about writing the goals makes them more real and gives them more force. Plus, having a visual reminder can be very motivating!*
- *USING THE S.M.A.R.T. APPROACH. This means you write goals that are **S**pecific, **M**easurable, **A**ttainable, **R**elevant (or **R**ealistic), and **T**ime-trackable. Using this approach forces you to set goals that aren't just daydreams or that are unrealistic.*

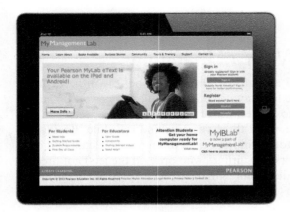

MyManagementLab®

⭐ **Improve Your Grade!**

When you see this icon, visit **www.mymanagementlab.com** for activities that are applied, personalized, and offer immediate feedback.

Learning Objectives

● SKILL OUTCOMES

1 **Define** the nature and purposes of planning.

2 **Classify** the types of goals organizations might have and the plans they use.

3 **Compare** and contrast approaches to goal-setting and planning.

- **Know how** to set goals personally and create a useful, functional to-do list.
- **Develop your skill** at helping your employees set goals.

4 **Discuss** contemporary issues in planning.

- *AVOIDING GOALS THAT ARE: ambiguous, overly ambitious or unrealistic, undocumented, and plan-less (without a plan).*

3. **Make your plans for reaching those goals.** *Setting goals is important, but so is deciding how you're going to achieve them. Your plans, just like your goals, need to be short-term and long-term. Having and using to-do lists can be productive. (Be sure to check out what this skill involves at the end of the chapter.)*

4. **Determine how you'll measure progress toward your goal.** *You need to think about how you will know you've achieved a goal. It's easy for some goals. For instance, getting your MBA degree. You*

measure progress by whether you're completing all necessary coursework and other requirements that will eventually lead to being awarded that degree. Other goals may not be quite that easy to measure for progress. However, having some way to assess progress is important to staying on track. It's also important that when you do achieve a goal (or goals) that you enjoy the satisfaction of having done so. Reward yourself appropriately!

5. **Review your goals periodically.** *Are the goals that you set still appropriate? Do they reflect your changing priorities or experiences? As your life and career circumstances change, change your goals to reflect that.*

You may think "planning" is relevant to large companies, but not something that's relevant to you right now. But when you figure out your class schedule for the next term or when you decide what you need to do to finish a class project on time, you're planning. And planning is something that all managers need to do. Although what they plan and how they plan may differ, it's still important that they do plan. In this text, we present the basics: what planning is, why managers plan, and how they plan.

THE WHAT AND WHY of Planning

L01 Boeing called its new 787 aircraft the Dreamliner, but the project turned into more of a nightmare for managers. The company's newest plane has been its most popular product ever, mostly because of its innovations, especially in fuel efficiency. However, the plane was delivered three years behind schedule. Boeing admitted the project's timeline was way too ambitious, even though every detail had been meticulously planned.[1] Some customers (the airlines who ordered the jets) got tired of waiting and canceled their orders. Could Boeing's managers have planned better?

What Is Planning?

planning

Management function that involves setting goals, establishing strategies for achieving those goals, and developing plans to integrate and coordinate work activities

Planning involves defining the organization's goals, establishing strategies for achieving those goals, and developing plans to integrate and coordinate work activities. It's concerned with both ends (what) and means (how).

When we use the term planning, we mean formal planning. In formal planning, specific goals covering a specific time period are defined. These goals are written and shared with organizational members to reduce ambiguity and create a common understanding about what needs to be done. Finally, specific plans exist for achieving these goals.

Why Do Managers Plan?

Planning seems to take a lot of effort. So why should managers plan? We can give you at least four reasons:

1. *Planning provides direction* to managers and nonmanagers alike. When employees know what their organization or work unit is trying to accomplish and what they must contribute to reach goals, they can coordinate their activities, cooperate with each other, and do what it takes to accomplish those goals. Without planning, departments and individuals might work at cross-purposes and prevent the organization from efficiently achieving its goals.
2. *Planning reduces uncertainty* by forcing managers to look ahead, anticipate change, consider the impact of change, and develop appropriate responses. Although planning won't eliminate uncertainty, managers plan so they can respond effectively.
3. *Planning minimizes waste and redundancy.* When work activities are coordinated around plans, inefficiencies become obvious and can be corrected or eliminated.
4. *Planning establishes the goals or standards* used in controlling. When managers plan, they develop goals and plans. When they control, they see whether the plans have been carried out and the goals met. Without planning, there would be no goals against which to measure work effort.

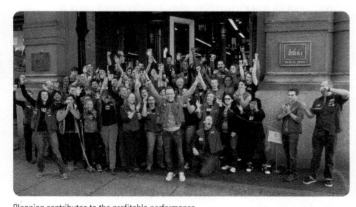

Planning contributes to the profitable performance of Recreational Equipment, Inc. Formal expansion plans have helped REI grow from one store in 1944 to become a major retailer of outdoor gear with more than 130 stores, 10,000 employees, and annual sales of $2 billion. Shown here are employees at an REI store opening in New York City's SoHo shopping district.
Source: Matt Peyton/AP Images

Planning and Performance

Is planning worthwhile? Numerous studies have looked at the relationship between planning and performance.[2] Although most have shown generally positive relationships, we can't say that organizations that formally plan always outperform those that don't plan. But *what* can we conclude?

First, generally speaking, formal planning is associated with positive financial results—higher profits, higher return on assets, and so forth. Second, it seems that doing a good job planning and implementing those plans play a bigger part in high performance than how much planning is done. Next, in those studies where formal planning didn't lead to higher performance, the external environment often was the culprit. When external forces—think governmental regulations or powerful labor unions—constrain managers' options, it reduces the impact planning has on an

organization's performance. Finally, the planning-performance relationship seems to be influenced by the planning time frame. It seems that at least four years of formal planning is required before it begins to affect performance.

GOALS and Plans

LO2 Planning is often called the primary management function because it establishes the basis for all the other things managers do as they organize, lead, and control. It involves two important aspects: goals and plans.

Goals (objectives) are desired outcomes or targets.[4] They guide management decisions and form the criterion against which work results are measured. That's why they're often described as the essential elements of planning. You have to know the desired target or outcome before you can establish plans for reaching it. **Plans** are documents that outline how goals are going to be met. They usually include resource allocations, schedules, and other necessary actions to accomplish the goals. As managers plan, they develop both goals and plans.

Types of Goals

It might seem that organizations have a single goal. Businesses want to make a profit and not-for-profit organizations want to meet the needs of some constituent group(s). However, a single goal can't adequately define an organization's success. And if managers emphasize only one goal, other goals essential for long-term success are ignored. Also, using a single goal such as profit may result in unethical behaviors because managers and employees will ignore other aspects of their jobs in order to look good on that one measure.[5] In reality, all organizations have multiple goals. For instance, businesses may want to increase market share, keep employees enthused about working for the organization, and work toward more environmentally sustainable practices. And a church provides a place for religious practices, but also assists economically disadvantaged individuals in its community and acts as a social gathering place for church members.

We can classify most company's goals as either strategic or financial. Financial goals are related to the financial performance of the organization, while strategic goals are related to all other areas of an organization's performance. For instance, Volkswagen states that its financial target (to be achieved by 2018) is to sell 10 million cars and trucks annually with a pretax profit margin over 8 percent.[6] And here's an example of a strategic goal from Uniqlo, Asia's biggest apparel chain: It wants to be the number-one apparel retailer in the United States.[7]

The goals just described are **stated goals**—official statements of what an organization says, and what it wants its stakeholders to believe, its goals are. However, stated goals—which can be found in an organization's charter, annual report, public relations announcements, or in public statements made by managers—are often conflicting and influenced by what various stakeholders think organizations should do. For instance, Nike's goal is "delivering inspiration and innovation to every athlete." Canadian company EnCana's vision is to "be the world's high performance benchmark independent oil and gas company." Deutsche Bank's goal is "to be the leading global provider of financial solutions, creating lasting value for our clients, our shareholders and people and the communities in which we operate."[8] Such statements are vague and probably better represent management's public relations skills than being meaningful guides to what the organization is actually trying to accomplish. It shouldn't be surprising then to find that an organization's stated goals are often irrelevant to what actually goes on.[9]

If you want to know an organization's **real goals**—those goals an organization actually pursues—observe what organizational members are doing. Actions define priorities. For example, universities may say their goal is limiting class sizes, facilitating

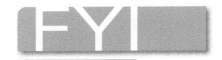

goals (objectives)
Desired outcomes or targets

plans
Documents that outline how goals are going to be met

stated goals
Official statements of what an organization says, and what it wants its various stakeholders to believe, its goals are

real goals
Goals that an organization actually pursues, as defined by the actions of its members

let's get REAL

The Scenario:

Tommy and Kate Larkin recently started a restaurant and specialty food store in Northern California. The store also sells wine and locally made crafts. Although the business does well during the summer tourist months, things get pretty lean from October to April when visitor numbers dwindle. The Larkins felt that the potential opportunities in this location were good.

What types of plans do the Larkins need to survive the off-season?

The slow season is a wonderful time for a business owner. This is the perfect opportunity for brand and business development. If a new Web site needs to be designed, this is the time to do it. If new recipes need to be tested, this would be the perfect time to run trials. Research and development during these months could make the busy season even more profitable. The "business development" season also presents a great opportunity to deepen ties in the community and it is the prime time to diversify business offerings. Perhaps the restaurant could focus on hosting events on site or catering off-site meals making themselves more valuable to the local community rather than depending so heavily on tourism. Finally, it is a great time for the owners to rest, recover and rejuvenate themselves from the last season and gear up for the next.

Prudence Rufus
Business Owner/Photographer

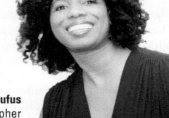

close student-faculty relations, and actively involving students in the learning process, but then they put students into 300+ student lecture classes! Knowing that real and stated goals may differ is important for recognizing what you might otherwise think are management inconsistencies.

Types of Plans

The most popular ways to describe organizational plans are breadth (strategic versus operational), time frame (short term versus long term), specificity (directional versus specific), and frequency of use (single use versus standing). As Exhibit 1 shows, these types of plans aren't independent. That is, strategic plans are usually long term, directional, and single use whereas operational plans are usually short term, specific, and standing. What does each include?

Strategic plans are plans that apply to the entire organization and establish the organization's overall goals. Plans that encompass a particular operational area of the organization are called **operational plans**. These two types of plans differ because strategic plans are broad while operational plans are narrow.

The number of years used to define short-term and long-term plans has declined considerably because of environmental uncertainty. Long-term used to mean anything over seven years. Try to imagine what you're likely to be doing in seven years, and you can begin to appreciate how difficult it would be for managers to establish plans that far in the future. We define **long-term plans** as those with a time frame beyond three years.[10] **Short-term plans** cover one year or less. Any time period in

strategic plans
Plans that apply to the entire organization and establish the organization's overall goals

operational plans
Plans that encompass a particular operational area of the organization

long-term plans
Plans with a time frame beyond three years

short-term plans
Plans covering one year or less

Exhibit 1
Types of Plans

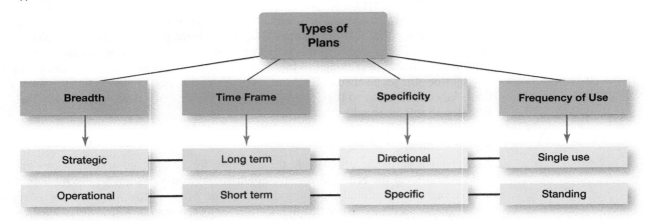

between would be an intermediate plan. Although these time classifications are fairly common, an organization can use any planning time frame it wants.

Intuitively, it would seem that specific plans would be preferable to directional, or loosely guided, plans. **Specific plans** are clearly defined and leave no room for interpretation. A specific plan states its objectives in a way that eliminates ambiguity and problems with misunderstanding. For example, a manager who seeks to increase his or her unit's work output by 8 percent over a given 12-month period might establish specific procedures, budget allocations, and schedules of activities to reach that goal.

However, when uncertainty is high and managers must be flexible in order to respond to unexpected changes, directional plans are preferable. **Directional plans** are flexible plans that set out general guidelines. They provide focus but don't lock managers into specific goals or courses of action. For example, Sylvia Rhone, president of Motown Records, said she has a simple goal—to "sign great artists."[11] So instead of creating a specific plan to produce and market 10 albums from new artists this year, she might formulate a directional plan to use a network of people around the world to alert her to new and promising talent so she can increase the number of new artists she has under contract. Keep in mind, however, that the flexibility of directional plans must be weighed against the lack of clarity of specific plans.

Some plans that managers develop are ongoing while others are used only once. A **single-use plan** is a one-time plan specifically designed to meet the needs of a unique situation. For instance, when Walmart wanted to expand the number of its stores in China, top-level executives formulated a single-use plan as a guide. In contrast, **standing plans** are ongoing plans that provide guidance for activities performed repeatedly. Standing plans include policies, rules, and procedures. An example of a standing plan is the non-discrimination and anti-harassment policy developed by the University of Arizona. It provides guidance to university administrators, faculty, and staff as they make hiring plans and do their jobs.

specific plans
Plans that are clearly defined and leave no room for interpretation

directional plans
Plans that are flexible and set out general guidelines

single-use plan
A one-time plan specifically designed to meet the needs of a unique situation

standing plans
Ongoing plans that provide guidance for activities performed repeatedly

Source: Kimberly White/Reuters Pictures

LEADER *making a* DIFFERENCE

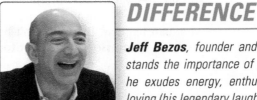

Jeff Bezos, *founder and CEO of Amazon.com, understands the importance of goals and plans. As a leader, he exudes energy, enthusiasm, and drive.[12] He's fun loving (his legendary laugh has been described as a flock of Canadian geese on nitrous oxide) but has pursued his vision for Amazon with serious intensity and has demonstrated an ability to inspire his employees through the ups and downs of a rapidly growing company. When Bezos founded the company as an online bookstore, his goal was to be the leader in online retailing. Now 20 years later, Amazon has become the world's general store, selling not only books, CDs, and DVDs, but LEGOs, power drills, and Jackalope Buck taxidermy mounts, to name a few of the millions of products you can buy.* What can you learn from this leader making a difference?

SETTING Goals and Developing Plans

LO3 Taylor Haines has just been elected president of her business school's honorary fraternity. She wants the organization to be more actively involved in the business school than it has been. Francisco Garza graduated from Tecnologico de Monterrey with a degree in marketing and computers three years ago and went to work for a regional consulting services firm. He recently was promoted to manager of an eight-person social media development team and hopes to strengthen the team's financial contributions to the firm. What should Taylor and Francisco do now? Their first step should be to set goals.

Approaches to Setting Goals

As we stated earlier, goals provide the direction for all management decisions and actions and form the criterion against which actual accomplishments are measured. Everything organizational members do should be oriented toward achieving goals. These goals can be set either through a traditional process or by using management by objectives.

traditional goal-setting
An approach to setting goals in which top managers set goals that then flow down through the organization and become subgoals for each organizational area

In **traditional goal-setting**, goals set by top managers flow down through the organization and become subgoals for each organizational area. This traditional perspective assumes that top managers know what's best because they see the "big picture." And the goals passed down to each succeeding level guide individual employees as they work to achieve those assigned goals. If Taylor were to use this approach, she would see what goals the dean or director of the school of business had set and develop goals for her group that would contribute to achieving those goals. Or take a manufacturing business, for example. The president tells the vice president of production what he expects manufacturing costs to be for the coming year and tells the marketing vice president what level he expects sales to reach for the year. These goals are passed to the next organizational level and written to reflect the responsibilities of that level, passed to the next level, and so forth. Then, at some later time, performance is evaluated to determine whether the assigned goals have been achieved. Although the process is supposed to happen in this way, in reality it doesn't always do so. Turning broad strategic goals into departmental, team, and individual goals can be a difficult and frustrating process.

Another problem with traditional goal-setting is that when top managers define the organization's goals in broad terms—such as achieving "sufficient" profits or increasing "market leadership"—these ambiguous goals have to be made more specific as they flow down through the organization. Managers at each level define the goals and apply their own interpretations and biases as they make them more specific. However, what often happens is that clarity is lost as the goals make their way down from the top of the organization to lower levels. Exhibit 2 illustrates what can happen. But it doesn't have to be that way. For example, at the Carrier-Carlyle Compressor Facility in Stone Mountain, Georgia, employees and managers

Exhibit 2
The Downside of Traditional Goal-Setting

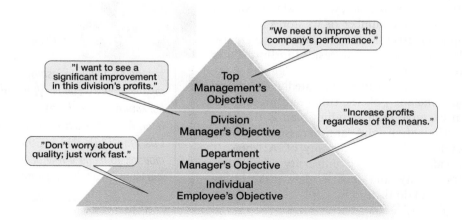

"We need to improve the company's performance."

"I want to see a significant improvement in this division's profits."

Top Management's Objective

Division Manager's Objective

"Increase profits regardless of the means."

"Don't worry about quality; just work fast."

Department Manager's Objective

Individual Employee's Objective

focus their work efforts around goals. Those goals encompass meeting and exceeding customer needs, concentrating on continuous improvement efforts, and engaging the workforce. To keep everyone focused on those goals, a "thermostat"—a 3-foot-by-4-foot metric indicator—found at the employee entrance communicates what factory performance is at any given time and where attention is needed. It identifies plant goals across a range of measures as well as how closely those goals are being met. Company executives say that good planning drives improved performance results. Does their goal approach work? In the past three years, the facility has experienced a nearly 76 percent reduction in customer reject rates and a 54.5 percent reduction in OSHA-recordable injury and illness cases.[13]

When the hierarchy of organizational goals is clearly defined, as it is at Carrier-Carlyle Compressor, it forms an integrated network of goals, or a **means-ends chain**. Higher-level goals (or ends) are linked to lower-level goals, which serve as the means for their accomplishment. In other words, the goals achieved at lower levels become the means to reach the goals (ends) at the next level. And the accomplishment of goals at that level becomes the means to achieve the goals (ends) at the next level and on up through the different organizational levels. That's how traditional goal-setting is supposed to work.

Instead of using traditional goal-setting, many organizations use **management by objectives (MBO)**, a process of setting mutually agreed-upon goals and using those goals to evaluate employee performance. If Francisco were to use this approach, he would sit down with each member of his team and set goals and periodically review whether progress was being made toward achieving those goals. MBO programs have four elements: goal specificity, participative decision making, an explicit time period,

means-ends chain
An integrated network of goals in which the accomplishment of goals at one level serves as the means for achieving the goals, or ends, at the next level

management by objectives (MBO)
A process of setting mutually agreed-upon goals and using those goals to evaluate employee performance

let's get REAL

The Scenario:

Geoff Vuleta, the CEO of Fahrenheit 212, an innovation consulting firm, has an interesting approach to planning. Every 100 days, the employees get together as a group and draw up a list of all the things they want to get done in the next 100 days. Then, each individual makes a list of commitments to how he or she is going to contribute to that list and sits down with the CEO and the company president to discuss the plan. The sum of everybody's plan becomes the focus of action.

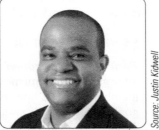

Source: Justin Kidwell

Justin Kidwell
Management Consultant

What do you think of this approach—good and bad?

This is an atypical planning approach, but has merit and should work well for a small company since this program would get more difficult to manage with a growing firm. Open communication among all employees, frequent "check-ins" and firm-wide planning sessions only serve to strengthen the organization by encouraging worker commitment and buy-in to the firm's direction. Two areas of concern with this approach are: 1) That the plans set during this process support the organization's strategic goals/philosophies and 2) that all employees have an equal voice in this dialogue. Without addressing these two concerns, these planning sessions may cause employees to disengage and/or work on initiatives that are inconsistent with corporate strategy.

Exhibit 3
Steps in MBO

Step 1: The organization's *overall objectives* and *strategies* are formulated.

Step 2: Major objectives are allocated among *divisional and departmental units*.

Step 3: Unit managers *collaboratively set specific objectives* for their units with their managers.

Step 4: Specific objectives are collaboratively set with *all department members*.

Step 5: *Action plans,* defining how objectives are to be achieved, are specified and agreed upon by managers and employees.

Step 6: The action plans are *implemented*.

Step 7: Progress toward objectives is *periodically reviewed,* and *feedback is provided*.

Step 8: Successful achievement of objectives is reinforced by *performance-based rewards*.

and performance feedback.[14] Instead of using goals to make sure employees are doing what they're supposed to be doing, MBO uses goals to motivate them as well. The appeal is that it focuses on employees working to accomplish goals they've had a hand in setting. Exhibit 3 lists the steps in a typical MBO program.

Does MBO work? Studies have shown that it can increase employee performance and organizational productivity. For example, one review of MBO programs found productivity gains in almost all of them.[15] But is MBO relevant for today's organizations? If it's viewed as a way of setting goals, then yes, because research shows that goal-setting can be an effective approach to motivating employees.[16]

CHARACTERISTICS OF WELL-WRITTEN GOALS   Goals aren't all written the same way. Some are better than others at making the desired outcomes clear. For instance, the CEO of Procter & Gamble said that he wants to see the company add close to 548,000 new customers a day, every day, for the next five years.[17] It's an ambitious but specific goal. Managers should be able to write well-written work goals. What makes a "well-written" work goal?[18] Exhibit 4 lists the characteristics.

STEPS IN GOAL-SETTING   Managers should follow five steps when setting goals.

1. *Review the organization's mission, or purpose.* A **mission** is a broad statement of an organization's purpose that provides an overall guide to what organizational members think is important. Managers should review the mission before writing goals because goals should reflect that mission.
2. *Evaluate available resources.* You don't want to set goals that are impossible to achieve given your available resources. Even though goals should be challenging, they should be realistic. After all, if the resources you have to work with won't allow you to achieve a goal no matter how hard you try or how much effort is exerted, you shouldn't set that goal. That would be like the person with a $50,000 annual income and no other financial resources setting a goal of building an investment portfolio worth $1 million in three years. No matter how hard he or she works at it, it's not going to happen.

mission
The purpose of an organization

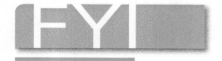

- 44 percent of employees say that leaders don't clearly communicate the organization's purpose and direction.[19]

Exhibit 4
Well-Written Goals

- Written in terms of outcomes rather than actions
- Measurable and quantifiable
- Clear as to a time frame
- Challenging yet attainable
- Written down
- Communicated to all necessary organizational members

FUTURE VISION | Stretch Goals—Setting Goals That Aren't Realistic

Jeff Bezos announces that Amazon is testing delivery by aerial drones. Elon Musk announces that Tesla Motors is investing $2 billion to build a factory that could produce 500,000 lithium-ion battery vehicle packs. On *Fast Company*'s most current list of the world's Top 10 Most Innovative Companies in Design are companies doing incredibly unique and daring things. We say that goals should be realistic, but is there room—and should there be room—for those outlandish, challenging, off-the-wall, *unrealistic* goals? What role should **stretch goals**, which we're defining as seemingly impossible goals, play in an organization's planning approach?

Although we're looking at this in a theme box called "Future Vision," the idea of stretch goals actually became popular when General Electric's then-CEO Jack Welch began promoting them back in the early 1990s.[20] He used the story of bullet trains in Japan and how if the goals had been only moderate (reasonable) improvements in speed and operating efficiency, the bullet train concept would never have gotten off the ground. Instead, the designers were challenged to think beyond what was realistic.

So, are stretch goals appropriate and will they be so in the future workplace? The lists below describe some benefits and challenges of stretch goals.[21]

Having goals is important to channeling work efforts in the appropriate direction. Considering the trade-offs here, maybe the *right* approach in your future workplace is to set the *right* goal(s) for each situation...whether stretch or realistic.

If your professor has chosen to assign this, go to **www.mymanagementlab.com** *to discuss the following questions:*

⭐ **TALK ABOUT IT 1:** *Are* stretch goals appropriate? Discuss.

⭐ **TALK ABOUT IT 2:** Take one "challenge" and discuss how managers could address it.

Benefits	Challenges
• Encourages exploration of new ideas, which can be critical for long-term survival	• Organizations/people have difficulty thinking beyond their current routines and processes
• Can make an organization more effective	• Can be demotivating if goals seem overwhelming and unachievable
• Can lead to personal growth and professional development	• Employees fear that failure will have negative consequences
• Can be highly motivating when goals are achieved	• Can lead to unethical behavior if individuals feel pressured to achieve the seemingly unachievable
• Shifts from a culture of "mediocrity" to a culture of "awesomeness"	• Can lead to excessive risk taking

3. *Determine the goals individually or with input from others.* The goals reflect desired outcomes and should be congruent with the organizational mission and goals in other organizational areas. These goals should be measurable, specific, and include a time frame for accomplishment.

4. *Write down the goals and communicate them to all who need to know.* Writing down and communicating goals forces people to think them through. The written goals also become visible evidence of the importance of working toward something.

5. *Review results and whether goals are being met.* If goals aren't being met, change them as needed.

Once the goals have been established, written down, and communicated, a manager is ready to develop plans for pursuing the goals.

stretch goals
Seemingly impossible goals

Goal Setting—If your instructor is using MyManagementLab, log onto mymanagementlab.com and test your *goal-setting knowledge.* **Be sure to refer back to the chapter opener!**

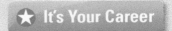
⭐ It's Your Career

Exhibit 5
Planning and Organizational Level

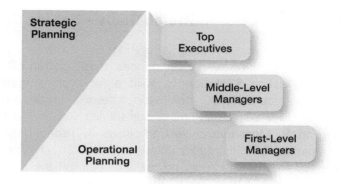

Strategic Planning

Top Executives

Middle-Level Managers

First-Level Managers

Operational Planning

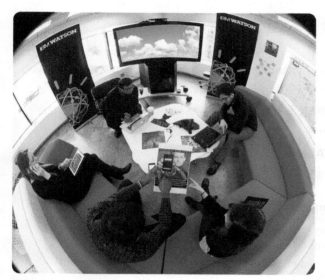

IBM replaced its traditional annual top-down planning process with an ongoing planning approach that involves employees from line managers to senior executives. The new approach enables IBM to explore and identify customer needs, new markets, technologies, and competitors from around the world and to create new ventures such as the IBM Watson Group for developing and commercializing cognitive computing innovations.
Source: Jon Simon/Newscom

commitment concept
Plans should extend far enough to meet those commitments made when the plans were developed

Developing Plans

The process of developing plans is influenced by three contingency factors and by the planning approach followed.

CONTINGENCY FACTORS IN PLANNING Three contingency factors affect the choice of plans: organizational level, degree of environmental uncertainty, and length of future commitments.[22]

Exhibit 5 shows the relationship between a manager's level in the organization and the type of planning done. For the most part, lower-level managers do operational planning while upper-level managers do strategic planning.

The second contingency factor is environmental uncertainty. When uncertainty is high, plans should be specific, but flexible. Managers must be prepared to change or amend plans as they're implemented. At times, they may even have to abandon the plans.[23] For example, prior to Continental Airlines' merger with United Airlines, the former CEO and his management team established a specific goal of focusing on what customers wanted most—on-time flights—to help the company become more competitive in the highly uncertain airline industry. Because of the high level of uncertainty, the management team identified a "destination, but not a flight plan," and changed plans as necessary to achieve that goal of on-time service.

The last contingency factor also is related to the time frame of plans. The **commitment concept** says that plans should extend far enough to meet those commitments made when the plans were developed. Planning for too long or too short a time period is inefficient and ineffective. For instance, Walmart, like many businesses during the economic recession, cut staff. Yet, it continued to add stores that need to be stocked and restocked with merchandise. With fewer employees, however, merchandise is piling up in stockrooms, shelves are going unstocked, checkout lines are longer, and fewer employees are in the store itself to help customers.[24] How does this illustrate the commitment concept? By deciding to cut staff, Walmart "committed" to the consequences of that decision—good and bad.

Approaches to Planning

Federal, state, and local government officials are working together on a plan to boost populations of wild salmon in the northwestern United States. Managers in the Global Fleet Graphics division of the 3M Company are developing detailed plans to satisfy increasingly demanding customers and to battle more aggressive competitors. Emilio Azcárraga Jean, chairman, president, and CEO of Grupo Televisa, gets input from many different people before setting company goals and then turns over the planning for achieving the goals to various executives. In each of these situations, planning is done a little differently. How an organization plans can best be understood by looking at who does the planning.

In the traditional approach, planning is done entirely by top-level managers who often are assisted by a **formal planning department**, a group of planning specialists whose sole responsibility is to help write the various organizational plans. Under this approach, plans developed by top-level managers flow down through other organizational levels, much like the traditional approach to goal-setting. As they flow down through the organization, the plans are tailored to the particular needs of each level. Although this approach makes managerial planning thorough, systematic, and coordinated, all too often the focus is on developing "the plan"—a thick binder (or binders) full of meaningless information that's stuck on a shelf and never used by anyone for guiding or coordinating work efforts. In fact, in a survey of managers about formal top-down organizational planning processes, more than 75 percent said their company's planning approach was unsatisfactory.[25] A common complaint was that, "plans are documents that you prepare for the corporate planning staff and later forget." Although this traditional top-down approach to planning is used by many organizations, it can be effective only if managers understand the importance of creating documents that organizational members actually use, not documents that look impressive but are ignored.

Another approach to planning is to involve more organizational members in the process. In this approach, plans aren't handed down from one level to the next, but instead are developed by organizational members at the various levels and in the various work units to meet their specific needs. For instance, at Dell, employees from production, supply management, and channel management meet weekly to make plans based on current product demand and supply. In addition, work teams set their own daily schedules and track their progress against those schedules. If a team falls behind, team members develop "recovery" plans to try to get back on schedule.[26] When organizational members are more actively involved in planning, they see that the plans are more than just something written down on paper. They can actually see that the plans are used in directing and coordinating work.

formal planning department
A group of planning specialists whose sole responsibility is helping to write organizational plans

---

If your professor has assigned this, go to **www.mymanagementlab.com** to watch a video titled: *Rudi's Bakery: Planning* and to respond to questions.

★ Watch It 1!

CONTEMPORARY Issues in Planning

LO4 The second floor of the 21-story Hyundai Motor headquarters buzzes with data 24 hours a day. That's where you'd find the company's Global Command and Control Center (GCCC), which is modeled after the CNN newsroom with numerous "computer screens relaying video and data keeping watch on Hyundai operations around the world." Managers get information on parts shipments from suppliers to factories. Cameras watch assembly lines and closely monitor the company's massive Ulsan, Korea, factory looking for competitors' spies and any hints of labor unrest. The GCCC also keeps tabs on the company's R&D activities in Europe, Japan, and North America. Hyundai can identify problems in an instant and react quickly. The company is all about aggressiveness and speed and is representative of how a successful twenty-first-century company approaches planning.[27]

We conclude this chapter by addressing two contemporary issues in planning. Specifically, we're going to look at planning effectively in dynamic environments and then at how managers can use environmental scanning, especially competitive intelligence.

If your professor has assigned this, go to **www.mymanagementlab.com** to complete the Simulation: Planning and get a better understanding of the challenges of planning in organizations.

 ★ Try It!

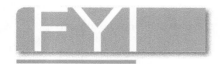

How Can Managers Plan Effectively in Dynamic Environments?

The external environment is continually changing. For instance, cloud computing storage is revolutionizing all kinds of industries from financial services to health care to engineering.[29] Social networking sites are used by companies to connect with customers, employees, and potential employees. Amounts spent on eating out instead of cooking at home are predicted to start rising after years of decline during the economic downturn. And experts believe that China and India are transforming the twenty-first-century global economy.

How can managers effectively plan when the external environment is continually changing? We already discussed uncertain environments as one of the contingency factors that affect the types of plans managers develop. Because dynamic environments are more the norm than the exception, let's look at how managers can effectively plan in such environments.

In an uncertain environment, managers should develop plans that are specific, but flexible. Although this may seem contradictory, it's not. To be useful, plans need some specificity, but the plans should not be set in stone. Managers need to recognize that planning is an ongoing process. The plans serve as a road map, although the destination may change due to dynamic market conditions. They should be ready to change directions if environmental conditions warrant. This flexibility is particularly important as plans are implemented. Managers need to stay alert to environmental changes that may impact implementation and respond as needed. Keep in mind, also, that even when the environment is highly uncertain, it's important to continue formal planning in order to see any effect on organizational performance. It's the persistence in planning that contributes to significant performance improvement. Why? It seems that, as with most activities, managers "learn to plan" and the quality of their planning improves when they continue to do it.[30] Finally, make the organizational hierarchy flatter to effectively plan in dynamic environments. This means allowing lower organizational levels to set goals and develop plans because there's little time for goals and plans to flow down from the top. Managers should teach their employees how to set goals and to plan and then trust them to do it. And you need look no further than Bangalore, India, to find a company that effectively understands this. Just a decade ago, Wipro Limited was "an anonymous conglomerate selling cooking oil and personal computers, mostly in India." Today, it's a $6.8 billion-a-year global company with much of its business coming from information-technology services.[31] Accenture, Hewlett-Packard, IBM, and the big U.S. accounting firms know all too well the competitive threat Wipro represents. Not only are Wipro's employees economical, they're knowledgeable and skilled. And they play an important role in the company's planning. Because the information services industry is continually changing, employees are taught to analyze situations and to define the scale and scope of a client's problems in order to offer the best solutions. These employees are on the front line with the clients, and it's their responsibility to establish what to do and how to do it. It's an approach that positions Wipro for success—no matter how the industry changes.

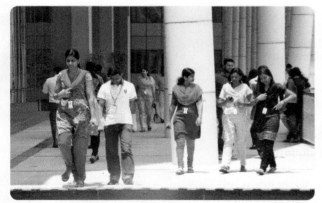

Knowledgeable and skilled employees play an important role in planning at Wipro, where managers teach them how to set goals and make plans. Employees help Wipro compete successfully in a dynamic environment by analyzing customers' ever-changing needs and devising solutions that help them function faster and more efficiently.
Source: Jagadeesh NV/Newscom

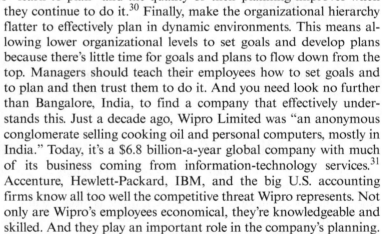

★ Watch It 2! If your professor has assigned this, go to **www.mymanagementlab.com** to watch a video titled: *CH2M Hill: Planning* and to respond to questions.

How Can Managers Use Environmental Scanning?

Crammed into a small Shanghai apartment that houses four generations of a Chinese family, Indra Nooyi, Chairman and CEO of PepsiCo Inc., asked the inhabitants several questions about "China's rapid development, their shopping habits, and how they

feel about Western brands." This visit was part of an "immersion" tour of China for Ms. Nooyi, who hoped to strengthen PepsiCo's business in emerging markets. She said, "I wanted to look at how people live, how they eat, what the growth possibilities are."[32] The information gleaned from her research—a prime example of environmental scanning up close and personal—will help in establishing PepsiCo's future goals and plans.

A manager's analysis of the external environment may be improved by **environmental scanning**, which involves screening information to detect emerging trends. One of the fastest-growing forms of environmental scanning is **competitor intelligence**, gathering information about competitors that allows managers to anticipate competitors' actions rather than merely react to them.[33] It seeks basic information about competitors: Who are they? What are they doing? How will what they're doing affect us?

Many who study competitive intelligence suggest that much of the competitor-related information managers need to make crucial strategic decisions is available and accessible to the public.[34] In other words, competitive intelligence isn't corporate espionage. Advertisements, promotional materials, press releases, reports filed with government agencies, annual reports, want ads, newspaper reports, information on the Internet, and industry studies are readily accessible sources of information. Specific information on an industry and associated organizations is increasingly available through electronic databases. Managers can literally tap into this wealth of competitive information by purchasing access to databases. Attending trade shows and debriefing your own sales staff also can be good sources of information on competitors. In addition, many organizations even regularly buy competitors' products and ask their own employees to evaluate them to learn about new technical innovations.[35]

In a changing global business environment, environmental scanning and obtaining competitive intelligence can be quite complex, especially since information must be gathered from around the world. However, one thing managers could do is subscribe to news services that review newspapers and magazines from around the globe and provide summaries to client companies.

Managers do need to be careful about the way information, especially competitive intelligence, is gathered to prevent any concerns about whether it's legal or ethical.[36] For instance, Starwood Hotels sued Hilton Hotels, alleging that two former employees stole trade secrets and helped Hilton develop a new line of luxury, trendy hotels designed to appeal to a young demographic.[37] The court filing said this was an obvious "case of corporate espionage, theft of trade secrets, unfair competition, and computer fraud." Competitive intelligence becomes illegal corporate spying when it involves the theft of proprietary materials or trade secrets by any means. The Economic Espionage Act makes it a crime in the United States to engage in economic espionage or to steal a trade secret. Difficult decisions about competitive intelligence arise because often there's a fine line between what's considered legal and ethical and what's considered legal but unethical. Although the top manager at one competitive intelligence firm contends that 99.9 percent of intelligence gathering is legal, there's no question that some people or companies will go to any lengths—some unethical—to get information about competitors.[38]

environmental scanning
Screening information to detect emerging trends

competitor intelligence
Gathering information about competitors that allows managers to anticipate competitors' actions rather than merely react to them

PREPARING FOR: Exams/Quizzes

CHAPTER SUMMARY by Learning Objectives

LO1 DEFINE the nature and purposes of planning.

Planning involves defining the organization's goals, establishing an overall strategy for achieving those goals, and developing plans for organizational work activities. The four purposes of planning include providing direction, reducing uncertainty,

minimizing waste and redundancy, and establishing the goals or standards used in controlling. Studies of the planning-performance relationship have concluded that formal planning is associated with positive financial performance, for the most part; it's more important to do a good job of planning and implementing the plans than doing more extensive planning; the external environment is usually the reason why companies that plan don't achieve high levels of performance; and the planning-performance relationship seems to be influenced by the planning time frame.

L02   CLASSIFY **the types of goals organizations might have and the plans they use.**

Goals are desired outcomes. Plans are documents that outline how goals are going to be met. Goals might be strategic or financial and they might be stated or real. Strategic plans apply to the entire organization while operational plans encompass a particular functional area. Long-term plans are those with a time frame beyond three years. Short-term plans cover one year or less. Specific plans are clearly defined and leave no room for interpretation. Directional plans are flexible and set out general guidelines. A single-use plan is a one-time plan designed to meet the needs of a unique situation. Standing plans are ongoing plans that provide guidance for activities performed repeatedly.

L03   COMPARE **and contrast approaches to goal-setting and planning.**

In traditional goal-setting, goals are set at the top of the organization and then become subgoals for each organizational area. MBO (management by objectives) is a process of setting mutually agreed-upon goals and using those goals to evaluate employee performance. Well-written goals have six characteristics: (1) written in terms of outcomes, (2) measurable and quantifiable, (3) clear as to time frame, (4) challenging but attainable, (5) written down, and (6) communicated to all organizational members who need to know them. Goal-setting involves these steps: review the organization's mission; evaluate available resources; determine the goals individually or with input from others; write down the goals and communicate them to all who need to know them; and review results and change goals as needed. The contingency factors that affect planning include the manager's level in the organization, the degree of environmental uncertainty, and the length of future commitments. The two main approaches to planning include the traditional approach, which has plans developed by top managers that flow down through other organizational levels and which may use a formal planning department. The other approach is to involve more organizational members in the planning process.

L04   DISCUSS **contemporary issues in planning.**

One contemporary planning issue is planning in dynamic environments, which usually means developing plans that are specific but flexible. Also, it's important to continue planning, even when the environment is highly uncertain. Finally, because there's little time in a dynamic environment for goals and plans to flow down from the top, lower organizational levels should be allowed to set goals and develop plans. Another contemporary planning issue involves using environmental scanning to help do a better analysis of the external environment. One form of environmental scanning, competitive intelligence, can be especially helpful in finding out what competitors are doing.

MyManagementLab

Go to **mymanagementlab.com** to complete the problems marked with this icon ⭐.

✪ REVIEW AND DISCUSSION QUESTIONS

1. Explain what studies have shown about the relationship between planning and performance.

2. Discuss the contingency factors that affect planning.

3. Will planning become more or less important to managers in the future? Why?

4. If planning is so crucial, why do some managers choose not to do it? What would you tell these managers?

5. Explain how planning involves making decisions today that will have an impact later.

6. How might planning in a not-for-profit organization such as the American Cancer Society differ from

planning in a for-profit organization such as Coca-Cola?

7. What types of planning do you do in your personal life? Describe these plans in terms of being (a) strategic or operational, (b) short term or long term, and (c) specific or directional.

8. Many companies have a goal of becoming more environmentally sustainable. One of the most important steps they can take is controlling paper waste. Choose a company—any type, any size. You've been put in charge of creating a program to do this for your company. Set goals and develop plans. Prepare a report for your boss (that is, your professor) outlining these goals and plans.

MyManagementLab

If your professor has assigned these, go to **mymanagementlab.com** for Auto-graded writing questions as well as the following Assisted-graded writing questions:

9. Describe how managers can effectively plan in today's dynamic environment.

10. The late Peter Drucker, an eminent management author, coined the SMART format for setting goals back in 1954: S (specific), M (measurable), A (attainable), R (relevant), and T (time-bound). Are these still relevant today? Discuss.

PREPARING FOR: My Career

✪ PERSONAL INVENTORY ASSESSMENTS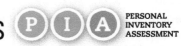

Tolerance of Ambiguity Scale

Managers often have to deal with ambiguous situations, which can make effective planning very challenging. In this PIA, you'll assess your level of tolerance for ambiguity.

✪ ETHICS DILEMMA

Rules are rules. Or are they? An incident at a Safeway store in Hawaii made international headlines after cops were called on a couple who failed to pay for two $2.50 sandwiches.[39] The couple had bought $50 worth of groceries and said they intended to pay for the sandwiches, which they'd eaten while shopping with their two-year-old daughter. The mother was about eight months pregnant and said she had felt lightheaded before eating one of the sandwiches. Despite the couple's request to just let them pay for the sandwiches, the store manager, trying to follow company policy, called the police, leading to the arrest of

both parents and their separation from their young daughter for more than 18 hours. Safeway did ultimately drop the shoplifting charges and apologized to the couple. But "by rigidly following a rule, the store may have turned a $5 theft into a much bigger dent in its reputation and bottom line."

11. What do you think? Was this a good business decision for Safeway?

12. What potential ethical issues do you see here?

13. If you were the store manager, what would you have done in this situation?

SKILLS EXERCISE Developing Your Goal-Setting Skill

About the Skill
Setting goals is a skill every manager needs to develop. Employees should have a clear understanding of what they're attempting to accomplish. Managers have the responsibility for seeing that this is done by helping employees set work goals.

Steps in Practicing the Skill
You can be more effective at setting goals for your employees if you use the following eight suggestions.

- *Identify an employee's key job tasks.* Goal-setting begins by defining what you want your employees to accomplish. The best source for this information is each employee's job description.

- *Establish specific and challenging goals for each key task.* Identify the level of performance expected of each employee. Specify the target toward which the employee is working.

- *Specify the deadlines for each goal.* Putting deadlines on each goal reduces ambiguity. Deadlines, however, should not be set arbitrarily. Rather, they need to be realistic given the tasks to be completed.

- *Allow the employee to actively participate.* When employees participate in goal-setting, they're more likely to accept the goals. However, it must be sincere participation. That is, employees must perceive that you are truly seeking their input, not just going through the motions.

- *Prioritize goals.* When you give someone more than one goal, it's important for you to rank the goals in order of importance. The purpose of prioritizing is to encourage the employee to take action and expend effort on each goal in proportion to its importance.

- *Rate goals for difficulty and importance.* Goal-setting should not encourage people to choose easy goals. Instead, goals should be rated for their difficulty and importance. When goals are rated, individuals can be given credit for trying difficult goals, even if they don't fully achieve them.

- *Build in feedback mechanisms to assess goal progress.* Feedback lets employees know whether their level of effort is sufficient to attain the goal. Feedback should be both self- and supervisor-generated. In either case, feedback should be frequent and recurring.

- *Link rewards to goal attainment.* It's natural for employees to ask, "What's in it for me?" Linking rewards to the achievement of goals will help answer that question.

Practicing the Skill
You worked your way through college while holding down a part-time job bagging groceries at the Food Town supermarket chain. You liked working in the food industry, and when you graduated, you accepted a position with Food Town as a management trainee. Three years have passed and you've gained experience in the grocery store industry and in operating a large supermarket. Several months ago, you received a promotion to store manager at one of the chain's locations. One of the things you've liked about Food Town is that it gives store managers a great deal of autonomy in running their stores. The company provides very general guidelines to its managers. Top management is concerned with the bottom line; for the most part, how you get there is up to you. Now that you're finally a store manager, you want to establish an MBO-type program in your store. You like the idea that everyone should have clear goals to work toward and then be evaluated against those goals.

Your store employs 70 people, although except for the managers, most work only 20 to 30 hours per week. You have six people reporting to you: an assistant manager; a weekend manager; and grocery, produce, meat, and bakery managers. The only highly skilled jobs belong to the butchers, who have strict training and regulatory guidelines. Other less-skilled jobs include cashier, shelf stocker, maintenance worker, and grocery bagger.

Specifically describe how you would go about setting goals in your new position. Include examples of goals for the jobs of butcher, cashier, and bakery manager.

SKILLS EXERCISE Making A To-Do List that Works and Using It

Do you have lots to do and limited time in which to do it? That sounds familiar, doesn't it! One tool that many successful people use is a to-do list. Lists can be useful because they: help organize and make sense of what needs to be done; keep details of work/life events; track progress; and help overcome procrastination. Making a to-do list that works and then using it is a skill that every manager needs to develop.

Steps in Practicing the Skill

- *Break project(s) into smaller tasks and prioritize those tasks.* When you have a major project to complete, spend some time up front identifying as many of the sequential tasks necessary to complete that project. Also, prioritize, prioritize, prioritize. It's the only way to get done what's most important.

- *Be realistic about your to-do list.* Whether your to-do list is daily, weekly, or monthly—or all of these—you've got to realize that interruptions will and do happen. Don't overestimate what you can get done. And you will face conflicting priorities. Re-prioritize when this happens.

- *Know and pay attention to your own time and energy.* Develop your own personal routines. You know when you're the most productive. Those are the times you need

to do your most important tasks. Or maybe you need to do the task you like least first. You'll want to get it done faster so you can move on to tasks that you enjoy doing.

- *Know your biggest time wasters and distractions.* We all have them, whether they're found online or on the television or elsewhere. (And you probably already know what yours are!) Also, realize you probably can't (nor do you want to) eliminate them. But do be leery of them, especially when you're trying to get something done or need to get something done.

- *Let technology be a tool, not a distraction.* Find an app (or written approach) that works FOR YOU. There are many available. And don't constantly try out new ones—that, in itself, wastes precious time. Find one that works for your needs and your personal situation and that you'll USE.

- *Conquer the e-mail/instant messaging challenge.* Although coworkers communicate in many ways in organizations, e-mail and instant messaging are popular *and* can be overwhelming to deal with when you're trying to accomplish work tasks. Again, you need to find what works best for you. Some ideas for "conquering" this distraction include:
  - Check only at certain times during the day.
  - Maybe avoid e-mail first thing in the morning because it's so easy to get sidetracked.

- Come up with a system for responding—if a response can be given in less than three minutes (or whatever time control you choose), respond immediately; if it can't, set the e-mail/message aside for later when you have more time. And a good rule: the faster your response time, the shorter the e-mail.

- Weed out any "subscriptions" that you're not reading/using. You know, those ones you thought sounded really interesting and you end up deleting immediately anyway. So, don't even get them—unsubscribe.

- Use your e-mail system tools—filters that move e-mails to folders, canned responses, auto-responders, and so forth—to manage your e-mail messages.

Practicing the Skill
The best way to practice this skill is to pick a project (school, work, personal) that you're facing and try to use the above suggestions. To get better at using to-do lists, you've just got to jump in, create them, and most importantly use them to guide what you do and when you do it. Discover what works for you and refine and tweak your approach as you learn more about getting things done efficiently and effectively.

WORKING TOGETHER Team Exercise

Form small groups of three to four individuals and read through the following scenario. Complete the work that's called for. Be sure your goals are well designed and your plans are descriptive.

Scenario
Facing budget shortfalls, many school districts are moving to a four-day week. Of nearly 15,000-plus districts nationwide, more than 300 have moved to the four-day system.[40] Suppose you are employed by a school district in San Antonio, Texas, that's moving to a four-day week by the start of the next school year. What type of planning would need to be done as your school district embarked on this process? Identify three or four primary goals for accomplishing this action. Then, describe what plans would be needed to ensure that those goals are met.

MY TURN TO BE A MANAGER

- Practice setting goals for various aspects of your personal life such as academics, career preparation, family, hobbies, and so forth. Set at least two short-term goals and at least two long-term goals for each area.

- For these goals that you have set, write out plans for achieving those goals. Think in terms of what you will have to do to accomplish each. For instance, if one of your academic goals is to improve your grade-point average, what will you have to do to reach it?

- Write a personal mission statement. Although this may sound simple to do, it's not going to be simple or easy. Our hope is that it will be something you'll want to keep,

use, and revise when necessary and that it will help you be the person you'd like to be and live the life you'd like to live. Start by doing some research on personal mission statements. There are some wonderful Web resources that can guide you. Good luck!

- Interview three managers about the types of planning they do. Ask them for suggestions on how to be a better planner. Write a report describing and comparing your findings.

- Choose two companies, preferably in different industries. Research the companies' Web sites and find examples of goals they have stated. (Hint: A company's

annual report is often a good place to start.) Evaluate these goals. Are they well-written? Rewrite those that don't exhibit the characteristics of well-written goals so that they do.

- What does it take to be a good planner? Do some research on this issue. As part of your research, talk to professors and other professionals. Make a bulleted list of suggestions. Be sure to cite your sources.

- In your own words, write down three things you learned in this text about being a good manager. Keep a copy of this for future reference.

Crisis Planning at Livestrong Foundation

In 1996, Lance Armstrong, the now-disgraced pro cyclist, was diagnosed with testicular cancer. Only 25 years old when he found out he had cancer, Armstrong chose to focus on being a survivor, not a victim. During his personal battle with cancer, he soon realized there was a critical lack of resources for individuals facing this disease. He decided to start a foundation devoted to helping others manage their lives on the cancer journey. Since 1998, the Livestrong Foundation has served millions of people affected by cancer. But in October 2012, everything turned upside down for the organization. That's when the U.S. Anti-Doping Agency released its report that "concluded once and for all that Lance Armstrong, the cancer charity's founder and chairman, was guilty of doping during his legendary cycling career."[41]

Doug Ulman, CEO and president of the Livestrong Foundation, said he remembers that day clearly. In fact, he had anticipated for months that this day would come. As good friends, Ulman had believed Armstrong's statements of innocence over the years. But now, "there was no more hiding."[42] After the news broke, Ulman called a meeting of every one of the foundation's 100-person staff, all squeezing into the foundation's boardroom. There, shoulder to shoulder and crammed together, the suspicions and tingling uncertainties all of a sudden became all too real. When Ulman announced that the organization could no longer "defend" its founder, it was a defining, watershed moment. Livestrong, the once high-flying charity that had raised half a billion dollars over the years, was now facing a crisis—maybe even a life or death crisis—of its own. Now, Livestrong would be operating in "life without Lance" mode.

Although it might be tempting to write off Livestrong as a hopeless case, Ulman and the rest of Livestrong's staff have worked hard to keep the foundation viable and focused on its purpose. It's not to ignore the challenges facing the organization, because those challenges are significant. But in managing through the crisis, Ulman had to keep staff morale up *and* make plans to transform and distance itself from Mr. Armstrong.[43] One piece of advice he received from a crisis-communications firm was to take the opportunity to get the foundation's message out. Like many of the cancer sufferers it helps, Livestrong wanted to come out on the other side stronger than ever. It's not been easy. The foundation has lost some of its biggest sponsors, including Nike and RadioShack. Revenues fell in 2012 and 2013. But in addition to his "crisis management" responsibilities, Ulman has been formulating plans and strategies. He says, "It's so ironic—we are in the business of survivorship, that's what we do. Now we find ourselves dealing with the same circumstances in a totally different place."[44]

⭐ DISCUSSION QUESTIONS

14. Could an organization even plan for this type of situation? If yes, how? If not, why not?

15. How would goals be useful in this type of situation? What types of goals might be necessary?

16. What types of plans will be useful to Live**strong**? Explain why you think these plans would be important.

17. What lessons about planning can managers learn from what Live**strong** has endured?

CASE APPLICATION 2 Shifting Direction

As the global leader in satellite navigation equipment, Garmin Ltd. recently hit a milestone number. It has sold more than 100 million of its products to customers—from motorists to runners to geocachers and more—who depend on the company's equipment to "help show them the way." Despite this milestone, the company's core business is in decline due to changing circumstances.[45] In response, managers at Garmin, the biggest maker of personal navigation devices, are shifting direction. Many of you probably have a dashboard-mounted navigation device in your car and chances are it might be a Garmin. However, a number of cars now have "dashboard command centers which combine smartphone docking stations with navigation systems." Sales of Garmin devices have declined as consumers increasingly use their smartphones for directions and maps. However, have you ever tried to use your smartphone navigation system while holding a phone to look at its display? It's dangerous to hold a phone and steer. Also, GPS apps can "crash" if multiple apps are running. That's why the Olathe, Kansas-based company is taking explicitly aggressive actions to team up with automakers to embed its GPS systems in car dashboards. Right now, its biggest in-dash contract is with Chrysler and its Uconnect dashboard system is found in several models of Jeep, Dodge, and Chrysler vehicles. Garmin also is working with Honda and Toyota for dashboard systems in the Asian market.

Despite these new market shifts, customers have gotten used to the GPS devices and it's become an essential part of their lives. That's why Garmin's executive team still believes there's a market for dedicated navigation systems. It's trying to breathe some life into the product with new features, better designs, and more value for the consumer's money. For instance, some of the new features include faster searching for addresses or points of interest, voice-activated navigation, and highlighting exit services such as gas stations and restaurants.

✪ DISCUSSION QUESTIONS

18. What role do you think goals would play in planning the change in direction for the company? List some goals you think might be important. (Make sure these goals have the characteristics of well-written goals.)

19. What types of plans would be needed in an industry such as this one? (For instance, long-term or short-term, or both?) Explain why you think these plans would be important.

20. What contingency factors might affect the planning Garmin executives have to do? How might those contingency factors affect the planning?

21. What planning challenges do you think Garmin executives face with continuing to be the global market leader? How should they cope with those challenges?

ENDNOTES

1. D. Gates and M. Allison, "Boeing, ANA Celebrate First 787 Delivery," *Seattle Times Online,* September 26, 2011; P. Sanders, "Boeing Says Flaw Slows 787 Assembly," *Wall Street Journal,* May 18, 2010, p. B1; Boeing News Release, "ANA Pilots First Customer Crew to Fly Boeing 787 Dreamliner" [boeingmediaroom.com], May 13, 2010; Seattle Times Business Staff, "25 More Orders Canceled for Boeing's New 787," *Seattle Times Online,* July 5, 2009; J. L. Lunsford, "Boeing Delays Dreamliner Delivery Again," *Wall Street Journal,* April 10, 2008, p. B3; and J. Teresko, "The Boeing 787: A Matter of Materials," *Industry Week,* December 2007, pp. 34–38.

2. See, for example, A. Ghobadian, N. O'Regan, H. Thomas, and J. Liu, "Formal Strategic Planning, Operating Environment, Size, Sector, and Performance," *Journal of General Management,* Winter 2008, pp. 1–19; F. Delmar and S. Shane, "Does Business Planning Facilitate the Development of New Ventures?" *Strategic Management Journal,* December 2003, pp. 1165–1185; R. M. Grant, "Strategic Planning in a Turbulent Environment: Evidence from the Oil Majors," *Strategic Management Journal,* June 2003, pp. 491–517; P. J. Brews and M. R. Hunt, "Learning to Plan and Planning to Learn: Resolving the Planning School/Learning School Debate," *Strategic Management Journal,* December 1999, pp. 889–913; C. C. Miller and L. B. Cardinal, "Strategic Planning and Firm Performance: A Synthesis of More Than Two Decades of Research," *Academy of Management Journal,* March 1994, pp. 1649–1685; N. Capon, J. U. Farley, and J. M. Hulbert, "Strategic Planning and Financial Performance: More Evidence," *Journal of Management Studies,* January 1994, pp. 22–38; D. K. Sinha, "The Contribution of Formal Planning to Decisions," *Strategic Management Journal,* October 1990, pp. 479–492; J. A. Pearce II, E. B. Freeman, and R. B. Robinson Jr., "The Tenuous Link between Formal Strategic Planning and Financial Performance," *Academy of Management Review,* October 1987, pp. 658–675; L. C. Rhyne, "Contrasting Planning Systems in High, Medium, and Low Performance Companies," *Journal of Management Studies,* July 1987, pp. 363–385; and J. A. Pearce II, K. K. Robbins, and R. B. Robinson, Jr., "The Impact of Grand Strategy and Planning Formality on Financial Performance," *Strategic Management Journal,* March–April 1987, pp. 125–134.

3. "As Q4 Approaches, Which of the Following Is Most Challenging for You As a Leader?" SmartBrief on Leadership, smartbrief.com/leadership, October 15, 2013.

4. R. Molz, "How Leaders Use Goals," *Long Range Planning,* October 1987, p. 91.

5. C. Hymowitz, "When Meeting Targets Becomes the Strategy, CEO Is on Wrong Path," *Wall Street Journal,* March 8, 2005, p. B1.

6. A. Taylor III, "Das Auto Giant," *Fortune,* July 23, 2012, pp. 150–155.

7. M. Negishi, D. Mattioli, and R. Dezember, "Japan's Uniqlo Sets Goal: No. 1 in the U.S.," *Wall Street Journal,* April 12, 2013, p. B7.

8. Nike [www.nikebiz.com/crreport/], Deutsche Bank [www.db.com/en/content/company/mission_and_brand.htm], and EnCana Corporate Constitution (2010) [www.encana.com].

9. See, for instance, J. Pfeffer, Organizational Design (Arlington Heights, IL: AHM Publishing, 1978), pp. 5–12; and C. K. Warriner, "The Problem of Organizational Purpose," *Sociological Quarterly,* Spring 1965, pp. 139–146.

10. J. D. Hunger and T. L. Wheelen, *Strategic Management and Business Policy,* 10th ed. (Upper Saddle River, NJ: Prentice Hall, 2006).

11. J. L. Roberts, "Signed. Sealed. Delivered?" *Newsweek,* June 20, 2005, pp. 44–46.

12. Leader Making a Difference box based on R. L. Brandt, "Birth of a Salesman," *Wall Street Journal,* October 15–16, 2012, pp. C1+; D. Lyons, "Jeff Bezos," *Newsweek,* December 28, 2009/January 4, 2010, pp. 85–86; B. Stone, "Can Amazon Be Wal-Mart of the Web?" *New York Times Online,* September 20, 2009; and K. Kelleher, "Why Amazon Is Bucking the Trend," CNNMoney.com, March 2, 2009.

13. J. Jusko, "Unwavering Focus," *Industry Week,* January 2010, p. 26.

14. P. N. Romani, "MBO by Any Other Name Is Still MBO," *Supervision,* December 1997, pp. 6–8; and A. W. Schrader and G. T. Seward, "MBO Makes Dollar Sense," *Personnel Journal,* July 1989, pp. 32–37.

15. R. Rodgers and J. E. Hunter, "Impact of Management by Objectives on Organizational Productivity," *Journal of Applied Psychology,* April 1991, pp. 322–336.

16. E. A. Locke and G. P. Latham, "Has Goal Setting Gone Wild, or Have Its Attackers Abandoned Good Scholarship?" *Academy of Management Perspectives,* February 2009, pp. 17–23; and G. P. Latham, "The Motivational Benefits of Goal-Setting," *Academy of Management Executive,* November 2004, pp. 126–129.

17. L. Wayne, "P&G Sees the World as Its Client," *New York Times Online,* December 12, 2009.

18. For additional information on goals, see, for instance, P. Drucker, *The Executive in Action* (New York: HarperCollins Books, 1996), pp. 207–214; and E. A. Locke and G. P. Latham, *A Theory of Goal Setting and Task Performance* (Upper Saddle River, NJ: Prentice Hall, 1990).

19. K. Ramaswamy and W. Youngdahl, "Are You Your Employees' Worst Enemy?" www.strategy-business.com, November 12, 2013.

20. S. Kerr and S. Landauer, "Using Stretch Goals to Promote Organizational Effectiveness and Personal Growth: General Electric and Goldman Sachs," *Academy of Management Executive,* November 2004, pp. 134–138.

21. D. Markovitz, "The Folly of Stretch Goals," *Management Science,* Winter 2012, pp. 34–35; S. Denning, "In Praise of Stretch Goals," www.forbes.com, April 23, 2012; S. B. Sitkin, K. E. See, C. C. Miller, M. W. Lawless, and A. M. Carton, "The Paradox of Stretch Goals: Organizations In Pursuit of the Seemingly Impossible," *Academy of Management Review,* July 2011, pp. 544–566; J. Zenger, J. Folkman, and S. K. Edinger, "Stretch Goals: How to Set and Hit Them," *Leadership Excellence,* July 2009, pp. 6–7; and S. Kerr and S. Landauer, "Using Stretch Goals to Promote Organizational Effectiveness and Personal Growth: General Electric and Goldman Sachs," *Academy of Management Executive,* November 2004, pp. 134–138.

22. Several of these factors were suggested by R. K. Bresser and R. C. Bishop, "Dysfunctional Effects of Formal Planning: Two Theoretical Explanations," *Academy of Management Review,* October 1983, pp. 588–599; and J. S. Armstrong, "The Value of Formal Planning for Strategic Decisions: Review of Empirical Research," *Strategic Management Journal,* July–September 1982, pp. 197–211.

23. Brews and Hunt, "Learning to Plan and Planning to Learn: Resolving the Planning School/Learning School Debate."

24. R. Dudley, "What Good Are Low Prices If the Shelves Are Empty?" *Bloomberg BusinessWeek,* April 1–7, 2013, pp. 23–24.

25. A. Campbell, "Tailored, Not Benchmarked: A Fresh Look at Corporate Planning," *Harvard Business Review,* March–April 1999, pp. 41–50.

26. J. H. Sheridan, "Focused on Flow," *IW,* October 18, 1999, pp. 46–51.

27. A. Taylor III, "Hyundai Smokes the Competition," *Fortune,* January 18, 2010, pp. 62–71.

28. "Disaster Alert," *CFO,* September 2012, p. 25.

29. J. Vance, "Ten Cloud Computing Leaders," *IT Management Online,* May 26, 2010; A. Rocadela, "Amazon Looks to Widen Lead in Cloud Computing," *Bloomberg BusinessWeek Online,* April 28, 2010; and S. Lawson, "Cloud Computing Could Be a Boon for Flash Storage," *Bloomberg BusinessWeek Online,* August 24, 2009.

30. Brews and Hunt, "Learning to Plan and Planning to Learn: Resolving the Planning School/Learning School Debate."

31. J. Ribeiro, "Wipro Sees Drop in Outsourcing Revenue," *Bloomberg BusinessWeek Online,* July 22, 2009; S. N. Mehta, "Schooled by China and India," *CNNMoney Online,* May 5, 2009; R. J. Newman, "Coming and Going," *US News and World Report,* January 23, 2006, pp. 50–52; T. Atlas, "Bangalore's Big Dreams," *US News and World Report,* May 2, 2005, pp. 50–52; and K. H. Hammonds, "Smart, Determined, Ambitious, Cheap: The New Face of Global Competition," *Fast Company,* February 2003, pp. 90–97.

32. G. Fairclough and V. Bauerlein, "Pepsi CEO Tours China to Get a Feel for Market," *Wall Street Journal,* July 1, 2009, p. B5.

33. See, for example, P. Tarraf and R. Molz, "Competitive Intelligence," *SAM Advanced Management Journal,* Autumn 2006, pp. 24–34; W.

M. Fitzpatrick, "Uncovering Trade Secrets: The Legal and Ethical Conundrum of Creative Competitive Intelligence," *SAM Advanced Management Journal,* Summer 2003, pp. 4–12; L. Lavelle, "The Case of the Corporate Spy," *BusinessWeek,* November 26, 2001, pp. 56–58; C. Britton, "Deconstructing Advertising: What Your Competitor's Advertising Can Tell You About Their Strategy," *Competitive Intelligence,* January/February 2002, pp. 15–19; and L. Smith, "Business Intelligence Progress in Jeopardy," *Information Week,* March 4, 2002, p. 74.

34. S. Greenbard, "New Heights in Business Intelligence," *Business Finance,* March 2002, pp. 41–46; K. A. Zimmermann, "The Democratization of Business Intelligence," *KN World,* May 2002, pp. 20–21; and C. Britton, "Deconstructing Advertising: What Your Competitor's Advertising Can Tell You About Their Strategy," *Competitive Intelligence,* January/February 2002, pp. 15–19.

35. L. Weathersby, "Take This Job and ***** It," *Fortune,* January 7, 2002, p. 122.

36. D. Leonard, "The Corporate Side of Snooping," *New York Times Online,* March 5, 2010; B. Acohido, "Corporate Espionage Surges in Tough Times," *USA Today,* July 29, 2009, pp. 1B+; and B. Rosner, "HR Should Get a Clue: Corporate Spying is Real," *Workforce,* April 2001, pp. 72–75.

37. P. Lattman, "Hotel Feud Prompts Probe by Grand Jury," *Wall Street Journal,* October 7, 2009, p. A1+; "Starwood vs. Hilton," *Hotels' Investment Outlook,* June 2009, p. 14; R. Kidder, "Hotel Industry Roiled by Corporate Espionage Claim," *Ethics Newsline* [www.globalethicslorg/newsline]; Reuters, "Hilton Hotels Is Subpoenaed in Espionage Case," *New York Times Online,* April 22, 2009; T. Audi, "U.S. Probes Hilton Over Theft Claims," *Wall Street Journal,* April 22, 2009, p. B1;

and T. Audi, "Hilton Is Sued Over Luxury Chain," *Wall Street Journal,* April 17, 2009, p. B1.

38. S. Bergsman, "Corporate Spying Goes Mainstream," *CFO,* December 1997, p. 24; and K. Western, "Ethical Spying," *Business Ethics,* September–October 1995, pp. 22–23.

39. "Wayward At Safeway," *Workforce.com,* November 8, 2011; S. Halzack, "Safeway Sandwich Theft Allegation: Charges Dropped; What Do You Think?" *Washingtonpost.com,* November 2, 2011; and "Couple Jailed, Lose Custody of Daughter, Over Stolen Sandwiches," Reuters.com, October 30, 2011.

40. K. Sheehy, "Educators at Some High Schools Tout Benefits of Four-Day Week," October 15, 2012, http://www.usnews.com/education/blogs/high-school-notes/2012/10/15/educators-at-some-high-schools-tout-benefits-of-4-day-week; and C. Herring, "Schools' New Math: The Four-Day Week," *Wall Street Journal,* March 8, 2010, pp. A1+.

41. I. Lapowsky, "Livestrong Without Lance," http://www.inc.com/magazine/201404/issie-lapowsky/what-livestrong-is-like-without-lance-armstrong.html, April 1, 2014.

42. Ibid.

43. V. O'Connell, "Livestrong Seeks Life After Lance Armstrong," *Wall Street Journal,* March 6, 2013, p. B7.

44. Ibid.

45. K. Naughton, "Recalculating Navigation Needs," *Bloomberg BusinessWeek,* July 29, 2013, pp. 35–36; "Garmin Finds Route Higher," *Forbes.com,* May 2, 2012; "Come on Baby, Drive My Car," *Tech Talk,* April 2012, pp. 24–28; E. Rhey, "A GPS Maker Shifts Gears," *Fortune,* March 19, 2012, p. 62; "Garmin® Arrives at a Milestone: 100 Million Products Sold," Garmin.com, May 2, 2012; and B. Charny, "Garmin's Positioning Comes Under Scrutiny," *Wall Street Journal,* April 2, 2008, p. A5.

Managing Strategy

It's Your Career

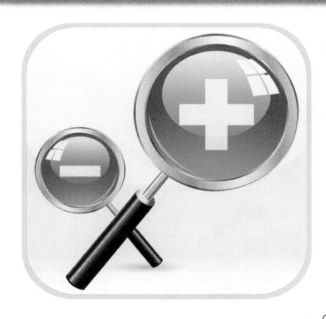

Source: Login/Fotolia

A key to success in management and in your career is knowing how to identify, evaluate, and make the best use of your personal strengths and weaknesses.

Learning Your Strengths and Weaknesses: Accentuate the Positive

Do you know your individual personal strengths and weaknesses? You need to! Why? One important reason is that interviewers commonly ask what you consider your strengths and weaknesses and you want to be prepared to answer those questions and demonstrate your level of self-knowledge and self-awareness. Another reason is that in today's knowledge-work world, you need to find, know, and leverage your workplace strengths so you can be the best employee possible. Finally, by knowing your strengths and weaknesses you can size up where you stand in your career and make good decisions about what you need to do to keep advancing. So, here are some suggestions to help you learn your strengths and weaknesses so you can accentuate your positive attributes and minimize or compensate for your weaknesses:

1. **Focus first on identifying your strengths.** Your strengths are your individual personal positive attributes and characteristics. As you look at your strengths, assess the following: skills (what you are good at), interests (what you enjoy doing), educational background (what qualifications you have), your values (what things are important to you), and your personality (what characteristics you have). As you evaluate these, think in terms of what sets you apart. What things do you like to do? What things do you do well? What things do you do better than others? It's also helpful to ask others you trust what they see as your strengths.

2. **Take a look at your weaknesses.** Your weaknesses are your individual personal negative attributes and characteristics, and it's never easy to look for those. Nobody likes to admit that they have weaknesses. But it is important to know the areas where you need improvement. What things could you improve

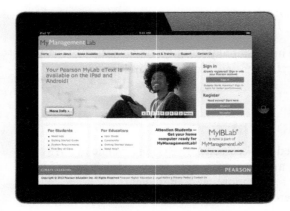

Learning Objectives

1   **Define** *strategic management and explain why it's important.*

2   **Explain** *what managers do during the six steps of the strategic management process.*

     ● **Know how** to identify your own personal strengths and weaknesses and deal with them.

     ● **Develop your skill** at strategic planning.

3   **Describe** *the three types of corporate strategies.*

4   **Describe** *competitive advantage and the competitive strategies organizations use to get it.*

5   **Discuss** *current strategic management issues.*

---

about yourself? What are your negative personal/ work habits? What things do you not like to do? What professional or career skills/training/education/ qualifications are you lacking that would make you a more valuable employee? Are you lacking career direction or focus? What things do others do better than you do? Again, it's helpful to ask others you trust what they see as your weaknesses.

*   **3. Develop a strategy to do something about your strengths and weaknesses.** What actions can you take to get the job you want or to best meet the requirements of your current job or a promotion you're seeking? Accentuate your positives! You want to leverage, emphasize, and capitalize on your strengths. This might involve strengthening a specific skill or attribute. Or it could mean following the great advice given in a commencement speech at MIT by Dropbox*

founder Drew Houston, "The most successful people are obsessed with solving an important problem, something that matters to them. They remind me of a dog chasing a tennis ball."[1] What's your tennis ball? What things grab your attention in a way you can't resist and how can you exploit those passions in your work life and career?

*   Minimize or compensate for your weaknesses. Improve upon your weaker skills, attitudes, habits, or qualifications to increase your present and future job opportunities.*

*   **4. Update your list of strengths and weaknesses periodically.** As you gain new experiences and as your life circumstances change, you'll want to revise your list of strengths and weaknesses. Sharpen your self-awareness so you can craft the kind of life— professionally and personally—you want to live.*

The importance of having good strategies can be seen daily if you pay attention to what's happening in the world of business. Managers must recognize market opportunities to exploit, take steps to correct company weaknesses, or formulate new and hopefully more effective strategies to be strong competitors. How they manage those

strategies will play an important role in a company's ability to reach its goals. An underlying theme in this text is that effective strategies can result in high organizational performance.

STRATEGIC Management

 • Domino's Pizza reported a 7.4 percent increase in revenue in 2013 (about $123.8 million), and most of it, surprisingly, didn't come from selling more pizzas but selling more pizza ingredients.
- Unilever and Procter & Gamble, fierce competitive rivals across many personal care product lines, are waging a shampoo price war.
- Zynga releases a mobile FarmVille game, a new and much-needed approach for the struggling video game maker.
- Taco Bell is launching a new fast-casual upscale concept restaurant chain called U.S. Taco, which will offer 10 kinds of premium tacos, spicy thick-cut fries, and shakes.
- Sony Corporation is downsizing at its two most troubled electronics units by eliminating 5,000 jobs.[2]

These are just a few of the business news stories from a single week, and each one is about a company's strategies. Strategic management is very much a part of what managers do. In this section, we want to look at what strategic management is and why it's important.

What Is Strategic Management?

The discount retail industry is a good place to see what strategic management is all about. Walmart and Kmart Corporation (now part of Sears Holdings) have battled for market dominance since 1962, the year both companies were founded. The two chains have other similarities: store atmosphere, names, markets served, and organizational purpose. Yet, Walmart's performance (financial and otherwise) has far surpassed that of Kmart. Walmart is the world's largest retailer and Kmart was the largest retailer ever to seek Chapter 11 bankruptcy protection. Why the difference in performance? Because of different strategies and competitive abilities.[3] Walmart has excelled by effectively managing strategies while Kmart has struggled by not effectively managing its strategies.

Strategic management is what managers do to develop the organization's strategies. It's an important task involving all the basic management functions—planning, organizing, leading, and controlling. What are an organization's **strategies**? They're the plans for how the organization will do whatever it's in business to do, how it will compete successfully, and how it will attract and satisfy its customers in order to achieve its goals.[4]

One term often used in strategic management is **business model**, which simply is how a company is going to make money. It focuses on two things: (1) whether customers will value what the company is providing and (2) whether the company can make any money doing that.[5] For instance, Jeff Bezos pioneered a new business model for selling books to consumers directly online instead of selling through bookstores. Did customers "value" that? Absolutely! Did Amazon make money doing it that way? Not at first, but now, absolutely! What began as the world's biggest bookstore is now the world's biggest everything store. As managers think about strategies, they need to think about the economic viability of their company's business model. (Check out the Developing Your Business Planning Skill at the end of the chapter.)

Why Is Strategic Management Important?

In the summer of 2002, a British television show spin-off called *American Idol* soon became one of the most-watched shows in American television history. But recently, its audience has been declining and there are a number of competitor shows airing, including NBC's popular *The Voice*. However, *American Idol's* executive producer

strategic management
What managers do to develop the organization's strategies

strategies
The plans for how the organization will do what it's in business to do, how it will compete successfully, and how it will attract and satisfy its customers in order to achieve its goals

business model
How a company is going to make money

says, "If we're smart about it, there's no reason why *Idol* wouldn't keep going. Just look at *Price is Right*. It's been on for over 35 years."[6] The managers behind *Idol* seem to understand the importance of strategic management. Now, their challenge is to keep the franchise a strong presence in the market by making strategic changes.

Why is strategic management so important? There are three reasons. The most significant one is that it can make a difference in how well an organization performs. Why do some businesses succeed and others fail, even when faced with the same environmental conditions? (Remember our Walmart and Kmart example.) Research has found a generally positive relationship between strategic planning and performance.[7] In other words, it appears that organizations that use strategic management do have higher levels of performance. And that fact makes it pretty important for managers!

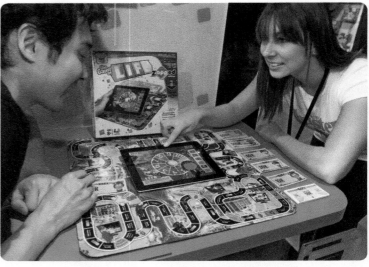

Hasbro achieves high organizational performance with a strategy focused on innovation in developing new toys and games and in growing its core brands to meet the changing demands of all age groups worldwide. Vital to Hasbro's continued success is launching app-enhanced classic board games such as *The Game of Life,* debuted by demonstrators at an international toy fair.
Source: Ray Stubblebine/AP Images

Another reason it's important has to do with the fact that managers in organizations of all types and sizes face continually changing situations. They cope with this uncertainty by using the strategic management process to examine relevant factors and decide what actions to take. For instance, as business executives across a wide spectrum of industries coped with the global recession, they focused on making their strategies more flexible. At Office Depot, for example, store managers throughout the company told corporate managers that cash-strapped consumers no longer wanted to buy pens or printer paper in bulk. So the company created special displays promoting single Sharpie pens and introduced five-ream packages of paper, half the size of the normal big box of paper.[8]

Finally, strategic management is important because organizations are complex and diverse. Each part needs to work together toward achieving the organization's goals; strategic management helps do this. For example, with more than 2.2 million employees worldwide working in various departments, functional areas, and stores, Walmart Stores, Inc., uses strategic management to help coordinate and focus employees' efforts on what's important as determined by its goals.

If your professor has assigned this, go to **www.mymanagementlab.com** to watch a video titled: *Rudi's Bakery: Strategic Management* and to respond to questions.

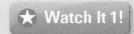
★ Watch It 1!

Today, both business organizations and not-for-profit organizations use strategic management. For instance, the U.S. Postal Service (USPS) is locked in competitive battles with overnight package delivery companies, telecommunications companies' e-mail and text messaging services, and private mailing facilities. In 2006, 213 billion pieces of mail were handled by the postal service. By 2013, that total had dropped to 158 billion, a decline of almost 26 percent.[9] Patrick Donahoe, USPS's CEO (the U.S. Postmaster General), is using strategic management to come up with a response. One possible action plan is a revised service level schedule: six-day package delivery and five-day mail delivery. Others include streamlining and consolidating mail processing facilities, and increasing the availability of self service in high-volume Post Offices. Such strategy changes are needed as the USPS faces losses of $238 billion over the next decade.[10] Strategic management will continue to be important to its operation. Check out the organization's *Five Year Business Plan,* which outlines its internal plan for the future.[11] Although strategic management in not-for-profits hasn't been as well researched as it has been for for-profit organizations, we know it's important for them as well.

Exhibit 1
Strategic Management Process

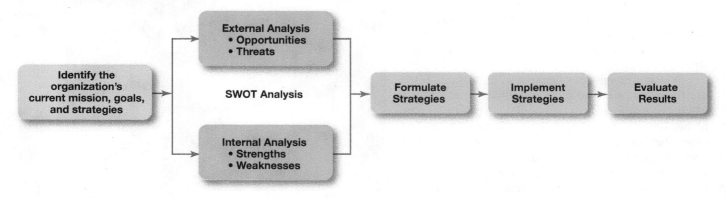

External Analysis
• Opportunities
• Threats

Internal Analysis
• Strengths
• Weaknesses

SWOT Analysis

Identify the organization's current mission, goals, and strategies

Formulate Strategies

Implement Strategies

Evaluate Results

THE STRATEGIC Management Process

LO2   The **strategic management process** (see Exhibit 1) is a six-step process that encompasses strategy planning, implementation, and evaluation. Although the first four steps describe the planning that must take place, implementation and evaluation are just as important! Even the best strategies can fail if management doesn't implement or evaluate them properly.

strategic management process
A six-step process that encompasses strategic planning, implementation, and evaluation

Step 1: Identifying the Organization's Current Mission, Goals, and Strategies

Every organization needs a **mission**—a statement of its purpose. Defining the mission forces managers to identify what it's in business to do. But sometimes that mission statement can be too limiting. For example, the cofounder of the leading Internet search engine Google says that while the company's purpose of providing a way to categorize and organize information and "making it universally accessible and useful" has served them well, they failed to see the whole social side of the Internet and have been playing catch-up.[12] What *should* a mission statement include? Exhibit 2 describes some typical components.

mission
The purpose of an organization

Exhibit 2
Components of a Mission Statement

Source: Based on *Strategic Management*, 13th edition, by Fred R. David. (Upper Saddle River: Pearson Education, Inc., 2011.)

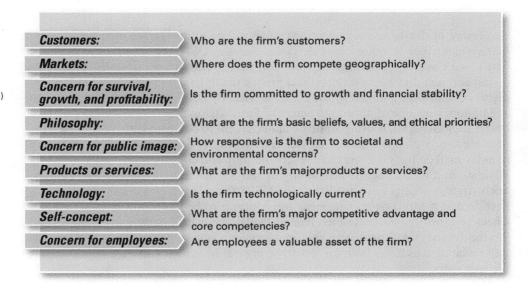

Customers: Who are the firm's customers?

Markets: Where does the firm compete geographically?

Concern for survival, growth, and profitability: Is the firm committed to growth and financial stability?

Philosophy: What are the firm's basic beliefs, values, and ethical priorities?

Concern for public image: How responsive is the firm to societal and environmental concerns?

Products or services: What are the firm's major products or services?

Technology: Is the firm technologically current?

Self-concept: What are the firm's major competitive advantage and core competencies?

Concern for employees: Are employees a valuable asset of the firm?

If your professor has assigned this, go to **www.mymanagementlab.com** to complete the Writing Assignment MGMT 11: Mission Statement.

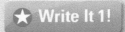

Step 2: Doing an External Analysis

What impact might the following trends have for businesses?

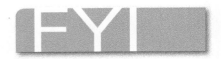

- With the passage of the national health care legislation, every big restaurant chain must now post calorie information on their menus and drive-through signs.
- Cell phones are now used by customers more for data transmittal and retrieval than for phone calls and the number of smartphones and tablet computers continues to soar.
- More young adults are earning college degrees according to data released from the U.S. Department of Education.[14]

- Only 41 percent of employees know what their company stands for.[13]

The external environment is an important constraint on a manager's actions. Analyzing that environment is a critical step in the strategic management process. Managers do an external analysis so they know, for instance, what the competition is doing, what pending legislation might affect the organization, or what the labor supply is like in locations where it operates. In an external analysis, managers should examine the economic, demographic, political/legal, sociocultural, technological, and global components to see the trends and changes.

Once they've analyzed the environment, managers need to pinpoint opportunities that the organization can exploit and threats that it must counteract or buffer against. **Opportunities** are positive trends in the external environment; **threats** are negative trends.

opportunities
Positive trends in the external environment

threats
Negative trends in the external environment

Step 3: Doing an Internal Analysis

Now we move to the internal analysis, which provides important information about an organization's specific resources and capabilities. An organization's **resources** are its assets—financial, physical, human, and intangible—that it uses to develop, manufacture, and deliver products to its customers. They're "what" the organization has. On the other hand, its **capabilities** are its skills and abilities in doing the work activities needed in its business—"how" it does its work. The major value-creating capabilities of the organization are known as its **core competencies**.[15] Both resources and core competencies determine the organization's competitive weapons.

After completing an internal analysis, managers should be able to identify organizational strengths and weaknesses. Any activities the organization does well or any unique resources that it has are called **strengths**. **Weaknesses** are activities the organization doesn't do well or resources it needs but doesn't possess.

resources
An organization's assets that are used to develop, manufacture, and deliver products to its customers

capabilities
An organization's skills and abilities in doing the work activities needed in its business

core competencies
The organization's major value-creating capabilities that determine its competitive weapons

strengths
Any activities the organization does well or its unique resources

weaknesses
Activities the organization does not do well or resources it needs but does not possess

Personal Strengths/Weaknesses—If your instructor is using MyManagementLab, log onto **mymanagementlab.com** and test your knowledge about learning your *personal strengths/weaknesses*. **Be sure to refer back to the chapter opener!**

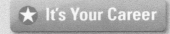

The combined external and internal analyses are called the **SWOT analysis**, an analysis of the organization's *s*trengths, *w*eaknesses, *o*pportunities, and *t*hreats. After completing the SWOT analysis, managers are ready to formulate appropriate strategies—that is, strategies that (1) exploit an organization's strengths and external opportunities, (2) buffer or protect the organization from external threats, or (3) correct critical weaknesses.

SWOT analysis
An analysis of the organization's strengths, weaknesses, opportunities, and threats

let's get REAL

The Scenario:

Johan Nilsson started his architectural firm in Stockholm more than 15 years ago. His business has grown to where he now employs eight architects in addition to himself and an office staff of four. Like many other companies, Johan's business suffered through the global economic downturn. However, now that things are starting to turn around, he feels it's important to re-establish his company's strategic direction. And he also believes that his job as a leader is to make sure his employees understand the strategic goals of the company.

What advice might you give Johan about sharing his organization's strategy and getting his employees to "buy into" the company's future?

The firm is small enough that Johan can take staff feedback into consideration as the new strategy is developed and get them involved in implementing that strategy. Buy-in is best achieved when stakeholders are kept informed throughout the process and it's even better when they can be part of the implementation.

Maribel Lara
Director, Account Management

Source: Maribel Lara

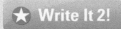 **Write It 2!** If your professor has assigned this, go to **www.mymanagementlab.com** to complete the Writing Assignment MKTG 2 - SWOT Analysis.

Step 4: Formulating Strategies

As managers formulate strategies, they should consider the realities of the external environment and their available resources and capabilities in order to design strategies that will help an organization achieve its goals. The three main types of strategies managers will formulate include corporate, competitive, and functional. We'll describe each shortly.

Step 5: Implementing Strategies

Once strategies are formulated, they must be implemented. No matter how effectively an organization has planned its strategies, performance will suffer if the strategies aren't implemented properly.

Step 6: Evaluating Results

The final step in the strategic management process is evaluating results. How effective have the strategies been at helping the organization reach its goals? What adjustments are necessary? For example, after assessing the results of previous strategies and determining that changes were needed, Xerox CEO Ursula Burns made strategic adjustments to regain market share and improve her company's bottom line. The company cut jobs, sold assets, and reorganized management.

 Write It 3! If your professor has assigned this, go to **www.mymanagementlab.com** to complete the Writing Assignment MGMT 7: Planning (Business Plan Research).

Exhibit 3

Types of Organizational Strategies

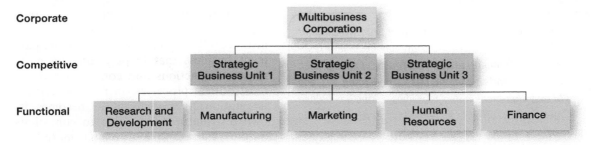

Corporate		Multibusiness Corporation
Competitive		Strategic Business Unit 1 / Strategic Business Unit 2 / Strategic Business Unit 3
Functional		Research and Development / Manufacturing / Marketing / Human Resources / Finance

CORPORATE Strategies

LO3 As we said earlier, organizations use three types of strategies: corporate, competitive, and functional. (See Exhibit 3.) Top-level managers typically are responsible for corporate strategies, middle-level managers for competitive strategies, and lower-level managers for the functional strategies. In this section, we'll look at corporate strategies.

What Is Corporate Strategy?

A **corporate strategy** is one that determines what businesses a company is in or wants to be in and what it wants to do with those businesses. It's based on the mission and goals of the organization and the roles that each business unit of the organization will play. We can see both of these aspects with PepsiCo, for instance. Its mission: To be the world's premier consumer products company focused on convenient foods and beverages. It pursues that mission with a corporate strategy that has put it in different businesses, including its PepsiCo Americas Beverage (beverage business), PepsiCo Americas Foods (snack and prepared foods businesses including Frito-Lay and Quaker Oats), and then its global businesses—PepsiCo Europe and PepsiCo Asia/Middle East/Africa. The other part of corporate strategy is when top managers decide what to do with those businesses: grow them, keep them the same, or renew them.

corporate strategy
An organizational strategy that determines what businesses a company is in or wants to be in, and what it wants to do with those businesses

What Are the Types of Corporate Strategy?

The three main types of corporate strategies are growth, stability, and renewal. Let's look at each type.

GROWTH Even though Walmart Stores is the world's largest retailer, it continues to grow internationally and in the United States. A **growth strategy** is when an organization expands the number of markets served or products offered, either through its current business(es) or through new business(es). Because of its growth strategy, an organization may increase revenues, number of employees, or market share. Organizations grow by using concentration, vertical integration, horizontal integration, or diversification.

An organization that grows using *concentration* focuses on its primary line of business and increases the number of products offered or markets served in this primary business. For instance, Beckman Coulter, Inc., a Fullerton, California-based organization has used concentration to become one of the world's largest medical diagnostics and research equipment companies. Another example of a company using concentration is Bose Corporation of Framingham, Massachusetts, which focuses on developing innovative audio products. It has become one of the world's leading manufacturers of speakers for home entertainment, automotive, and pro audio markets with annual sales of more than $1 billion.

growth strategy
A corporate strategy that's used when an organization wants to expand the number of markets served or products offered, either through its current business(es) or through new business(es)

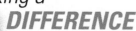

LEADER making a DIFFERENCE

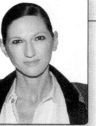

Under the guidance and leadership of Creative Director and President Jenna Lyons, J.Crew has become a fashion force. Positioned between fast-fashion chains such as Zara (see end-of-chapter Case Application #1) and H&M and high-fashion designer lines, Lyons has helped J.Crew find a profitable niche. Although it's not as big as Gap, J.Crew is making strategic inroads. Lyons's philosophy is that "Style is for everyone. We don't talk down to our customers. We want people to be excited about clothes."[16] As the company's creative visionary, her focus is not just on financial concerns (price, units sold, etc.) but on whether products are beautiful and whether she and her team love them. Financial decisions and creative decisions have equal weight. Following a strategic approach where design is supreme means running the business in a completely different way. Before Lyons, designers were told to develop products that would meet specific merchandising goals. Now, designers are free to, well, design. When their experiments don't work, all Lyons asks is for her staff to take responsibility. Then together, they try to fix it.[17] They've had steady growth—the company has over 446 stores in the United States and Canada, and 2014 revenues were up 9 percent. In late 2013, J.Crew's three new London stores opened. In 2014, J.Crew plans to continue developing its new store format—J.Crew Mercantile—targeted to budget-conscious shoppers.[18] The next global strategic push is Hong Kong, where J.Crew is opening two stores. This move presents its own unique set of problems as Asian consumers are extremely logo-conscious. That will be a real strategic test for Lyons and her team. What can you learn from this leader making a difference?

A company also might choose to grow by *vertical integration*, either backward, forward, or both. In backward vertical integration, the organization becomes its own supplier so it can control its inputs. For instance, eBay owns PayPal, an online payment business that helps it provide more secure transactions and control one of its most critical processes. In forward vertical integration, the organization becomes its own distributor and is able to control its outputs. For example, Apple has more than 400 retail stores worldwide to distribute its product.

In *horizontal integration*, a company grows by combining with competitors. For instance, French cosmetics giant L'Oreal acquired The Body Shop. Another example is Live Nation, the largest concert promoter in the United States, which combined operations with competitor HOB Entertainment, the operator of the House of Blues Clubs. Horizontal integration has been used in a number of industries in the last few years—financial services, consumer products, airlines, department stores, and software, among others. The U.S. Federal Trade Commission usually scrutinizes these combinations closely to see if consumers might be harmed by decreased competition. Other countries may have similar restrictions. For instance, the European Commission, the "watchdog" for the European Union, conducted an in-depth investigation into Unilever's acquisition of the body and laundry care units of Sara Lee.

Finally, an organization can grow through *diversification*, either related or unrelated. Related diversification happens when a company combines with other companies in different, but related, industries. For example, Google has acquired a number of businesses (some 150 total), including YouTube, DoubleClick, Nest, and Motorola Mobility. Although this mix of businesses may seem odd, the company's "strategic fit" is its information search capabilities and efficiencies. Unrelated diversification is when a company combines with firms in different and unrelated industries. For instance, the Tata Group of India has businesses in chemicals, communications and IT, consumer products, energy, engineering, materials, and services. Again, an odd mix. But in this case, there's no strategic fit among the businesses.

STABILITY   As the global recession dragged on and U.S. sales of candy and chocolate slowed down, Cadbury Schweppes—with almost half of its confectionary sales coming from chocolate—maintained things as they were. A **stability strategy** is a corporate strategy in which an organization continues to do what it is currently doing. Examples of this strategy include continuing to serve the same clients by offering the same product or service, maintaining market share, and sustaining the organization's current business operations. The organization doesn't grow, but doesn't fall behind, either.

stability strategy
A corporate strategy in which an organization continues to do what it is currently doing

RENEWAL   In 2013, AMR (American Airlines' parent) lost almost $1.8 billion. Hewlett-Packard lost $12 billion, JCPenney lost over $985 million, and many energy

and technology services companies faced serious financial issues with huge losses. When an organization is in trouble, something needs to be done. Managers need to develop strategies, called **renewal strategies**, that address declining performance. The two main types of renewal strategies are retrenchment and turnaround strategies. A *retrenchment strategy* is a short-run renewal strategy used for minor performance problems. This strategy helps an organization stabilize operations, revitalize organizational resources and capabilities, and prepare to compete once again. When an organization's problems are more serious, more drastic action—the *turnaround strategy*—is needed. Managers do two things for both renewal strategies: cut costs and restructure organizational operations. However, in a turnaround strategy, these measures are more extensive than in a retrenchment strategy.

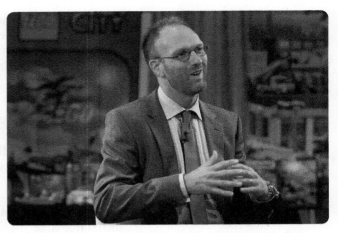

After nearly collapsing in 2003, the Danish firm Lego named Jorgen Vig Knudstorp as CEO to lead a new team of managers in developing a renewal strategy. Part of Knudstorp's successful turnaround strategy included cutting costs by trimming Lego's product line, restructuring its supply chain, and refocusing on the company's core product of unique plastic bricks.
Source: Edgar Su/Reuters Pictures

renewal strategy
A corporate strategy designed to address declining performance

BCG matrix
A strategy tool that guides resource allocation decisions on the basis of market share and growth rate of SBUs

How Are Corporate Strategies Managed?

When an organization's corporate strategy encompasses a number of businesses, managers can manage this collection, or portfolio, of businesses using a tool called a corporate portfolio matrix. This matrix provides a framework for understanding diverse businesses and helps managers establish priorities for allocating resources.[19] The first portfolio matrix—the **BCG matrix**—was developed by the Boston Consulting Group and introduced the idea that an organization's various businesses could be evaluated and plotted using a 2 × 2 matrix to identify which ones offered high potential and which were a drain on organizational resources.[20] The horizontal axis represents market share (low or high), and the vertical axis indicates anticipated market growth (low or high). A business unit is evaluated using a SWOT analysis and placed in one of the four categories, which are as follows:

• **Stars:** High market share/High anticipated growth rate
• **Cash Cows:** High market share/Low anticipated growth rate
• **Question Marks:** Low market share/High anticipated growth rate
• **Dogs:** Low market share/Low anticipated growth rate

What are the strategic implications of the BCG matrix? The dogs should be sold off or liquidated as they have low market share in markets with low growth potential. Managers should "milk" cash cows for as much as they can, limit any new investment in them, and use the large amounts of cash generated to invest in stars and question marks with strong potential to improve market share. Heavy investment in stars will help take advantage of the market's growth and help maintain high market share. The stars, of course, will eventually develop into cash cows as their markets mature and sales growth slows. The hardest decision for managers relates to the question marks. After careful analysis, some will be sold off and others strategically nurtured into stars.

COMPETITIVE Strategies

LO4 A **competitive strategy** is a strategy for how an organization will compete in its business(es). For a small organization in only one line of business or a large organization that has not diversified into different products or markets, its competitive strategy describes how it will compete in its primary or main market. For organizations in multiple businesses, however, each business will have its own competitive strategy that defines its competitive advantage, the products or services it will offer, the customers it wants to reach, and the like. For example, French company LVMH-Moët Hennessy Louis Vuitton SA has different competitive strategies for its businesses, which include Donna Karan fashions, Louis Vuitton leather

competitive strategy
An organizational strategy for how an organization will compete in its business(es)

goods, Guerlain perfume, TAG Heuer watches, Dom Perignon champagne, and other luxury products. When an organization is in several different businesses, those single businesses that are independent and that have their own competitive strategies are referred to as **strategic business units (SBUs)**.

strategic business unit (SBU)
The single independent businesses of an organization that formulate their own competitive strategies

The Role of Competitive Advantage

Michelin has mastered a complex technological process for making superior radial tires. Apple has created the world's best and most powerful brand using innovative design and merchandising capabilities.[21] The Ritz Carlton hotels have a unique ability to deliver personalized customer service. Each of these companies has created a competitive advantage.

Developing an effective competitive strategy requires an understanding of **competitive advantage**, which is what sets an organization apart—that is, its distinctive edge.[22] That distinctive edge can come from the organization's core competencies by doing something that others cannot do or doing it better than others can do it. For example, Southwest Airlines has a competitive advantage because of its skills at giving passengers what they want—convenient and inexpensive air passenger service. Or competitive advantage can come from the company's resources because the organization has something its competitors do not have. For instance, Walmart's state-of-the-art information system allows it to monitor and control inventories and supplier relations more efficiently than its competitors, which Walmart has turned into a cost advantage.

competitive advantage
What sets an organization apart; its distinctive edge

QUALITY AS A COMPETITIVE ADVANTAGE When W. K. Kellogg started manufacturing his cornflake cereal in 1906, his goal was to provide his customers with a high-quality, nutritious product that was enjoyable to eat. That emphasis on quality is still important today. Every employee has a responsibility to maintain the high quality of Kellogg products. If implemented properly, quality can be a way for an organization to create a sustainable competitive advantage.[23] That's why many organizations apply quality management concepts in an attempt to set themselves apart from competitors. If a business is able to continuously improve the quality and reliability of its products, it may have a competitive advantage that can't be taken away.[24]

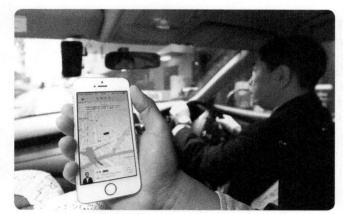

Giving customers the convenience of mobile payments is a competitive advantage for Uber Technologies, Inc., a transportation service firm that makes mobile application software to connect passengers with drivers of vehicles for hire and ridesharing services. Customers value Uber's mobile payment system, which also calculates and includes a tip, over the cash or credit transactions of traditional transportation service firms.
Source: Junko Kimura-Matsumoto/Bloomberg via Getty Images

DESIGN THINKING AS A COMPETITIVE ADVANTAGE In today's world, consumers can find just about anything they want online. And those consumers also expect a greater variety of choices and faster service when ordering online than ever before. One company that recognized the opportunities— and challenges—of this is Kiva Systems.[25] Kiva makes autonomous robots used in flexible automation systems that are critical to companies' strategic e-commerce efforts. By doing this efficiently, the company's robots can gather goods within minutes of an order and deliver them to warehouse pickworkers, who can then ship up to four times more packages in an hour. Kiva (which was recently acquired by Amazon) also has "taught" its robots to move cardboard boxes to the trash compactor and to assist in gift-wrapping.

Here's a company that understands the power of design thinking—defined as approaching management problems the way designers approach design problems. Using design thinking means thinking in unusual ways about what the business is and how it's doing what it's in business to do—or as one person said, "solving wicked problems with creative resolutions by thinking outside existing alternatives and creating new alternatives."[26] After all, who would have thought to "teach" robots to help wrap gifts so that e-commerce warehouse fulfillment could be made even more

FUTURE VISION | Big Data As a Strategic Weapon

Big data can be an effective counterpart to the information exchange generated through social media. All the enormous amounts of data collected about customers, partners, employees, markets, and other quantifiables can be used to respond to the needs of these same stakeholders. With big data, managers can measure and know more about their businesses and "translate that knowledge into improved decision making and performance."[27] Case in point: When Walmart began looking at its enormous database, it noticed that when a hurricane was forecasted, not only did sales of flashlights and batteries increase, but so did sales of Pop-Tarts. Now, when a hurricane is threatening, stores stock Pop-Tarts with other emergency storm supplies at the front entrance. This helps them

better serve customers *and* drive sales.[28] By helping a business do what it's in business to do—compete successfully—and attract and satisfy its customers in order to achieve its goals, big data is a critical strategic weapon for organizations in the future.

If your professor has chosen to assign this, go to **www.mymanagementlab.com** *to discuss the following questions.*

⭐ **TALK ABOUT IT 1:** What strategic connection(s) do you see between big data and social media?

⭐ **TALK ABOUT IT 2:** What ethical obstacles might big data present? How can managers overcome those obstacles?

---

efficient? However, as important as design thinking is to the design of amazing products, it also means recognizing that "design" isn't just for products or processes but for any organizational work problems that can arise. That's why a company's ability to use design thinking in the way its employees and managers strategically manage can be a powerful competitive tool.

SOCIAL MEDIA AS A COMPETITIVE ADVANTAGE When Red Robin Gourmet Burgers launched its Tavern Double burger line, everything about the introduction needed to be absolutely on target. So what did company executives do? Utilized social media.[29] Using an internal social network resembling Facebook, managers in the 475-restaurant chain were taught everything from the recipes to tips on efficiently making the burgers. That same internal network has been a great feedback tool. Company chefs have used tips and suggestions from customer feedback and from store managers to tweak the recipe.

Successful social media strategies should (1) help people—inside and outside the organization—connect; and (2) reduce costs or increase revenue possibilities or both. As managers look at how to strategically use social media, it's important to have goals and a plan. For instance, at global banking firm Wells Fargo & Co., executives realized that social media tools don't just "exist for their own sake" and that they wanted "…to know how we can use them to enhance business strategy."[30] Now Wells Fargo uses blogs, wikis, and other social media tools for a variety of specific needs that align with their business goals.

It's not just for the social connections that organizations are employing social media strategies. Many are finding that social media tools can boost productivity.[31] For example, many physicians are tapping into online postings and sharing technologies as part of their daily routines. Collaborating with colleagues and experts allows them to improve the speed and efficiency of patient care. At Trunk Club, an online men's clothes shopping service that sends out, on request, trunks to clients with new clothing items, the CEO uses a software tool called Chatter to let the company's personal shoppers know about hot new shipments of shoes or clothes. He says that when he "chats" that information out to the team, he immediately sees the personal shoppers putting the items into customers' "trunks."[32] When used strategically, social media can be a powerful competitive weapon!

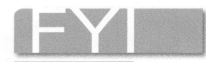

- 52 percent of managers say social media are important/somewhat important to their business.

SUSTAINING COMPETITIVE ADVANTAGE   Every organization has resources (assets) and capabilities (how work gets done). So what makes some organizations more successful than others? Why do some professional baseball teams consistently win championships or draw large crowds? Why do some organizations have consistent and continuous growth in revenues and profits? Why do some colleges, universities, or departments experience continually increasing enrollments? Why do some companies consistently appear at the top of lists ranking the "best," or the "most admired," or the "most profitable"? The answer is that not every organization is able to effectively exploit its resources and to develop the core competencies that can provide it with a competitive advantage. And it's not enough simply to create a competitive advantage. The organization must be able to sustain that advantage; that is, to keep its edge despite competitors' actions or evolutionary changes in the industry. But that's not easy to do! Market instabilities, new technology, and other changes can challenge managers' attempts at creating a long-term, sustainable competitive advantage. However, by using strategic management, managers can better position their organizations to get a sustainable competitive advantage.

Many important ideas in strategic management have come from the work of Michael Porter.[33] One of his major contributions was explaining how managers can create a sustainable competitive advantage. An important part of doing this is an industry analysis, which is done using the five forces model.

FIVE FORCES MODEL   In any industry, five competitive forces dictate the rules of competition. Together, these five forces determine industry attractiveness and profitability, which managers assess using these five factors:

1. *Threat of new entrants.* How likely is it that new competitors will come into the industry?
2. *Threat of substitutes.* How likely is it that other industries' products can be substituted for our industry's products?
3. *Bargaining power of buyers.* How much bargaining power do buyers (customers) have?
4. *Bargaining power of suppliers.* How much bargaining power do suppliers have?
5. *Current rivalry.* How intense is the rivalry among current industry competitors?

Choosing a Competitive Strategy

Once managers have assessed the five forces and done a SWOT analysis, they're ready to select an appropriate competitive strategy—that is, one that fits the competitive strengths (resources and capabilities) of the organization and the industry it's in. According to Porter, no firm can be successful by trying to be all things to all people. He proposed that managers select a strategy that will give the organization a competitive advantage, either from having lower costs than all other industry competitors or by being significantly different from competitors.

When an organization competes on the basis of having the lowest costs (costs or expenses, not prices) in its industry, it's following a *cost leadership strategy.* A low-cost leader is highly efficient. Overhead is kept to a minimum, and the firm does everything it can to cut costs. You won't find expensive art or interior décor at offices of low-cost leaders. For example, at Walmart's headquarters in Bentonville, Arkansas, office furnishings are functional, not elaborate, maybe not what you'd expect for the world's largest retailer. Although a low-cost leader doesn't place a lot of emphasis on "frills," its product must be perceived as comparable in quality to that offered by rivals or at least be acceptable to buyers.

A company that competes by offering unique products that are widely valued by customers is following a *differentiation strategy.* Product differences might come from exceptionally high quality, extraordinary service, innovative design, technological capability, or an unusually positive brand image. Practically any successful consumer product or service can be identified as an example of the differentiation strategy; for

instance, Nordstrom (customer service); 3M Corporation (product quality and innovative design); Coach (design and brand image); and Apple (product design).

Although these two competitive strategies are aimed at the broad market, the final type of competitive strategy—the *focus strategy*—involves a cost advantage (cost focus) or a differentiation advantage (differentiation focus) in a narrow segment or niche. Segments can be based on product variety, customer type, distribution channel, or geographical location. For example, Denmark's Bang & Olufsen, whose revenues exceed $490 million, focuses on high-end audio equipment sales. Whether a focus strategy is feasible depends on the size of the segment and whether the organization can make money serving that segment.

What happens if an organization can't develop a cost or a differentiation advantage? Porter called that being *stuck in the middle* and warned that's not a good place to be. An organization becomes stuck in the middle when its costs are too high to compete with the low-cost leader or when its products and services aren't differentiated enough to compete with the differentiator. Getting unstuck means choosing which competitive advantage to pursue and then doing so by aligning resources, capabilities, and core competencies.

Although Porter said you had to pursue either the low cost or the differentiation advantage to prevent being stuck in the middle, more recent research has shown that organizations *can* successfully pursue both a low cost and a differentiation advantage and achieve high performance.[34] Needless to say, it's not easy to pull off! You have to keep costs low *and* be truly differentiated. But companies such as Southwest Airlines, Google, and Coca-Cola have been able to do it.

If your professor has assigned this, go to **www.mymanagementlab.com** to complete the Writing Assignment MGMT 13: Strategic Decision Making (Competitive Marketing Strategy).

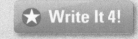

Before we leave this section, we want to point out the final type of organizational strategy, the **functional strategies**, which are the strategies used by an organization's various functional departments to support the competitive strategy. For example, when R. R. Donnelley & Sons Company, a Chicago-based printer, wanted to become more competitive and invested in high-tech digital printing methods, its marketing department had to develop new sales plans and promotional pieces, the production department had to incorporate the digital equipment in the printing plants, and the human resources department had to update its employee selection and training programs. We don't cover specific functional strategies in this book because you'll cover them in other business courses you take.

functional strategy
A strategy used by an organization's various functional departments to support the competitive strategy

If your professor has assigned this, go to **www.mymanagementlab.com** to complete the Simulation: Strategic Management and get a better understanding of the challenges of managing strategy in organizations.

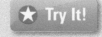

CURRENT Strategic Management Issues

L05 There's no better example of the strategic challenges faced by managers in today's environment than the recorded music industry. Overall, sales of CDs have plummeted in the last decade. As a *Billboard* magazine article title stated so plainly, "Is 2014 The Year Digital Takes Over?"[35] Not only has this trend

impacted music companies, but music retailers as well. Retailers have been forced to look to other products to replace the lost revenue. For instance, Best Buy, the national electronics retailer, experimented with selling musical instruments. Other major music retailers, such as Walmart, have shifted selling space used for CDs to other departments. Survival means finding ways to diversify. Managers are struggling to find strategies that will help their organizations succeed in such an environment. Many have had to shift into whole new areas of business.[36] But it isn't just the music industry that's dealing with strategic challenges. Managers everywhere face increasingly intense global competition and high performance expectations by investors and customers. How have they responded to these new realities? In this section, we look at three current strategic management issues, including the need for strategic leadership, the need for strategic flexibility, and how managers design strategies to emphasize e-business, customer service, and innovation.

The Need for Strategic Leadership

"Amazon is so serious about its next big thing that it hired three women to do nothing but try on size 8 shoes for its Web reviews. Full time." Hmmmm...now that sounds like a fun job! What exactly is Amazon's CEO Jeff Bezos thinking? Having conquered the book publishing, electronics, and toy industries (among others), his next target is high-end clothing. And he's doing it as he always does—all out."[37]

An organization's strategies are usually developed and overseen by its top managers. An organization's top manager is typically the CEO (chief executive officer). This individual usually works with a top management team that includes other executive or senior managers such as a COO (chief operating officer), CFO (chief financial officer), CIO (chief information officer), and other individuals who may have various titles. Traditional descriptions of the CEO's role in strategic management include being the "chief" strategist, structural architect, and developer of the organization's

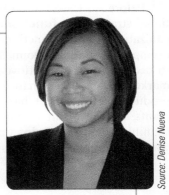

let's get REAL

The Scenario:

Caroline Fulmer was just promoted to executive director of a municipal art museum in a medium-sized city in the Midwest. Although she's very excited about her new position and what she hopes to accomplish there, she knows the museum's board is adamant about solidifying the organization's strategic future. Although she knows they feel she's capable of doing so since they hired her for the position, she wants to be an effective strategic leader.

Source: Denise Nueva

Denise Nueva
Art Director

What skills do you think Caroline will need to be an effective strategic leader?

To be an effective strategic leader, Caroline must be able to manage day-to-day processes of the museum while keeping in mind the big picture of the organization's mission. With this mission in mind, Caroline must align her team of likewise talented individuals to share her passion and commitment. Lastly, it is important for Caroline to remain an unbiased leader and quickly identify and work through issues that may arise.

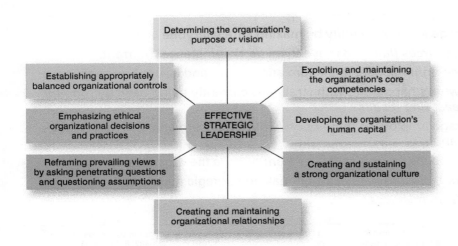

Exhibit 4
Effective Strategic Leadership

Sources: Based on J. P. Wallman, "Strategic Transactions and Managing the Future: A Druckerian Perspective," *Management Decision,* vol. 48, no. 4, 2010, pp. 485–499; D. E. Zand, "Drucker's Strategic Thinking Process: Three Key Techniques," *Strategy & Leadership,* vol. 38, no. 3, 2010, pp. 23–28; and R. D. Ireland and M. A. Hitt, "Achieving and Maintaining Strategic Competitiveness in the 21st Century: The Role of Strategic Leadership," *Academy of Management Executive,* February 1999, pp. 43–57.

information/control systems.[38] Other descriptions of the strategic role of the "chief executive" include key decision maker, visionary leader, political actor, monitor and interpreter of environment changes, and strategy designer.[39]

No matter how top management's job is described, you can be certain that from their perspective at the organization's upper levels, it's like no other job in the organization. By definition, top managers are ultimately responsible for every decision and action of every organizational employee. One important role that top managers play is that of strategic leader. Organizational researchers study leadership in relation to strategic management because an organization's top managers must provide effective strategic leadership. What is **strategic leadership**? It's the ability to anticipate, envision, maintain flexibility, think strategically, and work with others in the organization to initiate changes that will create a viable and valuable future for the organization.[40] How can top managers provide effective strategic leadership? Eight key dimensions have been identified.[41] (See Exhibit 4.) These dimensions include determining the organization's purpose or vision, exploiting and maintaining the organization's core competencies, developing the organization's human capital, creating and sustaining a strong organizational culture, creating and maintaining organizational relationships, reframing prevailing views by asking penetrating questions and questioning assumptions, emphasizing ethical organizational decisions and practices, and establishing appropriately balanced organizational controls. Each dimension encompasses an important part of the strategic management process.

strategic leadership
The ability to anticipate, envision, maintain flexibility, think strategically, and work with others in the organization to initiate changes that will create a viable and valuable future for the organization

The Need for Strategic Flexibility

Not surprisingly, the economic recession changed the way that many companies approached strategic planning.[42] For instance, at Spartan Motors, a maker of specialty vehicles, managers used to draft a one-year strategic plan and a three-year financial plan, reviewing each one every financial quarter. However, CEO John Sztykiel felt that type of fixed approach led to a drastic drop in sales and profits. Now, the company uses a three-year strategic plan that the top management team updates every month.[43] And at J. C. Penney Company, an ambitious five-year strategic growth plan rolled out in 2007 was put on hold as the economy floundered.[44] In its place, the CEO crafted a tentative "bridge" plan to guide the company. This plan worked as the company improved its profit margins and did not have to lay off any employees.

Jürgen Schrempp, former CEO of Daimler AG, stated, "My principle always was...move as fast as you can and [if] you indeed make mistakes, you have to correct them....It's much better to move fast, and make mistakes occasionally, than move too slowly."[45] You wouldn't think that smart individuals who are paid lots of money to manage organizations would make mistakes when it comes to strategic decisions.

Exhibit 5
Developing Strategic Flexibility

- *Encourage leadership unity* by making sure everyone is on the same page.
- *Keep resources fluid* and move them as circumstances warrant.
- *Have the right mindset* to explore and understand issues and challenges.
- Know what's happening with strategies currently being used by *monitoring and measuring results.*
- Encourage employees to *be open about disclosing and sharing negative information.*
- *Get new ideas and perspectives from outside* the organization.
- Have *multiple alternatives* when making strategic decisions.
- *Learn from mistakes.*

Sources: Based on Y. L. Doz and M. Kosonen, "Embedding Strategic Agility: A Leadership Agenda for Accelerating Business Model Renewal," *Long Range Planning,* April 2010, pp. 370–382; E. Lewis, D. Romanaggi, and A. Chapple, "Successfully Managing Change During Uncertain Times," *Strategic HR Review,* vol. 9, no. 2, 2010, pp. 12–18; and K. Shimizu and M. Hitt, "Strategic Flexibility: Organizational Preparedness to Reverse Ineffective Strategic Decisions," *Academy of Management Executive,* November 2004, pp. 44–59.

strategic flexibility
The ability to recognize major external changes, to quickly commit resources, and to recognize when a strategic decision was a mistake

But even when managers use the strategic management process, there's no guarantee that the chosen strategies will lead to positive outcomes. Reading any of the current business periodicals would certainly support this assertion! But the key is responding quickly when it's obvious the strategy isn't working. In other words, they need **strategic flexibility**—that is, the ability to recognize major external changes, to quickly commit resources, and to recognize when a strategic decision isn't working. Given the highly uncertain environment that managers face today, strategic flexibility seems absolutely necessary! Exhibit 5 provides suggestions for developing such strategic flexibility.

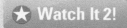 **Watch It 2!** If your professor has assigned this, go to **www.mymanagementlab.com** to watch a video titled: *CH2MHill: Strategic Management* and to respond to questions.

Important Organizational Strategies for Today's Environment

ESPN.com gets more than 16 million unique users a month. Sixteen million! That's almost twice the population of New York City. And its popular online business is just one of many of ESPN's businesses. Originally founded as a television channel, ESPN is now into original programming, radio, online, publishing, gaming, X Games, ESPY Awards, ESPN Zones, global, and is looking to move into more local sports coverage.[46] Company president John Skipper "runs one of the most successful and envied franchises in entertainment" and obviously understands how to successfully manage its various strategies in today's environment! We think three strategies are important in today's environment: e-business, customer service, and innovation.

E-BUSINESS STRATEGIES Managers use e-business strategies to develop a sustainable competitive advantage.[47] A cost leader can use e-business to lower costs in a variety of ways. For instance, it might use online bidding and order processing to eliminate the need for sales calls and to decrease sales force expenses; it could use Web-based inventory control systems that reduce storage costs; or it might use online testing and evaluation of job applicants.

A differentiator needs to offer products or services that customers perceive and value as unique. For instance, a business might use Internet-based knowledge

systems to shorten customer response times, provide rapid on-line responses to service requests, or automate purchasing and payment systems so that customers have detailed status reports and purchasing histories.

Finally, because the focuser targets a narrow market segment with customized products, it might provide chat rooms or discussion boards for customers to interact with others who have common interests, design niche Web sites that target specific groups with specific interests, or use Web sites to perform standardized office functions such as payroll or budgeting.

Research also has shown that an important e-business strategy might be a clicks-and-bricks strategy. A clicks-and-bricks firm is one that uses both online (clicks) and traditional stand-alone locations (bricks).[48] For example, Walgreens established an online site for ordering prescriptions, but some 90 percent of its customers who placed orders on the Web preferred to pick up their prescriptions at a nearby store rather than have them shipped to their home. So its "clicks-and-bricks" strategy has worked well! Other retailers, such as Walmart, The Container Store, and Home Depot, are transforming their stores into extensions of their online operations by adding Web return centers, pickup locations, free shipping outlets, and payment booths.[49]

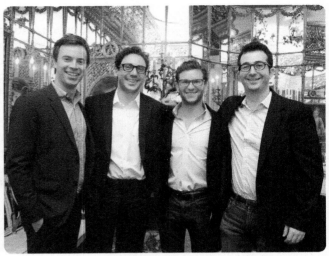

The four cofounders of Warby Parker developed a competitive advantage by launching an innovative and customer-focused eyeglass business. The company sells stylish eyewear quickly, easily, directly, and inexpensively at a uniform price of $95. Warby Parker sources and designs its own products and donates one pair of glasses to the needy for every pair purchased.
Source: Carly Otness/BFAnyc/Sipa USA/Newscom

CUSTOMER SERVICE STRATEGIES Companies emphasizing excellent customer service need strategies that cultivate that atmosphere from top to bottom. Such strategies involve giving customers what they want, communicating effectively with them, and providing employees with customer service training. Let's look first at the strategy of giving customers what they want.

It shouldn't surprise you that an important customer service strategy is giving customers what they want, which is a major aspect of an organization's overall marketing strategy. For instance, New Balance Athletic Shoes gives customers a truly unique product: shoes in varying widths. No other athletic shoe manufacturer has shoes for narrow or wide feet and in practically any size.[50]

Having an effective customer communication system is an important customer service strategy. Managers should know what's going on with customers. They need to find out what customers liked and didn't like about their purchase encounter—from their interactions with employees to their experience with the actual product or service. It's also important to let customers know if something is going on with the company that might affect future purchase decisions. Finally, an organization's culture is important to providing excellent customer service. This typically requires that employees be trained to provide exceptional customer service. For example, Singapore Airlines is well-known for its customer treatment. "On everything facing the customer, they do not scrimp," says an analyst based in Singapore.[51] Employees are expected to "get service right," leaving employees with no doubt about the expectations as far as how to treat customers.

INNOVATION STRATEGIES When Procter & Gamble purchased the Iams pet food business, it did what it always does—used its renowned research division to look for ways to transfer technology from its other divisions to make new products.[52] One outcome of this cross-divisional combination: a new tartar-fighting ingredient from toothpaste that's included in all of its dry adult pet foods.

As this example shows, innovation strategies aren't necessarily focused on just the radical, breakthrough products. They can include applying existing technology to new uses. And organizations have successfully used both approaches. What types of innovation strategies do organizations need in today's environment? Those strategies should reflect their innovation philosophy, which is shaped by two strategic decisions: innovation emphasis and innovation timing.

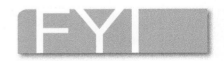

- Only 43 percent of companies have someone at the executive level who is formally accountable for innovation.

- Only 42 percent of organizations have an explicit innovation strategy.

- Only 25 percent of executives say that most of their company's innovation efforts have a positive impact on business results.[53]

Managers must first decide where the emphasis of their innovation efforts will be. Is the organization going to focus on basic scientific research, product development, or process improvement? Basic scientific research requires the most resource commitment because it involves the nuts-and-bolts work of scientific research. In numerous industries (for instance, genetics engineering, pharmaceuticals, information technology, or cosmetics), an organization's expertise in basic research is the key to a sustainable competitive advantage. However, not every organization requires this extensive commitment to scientific research to achieve high performance levels. Instead, many depend on product development strategies. Although this strategy also requires a significant resource investment, it's not in areas associated with scientific research. Instead, the organization takes existing technology and improves on it or applies it in new ways, just as Procter & Gamble did when it applied tartar-fighting knowledge to pet food products. Both of these first two strategic approaches to innovation (basic scientific research and product development) can help an organization achieve high levels of differentiation, which can be a significant source of competitive advantage.

Finally, the last strategic approach to innovation emphasis is a focus on process development. Using this strategy, an organization looks for ways to improve and enhance its work processes. The organization innovates new and improved ways for employees to do their work in all organizational areas. This innovation strategy can lead to lower costs, which, as we know, also can be a significant source of competitive advantage.

Once managers have determined the focus of their innovation efforts, they must decide their innovation timing strategy. Some organizations want to be the first with innovations whereas others are content to follow or mimic the innovations. An organization that's first to bring a product innovation to the market or to use a new process innovation is called a **first mover**. Being a first mover has certain strategic advantages and disadvantages, as shown in Exhibit 6. Some organizations pursue this route, hoping to develop a sustainable competitive advantage. Others have successfully developed a sustainable competitive advantage by being the followers in the industry. They let the first movers pioneer the innovations and then mimic their products or processes. Which approach managers choose depends on their organization's innovation philosophy and specific resources and capabilities.

first mover
An organization that's first to bring a product innovation to the market or to use a new process innovation

Exhibit 6
First Mover Advantages and Disadvantages

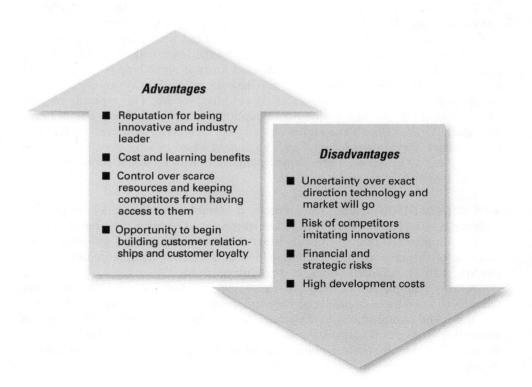

Advantages

- Reputation for being innovative and industry leader
- Cost and learning benefits
- Control over scarce resources and keeping competitors from having access to them
- Opportunity to begin building customer relationships and customer loyalty

Disadvantages

- Uncertainty over exact direction technology and market will go
- Risk of competitors imitating innovations
- Financial and strategic risks
- High development costs

CHAPTER SUMMARY by Learning Objectives

LO1 DEFINE strategic management and explain why it's important.

Strategic management is what managers do to develop the organization's strategies. Strategies are the plans for how the organization will do whatever it's in business to do, how it will compete successfully, and how it will attract and satisfy its customers in order to achieve its goals. A business model is how a company is going to make money. Strategic management is important for three reasons. First, it makes a difference in how well organizations perform. Second, it's important for helping managers cope with continually changing situations. Finally, strategic management helps coordinate and focus employee efforts on what's important.

LO2 EXPLAIN what managers do during the six steps of the strategic management process.

The six steps in the strategic management process encompass strategy planning, implementation, and evaluation. These steps include the following: (1) identify the current mission, goals, and strategies; (2) do an external analysis; (3) do an internal analysis (steps 2 and 3 collectively are known as SWOT analysis); (4) formulate strategies; (5) implement strategies; and (6) evaluate strategies. Strengths are any activities the organization does well or its unique resources. Weaknesses are activities the organization doesn't do well or resources it needs. Opportunities are positive trends in the external environment. Threats are negative trends.

LO3 DESCRIBE the three types of corporate strategies.

A growth strategy is when an organization expands the number of markets served or products offered, either through current or new businesses. The types of growth strategies include concentration, vertical integration (backward and forward), horizontal integration, and diversification (related and unrelated). A stability strategy is when an organization makes no significant changes in what it's doing. Both renewal strategies—retrenchment and turnaround—address organizational weaknesses leading to performance declines. The BCG matrix is a way to analyze a company's portfolio of businesses by looking at a business's market share and its industry's anticipated growth rate. The four categories of the BCG matrix are cash cows, stars, question marks, and dogs.

LO4 DESCRIBE competitive advantage and the competitive strategies organizations use to get it.

An organization's competitive advantage is what sets it apart, its distinctive edge. A company's competitive advantage becomes the basis for choosing an appropriate competitive strategy. Porter's five forces model assesses the five competitive forces that dictate the rules of competition in an industry: threat of new entrants, threat of substitutes, bargaining power of buyers, bargaining power of suppliers, and current rivalry. Porter's three competitive strategies are as follows: cost leadership (competing on the basis of having the lowest costs in the industry), differentiation (competing on the basis of having unique products that are widely valued by customers), and focus (competing in a narrow segment with either a cost advantage or a differentiation advantage).

L05 DISCUSS **current strategic management issues.**

Managers face three current strategic management issues: strategic leadership, strategic flexibility, and important types of strategies for today's environment. Strategic leadership is the ability to anticipate, envision, maintain flexibility, think strategically, and work with others in the organization to initiate changes that will create a viable and valuable future for the organization and includes eight key dimensions. Strategic flexibility—that is, the ability to recognize major external environmental changes, to quickly commit resources, and to recognize when a strategic decision isn't working—is important because managers often face highly uncertain environments. Managers can use e-business strategies to reduce costs, to differentiate their firm's products and services, to target (focus on) specific customer groups, or to lower costs by standardizing certain office functions. Another important e-business strategy is the clicks-and-bricks strategy, which combines online and traditional, stand-alone locations. Strategies managers can use to become more customer oriented include giving customers what they want, communicating effectively with them, and having a culture that emphasizes customer service. Strategies managers can use to become more innovative include deciding their organization's innovation emphasis (basic scientific research, product development, or process development) and its innovation timing (first mover or follower).

MyManagementLab

Go to **mymanagementlab.com** to complete the problems marked with this icon ⭐.

⭐ REVIEW AND DISCUSSION QUESTIONS

1. Describe the six steps in the strategic management process.

2. How could the Internet be helpful to managers as they follow the steps in the strategic management process?

3. How might the process of strategy formulation, implementation, and evaluation differ for (a) large businesses, (b) small businesses, (c) not-for-profit organizations, and (d) global businesses?

4. Should ethical considerations be included in analyses of an organization's internal and external environments? Why or why not?

5. Describe the three major types of corporate strategies and how the BCG matrix is used to manage those corporate strategies.

6. Describe the role of competitive advantage and how Porter's competitive strategies help an organization develop competitive advantage.

7. "The concept of competitive advantage is as important for not-for-profit organizations as it is for for-profit organizations." Do you agree or disagree with this statement? Explain, using examples to make your case.

8. Describe e-business, customer service, and innovation strategies.

MyManagementLab

If your professor has assigned these, go to **mymanagementlab.com** for Auto-graded writing questions as well as the following Assisted-graded writing questions:

9. Explain why strategic management is important.

10. Explain why strategic leadership and strategic flexibility are important.

PREPARING FOR: My Career

⭐ PERSONAL INVENTORY ASSESSMENTS 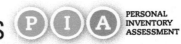 PERSONAL INVENTORY ASSESSMENT

Creative Style Indicator

Good strategic decision makers are creative in formulating and implementing strategies. Take this PIA and get a better feel for your creative style.

⭐ ETHICS DILEMMA

Do you shop? Well, you might be saying to yourself, that's kind of a stupid question ... of course I shop. Well, here's another question: Do you realize the extent to which retail stores are spying on you as you shop?[54] Although most of us "accept" the fact that when we shop online, we're "allowing" the online retailer to install its cookies and to track our every move and click. Now, however, technology is being used more frequently in the physical retail environment. And it's more than cameras watching us. Many retailers are using cell phone tracking technology, personalized advertising, and super spy cams. Why? To track your behavior and to get you (and all those other shoppers) to buy more. Results from a survey conducted in

March 2014 showed that 80 percent of consumers do not want stores to track their movements via smartphone. And 44 percent said that a tracking program would make them less likely to shop with that store.

11. What do you think? Are you more "accepting" of tracking shopping behavior online than you are of tracking shopping behavior in a physical store?

12. What ethical dilemmas are involved with this strategy of retail consumer tracking?

13. What factors would influence a business's decision to use it? (Think in terms of the various stakeholders who might be affected by this decision.)

SKILLS EXERCISE Developing Your Business Planning Skill

About the Skill

An important step in starting a business or in determining a new strategic direction is preparing a business plan.[55] Not only does the business plan aid in thinking about what to do and how to do it, but it can be a sound basis from which to obtain funding and resources.

Steps in Practicing the Skill

- *Describe your company's background and purpose.* Provide the history of the company. Briefly describe the company's history and what this company does that's unique. Describe what your product or service will be, how you intend to market it, and what you need to bring your product or service to the market.

- *Identify your short- and long-term goals.* What is your intended goal for this organization? Clearly, for a new company three broad objectives are relevant: creation, survival, and profitability. Specific objectives can include such things as sales, market share, product quality, employee morale, and social responsibility. Identify how you plan to achieve each objective, how you intend to

determine whether you met the objective, and when you intend the objective to be met (e.g., short or long term).

- *Do a thorough market analysis.* You need to convince readers that you understand what you are doing, what your market is, and what competitive pressures you'll face. In this analysis, you'll need to describe the overall market trends, the specific market you intend to compete in, and who the competitors are. In essence, in this section you'll perform your SWOT analysis.

- *Describe your development and production emphasis.* Explain how you're going to produce your product or service. Include time frames from start to finish. Describe the difficulties you may encounter in this stage as well as how much you believe activities in this stage will cost. Provide an explanation of what decisions (e.g., make or buy?) you will face and what you intend to do.

- *Describe how you'll market your product or service.* What is your selling strategy? How do you intend to reach your customers? In this section, describe your product or service in terms of your competitive advantage

and demonstrate how you'll exploit your competitors' weaknesses. In addition to the market analysis, provide sales forecasts in terms of the size of the market, how much of the market you can realistically capture, and how you'll price your product or service.

- *Put together your financial statements.* What's your bottom line? Investors want to know this information. In the financial section, provide projected profit-and-loss statements (income statements) for approximately three to five years, a cash flow analysis, and the company's projected balance sheets. In the financial section, give thought to how much start-up costs will be and develop a financial strategy—how you intend to use funds received from a financial institution and how you'll control and monitor the financial well-being of the company.

- *Provide an overview of the organization and its management.* Identify the key executives, summarizing their education, experience, and any relevant qualifications. Identify their positions in the organization and their job roles. Explain how much salary they intend to earn initially. Identify others who may assist the organization's management (e.g., company lawyer, accountant, board of directors). This section should also include, if relevant, a subsection on how you intend to deal with employees. For example, how will employees be paid, what benefits will be offered, and how will employee performance be assessed?

- *Describe the legal form of the business.* Identify the legal form of the business. For example, is it a sole proprietorship, a partnership, a corporation? Depending on the legal form, you may need to provide information regarding equity positions, shares of stock issued, and the like.

- *Identify the critical risks and contingencies facing the organization.* In this section, identify what you'll do if problems arise. For instance, if you don't meet sales forecasts, what then? Similar responses to such questions as problems with suppliers, inability to hire qualified employees, poor-quality products, and so on should be addressed. Readers want to see if you've anticipated potential problems and if you have contingency plans. This is the "what if" section.

- *Put the business plan together.* Using the information you've gathered from the previous nine steps, it's now

time to put the business plan together into a well-organized document. A business plan should contain a cover page that shows the company name, address, contact person, and numbers at which the individual can be reached. The cover page should also contain the date the business was established and, if one exists, the company logo. The next page of the business plan should be a table of contents. Here you'll want to list and identify the location of each major section and subsection in the business plan. Remember to use proper outlining techniques. Next comes the executive summary, the first section the readers will actually read. Thus, it's one of the more critical elements of the business plan, because if the executive summary is poorly done, readers may not read any further. In a two- to three-page summary, highlight information about the company, its management, its market and competition, the funds requested, how the funds will be used, financial history (if available), financial projections, and when investors can expect to get their money back (called the exit). Next come the main sections of your business plan; that is, the material you've researched and written about in steps 1 through 9. Close out the business plan with a section that summarizes the highlights of what you've just presented. Finally, if you have charts, exhibits, photographs, tables, and the like, you might want to include an appendix in the back of the business plan. If you do, remember to cross-reference this material to the relevant section of the report.

Practicing the Skill
You have a great idea for a business and need to create a business plan to present to a bank. Choose one of the following products or services and draft the part of your plan that describes how you will price and market it (see step 5).

1. Haircuts at home (you make house calls)
2. Olympic snowboarding computer game for consoles and mobile devices
3. Online apartment rental listing
4. Voice-activated house alarm

Now choose a different product or service from the list and identify critical risks and contingencies (see step 9).

WORKING TOGETHER Team Exercise

Organizational mission statements. Are they a promise, a commitment, or just a bunch of hot air? Form small groups of three to four individuals and find examples of three different organizational mission statements. Your first task is to evaluate the mission statements. How do they compare to the items listed in Exhibit 2? Would you describe

each as an effective mission statement? Why or why not? How might you rewrite each mission statement to make it better? Your second task is to use the mission statements to describe the types of corporate and competitive strategies each organization might use to fulfill that mission statement. Explain your rationale for choosing each strategy.

MY TURN TO BE A MANAGER

- Using current business periodicals, find two examples of each of the corporate and competitive strategies. Write a description of what these businesses are doing and how it represents that particular strategy.

- Pick five companies from the latest version of *Fortune*'s "Most Admired Companies" list. Research these companies and identify their (a) mission statement, (b) strategic goals, and (c) strategies used.

- Customer service, social media, and innovation strategies are particularly important to managers today. We described specific ways companies can pursue these strategies. Your task is to pick customer service, e-business, or innovation and find one example for each of the specific approaches in that category. For instance, if you choose customer service, find an example of (a) giving customers what they want, (b) communicating effectively with them, and (c) providing employees with customer service training. Write a report describing your examples.

- In your own words, write down three things you learned in this text about being a good manager. Keep a copy of this for future reference.

CASE APPLICATION 1 Fast Fashion

When Amancio Ortega, a former Spanish bathrobe maker, opened his first Zara clothing store, his business model was simple: sell high-fashion look-alikes to price-conscious Europeans.[56] After succeeding in this, he decided to tackle the outdated clothing industry in which it took six months from a garment's design to consumers being able to purchase it in a store. What Ortega envisioned was "fast fashion"—getting designs to customers quickly. And that's exactly what Zara has done!

The company has been described as having more style than Gap, faster growth than Target, and logistical expertise rivaling Walmart's. Zara, owned by the Spanish fashion retail group Inditex SA, recognizes that success in the fashion world is based on a simple rule—get products to market quickly. Accomplishing this, however, isn't so simple. It involves a clear and focused understanding of fashion, technology, and their market, *and* the ability to adapt quickly to trends.

Inditex, the world's largest fashion retailer by sales worldwide, has seven chains: Zara (including Zara Kids and Zara Home), Pull and Bear, Massimo Dutti, Stradivarius, Bershka, Oysho, and Uterqüe. The company has more than 6,340 stores in 87 countries, although Zara pulls in more than 60 percent of the company's revenues. Despite its global presence, Zara is not yet a household name in the United States, with just 45 stores open, including a flagship store in New York City.

What is Zara's secret to excelling at fast fashion? It takes approximately two weeks to get a new design from drawing board to store floor. And stores are stocked with new designs twice a week as clothes are shipped directly to the stores from the factory. Thus, each aspect of Zara's business contributes to the fast turnaround. Sales managers at "the Cube"—what employees call their futuristic-looking headquarters—sit at a long row of computers and scrutinize sales at every store. They see the hits and the misses almost instantaneously. They ask the in-house designers, who work in teams, sketching out new styles and deciding which fabrics will provide the best combination of style and price, for new designs. Once a design is drawn, it's sent electronically to Zara's factory across the street, where a clothing sample is made. To minimize waste, computer programs arrange and rearrange clothing patterns on the massive fabric rolls before a laser-guided machine does the cutting. Zara produces most of its designs close to home—in Morocco, Portugal, Spain, and Turkey. Finished garments are returned to the factory within a week. Finishing touches (buttons, trim, detailing, etc.) are added, and each garment goes through a quality check. Garments that don't pass

are discarded while those that do pass are individually pressed. Then, garment labels (indicating to which country garments will be shipped) and security tags are added. The bundled garments proceed along a moving carousel of hanging rails via a maze of tunnels to the warehouse, a four-story, 5-million-square-foot building (about the size of 90 football fields). As the merchandise bundles move along the rails, electronic bar code tags are read by equipment that send them to the right "staging area," where specific merchandise is first sorted by country and then by individual store, ensuring that each store gets exactly the shipment it's supposed to. From there, merchandise for European stores is sent to a loading dock and packed on a truck with other shipments in order of delivery. Deliveries to other locations go by plane. Some 60,000 items each hour—more than 2.6 million items a week—move through this ultrasophisticated distribution center. And this takes place with only a handful of workers, who monitor the entire process. The company's just-in-time production (an idea borrowed from the auto industry) gives it a competitive edge in terms of speed and flexibility.

Despite Zara's success at fast fashion, its competitors are working to be faster. But CEO Pablo Isla isn't standing still. To maintain Zara's leading advantage, he's introducing new methods that enable store managers to order and display merchandise faster and is adding new cargo routes for shipping goods. Also, the company recently announced that it's developing a new logistics hub that will be able to distribute almost half a million garments daily to its stores on five continents. Zara's CEO says that this new facility will lay the groundwork for continued rapid expansion worldwide. And the company has finally made the jump into online retailing. One analyst forecasts that the company could quadruple sales, with a majority of that coming from online sales.

⭐ DISCUSSION QUESTIONS

14. How is strategic management illustrated by this case story?

15. How might SWOT analysis be helpful to Inditex executives? To Zara store managers?

16. What competitive advantage do you think Zara is pursuing? How does it exploit that competitive advantage?

17. Do you think Zara's success is due to external or internal factors or both? Explain.

18. What strategic implications does Zara's move into online retailing have? (Hint: Think in terms of resources and capabilities.)

CASE APPLICATION 2 Rewind and Replay

There's no doubt that people like to watch movies, but *how* they watch is changing.[57] Although many people still prefer going to an actual movie theater, more and more are settling back in their easy chairs in front of home entertainment systems, especially now that technology has improved to the point where those systems are affordable and offer many of the same features as those found in movie theaters. Along with the changes in *where* people watch movies, *how* people get those movies has changed. For many, the weekend used to start with a trip to the video rental store to search the racks for something good to watch, an approach Blockbuster built its business on. Today's consumers can choose a movie by going to their computer and visiting an online DVD subscription and delivery site where the movies come to the customers—a model invented by Netflix.

Launched in 1999, Netflix's subscriber base grew rapidly. It now has more than 50 million subscribers and thousands of movie titles and other content from which to

choose. From the beginning, Netflix's goal was to provide the most extensive and all-inclusive selection of DVDs, a simple and fast way to select movies, and fast, free delivery.

Netflix founder and CEO Reed Hastings believed in the approach he pioneered and set some ambitious goals for his company: build the world's best Internet movie service and grow earnings per share (EPS) and subscribers every year. In 2011, though, Hastings made a decision that had customers complaining loudly. Netflix's troubles began when it announced it would charge separate prices for its DVDs-by-mail and streaming video plans. Then, it decided to rebrand its DVD service as Qwikster. Customers raged so much that Netflix reversed that decision and pulled the plug on the entire Qwikster plan. As Netflix regained its focus with customers, it was once again ready to refocus on its competitors.

Success ultimately attracts competition. Other businesses want a piece of the market. Trying to gain an edge in how customers get the movies they want, when and where they want them, has led to an all-out competitive war. Now, what Netflix did to Blockbuster, other competitors are doing to Netflix. Hastings said he has learned never to underestimate the competition. He says, "We erroneously concluded that Blockbuster probably wasn't going to launch a competitive effort when they hadn't by 2003. Then, in 2004, they did. We thought...well they won't put much money behind it. Over the past four years, they've invested more than $500 million against us." Not wanting to suffer the same fate as Blockbuster (it filed for bankruptcy protection in 2010 and was sold to Satellite TV service provider DISH Network in 2011), Netflix is bracing for other onslaughts. In fact, CEO Hastings, defending his misguided decisions in 2011, said, "We did so many difficult things this year that we got overconfident. Our big obsession for the year was streaming, the idea that 'let's not die with DVDs.'"

The in-home entertainment industry is intensely competitive and continually changing. Many customers have multiple providers (e.g., HBO, renting a DVD from Red Box, buying a DVD, streaming a movie or television series or original programming from providers such as Hulu, Apple, and Amazon Prime) and may use any or all of those services in the same month. Video-on-demand and streaming are becoming extremely competitive.

To counter such competitive challenges, Hastings is focusing the company's competitive strengths on a select number of initiatives. The most important initiative is continuing to improve its programming, its personalization technology, and its marketing to attract new customers. He says, "Streaming is the future; we're focused on it. DVD is going to do whatever it's going to do. We don't want to hurt it, but we're not putting much time or energy into it." Other strategic initiatives include embarking on a substantial European expansion, negotiating contracts with cable providers for direct connectivity, developing profitable partnerships with other content providers, controlling the cost and quality of streaming content, and even continuing to create original series. In fact, its first original series, called *House of Cards* and starring Kevin Spacey, won a Primetime Emmy Award in 2013. The company also premiered its newest hit series, *Orange Is the New Black*. With other companies hoping to get established in the market, the competition is intense. Does Netflix have the script it needs to be a dominant player? CEO Hastings says, "If it's true that you should be judged by the quality of your competitors, we must be doing pretty well."

⭐ DISCUSSION QUESTIONS

19. Using Porter's framework, describe Netflix's competitive strategy. Explain your choice.

20. What competitive advantage(s) do you think Netflix has? Have its resources, capabilities, or core competencies contributed to its competitive advantage(s)? Explain.

21. How will Netflix's functional strategies have to support its competitive strategy? Explain.

22. What do you think Netflix is going to have to do to maintain its competitive position, especially as its industry changes?

ENDNOTES

1. W. Berger, "Find Your Passion With These 8 Thought-Provoking Questions," www.fastcodesign.com, April 14, 2014; and **G. Anders, "MIT's Inspired Call: Graduation Talk by Dropbox CEO, Age 30," www.forbes. com, June 8, 2013.**

2. V. Wong, "Forget Pizza: Domino's Makes More Money Selling Ingredients," www.businessweek.com, February 27, 2014; P. Evans, "Unilever, P&G Wage Shampoo Price War," *Wall Street Journal,* February 25, 2014, p. B5; B. Molina, "Zynga Bets the Farm(Ville) on Mobile," *USA Today,* April 17, 2014, p. 2B; S. Berfield, "Taco Bell Is Going Upscale— Really," www.businessweek.com, April 24, 2014; and K. Inagaki, "Sony Jolts Its Electronics Businesses," *Wall Street Journal,* February 7, 2014, pp. B1+.

3. J. W. Dean, Jr. and M. P. Sharfman, "Does Decision Process Matter? A Study of Strategic Decision-Making Effectiveness," *Academy of Management Journal,* April 1996, pp. 368–396.

4. Based on A. A. Thompson Jr., A. J. Strickland III, and J. E. Gamble, *Crafting and Executing Strategy,* 14th ed. (New York: McGraw-Hill Irwin, 2005).

5. J. Magretta, "Why Business Models Matter," *Harvard Business Review,* May 2002, pp. 86–92.

6. B. Carter, "'American Idol' and Its Owner to Undergo a Retooling," *New York Times Online,* May 30, 2012; B. Keveney, "'Idol' May Be Down, But It's Not Out," *USA Today,* May 22, 2012, p. 1D; G. Levin and B. Keveney, "NBC Upstart 'The Voice' Calls Out 'American Idol'," *USA Today,* February 16, 2012, pp. 1B+; S. Schechner, "Fewer Viewers Tune in for Cowell's 'Idol' Finale," *Wall Street Journal,* May 28, 2010, p. B7; B. Keveny, "Idol Ratings Take A Tumble," *USA Today,* May 4, 2010, p. 1D; R. Bianco, "Time for Producers to Fix 'Idol' Franchise," *USA Today,* May 4, 2010, p. 7D; **D. J. Lang, "'Idol' top boss: Abdul isn't going anywhere," Associated Press, April 30, 2008.**

7. M. Song, S. Im, H. van der Bij, and L. Z. Song, "Does Strategic Planning Enhance or Impede Innovation and Firm Performance?" *Journal of Product Innovation Management,* July 2011, pp. 503–520; M. Reimann, O. Schilke, and J. S. Thomas, "Customer Relationship Management and Firm Performance: The Mediating Role of Business Strategy," *Journal of the Academy of Marketing Science,* Summer 2010, pp. 326–346; J. Aspara, J. Hietanen, and H. Tikkanen, "Business Model Innovation vs. Replication: Financial Performance Implications of Strategic Emphases," *Journal of Strategic Marketing,* February 2010, pp. 39–56; J. C. Short, D. J. Ketchen Jr., T. B. Palmer, and G. T. M. Hult, "Firm, Strategic Group, and Industry Influences on Performance," *Strategic Management Journal,* February 2007, pp. 147–167; H. J. Cho and V. Pucik, "Relationship Between Innovativeness, Quality, Growth, Profitability, and Market Value," *Strategic Management Journal,* June 2005, pp. 555–575; A. Carmeli and A. Tischler, "The Relationships Between Intangible Organizational Elements and Organizational Performance," *Strategic Management Journal,* December 2004, pp. 1257–1278; D. J. Ketchen, C. C. Snow, and V. L. Street, "Improving Firm Performance by Matching Strategic Decision-Making Processes to Competitive Dynamics," *Academy of Management Executive,* November 2004, pp. 29–43; E. H. Bowman and C. E. Helfat, "Does Corporate Strategy Matter?" *Strategic Management Journal,* 22 (2001), pp. 1–23; P. J. Brews and M. R. Hunt, "Learning to Plan and Planning to Learn: Resolving the Planning School-Learning School Debate," *Strategic Management Journal,* 20 (1999), pp. 889–913; D. J. Ketchen Jr., J. B. Thomas, and R. R. McDaniel Jr., "Process, Content and Context; Synergistic Effects on Performance," *Journal of Management,* 22, no. 2 (1996), pp. 231–257; C. C. Miller and L. B. Cardinal, "Strategic Planning and Firm Performance: A Synthesis of More Than Two Decades of Research," *Academy of Management Journal,* December 1994, pp. 1649–1665; and N. Capon, J. U. Farley, and J. M. Hulbert, "Strategic Planning and Financial Performance: More Evidence," *Journal of Management Studies,* January 1994, pp. 105–110.

8. J. S. Lublin and D. Mattioli, "Strategic Plans Lose Favor," *Wall Street Journal,* January 25, 2010, p. B7.

9. "Pieces of Mail Handled, Number of Post Offices, Income, and Expenses Since 1789," *Annual Report of the Postmaster General,* http://about.usps.com/who-we-are/postal-history/pieces-of-mail-since-1789.htm, April 27, 2014.

10. J. Liberto, "Postal Plants to Shrink, 28,000 Jobs at Stake," *CNN Money. com,* May 17, 2012; C. Boles, "Postal Rescue Passes Senate," *Wall Street Journal,* April 26, 2012, p. A2; J. Liberto, "Congress Ready to Tackle Postal Reform," *CNNMoney.com,* April 16, 2012; D. Leinwand, "Postal Service Seeks 5-Day Delivery," *USA Today,* March 2, 2010, p. 3A; and Wire Reports, "Postal Chief Calls for 5-Day Delivery to Save $3.5 Billion Yearly," *USA Today,* March 26, 2009, p. 4A.

11. You can see this document at http://about.usps.com/strategic-planning/five-year-business-plan-2012-2017.pdf.

12. B. Stone, "The Education of Larry Page," *Bloomberg BusinessWeek,* April 9–15, 2012, pp. 12–14.

13. C. Groscurth, "Why Your Company Must Be Mission-Driven," *Gallup Business Journal,* businessjournal.gallup.com, March 6, 2014.

14. C. Armario, "More Young Adults Earn College Degrees," Associated Press, *Springfield, Missouri, News-Leader,* July 13, 2012, p. 3A; A. R. Sorkin, "Angry Birds Maker Posted Revenue of $106.3 Million in 2011," *New York Times Online,* May 7, 2012; J. Wortham, "Cellphones Now Used More for Data Than for Calls," *New York Times Online,* May 13, 2010; and S. Rosenbloom, "Calorie Data to Be Posted at Most Chains," *New York Times Online,* March 23, 2010.

15. C. K. Prahalad and G. Hamel, "The Core Competence of the Corporation," *Harvard Business Review,* May–June 1990, pp. 79–91.

16. E. Rosenblum, "The J. Crew Invasion," *Bloomberg BusinessWeek,* November 27, 2013, pp. 50–54.

17. D. Sacks, "The Devil Wears J. Crew," *Fast Company,* May 2013, pp. 80+.

18. S. Kapner, "J.Crew Tailors New Stores to the Frugal," *Wall Street Journal,* May 2, 2014, p. B3.

19. H. Quarls, T. Pernsteiner, and K. Rangan, "Love Your Dogs," *Strategy & Business,* Spring 2006, pp. 58–65; and P. Haspeslagh, "Portfolio Planning: Uses and Limits," *Harvard Business Review,* January–February 1982, pp. 58–73.

20. *Perspective on Experience* (Boston: Boston Consulting Group, 1970).

21. "Global 500 2014: The World's Most Valuable Brands," http://brandirectory.com/league_Tables/table/global-500-2014.

22. J. B. Barney, "Looking Inside for Competitive Advantage," *Academy of Management Executive,* November 1995, pp. 49–61; M. A. Peteraf, "The Cornerstones of Competitive Advantage: A Resource-Based View," *Strategic Management Journal,* March 1993, pp. 179–191; J. Barney, "Firm Resources and Sustained Competitive Advantage," *Journal of Management* 17, No. 1 (1991), pp. 99–120; M. E. Porter, *Competitive Advantage: Creating and Sustaining Superior Performance* (New York: Free Press, 1985); and R. Rumelt, "Towards a Strategic Theory of the Firm," in R. Lamb (ed.), *Competitive Strategic Management* (Upper Saddle River, NJ: Prentice Hall, 1984), pp. 556–570.

23. R. D. Spitzer, "TQM: The Only Source of Sustainable Competitive Advantage," *Quality Progress,* June 1993, pp. 59–64; T. C. Powell, "Total Quality Management as Competitive Advantage: A Review and Empirical Study," *Strategic Management Journal,* January 1995, pp. 15–37; and N. A. Shepherd, "Competitive Advantage: Mapping Change and the Role of the Quality Manager of the Future," *Annual Quality Congress,* May 1998, pp. 53–60.

24. See special issue of *Academy of Management Review* devoted to TQM, July 1994, pp. 390–584; B. Voss, "Quality's Second Coming," *Journal of Business Strategy,* March–April 1994, pp. 42–46; R. Krishnan, A. B. Shani, R. M. Grant, and R. Baer, "In Search of Quality Improvement Problems of Design and Implementation," *Academy of Management Executive,* November 1993, pp. 7–20; C. A. Barclay, "Quality Strategy and TQM Policies: Empirical Evidence," *Management International Review,* Special Issue 1993, pp. 87–98; and R. Jacob, "TQM: More Than a Dying Fad?" *Fortune,* October 18, 1993, pp. 66–72; and R. J. Schonenberger, "Is Strategy Strategic? Impact of Total Quality Man-

agement on Strategy," *Academy of Management Executive*, August 1992, pp. 80–87.

25. "Executive Insight: An Interview with Peter Blair, Senior Director of Marketing, Kiva Systems," *Apparel Magazine*, June 2012, p. 24; A. Noto, "Amazon's Robotics Play Underscores Industry Trend," *Mergers & Acquisitions: The Dealmaker's Journal*, May 2012, p. 14; "Amazon to Acquire Kiva Systems for $775 Million," *Material Handling & Logistics*," April 2012, p. 7; and C. Chaey, "The World's 50 Most Innovative Companies: Kiva Systems," *FastCompany.com*, March 2012, p. 110.

26. D. Dunne and R. Martin, "Design Thinking and How It Will Change Management Education: An Interview and Discussion," *Academy of Management Learning & Education*, December 2006, pp. 512–523.

27. A. McAfee and E. Brynjolfsson, "Big Data: The Management Revolution," *Harvard Business Review*, October 2012, p. 62.

28. K. Cukier and V. Mayer-Schönberger, "The Financial Bonanza of Big Data," *Wall Street Journal*, March 8, 2013, p. A15.

29. T. Mullaney, "'Social Business' Launched This Burger," *USA Today*, May 17, 2012, pp. 1A+.

30. B. Roberts, "Social Media Gets Strategic," *HR Magazine*, October 2012, p. 30.

31. B. Acohido, "Social-Media Tools Boost Productivity," *USA Today*, August 13, 2012, pp. 1B+.

32. Ibid.

33. See, for example, A. Brandenburger, "Porter's Added Value: High Indeed!" *Academy of Management Executive*, May 2002, pp. 58–60; N. Argyres and A. M. McGahan, "An Interview with Michael Porter," *Academy of Management Executive*, May 2002, pp. 43–52; D. F. Jennings and J. R. Lumpkin, "Insights Between Environmental Scanning Activities and Porter's Generic Strategies: An Empirical Analysis," *Strategic Management Journal*, 18, No. 4 (1992), pp. 791–803; I. Bamberger, "Developing Competitive Advantage in Small and Medium-Sized Firms," *Long Range Planning*, October 1989, pp. 80–88; C. W. L. Hill, "Differentiation Versus Low Cost or Differentiation and Low Cost: A Contingency Framework," *Academy of Management Review*, July 1988, pp. 401–412; A. I. Murray, "A Contingency View of Porter's 'Generic Strategies,'" *Academy of Management Review*, July 1988, pp. 390–400; M. E. Porter, "From Competitive Advantage to Corporate Strategy," *Harvard Business Review*, May–June 1987, pp. 43–59; G. G. Dess and P. S. Davis, "Porter's (1980) Generic Strategies and Performance: An Empirical Examination with American Data—Part II: Performance Implications," *Organization Studies*, No. 3 (1986), pp. 255–261; G. G. Dess and P. S. Davis, "Porter's (1980) Generic Strategies and Performance: An Empirical Examination with American Data—Part I: Testing Porter," *Organization Studies*, no. 1 (1986), pp. 37–55; G. G. Dess and P. S. Davis, "Porter's (1980) Generic Strategies as Determinants of Strategic Group Membership and Organizational Performance," *Academy of Management Journal*, September 1984, pp. 467–488; Porter, *Competitive Advantage: Creating and Sustaining Superior Performance*; and M. E. Porter, *Competitive Strategy: Techniques for Analyzing Industries and Competitors* (New York: Free Press, 1980).

34. J. W. Bachmann, "Competitive Strategy: It's O.K. to Be Different," *Academy of Management Executive*, May 2002, pp. 61–65; S. Cappel, P. Wright, M. Kroll, and D. Wyld, "Competitive Strategies and Business Performance: An Empirical Study of Select Service Businesses," *International Journal of Management*, March 1992, pp. 1–11; D. Miller, "The Generic Strategy Trap," *Journal of Business Strategy*, January–February 1991, pp. 37–41; R. E. White, "Organizing to Make Business Unit Strategies Work," in H. E. Glass (ed.), *Handbook of Business Strategy*, 2d ed. (Boston: Warren Gorham and Lamont, 1991), pp. 1–24; and Hill, "Differentiation Versus Low Cost or Differentiation and Low Cost: A Contingency Framework."

35. K. Caulfield, "CD Album Sales Fall Behind Album Downloads, Is 2014 The Year Digital Takes Over?" www.billboard.com, February 11, 2014.

36. B. Sisario, "Out to Shake Up Music, Often with Sharp Words," *New York Times Online*, May 6, 2012; and J. Plambeck, "As CD Sales Wane, Music Retailers Diversify," *New York Times Online*, May 30, 2010.

37. J. Greene, "Amazon Woos Fashion Industry as New Studio Opens in N.Y.," seattletimes.com, October 21, 2013; S. Clifford, "Amazon Leaps

38. into High End of the Fashion Pool," *New York Times Online*, May 7, 2012; and "Can Amazon Be A Fashion Player?" *Women's Wear Daily*, May 4, 2012, p. 1.

38. S. Ghoshal and C. A. Bartlett, "Changing the Role of Top Management: Beyond Structure to Process," *Harvard Business Review*, January–February 1995, pp. 86–96.

39. R. Calori, G. Johnson, and P. Sarnin, "CEO's Cognitive Maps and the Scope of the Organization," *Strategic Management Journal*, July 1994, pp. 437–457.

40. R. D. Ireland and M. A. Hitt, "Achieving and Maintaining Strategic Competitiveness in the 21st Century: The Role of Strategic Leadership," *Academy of Management Executive*, February 1999, pp. 43–57.

41. J. P. Wallman, "Strategic Transactions and Managing the Future: A Druckerian Perspective," *Management Decision*, vol. 48, no. 4, 2010, pp. 485–499; D. E. Zand, "Drucker's Strategic Thinking Process: Three Key Techniques," *Strategy & Leadership*, vol. 38, no. 3, 2010, pp. 23–28; and R. D. Ireland and M. A. Hitt, "Achieving and Maintaining Strategic Competitiveness in the 21st Century: The Role of Strategic Leadership."

42. Lublin and Mattioli, "Strategic Plans Lose Favor."

43. Based on J. S. Lublin and D. Mattioli, "Strategic Plans Lose Favor: Slump Showed Bosses Value of Flexibility, Quick Decisions," *Wall Street Journal*, January 25, 2010, p. B7.

44. Ibid.

45. K. Shimizu and M. A. Hitt, "Strategic Flexibility: Organizational Preparedness to Reverse Ineffective Decisions," *Academy of Management Executive*, November 2004, p. 44.

46. B. Barnes, "Across U.S., ESPN Aims to Be the Home Team," *New York Times Online*, July 20, 2009; P. Sanders and M. Futterman, "Competition Pushes Up Content Costs for ESPN," *Wall Street Journal*, February 23, 2009, pp. B1+; T. Lowry, "ESPN's Cell-Phone Fumble," *BusinessWeek Online*, October 30, 2006; and T. Lowry, "In the Zone," *BusinessWeek*, October 17, 2005, pp. 66–77.

47. E. Kim, D. Nam, and J. L. Stimpert, "The Applicability of Porter's Generic Strategies in the Digital Age: Assumptions, Conjectures, and Suggestions," *Journal of Management*, vol. 30, no. 5 (2004), pp. 569–589; and G. T. Lumpkin, S. B. Droege, and G. G. Dess, "E-Commerce Strategies: Achieving Sustainable Competitive Advantage and Avoiding Pitfalls," *Organizational Dynamics*, Spring 2002, pp. 325–340.

48. Kim, Nam, and Stimpert, "The Applicability of Porter's Generic Strategies in the Digital Age: Assumptions, Conjectures, and Suggestions."

49. S. Clifford, "Luring Online Shoppers Offline," *New York Times Online*, July 4, 2012.

50. J. Gaffney, "Shoe Fetish," *Business 2.0*, March 2002, pp. 98–99.

51. D. Fickling, "The Singapore Girls Aren't Smiling Anymore," *Bloomberg BusinessWeek*, May 21–27, 2012, pp. 25–26; L. Heracleous and J. Wirtz, "Singapore Airlines' Balancing Act," *Harvard Business Review*, July–August 2010, pp. 145–149; and J. Doebele, "The Engineer," *Forbes*, January 9, 2006, pp. 122–124.

52. "Innovation at Work: Is Anyone In Charge?" *Wall Street Journal*, January 22, 2013, p. B14.

53. S. Ellison, "P&G to Unleash Dental Adult-Pet Food," *Wall Street Journal*, December 12, 2002, p. B4.

54. "In-Store Cell Phone Tracking Pits Consumers Against Retailers: Transparency Is Vital if Retailers Want to Build Trust with Customers," adage.com, April 17, 2014; "New Study: Consumers Overwhelmingly Reject In-Store Tracking by Retailers," www.prweb.com, March 27, 2014; A. Farnham, "Retailers Snooping on Holiday Shoppers Raises Privacy Concerns," abcnews.go.com/Business/, December 10, 2013; V. Kopytoff, "Stores Sniff Out Smartphones to Follow Shoppers," *MIT Technology Review*, www.technologyreview.com, November 12, 2013; "How Stores Spy on You," www.consumerreports.org, March 2013; J. O'Donnell and S. Meehan, "Retailers Want to Read Your Mind," *USA Today*, March 2, 2012, pp. 1B+; and C. Duhigg, "How Companies Learn Your Secrets," *New York Times Online*, February 16, 2012.

55. Materials for developing a business plan can be found at Small Business Administration, *The Business Plan Workbook* (Washington, DC, May 17, 2001); and on the Small Business Administration

Web site [www.sba.gov]. In addition, readers may find software such as Business Plan Pro Software, available at [www.businessplanpro.com], useful.

56. C. Bjork, "Zara Owner Lays Ground for Rapid Expansion," *Wall Street Journal,* March 20, 2014, p. B9; C. Moon, "The Secret World of Fast Fashion," www.psmag.com, March 17, 2014; V. Walt, "Meet the Third-Richest Man in the World," *Fortune,* January 14, 2013, pp. 74–79; S. Hansen, "How Zara Grew into the World's Largest Fashion Retailer," *New York Times Online,* November 9, 2012; D. Roman and W. Kemble-Diaz, "Owner of Fast-Fashion Retailer Zara Keeps Up Emerging-Markets Push," *Wall Street Journal,* June 14, 2012, p. B3; Press Releases, "Inditex Achieves Net Sales of 9,709 Million Euros, an Increase of 10 percent," [www.inditex.com], February 22, 2012; C. Bjork, "'Cheap Chic' Apparel Sellers Heat Up U.S. Rivalry on Web," *Wall Street Journal,* September 6, 2011, pp. B1+; A. Kenna, "Zara Plays Catch-up With Online Shoppers," *Bloomberg BusinessWeek,* August 29–September 4, 2011, pp. 24–25; K. Girotra and S. Netessine, "How to Build Risk into Your Business Model," *Harvard Business Review,* May 2011, pp. 100–105; M. Dart and R. Lewis, "Break the Rules the Way Zappos and Amazon Do," *Bloomberg BusinessWeek Online,* April 29, 2011; K. Cappell, "Zara Thrives by Breaking All the Rules," *BusinessWeek,* October 20, 2008, p. 66; and C. Rohwedder and K. Johnson, "Pace-Setting Zara Seeks More Speed to Fight Its Rising Cheap-Chic Rivals," *Wall Street Journal,* February 20, 2008, pp. B1+.

57. E. Steel, "Netflix, Growing, Envisions Expansion Abroad," *New York Times Online,* July 21, 2014; K. Opam, "The Streaming Service Cuts Deals While Net Neutrality Hangs in the Balance," www.theverge.com, April 28, 2014; D. Carr and R. Somaiya, "Punching Above Its Weight, Upstart Netflix Pokes at HBO," *New York Times Online,* February 16, 2014; J. Kell and A. Sharma, "Netflix Subscriber Ranks Grow," *Wall Street Journal,* January 23, 2014, p. B4; C. Edwards, A. Pringle, and N. Summers, "The Battle Over Netflix," *Bloomberg BusinessWeek,* November 11–17, 2013, pp. 49–50; B. Stelter, "Netflix Hits Milestone and Raises Its Sights," *New York Times Online,* October 24, 2013; D. Reisinger, "Dark Days Ahead for Netflix?" *Fortune.com,* July 12, 2012; S. Woo and I. Sherr, "Netflix's Growth Disappoints," *Wall Street Journal,* April 24, 2012, pp. B1+; S. Woo and I. Sherr, "Netflix Recovers Subscribers," *Wall Street Journal,* January 26, 2012, pp. B1+; **J. Pepitone, "Netflix CEO: We Got Overconfident," *CNNMoney.com,* December 6, 2011**; D. McDonald, "Netflix: Down, But Not Out," *CNN.com,* November 23, 2011; H. W. Jenkins, Jr., "Netflix Isn't Doomed," *Wall Street Journal,* October 26, 2011, p. A13; C. Edwards, "Netflix Drops Most Since 2004 After Losing 800,000 Customers," *BusinessWeek.com,* October 25, 2011; N. Wingfield and B. Stelter, "How Netflix Lost 800,000 Members and Good Will," *New York Times Online,* October 24, 2011; C. Edwards and R. Grover, "Can Netflix Regain Lost Ground," *BusinessWeek.com,* October 19, 2011; and R. Grover, C. Edwards, and A. Fixmer, "Can Netflix Find Its Future by Abandoning the Past?" *Bloomberg BusinessWeek,* September 26–October 2, 2011, pp. 29–30.

Management Practice: Part 3

Management Practice

A Manager's Dilemma

Habitat for Humanity is a nonprofit, ecumenical Christian housing ministry dedicated to building affordable housing for individuals dealing with poverty or homelessness. Habitat's approach is simple. Families in need of decent housing apply to a local Habitat affiliate. Homeowners are chosen based on their level of need, their willingness to become partners in the program, and their ability to repay the loan. And that's the unique thing about Habitat's approach. It's not a giveaway program. Families chosen to become homeowners have to make a down payment and monthly mortgage payments, and invest hundreds of hours of their own labor into building their Habitat home. And they have to commit to helping build other Habitat houses. Habitat volunteers (maybe you've been involved on a Habitat build) provide labor and donations of money and materials as well.

Social service organizations often struggle financially to provide services that are never enough to meet the overwhelming need. Habitat for Humanity, however, was given an enormous financial commitment—$100 million—from an individual who had worked with Habitat and seen the gift it offers to families in poverty. That amount of money means that Habitat can have a huge impact now and in the future. But the management team wants to use the gift wisely—a definite planning, strategy, and control challenge.

Pretend you're part of that management team. Using what you've learned about planning and strategic management, what five things would you suggest the team focus on? Think carefully about your suggestions to the team.

Global Sense

Manufacturers have spent years building low-cost global supply chains. However, when those businesses are dependent on a global supply chain, any unplanned disruptions (political, economic, weather, natural disaster, etc.) can wreak havoc on plans, schedules, and budgets. The Icelandic Eyjafjallajokull volcano in 2010 and the Japanese earthquake/tsunami and Thailand flooding in 2011 are still fresh in the minds of logistics, transportation, and operations managers around the globe. Although unexpected problems in the supply chain have always existed, now the far-reaching impact of something happening not in your own facility but thousands of miles away has created additional volatility and risk for managers and organizations. For instance, when the Icelandic volcano erupted, large portions of European airspace were shut down for more than a week, which affected air traffic worldwide. At BMW's plant in Spartanburg, South Carolina, air shipments of car components were delayed and workers' hours had to be scaled back and plans made for a possible shutdown of the entire facility. During the Thailand floods in late 2011, industrial parks that manufactured semiconductors for companies like Apple and Samsung were underwater and crawling with crocodiles. After the 2011 Japanese earthquake and tsunami shut down dozens of contractors and subcontractors that supply many parts to the auto and technology industries, companies like Toyota, Honda, and Hewlett-Packard had to adjust to critical parts shortages.

Discuss the following questions in light of what you learned in Part 3:

- *You see the challenges associated with a global supply chain; what are some of the benefits of it? What can managers do to minimize the impact of such disruptions?*
- *What types of plans would be best in these unplanned events?*
- *How can managers plan effectively in dynamic environments?*
- *Could SWOT analysis be useful in these instances? Explain.*
- *How might managers use scenario planning in preparing for such disasters?*

Sources: R. Teijken, "Local Issues in Global Supply Chains," Logistics & Transport Focus, April 2012, pp. 41–43; J. Beer, "Sighted: The Ends of the Earth," Canadian Business, Winter 2011/2012, pp. 19–22; B. Powell, "When Supply Chains Break," Fortune, December 26, 2011, pp. 29–32; A. H. Merrill, R. E. Scale, and M. D. Sullivan, "Post-Natural Disaster Appraisal and Valuation: Lessons from the Japan Experience," The Secured Lender, November/December 2011, pp. 30–33; J. Rice, "Alternate Supply," Industrial Engineer, May 2011, p. 10; and "Risk Management: An Increasingly Small World," Reactions, April 2011, p. 252.

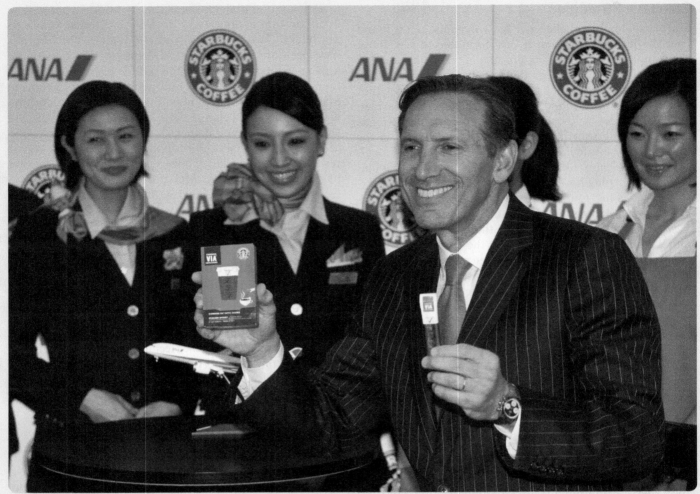

Starbucks CEO Howard Schultz introduced the company's innovative VIA Ready Brew instant coffee during a product launch ceremony with personnel of Japan's All Nippon Airways. VIA is a product innovation available not only in Starbucks stores but also in global distribution channels including airlines, grocery stores, and e-commerce. Developing innovations like VIA helps Starbucks achieve its financial goals and its goal of maintaining its standing as one of the most recognized brands in the world.

Source: Yoshikazu TSUNO/Newscom

Continuing Case

Starbucks—Planning

All managers plan. The planning they do may be extensive or it may be limited. It might be for the next week or month or it might be for the next couple of years. It might cover a work group or it might cover an entire division or the entire organization. No matter what type or extent of planning a manager does, the important thing is that planning takes place. Without planning, there would be nothing for managers to organize, lead, or control.

Based on Starbucks' numerous achievements, there's no doubt that managers have done their planning. Let's take a look.

Company Goals

At the end of 2013, Starbucks had over 19,000 stores in more than 62 countries. The company's goal for 2014–15 is 1,500 net new stores (new stores opened minus existing stores closed). Starbucks' financial goals include revenue growth of 10 percent to 13 percent and earnings per share growth of 15 percent to 20 percent. In addition to the quantitative/fiscal goals, Starbucks focuses on continuing to develop new coffee/tea/juice/bakery products in multiple forms and staying true to its global social responsibilities. Starbucks' ambition is to rank among the world's most admired brands and enduring companies through its "laser focus on disciplined execution and robust innovation" and to maintain Starbucks' standing as one of the most recognized brands in the world.

Company Strategies

Starbucks has been called the most dynamic retail brand over the last two decades. It has been able to rise above the commodity nature of its product and become a global brand leader by reinventing the coffee experience. Over 60 million times a week, a customer receives a product (hot drink, chilled drink, food, etc.) from a Starbucks partner. It's a reflection of the success that Howard Schultz has had in creating something that never really existed in the United States—café life. And in so doing, he created a cultural phenomenon. Starbucks is changing what we eat and drink. It's shaping how we spend our time and money.

Starbucks has found a way to appeal to practically every customer demographic, as its customers cover a broad base. It's not just the affluent or the urban professionals and it's not just the intellectuals or the creative types who frequent Starbucks. You'll find soccer moms, construction workers, bank tellers, and office assistants at Starbucks. And despite the high price of its products, customers pay it because they think it's worth it. What they get for that price is some of the finest coffee available commercially, custom preparation, and, of course, that Starbucks ambiance—the comfy chairs, the music, the aromas, the hissing steam from the espresso machine—all invoking that warm feeling of community and connection that Schultz experienced on his first business trip to Italy and knew instinctively could work elsewhere.

As the world's number one specialty coffee retailer, Starbucks' portfolio includes goods and services under its flagship Starbucks brand and the Teavana, Tazo, Seattle's Best Coffee, Starbucks VIA, Starbucks Refreshers, Evolution Fresh, La Boulange, and Verismo brands. Recent product introductions include a Hazelnut Macchiato, a single-origin coffee from Ethiopia, and a Starbucks Reserve® coffee from Colombia.

Here's something you might be surprised at. You can expect to get carded at your neighborhood Starbucks soon. What? Starbucks is making a more intentional move into wine and beer sales. The company tested the concept at a single Seattle store in 2010 and now offers alcohol at 26 locations, where store sales have shown a significant increase during the time of day when alcohol is offered. The "Starbucks' Evenings" concept offers selected adult beverages (beer and wine...tailored to regional taste preferences) and an expanded food menu after 4 P.M. So, the plan is to roll out Starbucks' Evenings to thousands of stores over the next several years.

Starbucks' loyalty program continues to distinguish it from competitors. Its My Starbucks Rewards™ has almost 7 million active members with more than $4 billion loaded onto the cards. And the company has made a huge investment in mobile payments, accounting for more than 4 million transactions every week in the United States. Its Starbucks Card apps for Android phones and iPhones have been hugely popular. The company also announced a partnership with Square, the mobile payments start-up. Square processes all credit and debit card transactions at Starbucks stores in the United States. Eventually, customers will be able to charge their order to their credit card simply by saying their names.

Starbucks' primary competition comes from quick-service restaurants and specialty coffee shops. McDonalds, for one, has invested heavily in its McCafé concept, which offers coffee, real fruit smoothies, shakes, and frappés. And there are numerous specialty coffee shops, but most of these tend to be in local markets only.

Discussion Questions

1. Make a list of Starbucks' goals. Describe what type of goal each is. Then, describe how that stated goal might affect how the following employees do their job: (a) a part-time store employee—a barista—in Omaha; (b) a quality assurance technician at the company's roasting plant in Amsterdam; (c) a regional sales manager; (d) the executive vice president of global supply chain operations; and (e) the CEO.
2. Discuss the types of growth strategies that Starbucks has used. Be specific.
3. What competitive advantages do you think Starbucks has? What will it have to do to maintain those advantages?
4. Do you think the Starbucks brand can become too saturated—that is, extended to too many different products? Why or why not?
5. What companies might be good benchmarks for Starbucks? Why? What companies might want to benchmark Starbucks? Why?
6. Describe how the following Starbucks managers might use forecasting, budgeting, and scheduling (be specific): (a) a retail store manager; (b) a regional marketing manager; (c) the manager for global development; and (d) the CEO.
7. Describe Howard Schultz as a strategic leader.
8. Is Starbucks "living" its mission? (You can find the company mission on its Web site at www.starbucks.com.) Discuss.
9. What ethical and social responsibility issues can you see with Starbucks' decision to sell alcohol after 4 P.M.? Think in terms of the various stakeholders and how those stakeholders might respond to this strategy?

Notes for the Continuing Case

Information from Starbucks Corporation 2013 Annual Report, www.investor.starbucks.com, May 2014; R. Dooley, "Will Starbucks Alcohol 'Infect' Other Products?" www.forbes.com, April 9, 2014; V. Wong, "What to Expect from Starbucks' New Booze Menu," www.businessweek.com, March 20, 2014; C. Cain Miller, "Starbucks and Square to Team Up," *New York Times Online,* August 8, 2012; R. Ahmed, "Tata Setting Up Starbucks Coffee Roasting Facility," www.online.wsj.com, July 26, 2012; B. Horovitz, "Starbucks Rolling Out Pop with Pep," *USA Today,* March 22, 2012, p. 1B; Starbucks News Release, "Starbucks Spotlights Connection Between Record Performance, Shareholder Value, and Company Values at Annual Meeting of Shareholders," news.starbucks.com, March 21, 2012; D. A. Kaplan, "Strong Coffee," *Fortune,* December 12, 2011, pp. 100–116; J. A. Cooke, Editor, "From Bean to Cup: How Starbucks Transformed Its Supply Chain," www.supplychainquarterly.com, Quarter 4, 2010; R. Ruggless, "Starbucks Exec: Security from Employee Theft Important When Implementing Gift Card Strategies," *Nation's Restaurant News,* December 12, 2005, p. 24; and R. Ruggless, "Transaction Monitoring Boosts Safety, Perks Up Coffee Chain Profits," *Nation's Restaurant News,* November 28, 2005, p. 35.

Designing Organizational Structure—Basic Designs

From Chapter 10 of *Management*, Thirteenth Edition. Stephen P. Robbins and Mary Coulter. Copyright © 2016 by Pearson Education, Inc. All rights reserved.

It's Your Career

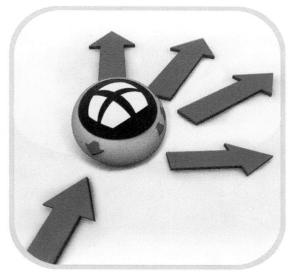

A key to success in management and in your career is knowing how to delegate work tasks to others.

You Can't Do It All: The Importance of Delegating

One of the most difficult tasks for individuals in their first management or team leadership position is accepting that they can't do everything. There are not enough hours in a day or days in a week to compensate for not delegating to others. Even if you're able to do a better job than any of those people reporting to you, the reality is that you have to give up some control and assign the authority and responsibility for work to others. Here's what you need to know to successfully delegate:

1. **Clarify the assignment.** The place to begin is determining what is to be delegated and to whom. Identify the person that's most capable of doing the task and if they're able and willing. Then, ideally, you should delegate only the end result—what is to be accomplished—and let your employee choose the means.

2. **Specify the employee's range of discretion.** Every situation of delegation comes with constraints. When you delegate to an employee, you're delegating the authority to act on certain issues and within certain parameters pertaining to those issues. Specify how far the person can go without checking further with you.

3. **Allow the employee to participate.** Individual motivation and accountability increase when you allow employees to participate in determining what is delegated, how much authority is needed to get the job done, and the standard by which they'll be judged.

4. **Inform others that delegation has occurred.** Delegation shouldn't take place behind the scenes. Anyone who might be affected by what's being delegated also needs to know what has been delegated and how much authority has been granted.

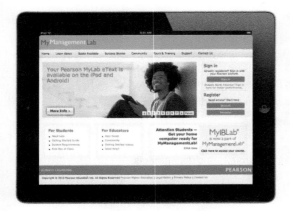

MyManagementLab®

⭐ Improve Your Grade!

When you see this icon, visit **www.mymanagementlab.com** for activities that are applied, personalized, and offer immediate feedback.

Learning Objectives

1 **Describe** *six key elements in organizational design.*

• **Know how** to delegate work to others and develop your skill at delegating.

2 **Contrast** *mechanistic and organic structures.*

3 **Discuss** *the contingency factors that favor either the mechanistic model or the organic model of organizational design.*

4 **Describe** *traditional organizational designs.*

---

*5. **Establish feedback controls to monitor progress.** Delegating without establishing feedback controls is inviting problems. Establishing feedback controls increases the likelihood that important problems will be identified early and that the task will be completed on time and to the desired specifications. Agree on a specific time for the completion of the task and then set progress dates when the employee will report back on how well he or she is doing and any major problems that may have come up. In addition, you can periodically check to ensure that authority guidelines aren't being*

abused, organizational policies are being followed, proper procedures are being met, and the like.

*6. **Recognize key performance milestones and accomplishments.** When an individual who has been delegated a task successfully completes that task, take the time to recognize his or her performance. A simple "thank you" or some other type of recognition can go a long way in reinforcing to your employees that you appreciate their efforts when you delegate tasks to them. And, it reinforces that you must have done a pretty good job at delegating!*

Welcome to the fascinating world of organizational structure and design. In this text, we present the basics of organizing. We define the key organizing concepts and their components and how managers use these to create a structured environment in which organizational members can do their work efficiently and effectively. Once the organization's goals, plans, and strategies are in place, managers must develop a structure that will best facilitate the attainment of those goals.

DESIGNING Organizational Structure

LO1   A short distance south of McAlester, Oklahoma, employees in a vast factory complex make products that must be perfect. These people "are so good at what they do and have been doing it for so long that they have a

Exhibit 1
Purposes of Organizing

- Divides work to be done into specific jobs and departments.
- Assigns tasks and responsibilities associated with individual jobs.
- Coordinates diverse organizational tasks.
- Clusters jobs into units.
- Establishes relationships among individuals, groups, and departments.
- Establishes formal lines of authority.
- Allocates and deploys organizational resources.

organizing
Management function that involves arranging and structuring work to accomplish the organization's goals

organizational structure
The formal arrangement of jobs within an organization

organizational chart
The visual representation of an organization's structure

organizational design
Creating or changing an organization's structure

work specialization
Dividing work activities into separate job tasks

100 percent market share."[1] They make bombs for the U.S. military and doing so requires a work environment that's an interesting mix of the mundane, structured, and disciplined, coupled with high levels of risk and emotion. The work gets done efficiently and effectively here. Work also gets done efficiently and effectively at Cisco Systems, although not in such a structured and formal way. At Cisco, some 70 percent of the employees work from home at least 20 percent of the time.[2] Both of these organizations get needed work done, although each does so using a different structure.

Few topics in management have undergone as much change in the past few years as that of organizing and organizational structure. Managers are reevaluating traditional approaches to find new structural designs that best support and facilitate employees' doing the organization's work—designs that can achieve efficiency but are also flexible.[3]

The basic concepts of organization design formulated by early management writers, such as Henri Fayol and Max Weber, offered structural principles for managers to follow. Over 90 years have passed since many of those principles were originally proposed. Given that length of time and all the changes that have taken place, you'd think that those principles would be pretty worthless today. Surprisingly, they're not. For the most part, they still provide valuable insights into designing effective and efficient organizations. Of course, we've also gained a great deal of knowledge over the years as to their limitations.

We define **organizing** as arranging and structuring work to accomplish organizational goals. It's an important process during which managers design an organization's structure. **Organizational structure** is the formal arrangement of jobs within an organization. This structure, which can be shown visually in an **organizational chart**, also serves many purposes. (See Exhibit 1.) When managers create or change the structure, they're engaged in **organizational design**, a process that involves decisions about six key elements: work specialization, departmentalization, chain of command, span of control, centralization and decentralization, and formalization.[4]

Work Specialization

At the Wilson Sporting Goods factory in Ada, Ohio, 150 workers (with an average work tenure exceeding 20 years) make every football used in the National Football League and most of those used in college and high school football games. To meet daily output goals, the workers specialize in job tasks such as molding, stitching and sewing, lacing, and so forth.[5] This is an example of **work specialization**, which is dividing work activities into separate job tasks. Individual employees "specialize" in doing part of an activity rather than the entire activity in order to increase work

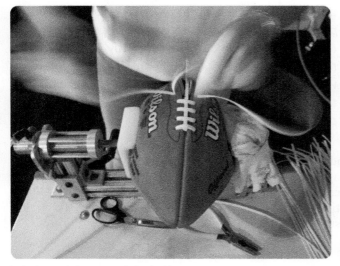

Lacing is one of 13 separate tasks involved in hand-crafting a Wilson Sporting Goods football. The company uses work specialization in dividing job activities as an organizing mechanism that helps employees boost their productivity and makes efficient use of workers' diverse skills.
Source: Jeff Haynes/AFP/Getty Images/Newscom

output. It's also known as division of labor, a concept we introduced in the management history module.

Work specialization makes efficient use of the diversity of skills that workers have. In most organizations, some tasks require highly developed skills; others can be performed by employees with lower skill levels. If all workers were engaged in all the steps of, say, a manufacturing process, all would need the skills necessary to perform both the most demanding and the least demanding jobs. Thus, except when performing the most highly skilled or highly sophisticated tasks, employees would be working below their skill levels. In addition, skilled workers are paid more than unskilled workers, and, because wages tend to reflect the highest level of skill, all workers would be paid at highly skilled rates to do easy tasks—an inefficient use of resources. This concept explains why you rarely find a cardiac surgeon closing up a patient after surgery. Instead, doctors doing their residencies in open-heart surgery and learning the skill usually stitch and staple the patient after the surgeon has finished the surgery.

Early proponents of work specialization believed it could lead to great increases in productivity. At the beginning of the twentieth century, that generalization was reasonable. Because specialization was not widely practiced, its introduction almost always generated higher productivity. But, as Exhibit 2 illustrates, a good thing can be carried too far. At some point, the human diseconomies from division of labor—boredom, fatigue, stress, low productivity, poor quality, increased absenteeism, and high turnover—exceed the economic advantages.[6]

TODAY'S VIEW Most managers today continue to see work specialization as important because it helps employees be more efficient. For example, McDonald's uses high work specialization to get its products made and delivered to customers efficiently and quickly—that's why it's called "fast" food. One person takes orders at the drive-through window, others cook and assemble the hamburgers, another works the fryer, another gets the drinks, another bags orders, and so forth. Such single-minded focus on maximizing efficiency has contributed to increasing productivity. In fact, at many McDonald's, you'll see a clock that times how long it takes employees to fill the order; look closer and you'll probably see posted somewhere an order fulfillment time goal. At some point, however, work specialization

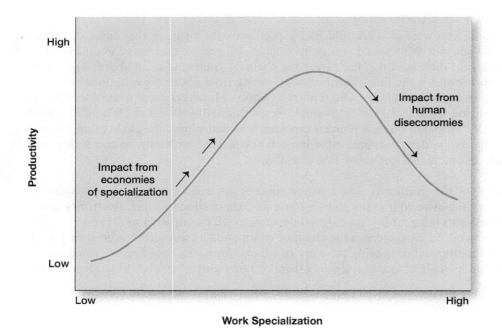

Exhibit 2
Economies and Diseconomies of Work Specialization

no longer leads to productivity. That's why companies such as Avery-Dennison, Ford Australia, Hallmark, and American Express use minimal work specialization and instead give employees a broad range of tasks to do.

Departmentalization

departmentalization
The basis by which jobs are grouped together

Does your college have a department of student services or financial aid department? Are you taking this course through a management department? After deciding what job tasks will be done by whom, common work activities need to be grouped back together so work gets done in a coordinated and integrated way. How jobs are grouped together is called **departmentalization**. Five common forms of departmentalization are used, although an organization may develop its own unique classification. (For instance, a hotel might have departments such as front desk operations, sales and catering, housekeeping and laundry, and maintenance.) Exhibit 3 illustrates each type of departmentalization as well as the advantages and disadvantages of each.

TODAY'S VIEW   Most large organizations continue to use combinations of most or all of these types of departmentalization. For example, a major Japanese electronics firm organizes its divisions along functional lines, its manufacturing units around processes, its sales units around seven geographic regions, and its sales regions into four customer groupings. Black & Decker organizes its divisions along functional lines, its manufacturing units around processes, its sales around geographic regions, and its sales regions around customer groupings.

One popular departmentalization trend is the increasing use of customer departmentalization. Because getting and keeping customers is essential for success, this approach works well because it emphasizes monitoring and responding to changes in customers' needs. Another popular trend is the use of teams, especially as work tasks have become more complex and diverse skills are needed to accomplish those tasks. One specific type of team that more organizations are using is a **cross-functional team**, a work team composed of individuals from various functional specialties. For instance, at Ford's material planning and logistics division, a cross-functional team of employees from the company's finance, purchasing, engineering, and quality control areas, along with representatives from outside logistics suppliers, has developed several work improvement ideas.[7]

cross-functional team
A work team composed of individuals from various functional specialties

Chain of Command

chain of command
The line of authority extending from upper organizational levels to the lowest levels, which clarifies who reports to whom

Suppose you were at work and had a problem with an issue that came up. What would you do? Who would you go to to help you resolve that issue? People need to know who their boss is. That's what the chain of command is all about. The **chain of command** is the line of authority extending from upper organizational levels to lower levels, which clarifies who reports to whom. Managers need to consider it when organizing work because it helps employees with questions such as "Who do I report to?" or "Who do I go to if I have a problem?" To understand the chain of command, you have to understand three other important concepts: authority, responsibility, and unity of command. Let's look first at authority.

authority
The rights inherent in a managerial position to tell people what to do and to expect them to do it

AUTHORITY   Authority was a major concept discussed by the early management writers; they viewed it as the glue that held an organization together. **Authority** refers to the rights inherent in a managerial position to tell people what to do and to expect them to do it.[8] Managers in the chain of command had authority to do their job of coordinating and overseeing the work of others. Authority could be delegated downward to lower-level managers, giving them certain rights while also prescribing certain

FUNCTIONAL DEPARTMENTALIZATION—Groups Jobs According to Function

Exhibit 3
The Five Common Forms
of Departmentalization

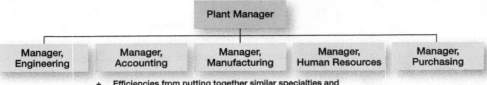

```
                        Plant Manager

Manager,      Manager,      Manager,        Manager,         Manager,
Engineering   Accounting    Manufacturing   Human Resources  Purchasing
```

+ Efficiencies from putting together similar specialties and
  people with common skills, knowledge, and orientations
+ Coordination within functional area
+ In-depth specialization
– Poor communication across functional areas
– Limited view of organizational goals

GEOGRAPHICAL DEPARTMENTALIZATION—Groups Jobs According to Geographic Region

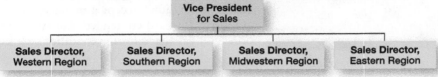

```
                     Vice President
                       for Sales

Sales Director,   Sales Director,   Sales Director,     Sales Director,
Western Region    Southern Region   Midwestern Region   Eastern Region
```

+ More effective and efficient handling of specific regional
  issues that arise
+ Serve needs of unique geographic markets better
– Duplication of functions
– Can feel isolated from other organizational areas

PRODUCT DEPARTMENTALIZATION—Groups Jobs by Product Line

Source: Bombardier Annual Report.

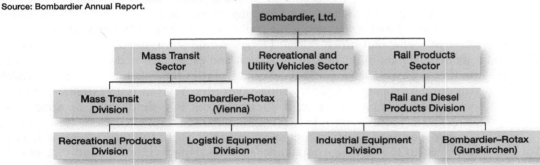

```
                        Bombardier, Ltd.

        Mass Transit      Recreational and      Rail Products
          Sector          Utility Vehicles Sector    Sector

    Mass Transit    Bombardier–Rotax          Rail and Diesel
      Division         (Vienna)              Products Division

Recreational Products  Logistic Equipment   Industrial Equipment   Bombardier–Rotax
      Division            Division               Division          (Gunskirchen)
```

+ Allows specialization in particular products and services
+ Managers can become experts in their industry
+ Closer to customers
– Duplication of functions
– Limited view of organizational goals

PROCESS DEPARTMENTALIZATION—Groups Jobs on the Basis of Product or Customer Flow

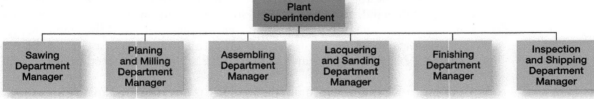

```
                            Plant
                        Superintendent

Sawing        Planing       Assembling    Lacquering     Finishing     Inspection
Department    and Milling   Department    and Sanding    Department    and Shipping
Manager       Department    Manager       Department     Manager       Department
              Manager                     Manager                      Manager
```

+ More efficient flow of work activities
– Can only be used with certain types of products

CUSTOMER DEPARTMENTALIZATION—Groups Jobs on the Basis of Specific and Unique Customers Who Have Common Needs

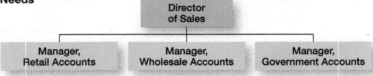

```
                     Director
                     of Sales

Manager,           Manager,             Manager,
Retail Accounts    Wholesale Accounts   Government Accounts
```

+ Customers' needs and problems can be met by specialists
– Duplication of functions
– Limited view of organizational goals

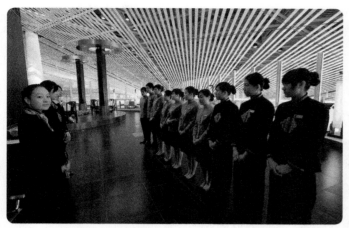

Managers of a restaurant at the Beijing Airport have the authority to give waiters and waitresses instructions for their work day. Such authority is an inherent right in a manager's position to tell people what to do and to expect them to do it. Authority is part of the chain of command that extends from higher organizational levels to lower levels and clarifies who reports to whom.
Source: Lou Linwei/Alamy

acceptance theory of authority
The view that authority comes from the willingness of subordinates to accept it

line authority
Authority that entitles a manager to direct the work of an employee

staff authority
Positions with some authority that have been created to support, assist, and advise those holding line authority

limits within which to operate. These writers emphasized that authority was related to one's position within an organization and had nothing to do with the personal characteristics of an individual manager. They assumed that the rights and power inherent in one's formal organizational position were the sole source of influence and that if an order was given, it would be obeyed.

Another early management writer, Chester Barnard, proposed another perspective on authority. This view, the **acceptance theory of authority**, says that authority comes from the willingness of subordinates to accept it.[9] If an employee didn't accept a manager's order, there was no authority. Barnard contended that subordinates *will* accept orders only if the following conditions are satisfied:

1. They understand the order.
2. They feel the order is consistent with the organization's purpose.
3. The order does not conflict with their personal beliefs.
4. They are able to perform the task as directed.

Barnard's view of authority seems to make sense, especially when it comes to an employee's ability to do what he or she is told to do. For instance, if my manager (my department chair) came into my classroom and told me to do open-heart surgery on one of my students, the traditional view of authority said that I would have to follow that order. Barnard's view would say, instead, that I would talk to my manager about my lack of education and experience to do what he's asked me to do and persuade him that it's probably not in the best interests of the student (or our department) for me to follow that order. Yes, this is an extreme and highly unrealistic example. However, it does point out that simply viewing a manager's authority as total control over what an employee does or doesn't do is unrealistic also—except in certain circumstances, such as the military, where soldiers are expected to follow their commander's orders. However, understand that Barnard believed most employees would do what their managers asked them to do if they were able to do so.

The early management writers also distinguished between two forms of authority: line authority and staff authority. **Line authority** entitles a manager to direct the work of an employee. It is the employer–employee authority relationship that extends from the top of the organization to the lowest echelon, according to the chain of command, as shown in Exhibit 4. As a link in the chain of command, a manager with line authority has the right to direct the work of employees and to make certain decisions without consulting anyone. Of course, in the chain of command, every manager is also subject to the authority or direction of his or her superior.

Keep in mind that sometimes the term *line* is used to differentiate line managers from staff managers. In this context, *line* refers to managers whose organizational function contributes directly to the achievement of organizational objectives. In a manufacturing firm, line managers are typically in the production and sales functions, whereas managers in human resources and payroll are considered staff managers with staff authority. Whether a manager's function is classified as line or staff depends on the organization's objectives. For example, at Staff Builders, a supplier of temporary employees, interviewers have a line function. Similarly, at the payroll firm of ADP, payroll is a line function.

As organizations get larger and more complex, line managers find that they do not have the time, expertise, or resources to get their jobs done effectively. In response, they create **staff authority** functions to support, assist, advise, and generally reduce some of their informational burdens. For instance, a hospital administrator who cannot effectively handle the purchasing of all the supplies

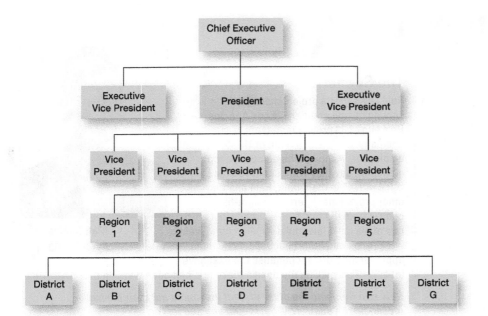

Exhibit 4
Chain of Command and
Line Authority

the hospital needs creates a purchasing department, which is a staff function. Of course, the head of the purchasing department has line authority over the purchasing agents who work for him. The hospital administrator might also find that she is overburdened and needs an assistant, a position that would be classified as a staff position. Exhibit 5 illustrates line and staff authority.

RESPONSIBILITY   When managers use their authority to assign work to employees, those employees take on an obligation to perform those assigned duties. This obligation or expectation to perform is known as **responsibility**. And employees should be held accountable for their performance! Assigning work authority without responsibility and accountability can create opportunities for abuse. Likewise, no one should be held responsible or accountable for work tasks over which he or she has no authority to complete those tasks.

responsibility
The obligation or expectation to perform any assigned duties

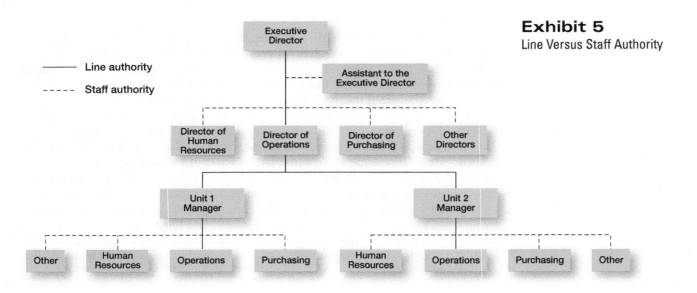

Exhibit 5
Line Versus Staff Authority

let's get REAL

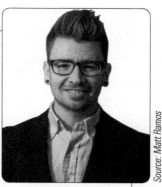

Matt Ramos
Director of Marketing

Source: Matt Ramos

The Scenario:

Reid Lawson is a project manager for a lighting design company in Los Angeles. He's one of 30 project managers in the company, each with a team of 10–15 employees. Although the company's top managers say they want employees to be "innovative" in their work, Reid and the other project managers face tight-fisted control from the top. Reid's already lost two of his most talented designers (who went to work for a competitor) because he couldn't get approval for a project because the executive team kept nit-picking the design these two had been working on.

How can Reid and the other project managers get their bosses to loosen up the control? What would you suggest?

Losing top notch talent is bad. Losing top notch talent to a direct competitor is killer, especially when it's avoidable. Reid's first step should be an honest meeting with his boss. The evidence is fairly clear that something needs to change, so it should be a simple conversation to get the ball rolling. If that doesn't produce results, he should turn to HR and recruiting as his biggest advocate. They almost always have the ear of the executive team. With their help, this is a very resolvable situation.

unity of command
The management principle that each person should report to only one manager

UNITY OF COMMAND Finally, the **unity of command** principle (one of Fayol's 14 management principles) states that a person should report to only one manager. Without unity of command, conflicting demands from multiple bosses may create problems as it did for Damian Birkel, a merchandising manager in the Fuller Brands division of CPAC, Inc. He found himself reporting to two bosses—one in charge of the department-store business and the other in charge of discount chains. Birkel tried to minimize the conflict by making a combined to-do list that he would update and change as work tasks changed.[10]

TODAY'S VIEW Although early management theorists (Fayol, Weber, Taylor, Barnard, and others) believed that chain of command, authority (line and staff), responsibility, and unity of command were essential, times have changed.[11] Those elements are far less important today. For example, at the Michelin plant in Tours, France, managers have replaced the top-down chain of command with "birdhouse" meetings, in which employees meet for five minutes at regular intervals throughout the day at a column on the shop floor and study simple tables and charts to identify production bottlenecks. Instead of being bosses, shop managers are enablers.[12] Information technology also has made such concepts less relevant today. Employees can access information that used to be available only to managers in a matter of a few seconds. It also means that employees can communicate with anyone else in the organization without going through the chain of command. Also, many employees, especially in organizations where work revolves around projects, find themselves reporting to more than one boss, thus violating the unity-of-command principle. However, such arrangements can and do work if communication, conflict, and other issues are managed well by all involved parties.

Span of Control

How many employees can a manager efficiently and effectively manage? That's what **span of control** is all about. The traditional view was that managers could not—and should not—directly supervise more than five or six subordinates. Determining the span of control is important because to a large degree, it determines the number of levels and managers in an organization—an important consideration in how efficient an organization will be. All other things being equal, the wider or larger the span, the more efficient the organization. Here's why.

Assume two organizations both have approximately 4,100 employees. As Exhibit 6 shows, if one organization has a span of four and the other a span of eight, the organization with the wider span will have two fewer levels and approximately 800 fewer managers. At an average manager's salary of $42,000 a year, the organization with the wider span would save over $33 million a year! Obviously, wider spans are more efficient in terms of cost. However, at some point, wider spans may reduce effectiveness if employee performance worsens because managers no longer have the time to lead effectively.

TODAY'S VIEW The contemporary view of span of control recognizes there is no magic number. Many factors influence the number of employees a manager can efficiently and effectively manage. These factors include the skills and abilities of the manager and the employees and the characteristics of the work being done. For instance, managers with well-trained and experienced employees can function well with a wider span. Other contingency variables that determine the appropriate span include similarity and complexity of employee tasks, the physical proximity of subordinates, the degree to which standardized procedures are in place, the sophistication of the organization's information system, the strength of the organization's culture, and the preferred style of the manager.[14]

The trend in recent years has been toward larger spans of control, which is consistent with managers' efforts to speed up decision making, increase flexibility, get closer to customers, empower employees, and reduce costs. Managers are beginning to recognize that they can handle a wider span when employees know their jobs well and when those employees understand organizational processes. For instance, at PepsiCo's Gamesa cookie plant in Mexico, 56 employees now report to each manager. However, to ensure that performance doesn't suffer because of these wider spans, employees were thoroughly briefed on company goals and processes. Also, new pay systems reward quality, service, productivity, and teamwork.[15]

Centralization and Decentralization

One of the questions that needs to be answered when organizing is "At what organizational level are decisions made?" **Centralization** is the degree to which decision making takes place at upper levels of the organization. If top managers make key

span of control
The number of employees a manager can efficiently and effectively manage

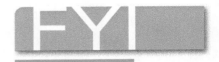

- 80 percent—the percentage of a company's workforce that typical frontline managers directly supervise.[13]

centralization
The degree to which decision making is concentrated at upper levels of the organization

Exhibit 6
Contrasting Spans of Control

Organizational Level	Members at Each Level	
	Assuming Span of 4	Assuming Span of 8
1 (Highest)	1	1
2	4	8
3	16	64
4	64	512
5	256	4,096
6	1,024	
7 (Lowest)	4,096	

Span of 4:
Employees: = 4,096
Managers (level 1–6) = 1,365

Span of 8:
Employees: = 4,096
Managers (level 1–4) = 585

decentralization
The degree to which lower-level employees provide input or actually make decisions

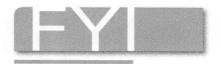

employee empowerment
Giving employees more authority (power) to make decisions

decisions with little input from below, then the organization is more centralized. On the other hand, the more that lower-level employees provide input or actually make decisions, the more **decentralization** there is. Keep in mind that centralization-decentralization is not an either-or concept. The decision is relative, not absolute—that is, an organization is never completely centralized or decentralized.

Early management writers proposed that the degree of centralization in an organization depended on the situation.[16] Their goal was the optimum and efficient use of employees. Traditional organizations were structured in a pyramid, with power and authority concentrated near the top of the organization. Given this structure, historically, centralized decisions were the most prominent, but organizations today have become more complex and responsive to dynamic changes in their environments. As such, many managers believe decisions need to be made by those individuals closest to the problems, regardless of their organizational level. In fact, the trend over the past several decades—at least in U.S. and Canadian organizations—has been a movement toward more decentralization in organizations.[17] Exhibit 7 lists some of the factors that affect an organization's use of centralization or decentralization.[18]

TODAY'S VIEW Today, managers often choose the amount of centralization or decentralization that will allow them to best implement their decisions and achieve organizational goals.[20] What works in one organization, however, won't necessarily work in another, so managers must determine the appropriate amount of decentralization for each organization and work units within it.

As organizations have become more flexible and responsive to environmental trends, there's been a distinct shift toward decentralized decision making.[21] This trend, also known as **employee empowerment**, gives employees more authority (power) to make decisions. In large companies especially, lower-level managers are "closer to the action" and typically have more detailed knowledge about problems and how best to solve them than top managers. For instance, at Terex Corporation, CEO Ron Defeo, a big proponent of decentralized management, tells his managers that, "You gotta' run the company you're given." And they have! The company generated revenues of more than $4 billion in 2009 with about 16,000 employees worldwide and a small corporate headquarters staff.[22] Another example can be seen at the General Cable plant in Piedras Negras, Coahuila, Mexico, where employees are responsible for managing nearly 6,000 active raw material SKUs (stock-keeping units) in inventory and on the plant floor. And company managers continue to look for ways to place more responsibility in the hands of workers.[23]

Exhibit 7
Centralization or Decentralization

More Centralization	More Decentralization
• Environment is stable.	• Environment is complex, uncertain.
• Lower-level managers are not as capable or experienced at making decisions as upper-level managers.	• Lower-level managers are capable and experienced at making decisions.
• Lower-level managers do not want a say in decisions.	• Lower-level managers want a voice in decisions.
• Decisions are relatively minor.	• Decisions are significant.
• Organization is facing a crisis or the risk of company failure.	• Corporate culture is open to allowing managers a say in what happens.
• Company is large.	• Company is geographically dispersed.
• Effective implementation of company strategies depends on managers retaining say over what happens.	• Effective implementation of company strategies depends on managers having involvement and flexibility to make decisions.

let's get REAL

The Scenario:

An old saying goes like this: "If you want something done right, do it yourself." But Alicia Nunez, customer service manager at a party imports company in Guadalajara, Mexico, wants to do just the opposite! She wants to delegate tasks to her team of 25 customer service representatives. But she also wants to do it in such a way that her team is still productive and functional.

What can Alicia do to make sure her employee delegation is successful?

There are several steps that will allow you to delegate successfully:

1. *Choose the appropriate employee by interviewing them and consider his/her time, interest, and capabilities.*
2. *Explain to the employee why they were selected for this task.*
3. *Discuss the task being assigned; discuss ideas; mutually set goals and objectives.*
4. *Define clearly the responsibilities being delegated to each employee. The end result is important, not the various steps. Everyone accomplishes tasks differently.*
5. *Give accurate and honest feedback. Employees want and deserve to know how they are doing. This is both an opportunity for giving satisfaction and encouraging growth. Allow for risk-taking and mistakes.*
6. *As a leader, it can be hard for you to let go; but delegating does not eliminate work. As you delegate appropriately, a multiplier effect occurs.*
7. *Follow up. This will also let you know how that individual is progressing on the task.*
8. *Evaluate. One of your most important roles as a leader is to help your employees to learn and grow through both their successes and their failures! Your employees are your greatest resource. Let them create and turn their creativity into action!*

Claudia Gutierrez
Service Manager

Source: Claudia Gutierrez

Delegating Knowledge—If your instructor is using MyManagementLab, log onto **mymanagementlab.com** and test your *delegating knowledge*. **Be sure to refer back to the chapter opener!**

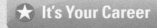 ★ It's Your Career

Formalization

Formalization refers to how standardized an organization's jobs are and the extent to which employee behavior is guided by rules and procedures. In highly formalized organizations, there are explicit job descriptions, numerous organizational rules, and clearly defined procedures covering work processes. Employees have little discretion over what's done, when it's done, and how it's done. However, where there is less formalization, employees have more discretion in how they do their work.

TODAY'S VIEW   Although some formalization is necessary for consistency and control, many organizations today rely less on strict rules and standardization to guide and regulate employee behavior. For instance, consider the following situation:

A customer comes into a branch of a large national drug store and drops off a roll of film for same-day developing 37 minutes after the store policy cut-off time.

formalization
How standardized an organization's jobs are and the extent to which employee behavior is guided by rules and procedures

Although the sales clerk knows he's supposed to follow rules, he also knows he could get the film developed with no problem and wants to accommodate the customer. So he accepts the film, violating policy, hoping that his manager won't find out.[24]

Has this employee done something wrong? He did "break" the rule. But by "breaking" the rule, he actually brought in revenue and provided good customer service.

Considering there are numerous situations where rules may be too restrictive, many organizations have allowed employees some latitude, giving them sufficient autonomy to make those decisions that they feel are best under the circumstances. It doesn't mean throwing out all organizational rules because there *will* be rules that are important for employees to follow—and these rules should be explained so employees understand why it's important to adhere to them. But for other rules, employees may be given some leeway.[25]

MECHANISTIC and Organic Structures

LO2 Stocking extra swimsuits in retail stores near water parks seems to make sense, right? And if size 11 women's shoes have been big sellers in Chicago, then stocking more size 11s seems to be a no-brainer. After suffering through 16 months of declining same-store sales, Macy's CEO Terry Lundgren decided it was time to restructure the organization to make sure these types of smart retail decisions are made.[26] He's making the company both more centralized and more locally focused. Although that may seem a contradiction, the redesign seems to be working. Lundgren centralized Macy's purchasing, planning, and marketing operations from seven regional offices to one office at headquarters in New York. He also replaced regional merchandise managers with more local managers—each responsible for a dozen stores—who spend more time figuring out what's selling. Designing (or redesigning) an organizational structure that works is important. Basic organizational design revolves around two organizational forms, described in Exhibit 8.[27]

mechanistic organization
An organizational design that's rigid and tightly controlled

The **mechanistic organization** (or bureaucracy) was the natural result of combining the six elements of structure. Adhering to the chain-of-command principle ensured the existence of a formal hierarchy of authority, with each person controlled and supervised by one superior. Keeping the span of control small at increasingly higher levels in the organization created tall, impersonal structures. As the distance between the top and the bottom of the organization expanded, top management would increasingly impose rules and regulations. Because top managers couldn't control lower-level activities through direct observation and ensure the use of standard practices, they substituted rules and regulations. The early management writers' belief in a high degree of work specialization created jobs that were simple, routine, and standardized. Further specialization through the use of departmentalization increased impersonality and the need for multiple layers of management to coordinate the specialized departments.[28]

organic organization
An organizational design that's highly adaptive and flexible

The **organic organization** is a highly adaptive form that is as loose and flexible as the mechanistic organization is rigid and stable. Rather than having standardized jobs and regulations, the organic organization's loose structure allows it to change rapidly, as required.[29] It has division of labor, but the jobs people do are

Exhibit 8
Mechanistic Versus Organic Organizations

Mechanistic	Organic
• High specialization	• Cross-functional teams
• Rigid departmentalization	• Cross-hierarchical teams
• Clear chain of command	• Free flow of information
• Narrow spans of control	• Wide spans of control
• Centralization	• Decentralization
• High formalization	• Low formalization

not standardized. Employees tend to be professionals who are technically proficient and trained to handle diverse problems. They need few formal rules and little direct supervision because their training has instilled in them standards of professional conduct. For instance, a petroleum engineer doesn't need to follow specific procedures on how to locate oil sources miles offshore. The engineer can solve most problems alone or after conferring with colleagues. Professional standards guide his or her behavior. The organic organization is low in centralization so that the professional can respond quickly to problems and because top-level managers cannot be expected to possess the expertise to make necessary decisions.

If your professor has assigned this, go to **www.mymanagementlab.com** to watch a video titled: *Elm City Market: Organizational Structure* and to respond to questions.

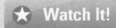 ★ **Watch It!**

CONTINGENCY Factors Affecting Structural Choice

L03 When Carol Bartz took over the CEO position at Yahoo! from co-founder Jerry Yang, she found a company "hobbled by slow decision making and ineffective execution on those decisions."[30] For a company that was once the darling of Web search, Yahoo! seemed to have lost its way, a serious misstep in an industry where change is continual and rapid. Bartz (who is no longer the CEO) implemented a new streamlined structure intended to speed up decision making, which would allow the company to respond more quickly to changing conditions. Marissa Mayer—formerly a top executive at Google—is now Yahoo's CEO, and she has put her own stamp on the organization's structure. Top managers typically put a lot of thought into designing an appropriate organizational structure. What that appropriate structure is depends on four contingency variables: the organization's strategy, size, technology, and degree of environmental uncertainty.

Strategy and Structure

An organization's structure should facilitate goal achievement. Because goals are an important part of the organization's strategies, it's only logical that strategy and structure are closely linked. Alfred Chandler initially researched this relationship.[31] He studied several large U.S. companies and concluded that changes in corporate strategy led to changes in an organization's structure that support the strategy.

Research has shown that certain structural designs work best with different organizational strategies.[32] For instance, the flexibility and free-flowing information of the organic structure works well when an organization is pursuing meaningful and unique innovations. The mechanistic organization with its efficiency, stability, and tight controls works best for companies wanting to tightly control costs.

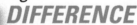

LEADER *making a* DIFFERENCE

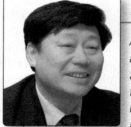

Source: Wang Jun/EyePress EPN/Newscom

As chairman and CEO of Haier Group, Zhang Ruimin runs a successful enterprise with annual revenues of almost $30 billion, and he has turned Haier into one of China's first global brands.[33] Zhang is considered by many to be China's leading corporate executive. When he took over a floundering refrigerator plant in Qingdao, he quickly found out it produced terrible refrigerators. The story goes that he gave the workers sledgehammers and ordered them to destroy every one. His message: Poor quality would no longer be tolerated. Using his business training, Zhang successfully organized Haier for efficient mass production. But here in the twenty-first century, Zhang believes success requires a different competency. So he reorganized the company into self-managed groups, each devoted to a customer or group of similar customers. Zhang gets it! He understands clearly how an organization's design can help it be successful. What can you learn from this leader making a difference?

Size and Structure

There's considerable evidence that an organization's size affects its structure.[34] Large organizations—typically considered to be those with more than 2,000 employees—tend to have more specialization, departmentalization, centralization, and rules and regulations than do small organizations. However, once an organization grows past a certain size, size has less influence on structure. Why? Essentially, once there are around 2,000 employees, it's already fairly mechanistic. Adding another 500 employees won't impact the structure much. On the other hand, adding 500 employees to an organization with only 300 employees is likely to make it more mechanistic.

Technology and Structure

unit production
The production of items in units or small batches

mass production
The production of items in large batches

process production
The production of items in continuous processes

Every organization uses some form of technology to convert its inputs into outputs. For instance, workers at Whirlpool's Manaus, Brazil, facility build microwave ovens and air conditioners on a standardized assembly line. Employees at FedEx Kinko's Office and Print Services produce custom design and print jobs for individual customers. And employees at Bayer's facility in Karachi, Pakistan, are involved in producing pharmaceuticals on a continuous-flow production line.

The initial research on technology's effect on structure can be traced to Joan Woodward, who studied small manufacturing firms in southern England to determine the extent to which structural design elements were related to organizational success.[35] She couldn't find any consistent pattern until she divided the firms into three distinct technologies that had increasing levels of complexity and sophistication. The first category, **unit production**, described the production of items in units or small batches. The second category, **mass production**, described large-batch manufacturing. Finally, the third and most technically complex group, **process production**, included continuous-process production. A summary of her findings is shown in Exhibit 9.

Other studies also have shown that organizations adapt their structures to their technology depending on how routine their technology is for transforming inputs into outputs.[36] In general, the more routine the technology, the more mechanistic the structure can be, and organizations with more nonroutine technology are more likely to have organic structures.[37]

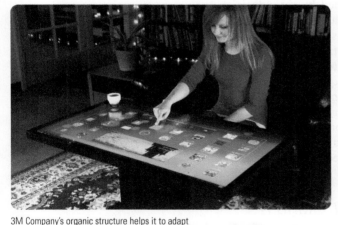

3M Company's organic structure helps it to adapt quickly to dynamic environmental forces of global competition and product innovation. With a flexible structure, 3M can satisfy customers' fast-growing demand for touch-screen products such as Ideum's new coffee table PC shown here that incorporates 3M's multitouch technology, an application that is key to expanding the reach of 3M's interactive systems and displays.
Source: Ideum/REX/AP Images

Environmental Uncertainty and Structure

Some organizations face stable and simple environments with little uncertainty; others face dynamic and complex environments with a lot of uncertainty. Managers try to minimize environmental uncertainty by adjusting the organization's structure.[38] In stable and simple environments, mechanistic designs can be more effective. On the other hand, the greater the uncertainty, the more an organization needs the flexibility of an organic design. For example, the uncertain nature of the oil industry means that

Exhibit 9
Woodward's Findings on Technology and Structure

	Unit Production	Mass Production	Process Production
Structural characteristics:	Low vertical differentiation	Moderate vertical differentiation	High vertical differentiation
	Low horizontal differentiation	High horizontal differentiation	Low horizontal differentiation
	Low formalization	High formalization	Low formalization
Most effective structure:	Organic	Mechanistic	Organic

oil companies need to be flexible. Soon after he was named CEO of Royal Dutch Shell PLC, Jeroen van der Veer (now the former CEO) streamlined the corporate structure to counteract some of the industry volatility. One thing he did was eliminate the company's cumbersome, overly analytical process of making deals with OPEC countries and other major oil producers.[39]

TODAY'S VIEW The evidence on the environment-structure relationship helps explain why so many managers today are restructuring their organizations to be lean, fast, and flexible. Worldwide economic downturns, global competition, accelerated product innovation by competitors, and increased demands from customers for high quality and faster deliveries are examples of dynamic environmental forces. Mechanistic organizations are not equipped to respond to rapid environmental change and environmental uncertainty. As a result, we're seeing organizations become more organic.

If your professor has assigned this, go to **www.mymanagementlab.com** to complete the Simulation: Organizational Structure and get a better understanding of the challenges of designing appropriate organizational structures.

 ★ Try It!

FUTURE VISION | Workplace Hierarchy: Why It's Still Important

Is organizational hierarchy important? Are the concepts of chain of command and authority still relevant? Do employees really need to know who reports to whom and who is responsible for what?[40] Here are some arguments "why" and "why not."

Why Hierarchy IS Relevant:	**Why Hierarchy ISN'T Relevant:**
• Hierarchy is a fundamental structural principle of all organizational systems from biological to social. Hierarchies can be found even among communities of animals and fish.	• A hierarchical system can inhibit innovation and employee engagement because of intrusive, irrelevant controls.
• Humans have a deep-seated need for order and security.	• In today's connected world of social networks, crowdsourcing, and readily-available communication technology, there's no need for a hierarchy.
• Hierarchy is important for accomplishing work tasks.	• Managers don't need to "control" employees since technology makes collaboration and computer-aided monitoring of work easier.
• Both internal *and* external stakeholders need to know who's in charge.	
• Organizations function better when there's a hierarchy in place.	

What's the bottom line? Even "in a world where a junior staffer" can message or tweet the company CEO and in more open/adaptive organizations, organizational hierarchy is important for getting work done efficiently and effectively. Although twenty-first-century organizations may not be as tightly structured or controlled as twentieth-century organizations, you'll still find some hierarchical mechanisms are necessary.

If your professor has chosen to assign this, go to **www.mymanagementlab.com** *to discuss the following questions.*

⭐ **TALK ABOUT IT 1:** What do YOU think? Will organizational hierarchy continue to be relevant and important in future workplaces?

⭐ **TALK ABOUT IT 2:** From a manager's perspective, discuss why employees need to know who reports to whom and who is responsible for what.

TRADITIONAL Organizational Designs

LO4 They're a big hit with the elementary-school crowd, and millions of them were sold every month. Ever heard of Silly Bandz?[41] If you're over the age of 10, you probably haven't! These colorful rubber bands retain the shapes they're twisted into and kids love them. The small business that created Silly Bandz—BCP Imports of Toledo, Ohio—increased its employee count from 20 to 200 and added 22 phone lines to keep up with inquiries. The person behind those organizing decisions is company president Robert Croak. In making structural decisions, managers have some common designs from which to choose. In this text, we're describing the traditional organizational designs.

When designing a structure, managers may choose one of the traditional organizational designs. These structures tend to be more mechanistic in nature. A summary of the strengths and weaknesses of each can be found in Exhibit 10.

Simple Structure

simple structure
An organizational design with little departmentalization, wide spans of control, centralized authority, and little formalization

Most companies start as entrepreneurial ventures using a **simple structure**, an organizational design with little departmentalization, wide spans of control, authority centralized in a single person, and little formalization.[42] As employees are added, however, most don't remain as simple structures. The structure tends to become more specialized and formalized. Rules and regulations are introduced, work becomes specialized, departments are created, levels of management are added, and the organization becomes increasingly bureaucratic. At this point, managers might choose a functional structure or a divisional structure.

Exhibit 10
Traditional Organizational Designs

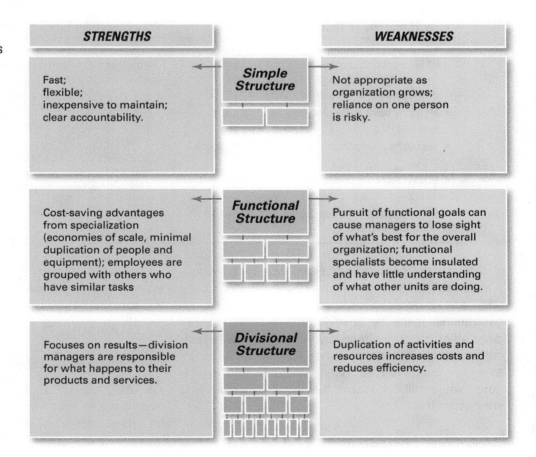

STRENGTHS		WEAKNESSES
Fast; flexible; inexpensive to maintain; clear accountability.	**Simple Structure**	Not appropriate as organization grows; reliance on one person is risky.
Cost-saving advantages from specialization (economies of scale, minimal duplication of people and equipment); employees are grouped with others who have similar tasks	**Functional Structure**	Pursuit of functional goals can cause managers to lose sight of what's best for the overall organization; functional specialists become insulated and have little understanding of what other units are doing.
Focuses on results—division managers are responsible for what happens to their products and services.	**Divisional Structure**	Duplication of activities and resources increases costs and reduces efficiency.

Functional Structure

A **functional structure** is an organizational design that groups similar or related occupational specialties together. You can think of this structure as functional departmentalization applied to the entire organization.

functional structure
An organizational design that groups together similar or related occupational specialties

Divisional Structure

The **divisional structure** is an organizational structure made up of separate business units or divisions.[43] In this structure, each division has limited autonomy, with a division manager who has authority over his or her unit and is responsible for performance. In divisional structures, however, the parent corporation typically acts as an external overseer to coordinate and control the various divisions, and often provides support services such as financial and legal. Walmart, for example, has two divisions: retail (Walmart Stores, International, Sam's Clubs, and others) and support (distribution centers).

divisional structure
An organizational structure made up of separate, semiautonomous units or divisions

Hopefully, you've seen in this text that organizational structure and design (or redesign) are important managerial tasks. Also, we hope that you recognize that organizing decisions aren't only important for upper-level managers. Managers at all levels may have to deal with work specialization or authority or span-of-control decisions.

PREPARING FOR: Exams/Quizzes

CHAPTER SUMMARY by Learning Objectives

LO1

DESCRIBE six key elements in organizational design.

The key elements in organizational design are work specialization, chain of command, span of control, departmentalization, centralization-decentralization, and formalization. Traditionally, work specialization was viewed as a way to divide work activities into separate job tasks. Today's view is that it is an important organizing mechanism but it can lead to problems. The chain of command and its companion concepts—authority, responsibility, and unity of command—were viewed as important ways of maintaining control in organizations. The contemporary view is that they are less relevant in today's organizations. The traditional view of span of control was that managers should directly supervise no more than five to six individuals. The contemporary view is that the span of control depends on the skills and abilities of the manager and the employees and on the characteristics of the situation.

The various forms of departmentalization are as follows: *Functional* groups jobs by functions performed; *product* groups jobs by product lines; *geographical* groups jobs by geographical region; *process* groups jobs on product or customer flow; and *customer* groups jobs on specific and unique customer groups.

Authority refers to the rights inherent in a managerial position to tell people what to do and to expect them to do it. The acceptance view of authority says that authority comes from the willingness of subordinates to accept it. Line authority entitles a manager to direct the work of an employee. Staff authority refers to functions that support, assist, advise, and generally reduce some of managers' informational burdens. Responsibility is the obligation or expectation to perform assigned duties. Unity of command states that a person should report to only one manager. Centralization-decentralization is a structural decision about who makes decisions—upper-level managers or lower-level employees. Formalization concerns the organization's use of standardization and strict rules to provide consistency and control.

LO2

CONTRAST mechanistic and organic structures.

A mechanistic organization is a rigid and tightly controlled structure. An organic organization is highly adaptive and flexible.

LO3

DISCUSS the contingency factors that favor either the mechanistic model or the organic model of organizational design.

An organization's structure should support the strategy. If the strategy changes, the structure also should change. An organization's size can affect its structure up to a certain point. Once an organization reaches a certain size (usually around 2,000 employees), it's fairly mechanistic. An organization's technology can affect its structure. An organic structure is most effective with unit production and process production technology. A mechanistic structure is most effective with mass production technology. The more uncertain an organization's environment, the more it needs the flexibility of an organic design.

LO4

DESCRIBE traditional organizational designs.

A simple structure is one with little departmentalization, wide spans of control, authority centralized in a single person, and little formalization. A functional structure groups similar or related occupational specialties together. A divisional structure is made up of separate business units or divisions.

MyManagementLab

Go to mymanagementlab.com to complete the problems marked with this icon ⭐.

⭐ REVIEW AND DISCUSSION QUESTIONS

1. Discuss the traditional and contemporary views of each of the six key elements of organizational design.

2. Contrast mechanistic and organic organizations.

3. Would you rather work in a mechanistic or an organic organization? Why?

4. Contrast the three traditional organizational designs.

5. With the availability of advanced information technology that allows an organization's work to be done anywhere at any time, is organizing still an important managerial function? Why or why not?

6. Researchers are now saying that efforts to simplify work tasks actually have negative results for both companies and their employees. Do you agree? Why or why not?

MyManagementLab

If your professor has assigned these, go to **mymanagementlab.com** for Auto-graded writing questions as well as the following Assisted-graded writing questions:

7. Can an organization's structure be changed quickly? Why or why not? Should it be changed quickly? Explain.

8. Explain the contingency factors that affect organizational design.

PREPARING FOR: My Career

⭐ PERSONAL INVENTORY ASSESSMENTS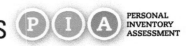

Delegation Self Assessment

You've seen why delegating is an important part of designing organizational structure. Use this PIA to assess your delegation ability and how comfortable you are with delegating.

⭐ ETHICS DILEMMA

Thomas Lopez, a lifeguard in the Miami area, was fired for leaving his assigned area to save a drowning man.[44] His employer, Jeff Ellis and Associates, which has a contract with the Florida city of Hallandale, said that by leaving his assigned patrol area uncovered, Lopez opened the company up to possible legal action. Lopez said he had no choice but to do what he did. He wasn't putting his job rules first over helping someone who desperately needed help. "I'm going to do what I felt was right, and I did." After this story hit the media, the company offered Lopez his job back, but he declined.

9. What do you think? What ethical concerns do you see in this situation?

10. What lessons can be applied to organizational design from this story?

SKILLS EXERCISE Developing Your Empowering People (Delegating) Skill

About the Skill

As a manager, your boss expects you to spend time doing things appropriate to what you've been hired to do. Managers get things done through other people. Because there are limits to any manager's time and knowledge, effective managers need to understand how to delegate and then do it. Delegation is the assignment of authority to another person to carry out specific duties. It allows an employee to make decisions. Delegation should not be confused with participation. In participative decision making, authority is shared. In delegation, employees make decisions on their own.

Steps in Practicing the Skill

As you saw in the chapter-opening, *It's Your Career*, a number of actions differentiate the effective delegator from the ineffective delegator. Here, we want to share some additional thoughts and suggestions on becoming a more effective delegator:

- *Don't be a "helicopter boss."* When you delegate a work task to one of your employees, don't hover over them. If you've properly delegated (following the suggested actions), there's no need for you to constantly and continually check on your people.

- *Let go of your need to have things done just so.* Be a guide. Ask your employees what they think they need to do and how they'll do it. Listen to what they have to say. Encourage them and tell them how much you're counting on them to get the job done efficiently and effectively.

- *Ignore that temptation to not delegate because "it's easier to do it myself."* Although that might well be true, you likely have your own tasks and responsibilities to handle. And yes, it does take time to delegate properly. However, by delegating in the correct way, wouldn't it be nice to free up some time to get your tasks done?

- *Don't let a bad delegating experience stop you from doing it again.* Alright, you tried delegating a task once and someone screwed up. Was it because of something *you* did: the direction you provided was unclear; you didn't establish appropriate feedback controls to monitor progress; or you had unrealistic expectations and the person didn't complete the task exactly how you wanted? Or was it because *this individual* wasn't particularly well-suited to the specific work task you delegated? Uncover the reason and do a better job of delegating next time.

Practicing the Skill

Read through the following scenario. Write a paper describing how you would handle the situation described. Be sure to refer to the six behaviors described for delegating in the chapter-opening *It's Your Career* and the suggestions included above.

Scenario

Ricky Lee is the manager of the contracts group of a large regional office supply distributor. His boss, Anne Zumwalt, has asked him to prepare by the end of the month the department's new procedures manual that will outline the steps followed in negotiating contracts with office products manufacturers who supply the organization's products. Because Ricky has another major project he's working on, he went to Anne and asked her if it would be possible to assign the rewriting of the procedures manual to Bill Harmon, one of his employees who's worked in the contracts group for about three years. Anne said she had no problems with Ricky reassigning the project as long as Bill knew the parameters and the expectations for the completion of the project. Ricky is preparing for his meeting in the morning with Bill regarding this assignment.

WORKING TOGETHER Team Exercise

An organizational chart can be a useful tool for understanding certain aspects of an organization's structure. Form small groups of three to four individuals. Among yourselves, choose an organization with which one of you is familiar (where you work, a student organization to which you belong, your college or university, etc.). Draw an organizational chart of this organization. Be careful to show departments (or groups) and especially be careful to get the chain of command correct. Be prepared to share your chart with the class.

MY TURN TO BE A MANAGER

- Find three different examples of an organizational chart. (A company's annual reports are a good place to look.) In a report, describe each of these. Try to decipher the organization's use of organizational design elements, especially departmentalization, chain of command, centralization-decentralization, and formalization.

- Survey at least 10 different managers as to how many employees they supervise. Also ask them whether they feel they could supervise more employees or whether they feel the number they supervise is too many. Graph your survey results and write a report describing what you found. Draw some conclusions about span of control.

- Using the organizational chart you created in the team exercise, redesign the structure. What structural changes might make this organization more efficient and effective? Write a report describing what you would do and why. Be sure to include an example of the original organizational chart as well as a chart of your proposed revision of the organizational structure.

- In your own words, write down three things you learned in this text about being a good manager. Keep a copy of this (along with the ones you do for other chapters) for future reference.

CASE APPLICATION 1 Ask Chuck

The Charles Schwab Corporation (Charles Schwab) is a San Francisco-based financial services company.[45] Like many companies in that industry, Charles Schwab struggled during the economic recession.

Founded in 1971 by its namesake as a discount brokerage, the company has now "grown up" into a full-service traditional brokerage firm, with more than 300 offices in some 45 states and in London and Hong Kong. It still offers discount brokerage services, but also financial research, advice, and planning; retirement plans; investment management; and proprietary financial products including mutual funds, mortgages, CDs, and other banking products through its Charles Schwab Bank unit. However, its primary business is still making stock trades for investors who make their own financial decisions. The company has a reputation for being conservative, which helped it avoid the financial meltdown suffered by other investment firms. Founder Charles R. Schwab has a black bowling ball perched on his desk. It's a reminder of another long-ago stock market bubble, when "shares of bowling-pin companies, shoemakers, chalk manufacturers, and lane operators were thought to be" sure bets because of the "limitless potential of suburbia." And guess what, they weren't. He keeps the ball as a reminder not to listen to the "hype or take excessive risks."

Like many companies, Charles Schwab is fanatical about customer service. By empowering front-line employees to respond fast to customer issues and concerns, Cheryl Pasquale, a manager at one of Schwab's branches, is on the front line of Schwab's efforts to prosper in a struggling economy. Every workday morning, she pulls up a customer feedback report for her branch generated by a brief survey the investment firm e-mails out daily. The report allows her to review how well her six financial consultants handled the previous day's transactions. She's able to see comments of customers who gave both high and low marks and whether a particular transaction garnered praise or complaint. On one particular day, she notices that several customers commented on how difficult it was to use the branch's in-house information kiosks. Wanting to know more, she decides to "ask her team for insights about this in their weekly meeting." One thing that she pays particular attention to is a "manager alert—a special notice triggered by a client who has given Schwab a poor rating for a delay in posting a transaction to his account." And she's not alone. Every day, Pasquale and the managers at all the company's branches receive this type of customer feedback. It's been particularly important to have this information in the economic climate of the last few years.

⭐ DISCUSSION QUESTIONS

11. Describe and evaluate what Charles Schwab is doing.

12. How might the company's culture of not buying into hype and not taking excessive risks affect its organizational structural design?

13. What structural implications—good and bad—might Schwab's intense focus on customer feedback have?

14. Do you think this arrangement would work for other types of organizations? Why or why not?

CASE APPLICATION 2 A New Kind of Structure

Admit it. Sometimes the projects you're working on (school, work, or both) can get pretty boring and monotonous. Wouldn't it be great to have a magic button you could push to get someone else to do that boring, time-consuming stuff? At Pfizer, that "magic button" is a reality for a large number of employees.[46]

As a global pharmaceutical company, Pfizer is continually looking for ways to help employees be more efficient and effective. The company's senior director of organizational effectiveness found that the highly educated MBAs it hired to "develop strategies and innovate were instead Googling and making PowerPoints" (A. Cohen, "Scuttling Scut Work," *Fast Company,* February 1, 2008, pp. 42–43). Indeed, internal studies conducted to find out just how much time its valuable talent was spending on menial tasks was startling. The average Pfizer employee was spending 20 percent to 40 percent of his or her time on support work (creating documents, typing notes, doing research, manipulating data, scheduling meetings) and only 60 percent to 80 percent on knowledge work (strategy, innovation, networking, collaborating, critical thinking). And the problem wasn't just at lower levels. Even the highest-level employees were affected. Take, for instance, David Cain, an executive director for global engineering. He enjoys his job—assessing environmental real estate risks, managing facilities, and controlling a multimillion-dollar budget. But he didn't so much enjoy having to go through spreadsheets and put together PowerPoints. Now, however, with Pfizer's "magic button," those tasks are passed off to individuals outside the organization.

Just what is this "magic button"? Originally called the Office of the Future (OOF), the renamed PfizerWorks allows employees to shift tedious and time-consuming tasks with the click of a single button on their computer desktop. They describe what they need on an online form, which is then sent to one of two Indian service-outsourcing firms. When a request is received, a team member in India calls the Pfizer employee to clarify what's needed and by when. The team member then e-mails back a cost specification for the requested work. If the Pfizer employee decides to proceed, the costs involved are charged to the employee's department. About this unique arrangement, Cain said that he relishes working with what he prefers to call his "personal consulting organization."

The number 66,500 illustrates just how beneficial PfizerWorks has been for the company. That's the number of work hours estimated to have been saved by employees who've used PfizerWorks. What about David Cain's experiences? When he gave the Indian team a complex project researching strategic actions that worked when consolidating company facilities, the team put the report together in a month, something that would have taken him six months to do alone. "Pfizer pays me not to work tactically, but to work strategically," he says (J. McGregor, "Outsourcing Tasks Instead of Jobs," *Bloomberg BusinessWeek,* March 11, 2009).

⭐ DISCUSSION QUESTIONS

15. Describe and evaluate what Pfizer is doing with its PfizerWorks.

16. What structural implications—good and bad—does this approach have? (Think in terms of the six organizational design elements.)

17. Do you think this arrangement would work for other types of organizations? Why or why not? What types of organizations might it also work for?

18. What role do you think organizational structure plays in an organization's efficiency and effectiveness? Explain.

ENDNOTES

1. B. Fenwick, "Oklahoma Factory Turns Out U.S. Bombs Used in Iraq," *Planet Ark* [www.planetark.com], November 4, 2003; A. Meyer, "Peeking Inside the Nation's Bomb Factory," *KFOR TV* [www.kfor.com], February 27, 2003; G. Tuchman, "Inside America's Bomb Factory," *CNN* [articles.cnn.com], December 5, 2002; and C. Fishman, "Boomtown, U.S.A.," *Fast Company,* June 2002, pp. 106–114.

2. D. Hudepohl, "Finesse a Flexible Work Schedule," *Wall Street Journal,* February 19, 2008, p. B8.

3. J. Nickerson, C. J. Yen, and J. T. Mahoney, "Exploring the Problem-Finding and Problem-Solving Approach for Designing Organizations," *Academy of Management Perspectives,* February 2012, pp. 52–72; R. Greenwood and D. Miller, "Tackling Design Anew: Getting Back to the Heart of Organizational Theory," *Academy of Management Perspectives,* November 2010, pp. 78–89.

4. See, for example, R. L. Daft, *Organization Theory and Design,* 10th ed. (Mason, OH: South-Western College Publishing, 2009).

5. S. Peterson, Associated Press, "Wilson Sporting Goods Football Factory," [www.chron.com], February 3, 2010; T. Arbel, Associated Press, "Factory Activity Fuels Economic Recovery," *OnlineAthens Banner-Herald* [www.onlineathens.com], February 2, 2010; and M. Hiestand, "Making a Stamp on Football," *USA Today,* January 25, 2005, pp. 1C+.

6. C. Dougherty, "Workforce Productivity Falls," *Wall Street Journal,* May 4, 2012, p. A5; and S. E. Humphrey, J. D. Nahrgang, and F. P. Morgeson, "Integrating Motivational, Social, and Contextual Work Design Features: A Meta-Analytic Summary and Theoretical Expansion of the Work Design Literature," *Journal of Applied Psychology,* September 2007, pp. 1332–1356.

7. D. Drickhamer, "Moving Man," *IW,* December 2002, pp. 44–46.

8. For a discussion of authority, see W. A. Kahn and K. E. Kram, "Authority at Work: Internal Models and Their Organizational Consequences," *Academy of Management Review,* January 1994, pp. 17–50.

9. C. I. Barnard, *The Functions of the Executive,* 30th Anniversary Edition (Cambridge, MA: Harvard University Press, 1968), pp. 165–166.

10. E. P. Gunn, "Who's the Boss?" *Smart Money,* April 2003, p. 121.

11. R. Ashkenas, "Simplicity-Minded Management," *Harvard Business Review,* December 2007, pp. 101–109; and P. Glader, "It's Not Easy Being Lean," *Wall Street Journal,* June 19, 2006, pp. B1+.

12. R. C. Morais, "The Old Lady Is Burning Rubber," *Forbes,* November 26, 2007, pp. 146–150.

13. F. Hassan, "The Frontline Advantage," *Harvard Business Review,* May 2011, p. 109.

14. G. L. Neilson and J. Wulf, "How Many Direct Reports?" *Harvard Business Review,* April 2012, pp. 112–119; and D. Van Fleet, "Span of Management Research and Issues," *Academy of Management Journal,* September 1983, pp. 546–552.

15. G. Anders, "Overseeing More Employees—With Fewer Managers," *Wall Street Journal,* March 24, 2008, p. B6.

16. H. Fayol, *General and Industrial Management,* trans. C. Storrs (London: Pitman Publishing, 1949), pp. 19–42.

17. J. Zabojnik, "Centralized and Decentralized Decision Making in Organizations," *Journal of Labor Economics,* January 2002, pp. 1–22.

18. See, for example, H. Mintzberg, *Power In and Around Organizations* (Upper Saddle River, NJ: Prentice Hall, 1983); and J. Child, *Organization: A Guide to Problems and Practices* (London: Kaiser & Row, 1984).

19. M. Weinstein, "It's A Balancing Act," *Training,* May 2009, p. 10.

20. See P. Kenis and D. Knoke, "How Organizational Field Networks Shape InterOrganizational Tie-Formation Rates," *Academy of Management Review,* April 2002, pp. 275–293.

21. A. D. Amar, C. Hentrich, and V. Hlupic, "To Be a Better Leader, Give Up Authority," *Harvard Business Review,* December 2009, pp. 22–24.

22. P. Siekman, "Dig It! A maker of monster machines, Terex has been scraping by for years—until now," *Fortune,* February 23, 2006.

23. J. Cable, "Operators Lead the Way," *Industry Week,* January 2010, p. 31.

24. E. W. Morrison, "Doing the Job Well: An Investigation of Pro-Social Rule Breaking," *Journal of Management,* February 2006, Volume 32(1).

25. Ibid.

26. M. Boyle, "A Leaner Macy's Tries Catering to Local Tastes," *Bloomberg BusinessWeek,* September 14, 2009, p. 13.

27. D. A. Morand, "The Role of Behavioral Formality and Informality in the Enactment of Bureaucratic Versus Organic Organizations," *Academy of Management Review,* October 1995, pp. 831–872; and T. Burns and G. M. Stalker, *The Management of Innovation* (London: Tavistock, 1961).

28. C. Feser, "Long Live Bureaucracy!" *Leader to Leader,* Summer 2012, pp. 57–62.

29. "How to Bust Corporate Barriers," *Gallup Management Journal Online,* August 18, 2011; and D. Dougherty, "Re-imagining the Differentiation and Integration of Work for Sustained Product Innovation," *Organization Science* (September–October 2001), pp. 612–631.

30. **R. D. Hof, "Yahoo's Bartz Shows Who's Boss," *BusinessWeek Online,* February 27, 2009**; and J. E. Vascellaro, "Yahoo CEO Set to Install Top-Down Management," *Wall Street Journal,* February 23, 2009, p. B1.

31. A. D. Chandler, Jr., *Strategy and Structure: Chapters in the History of the Industrial Enterprise* (Cambridge, MA: MIT Press, 1962).

32. See, for instance, W. Chan Kim and R. Mauborgne, "How Strategy Shapes Structure," *Harvard Business Review,* September 2009, pp. 73–80; L. L. Bryan and C. I. Joyce, "Better Strategy Through Organizational Design," *The McKinsey Quarterly,* 2007, Number 2, pp. 21–29; D. Jennings and S. Seaman, "High and Low Levels of Organizational Adaptation: An Empirical Analysis of Strategy, Structure, and Performance," *Strategic Management Journal,* July 1994, pp. 459–475; D. C. Galunic and K. M. Eisenhardt, "Renewing the Strategy-Structure-Performance Paradigm," in B. M. Staw and L. L. Cummings (eds.), *Research in Organizational Behavior,* vol. 16 (Greenwich, CT: JAI Press, 1994), pp. 215–255; R. Parthasarthy and S. P. Sethi, "Relating Strategy and Structure to Flexible Automation: A Test of Fit and Performance Implications," *Strategic Management Journal,* 14, no. 6 (1993), pp. 529–549; H. A. Simon, "Strategy and Organizational Evolution," *Strategic Management Journal,* January 1993, pp. 131–142; H. L. Boschken, "Strategy and Structure: Re-conceiving the Relationship," *Journal of Management,* March 1990, pp. 135–150; D. Miller, "The Structural and Environmental Correlates of Business Strategy," *Strategic Management Journal,* January–February 1987, pp. 55–76; and R. E. Miles and C. C. Snow, *Organizational Strategy, Structure, and Process* (New York: McGraw-Hill, 1978).

33. Leader Making a Difference box based on M. Schuman, "Zhang Ruimin's Haier Power," time.com, April 4, 2014; "Fortune Names Haier Group Chairman & CEO Zhang Ruimin Among 'The World's 50 Greatest Leaders,'" globenewswire.com, March 21, 2014; P. Day, "Smashing Way to Start a Global Business," www.bbc.news, October 22, 2013; "Haier and Higher," www.economist.com, October 12, 2013; R. Gluckman, "Every Customer Is Always Right," *Forbes,* May 21, 2012, pp. 38–40; G. Colvin, "The Next Management Icon: Would You Believe He's From China?" *Fortune,* July 25, 2011, p. 77; and D. J. Lynch, "CEO Pushes China's Haier as Global Brand," *USA Today,* January 3, 2003, pp. 1B+.

34. See, for instance, R. Z. Gooding and J. A. Wagner III, "A Meta-Analytic Review of the Relationship between Size and Performance: The Productivity and Efficiency of Organizations and Their Subunits," *Administrative Science Quarterly,* December 1985, pp. 462–481; D. S. Pugh, "The Aston Program of Research: Retrospect and Prospect," in A. H. Van de Ven and W. F. Joyce (eds.), *Perspectives on Organization Design and Behavior* (New York: John Wiley, 1981), pp. 135–166; and P. M. Blau and R. A. Schoenherr, *The Structure of Organizations* (New York: Basic Books, 1971).

35. J. Woodward, *Industrial Organization: Theory and Practice* (London: Oxford University Press, 1965).

36. See, for instance, J. Zhang and C. Baden-Fuller, "The Influence of Technological Knowledge Base and Organizational Structure on Technology Collaboration," *Journal of Management Studies,* June 2010, pp. 679–704; C. C. Miller, W. H. Glick, Y. D. Wang, and G. Huber, "Understanding Technology-Structure Relationships: Theory Development and Meta-Analytic Theory Testing," *Academy of Management Journal,* June 1991, pp. 370–399; J. Hage and

M. Aiken, "Routine Technology, Social Structure, and Organizational Goals," *Administrative Science Quarterly*, September 1969, pp. 366–377; J. D. Thompson, *Organizations in Action* (New York: McGraw-Hill, 1967); and C. Perrow, "A Framework for the Comparative Analysis of Organizations," *American Sociological Review*, April 1967, pp. 194–208.

37. D. M. Rousseau and R. A. Cooke, "Technology and Structure: The Concrete, Abstract, and Activity Systems of Organizations," *Journal of Management*, Fall–Winter 1984, pp. 345–361; and D. Gerwin, "Relationships between Structure and Technology," in P. C. Nystrom and W. H. Starbuck (eds.), *Handbook of Organizational Design*, vol. 2 (New York: Oxford University Press, 1981), pp. 3–38.

38. S. Rausch and J. Birkinshaw, "Organizational Ambidexterity: Antecedents, Outcomes, and Moderators," *Journal of Management*, June 2008, pp. 375–409; M. Yasai-Ardekani, "Structural Adaptations to Environments," *Academy of Management Review*, January 1986, pp. 9–21; P. Lawrence and J. W. Lorsch, *Organization and Environment: Managing Differentiation and Integration* (Boston: Harvard Business School, Division of Research, 1967); and F. E. Emery and E. Trist, "The Causal Texture of Organizational Environments," *Human Relations*, February 1965, pp. 21–32.

39. S. Reed, "He's Brave Enough to Shake Up Shell," *BusinessWeek*, July 18, 2005, p. 53.

40. E. Zimmerman, "The Case for Workplace Hierarchy," qz.com, March 26, 2014; J. Pfeffer, "You're Still the Same: Why Theories of Power Hold Over Time and Across Contexts," *Academy of Management Perspectives*, November 2013, pp. 269–280; S. Grobart, "Hooray for Hierarchy," *Bloomberg BusinessWeek*, January 14–20, 2013, p. 74; J. P. Kotter, "Hierarchy and Network: Two Structures, One Organization," blogs.hbr.org, May 23, 2011; and C. Anderson and C. E. Brown, "The Functions and Dysfunctions of Hierarchy," *Research in Organizational Behavior*, 2010, vol. 30, pp. 55–89.

41. B. Rochman, "Banning the Bandz," *Time*, June 14, 2010, p. 99; and S. Berfield, "The Man Behind the Bandz," *Bloomberg BusinessWeek Online*, June 10, 2010.

42. H. Mintzberg, *Structure in Fives: Designing Effective Organizations* (Upper Saddle River, NJ: Prentice Hall, 1983), p. 157.

43. R. J. Williams, J. J. Hoffman, and B. T. Lamont, "The Influence of Top Management Team Characteristics on M-Form Implementation Time," *Journal of Managerial Issues*, Winter 1995, pp. 466–480.

44. C. Hausman, "Lifeguard Fired for Leaving Patrol Zone to Save Drowning Man," *Ethics Newsline Online*, July 9, 2012; S. Grossman, "Lifeguard Who Got Fired for Saving Drowning Swimmer Declines Offer to Return," *newsfeed.time.com*, July 6, 2012; E. Illades and C. Teproff, "Fired Lifeguard Says 'No Thanks' When He's Re-offered Job," *MiamiHerald.com*, July 5, 2012; and W. Lee, "Florida Lifeguard Helps Save Life, Gets Fired," *USA Today Online*, July 4, 2012.

45. B. Philbin, "Schwab's Net Drops 20%," *Wall Street Journal*, April 17, 2012, p. C9; M. Tian, "Charles Schwab—An Unnoticed Transformation," *Morningstar OpportunisticInvestor*, March 2012, pp. 6–9; B. Morris, "Chuck Schwab Is Worried About the Small Investor," *Bloomberg BusinessWeek*, May 31–June 6, 2010, pp. 58–64; L. Gibbs, "Chuck Would Like a Word with You," *Money*, January/February 2010, pp. 98–103; R. Markey, F. Reichheld, and A. Dullweber, "Closing the Customer Feedback Loop," *Harvard Business Review*, December 2009, pp. 43–47; and R. Farzad and C. Palmeri, "Can Schwab Seize the Day?" *Bloomberg BusinessWeek*, July 27, 2009, pp. 36–39.

46. S. Silbermann, "How Culture and Regulation Demand New Ways to Sell," *Harvard Business Review*, July/August 2012, pp. 104–105; P. Miller and T. Wedell-Wedellsborg, "How to Make an Offer That Managers Can't Refuse?" *IESE Insight*, 2011 (second quarter), issue 9, pp. 66–67; S. Hernández, "Prove Its Worth," *IESE Insight*, 2011 (second quarter), issue 9, p. 68; T. Koulopoulos, "Know Thyself," *IESE Insight*, 2011 (second quarter), issue 9, p. 69; M. Weinstein, "Retrain and Restructure Your Organization," *Training*, May 2009, p. 36; J. McGregor, "Outsourcing Tasks Instead of Jobs," *Bloomberg BusinessWeek*, March 11, 2009; "Pfizer: Making It 'Leaner, Meaner, More Efficient,'" *BusinessWeek Online*, March 2, 2009; and A. Cohen, "Scuttling Scut Work," *Fast Company*, February 1, 2008, pp. 42–43.

Designing Organizational Structure—Adaptive Designs

From Chapter 11 of *Management*, Thirteenth Edition. Stephen P. Robbins and Mary Coulter. Copyright © 2016 by Pearson Education, Inc. All rights reserved.

It's Your Career

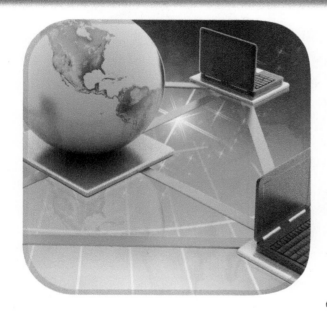

Source: RAJ CREATIONZS/Shutterstock

A key to success in management and in your career is knowing how to stay connected and in the organizational loop when you're in a nontraditional working arrangement.

Staying Connected

The odds are good that at some point in your career, you'll be offered the opportunity to telecommute/work at home. (According to a recent survey, 37 percent of workers say their company offers that option.[1]) And working from home can be a good thing. (A recent study showed that an employee's efficiency can improve by 13 percent.[2]) Although you might be efficient, not being physically at the workplace can make it seem like you're totally disconnected from what's going on. (Another recent study showed that telecommuters move up more slowly than their in-office peers.[3]) When working as a remote employee—or even if you, at some point, manage someone in that kind of work arrangement—it's important to find ways to make the work relationship, well . . . work. And work well! Here are some suggestions for staying in the organizational loop and making yourself a valuable employee:

*1.   **Stay focused and productive.** Time management is absolutely critical. Plan ahead using goal setting and to-do lists. Control—or even better, eliminate—interruptions and distractions. When you have work appointments (online, phone, Skype, etc.), keep them; and make sure you're prepared by having the materials you will need for the conversation. Respect the schedules and time requirements of your colleagues. Finally, build in the kind of accountability you'd have in a traditional work arrangement. Recruit your manager or a colleague to be your accountability partner. Let them know what you intend to accomplish that day (or week) and check in daily (or weekly) to discuss what you've accomplished.*

*2.   **Communicate. Communicate. Communicate.** Communication is always important— regardless of where you do your work—but especially so when face-to-face exchanges are minimal or nonexistent. It's critical to think*

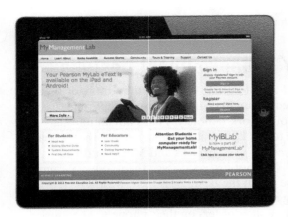

MyManagementLab®

⭐ **Improve Your Grade!**

When you see this icon, visit
www.mymanagementlab.com for activities that are
applied, personalized, and offer immediate feedback.

Learning Objectives

1 **Describe** *contemporary organizational designs.*

- **Develop your skill** at acquiring and using power.

2 **Discuss** *how organizations organize for collaboration.*

3 **Explain** *flexible work arrangements used by organizations.*

- **Know how** to stay connected and "in the loop" when working remotely.

4 **Discuss** *organizing issues associated with a contingent workforce.*

5 **Describe** *today's organizational design challenges.*

---

before you communicate. Choose your communication approach carefully. There are times when a more matter-of-fact approach is the best and times when a more personal touch is appropriate. Watch your "tone" (even in written communications) and be courteous. Hone your listening and "interpretation" skills. Try to understand the meaning behind what someone is saying in writing or when speaking.

3. ***Choose appropriate technology.*** *Know and choose the tools that are most appropriate for your situation. Will you need to collaborate with others*

or will your work be mainly solitary? What type of communication will be necessary—e-mail, instant messaging, video messaging, etc.? Choose your tech tools wisely.

4. ***Be aware of the "people" aspects of*** ***remote work arrangements.*** *When a person is not physically at a workplace, it is hard to build closeness and camaraderie. But those things are still important. Find ways to combat the isolation and loneliness. Get to know your other team members (remote and in-the-workplace).*

Welcome to the fascinating world of organizational structure and design in the twenty-first century! Included in the basic concepts of traditional organizational design are the six building blocks of an organization's structure: work specialization, departmentalization, chain of command, span of control, centralization and decentralization, and formalization. In this text, we're going to explore contemporary aspects of organizational design as organizations adapt to the demands of today's environment. We're going to first look at some contemporary organizational designs and then move on to discussing how organizations are coping with those demands through collaborative work efforts, flexible work arrangements, and a contingent workforce. We'll wrap up the chapter by describing some organizational design challenges facing today's managers.

CONTEMPORARY Organizational Designs

LO1

• Late last fall, as part of a cost-cutting initiative, the editors of the *Arizona Republic* informed about 20 of its community reporters that they were getting laptops so they could work remotely. That's not an unusual decision for organizations to make today, but what *was* unusual was the company's recommendation that these employees go to Starbucks and McDonald's as unofficial places to do their work.[4] Why not just encourage them to work from home? Because reporters need to be out in the field.

• At Panera, the task of order taking is being shifted from cashiers to kiosks. Its new store design allows customers to place their orders on their phone or at a kiosk.[5] Although there will be fewer cashiers, employees will still bring orders to tables and help as needed in the kitchen.

Many organizations, like Panera and the *Arizona Republic,* are finding that the traditional organizational designs often aren't appropriate for today's increasingly dynamic and complex environment. Instead, organizations need to be lean, flexible, and innovative; that is, they need to be more organic. So managers are finding creative ways to structure and organize work. These contemporary designs include team structures, matrix and project structures, boundaryless organizations, and learning organizations. (See Exhibit 1 for a summary of these designs.)

Team Structures

team structure
An organizational structure in which the entire organization is made up of work teams

matrix structure
An organizational structure that assigns specialists from different functional departments to work on one or more projects

project structure
An organizational structure in which employees continuously work on projects

Larry Page and Sergey Brin, cofounders of Google, created a corporate structure that organized projects around "small, tightly focused teams."[6] A **team structure** is one in which the entire organization is made up of work teams that do the organization's work.[7] In this structure, employee empowerment is crucial because no line of managerial authority flows from top to bottom. Rather, employee teams design and do work in the way they think is best, but the teams are also held responsible for all work performance results in their respective areas.

In large organizations, the team structure complements what is typically a functional or divisional structure and allows the organization to have the efficiency of a bureaucracy *and* the flexibility that teams provide. Companies such as Amazon, Boeing, Hewlett-Packard, Louis Vuitton, Motorola, and Xerox, for instance, extensively use employee teams to improve productivity.

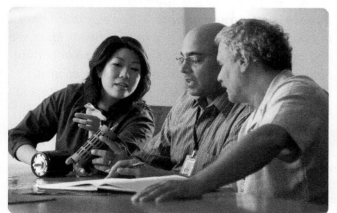

W. L. Gore & Associates has been a team-based organization since Bill Gore founded the company in 1958. All 9,000 Gore associates located in 30 countries work in cross-functional and self-managed teams. The team corporate structure is key to Gore's success as an innovative, technology-driven firm and contributes to its high associate satisfaction and retention.
Source: PRNewsFoto/W. L. Gore & Associates, Pete Stone

Matrix and Project Structures

Other popular contemporary designs are the matrix and project structures. The **matrix structure** assigns specialists from different functional departments to work on projects being led by a project manager. (See Exhibit 2.) One unique aspect of this design is that it creates a *dual chain of command* because employees in a matrix organization have two managers: their functional area manager and their product or project manager, who share authority. The project manager has authority over the functional members who are part of his or her project team in areas related to the project's goals. However, any decisions about promotions, salary recommendations, and annual reviews typically remain the functional manager's responsibility. The matrix design "violates" the unity of command principle, which says that each person should report to only one boss; however, it can—and does—work effectively if both managers communicate regularly, coordinate work demands on employees, and resolve conflicts together.[8]

Many organizations use a **project structure**, in which employees continuously work on projects. Unlike the matrix structure, a project structure has no formal

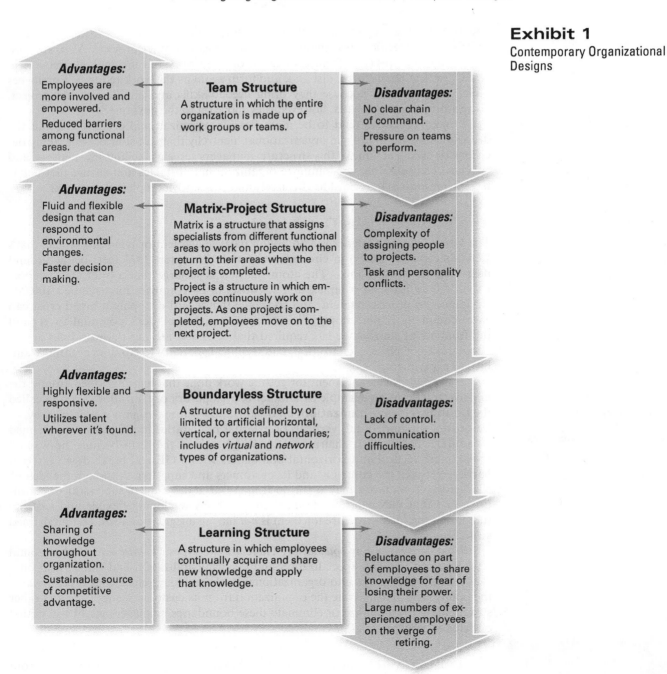

Exhibit 1
Contemporary Organizational Designs

Team Structure
A structure in which the entire organization is made up of work groups or teams.

Advantages:
Employees are more involved and empowered.
Reduced barriers among functional areas.

Disadvantages:
No clear chain of command.
Pressure on teams to perform.

Matrix-Project Structure
Matrix is a structure that assigns specialists from different functional areas to work on projects who then return to their areas when the project is completed.
Project is a structure in which employees continuously work on projects. As one project is completed, employees move on to the next project.

Advantages:
Fluid and flexible design that can respond to environmental changes.
Faster decision making.

Disadvantages:
Complexity of assigning people to projects.
Task and personality conflicts.

Boundaryless Structure
A structure not defined by or limited to artificial horizontal, vertical, or external boundaries; includes *virtual* and *network* types of organizations.

Advantages:
Highly flexible and responsive.
Utilizes talent wherever it's found.

Disadvantages:
Lack of control.
Communication difficulties.

Learning Structure
A structure in which employees continually acquire and share new knowledge and apply that knowledge.

Advantages:
Sharing of knowledge throughout organization.
Sustainable source of competitive advantage.

Disadvantages:
Reluctance on part of employees to share knowledge for fear of losing their power.
Large numbers of experienced employees on the verge of retiring.

Exhibit 2
Example of a Matrix Organization

R&D	Marketing	Customer Services (CS)	Human Resources (HR)	Finance	Information Systems (IS)
Product 1 R&D Group	Marketing Group	CS Group	HR Group	Finance Group	IS Group
Product 2 R&D Group	Marketing Group	CS Group	HR Group	Finance Group	IS Group
Product 3 R&D Group	Marketing Group	CS Group	HR Group	Finance Group	IS Group

275

departments where employees return at the completion of a project. Instead, employees take their specific skills, abilities, and experiences to other projects. Also, all work in project structures is performed by teams of employees. For instance, at design firm IDEO, project teams form, disband, and form again as the work requires. Employees "join" project teams because they bring needed skills and abilities to that project. Once a project is completed, however, they move on to the next one.[9]

Project structures tend to be more flexible organizational designs, without the departmentalization or rigid organizational hierarchy that can slow down making decisions or taking action. In this structure, managers serve as facilitators, mentors, and coaches. They eliminate or minimize organizational obstacles and ensure that teams have the resources they need to effectively and efficiently complete their work.

The Boundaryless Organization

The Large Hadron Collider is a $6 billion particle accelerator lying in a tunnel that's 27 kilometers (17 miles) in circumference and 175 meters (574 feet) below ground near Geneva, Switzerland. "The atom smasher is so large that a brief status report lists 2,900 authors, so complex that scientists in 34 countries have readied 100,000 computers to process its data, and so fragile that a bird dropping a bread crust can short-circuit its power supply."[10] But exploiting the collider's potential to expand the frontiers of knowledge has required that scientists around the world cut across "boundaries of place, organization, and technical specialty to conduct ever more ambitious experiments."

The structural arrangement for getting work done that has developed around the massive collider is an example of another contemporary organizational design called the **boundaryless organization**, an organization whose design is not defined by, or limited to, the horizontal, vertical, or external boundaries imposed by a predefined structure.[11] Former GE chairman Jack Welch coined the term because he wanted to eliminate vertical and horizontal boundaries within GE and break down external barriers between the company and its customers and suppliers. Although the idea of eliminating boundaries may seem odd, many of today's most successful organizations find that they can operate most effectively by remaining flexible and *un*structured: that the ideal structure for them is *not* having a rigid, bounded, and predefined structure.[12]

What do we mean by *boundaries*? There are two types: (1) *internal*—the horizontal ones imposed by work specialization and departmentalization and the vertical ones that separate employees into organizational levels and hierarchies; and (2) *external*—the boundaries that separate the organization from its customers, suppliers, and other stakeholders. To minimize or eliminate these boundaries, managers might use virtual or network structural designs.

VIRTUAL ORGANIZATIONS Is an internship something you've ever thought about doing (or maybe have done)? How about an internship that you could do, not in a workplace cubicle, but from your couch using your computer?[13] Such virtual internships are becoming quite popular, especially with smaller and midsize companies and, of course, with online businesses. The type of work virtual interns do typically involves "researching, sales, marketing, and social media development"—tasks that can be done anywhere with a computer and online access. Some organizations are structured in a way that allows most employees to be virtual employees.

A **virtual organization** typically consists of a small core of full-time employees and outside specialists temporarily hired as needed to work on projects.[15] An example is when Second Life, a company creating a virtual world of colorful online avatars, was building its software. Founder Philip Rosedale hired programmers from around the world and divided up the work into about 1,600 individual tasks, "from setting up databases to fixing bugs." The process worked so well, the company used it for all sorts of work.[16] Another example is Nashville-based Emma Inc., an e-mail marketing

boundaryless organization
An organization whose design is not defined by, or limited to, the horizontal, vertical, or external boundaries imposed by a predefined structure

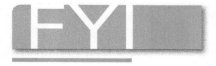

- 64 percent of people said if given a choice, they'd rather work virtually than in an office.[14]

virtual organization
An organization that consists of a small core of full-time employees and outside specialists temporarily hired as needed to work on projects

firm with 100 employees who work from home or offices in Austin, Denver, New York, and Portland.[17] The biggest challenge they've faced is creating a "virtual" culture, a task made more challenging by the fact that the organization is virtual.

If your professor has assigned this, go to **www.mymanagementlab.com** to watch a video titled: *Rudi's Bakery: Adaptive Organizational Design* and to respond to questions.

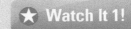 ★ **Watch It 1!**

NETWORK ORGANIZATIONS Food marketer Smart Balance Inc. helps people stay trim and lean with its heart-healthy products.[18] The company's organizational structure is also trim and lean. With only 67 employees, the company outsources almost every other organizational function, including manufacturing, product distribution, and sales. Smart Balance's structural approach is one that also eliminates organizational boundaries and can be described as a **network organization**, which uses its own employees to do some work activities and networks of outside suppliers to provide other needed product components or work processes.[19] This organizational form is sometimes called a modular organization by manufacturing firms.[20] Such an approach allows organizations to concentrate on what they do best by contracting out other activities to companies that do those activities best. For instance, the strategy of British company ARM, a microchip designer, is to find a lot of partners. It contracts with those partners for manufacturing and sales. Because ARM doesn't manufacture, it can encourage its customers (ARM's chip designs serve as the brains of 98 percent of the world's cell phones) to request whatever they like. Such flexibility is particularly valuable in the cell phone market, where having custom chips and software can provide an edge.[21] At Boeing, the company's head

network organization
An organization that uses its own employees to do some work activities and networks of outside suppliers to provide other needed product components or work processes

FUTURE VISION | **Flexible Organizations**

By 2025, a considerably smaller proportion of the labor force will hold full-time jobs. Organizations will increasingly rely on contract employees and part-timers to get the work done, giving the organization greater flexibility. Many workers will be doing pieces of what is today a single job. From the employee's standpoint, it will mean greater individual control of the employee's future rather than being dependent on a single employer.

Future workers will be more like outside consultants than full-time employees. Assignments will be temporary. They might last a few weeks or a few years, but the presumption is—on the part of both workers and employers—that the relationship will not become permanent. As such, you will find yourself consistently working on new projects with a different group of coworkers.

Additionally, expect to see fewer large corporate headquarter buildings and centralized corporate centers. Work demands will not require organizations to house large numbers of workers in one place.

"Headquarter" cities such as New York, Toronto, or London will find themselves with lots of empty office space. Conversely, job opportunities will be geographically dispersed, and in many cases, not dependent at all on where employees reside. An increasing proportion of the labor force will work from home. And many organizations will create regional satellite centers where employees meet or work. These centers will be less costly to operate than centralized offices and will cut down on commuting distances for workers.

If your professor has chosen to assign this, go to ***www.mymanagementlab.com*** *to discuss the following questions.*

★ **TALK ABOUT IT 1:** What are the challenges of "flexibility" for organizations and managers? For workers?

★ **TALK ABOUT IT 2:** What about you? How do you feel about working like this?

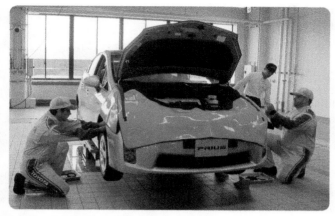

A guiding principle at Toyota Motor Corporation is to "become a learning organization through relentless reflection and continuous improvement." This principle motivates Toyota's managers and employees to reflect on weaknesses and mistakes, devise and apply ways to constantly improve products and processes, and disseminate that information throughout the organization.
Source: AP Photo/Yuri Kageyama

learning organization
An organization that has developed the capacity to continuously learn, adapt, and change

of development for the 787 Dreamliner manages thousands of employees and some 100 suppliers at more than 100 sites in different countries.[22] Sweden's Ericsson contracts its manufacturing and even some of its research and development to more cost-effective contractors in New Delhi, Singapore, California, and other global locations.[23] And at Penske Truck Leasing, dozens of business processes, such as securing permits and titles, entering data from drivers' logs, and processing data for tax filings and accounting, have been outsourced to Mexico and India.[24]

Learning Organizations

Doing business in an intensely competitive global environment, British retailer Tesco realizes how important it is for its stores to run well behind the scenes.[25] And it does so using a proven "tool" called Tesco in a Box, a self-contained complete IT system and matching set of business processes that provides the model for all of Tesco's international business operations. This approach promotes consistency in operations and is a way to share innovations.[26] Tesco is an example of a **learning organization**, an organization that has developed the capacity to continuously learn, adapt, and change. "Today's managerial challenge is to inspire and enable knowledge workers to solve, day in and day out, problems that cannot be anticipated."[27] In a learning organization, employees continually acquire and share new knowledge and apply that knowledge in making decisions or doing their work. Some organizational theorists even go so far as to say that an organization's ability to do this—that is, to learn and to apply that learning—may be the only sustainable source of competitive advantage.[28] What structural characteristics does a learning organization need?

Employees throughout the entire organization—across different functional specialties and even at different organizational levels—must share information and collaborate on work activities. Such an environment requires minimal structural and physical barriers, which allows employees to work together in doing the organization's work the best way they can and, in the process, learn from each other. Finally, empowered work teams tend to be an important feature of a learning organization's structural design. These teams make decisions about doing whatever work needs to be done or resolving issues. With empowered employees and teams, there's little need for "bosses" to direct and control. Instead, managers serve as facilitators, supporters, and advocates.

ORGANIZING for Collaboration

LO2 In 3M's dental products division, Sumita Mitra, a research scientist, helped develop coatings that prevent tooth plaque and innovative cement bonding materials that could be set by light.[29] However, as cosmetic dentistry's popularity increased, she sensed an opportunity for developing a product that had both the strength and the natural appearance that dentists wanted. Finding that product meant venturing outside the realm of traditional dental materials. Mitra first turned to 3M's database of technical reports written by the company's approximately 7,000 scientists. Although this database is invaluable for spreading knowledge throughout the company, "the real work of collaboration happens face-to-face, often at events sponsored by TechForum, an employee-run organization designed to foster communications between scientists in different labs or divisions." There, Mitra found valuable information and guidance from other scientists in different divisions of the company. 3M also has an R&D Workcenter networking Web site, which Mitra describes as "a LinkedIn for 3M scientists." It also proved to be a valuable collaborative tool. Both the TechForum and the R&D Workcenter proved beneficial for Mitra's research efforts. Three years after starting her research, 3M introduced Filtek Supreme Plus, a strong, polishable dental material and the first to include

Benefits	Drawbacks
• Increased communication and coordination • Greater innovative output • Enhanced ability to address complex problems • Sharing of information and best practices	• Potential interpersonal conflict • Different views and competing goals • Logistics of coordinating

Exhibit 3
Benefits and Drawbacks of Collaborative Work

Sources: Based on R. Wagner and G. Muller, "The Pinnacle of Partnership: Unselfishness," *Gallup Management Journal Online* [http://gmj.gallup.com], February 18, 2010; M.T. Hansen, "When Internal Collaboration Is Bad for Your Company," *Harvard Business Review*, April 2009, pp. 83–88; G. Ahuja, "Collaboration Networks, Structural Holes and Innovation: A Longitudinal Study," *Academy of Management Proceedings Online*, 1998; and M. Pincher, "Collaboration: Find a New Strength in Unity," *Computer Weekly*, November 27, 2007, p. 18.

nanoparticles. At 3M, employees are expected to collaborate and are evaluated on their success. Such collaborations among the company's scientists have led to several breakthroughs in product technology.

It's fair to say that the world of work has changed. Organizations need to be more flexible in how work gets done, although it still needs to get done efficiently and effectively. Throw in the fact that innovation and the ability to bring innovations to market quickly is critical, and you can begin to appreciate how traditional top-down decision making that strictly follows the chain of command and narrowly defined functional arrangements might not be the best structural mechanisms to do this. Many organizations, like 3M, are encouraging collaborative work among employees. Exhibit 3 lists some of the benefits and drawbacks of working collaboratively. An organization's collaboration efforts can be internal—that is, among employees within the organization. Or those efforts can be external collaborations with any stakeholders. In both types, it's important that managers recognize how such collaborative efforts "fit" with the organization's structure and the challenges of making all the pieces work together successfully. Let's take a look at each of these types of collaboration.

Internal Collaboration

When managers believe collaboration among employees is needed for more coordinated and integrated work efforts, they can use several different structural options. Some of the more popular include cross-functional teams, task forces, and communities of practice.

CROSS-FUNCTIONAL TEAMS You'd probably agree that hospitals would be challenging organizations to manage. When Wright L. Lassiter took on the job as CEO of the Alameda County Medical Center in Oakland, California, he had a massive challenge on his hands. Nurses followed doctors' orders only when they felt like it, a doctor was beaten and strangled to death by a patient and his body left on the floor for 30 minutes until a janitor found it, the organization lost millions of dollars every year, and so on. However, Lassiter turned a "shockingly mismanaged urban safety-net hospital system in one of America's most violent cities into a model for other public hospitals." And one of the approaches he took was what he called "odd-couple arrangements"—what we would call cross-functional teams—of doctors, nurses, technicians, and other managers and made them responsible for finding ways to be more efficient and effective.[30]

Organizations use team-based structures because they've found that teams are more flexible and responsive to changing events than traditional departments or

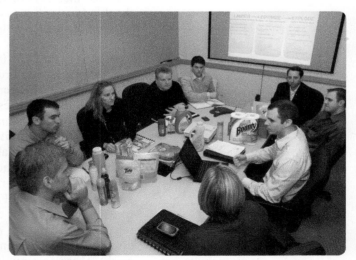

Procter & Gamble's cross-functional teams that include employees from research and development, marketing, engineering, logistics, and other functional areas enable P&G to organize and use its resources effectively and efficiently on a global basis. Team members shown here meet to launch e-Store, an online shopping service for P&G consumer brands.
Source: AP Photo/Al Behrman

cross-functional team
A work team composed of individuals from various functional specialties

other permanent work groups. Teams have the ability to quickly assemble, deploy, refocus, and disband. A **cross-functional team** is one of the various forms of departmentalization. Remember that it's a work team composed of individuals from various functional specialties. When a cross-functional team is formed, team members are brought together to collaborate on resolving mutual problems that affect the respective functional areas. Ideally, the artificial boundaries that separate functions disappear, and the team focuses on working together to achieve organizational goals. For instance, at ArcelorMittal, the world's biggest steel company, cross-functional teams of scientists, plant managers, and salespeople review and monitor product innovations.[31] The concept of cross-functional teams is being applied in health care, as we noted in the example at the beginning of this section. And, at Suburban Hospital in Bethesda, Maryland, intensive care unit (ICU) teams composed of a doctor trained in intensive care medicine, a pharmacist, a social worker, a nutritionist, the chief ICU nurse, a respiratory therapist, and a chaplain meet daily with every patient's bedside nurse to discuss and debate the best course of treatment. The hospital credits this team care approach with reducing errors, shortening the amount of time patients spent in ICU, and improving communication between families and the medical staff.[32]

task force (or ad hoc committee)
A temporary committee or team formed to tackle a specific short-term problem affecting several departments

TASK FORCES Another structural option organizations might use is a **task force** (also called an **ad hoc committee**), a temporary committee or team formed to tackle a specific short-term problem affecting several departments. The temporary nature of a task force is what differentiates it from a cross-functional team. Task force members usually perform many of their normal work tasks while serving on the task force; however, the members of a task force must collaborate to resolve the issue that's been assigned to them. When the issue or problem is solved, the task force is no longer needed and members return to their regular assignments. Many organizations, from government agencies to universities to businesses, use task forces. For instance, at San Francisco–based accounting firm Eichstaedt & Devereaux, employee task forces have helped develop formal recruiting, mentoring, and training programs. And at Frito-Lay, a subsidiary of PepsiCo, Inc., a task force that included members of the company's Hispanic employees' resource group helped in the development of two products: Lay's Cool Guacamole potato chips and Doritos Guacamole tortilla chips.[33]

communities of practice
Groups of people who share a concern, a set of problems, or a passion about a topic and who deepen their knowledge and expertise in that area by interacting on an ongoing basis

COMMUNITIES OF PRACTICE American soldiers training Afghan and Iraqi armies were having problems using a rocket-propelled grenade launcher. The frustrated unit commander posted a question to one of the U.S. Army's online forums where soldiers ask questions and share ideas with peers around the world. Within a few days, someone who had a similar experience with the launcher posted a simple solution on the Web site on how to safely prevent misfiring. Problem solved![34] Such types of internal collaborations are called **communities of practice**, which are "groups of people who share a concern, a set of problems, or a passion about a topic, and who deepen their knowledge and expertise in that area by interacting on an ongoing basis."[35] For example, repair technicians at Xerox share "war stories" to communicate their experiences and to help others solve difficult problems with repairing machines.[36] At pharmaceutical firm Pfizer, communities of practice are integrated into the company's formal structure. Called employee councils and networks, these communities share knowledge and help product development teams on difficult issues such as safety.[37] Pfizer's more structured approach to recognizing the value of such collaboration is becoming more common. But how effective are these communities of practice? Research studies have found that communities of practice can "create value by contributing to increased effectiveness in employees' job performance through greater access that they provide to the ideas, knowledge, and best practices shared among community members."[38] Exhibit 4 lists some suggestions for making such communities work.

- Have top management support and set clear expectations.
- Create an environment that will attract people and make them want to return for advice, conversation, and knowledge sharing.
- Encourage regular meetings of the community, whether in person or online.
- Establish regular communication among community members.
- Focus on real problems and issues important to the organization.
- Have clear accountability and managerial oversight.

Sources: Based on R. McDermott and D. Archibald, "Harnessing Your Staff's Informal Networks," *Harvard Business Review,* March 2010, pp. 82–89; S. F. Gale, "The Power of Community," *Workforce Management Online,* March 2009; and E. Wenger, R. McDermott, and W. Snyder, *Cultivating Communities of Practice: A Guide to Managing Knowledge* (Boston: Harvard Business School Press, 2002).

Exhibit 4
Making Communities of Practice Work

External Collaboration

Intuit has figured out a way to get its customers involved. Devoted users of QuickBooks can access a site—QuickBooks Live Community—and exchange helpful information with others. For customers, that often means faster answers to problems. And for the company, this "volunteer army" means less investment in paid technicians.[39] External collaboration efforts have become quite popular for organizations, especially in the area of product innovation. We're going to look at two forms of external collaboration: open innovation and strategic partnerships. Each of these can provide organizations with needed information, support, and contributions to getting work done and achieving organizational goals. But it's important that managers understand the challenges of how each might fit into the organization's structural design.

OPEN INNOVATION Frito Lay offered a cool $1 million to the winner of the company's contest for a new potato chip flavor. The winner was selected by a Facebook

let's get REAL

The Scenario:

Leann Breur is the human resources (HR) manager at a large grocery supply company that has locations in four Midwestern states and more than 800 employees. Leann's team, which includes all four locations, has 18 people. At the home office, she sees her staff being quite innovative in getting their work done, and she's certain the HR offices at the other offices have great ideas, too. How can Leann get her employees to share their knowledge with each other?

What advice would you give to Leann?

Leann should first work with her group to identify what has been successful for them and why. She should then set up weekly conference calls so teams at all locations can discuss best practices, success stories, and challenges. A shared network folder will allow all teams to exchange ideas and documents quickly and efficiently. Periodic conferences can be motivating and engaging, and can elevate relationships while improving the flow of ideas.

ToniAnn Petrella-Diaz
Retail Manager

Source: ToniAnn Petrella-Diaz

vote. Pharmaceutical giant GlaxoSmithKline PLC opened to the public the designs behind 13,500 chemical compounds associated with the parasite that causes malaria. Glaxo "hopes that sharing information and working together will lead scientists to come up with a drug for treating the mosquito-borne disease faster than the company could do on its own."[40]

The days may be numbered when businesses generate their own product development ideas and develop, manufacture, market, and deliver those products to customers. Today, many companies are trying **open innovation**, opening up the search for new ideas beyond the organization's boundaries and allowing innovations to easily transfer inward and outward. For instance, Procter & Gamble, Starbucks, Dell, Best Buy, and Nike have all created digital platforms that allow customers to help them create new products and messages.[41] As you can see, many of today's successful companies are collaborating directly with customers in the product development process. Others are partnering with suppliers, other outsiders, and even competitors. Exhibit 5 describes some of the benefits and drawbacks of open innovation.

STRATEGIC PARTNERSHIPS Companies worldwide are finding ways to connect to each other. Once bitter rivals, Nokia and Qualcomm formed a cooperative agreement to develop next-generation cell phones for North America. Nokia also collaborated with Microsoft in a partnership where Microsoft's software powers e-mail and chat services on most Nokia phones.[42]

In today's environment, organizations are looking for advantages wherever they can get them. One way they can do this is with **strategic partnerships**, collaborative relationships between two or more organizations in which they combine their resources and capabilities for some business purpose. Here are some reasons why such partnerships make sense: flexibility and informality of arrangements promote efficiencies, provide access to new markets and technologies, and entail less paperwork

open innovation
Opening up the search for new ideas beyond the organization's boundaries and allowing innovations to easily transfer inward and outward

strategic partnerships
Collaborative relationships between two or more organizations in which they combine their resources and capabilities for some business purpose

Exhibit 5
Benefits and Drawbacks of Open Innovation

Sources: Based on S. Lindegaard, "The Side Effects of Open Innovation," *Bloomberg BusinessWeek Online,* June 7, 2010; H. W. Chesbrough and A. R. Garman, "How Open Innovation Can Help You Cope in Lean Times," *Harvard Business Review,* December 2009, pp. 68–76; A. Gabor, "The Promise [and Perils] of Open Collaboration," *Strategy & Business Online,* Autumn 2009; and J. Winsor, "Crowdsourcing: What It Means for Innovation," *BusinessWeek Online,* June 15, 2009.

Benefits
- Gives customers what they want—a voice
- Allows organizations to respond to complex problems
- Nurtures internal and external relationships
- Brings focus back to marketplace
- Provides way to cope with rising costs and uncertainties of product development

Drawbacks
- High demands of managing the process
- Extensive support needed
- Cultural challengess
- Greater need for flexibility
- Crucial changes required in how knowledge is controlled and shared

when creating and disbanding projects; risks and expenses are shared by multiple parties; independent brand identification is kept and can be exploited; working with partners possessing multiple skills can create major synergies; rivals can often work together harmoniously; partnerships can take on varied forms from simple to complex; dozens of participants can be accommodated in partnership arrangements; and antitrust laws can protect R&D activities.[43] Strategic partnerships are growing in popularity. However, as with all the collaborative arrangements we've described—external and internal—the challenge for managers is finding ways to exploit the benefits of such collaboration while incorporating the collaborative efforts seamlessly into the organization's structural design.

FLEXIBLE Work Arrangements

LO3   Accenture consultant Keyur Patel's job arrangement is becoming the norm, rather than the exception.[44] During his recent consulting assignment, he had three clocks on his desk: one set to Manila time (where his software programmers were), one to Bangalore (where another programming support team worked), and the third for San Francisco, where he was spending four days a week helping a major retailer implement IT systems to track and improve sales. And his cell phone kept track of the time in Atlanta, his home, where he headed on Thursday evenings.

For this new breed of professionals, life is a blend of home and office, work and leisure. Thanks to technology, work can now be done anywhere, anytime. As organizations adapt their structural designs to these new realities, we see more of them adopting flexible working arrangements. Such arrangements not only exploit the power of technology, but give organizations the flexibility to deploy employees when and where needed. In this section, we're going to take a look at some different types of flexible work arrangements, including telecommuting and compressed workweeks, flextime, and job sharing. As with the other structural options we've looked at, managers must evaluate these types in light of the implications for decision making, communication, authority relationships, work task accomplishment, and so forth.

FedEx jobs involved in the physical transport of packages are not suitable for telecommuting. But in operating one of the world's largest telecommunications networks for recording and tracking shipments to more than 220 countries and territories, FedEx offers many computer-based jobs for telecommuters who help process more than 100 million electronic transactions every day.
Source: Russell Gordon/DanitaDelimont.com "Danita Delimont Photography"/Newscom

Telecommuting

Eve Gelb used to endure hour-and-a-half commutes morning and evening on the 405 freeway in Los Angeles to her job as a project manager at SCAN Health Plan.[45] Now, she's turned her garage into an office and works from home as a telecommuter. On the days when she does have to go in to the corporate office, she shares a space with her three subordinates who also work flexibly. Information technology has made telecommuting possible, and external environmental changes have made it necessary for many organizations. **Telecommuting** is a work arrangement in which employees work at home and are linked to the workplace by computer. Needless to say, not every job is a candidate for telecommuting, but many are.

Working from home used to be considered a "cushy perk" for a few lucky employees, and such an arrangement wasn't allowed very often. Now, many businesses view telecommuting as a business necessity. For instance, at SCAN Health Plan, the company's chief financial officer said that getting more employees to telecommute provided the company a way to grow without having to incur any additional fixed costs such as office buildings, equipment, or parking lots. In addition, some companies view the arrangement as a way to combat high gas prices and to attract talented employees who want more freedom and control over their work.

Despite its apparent appeal, many managers are reluctant to have their employees become "laptop hobos."[47] They argue that employees will waste time surfing the

telecommuting
A work arrangement in which employees work at home and are linked to the workplace by computer

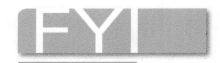

- 70 percent of employees say they would rather telecommute than work in their office.[46]

Internet or playing online games instead of working, that they'll ignore clients, and that they'll desperately miss the camaraderie and social exchanges of the workplace. In addition, managers wonder how they'll "manage" these employees. How do you interact with an employee and gain his or her trust when they're not physically present? And what if their work performance isn't up to par? How do you make suggestions for improvement? Another significant challenge is making sure that company information is kept safe and secure when employees are working from home.

Employees often express the same concerns about working remotely, especially when it comes to the isolation of not being "at work." At Accenture, where employees are scattered around the world, the chief human resources officer says it isn't easy to maintain that esprit de corps.[48] However, the company has put in place a number of programs and processes to create that sense of belonging for its workforce, including Web-conferencing tools, assigning each employee to a career counselor, and holding quarterly community events at its offices. In addition, the telecommuter employee may find that the line between work and home becomes even more blurred, which can be stressful.[49] Managers and organizations must address these important organizing issues as they move toward having employees telecommute.

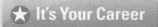 **It's Your Career**

Staying Connected Knowledge—If your instructor is using MyManagementLab, log onto **mymanagementlab.com** and test your *staying connected knowledge*. **Be sure to refer back to the chapter opener!**

let's get REAL

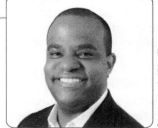

Source: Justin Kidwell

Justin Kidwell
Management Consultant

The Scenario:

Isabella Castillo, vice president of professional services at a consulting company that helps IT organizations deliver better service to their customers, needs help with her professional staff of 16 consultants, who all work from home. Her problem: dealing with the realities of telecommuting—lack of direct interaction, lack of camaraderie, feeling isolated and out-of-the-loop, etc. For their type of business, remote work makes good business sense, but how can she connect and engage her employees?

What advice would you give Isabella?

I would focus on a few things:

1. *Making people development a strategic goal*
2. *Semi-annual retreats*
3. *Leveraging technology*

Embedding people development into the performance measurement equation ensures interaction and teaming. The semiannual retreats provide a bonding environment and opportunity to gain buy-in to management priorities. Collaborative tools make phone only meetings obsolete.

So, once an organization decides that it wants to establish telecommuting opportunities for employees, what needs to happen next? One of the first issues to address is encouraging employees to make that decision to become remote workers. For instance, at SCAN Health Plan, the company offered free high-speed Internet access and free office furniture, along with help in setting it up, to encourage more of its workforce to work from home. Other companies have encouraged employees to work anywhere but at the office by pointing to the pay "increase" employees would receive from money saved on gas, dry cleaning, and eating out at lunch. Other companies have used the "green" angle, emphasizing the carbon-free aspect of not driving long distances to and from the workplace. Managing the telecommuters then becomes a matter of keeping employees feeling like they're connected and engaged—a topic we delve into at the end of the chapter as we look at today's organizational design challenges.

Compressed Workweeks, Flextime, and Job Sharing

During the global economic crisis in the United Kingdom, accounting firm KPMG needed to reduce costs. It decided to use flexible work options as a way of doing so. The company's program, called Flexible Futures, offered employees four options to choose from: a four-day workweek with a 20 percent salary reduction; a two- to twelve-week sabbatical at 30 percent of pay; both options; or continue with their regular schedule. Some 85 percent of the U.K. employees agreed to the reduced-workweek plan. "Since so many people agreed to the flexible work plans, KPMG was able to cap the salary cut at about 10 percent for the year in most cases." The best thing, though, was that as a result of the plan, KPMG didn't have to do large-scale employee layoffs.[50]

As this example shows, organizations may sometimes find they need to restructure work using forms of flexible work arrangements. One approach is a **compressed workweek**, a workweek where employees work longer hours per day but fewer days per week. The most common arrangement is four 10-hour days (a 4–40 program). For example, in Utah, state employees have a mandated (by law) four-day workweek, with offices closed on Fridays in an effort to reduce energy costs. After a year's time, the state found that its compressed workweek resulted in a 13 percent reduction in energy use and estimated that state employees saved as much as $6 million in gasoline costs.[51] Another alternative is **flextime** (also known as **flexible work hours**), a scheduling system in which employees are required to work a specific number of hours a week but are free to vary those hours within certain limits. A flextime schedule typically designates certain common core hours when all employees are required to be on the job, but allows starting, ending, and lunch-hour times to be flexible. According to a survey of companies by the Families and Work Institute, 81 percent of the respondents now offer flextime benefits. Another survey by Watson Wyatt of mid- and large-sized companies found that a flexible work schedule was the most commonly offered benefit.[52]

In Great Britain, McDonald's experimented with an unusual program—dubbed the Family Contract—to reduce absenteeism and turnover at some of its restaurants. Under this Family Contract, employees from the same immediate family can fill in for one another for any work shift without having to clear it first with their manager.[53] This type of job scheduling is called **job sharing**—the practice of having two or more people split a full-time job. Although something like McDonald's Family Contract may be appropriate for a low-skilled job, other organizations might offer job sharing to professionals who want to work but don't want the demands and hassles of a full-time position. For instance, at Ernst & Young, employees in many of the company's

compressed workweek
A workweek where employees work longer hours per day but fewer days per week

flextime (or flexible work hours)
A scheduling system in which employees are required to work a specific number of hours a week but are free to vary those hours within certain limits

job sharing
The practice of having two or more people split a full-time job

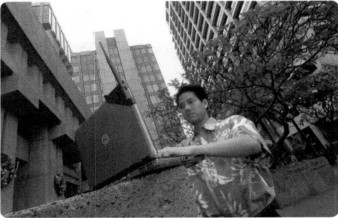

Flexible work arrangements that allow employees to schedule their jobs around life events are part of the "People First" culture at accounting firm Ernst & Young. The EY advanced security operations employee in this photo may choose from initiatives such as day to-day work hour flexibility, compressed workweeks, job sharing, and reduced work-hour schedules.
Source: The Honolulu Advertiser, Bruce Asato/ Associated Press

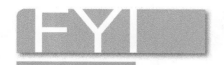

contingent workers
Temporary, freelance, or contract workers whose employment is contingent on demand for their services

locations can choose from a variety of flexible work arrangements, including job sharing. Also, many companies have used job sharing during the economic downturn to avoid employee layoffs.[54]

CONTINGENT Workforce

LO4   At Conrad & Co., a small private accounting firm in Spartanburg, South Carolina, Diana Galvin started as a temporary, part-time employee before moving into a full-time staff accountant position. She got her full-time job by learning how to do and then doing her assignments well and offering suggestions on how the company could improve.[56] But not every temporary worker gets offered a full-time job (or wants to be offered one). Prior to her full-time employment, Diana was part of what has been called the contingent workforce. **Contingent workers** are temporary, freelance, or contract workers whose employment is *contingent* on demand for their services. Some are now referring to these workers as the *independent* work force, since there's no dependent relationship between worker and organization.[57]

"Companies are starting to rethink the way they get work done."[58] As full-time jobs are eliminated through downsizing and other organizational restructurings, managers often rely on a contingent workforce to fill in as needed. One of the top-ranking forecasts in a survey that asked HR experts to look ahead to 2018 was that "Firms will become adept at sourcing and engaging transient talent around short-term needs, and will focus considerable energy on the long-term retention of smaller core talent groups."[59] The model for the contingent worker structural approach can be seen in the film industry. There, people are essentially "free agents" who move from project to project applying their skills—directing, talent casting, costuming, makeup, set design, and so forth—as needed. They assemble for a movie, then disband once it's finished and move on to the next project. This type of contingent worker is common in project organizations. But contingent workers can also be temporary employees brought in to help with special needs such as seasonal work. Let's look at some of the organizational issues associated with contingent workers.

One of the main issues businesses face with their contingent workers, especially those who are independent contractors or freelancers, is classifying who actually qualifies as one.[60] The decision on who is and who isn't an independent contractor isn't as easy or as unimportant as it may seem. Companies don't have to pay Social Security, Medicare, or unemployment insurance taxes on workers classified as independent contractors. And those individuals also aren't covered by most workplace laws. So it's an important decision. For instance, FedEx treats some 12,000 of its package deliverers in its FedEx Ground Division as contractors. Their classification of these workers as independent contractors has caused battles with the Internal Revenue Service and state governments and riled competitor UPS, whose drivers are unionized employees and argues that FedEx's policy is "unfair to taxpayers, competitors, and the workers themselves."[61] The federal government is also looking at increased power to penalize employers that misclassify workers. So, there is an incentive to be totally above board in classifying who is and who is not an independent contractor. The legal definition of a contract worker depends on how much control a company has over the person; that is, does the company control what the worker does and how the worker does his or her job? When a company has more control, the individual is more likely to be considered an employee, not an independent contractor. And it isn't just the legal/tax issues that are important in how workers are classified. The structural implications, especially in terms of getting work done and how performance problems are resolved, are important as well.

Another issue with contingent workers is the process for recruiting, screening, and placing these contingent workers where their work skills and efforts are needed.[62] These important steps help ensure that the right people are in the right places at the right times in order to get work done efficiently and effectively. Any organization that wants to minimize potential problems with its contingent workers needs to pay attention to hiring.

The final issue we want to look at is the importance of a contingent employee's performance. Just like a regular employee, a contingent employee is brought on board to do some specific work task(s). It's important that managers have a method of establishing goals, schedules, and deadlines with the contingent employees.[63] And it's also important that mechanisms be in place to monitor work performance and goal achievement, especially if the contingent employee is working off-site.

If your professor has assigned this, go to **www.mymanagementlab.com** to complete the Writing Assignment MGMT 2: Organizational Structures.

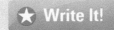

★ Write It!

TODAY'S Organizational Design Challenges

L05 As managers look for organizational designs that will best support and facilitate employees doing their work efficiently and effectively, they must contend with certain challenges. These challenges include keeping employees connected and managing global structural issues.

Keeping Employees Connected

Many organizational design concepts were developed during the twentieth century, when work was done at an employer's place of business under a manager's supervision, work tasks were fairly predictable and constant, and most jobs were full-time and continued indefinitely.[65] But that's not the way it is today at many companies. For instance, thousands of Cisco Systems employees sit at unassigned desks in team rooms interspersed with communal break areas. At some IBM divisions, only a small percentage of employees—mostly top managers and their assistants—have fixed desks or offices. All others are either mobile employees or they share desks when they need to be at work. At Sabre Holdings, teams are assigned to neighborhoods of workspaces and employees find places for themselves when they arrive.[66]

As these examples show, a major structural design challenge for managers is finding a way to offer flexibility while also keeping widely dispersed and mobile employees connected to the organization. Mobile computing and communication technology have given organizations and employees ways to stay connected and to be more productive. For instance, handheld devices have e-mail, calendars, and contacts that can be used anywhere there's a wireless network. And these devices can be used to log into corporate databases and company intranets. Employees can videoconference using broadband networks and Webcams. Many companies are giving employees key fobs with constantly changing encryption codes that allow them to log onto the corporate network to access e-mail and company data from any computer hooked up to the Internet. Cell phones switch seamlessly between cellular networks and corporate Wi-Fi connections. The biggest

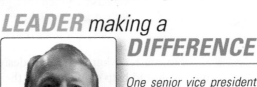

LEADER making a DIFFERENCE

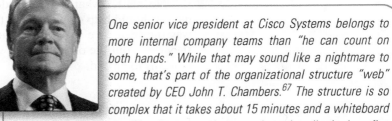

Source: Daniel Barry/Newscom

One senior vice president at Cisco Systems belongs to more internal company teams than "he can count on both hands." While that may sound like a nightmare to some, that's part of the organizational structure "web" created by CEO John T. Chambers.[67] The structure is so complex that it takes about 15 minutes and a whiteboard to explain it. However, Chambers uses three words to describe its benefits: "speed, skill, and flexibility." His idea for the company's structure originated at the end of the 2001 downturn after Cisco wrote off some $2.2 billion in losses. Chambers realized that the "company's hierarchical structure precluded it from moving quickly into new markets." So he began grouping executives into cross-functional teams figuring that this would help break down traditional silos and lead to faster decision making. At first, the executives didn't like it. Some couldn't handle working with unfamiliar colleagues; others were upset with the new team-based compensation structure. However, the company's decision making has accelerated—it took executives only eight days to figure out that it made sense to acquire Web-conferencing company WebEx. And as the chaotic tech industry continues to evolve, it's important for Chambers's organization to stay on top of things, and its structural arrangement contributes to being able to do that. What can you learn from this leader making a difference?

issue in doing work anywhere, anytime, however, is security. Companies must protect their important and sensitive information. Fortunately, software and other disabling devices have minimized security issues considerably. Even insurance providers are more comfortable giving their mobile employees access to information. For instance, Health Net Inc. gave BlackBerry phones to many of its managers so they can tap into customer records from anywhere.

Managing Global Structural Issues

Are there global differences in organizational structures? Are Australian organizations structured like those in the United States? Are German organizations structured like those in France or Mexico? Given the global nature of today's business environment, managers need to be familiar with this issue. Researchers have concluded that the structures and strategies of organizations worldwide are similar, "while the behavior within them is maintaining its cultural uniqueness."[68] What does this distinction between strategy and culture mean for designing effective and efficient structures? When designing or changing structure, managers may need to think about the cultural implications of certain design elements. For instance, one study showed that formalization—rules and bureaucratic mechanisms—may be more important in less economically developed countries and less important in more economically developed countries where employees may have higher levels of professional education and skills.[69] Another study found that organizations with people from high power-distance countries (such as Greece, France, and most of Latin America) find that their employees are much more accepting of mechanistic structures than are employees from low power-distance countries. Other structural design elements may be affected by cultural differences as well.

★ Watch It 2! If your professor has assigned this, go to **www.mymanagementlab.com** to watch a video titled: *CH2MHill: Adaptive Organizational Design* and to respond to questions.

No matter what structural design managers choose for their organizations, the design should help employees do their work in the best—most efficient and effective— way they can. The structure should support and facilitate organizational members as they carry out the organization's work. After all, an organization's structure is simply a means to an end.

PREPARING FOR: Exams/Quizzes

CHAPTER SUMMARY by Learning Objectives

LO1 — DESCRIBE **contemporary organizational designs.**

In a team structure, the entire organization is made up of work teams. The matrix structure assigns specialists from different functional departments to work on one or more projects being led by project managers. A project structure is one in which employees continuously work on projects. A virtual organization consists of a small core of full-time employees and outside specialists temporarily hired as needed to work on projects. A network organization is an organization that uses its own employees to do some work activities and networks of outside suppliers to provide other needed product components or work processes. A learning organization is one that has developed the capacity to continuously learn, adapt, and change. It has certain structural characteristics, including an emphasis on sharing information and collaborating on work activities, minimal structural and physical barriers, and empowered work teams.

LO2 — DISCUSS **how organizations organize for collaboration.**

An organization's collaboration efforts can be internal or external. Internal collaborative structural options include cross-functional teams, task forces, and communities of practice. A cross-functional team is a work team composed of individuals from various functional specialties. A task force is a temporary committee or team formed to tackle a specific short-term problem affecting several departments. Communities of practice are groups of people who share a concern, a set of problems, or a passion about a topic and who deepen their knowledge and expertise in that area by interacting on an ongoing basis. External collaborative options include open innovation and strategic partnerships. Open innovation expands the search for new ideas beyond the organization's boundaries and allows innovations to easily transfer inward and outward. Strategic partnerships are collaborative relationships between two or more organizations in which they combine resources and capabilities for some business purpose.

LO3 — EXPLAIN **flexible work arrangements used by organizations.**

Flexible work arrangements give organizations the flexibility to deploy employees when and where they're needed. Structural options include telecommuting, compressed workweeks, flextime, and job sharing. Telecommuting is a work arrangement in which employees work at home and are linked to the workplace by computer. A compressed workweek is one in which employees work longer hours per day but fewer days per week. Flextime is a scheduling system in which employees are required to work a specific number of hours a week but are free to vary those hours within certain limits. Job sharing is when two or more people split a full-time job.

LO4 — DISCUSS **organizing issues associated with a contingent workforce.**

Contingent workers are temporary, freelance, or contract workers whose employment is contingent on demand for their services. Organizing issues include classifying who actually qualifies as an independent contractor; setting up a process for recruiting, screening, and placing contingent workers; and having a method in place for establishing goals, schedules, and deadlines and for monitoring work performance.

LO5 — DESCRIBE **today's organizational design challenges.**

The two main organizational design challenges for today include keeping employees connected and managing global structural issues.

MyManagementLab

Go to **mymanagementlab.com** to complete the problems marked with this icon ✪.

✪ REVIEW AND DISCUSSION QUESTIONS

1. Describe the four contemporary organizational designs. How are they similar? Different?

2. Differentiate between matrix and project structures.

3. How can an organization operate without boundaries?

4. What types of skills would a manager need to effectively work in a project structure? In a boundaryless organization? In a learning organization?

5. How does each of the different types of collaboration (both internal and external)

contribute to more coordinated and integrated work efforts?

6. What structural issues might arise in managing employees' flexible work arrangements? Think about what you've learned about organizational design. How might that information help a manager address those issues?

7. Does the idea of a flexible work arrangement appeal to you? Why or why not?

8. Why is it a challenge to "keep employees connected" in today's organizations?

MyManagementLab

If your professor has assigned these, go to **mymanagementlab.com** for Auto-graded writing questions as well as the following Assisted-graded writing questions:

9. The boundaryless organization has the potential to create a major shift in the way we work. Do you agree or disagree? Explain.

10. What structural issues might arise in managing employees' flexible work arrangements? Think about what you've learned about organizational design. How might that information help a manager address those issues?

PREPARING FOR: My Career

✪ PERSONAL INVENTORY ASSESSMENTS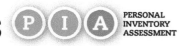

Organizational Structure Assessment

As this text described, there are many different approaches to designing organizational structure. What type of structure appeals to you? Take this PIA and find out.

⭐ ETHICS DILEMMA

"Ethical hacking." It's probably an understatement to say that people were excited about the introduction of Apple's iPad.[70] Then the news broke that a small group of computer experts calling themselves Goatse Security had hacked into AT&T's Web site and found numbers that identified iPads connected to AT&T's mobile network. Those numbers allowed the group to uncover 114,000 e-mail addresses of thousands of first-adopter iPad customers, including prominent officials in companies, politics, and the military. AT&T called it an act of malice, condemned the hackers, and apologized to its affected customers. The group that exposed the flaw said that it did a "public service."

One analyst for CNET also said that the group did a good thing. "Security researchers often disclose holes to keep vendors honest. Many sources complain that they notify companies of security vulnerabilities and that the companies take months, or even years, to provide a fix to customers. In the meantime, malicious hackers may have discovered the same hole and may be using it to steal data, infect computers, or attack systems without the computer owner knowing there is even a risk."[71]

11. What do you think? Is there such a thing as "ethical hacking?"

12. What ethical issues do you see here? What are the implications for various stakeholders in this situation?

SKILLS EXERCISE Developing Your Acquiring Power Skill

About the Skill

Power is a natural process in any group or organization, and to perform their jobs effectively, managers need to know how to acquire and use power.[72] Why is having power important? Because power makes you less dependent on others. When a manager has power, he or she is not as dependent on others for critical resources. And if the resources a manager controls are important, scarce, and nonsubstitutable, her power will increase because others will be more dependent on her for those resources.

Steps in Practicing the Skill

You can be more effective at acquiring and using power if you use the following eight behaviors.

- *Frame arguments in terms of organizational goals.* To be effective at acquiring power means camouflaging your self-interests. Discussions over who controls what resources should be framed in terms of the benefits that will accrue to the organization; do not point out how you personally will benefit.

- *Develop the right image.* If you know your organization's culture, you already understand what the organization wants and values from its employees in terms of dress, associates to cultivate and those to avoid, whether to appear risk taking or risk aversive, the preferred leadership style, the importance placed on getting along well with others, and so forth. With this knowledge, you're equipped to project the appropriate image. Because

the assessment of your performance isn't always a fully objective process, you need to pay attention to style as well as substance.

- *Gain control of organizational resources.* Controlling organizational resources that are scarce *and* important is a source of power. Knowledge and expertise are particularly effective resources to control. They make you more valuable to the organization and therefore more likely to have job security, chances for advancement, and a receptive audience for your ideas.

- *Make yourself appear indispensable.* Because we're dealing with appearances rather than objective facts, you can enhance your power by appearing to be indispensable. You don't really have *to be* indispensable, as long as key people in the organization believe that you are.

- *Be visible.* If you have a job that brings your accomplishments to the attention of others, that's great. However, if you don't have such a job, you'll want to find ways to let others in the organization know what you're doing by highlighting successes in routine reports, having satisfied customers relay their appreciation to senior executives, being seen at social functions, being active in your professional associations, and developing powerful allies who speak positively about your accomplishments. Of course, you'll want to be on the lookout for those projects that will increase your visibility.

- *Develop powerful allies.* To get power, it helps to have powerful people on your side. Cultivate contacts with potentially influential people above you, at your own level, and at lower organizational levels. These allies often can provide you with information that's otherwise not readily available. In addition, having allies can provide you with a coalition of support—if and when you need it.

- *Avoid "tainted" members.* In almost every organization, there are fringe members whose status is questionable. Their performance and/or loyalty may be suspect. Keep your distance from such individuals.

- *Support your boss.* Your immediate future is in the hands of your current boss. Because he or she evaluates your performance, you'll typically want to do whatever is necessary to have your boss on your side. You should make every effort to help your boss succeed, make her look good, support her if she is under siege, and spend the time to find out the criteria she will use to assess your effectiveness. Don't undermine your boss. And don't speak negatively of her to others.

Practicing the Skill

The following suggestions are activities you can do to practice the behaviors associated with acquiring power.

1. Keep a one-week journal of your behavior describing incidences when you tried to influence others around you. Assess each incident by asking: Were you successful at these attempts to influence them? Why or why not? What could you have done differently?

2. Review recent issues of a business periodical (such as *Bloomberg BusinessWeek, Fortune, Forbes, Fast Company, Industry Week,* or the *Wall Street Journal*). Look for articles on reorganizations, promotions, or departures from management positions. Find at least two articles where you believe power issues are involved. Relate the content of the articles to the concepts introduced in this skill module.

WORKING TOGETHER Team Exercise

A company's future may well depend on how well it's able to learn.

Form small groups of three to four individuals. Your team's "job" is to find some current information on learning organizations. You'll probably be able to find numerous articles about the topic, but limit your report to five of what you consider to be the best sources of information on the topic. Using this information, write a one-page bulleted list discussing your reactions to the statement set in bold at the beginning of this exercise. Be sure to include bibliographic information for your five chosen articles at the end of your one-page bulleted list.

MY TURN TO BE A MANAGER

- Since you may be a telecommuter sometime during your career (or may manage employees who are telecommuters), do some research on tips for making telecommuting work.

- Find the most current list of *Fortune*'s Best Companies to Work For (usually published in early February). Look through the list, and tally how many of the top 50 provide some type of flexible work arrangements for their employees and the type of flexible work arrangements they use.

- Using current business periodicals, do some research on open innovation efforts by companies. Choose three examples of businesses using this and describe and evaluate what each is doing.

- Create a chart describing each adaptive organizational design discussed in this text along with what you perceive as potential advantages and disadvantages of each.

- In your own words, write down three things you learned in this text about being a good manager. Keep a copy of this for future reference.

CASE APPLICATION 1 You Work Where?

Where IS work done most efficiently and effectively? Yahoo!, a pioneer in Web search and navigation, struggles to remain relevant in the face of competition from the likes of Google, Facebook, and Twitter.[73] It missed the two biggest Internet trends—social networking and mobile. However, in July 2012, after the company did its own search, it snagged a gem as the company's new CEO—Marissa Mayer, one of Goggle's top executives. Mayer had been one of the few public faces of Google and was responsible for the look and feel of Google's most popular products. Guiding Yahoo! as it tries to regain its former prominence is proving to be the challenge that experts predicted, but they're also saying that if anyone could take on the challenge of making Yahoo! an innovator once again, Mayer is the person.

Two of her initial decisions included free food at the office and new smartphones for every employee, something that Google does. However, in early 2013, Mayer launched an employee initiative that generated lots of discussion—positive and negative. She decided that as of mid-2013, Yahoo! employees who worked remotely had to come back to the office. The memo from the vice president of people and development (code for head of Human Resources) clarified that the new initiative was a response to productivity issues that often arise when employees work from home. With a new boss and a renewed commitment to making Yahoo! a strong company in a challenging industry, employees were expected to be physically present in the workplace, hopefully leading to developing a strong common bond and greater productivity. The announcement affected not only those who worked from home full time—mainly customer service reps—but also those employees who had arranged to work from home one or two days a week. Yahoo! isn't the only company asking remote workers to return. Bank of America, which had a popular remote work program, decided late in 2012 that employees in certain roles had to come back to the office. And Best Buy Co. recently cut its longtime telecommuting program.

Before Mayer became CEO at Yahoo!, it's a wonder anything ever got done. What she found wasn't even remotely like the way employees functioned at Google. At Yahoo!, few people were physically at work in the office cubicles throughout the building. Few cars or bikes or other vehicles could be found in the facility's parking lots. Even more disturbing, some of the employees who *were* physically present did as little work as needed and then took off early. She also discovered that other employees who worked from home did little but collect a paycheck or maybe worked on a sideline business they had started. Even at the office, one former manager described morale as low as it could be because employees thought the company was failing—that they were on a sinking ship. These were some of the reasons that Mayer abolished Yahoo!'s work-from-home policy. If Yahoo! was to again become the nimble company it had once been, a new culture of innovation, communication, and collaboration was needed. And that meant employees had to be at work—physically at work, together. Restoring Yahoo!'s "cool" factor—from its products to its deteriorating morale and culture—would be difficult if the organization's people weren't there. That's why Mayer's decision created such an uproar. Yahoo!'s only official statement on the new policy said, "This isn't a broad industry view on working from home. This is about what is right for Yahoo!, right now" (Yahoo! Press Release, February 26, 2013).

Where work is done most efficiently and effectively—office, home, combination—is an important workplace issue. The three main managerial concerns are productivity, innovation, and collaboration. Do flexible arrangements lead to greater productivity or inhibit innovation and collaboration? Another concern is that employees, especially younger ones, expect to be able to work remotely. Yes, the trend has been toward greater workplace flexibility, but does that flexibility lead to a bloated, lazy, and unproductive remote workforce? These are the challenges of designing organizational structures.

⭐ **DISCUSSION QUESTIONS**

13. Evaluate Yahoo!'s new work initiative. Did it have to be an "all or nothing" proposition? Discuss.

14. What can managers and organizations do to help employees who work from home be efficient and productive?

15. Take the three main concerns—productivity, innovation, and collaboration. From the perspective of management, how do you think flexible arrangements stack up? How about from the employee's perspective?

16. Is face time (that is, showing up at work to be seen by your boss and others) critical to one's career? Discuss.

17. Is being able to work remotely important to you? Why or why not?

CASE APPLICATION 2 Organizational Volunteers

They're individuals you might never have thought of as being part of an organization's structure, but for many organizations, volunteers provide a much-needed source of labor.[74] Maybe you've volunteered at a Habitat for Humanity build, a homeless shelter, or some nonprofit organization. However, what if the volunteer assignment was at a for-profit business and the job description read like this: "Spend a few hours a day at your computer, supplying answers online to customer questions about technical matters like how to set up an Internet home network or how to program a new high-definition television," all for no pay. Many large corporations, start-up companies, and venture capitalists are betting that this "emerging corps of Web-savvy helpers will transform the field of customer service."

Self check-outs. Self check-ins. Self order-placing. Pumping your own gas (although most of you are probably too young to remember having an attendant that pumped your gas, checked your oil, and washed your windshield). Filling out online forms. Businesses have become very good at getting customers to do free work. Now, they're taking the concept even further, especially in customer service settings, by getting "volunteers" to perform specialized work tasks.

The role that these volunteer "enthusiasts" have played, especially in contributing innovations to research and development efforts, has been closely researched in recent years. For example, case studies highlight the product tweaks made by early skateboarders and mountain bikers to their gear. Researchers have also studied the programmers behind open-source software like the Linux operating system. It seems that individuals who do this type of "volunteering" are motivated mainly by a payoff in enjoyment and respect among their peers and to some extent the skills they're able to develop. Now, as the concept of individuals volunteering for work tasks moves to the realm of customer service, can it work and what does it mean for managers?

For instance, at Verizon's high-speed fiber optic Internet, television, and telephone service, "volunteers" are answering customer questions about technical matters on a company-sponsored customer-service Web site for no pay. Mark Studness, director of Verizon's e-commerce unit, was familiar with sites where users offered tips and answered questions. His challenge? Find a way to use that potential resource for customer service. His solution? "Super," or lead, users—that is, users who provided the best answers and dialogue in Web forums.

The experiment at Verizon seems to be working well and these online "volunteers" can be an important addition to a company's customer service efforts. Studness says that creating an atmosphere that these super users find desirable is a key consideration because without that, you have nothing. A company that worked with Verizon to set up its structure said that these super or lead users are driven by the same online challenges and aspects as fervent gamers are. So they set up the structure with an elaborate rating system for contributors with ranks, badges, and "kudos counts." So far, Studness is happy with how it's gone. He says the company-sponsored customer-service site has been extremely useful and cost efficient in redirecting thousands of questions that would have been answered by staff at a Verizon call center.

⭐ DISCUSSION QUESTIONS

18. What do you think about using "volunteers" to do work that other people get paid to do?

19. If you were in Mark Studness's position, what would you be most concerned about in this arrangement? How would you "manage" that concern?

20. How do these "volunteers" fit into an organization's structure? Take each of the six elements of organizational design and discuss how each would affect this structural approach.

21. Do you think this approach could work for other types of work being done or in other types of organizations? Explain.

ENDNOTES

1. A. R. Carey and P. Trap, "Fewer Hours at the Office," *USA Today,* October 17, 2013, p. 1A.

2. "The Simple List," *Real Simple,* September 2013, p. 14.

3. Ibid.

4. V. Wong, "Sending Employees Out to Starbucks—And Telling Them to Stay," *Bloomberg BusinessWeek Online,* October 7, 2013.

5. V. Wong, "More Kiosks, Fewer Cashiers Coming Soon to Panera," *Bloomberg BusinessWeek Online,* May 2, 2014.

6. Q. Hardy, "Google Thinks Small," *Forbes,* November 14, 2005, pp. 198–202.

7. See, for example, A. C. Edmondson, "Teamwork On the Fly," *Harvard Business Review,* April 2012, pp. 72–80; D. R. Denison, S. L. Hart, and J. A. Kahn, "From Chimneys to Cross-Functional Teams: Developing and Validating a Diagnostic Model," *Academy of Management Journal,* December 1996, pp. 1005–1023; D. Ray and H. Bronstein, *Teaming Up: Making the Transition to a Self-Directed Team-Based Organization* (New York: McGraw Hill, 1995); J. R. Katzenbach and D. K. Smith, *The Wisdom of Teams* (Boston: Harvard Business School Press, 1993); J. A. Byrne, "The Horizontal Corporation," *BusinessWeek,* December 20, 1993, pp. 76–81; B. Dumaine, "Payoff from the New Management," *Fortune,* December 13, 1993, pp. 103–110; and H. Rothman, "The Power of Empowerment," *Nation's Business,* June 1993, pp. 49–52.

8. E. Krell, "Managing the Matrix," *HR Magazine,* April 2011, pp. 69–71.

9. J. Hyatt, "Engineering Inspiration," *Newsweek,* June 14, 2010, p. 44; T. McKeough, "Blowing Hot and Cold," *Fast Company,* December 2009–January 2010, p. 66; H. Walters, "Inside the Design Thinking Process," *BusinessWeek Online,* December 15, 2009; P. Kaihla, "Best-Kept Secrets of the World's Best Companies," *Business 2.0,* April 2006, p. 83; C. Taylor, "School of Bright Ideas," *Time Inside Business,* April 2005, pp. A8–A12; and B. Nussbaum, "The Power of Design," *BusinessWeek,* May 17, 2004, pp. 86–94.

10. R. L. Hotz, "More Scientists Treat Experiments as a Team Sport," *Wall Street Journal,* November 20, 2009, p. A23.

11. See, for example, G. G. Dess, A. M. A. Rasheed, K. J. McLaughlin, and R. L. Priem, "The New Corporate Architecture," *Academy of Management Executive,* August 1995, pp. 7–20.

12. For additional readings on boundaryless organizations, see Rausch and Birkinshaw, June 2008; M. F. R. Kets de Vries, "Leadership Group Coaching in Action: The Zen of Creating High-Performance Teams," *Academy of Management Executive,* February 2005, pp. 61–76; J. Child and R. G. McGrath, "Organizations Unfettered: Organizational Form in an Information-Intensive Economy," *Academy of Management Journal,* December 2001, pp. 1135–1148; M. Hammer and S. Stanton, "How Process Enterprises Really Work," *Harvard Business Review,* November–December 1999, pp. 108–118; T. Zenger and W. Hesterly, "The Disaggregation of Corporations: Selective Intervention, High-Powered Incentives, and Modular Units," *Organization Science,* 1997, vol. 8, pp. 209–222; R. Ashkenas, D. Ulrich, T. Jick, and S. Kerr, *The Boundaryless Organization: Breaking the Chains of Organizational Structure* (San Francisco: Jossey-Bass, 1997); R. M. Hodgetts, "A Conversation with Steve Kerr," *Organizational Dynamics,* Spring 1996, pp. 68–79; and J. Gebhardt, "The Boundaryless Organization," *Sloan Management Review,* Winter 1996, pp. 117–119. For another view of boundaryless organizations, see B. Victor, "The Dark Side of the New Organizational Forms: An Editorial Essay," *Organization Science,* November 1994, pp. 479–482.

13. J. Marte, "An Internship from Your Couch," *Wall Street Journal,* September 9, 2009, pp. D1+.

14. J. Yang and A. Gonzalez, "If Given A Choice, I'd Rather Work ..." *USA Today,* January 22, 2013, p. 1B.

15. See, for instance, R. J. King, "It's a Virtual World," *Strategy+Business* [www.strategy-business.com], April 21, 2009; Y. Shin, "A Person-Environment Fit Model for Virtual Organizations," *Journal of Management,* December 2004, pp. 725–743; D. Lyons, "Smart and Smarter," *Forbes,* March 18, 2002, pp. 40–41; W. F. Cascio, "Managing a Virtual Workplace," *Academy of Management Executive,* August 2000, pp. 81–90; G. G. Dess, A. M. A. Rasheed, K. J. McLaughlin, and R. L. Priem,

"The New Corporate Architecture"; H. Chesbrough and D. Teece, "When Is Virtual Virtuous: Organizing for Innovation," *Harvard Business Review,* January–February 1996, pp. 65–73; and W. H. Davidow and M. S. Malone, *The Virtual Corporation* (New York: Harper Collins, 1992).

16. Q. Hardy, "Bit by Bit, Work Exchange Site Aims to Get Jobs Done," *New York Times Online,* November 6, 2011.

17. M. V. Rafter, "Cultivating A Virtual Culture," *Workforce Management Online,* April 5, 2012.

18. R. Reisner, "A Smart Balance of Staff and Contractors," *BusinessWeek Online,* June 16, 2009; and J. S. Lublin, "Smart Balance Keeps Tight Focus on Creativity," *Wall Street Journal,* June 8, 2009, p. B4.

19. R. Merrifield, J. Calhoun, and D. Stevens, "The Next Revolution in Productivity," *Harvard Business Review,* June 2008, pp. 73–80; R. E. Miles et al., "Organizing in the Knowledge Age: Anticipating the Cellular Form," *Academy of Management Executive,* November 1997, pp. 7–24; C. Jones, W. Hesterly, and S. Borgatti, "A General Theory of Network Governance: Exchange Conditions and Social Mechanisms," *Academy of Management Review,* October 1997, pp. 911–945; R. E. Miles and C. C. Snow, "The New Network Firm: A Spherical Structure Built on Human Investment Philosophy," *Organizational Dynamics,* Spring 1995, pp. 5–18; and R. E. Miles and C. C. Snow, "Causes of Failures in Network Organizations," *California Management Review,* 1992, vol. 34, no. 4, pp. 53–72.

20. G. Hoetker, "Do Modular Products Lead to Modular Organizations?" *Strategic Management Journal,* June 2006, pp. 501–518; C. H. Fine, "Are You Modular or Integral?" *Strategy & Business,* Summer 2005, pp. 44–51; D. A. Ketchen, Jr. and G. T. M. Hult, "To Be Modular or Not to Be? Some Answers to the Question," *Academy of Management Executive,* May 2002, pp. 166–167; M. A. Schilling, "The Use of Modular Organizational Forms: An Industry-Level Analysis," *Academy of Management Journal,* December 2001, pp. 1149–1168; D. Lei, M. A. Hitt, and J. D. Goldhar, "Advanced Manufacturing Technology: Organizational Design and Strategic Flexibility," *Organization Studies,* 1996, vol. 17, pp. 501–523; R. Sanchez and J. Mahoney, "Modularity Flexibility and Knowledge Management in Product and Organization Design," *Strategic Management Journal,* 1996, vol. 17, pp. 63–76; and R. Sanchez, "Strategic Flexibility in Product Competition," *Strategic Management Journal,* 1995, vol. 16, pp. 135–159.

21. J. Fortt, "The Chip Company That Dares to Battle Intel," *Fortune,* July 20, 2009, pp. 51–56.

22. C. Hymowitz, "Have Advice, Will Travel," *Wall Street Journal,* June 5, 2006, pp. B1+.

23. S. Reed, A. Reinhardt, and A. Sains, "Saving Ericsson," *BusinessWeek,* November 11, 2002, pp. 64–68.

24. P. Engardio, "The Future of Outsourcing," *BusinessWeek,* January 30, 2006, pp. 50–58.

25. P. Sonne, "Tesco's CEO-to-Be Unfolds Map for Global Expansion," *Wall Street Journal,* June 9, 2010, p. B1; T. Shifrin, "Grocery Giant Tesco Is Creating a Storm in the US Market with Its Tesco in a Box Set of Systems," [www.computerworlduk.com], January 14, 2008; P. Olson, "Tesco's Landing," *Forbes,* June 4, 2007, pp. 116–118; and P. M. Senge, *The Fifth Discipline: The Art and Practice of Learning Organizations* (New York: Doubleday, 1990).

26. J. J. Salopek, "Keeping Learning Well-Oiled," *T&D,* October 2011, pp. 32–35.

27. A. C. Edmondson, "The Competitive Imperative of Learning," *Harvard Business Review,* July–August 2008, pp. 60–67.

28. S. A. Sackmann, P. M. Eggenhofer-Rehart, and M. Friesl, "Long-Term Efforts Toward Developing a Learning Organization," *Journal of Applied Behavioral Science,* December 2009, pp. 521–549; D. A. Garvin, A. C. Edmondson, and F. Gino, "Is Yours a Learning Organization?" *Harvard Business Review,* March 2008, pp. 109–116; A. N. K. Chen and T. M. Edgington, "Assessing Value in Organizational Knowledge Creation: Considerations for Knowledge Workers," *MIS Quarterly,* June 2005, pp. 279–309; K. G. Smith, C. J. Collins, and K. D. Clark, "Existing Knowledge, Knowledge Creation Capability, and the Rate of New Product Introduction in High-Technology Firms," *Academy of Management Journal,* April 2005,

pp. 346–357; R. Cross, A. Parker, L. Prusak, and S. P. Borgati, "Supporting Knowledge Creation and Sharing in Social Networks," *Organizational Dynamics*, Fall, 2001, pp. 100–120; M. Schulz, "The Uncertain Relevance of Newness: Organizational Learning and Knowledge Flows," *Academy of Management Journal*, August 2001, pp. 661–681; G. Szulanski, "Exploring Internal Stickiness: Impediments to the Transfer of Best Practice within the Firm," *Strategic Management Journal*, Winter Special Issue, 1996, pp. 27–43; and J. M. Liedtka, "Collaborating across Lines of Business for Competitive Advantage," *Academy of Management Executive*, April 1996, pp. 20–37.

29. J. Scanlon, "How 3M Encourages Collaboration," *BusinessWeek Online*, September 2, 2009.

30. R. Mitchell, "The Cure," *Fast Company.com*, May 2011, pp. 108+.

31. "Meet the New Steel," *Fortune*, October 1, 2007, pp. 68–71.

32. J. Appleby and R. Davis, "Teamwork Used to Save Money; Now It Saves Lives," *USA Today* [www.usatoday.com], March 1, 2001.

33. C. Kauffman, "Employee Involvement: A New Blueprint for Success," *Journal of Accountancy*, May 2010, pp. 46–49; and R. L. Daft, *Management*, 9th ed. (Mason, OH: South-Western Cengage Learning, 2010), p. 262.

34. S. F. Gale, "The Power of Community," *Workforce Management Online*, March 2009.

35. C. G. Cataldo, "Book Review," *Academy of Management Learning & Education*, June 2009, pp. 301–303; E. Wenger, R. McDermott, and W. Snyder, *Cultivating Communities of Practice: A Guide to Managing Knowledge* (Boston: Harvard Business School Press, 2002), p. 4.

36. E. Wenger, R. McDermott, and W. Snyder, *Cultivating Communities of Practice: A Guide to Managing Knowledge* (Boston: Harvard Business School Press, 2002), p. 39.

37. R. McDermott and D. Archibald, "Harnessing Your Staff's Informal Networks," *Harvard Business Review*, March 2010, pp. 82–89.

38. T. L. Griffith and J. E. Sawyer, "Multilevel Knowledge and Team Performance," *Journal of Organizational Behavior*, October 2010, pp. 1003–1031; and M. Hemmasi and C. M. Csanda, "The Effectiveness of Communities of Practice: An Empirical Study," *Journal of Managerial Issues*, Summer 2009, pp. 262–279.

39. R. Jana, "How Intuit Makes a Social Network Pay," *BusinessWeek Online*, July 2, 2009.

40. B. Horovitz, "Tasty Potato Chip Offer: $1 Million Prize," *USA Today*, July 19, 2012, p. 1A; and **R. A. Guth, "Glaxo Tries a Linux Approach," *Wall Street Journal*, May 26, 2010, p. B4.**

41. J. Winsor, "Crowdsourcing: What It Means for Innovation," *BusinessWeek Online*, June 15, 2009.

42. K. J. O'Brien, "One Year Later, Nokia and Microsoft Deliver," *New York Times Online*, February 27, 2012.

43. D. Lavie, U. Stettner, and M. L. Tushman, "Exploration and Exploitation Within and Across Organizations," *Academy of Management Annals*, June 2010, pp. 109–155; H. Mitsuhashi and H. R. Greve, "A Matching Theory of Alliance Formation and Organizational Success: Complementarity and Compatibility," *Academy of Management Journal*, October 2009, pp. 975–995; D. Durfee, "Try Before You Buy," *CFO*, May 2006, pp. 48–54; B. McEvily and A. Marcus, "Embedded Ties and the Acquisition of Competitive Capabilities," *Strategic Management Journal*, November 2005, pp. 1033–1055; R. D. Ireland, M. A. Hitt, and D. Vaidyanath, "Alliance Management as a Source of Competitive Advantage," *Journal of Management*, 2002, vol. 28, no. 3, pp. 413–446; E. Krell, "The Alliance Advantage," *Business Finance*, July 2002, pp. 16–23; D. Sparks, "Partners," *BusinessWeek*, October 25, 1999, pp. 106–112; and D. Brady, "When Is Cozy Too Cozy?" *BusinessWeek*, October 25, 1999, pp. 127–130.

44. J. Marquez, "Connecting a Virtual Workforce," *Workforce Management Online*, February 3, 2009.

45. M. Conlin, "Home Offices: The New Math," *BusinessWeek*, March 9, 2009, pp. 66–68.

46. M. Mihelich, "Hey, Jealousy: Envy Blossoms Among In-House Workers," www.workforce.com, October 11, 2013.

47. M. Conlin, "Home Offices: The New Math."

48. J. Marquez, "Connecting a Virtual Workforce."

49. S. Jayson, "Working At Home: Family-Friendly," *USA Today*, April 15, 2010, pp. 1A+; T. D. Hecht and N. J. Allen, "A Longitudinal Examination of the Work-Nonwork Boundary Strength Construct,"

Journal of Organizational Behavior, October 2009, pp. 839–862; and G. E. Kreiner, E. C. Hollensbe, and M. L. Sheep, "Balancing Borders and Bridges: Negotiating the Work-Home Interface via Boundary Work Tactics," *Academy of Management Journal*, August 2009, pp. 704–730.

50. J. T. Marquez, "The Future of Flex," *Workforce Management Online*, January 27, 2010.

51. B. Walsh, "Thank God It's Thursday," *Time*, September 7, 2009, p. 58.

52. J. Sahadi, "Flex-time, Time Off—Who's Getting These Perks?" *CNNMoney.com*, June 25, 2007.

53. M. Arndt, "The Family That Flips Together …" *BusinessWeek*, April 17, 2006, p. 14.

54. S. Greenhouse, "Work-Sharing May Help Companies Avoid Layoffs," *New York Times Online*, June 16, 2009.

55. J. Yang and A. Gonzalez, "Would Asking for Flexible Work Options Hurt Your Career Advancement?" *USA Today*, October 2, 2013, p. 1B.

56. M. Korn, "Making a Temporary Stint Stick," *Wall Street Journal*, February 9, 2010, p. D6.

57. A. Levit, "The Rise of the Independent Work Force," *New York Times Online*, April 14, 2012.

58. I. Speizer, "Special Report on Contingency Staffing—The Future of Contingent Staffing Could Be Like Something Out of a Movie," *Workforce Management Online*, October 19, 2009.

59. E. Frauenheim, "Special Report on HR Technology: Tracking the Contingents," *Workforce Management Online*, April 2010.

60. S. G. Hauser, "Independent Contractors Helping to Shape the New World of Work," *Workforce Management Online*, February 3, 2012; S. Greenhouse, "U.S. Cracks Down on 'Contractors' as a Tax Dodge," *New York Times Online*, February 18, 2010; and M. Orey, "FedEx: They're Employees. No, They're Not," *Bloomberg BusinessWeek*, November 5, 2009, pp. 73–74.

61. M. Orey, "FedEx: They're Employees. No, They're Not," *Bloomberg BusinessWeek*, November 5, 2009, pp. 73–74.

62. V. Smith and E. B. Neuwirth, "Temporary Help Agencies and the Making of a New Employment Practice," *Academy of Management Perspectives*, February 2009, pp. 56–72.

63. E. Frauenheim, "Special Report on HR Technology: Tracking the Contingents."

64. J. Yang and A. Gonzalez, "Will Mobile Computing Kill the Traditional Office in 50 Years?" *USA Today*, March 8, 2013, p. 1B.

65. C. E. Connelly and D. G. Gallagher, "Emerging Trends in Contingent Work Research," *Journal of Management*, November 2004, pp. 959–983.

66. K. Holland, "The Anywhere, Anytime Office," *New York Times Online*, September 28, 2008; C. Edwards, "Wherever You Go, You're On The Job," *Bloomberg BusinessWeek*, June 19, 2005.

67. Leader Making a Difference box based on C. Rose, "Charlie Rose Talks to Cisco's John Chambers," *Bloomberg BusinessWeek*, April 23, 2012, p. 41; M. T. Hansen et al., "The Best-Performing CEOs in the World," *Harvard Business Review*, January–February 2010, pp. 104–113; P. Burrows, "Cisco's Extreme Ambitions," *BusinessWeek*, November 30, 2009, pp. 26–27; P. Burrows and A. Ricadela, "Cisco Seizes the Moment," *BusinessWeek*, May 25, 2009, pp. 46–48; and "Cisco Systems Layers It On," *Fortune*, December 8, 2008, p. 24.

68. N. M. Adler, *International Dimensions of Organizational Behavior*, 5th ed. (Cincinnati, OH: South-Western, 2008), p. 62.

69. P. B. Smith and M. F. Peterson, "Demographic Effects on the Use of Vertical Sources of Guidance by Managers in Widely Differing Cultural Contexts," *International Journal of Cross Cultural Management*, April 2005, pp. 5–26.

70. C. Hausman, "Was AT&T's iPad Security Breach 'Ethical' Hacking?" *Ethics Newsline* [www.globalethics.org], June 21, 2010; S. E. Ante and B. Worthen, "FBI to Probe iPad Breach—Group That Exposed AT&T Flaw to See Addresses Says It Did a Public Service," *Wall Street Journal*, June 11, 2010, p. B1; and S. E. Ante, "AT&T Discloses Breach of iPad Owner Data," *Wall Street Journal Online*, June 9, 2010.

71. E. Mills, "Hackers Were Right to Disclose AT&T-iPad Site Hole," *CNET*, June 14, 2010.

72. Based on H. Mintzberg, *Power In and Around Organizations* (Upper Saddle River, NJ: Prentice Hall, 1983), p. 24; P. L. Hunsaker, *Training in Management Skills* (Upper Saddle River, NJ: Prentice Hall, 2001),

pp. 339–364; G. Ferris, S. Davidson, and P. Perrewé, "Developing Political Skill at Work," *Training,* November 2005, pp. 40–45; B. Uzzi and S. Dunlap, "How to Build Your Network," *Harvard Business Review,* December 2005, pp. 53–60; and B. Brim, "The Best Way to Influence Others," *Gallup Management Journal* [http://gmj.gallup.com], February 9, 2006.

73. E. Frauenheim, "Research Backs Benefits of Flex Work for Workers—and Companies," www.workforce.com, May 29, 2013; R. E. Silverman, "Telecommuting Boosts Firms' Revenue Growth," *Wall Street Journal,* April 17, 2013, p. B8; C. C. Miller and N. Perlroth, "Yahoo Says New Policy Is Meant to Raise Morale," *New York Times Online,* March 5, 2013; C. Suddath, "Work-From-Home Truths, Half-Truths, and Myths," *Bloomberg BusinessWeek,* March 4–10, 2013, p. 75; Q. Fottrell, "The Home Office in the Spotlight," *Wall Street Journal,* February 27, 2013, p. B6; E. Weise, "Telecommuters to Yahoo: Boo." *USA Today,* February 26, 2013, p. 1A; R. E. Silverman and R. Bell, "Examining Marissa Mayer's Out-of-Office Message to Yahoo Employees," www.workforce.com, February 26, 2013; C. C. Miller and C. Rampell, "Yahoo Orders Home Workers Back to the Office," *New York Times Online,* February 25, 2013; and K. Swisher, "'Physically Together': Here's the Internal Yahoo No-Work-From-Home Memo for Remote Workers and Maybe More," allthingsd.com, February 22, 2013.

74. J. Graham, "Product Fans Can Become Customer Service Reps," *USA Today,* May 31, 2012, p. 3B; A. Fox, "Pave the Way for Volunteers," *HR Magazine,* June 2010, pp. 70–74; G. Morse, "The Power of Unwitting Workers," *Harvard Business Review,* October 2009, p. 27; **S. Lohr, "Customer Service? Ask A Volunteer," *New York Times Online,* April 26, 2009;** and B. Xu, D. R. Jones, and B. Shao, "Volunteers' Involvement in Online Community Based Software Development," *Information & Management,* April 2009, pp. 151–158.

Managing Human Resources

From Chapter 12 of *Management*, Thirteenth Edition. Stephen P. Robbins and Mary Coulter. Copyright © 2016 by Pearson Education, Inc. All rights reserved.

It's Your Career

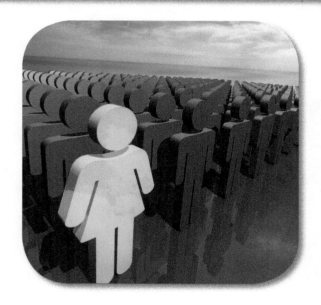

Source: Kyu Oh/Getty

A key to success in management and in your career is knowing how to interview for a job effectively.

Acing Your Interviews

Although it may feel that way, you're actually not going to be in college forever. Graduation is coming soon (hopefully) and you'll be looking for a job. A big hurdle in that search is the job interview. *An interview allows potential employers to solicit information about you and to see you "in action." You want to put your best foot forward and show that you're a good catch! Here are some suggestions for helping you "ace" that interview:*

1. Research the company ahead of time. *You already know you need to do this, but do you know what to look for? Know the company's competitive advantages—what makes this company unique. Look closely at its financial "health." Know the company's strategic initiatives. Find out what you can about the company's culture. Where do you find this information? Check the company's Web site, especially the "About Us" and financial sections. Check the company's social media presence: blogs, Facebook and LinkedIn profiles, Twitter. Check out information on other Web sites such as Glassdoor and The Muse, and business news sites.*

2. Research the industry and competitors. *Familiarize yourself with this industry and the main competitors, but only the big-picture stuff, not minute details.*

3. Decide ahead of time how you will answer certain "standard" interview questions.

- *The "Tell me about yourself" question: Although this question seems easy enough, you want to show how you're the perfect fit for the job. One expert suggests a "present-past-future" approach.[1] Describe where you are right now, describe a little about your past experiences and the skills you've gained, finish with describing the future and why you're excited about this particular job opportunity.*

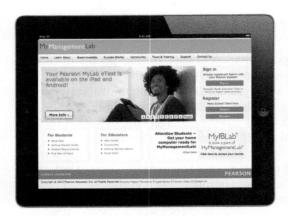

MyManagementLab®

⭐ **Improve Your Grade!**

When you see this icon, visit
www.mymanagementlab.com for activities that are
applied, personalized, and offer immediate feedback.

Learning Objectives

1 **Explain** the importance of the human resource management process and the external
influences that might affect that process.

2 **Discuss** the tasks associated with identifying and selecting competent employees.

- **Know how** to be a good interviewee.
- **Develop your skill** at being a good interviewer.

3 **Explain** the different types of orientation and training.

4 **Describe** strategies for retaining competent, high-performing employees.

5 **Discuss** contemporary issues in managing human resources.

- The "What's your greatest weakness" question: If you're not prepared, this question can trip you up. You don't want to give the cliché answers of "I'm a perfectionist" or "I work too hard." All these do is show you're not prepared with a good answer. One expert suggests talking about weaknesses that don't relate to the job (e.g., if you know the job doesn't require public speaking and public speaking is one of your weaknesses, talk about that). This shows you're self-aware and realize you have weaknesses, like all of us do.[2] Another approach is to talk about past weaknesses and how you dealt with them by getting advice or additional training. This expert also said never mention these weaknesses: "I'm not a team player, I'm not trustworthy, I'm not reliable, I have difficulty accepting feedback, I'm not able to take initiative and work independently." We would agree 100 percent with that!

  4. **Watch your body language.**[3] You want to present a polished, poised, and professional demeanor. So, NO: bad posture, too weak/too forceful handshake, lack of eye contact, fidgeting, appearing distracted or uninterested, not smiling. And definitely no cell phone going off in the middle of your interview!

  5. **Review the job description carefully.** Pay particular attention to stated requirements outside the standard "various duties as assigned." Come up with possible questions an interviewer might ask about those requirements and think about how you would answer those questions.

  6. **Review your résumé with the critical eye of an interviewer.** What stands out? What would you ask a person who had those statements/descriptions on their résumé?

With the organization's structure in place, managers have to find people to fill the jobs that have been created or to remove people from jobs if business circumstances require. That's where human resource management (HRM) comes in. It's an important task that involves having the right number of the right people in the right place at the right time. In this text, we'll look at the process managers use to do just that. In addition, we'll look at some contemporary HRM issues facing managers.

A major HRM challenge for managers is ensuring that their company has a high-quality workforce. Getting and keeping competent and talented employees is critical to the success of every organization, whether an organization is just starting or has been in business for years. If an organization doesn't take its HRM responsibilities seriously, performance may suffer. Therefore, part of every manager's job when organizing is human resource management. Research has shown that when line managers are responsible for recruiting, performance management, and retention, their companies are 29 percent more successful.[4] That's a good reason for all managers to engage in some HRM activities, such as interviewing job candidates, orienting new employees, and evaluating their employees' work performance, even if there is a separate HRM department.

THE HUMAN Resource Management Process

LO1 Many organizations profess that their people are their most important asset and acknowledge the important role that employees play in organizational success. However, why is HRM important, and what external factors influence the HRM process?

Why Is HRM Important?

HRM is important for three reasons. First, as various studies have concluded, it can be a significant source of competitive advantage.[5] And that's true for organizations around the world, not just U.S. firms. The Human Capital Index, a comprehensive study of more than 2,000 global firms, concluded that people-oriented HR gives an organization an edge by creating superior shareholder value.[6] Another study found that 71 percent of CEOs say that their "human capital" is the key source of sustained economic value.[7]

Second, HRM is an important part of organizational strategies. Achieving competitive success through people means managers must change how they think about their employees and how they view the work relationship. They must work with people and treat them as partners, not just as costs to be minimized or avoided. That's what people-oriented organizations such as Southwest Airlines and W. L. Gore do.

Finally, the way organizations treat their people has been found to significantly impact organizational performance.[8] For instance, one study reported that improving work practices could increase market value by as much as 30 percent.[9] Another study that tracked average annual shareholder returns of companies on *Fortune's* list of 100 Best Companies to Work For found that these companies significantly beat the S&P 500 over 10-year, 5-year, 3-year, and 1-year periods.[10] Another study found a positive relationship between companies' high- performance work practices and the ability of the organization to efficiently adapt to changing and challenging markets.[11] Work practices that lead to both high individual and high organizational performance are known as **high-performance work practices**. (See some examples in Exhibit 1.) The common thread among these practices seems to be a commitment to involving employees; improving the knowledge, skills, and abilities of an organization's employees; increasing their motivation; reducing loafing on the job; and enhancing the retention of quality employees while encouraging low performers to leave.

Even if an organization doesn't use high-performance work practices, other specific HRM activities must be completed in order to ensure that the organization has qualified people to perform the work that needs to be done—activities that comprise the HRM process. Exhibit 2 shows the eight activities in this process. The first

high-performance work practices
Work practices that lead to both high individual and high organizational performance

Exhibit 1
High-Performance Work Practices

- Self-managed teams
- Decentralized decision making
- Training programs to develop knowledge, skills, and abilities
- Flexible job assignments
- Open communication
- Performance-based compensation
- Staffing based on person–job and person–organization fit
- Extensive employee involvement
- Giving employees more control over decision making
- Increasing employee access to information

Sources: C. H. Chuang and H. Liao, "Strategic Human Resource Management in Service Context: Taking Care of Business by Taking Care of Employees and Customers," *Personnel Psychology,* Spring 2010, pp. 153–196; M. Subramony, "A Meta-Analytic Investigation of the Relationship Between HRM Bundles and Firm Performance," *Human Resource Management,* September–October 2009, pp. 745–768; M. M. Butts et al., "Individual Reactions to High Involvement Work Practices: Investigating the Role of Empowerment and Perceived Organizational Support," *Journal of Occupational Health Psychology,* April 2009, pp. 122–136; and W. R. Evans and W. D. Davis, "High-Performance Work Systems and Organizational Performance: The Mediating Role of Internal Social Structure," *Journal of Management,* October 2005, p. 760.

three activities ensure that competent employees are identified and selected; the next two involve providing employees with up-to-date knowledge and skills; and the final three ensure that the organization retains competent and high-performing employees. Before we discuss those specific activities, we need to look at external factors that affect the HRM process.

External Factors That Affect the HRM Process

An administrative assistant job opening paying $13 an hour at a Burns Harbor, Indiana, truck driver training school for C. R. England, a nationwide trucking company, was posted on a Friday afternoon.[12] By the time the company's head of corporate recruiting arrived at work on Monday morning, there were about 300 applications

Exhibit 2
HRM Process

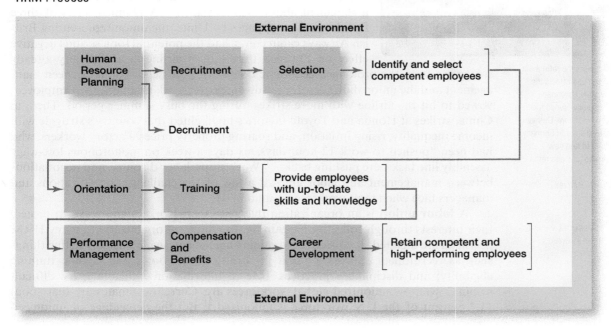

in the company's e-mail inbox. And an inch-and-a-half stack of résumés was piled up by the now out-of-paper fax machine. Out of those 500-plus applicants, one person, who had lost her job four months earlier, impressed the hiring manager so much that the job was hers, leaving the remaining 499-plus people—including a former IBM analyst with 18 years of experience, a former director of human resources, and someone with a master's degree and 12 years of experience at accounting firm Deloitte & Touche—still searching for a job. During the economic slowdown, filling job openings was an almost mind-boggling exercise.

As you can see, the entire HRM process is influenced by the external environment. Those factors most directly influencing it include the economy, employee labor unions, governmental laws and regulations, and demographic trends.

THE ECONOMY'S EFFECT ON HRM The global economic downturn has left what many experts believe to be an enduring mark on HRM practices worldwide. For instance, in Japan, workers used to count on two things: a job for life and a decent pension. Now, lifetime employment is long gone and corporate pension plans are crumbling.[13] In the European Union, the early 2014 jobless rate was 11.9 percent, with Greece and Spain being hit hardest with an unemployment rate of 27.5 percent and 25.6 percent respectively.[14] And in Thailand, employees in the automotive industry dealt with reduced work hours, which affected their pay and their skill upgrades.[15] In the United States, labor economists say that jobs are coming back slowly but aren't the same ones employees were used to. Many of these jobs are temporary or contract positions, rather than full-time jobs with benefits. And many of the more than 8.4 million jobs lost during the recession aren't coming back at all, but they may be replaced by other types of work in growing industries.[16] All of these changes have affected employers and workers. A Global Workforce Study survey by global professional services company Towers Watson confirmed that the recession has "fundamentally altered the way U.S. employees view their work and leaders.... U.S. workers have dramatically lowered their career and retirement expectations for the foreseeable future."[17] Such findings have profound implications for how an organization manages its human resources.

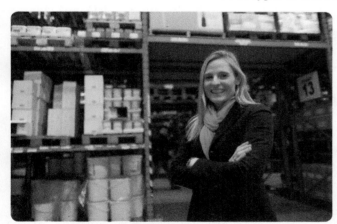

A new law in Germany that lowers the retirement age from 67 to 63 for some workers affects the HRM practices of Marie-Christine Ostermann, general manager of Rullko, a family-owned food and kitchen supply wholesaler in Hamm, Germany. Along with a shortage of skilled labor in Germany, the law challenges Ostermann to find new employees to replace those who now can retire earlier than they planned.
Source: Ina Fassbender/Reuters Pictures

labor union
An organization that represents workers and seeks to protect their interests through collective bargaining

EMPLOYEE LABOR UNIONS Hundreds of workers at Amazon's two fulfillment centers in Germany used a series of wildcat strikes—the first of any kind against the company—to make a statement about their demands.[18] A planned series of three five-day work stoppages by Unite, the union representing British Airways cabin crews, had the potential for a serious negative effect on Europe's third-largest airline in an industry already struggling from the prolonged economic downturn.[19] If negotiations between management and the union didn't resolve the disputes over work practices, then employees vowed to hit the airline with more strikes during the busy summer period. Then, in China, strikes at Honda and Toyota factories highlighted that country's struggle with income inequality, rising inflation, and soaring property prices. Factory workers, who had been "pushed to work 12-hour days, six days a week on monotonous low-wage assembly line tasks, are pushing back."[20] Work stops, labor disputes, and negotiations between management and labor are just a few of the challenges organizations and managers face when their workforce is unionized.

A **labor union** is an organization that represents workers and seeks to protect their interests through collective bargaining. In unionized organizations, many HRM decisions are dictated by collective bargaining agreements, which usually define things such as recruitment sources; criteria for hiring, promotions, and layoffs; training eligibility; and disciplinary practices. Due to information availability, it's difficult to pin down how unionized global workforces are. Current estimates are that about 11.3 percent of the U.S. workforce is unionized.[21] But the percentage of unionized

workers tends to be higher in other countries, except in France, where some 7.8 percent of workers are unionized. For instance, in Japan, some 18 percent of the labor force belongs to a union; in Germany, 18 percent; in Denmark, 68.5 percent; in Australia, 17.9 percent; in Canada, 26.8 percent; and in Mexico, 13.6 percent.[22] One union membership trend we're seeing, especially in the more industrialized countries, is that the rate in private enterprise is declining while that in the public sector (which includes teachers, police officers, firefighters, and government workers) is climbing. Although labor unions can affect an organization's HRM practices, the most significant environmental constraint is governmental laws, especially in North America.

LEGAL ENVIRONMENT OF HRM Two hundred fifty million dollars. That's the amount a New York City jury awarded in punitive damages to plaintiffs who claim drug company Novartis AG discriminated against women.[23] As this example shows, an organization's HRM practices are governed by a country's laws and not following those laws can be costly. (See Exhibit 3 for some of the important U.S. laws that affect the HRM process.) For example, decisions regarding who will be hired or which

Exhibit 3
Major HRM Laws

LAW OR RULING	YEAR	DESCRIPTION
Equal Employment Opportunity and Discrimination		
Equal Pay Act	1963	Prohibits pay differences for equal work based on gender
Civil Rights Act, Title VII	1964 (amended in 1972)	Prohibits discrimination based on race, color, religion, national origin, or gender
Age Discrimination in Employment Act	1967 (amended in 1978)	Prohibits discrimination against employees 40 years and older
Vocational Rehabilitation Act	1973	Prohibits discrimination on the basis of physical or mental disabilities
Americans with Disabilities Act	1990	Prohibits discrimination against individuals who have disabilities or chronic illnesses; also requires reasonable accommodations for these individuals
Compensation/Benefits		
Worker Adjustment and Retraining Notification Act	1990	Requires employers with more than 100 employees to provide 60 days' notice before a mass layoff or facility closing
Family and Medical Leave Act	1993	Gives employees in organizations with 50 or more employees up to 12 weeks of unpaid leave each year for family or medical reasons
Health Insurance Portability and Accountability Act	1996	Permits portability of employees' insurance from one employer to another
Lilly Ledbetter Fair Pay Act	2009	Changes the statute of limitations on pay discrimination to 180 days from each paycheck
Patient Protection and Affordable Care Act	2010	Health care legislation that puts in place comprehensive health insurance reforms
Health/Safety		
Occupational Safety and Health Act (OSHA)	1970	Establishes mandatory safety and health standards in organizations
Privacy Act	1974	Gives employees the legal right to examine personnel files and letters of reference
Consolidated Omnibus Reconciliation Act (COBRA)	1985	Requires continued health coverage following termination (paid by employee)

Source: United States Equal Employment Opportunity Commission, www.eeoc.gov; United States Department of Labor, www.dol.gov; United States Occupational Safety and Health Administration, www.osha.gov.

employees will be chosen for a training program or what an employee's compensation will be must be made without regard to race, sex, religion, age, color, national origin, or disability. Exceptions can occur only in special circumstances. For instance, a community fire department can deny employment to a firefighter applicant who is confined to a wheelchair; but if that same individual is applying for a desk job, such as a dispatcher, the disability cannot be used as a reason to deny employment. The issues, however, are rarely that clear-cut. For example, employment laws protect most employees whose religious beliefs require a specific style of dress—robes, long shirts, long hair, and the like. However, if the specific style of dress may be hazardous or unsafe in the work setting (such as when operating machinery), a company could refuse to hire a person who won't adopt a safer dress code.

As you can see, a number of important laws and regulations affect what you can and cannot do legally as a manager. Because workplace lawsuits are increasingly targeting supervisors, as well as their organizations, managers must know what they can and cannot do by law.[24] Trying to balance the "shoulds" and "should nots" of many laws often falls within the realm of **affirmative action**. Many U.S. organizations have affirmative action programs to ensure that decisions and practices enhance the employment, upgrading, and retention of members from protected groups such as minorities and females. That is, an organization refrains from discrimination and actively seeks to enhance the status of members from protected groups. However, U.S. managers are not completely free to choose whom they hire, promote, or fire, or free to treat employees any way they want. Although laws have helped reduce employment discrimination and unfair work practices, they have, at the same time, reduced managers' discretion over HRM decisions.

We do want to mention some U.S. laws that will and some that are likely to affect future HRM practices. The first of these, the Patient Protection and Affordable Care Act (PPACA and commonly called the Health Care Reform Act), was signed into law in March 2010 and upheld by the Supreme Court of the United States in 2012.[25] This law is affecting current HRM practices as employers are beginning to sort through the requirements and the deadlines for compliance. Other proposed legislation that is likely to affect HRM practices includes (1) the Social Networking Online Protection Act (SNOPA), which has been introduced and would prohibit employers from requiring a username, password, or other access to online content;[26] and (2) immigration reform, which is aimed at providing a way for undocumented individuals to become legal citizens.[27] The best source of advice about these and other important legal issues will be your company's HR department.

What about HRM laws globally? It's important that managers in other countries be familiar with the specific laws that apply there. Let's take a look at some of the federal legislation in countries such as Canada, Mexico, Australia, and Germany.

Canadian laws pertaining to HRM practices closely parallel those in the United States. The Canadian Human Rights Act prohibits discrimination on the basis of race, religion, age, marital status, sex, physical or mental disability, or national origin. This act governs practices throughout the country. Canada's HRM environment, however, is somewhat different from that in the United States in that it involves more decentralization of lawmaking to the provincial level. For example, discrimination on the basis of language is not prohibited anywhere in Canada except in Quebec.

In Mexico, employees are more likely to be unionized than they are in the United States. Labor matters in Mexico are governed by the Mexican Federal Labor Law. One hiring law states that an employer has 28 days to evaluate a new employee's work performance. After that period, the employee is granted job security and termination is quite difficult and expensive. Those who violate the Mexican Federal Labor Law are subject to severe penalties, including criminal action that can result in steep fines and even jail sentences for employers who fail to pay, for example, the minimum wage. Recently, Mexican labor laws underwent a major overhaul. Some of the important new changes include controls on outsourcing jobs, hiring and firing, wrongful discharge, and additional antidiscrimination requirements.[28]

affirmative action
Organizational programs that enhance the status of members of protected groups

Australia's discrimination laws were not enacted until the 1980s and generally apply to discrimination and affirmative action for women. Yet, gender opportunities for women in Australia appear to lag behind those in the United States. In Australia, however, a significant proportion of the workforce is unionized. The higher percentage of unionized workers has placed increased importance on industrial relations specialists in Australia and reduced the control of line managers over workplace labor issues. In 1997, Australia overhauled its labor and industrial relations laws with the objective of increasing productivity and reducing union power. The Workplace Relations Bill gives employers greater flexibility to negotiate directly with employees on pay, hours, and benefits. It also simplifies federal regulation of labor–management relations.

Our final example, Germany, is similar to most Western European countries when it comes to HRM practices. Legislation requires companies to practice representative participation, in which the goal is to redistribute power within the organization, putting labor on a more equal footing with the interests of management and stockholders. The two most common forms of representative participation are work councils and board representatives. **Work councils** link employees with management. They are groups of nominated or elected employees who must be consulted when management makes decisions involving personnel. **Board representatives** are employees who sit on a company's board of directors and represent the interests of the firm's employees.

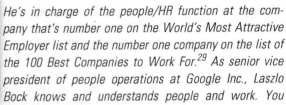

LEADER *making a* DIFFERENCE

He's in charge of the people/HR function at the company that's number one on the World's Most Attractive Employer list and the number one company on the list of the 100 Best Companies to Work For.[29] As senior vice president of people operations at Google Inc., Laszlo Bock knows and understands people and work. You shouldn't be surprised that the comprehensive (and complicated) analysis that goes into Google search efforts also characterizes its approach to managing its human resources. Bock's current pursuit is a long-term study of work (patterned after the long-running Framingham Heart Study that transformed what we know about heart disease). Bock says, "I believe that the experience of work can be—should be—so much better."[30] He and his team hope to learn more about work-life balance, improving employee well-being, cultivating better leaders, doing a better job of engaging Googlers (the name for Google employees) long term, and how happiness and work impact each other. Undoubtedly, there will be some interesting insights that result! (P.S. If you'd like to work at Google and want to know more about getting hired, check out the references cited above! There are good tips in there!) What can you learn from this leader making a difference?

work councils
Groups of nominated or elected employees who must be consulted when management makes decisions involving personnel

board representatives
Employees who sit on a company's board of directors and represent the interests of the firm's employees

DEMOGRAPHIC TRENDS A few years back, the head of BMW's 2,500-employee power train plant in Dingolfing, Lower Bavaria, was worried about the potential inevitable future decline in productivity due to an aging workforce.[31] That's when company executives decided to redesign its factory for older workers. With input from employees, they implemented physical changes to the workplace—for instance, new wooden floors to reduce joint strain and special chairs for sitting down or relaxing for short periods—that would reduce wear and tear on workers' bodies. Other organizations worldwide are preparing for a shift as baby boomers retire. Many older workers delayed their retirement during the recession, reducing the threat of mass turnover for a few years. "But now it's sneaking up on companies." Companies are responding by creating succession plans, bringing retirees on as consultants, and increasing cross-training efforts to prepare younger workers to fill the void. Almost half of HR professionals surveyed said this potential loss of talent over the next decade is a problem for their organizations.[32] As these examples show, demographic trends impact HRM practices worldwide.

Much of the change in the U.S. workforce over the last 50 years can be attributed to federal legislation enacted in the 1960s that prohibited employment discrimination. With these laws, avenues opened up for minority and female job applicants. These two groups dramatically changed the workplace in the latter half of the twentieth century. Women, in particular, have changed the composition of the workforce as they now hold some 49.1 percent of jobs. And because women tend to be employed

in education and health care industries, their jobs are less sensitive to economic ups and downs.[33] If this trend continues, women may, at some point, become the majority group in the workforce.

Workforce trends in the first half of the twenty-first century will be notable for three reasons: (1) changes in racial and ethnic composition, (2) an aging baby boom generation, and (3) an expanding cohort of Gen Y workers. By 2050, Hispanics will grow from today's 13 percent of the workforce to 24 percent, blacks will increase from 12 percent to 14 percent, and Asians will increase from 5 percent to 11 percent. Meanwhile, the labor force is aging. The 55-and-older age group, which currently makes up 13 percent of the workforce, will increase to 20 percent by 2014. Another group that's having a significant impact on today's workforce is Gen Y, a population group that includes individuals born from about 1978 to 1994. Gen Y has been the fastest-growing segment of the workforce—increasing from 14 percent to more than 24 percent. With Gen Y now in the workforce, analysts point to the four generations that are working side-by-side in the workplace[34]:

- The oldest, most experienced workers (those born before 1946) make up 6 percent of the workforce.
- The baby boomers (those born between 1946 and 1964) make up 41.5 percent of the workforce.
- Gen Xers (those born 1965 to 1977) make up almost 29 percent of the workforce.
- Gen Yers (those born 1978 to 1994) make up almost 24 percent of the workforce.

These and other demographic trends are important because of the impact they're having on current and future HRM practices.

IDENTIFYING and Selecting Competent Employees

LO2 Executives at Texas-based global engineering giant Fluor are expected to recognize and mentor high-performing employees. The company's senior vice president of human resources and administration says such efforts are necessary because "you can't create a senior mechanical engineer overnight. It takes years." Here's a company that understands the importance of tracking talent on a global scale.[35] Is a job in the insurance industry on your list of jobs you'll apply for after graduation? Unfortunately for the insurance industry, it's not for many college graduates. Like many other nonglamorous industries, including transportation, utilities, and manufacturing, the insurance industry is not "particularly attractive to the so-called 'millennials'—people who turned 21 in 2000 or later." In all these industries, the number of skilled jobs is already starting to overtake the number of qualified people available to fill them.[36]

Every organization needs people to do whatever work is necessary for doing what the organization is in business to do. How do they get those people? And more importantly, what can they do to ensure they get competent, talented people? This first phase of the HRM process involves three tasks: human resource planning, recruitment and decruitment, and selection.

Human Resource Planning

Human resource planning is the process by which managers ensure that they have the right number and kinds of capable people in the right places and at the right times. Through planning, organizations avoid sudden people shortages and surpluses.[37] HR planning entails two steps: (1) assessing current human resources and (2) meeting future HR needs.

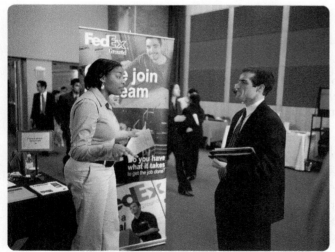

Recruiting good people who become loyal employees and are happy with their jobs is an important part of Federal Express Corporation's human resource planning and plays a major role in maintaining an employee turnover rate of just one percent. The company operates recruiting centers at 25 locations in the United States that help process and screen applicants.
Source: Robert Nickelsberg/Alamy

human resource planning
Ensuring that the organization has the right number and kinds of capable people in the right places and at the right times

CURRENT ASSESSMENT   Managers begin HR planning by inventorying current employees. This inventory usually includes information on employees such as name, education, training, prior employment, languages spoken, special capabilities, and specialized skills. Sophisticated databases make getting and keeping this information quite easy. For example, Stephanie Cox, Schlumberger's director of personnel for North and South America, uses a company planning program called PeopleMatch to help pinpoint managerial talent. Suppose she needs a manager for Brazil. She types in the qualifications: someone who can relocate, speak Portuguese, and is a "high potential" employee. Within a minute, 31 names of possible candidates pop up.[38] At Hoover's Inc., a Dun & Bradstreet subsidiary, getting a clear picture of employees' skills and finding the right people for projects is done through a sophisticated software program and an internally developed employee appraisal system that charts employees' progress along their career paths.[39] That's what good HR planning should do—help managers identify the people they need.

An important part of a current assessment is **job analysis**, an assessment that defines a job and the behaviors necessary to perform it. For instance, what are the duties of a level 3 accountant who works for General Motors? What minimal knowledge, skills, and abilities are necessary to adequately perform this job? How do these requirements compare with those for a level 2 accountant or for an accounting manager? Information for a job analysis is gathered by directly observing individuals on the job, interviewing employees individually or in a group, having employees complete a questionnaire or record daily activities in a diary, or having job "experts" (usually managers) identify a job's specific characteristics.

Using this information from the job analysis, managers develop or revise job descriptions and job specifications. A **job description** (or **position description**) is a written statement describing a job—typically job content, environment, and conditions of employment. A **job specification** states the minimum qualifications that a person must possess to successfully perform a given job. It identifies the knowledge, skills, and attitudes needed to do the job effectively. Both the job description and job specification are important documents when managers begin recruiting and selecting.

job analysis
An assessment that defines jobs and the behaviors necessary to perform them

job description (position description)
A written statement that describes a job

job specification
A written statement of the minimum qualifications a person must possess to perform a given job successfully

MEETING FUTURE HR NEEDS   Future HR needs are determined by the organization's mission, goals, and strategies. Demand for employees results from demand for the organization's products or services. After assessing both current capabilities and future needs, managers can estimate areas in which the organization will be understaffed or overstaffed. Then they're ready to proceed to the next step in the HRM process.

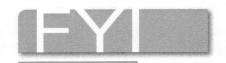

- 28 percent of executives said that identifying good interpersonal skills was the biggest challenge when developing job descriptions.[40]

Recruitment and Decruitment

Competition for talent by India's two largest technology outsourcing companies has led to an all-out recruiting war. In the United States, the tech sector is also in a hiring push, pitting start-up companies against giants such as Google and Intel in the hunt for employees.[41] At CH2MHill, a global engineering firm based in Colorado, it's a real struggle to recruit foreign employees. To be successful at global talent acquisition, its company's talent acquisition director has a plan for dealing with different recruiting cultures in different parts of the world.[42]

If your professor has assigned this, go to **www.mymanagementlab.com** to watch a video titled: *CH2MHill: Human Resource Management* and to respond to questions.

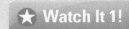

If employee vacancies exist, managers should use the information gathered through job analysis to guide them in **recruitment**—that is, locating, identifying, and attracting capable applicants.[43] On the other hand, if HR planning shows a surplus of employees, managers may want to reduce the organization's workforce through **decruitment**.[44]

recruitment
Locating, identifying, and attracting capable applicants

decruitment
Reducing an organization's workforce

Exhibit 4
Recruiting Sources

Source	Advantages	Disadvantages
Internet	Reaches large numbers of people; can get immediate feedback	Generates many unqualified candidates
Employee referrals	Knowledge about the organization provided by current employee; can generate strong candidates because a good referral reflects on the recommender	May not increase the diversity and mix of employees
Company Web site	Wide distribution; can be targeted to specific groups	Generates many unqualified candidates
College recruiting	Large centralized body of candidates	Limited to entry-level positions
Professional recruiting organizations	Good knowledge of industry challenges and requirements	Little commitment to specific organization

RECRUITMENT Some organizations have interesting approaches to finding employees. For instance, McDonald's, the world's largest hamburger chain, held a National Hiring Day hoping to hire 50,000 people. The chain and its franchisees actually hired 62,000 workers.[45] Microsoft launched a new Web site that integrated 103 country sites into one career-related site. There, potential applicants find employee blogs on everything from interview tips to whether a failed start-up on a résumé hurts in applying for a job at the company.[46] Accounting firm Deloitte & Touche created its Deloitte Film Festival to get employee team-produced films about "life" at Deloitte to use in college recruiting.[47] Even the U.S. Army is getting social by seeking recruits using social media.[48] A survey of what organizations are using to recruit potential job applicants reported that 77 percent of organizations were using social networking sites.[49] Exhibit 4 explains different recruitment sources managers can use to find potential job candidates.[50]

Although online recruiting is popular and allows organizations to identify applicants cheaply and quickly, applicant quality may not be as good as other sources. Research has found that employee referrals generally produce the best candidates.[51] Why? Because current employees know both the job and the person being recommended, they tend to refer applicants who are well qualified. Also, current employees often feel their reputation is at stake and refer others only when they're confident that the person will not make them look bad.

DECRUITMENT The other approach to controlling labor supply is decruitment, which is not a pleasant task for any manager. Decruitment options are shown in Exhibit 5. Although employees can be fired, other choices may be better. However, no matter how you do it, it's never easy to reduce an organization's workforce.

Selection

selection
Screening job applicants to ensure that the most appropriate candidates are hired

Once you have a pool of candidates, the next step in the HRM process is **selection**, screening job applicants to determine who is best qualified for the job. Managers need to "select" carefully since hiring errors can have significant implications. For instance, a driver at Fresh Direct, an online grocer that delivers food to masses of apartment-dwelling New Yorkers, was charged with, and later pled guilty to, stalking and harassing female customers.[52] At T-Mobile, lousy customer service led to its last-place ranking in the J.D. Power's customer-satisfaction survey. The first step in a total overhaul of

Option	Description
Firing	Permanent involuntary termination
Layoffs	Temporary involuntary termination; may last only a few days or extend to years
Attrition	Not filling openings created by voluntary resignations or normal retirements
Transfers	Moving employees either laterally or downward; usually does not reduce costs but can reduce intraorganizational supply–demand imbalances
Reduced workweeks	Having employees work fewer hours per week, share jobs, or perform their jobs on a part-time basis
Early retirements	Providing incentives to older and more senior employees for retiring before their normal retirement date
Job sharing	Having employees share one full-time position

Exhibit 5
Decruitment Options

the customer service area was revamping the company's hiring practices to increase the odds of hiring employees who would be good at customer service.[53]

WHAT IS SELECTION? At Boston's Seaport Hotel & World Trade Center, the HR team decided to integrate an online application with a 20-minute behavioral assessment. After implementing this approach, the company's two-digit turnover rate fell to a single-digit rate.[54] That's the kind of result organizations—and managers—like to see from their hiring process. Selection involves predicting which applicants will be successful if hired. For example, in hiring for a sales position, the selection process should predict which applicants will generate a high volume of sales. As shown in Exhibit 6, any selection decision can result in four possible outcomes—two correct and two errors.

A decision is correct when the applicant was predicted to be successful and proved to be successful on the job, or when the applicant was predicted to be unsuccessful and was not hired. In the first instance, we have successfully accepted; in the second, we have successfully rejected.

Problems arise when errors are made in rejecting candidates who would have performed successfully on the job (reject errors) or accepting those who ultimately perform poorly (accept errors). These problems can be significant. Given today's HR laws and regulations, reject errors can cost more than the additional screening needed to find acceptable candidates. Why? Because they can expose the organization to discrimination charges, especially if applicants from protected groups are disproportionately rejected. For instance, two written firefighter exams used by the New York City Fire Department were found to have had a disparate impact on black and Hispanic candidates.[55] On the other hand, the costs of accept errors include the cost of training the employee, the profits lost because of the employee's incompetence, the cost of severance, and the subsequent costs of further recruiting and screening. The major emphasis of any selection activity should be reducing the probability of reject errors or accept errors while increasing the probability of making correct decisions. Managers do this by using selection procedures that are both valid and reliable.

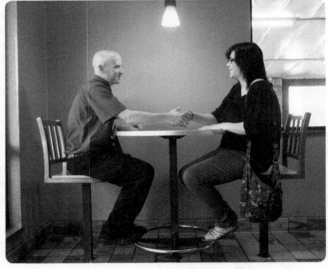

The job interview is a selection tool McDonald's uses for job candidates in both entry-level and professional positions at its 34,000 locations worldwide. During personal interviews, the store manager shown here looks for applicants who possess good communication skills, would qualify in meeting McDonald's customer-service standards, and work well as a team member.
Source: The Idaho Statesman, Joe Jaszewski/ Associated Press

Exhibit 6
Selection Decision Outcomes

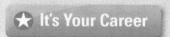

	Selection Decision	
	Accept	**Reject**
Successful	Correct Decision	Reject Error
Unsuccessful	Accept Error	Correct Decision

(Left axis label: Later Job Performance)

VALIDITY AND RELIABILITY A valid selection device is characterized by a proven relationship between the selection device and some relevant criterion. Federal employment laws prohibit managers from using a test score to select employees unless clear evidence shows that, once on the job, individuals with high scores on this test outperform individuals with low test scores. The burden is on managers to support that any selection device they use to differentiate applicants is validly related to job performance.

A reliable selection device indicates that it measures the same thing consistently. On a test that's reliable, any single individual's score should remain fairly consistent over time, assuming that the characteristics being measured are also stable. No selection device can be effective if it's not reliable. Using such a device would be like weighing yourself every day on an erratic scale. If the scale is unreliable—randomly fluctuating, say, 5 to 10 pounds every time you step on it—the results don't mean much.

A growing number of companies are adopting a new measure of recruitment effectiveness called "quality of fill."[56] This measure looks at the contributions of good hires versus those of hires who have failed to live up to their potential. Five key factors are considered in defining this quality measure: employee retention, performance evaluations, number of first-year hires who make it into high-potential training programs, number of employees who are promoted, and what surveys of new hires indicate. Such measures help an organization assess whether its selection process is working well.

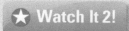 **It's Your Career**

Interviewing—If your instructor is using MyManagementLab, log onto **mymanagementlab.com** and test your *interviewing knowledge*. **Be sure to refer back to the chapter opener!**

TYPES OF SELECTION TOOLS The best-known selection tools include application forms, written and performance-simulation tests, interviews, background investigations, and in some cases, physical exams. Exhibit 7 lists the strengths and weaknesses of each.[57] Because many selection tools have limited value for making selection decisions, managers should use those that effectively predict performance for a given job.

★ **Watch It 2!**

If your professor has assigned this, go to **www.mymanagementlab.com** to watch a video titled: *Rudi's Bakery: Human Resource Management* and to respond to questions.

Exhibit 7
Selection Tools

Application Forms

- Almost universally used
- Most useful for gathering information
- Can predict job performance but not easy to create one that does

Written Tests

- Must be job related
- Include intelligence, aptitude, ability, personality, and interest tests
- Are popular (e.g., personality tests; aptitude tests)
- Relatively good predictor for supervisory positions

Performance-Simulation Tests

- Use actual job behaviors
- Work sampling—test applicants on tasks associated with that job; appropriate for routine or standardized work
- Assessment center—simulate jobs; appropriate for evaluating managerial potential

Interviews

- Almost universally used
- Must know what can and cannot be asked
- Can be useful for managerial positions

Background Investigations

- Used for verifying application data—valuable source of information
- Used for verifying reference checks—not a valuable source of information

Physical Examinations

- Are for jobs that have certain physical requirements
- Mostly used for insurance purposes

REALISTIC JOB PREVIEWS At the Hilton Baltimore BWI Airport, housekeeping job prospects are taken to a guest room and asked to make a bed with the precision that the interviewer demonstrated. By introducing applicants to what's involved in doing the job they're seeking, the hotel is hoping to eliminate misconceptions or surprises.[58] One thing managers need to carefully watch is how they portray the organization and the work an applicant will be doing. If they tell applicants only the good aspects, they're likely to have a workforce that's dissatisfied and prone to high turnover.[59] Negative things can happen when the information an applicant receives is excessively inflated. First, mismatched applicants probably won't withdraw from the selection process. Second, inflated information builds unrealistic expectations, so new employees may quickly become dissatisfied and leave the organization. Third, new hires become disillusioned and less committed to the organization when they face the unexpected harsh realities of the job. In addition, these individuals may feel they were misled during the hiring process and then become problem employees.

To increase employee job satisfaction and reduce turnover, managers should consider a **realistic job preview (RJP)**, one that includes both positive and negative information about the job and the company. For instance, in addition to the positive comments typically expressed during an interview, the job applicant might be told there are limited opportunities to talk to coworkers during work hours,

realistic job preview (RJP)
A preview of a job that provides both positive and negative information about the job and the company

let's get REAL

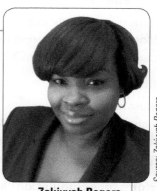

The Scenario:

José Salinas is the HR director at a large food processor. Within the last couple of years, he has seen more frequent parental involvement in their adult child's job hunt. In fact, one candidate's parents actually contacted the company after their child got a job offer wanting to discuss their daughter's salary, relocation package, and educational reimbursement opportunities. He's not sure how to handle these occurrences.

What advice would you give José?

You may understand a parent's concern but we cannot discuss company information with them. Our relationship is with the potential employee. Let the parent know you are willing to speak directly to their child and answer any questions they may have.

Zakiyyah Rogers
Department Manager,
Human Resources

that promotional advancement is unlikely, or that work hours are erratic and they may have to work weekends. Research indicates that applicants who receive an RJP have more realistic expectations about the jobs they'll be performing and are better able to cope with the frustrating elements than applicants who receive only inflated information.

PROVIDING Employees with Needed Skills and Knowledge

L03 As one of the nation's busiest airports, Miami International Airport served more than 40.5 million passengers in 2013. But Miami International is doing something that no other airport has done. It's asked different groups of employees to "think and act as ambassadors for regional tourism." These airport workers are discovering how important it is to help travelers find solutions to the frustrating issues they face as they travel into and out of Miami. Accomplishing that means that all employees who work on airport grounds are required to thoroughly learn and understand customer service through a series of tourism training efforts. The required training is tied to renewal of airport ID badges, providing a critical incentive for employees to participate.[60]

If recruiting and selecting are done properly, we should have hired competent individuals who can perform successfully on the job. But successful performance requires more than possessing certain skills. New hires must be acclimated to the organization's culture and be trained and given the knowledge to do the job in a manner consistent with the organization's goals. Current employees, like those at Miami International Airport, may have to complete training programs to improve or update their skills. For these acclimation and skill improvement tasks, HRM uses orientation and training.

Orientation

Did you participate in some type of organized "introduction to college life" when you started school? If so, you may have been told about your school's rules and the procedures for activities such as applying for financial aid, cashing a check, or registering

for classes, and you were probably introduced to some of the college administrators. A person starting a new job needs the same type of introduction to his or her job and the organization. This introduction is called **orientation**.

orientation
Introducing a new employee to his or her job and the organization

There are two types of orientation. *Work unit orientation* familiarizes the employee with the goals of the work unit, clarifies how his or her job contributes to the unit's goals, and includes an introduction to his or her new coworkers. *Organization orientation* informs the new employee about the company's goals, history, philosophy, procedures, and rules. It should also include relevant HR policies and maybe even a tour of the facilities.

Many organizations have formal orientation programs, while others use a more informal approach in which the manager assigns the new employee to a senior member of the work group who introduces the new hire to immediate coworkers and shows him or her where important things are located. And then there are intense orientation programs like that at Randstad USA, a staffing company based in Atlanta. The company's 16-week program covers everything from the company's culture to on-the-job training. The executive in charge of curriculum development says it's a comprehensive process that covers what new employees have to learn and do and what the managers of these new employees are expected to do."[61] And managers do have an obligation to effectively and efficiently integrate any new employee into the organization. They should openly discuss mutual obligations of the organization and the employee.[62] It's in the best interests of both the organization and the new employee to get the person up and running in the job as soon as possible. Successful orientation results in an outsider-insider transition that makes the new employee feel comfortable and fairly well adjusted, lowers the likelihood of poor work performance, and reduces the probability of a surprise resignation only a week or two into the job.

Employee Training

On the whole, planes don't cause airline accidents, people do. Most collisions, crashes, and other airline mishaps—nearly three-quarters of them—result from errors by the pilot or air traffic controller, or from inadequate maintenance. Weather and structural failures typically account for the remaining accidents.[63] We cite these statistics to illustrate the importance of training in the airline industry. Such maintenance and human errors could be prevented or significantly reduced by better employee training, as shown by the amazing "landing" of US Airways Flight 1549 in the Hudson River in January 2009 with no loss of life. Pilot Captain Chesley Sullenberger attributed the positive outcome to the extensive and intensive training that all pilots and flight crews undergo.[64] At management and technology consulting firm BearingPoint, the ethics and compliance training program became a series of fictional films modeled after *The Office*, even with a "Michael Scott-esque leader."[65] The film episodes were an immediate sensation in the company, with employees commenting that this training was the best ever or that this training topic totally described challenges faced by their team. The new episodes became so popular that employees started tracking them down on the company's staging server, which is pretty amazing considering these training videos covered issues that most employees find boring, even though it's critical information. Everything that employees at Ruth's Chris Steak House restaurants need to know can be found on sets of 4 × 8½-inch cards. Whether it's a recipe for caramelized banana cream pie or how to acknowledge customers, it's on the cards. And since the cards for all jobs are readily available, employees know the behaviors and skills it takes to get promoted. It's a unique approach to employee training, but it seems to work. Since the card system was implemented, employee turnover has decreased, something that's not easy to accomplish in the restaurant industry.[66] Training is just as important at other restaurants, with servers trained to "read" diners and make the service more personal.[67]

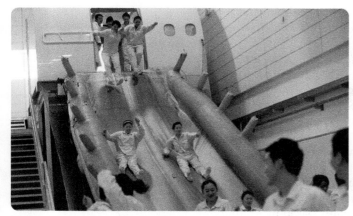

Pilots and cabin crew members of China's Hainan Airlines learn how to use an escape slide in evacuating an airplane quickly during emergency situations. Training for emergencies and evacuations such as the operation of escape slides and life rafts and the mechanical workings of aircraft doors is a top priority of airlines' intensive safety training programs.
Source: Wang Jianhua/Newscom

Employee training is an important HRM activity. As job demands change, employee skills have to change. In 2012, U.S. business firms spent more than $164 billion on formal employee training.[68] Managers, of course, are responsible for deciding what type of training employees need, when they need it, and what form that training should take.

TYPES OF TRAINING Exhibit 8 describes the major types of training that organizations provide. Some of the most popular types include profession/industry-specific training, management/supervisory skills, mandatory/compliance information (such as sexual harassment, safety, etc.), and customer service training. For many organizations, employee interpersonal skills training—communication, conflict resolution, team building, customer service, and so forth—is a high priority. For example, the director of training and development for Vancouver-based Boston Pizza International said, "Our people know the Boston Pizza concept; they have all the hard skills. It's the soft skills they lack."[69] So the company launched Boston Pizza College, a training program that uses hands-on, scenario-based learning about many interpersonal skills topics. For Canon, Inc., it's the repair personnel's technical skills that are important.[70] As part of their training, repair people play a video game based on the familiar kids' board game Operation in which "lights flashed and buzzers sounded if copier parts were dragged and dropped poorly." The company found that comprehension levels were 5 to 8 percent higher than when traditional training manuals were used.

TRAINING METHODS Although employee training can be done in traditional ways, many organizations are relying more on technology-based training methods because of their accessibility, cost, and ability to deliver information. Exhibit 9 provides a description of the various traditional and technology-based training methods that managers might use. Of all these training methods, experts believe that organizations will increasingly rely on e-learning and mobile applications to deliver important information and to develop employees' skills.

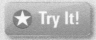

If your professor has assigned this, go to **www.mymanagementlab.com** to complete the Simulation: Human Resource Management and get a better understanding of the challenges of training in organizations.

Exhibit 8
Types of Training

Source: Based on "2005 Industry Report—Types of Training," *Training*, December 2005, p. 22.

TYPE	INCLUDES
General	Communication skills, computer systems application and programming, customer service, executive development, management skills and development, personal growth, sales, supervisory skills, and technological skills and knowledge
Specific	Basic life–work skills, creativity, customer education, diversity/cultural awareness, remedial writing, managing change, leadership, product knowledge, public speaking/presentation skills, safety, ethics, sexual harassment, team building, wellness, and others

Exhibit 9
Traditional Training Methods

On-the-job—Employees learn how to do tasks simply by performing them, usually after an initial introduction to the task.

Job rotation—Employees work at different jobs in a particular area, getting exposure to a variety of tasks.

Mentoring and coaching—Employees work with an experienced worker who provides information, support, and encouragement; also called apprenticeships in certain industries.

Experiential exercises—Employees participate in role-playing, simulations, or other face-to-face types of training.

Workbooks/manuals—Employees refer to training workbooks and manuals for information.

Classroom lectures—Employees attend lectures designed to convey specific information.

Technology-Based Training Methods

CD-ROM/DVD/videotapes/audiotapes/podcasts—Employees listen to or watch selected media that convey information or demonstrate certain techniques.

Videoconferencing/teleconferencing/satellite TV—Employees listen to or participate as information is conveyed or techniques demonstrated.

E-learning—Internet-based learning where employees participate in multimedia simulations or other interactive modules.

Mobile learning—Learning delivered via mobile devices.

RETAINING Competent, High-Performing Employees

LO4 At Procter & Gamble, mid-year employee evaluations were used to adjust work goals to reflect more accurately what could be achieved in such a challenging economic environment. The company has directed managers to focus on employees' achievements rather than just to point out areas that need improvement. P&G's director of human resources said, "Particularly in this economy, people are living in the survival zone. Setting attainable targets was important to keeping up morale."[71]

Once an organization has invested significant dollars in recruiting, selecting, orienting, and training employees, it wants to keep them, especially the competent, high-performing ones! Two HRM activities that play a role in this area are managing employee performance and developing an appropriate compensation and benefits program.

Employee Performance Management

A survey found that two-thirds of surveyed organizations felt they had inefficient performance management processes in place.[72] That's scary because managers need to know whether their employees are performing their jobs efficiently and effectively. That's what a **performance management system** does—establishes performance standards used to evaluate employee performance. How do managers evaluate employees' performance? That's where the different performance appraisal methods come in.

performance management system
Establishes performance standards used to evaluate employee performance

PERFORMANCE APPRAISAL METHODS More than 70 percent of managers admit they have trouble giving a critical performance review to an underachieving employee.[73] It's particularly challenging when managers and employees alike sense

Exhibit 10
Performance Appraisal Methods

Written Essay
Evaluator writes a description of employee's strengths and weaknesses, past performance, and potential; provides suggestions for improvement.

+ Simple to use
− May be better measure of evaluator's writing ability than of employee's actual performance

Critical Incident
Evaluator focuses on critical behaviors that separate effective and ineffective performance.

+ Rich examples, behaviorally based
− Time-consuming, lacks quantification

Graphic Rating Scale
Popular method that lists a set of performance factors and an incremental scale; evaluator goes down the list and rates employee on each factor.

+ Provides quantitative data; not time-consuming
− Doesn't provide in-depth information on job behavior

BARS (Behaviorally Anchored Rating Scale)
Popular approach that combines elements from critical incident and graphic rating scale; evaluator uses a rating scale, but items are examples of actual job behaviors.

+ Focuses on specific and measurable job behaviors
− Time-consuming; difficult to develop

Multiperson Comparison
Employees are rated in comparison to others in work group.

+ Compares employees with one another
− Difficult with large number of employees; legal concerns

MBO
Employees are evaluated on how well they accomplish specific goals.

+ Focuses on goals; results oriented
− Time-consuming

360-Degree Appraisal
Utilizes feedback from supervisors, employees, and coworkers.

+ Thorough
− Time-consuming

they're not beneficial.[74] And some companies—about 1 percent—are eliminating the formal performance review entirely.[75] Although appraising someone's performance is never easy, especially with employees who aren't doing their jobs well, managers can be better at it by using any of the seven different performance appraisal methods. A description of each of these methods, including advantages and disadvantages, is shown in Exhibit 10.

Compensation and Benefits
Executives at Discovery Communications Inc. had an employee morale problem on their hands. Many of the company's top performers were making the same salaries as the poorer performers, and the company's compensation program didn't allow for

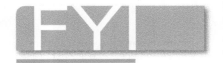

giving raises to people who stayed in the same position. The only way for managers to reward the top performers was to give them a bonus or promote them to another position. Executives were discovering that not only was that unfair, it was counterproductive. So they overhauled the program.[77]

Just in case you think that compensation and benefits decisions aren't important, a survey showed that 71 percent of workers surveyed said their benefits package would influence their decision to leave their job.[78] Most of us expect to receive appropriate compensation from our employer. Developing an effective and appropriate compensation system is an important part of the HRM process.[79] It can help attract and retain competent and talented individuals who help the organization accomplish its mission and goals. In addition, an organization's compensation system has been shown to have an impact on its strategic performance.[80]

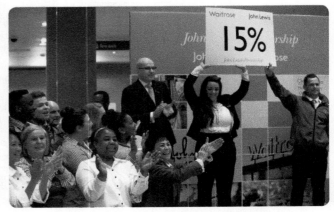

Employees of British retailer John Lewis Partnership cheer as they celebrate receiving an annual bonus of 15 percent of their salary based on the company's almost 10 percent increase in profits. A bonus is one example of a variable pay system that compensates employees on the basis of some performance measure.
Source: Andrew Winning/Reuters Pictures

Managers must develop a compensation system that reflects the changing nature of work and the workplace in order to keep people motivated. Organizational compensation can include many different types of rewards and benefits such as base wages and salaries, wage and salary add-ons, incentive payments, and other benefits and services. Some organizations offer employees some unusual, but popular, benefits. For instance, at Qualcomm, employees can receive surfing lessons, kayaking tours, and baseball game tickets. Employees at CHG Healthcare Services enjoy an on-site fitness center, fresh fruit baskets every morning, and an annual wellness fair. And at J. M. Smucker, new hires get a gift basket sent to their homes and all employees enjoy softball games and bowling nights.[81]

How do managers determine who gets paid what? Several factors influence the compensation and benefit packages that different employees receive. Exhibit 11 on the next page summarizes these factors, which are job-based and business- or industry-based. Many organizations, however, are using alternative approaches to determining compensation: skill-based pay and variable pay.

Skill-based pay systems reward employees for the job skills and competencies they can demonstrate. Under this type of pay system, an employee's job title doesn't define his or her pay category, skills do.[82] Research shows these types of pay systems tend to be more successful in manufacturing organizations than in service organizations and organizations pursuing technical innovations.[83] On the other hand, many organizations use **variable pay** systems, in which an individual's compensation is contingent on performance—90 percent of U.S. organizations use some type of variable pay plans, and 81 percent of Canadian and Taiwanese organizations do.[84]

skill-based pay
A pay system that rewards employees for the job skills they can demonstrate

variable pay
A pay system in which an individual's compensation is contingent on performance

Although many factors influence the design of an organization's compensation system, flexibility is a key consideration. The traditional approach to paying people reflected a more stable time when an employee's pay was largely determined by seniority and job level. Given the dynamic environments that many organizations face, the trend is to make pay systems more flexible and to reduce the number of pay levels. However, whatever approach managers use, they must establish a fair, equitable, and motivating compensation system that allows the organization to recruit and keep a talented and productive workforce.

If your professor has assigned this, go to **www.mymanagementlab.com** to complete the Writing Assignment MGMT 9: Management & Human Resources (HR Decision Making).

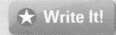

Exhibit 11
What Determines Pay
and Benefits

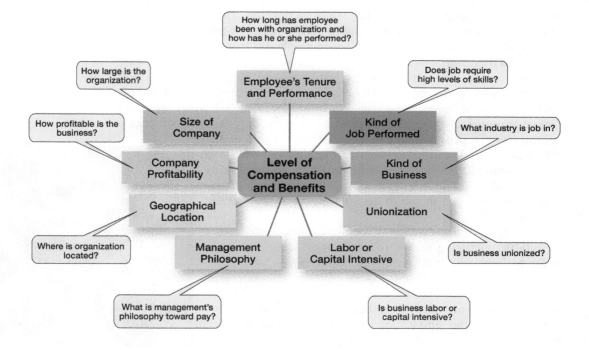

CONTEMPORARY Issues in Managing Human Resources

L05 We'll conclude this text by looking at some contemporary HR issues facing today's managers. These concerns include managing downsizing, sexual harassment, work–life balance, and controlling HR costs.

Managing Downsizing

"Before 1981, the word 'layoff' in the sense of permanent separation from a job with no prospects for recall, was so uncommon that the U.S. Bureau of Labor Statistics didn't even keep track of such cuts."[85] How things have changed!

downsizing
The planned elimination of jobs in an organization

Downsizing (or layoffs) is the planned elimination of jobs in an organization. When an organization has too many employees—which can happen when it's faced with an economic recession, declining market share, overly aggressive growth, or poorly managed operations—one option for improving profits is to eliminate some of those excess workers. During the most current economic recession, many well-known companies downsized—including, among others, Boeing, Nokia, Procter & Gamble, Hewlett-Packard, Volkswagen, Dell, General Motors, Unisys, Siemens, Merck, Honeywell, and eBay. And layoffs continue, although not as frequently. Some HR experts suggest that a "cost" associated with mass layoffs is the damage they can cause to long-term growth prospects.[86]

How can managers best manage a downsized workplace? Disruptions in the workplace and in employees' personal lives should be expected. Stress, frustration, anxiety, and anger are typical reactions of both individuals being laid off and the job survivors. Exhibit 12 lists some ways that managers can lessen the trauma both for the employees being laid off and for the survivors.[87]

Managing Sexual Harassment

A Kentucky appeals court said that McDonald's Corporation is liable in the sexual assault case of an employee detained by supervisors who were following the instructions of a prank caller pretending to be a police officer. The ruling said that McDonald's knew of 30 hoax telephone calls made to its restaurants from 1994 to

Exhibit 12
Tips for Managing Downsizing

- Treat everyone with respect.
- Communicate openly and honestly:
  - Inform those being let go as soon as possible.
  - Tell surviving employees the new goals and expectations.
  - Explain impact of layoffs.
- Follow any laws regulating severance pay or benefits.
- Provide support/counseling for surviving (remaining) employees.
- Reassign roles according to individuals' talents and backgrounds.
- Focus on boosting morale:
  - Offer individualized reassurance.
  - Continue to communicate, especially one-on-one.
  - Remain involved and available.
- Have a plan for the empty office spaces/cubicles so it isn't so depressing for surviving employees.

2004, including several calls to Kentucky restaurants in which the caller persuaded managers and employees to conduct strip searches and sexual assaults.[88]

Sexual harassment is a serious issue in both public and private sector organizations. During 2013 (the latest data available), more than 7,200 complaints were filed with the Equal Employment Opportunity Commission (EEOC), a drop from 7,944 in 2010, 7,809 in 2011, and 7,571 in 2012.[89] Although most complaints are filed by women, the percentage of charges filed by males were 17.6 percent. The costs of sexual harassment are high. Almost all *Fortune* 500 companies in the United States have had complaints lodged by employees, and at least a third have been sued.[90] Settlements can range from low thousands to millions.[91] Sexual harassment isn't a problem just in the United States. It's a global issue. For instance, data collected by the European Commission found that 30 to 50 percent of female employees in European Union countries had experienced some form of sexual harassment.[92] And sexual harassment charges have been filed against employers in other countries such as Japan, Australia, New Zealand, and Mexico.[93]

Even though discussions of sexual harassment cases often focus on the large awards granted by a court, there are other concerns for employers. It creates an unpleasant, oftentimes hostile, work environment and undermines workers' ability to perform their job.

So what is **sexual harassment**? It's defined as any unwanted action or activity of a sexual nature that explicitly or implicitly affects an individual's employment, performance, or work environment. And as we indicated earlier, it can occur between members of the opposite sex or of the same sex.

Many problems associated with sexual harassment involve determining exactly what constitutes this illegal behavior. The EEOC defines sexual harassment this way: "Unwelcome sexual advances, requests for sexual favors, and other verbal or physical conduct of a sexual nature constitute sexual harassment when this conduct explicitly or implicitly affects an individual's employment, unreasonably interferes with an individual's work performance, or creates an intimidating, hostile or offensive work environment."[94] The EEOC has added that sexual harassment can include offensive remarks about a person's sex. For many organizations, it's the offensive or hostile environment issue that is problematic. Managers must be aware of what constitutes such an environment. Another thing that managers must understand is that the victim doesn't necessarily have to be the person harassed but could be anyone affected by the offensive conduct.[95] The key is being attuned to what makes fellow employees uncomfortable—and if we don't know, we should ask![96]

What can an organization do to protect itself against sexual harassment claims?[97] The courts want to know two things: First, did the organization know about, or

sexual harassment
Any unwanted action or activity of a sexual nature that explicitly or implicitly affects an individual's employment, performance, or work environment

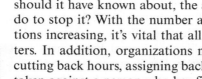

let's get REAL

The Scenario:

Lisa Brown is the HR director at a health care facility. She says, "I have a great employee who has a troubling habit of being 'touchy' in the workplace. Whenever this person is standing next to someone, she likes to touch the person's arm, hand, or shoulder. Just last week, I saw her talking to a male employee and she had her hand on his chest. Other than this habit, she's an outstanding worker."

What advice would you give Lisa?

My advice to Lisa would be to first, gently remind her employee that while she may think nothing of her affection, others may be uncomfortable or uneasy with such displays. If her behavior continues, the employee should be written up and spoken to again before the situation becomes more serious when she approaches someone who is upset by her communication "style."

Katie Pagan
Accounting & HR Manager

Source: Katie Pagan

should it have known about, the alleged behavior? And secondly, what did managers do to stop it? With the number and dollar amounts of the awards against organizations increasing, it's vital that all employees be educated on sexual harassment matters. In addition, organizations need to ensure that no retaliatory actions—such as cutting back hours, assigning back-to-back work shifts without a rest break, etc.—are taken against a person who has filed harassment charges, especially in light of a U.S. Supreme Court ruling that broadened the definition of retaliation.[98] One final area of interest we want to discuss in terms of sexual harassment is workplace romances.

WORKPLACE ROMANCES If you're employed, have you ever dated someone at work? If not, have you ever been attracted to someone in your workplace and thought about pursuing a relationship? Such situations are more common than you might think—40 percent of employees surveyed by the *Wall Street Journal* said they have had an office romance.[100] And another survey found that 43 percent of single men and 28 percent of single women said they would be open to dating a coworker.[101] The environment in today's organizations with mixed-gender work teams and long work hours has likely contributed to this situation. "People realize they're going to be at work such long hours, it's almost inevitable that this takes place," said one survey director.[102] And some 67 percent of employees feel there's no need to hide their office relationships.[103]

But workplace romances can potentially become big problems for organizations.[104] In addition to the potential conflicts and retaliation between coworkers who decide to stop dating or to end a romantic relationship, more serious problems stem from the potential for sexual harassment accusations, especially when it's between supervisor and subordinate. The standard used by judicial courts has been that workplace sexual conduct is prohibited sexual harassment *if* it is unwelcome. If it's welcome, it still may be inappropriate, but usually is not unlawful. However, a ruling by the California Supreme Court concerning specifically a supervisor–subordinate relationship that got out of hand is worth noting. That ruling said "completely consensual workplace romances can create a hostile work environment for others in the workplace."[105]

What should managers do about workplace romances? Over the last decade, companies have become more flexible about workplace romances. People spend so much time at the office that coworker romances are almost inevitable.[106] However,

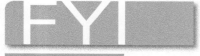

it's important to educate employees about the potential for sexual harassment. A survey of organizations showed that 42 percent have written or verbal policies on office romances.)[107] And because the potential liability is more serious when it comes to supervisor–subordinate relationships, a more proactive approach is needed in terms of discouraging such relationships and perhaps even requiring supervisors to report any such relationships to the HR department. At some point, the organization may even want to consider banning such relationships, although an outright ban may be difficult to put into practice.

Managing Work–Life Balance

In 2009, Verizon employees contacted VZ-LIFE, the company's employee assistance program, more than 1,100 times a month by phone and logged more than 35,000 visits a month to the Web site. This program provides resources on parenting and childcare, adult care, health and wellness, moving and relocation, and much more.[108]

Smart managers recognize that employees don't leave their families and personal lives behind when they come to work. Although managers can't be sympathetic with every detail of an employee's family life, organizations are becoming more attuned to the fact that employees have sick children, elderly parents who need special care, and other family issues that may require special arrangements. In response, many organizations are offering **family-friendly benefits**, which accommodate employees' needs for work–family life balance. They've introduced programs such as on-site child care, summer day camps, flextime, job sharing, time off for school functions, telecommuting, and part-time employment. Work–family life conflicts are as relevant to male workers with children and women without children as they are for female employees with children. Heavy workloads and increased travel demands have made it hard for many employees to satisfactorily juggle both work and personal responsibilities. A *Fortune* survey found that 84 percent of male executives surveyed said that "they'd like job options that let them realize their professional aspirations while having more time for things outside work."[109] Also, 87 percent of these executives believed that any company that restructured top-level management jobs in ways that would both increase productivity and make more time available for life outside the office would have a competitive advantage in attracting talented employees. Younger employees, particularly, put a higher priority on family and a lower priority on jobs and are looking for organizations that give them more work flexibility.[110]

Today's progressive workplaces must accommodate the varied needs of a diverse workforce. How? By providing a wide range of scheduling options and benefits that allow employees more flexibility at work and to better balance or integrate their work and personal lives. Despite these organizational efforts, work–family life programs certainly have room for improvement. One survey showed that more than 31 percent of college-educated male workers spend 50 or more hours a week at work (up from 22 percent in 1980) and that about 40 percent of American adults get less than seven hours of sleep on weekdays (up from 34 percent in 2001).[111] What about women? Another survey showed that the percentage of American women working 40 hours or more per week had increased. By the way, this same survey showed that the percentage of European women working 40 hours or more had actually declined.[112] Other workplace surveys still show high levels of employee stress stemming from work–family life conflicts. And large groups of women and minority workers remain unemployed or underemployed because of family responsibilities and bias in the workplace.[113] So what can managers do?

Research on work–family life balance has shown positive outcomes when individuals are able to combine work and family roles.[114] As one study participant noted, "I think being a mother and having patience and watching someone else grow has made me a better manager. I am better able to be patient with other people and let them grow and develop in a way that is good for them."[115] In addition, individuals who have

family-friendly benefits
Benefits that accommodate employees' needs for work–life balance

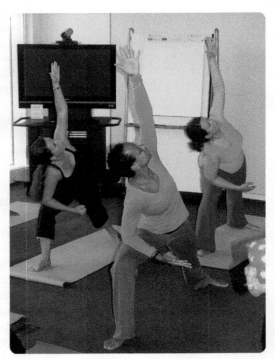

Discovery Communications provides flexible work arrangements, work-life initiatives, and wellness programs such as yoga classes to accommodate employees' different life styles, life stages, and life events. To help employees balance work and personal responsibilities, the media company offers telework, compressed work weeks, job sharing, and a summer-hours program.
Source: Susan Heavey/Reuters Pictures

FUTURE VISION | 24/7 Work Life

Technology and globalization have played major roles in blurring the lines between work and leisure time. It's increasingly expected that today's professional worker be available 24/7. So employees regularly check their e-mail before going to bed, take calls from the boss during dinner, participate in global conference calls at 6 A.M., and read tweets from colleagues on weekends.

The 24/7 work life eventually undermines real social relationships. Face-to-face interactions with family and friends suffer and people are likely to feel stressed out and emotionally empty. In response, employees are likely to demand real and virtual barriers that can separate their work and personal lives. For instance, you'll set up separate accounts, Web sites, and networks for work and friends. Employers will find that employees balk at work demands outside defined work hours. In order to get and keep good employees, organizations will need to restructure work communications so as to confine them to more traditional hours.

If your professor has chosen to assign this, go to **www.mymanagementlab.com** *to discuss the following questions.*

⭐ **TALK ABOUT IT 1:** As the title says, *is* work life 24/7? Why or why not?

⭐ **TALK ABOUT IT 2:** Why is this an HRM issue? Or is it? Discuss.

family-friendly workplace support appear to be more satisfied on the job.[116] This finding seems to strengthen the notion that organizations benefit by creating a workplace in which employee work–family life balance is possible. And the benefits are financial as well. Research has shown a significant, positive relationship between work–family life initiatives and an organization's stock price.[117] However, managers need to understand that people do differ in their preferences for work–family life scheduling options and benefits.[118] Some prefer organizational initiatives that better *segment* work from their personal lives. Others prefer programs that facilitate *integration*. For instance, flextime schedules segment because they allow employees to schedule work hours that are less likely to conflict with personal responsibilities. On the other hand, on-site child care integrates the boundaries between work and family responsibilities. People who prefer segmentation are more likely to be satisfied and committed to their jobs when offered options such as flextime, job sharing, and part-time hours. People who prefer integration are more likely to respond positively to options such as on-site child care, gym facilities, and company-sponsored family picnics.

Controlling HR Costs

It's estimated that worker obesity costs U.S. companies as much as $153 billion annually.[119] HR costs are skyrocketing, especially employee health care and employee pensions. Organizations are looking for ways to control these costs.

EMPLOYEE HEALTH CARE COSTS At AOL, almost 1,000 employees enrolled in an 11-week activity challenge to take as many steps as possible. By the end of the challenge, those employees had taken more than 530 million total steps—equivalent to walking around the globe more than 10 times. Employees at Paychex who undergo a confidential health screening and risk assessment, and those who smoke who agree to enroll in a smoking cessation program, can get free annual physicals, colonoscopies, and 100 percent coverage of preventive care as well as lower deductibles and costs. At Black and Decker Corporation, employees and dependents who certify in an honor system that they have been tobacco-free for at least six months pay $75 less per month for their medical and dental coverage. At Amerigas Propane, employees were given an ultimatum: get their medical check-ups or lose their health insurance.[120]

All these examples illustrate how companies are trying to control skyrocketing employee health care costs. Since 2002, health care costs have risen an average of

15 percent a year and are expected to double by the year 2016 from the $2.2 trillion spent in 2007.[121] And smokers cost companies even more—about 25 percent more for health care than nonsmokers.[122] However, the biggest health care cost for companies—estimated at $153 billion a year—is obesity and its related costs arising from medical expenditures and absenteeism.[123] A study of manufacturing organizations found that presenteeism, defined as employees not performing at full capacity, was 1.8 percent higher for workers with moderate to severe obesity than for all other employees.[124] The reason for the lost productivity is likely the result of reduced mobility because of body size or pain problems such as arthritis. Is it any wonder that organizations are looking for ways to control their health care costs? How? First, many organizations are providing opportunities for employees to lead healthy lifestyles. From financial incentives to company-sponsored health and wellness programs, the goal is to limit rising health care costs. About 41 percent of companies use some type of positive incentives aimed at encouraging healthy behavior, up from 34 percent in 1996.[125] Another study indicated that nearly 90 percent of companies surveyed planned to aggressively promote healthy lifestyles to their employees during the next three to five years.[126] Many are starting sooner: Google, Yamaha Corporation of America, Caterpillar, and others are putting health food in company break rooms, cafeterias, and vending machines; providing deliveries of fresh organic fruit; and putting "calorie taxes" on fatty foods.[127] In the case of smokers, however, some companies have taken a more aggressive stance by increasing the amount smokers pay for health insurance or by firing them if they refuse to stop smoking.

EMPLOYEE PENSION PLAN COSTS   The other area where organizations are looking to control costs is employee pension plans. Corporate pensions have been around since the nineteenth century.[128] But the days when companies could afford to give employees a broad-based pension that provided them a guaranteed retirement income have changed. Pension commitments have become such an enormous burden that companies can no longer afford them. In fact, the corporate pension system has been described as "fundamentally broken."[129] Many companies no longer provide pensions. Even IBM, which closed its pension plan to new hires in December 2004, told employees that their pension benefits would be frozen.[130] A survey found that only 57 percent of employers surveyed offered both a traditional pension plan and a defined contribution plan (down from 64 percent in 2009). Of those with traditional pension plans, only 44 percent remained open to new hires.[131] Obviously, the pension issue is one that directly affects HR decisions. On the one hand, organizations want to attract talented, capable employees by offering them desirable benefits such as pensions. But on the other hand, organizations have to balance offering benefits with the costs of providing such benefits.

PREPARING FOR: Exams/Quizzes

CHAPTER SUMMARY by Learning Objectives

LO1

EXPLAIN the importance of the human resource management process and the external influences that might affect that process.

HRM is important for three reasons. First, it can be a significant source of competitive advantage. Second, it's an important part of organizational strategies. Finally, the way organizations treat their people has been found to significantly impact organizational performance.

The external factors that most directly affect the HRM process are the economy, labor unions, legal environment, and demographic trends.

LO2 DISCUSS **the tasks associated with identifying and selecting competent employees.**

A job analysis is an assessment that defines a job and the behaviors necessary to perform it. A job description is a written statement describing a job, and typically includes job content, environment, and conditions of employment. A job specification is a written statement that specifies the minimum qualifications a person must possess to successfully perform a given job.

The major sources of potential job candidates include the Internet, employee referrals, company Web site, college recruiting, and professional recruiting organizations.

The different selection devices include application forms (best used for gathering employee information), written tests (must be job-related), work sampling (appropriate for complex nonmanagerial and routine work), assessment centers (most appropriate for top-level managers), interviews (widely used, but most appropriate for managerial positions, especially top-level managers), background investigations (useful for verifying application data, but reference checks are essentially worthless), and physical exams (useful for work that involves certain physical requirements and for insurance purposes).

A realistic job preview is important because it gives an applicant more realistic expectations about the job, which in turn should increase employee job satisfaction and reduce turnover.

LO3 EXPLAIN **the different types of orientation and training.**

Orientation is important because it results in an outsider-insider transition that makes the new employee feel comfortable and fairly well-adjusted, lowers the likelihood of poor work performance, and reduces the probability of an early surprise resignation.

The two types of training are general (includes communication skills, computer skills, customer service, personal growth, etc.) and specific (includes basic life/work skills, customer education, diversity/cultural awareness, managing change, etc.). This training can be provided using traditional training methods (on-the-job, job rotation, mentoring and coaching, experiential exercises, workbooks/manuals, and classroom lectures) or by technology-based methods (CD/DVD/videotapes/audiotapes, video-conferencing or teleconferencing, or e-learning).

LO4 DESCRIBE **strategies for retaining competent, high-performing employees.**

The different performance appraisal methods are written essays, critical incidents, graphic rating scales, BARS, multiperson comparisons, MBO, and 360-degree appraisals.

The factors that influence employee compensation and benefits include the employee's tenure and performance, kind of job performed, kind of business/industry, unionization, labor or capital intensive, management philosophy, geographical location, company profitability, and size of company.

Skill-based pay systems reward employees for the job skills and competencies they can demonstrate. In a variable pay system, an employee's compensation is contingent on performance.

LO5 DISCUSS **contemporary issues in managing human resources.**

Managers can manage downsizing by communicating openly and honestly, following appropriate laws regarding severance pay or benefits, providing support/counseling for surviving employees, reassigning roles according to individuals' talents and backgrounds, focusing on boosting morale, and having a plan for empty office spaces.

Sexual harassment is any unwanted action or activity of a sexual nature that explicitly or implicitly affects an individual's employment, performance, or work environment. Managers need to be aware of what constitutes an offensive or hostile work environment, educate employees on sexual harassment, and ensure that no retaliatory actions are taken against any person who files harassment charges. Also, they may need to have a policy in place for workplace romances.

Organizations are dealing with work–family life balance issues by offering family-friendly benefits such as on-site child care, flextime, telecommuting, and so on. Managers need to understand that people may prefer programs that segment work and personal lives, while others prefer programs that integrate their work and personal lives.

Organizations are controlling HR costs by controlling employee health care costs through employee health initiatives (encouraging healthy behavior and penalizing unhealthy behaviors) and controlling employee pension plans by eliminating or severely limiting them.

MyManagementLab

Go to **mymanagementlab.com** to complete the problems marked with this icon ⭐.

⭐ REVIEW AND DISCUSSION QUESTIONS

1. Discuss the external environmental factors that most directly affect the HRM process.

2. Some critics claim that corporate HR departments have outlived their usefulness and are not there to help employees, but to keep the organization from legal problems. What do you think? What benefits are there to having a formal HRM process? What drawbacks?

3. Describe the different selection devices and which work best for different jobs.

4. What are the benefits and drawbacks of realistic job previews? (Consider this question from the perspective of both the organization and the employee.)

5. Describe the different types of orientation and training and how each of the types of training might be provided.

6. List the factors that influence employee compensation and benefits.

7. Describe the different performance appraisal methods.

8. What, in your view, constitutes sexual harassment? Describe how companies can minimize sexual harassment in the workplace.

MyManagementLab

If your professor has assigned these, go to **mymanagementlab.com** for Auto-graded writing questions as well as the following Assisted-graded writing questions:

9. How does HRM affect all managers?

10. Should an employer have the right to choose employees without governmental interference? Support your conclusion.

PREPARING FOR: My Career

⭐ PERSONAL INVENTORY ASSESSMENTS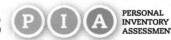

Work Performance Assessment

As this text indicated, performance assessment is an important HR function. Use this PIA to assess work performance.

⭐ ETHICS DILEMMA

It's likely to be a challenging issue for HR managers.[132] "It" is the use of medical marijuana by employees. Seventeen states and the District of Columbia have laws or constitutional amendments that allow patients with certain medical conditions such as cancer, glaucoma, or chronic pain to use marijuana without fear of being prosecuted. Federal prosecutors have been directed by the Obama administration not to bring criminal charges against marijuana users who follow their states' laws. However, that puts employers in a difficult position as they try to accommodate state laws on medical marijuana use while having to enforce federal rules or company drug-use policies based on federal law. Although courts have generally ruled that companies do not have to accommodate medical marijuana users, legal guidance is still not all that clear. Legal experts have warned employers to "not run afoul of disability and privacy laws." In addition to the legal questions, employers are concerned about the challenge of maintaining a safe workplace.

11. What ethical issues do you see here?

12. How might this issue affect HR processes such as recruitment, selection, performance management, compensation and benefits, and safety and health?

13. What other stakeholders might be impacted by this? In what ways might they be impacted?

SKILLS EXERCISE Developing Your Interviewing Skills

About the Skill

In the chapter-opening *It's Your Career,* we discussed ways for you to be a good interviewee. Now, we need to switch roles. As a manager, you need to develop your interviewing skills. The following discussion highlights the key behaviors associated with this skill.

Steps in Practicing the Skill

- *Review the job description and job specification.* Reviewing pertinent information about the job provides valuable information about how to assess the candidate. Furthermore, relevant job requirements help to eliminate interview bias.

- *Prepare a structured set of questions to ask all applicants for the job.* By having a set of prepared questions, you ensure that the information you wish to elicit is attainable. Furthermore, if you ask all applicants similar questions, you're better able to compare their answers against a common base.

- *Before meeting an applicant, review his or her application form and résumé.* Doing so helps you to create a complete picture of the applicant in terms of what is represented on the résumé or application and what the job requires. You will also begin to identify areas to explore in the interview. That is, areas not clearly defined on the résumé or application but essential for the job will become a focal point of your discussion with the applicant.

- *Open the interview by putting the applicant at ease and by providing a brief preview of the topics to be discussed.* Interviews are stressful for job applicants. By opening with small talk (e.g., the weather), you give the person time to adjust to the interview setting. By providing a preview of topics to come, you're giving the applicant an agenda that helps the individual begin framing what he or she will say in response to your questions.

- *Ask your questions and listen carefully to the applicant's answers.* Select follow-up questions that naturally flow from the answers given. Focus on the responses as they relate to information you need to ensure that the applicant meets your job requirements. Any uncertainty you may still have requires a follow-up question to probe further for the information.

- *Close the interview by telling the applicant what's going to happen next.* Applicants are anxious about the status of your hiring decision. Be honest with the applicant regarding others who will be interviewed and the remaining steps in the hiring process. If you plan to make a decision in two weeks or so, let the individual know what you intend to do. In addition, tell the applicant how you will let him or her know about your decision.

- *Write your evaluation of the applicant while the interview is still fresh in your mind.* Don't wait until the end of your day, after interviewing several applicants, to write your analysis of each one. Memory can fail you. The sooner you complete your write-up after an interview, the better chance you have of accurately recording what occurred in the interview.

Practicing the Skill

Review and update your résumé. Then have several friends critique it who are employed in management-level positions or in management training programs. Ask them to explain their comments and make any changes to your résumé they think will improve it.

Now inventory your interpersonal and technical skills and any practical experiences that do not show up in your résumé. Draft a set of leading questions you would like to be asked in an interview that would give you a chance to discuss the unique qualities and attributes you could bring to the job.

WORKING TOGETHER Team Exercise

The increasing popularity of body art is posing challenges for employers and HR departments in every profession and industry.[133] A Pew Research Center survey reported that 36 percent of 18- to 25-year-olds and 40 percent of 26- to 40-year-olds have at least one tattoo. In those same age groups, 30 percent and 22 percent, respectively, have a piercing somewhere other than their ears. The same survey found that even in the 40- to 60-year-old age group, more than 10 percent had tattoos or piercings outside of their ears.

Form small groups of three to four individuals. Your team's task is to come up with a dress code and grooming policy that clearly spells out guidelines regarding body art and what is permitted. You can do this in the form of a bulleted list. Be prepared to share your proposed policy with the class.

MY TURN TO BE A MANAGER

- Studies show that women's salaries still lag behind men's and, even with equal opportunity laws and regulations, women are paid about 82 percent of what men are paid.[134] Do some research on designing a compensation system that would address this issue. Write up your findings in a bulleted list format.

- Go to the Society for Human Resource Management Web site [www.shrm.org] and look for the HR News. Pick one of the news stories to read. (Note: Some of these may be available only to SHRM members, but others should be generally available.) Write a summary of the information. At the end of your summary, discuss the implications of the topic for managers.

- Use the Internet to research five different companies that interest you and check out what they say about careers or their people. Put this information in a bulleted-format report. Be prepared to make a presentation to the class on your findings.

- Work on your résumé. If you don't have one already, research what a good résumé should include. If you have one already, make sure it provides specific information that explicitly describes your work skills and experience rather than meaningless phrases such as "results-oriented."

- If you're working, note what types of HRM activities your managers do (such as interview, appraise performance, etc.). Ask them what they've found to be effective in getting and keeping good employees. What hasn't been effective? What can you learn from this? If you're not working, interview three different managers as to what HRM activities they do and which they've found to be effective or not effective.

- Research your chosen career by finding out what it's going to take to be successful in that career in terms of education, skills, experience, and so forth. Write a Personal Career Guide detailing this information.

- Pick one of the four topics in the section on contemporary issues in managing human resources. Research this topic and write a paper about it. Focus on finding current information and current examples of companies dealing with these issues.

- In your own words, write down three things you learned in this text about being a good manager. Keep a copy of this for future reference.

CASE APPLICATION 1 Thinking Outside the Box

It's the world's largest package delivery company with the instantly recognizable brown trucks.[135] Every day United Parcel Service (UPS) transports more than 15 million packages and documents throughout the United States to more than 220 countries and territories. Delivering those packages efficiently is what it gets paid to do, and that massive effort wouldn't be possible without its 102,000-plus drivers. UPS recognizes that it has an HR challenge: hiring and training some 25,000 drivers over the next five years to replace retiring baby boomers. But the company has a plan in place that combines its tested business model of uniformity

and efficiency (for instance, drivers are trained to hold their keys on a pinky finger so they don't waste time fumbling in their pockets for the keys) with a new approach to driver training.

UPS's traditional classroom driver training obviously wasn't working, as some 30 percent of its driver candidates didn't make it. The company was convinced that the twentysomethings—the bulk of its driver recruits—responded best to high-tech instruction instead of books and lectures. Now, trainees use videogames, a "slip and fall simulator which combines a greased floor with slippery shoes," and an obstacle course around a mock village.

At a UPS training center outside of Washington, D.C., applicants for a driver's job, which pays an average of $74,000 annually, spend one week practicing and training to be a driver. They move from one station to the next practicing the company's "340 Methods," techniques developed by industrial engineers "to save seconds and improve safety in every task from lifting and loading boxes to selecting a package from a shelf in the truck." Applicants play a videogame where they're in the driver's seat and must identify obstacles. From computer simulations, they move to "Clarksville," a mock village with miniature houses and faux businesses. There, they drive a real truck and "must successfully execute five deliveries in 19 minutes." And, in the interest of safety and efficiency, trainees learn to carefully walk on ice with the slip and fall simulator.

How are the new training methods working? So far, so good. Of the 1,629 trainees who have completed it, "only 10 percent have failed the training program, which takes a total of six weeks overall, including 30 days of driving a truck in the real world."

⭐ DISCUSSION QUESTIONS

14. What external factors were affecting UPS's HR practices? How did UPS respond to these trends?

15. Why is efficiency and safety so important to UPS? What role do the company's industrial engineers play in how employees do their work?

16. What changes did the company make to its driver training program? What do you think of these changes?

17. What advantages and drawbacks do you see to this training approach for (a) the trainee and (b) the company?

CASE APPLICATION 2 Stopping Traffic

Things weren't turning out so good for J. C. Penney Co. and its CEO, Ron Johnson (now the former CEO, as he was let go in April 2013).[136] Johnson arrived with much acclaim from being the head of Apple's successful retail operations. At Penney's, he immediately began one of retailing's most ambitious overhauls, trying to position the company for success in a very challenging and difficult industry. His plans included a "stores-within-a store" concept, no sales or promotions, and a three-tiered pricing plan. He suggested that "Penney needed a little bit of Apple's magic." From the start, analysts and experts questioned whether Penney's customers, who were used to sales and coupons, would accept this new approach. Long story short...customers didn't. For the full fiscal year of 2012, Penney had a loss of $985 million (compared to a loss of $152 million in 2011). Now, you may be asking yourself, what does this story have to do with HRM? Well, a lot it turns out! When a company is struggling financially, it *is* going to impact its people.

And for JCPenney employees, that impact came in the form of a "traffic light" color-coded performance appraisal system. In a companywide broadcast, supervisors were told that they should categorize their employees by one of three colors: Green—their performance is okay; Yellow—they need some coaching to improve performance; and Red—their performance is not up to par and they need to leave. Many employees weren't even aware of the system and supervisors were given no guidance one way or the other regarding whether to tell them about it, although company headquarters chose not to disclose the light system to employees.

Although the uncertainties over how to inform or even whether to inform employees about this HR initiative is troubling, communication and HR experts say there are other problems with this green/yellow/red approach. One is that it's insensitive to "approach the livelihoods of human beings" this way. The easy-to-understand simplistic nature of green, yellow, and red colors doesn't translate well to what will be a tremendously personal and difficult situation for many employees, especially those with a "red" appraisal. Another problem is that labeling employees can create difficult interpersonal situations. The labels can become a source of humor and teasing, which can deteriorate into hurt feelings and even feelings of being discriminated against. "No matter how benign a color-coding system may seem, it's never going to work." This doesn't mean that employers don't evaluate employees. But companies should be open about it. Employees should know that they're being rated, what the criteria are, and if they have a poor rating, what options they have for improving. There should also be a fair process of appeal or protest if an employee feels the rating was unfair.

⭐ DISCUSSION QUESTIONS

18. Many managers say that evaluating an employee's performance is one of their most difficult tasks. Why do you think they feel this way? What can organizations (and managers) do to make it an effective process?

19. What's your impression of the color-coded system suggested by the former CEO? As a store department supervisor, how would you have approached that?

20. What could JCPenney executives have done to make this process more effective?

ENDNOTES

1. Daily Muse Editor, "A Simple Formula for Answering 'Tell Me About Yourself'," www.themuse.com, May 2, 2014.
2. J. Smith, "Here's How to Answer the Dreaded 'What's Your Greatest Weakness' Interview Question," www.businessinsider.com, March 18, 2014.
3. J. Smith, "The 7 Worst Body Language Mistakes Job Seekers Make," www.businessinsider.com, April 28, 2014.
4. P. Cappelli, "HR for Neophytes," *Harvard Business Review*, October 2013, pp. 25–27.
5. A. Carmeli and J. Shaubroeck, "How Leveraging Human Resource Capital with Its Competitive Distinctiveness Enhances the Performance of Commercial and Public Organizations," *Human Resource Management*, Winter 2005, pp. 391–412; L. Bassi and D. McMurrer, "How's Your Return on People?" *Harvard Business Review*, March 2004, p. 18; C. J. Collins and K. D. Clark, "Strategic Human Resource Practices, Top Management Team Social Networks, and Firm Performance: The Role of Human Resource Practices in Creating Organizational Competitive Advantage," *Academy of Management Journal*, December 2003, pp. 740–751; J. Pfeffer, *The Human Equation* (Boston: Harvard Business School Press, 1998); J. Pfeffer, *Competitive Advantage Through People* (Boston: Harvard Business School Press, 1994); A. A. Lado and M. C. Wilson, "Human Resource Systems and Sustained Competitive Advantage," *Academy of Management Review*, October 1994, pp. 699–727; and P. M. Wright and G. C. McMahan, "Theoretical Perspectives for Strategic Human Resource Management," *Journal of Management* 18, no. 1, 1992, pp. 295–320.
6. "Maximizing the Return on Your Human Capital Investment: The 2005 Watson Wyatt Human Capital Index® Report," "WorkAsia 2004/2005: A Study of Employee Attitudes in Asia," and "European Human Capital Index 2002," Watson Wyatt Worldwide (Washington, DC).
7. "Leading Through Connections: Highlights of the Global Chief Executive Officer Study," ibm.com/ceostudy 2012, 2012.
8. See, for example, C. H. Chuang and H. Liao, "Strategic Human Resource Management in Service Context: Taking Care of Business by Taking Care of Employees and Customers," *Personnel Psychology*, Spring 2010, pp. 153–196; M. Subramony, "A Meta-Analytic Investigation of the Relationship Between HRM Bundles and Firm Performance," *Human Resource Management*, September–October 2009, pp. 745–768; M. M. Butts et al., "Individual Reactions to High Involvement Work Practices: Investigating the Role of Empowerment and Perceived Organizational Support," *Journal of Occupational Health Psychology*, April 2009, pp. 122–136; L. Sun, S. Aryee, and K. S. Law, "High-Performance Human Resource Practices, Citizenship Behavior, and Organizational Performance: A Relational Perspective," *Academy of Management Journal*, June 2007, pp. 558–577; A. Carmeli and J. Shaubroeck, "How Leveraging Human Resource Capital with Its

Competitive Distinctiveness Enhances the Performance of Commercial and Public Organizations," 2005; Y. Y. Kor and H. Leblebici, "How Do Interdependencies Among Human-Capital Deployment, Development, and Diversification Strategies Affect Firms' Financial Performance?" *Strategic Management Journal,* October 2005, pp. 967–985; D. E. Bowen and C. Ostroff, "Understanding HRM–Firm Performance Linkages: The Role of the 'Strength' of the HRM System," *Academy of Management Review,* April 2004, pp. 203–221; A. S. Tsui, J. L. Pearce, L. W. Porter, and A. M. Tripoli, "Alternative Approaches to the Employee-Organization Relationship: Does Investment in Employees Pay Off?" *Academy of Management Journal,* October 1997, pp. 1089–1121; M. A. Huselid, S. E. Jackson, and R. S. Schuler, "Technical and Strategic Human Resource Management Effectiveness as Determinants of Firm Performance," *Academy of Management Journal,* January 1997, pp. 171–188; J. T. Delaney and M. A. Huselid, "The Impact of Human Resource Management Practices on Perceptions of Organizational Performance," *Academy of Management Journal,* August 1996, pp. 949–969; B. Becker and B. Gerhart, "The Impact of Human Resource Management on Organizational Performance: Progress and Prospects," *Academy of Management Journal,* August 1996, pp. 779–801; M. J. Koch and R. G. McGrath, "Improving Labor Productivity: Human Resource Management Policies Do Matter," *Strategic Management Journal,* May 1996, pp. 335–354; and M. A. Huselid, "The Impact of Human Resource Management Practices on Turnover, Productivity, and Corporate Financial Performance," *Academy of Management Journal,* June 1995, pp. 635–672.

9. "Human Capital a Key to Higher Market Value," *Business Finance,* December 1999, p. 15.

10. M. Boyle, "Happy People, Happy Returns," *Fortune,* January 11, 2006, p. 100.

11. P. C. Patel, J. G. Messersmith, and D. P. Lepak, "Walking the Tightrope: An Assessment of the Relationship Between High-Performance Work Systems and Organizational Ambidexterity," *Academy of Management Journal,* October 2013, pp. 1420–1442.

12. M. Luo, "$13 an Hour? 500 Sign Up, 1 Wins a Job," *New York Times Online,* October 22, 2009.

13. J. Clenfield, "A Tear in Japan's Safety Net," *Bloomberg BusinessWeek,* April 12, 2010, pp. 60–61.

14. A. Kashyap, "Europe Unemployment Dips; Lowest Rates Recorded in Austria, Germany and Luxembourg; Highest in Greece and Spain," www.ibtimes.com, April 1, 2014.

15. A. Kohpaiboon et al., "Global Recession: Labour Market Adjustment and International Production Networks," *ASEAN Economic Bulletin,* April 2010, pp. 98–120.

16. J. Schramm, "Tomorrow's Workforce," *HR Magazine,* March 2012, p. 112; C. Isidore, "Say Goodbye to Full-Time Jobs with Benefits," *CNNMoney.com,* June 1, 2010; C. Rampell, "In a Job Market Realignment, Some Left Behind," *New York Times Online,* May 12, 2010; and P. Izzo, "Economists Expect Shifting Work Force," *Wall Street Journal Online,* February 11, 2010.

17. F. Hansen, "Jobless Recovery Is Leaving a Trail of Recession-Weary Employees in Its Wake," *Compensation & Benefits Review,* May/June 2010, pp. 135–136; J. Hollon, "Worker 'Deal' Is Off," *Workforce Management,* April 2010, p. 42; and "The New Employment Deal: How Far, How Fast, and How Enduring? The 2010 Global Workforce Study," *Towers Watson* [www.towerswatson.com], April 2010.

18. D. Streitfeld, "Amazon Strikers Take Their Fight to Seattle," *New York Times Online,* December 16, 2013.

19. K. Niththyananthan, "BA, Union Set to Restart Talks," *Wall Street Journal Online,* June 1, 2010; The Associated Press, "No Deal in Talks on British Airway," *MSNBC.com,* May 27, 2010; D. Cameron and D. Michaels, "BA Crews Begin Walkout," *Wall Street Journal,* May 25, 2010, p. B2; and J. Brustein, "British Airways Cabin Crew Walks Out," *New York Times Online,* May 24, 2010.

20. K. Bradsher and D. Barboza, "Strike in China Highlights Gap in Workers' Pay," *New York Times Online,* May 28, 2010.

21. A. Smith, "Union Membership Inches Up," www.shrm.org, January 27, 2012.

22. "Trade Union Density," OECD.Stat Extracts, http://stats.oecd.org/Index.aspx?DataSetCode=UN_DEN, May 9, 2014.

23. C. Hausman, "Novartis Hit with Punitive Damages in Sex Discrimination Case," *Ethics Newsline* [www.globalethics.org/newsline], May 24, 2010.

24. S. Armour, "Lawsuits Pin Target on Managers," *USA Today* [www.usatoday.com], October 1, 2002.

25. G. B. Kushner, "Special Report: What HR Professionals Should Do Now," www.shrm.org, June 28, 2012; and S. G. Stolberg and R. Pear, "Obama Signs Health Care Overhaul Bill, with a Flourish," *New York Times Online,* March 23, 2010.

26. A. Smith, "Social Networking Online Protection Act Introduced," www.shrm.org, May 1, 2012.

27. B. Sarlin, "Obama Demands House GOP Vote on Immigration Reform," www.msnbc.com, April 16, 2014.

28. D. Cadrain, "Mexico Adapts to Labor Reform," *HR Management,* June 2013, pp. 83–88.

29. Leader Making a Difference box based on T. L. Friedman, "How to Get a Job at Google, Part 2," *New York Times Online,* April 19, 2014; L. Bock, "Google's Scientific Approach to Work-Life Balance (and Much More)," blogs.hbr.org, March 27, 2014; T. L. Friedman, "How to Get a Job at Google," *New York Times Online,* February 22, 2014; M. Moskowitz, R. Levering, C. Bessette, C. Dunn, C. Fairchild, and B. Southward, "The 100 Best Companies to Work For," *Fortune,* February 3, 2014, pp. 108+; M. Niesen, "The 50 Companies Young People Want to Work For the Most," www.businessinsider.com, September 20, 2013; M. Niesen, "Google HR Boss Explains Why GPA and Most Interviews Are Useless," www.businessinsider.com, June 19, 2013; and L. Bock, "Passion, Not Perks," www.thinkwithgoogle.com/articles/, September 2011.

30. L. Bock, "Google's Scientific Approach to Work-Life Balance (and Much More)."

31. C. H. Loch, F. J. Sting, N. Bauer, and J. Mauermann, "How BMW Is Defusing the Demographic Time Bomb," *Harvard Business Review,* March 2010, pp. 99–102.

32. M. Korn, "As Baby Boomers Retire, Firms Prepare for Shift," *Wall Street Journal,* April 18, 2012, p. B8; and T. Minton-Eversole, "Concerns Grow Over Workforce Retirements and Skills Gaps," [www.shrm.org], April 9, 2012.

33. C. Rampell, "As Layoffs Surge, Women May Pass Men in Job Force," *New York Times Online,* February 6, 2009.

34. B. Tulgan, "Generation Y Defined: The New Young Workforce," *HR Tools Online* [www.hrtools.com/insights/bruce_tulgan], February 25, 2009.

35. S. F. Gale, "From Texas to Timbuktu—How Fluor Tracks Talent on a Global Scale," *Workforce Management Online,* March 7, 2012.

36. M. A. Costonis and R. Salkowitz, "The Tough Match of Young Workers and Insurance," *New York Times Online,* June 11, 2010.

37. E. Seubert, "What Are Your Organization's Critical Positions," *Workforce Management Online,* December 2009; F. Hansen, "Strategic Workforce Planning in an Uncertain World," *Workforce Management Online,* July 2009; and J. Sullivan, "Workforce Planning: Why to Start Now," *Workforce,* September 2002, pp. 46–50.

38. N. Byrnes, "Star Search," *BusinessWeek,* October 10, 2005, pp. 68–78.

39. D. Robb, "Sizing Up Talent," *HR Magazine,* April 2011, p. 77.

40. J. Yang and P. Trap, "What Challenges Do You Have When Developing Job Descriptions?" *USA Today,* December 3, 2013, p. 1B.

41. J. Swartz, "Tech Firms Go On A Hiring Binge Again," *USA Today,* April 21, 2011, pp. 1B+; B. Einhorn and K. Gokhale, "Bangalore's Paying Again to Keep the Talent," *Bloomberg BusinessWeek,* May 24–30, 2010, pp. 14–16; D. A. Thoppil, "Pay War Breaks Out as India's Tech Firms Vie for Talent," *Wall Street Journal,* April 27, 2010, p. B8; and C. Tuna, J. E. Vascellaro, and P-W. Tam, "Tech Sector in Hiring Drive," *Wall Street Journal,* April 16, 2010, pp. A1+.

42. S. F. Gale, "Companies Struggle to Recruit Internationally," www.workforce.com, March 4, 2013.

43. A. S. Bargerstock and G. Swanson, "Four Ways to Build Cooperative Recruitment Alliances," *HRMagazine,* March 1991, p. 49; and T. J. Bergmann and M. S. Taylor, "College Recruitment: What Attracts Students to Organizations?" *Personnel,* May–June 1984, pp. 34–46.

44. J. R. Gordon, *Human Resource Management: A Practical Approach* (Boston: Allyn and Bacon, 1986), p. 170.

45. C. Reynolds, "McDonald's Hiring Day Draws Crowds, High Hopes," AP Business Writer, *Springfield, Missouri News-Leader,* April 20, 2011,

p. 6A; and A. Gasparro, "Fast-Food Chain Aims to Alter 'McJob' Image," *Wall Street Journal*, April 5, 2011, p. B9.

46. J. Walker, "Firms Invest Big in Career Sites," *Wall Street Journal Online*, June 8, 2010.

47. K. Plourd, "Lights, Camera, Audits!" *CFO*, November 2007, p. 18.

48. S. Elliott, "Army Seeks Recruits in Social Media," *New York Times Online*, May 24, 2011.

49. S. Horrigan, "Social Media Clout—A New Job Criteria?" *HR Magazine*, June 2013, p. 11.

50. S. Burton and D. Warner, "The Future of Hiring—Top 5 Sources for Recruitment Today," *Workforce Vendor Directory 2002*, p. 75.

51. See, for example, L. G. Klaff, "New Internal Hiring Systems Reduce Cost and Boost Morale," *Workforce Management*, March 2004, pp. 76–79; M. N. Martinez, "The Headhunter Within," *HR Magazine*, August 2001, pp. 48–55; R. W. Griffeth, P. W. Hom, L. S. Fink, and D. J. Cohen, "Comparative Tests of Multivariate Models of Recruiting Sources Effects," *Journal of Management*, vol. 23, no. 1, 1997, pp. 19–36; and J. P. Kirnan, J. E. Farley, and K. F. Geisinger, "The Relationship between Recruiting Source, Applicant Quality, and Hire Performance: An Analysis by Sex, Ethnicity, and Age," *Personnel Psychology*, Summer 1989, pp. 293–308.

52. J. McGregor, "Background Checks That Never End," *Business Week*, March 20, 2006, p. 40.

53. A. Fisher, "For Happier Customers, Call HR," *Fortune*, November 28, 2005, p. 272.

54. B. Roberts, "Most Likely to Succeed," *HR Magazine*, April 2014, pp. 69–71.

55. J. Greenwald, "Judge Rules New York City Fire Department Exams Showed Racial Bias," *Workforce Management Online*, July 28, 2009.

56. A. Douzet, "Quality of Fill an Emerging Recruitment Metric," *Workforce Management Online*, June 24, 2010; and "Quality of Hire Metrics Help Staffing Unit Show Its Contribution to Bottom Line," *Society for Human Resource Management Online*, January 25, 2009.

57. A. Shadday, "Assessments 101: An Introduction to Candidate Testing," *Workforce Management Online*, January 2010; A. M. Ryan and R. E. Ployhart, "Applicants' Perceptions of Selection Procedures and Decisions: A Critical Review and Agenda for the Future," *Journal of Management*, vol. 26, no. 3, 2000, pp. 565–606; C. Fernandez-Araoz, "Hiring Without Firing," *Harvard Business Review*, July–August 1999, pp. 108–120; A. K. Korman, "The Prediction of Managerial Performance: A Review," *Personnel Psychology*, Summer 1986, pp. 295–322; G. C. Thornton, *Assessment Centers in Human Resource Management* (Reading, MA: Addison-Wesley, 1992); I. T. Robertson and R. S. Kandola, "Work Sample Tests: Validity, Adverse Impact, and Applicant Reaction," *Journal of Occupational Psychology*, vol. 55, no. 3, 1982, pp. 171–183; E. E. Ghiselli, "The Validity of Aptitude Tests in Personnel Selection," *Personnel Psychology*, Winter 1973, p. 475; G. Grimsley and H. F. Jarrett, "The Relation of Managerial Achievement to Test Measures Obtained in the Employment Situation: Methodology and Results," *Personnel Psychology*, Spring 1973, pp. 31–48; J. J. Asher, "The Biographical Item: Can It Be Improved?" *Personnel Psychology*, Summer 1972, p. 266; and G. W. England, *Development and Use of Weighted Application Blanks*, rev. ed. (Minneapolis: Industrial Relations Center, University of Minnesota, 1971).

58. M. A. Tucker, "Show and Tell," *HR Magazine*, January 2012, pp. 51–53.

59. See, for example, P. Sweeney, "Sometimes, the Boss Is the One Lying in the Job Interview," qz.com, March 10, 2014; G. Kranz, "New Employees: 'We Were Jobbed About This Job,'" www.workforce.com, February 1, 2013; Y. Ganzach, A. Pazy, Y. Ohayun, and E. Brainin, "Social Exchange and Organizational Commitment: Decision-Making Training for Job Choice as an Alternative to the Realistic Job Preview," *Personnel Psychology*, Autumn 2002, pp. 613–637; B. M. Meglino, E. C. Ravlin, and A. S. DeNisi, "A Meta-Analytic Examination of Realistic Job Preview Effectiveness: A Test of Three Counterintuitive Propositions," *Human Resource Management Review*, vol. 10, no. 4, 2000, pp. 407–434; J. A. Breaugh and M. Starke, "Research on Employee Recruitment: So Many Studies, So Many Remaining Questions," *Journal of Management*, vol. 26, no. 3, 2000, pp. 405–434; and S. L. Premack and J. P. Wanous, "A Meta-Analysis of Realistic Job Preview Experiments," *Journal of Applied Psychology*, November 1985, pp. 706–720.

60. G. Kranz, "Tourism Training Takes Flight in Miami," *Workforce Management Online*, May 2010.

61. K. Gustafson, "A Better Welcome Mat," *Training*, June 2005, pp. 34–41.

62. M. Jokisaari and J-E. Nurmi, "Change in Newcomers' Supervisor Support and Socialization Outcomes After Organizational Entry," *Academy of Management Journal*, June 2009, pp. 527–544; D. G. Allen, "Do Organizational Socialization Tactics Influence Newcomer Embeddedness and Turnover?" *Journal of Management*, April 2006, pp. 237–256; C. L. Cooper, "The Changing Psychological Contract at Work: Revisiting the Job Demands-Control Model," *Occupational and Environmental Medicine*, June 2002, p. 355; D. M. Rousseau and S. A. Tijoriwala, "Assessing Psychological Contracts: Issues, Alternatives and Measures," *Journal of Organizational Behavior*, vol. 19, 1998, pp. 679–695; S. L. Robinson, M. S. Kraatz, and D. M. Rousseau, "Changing Obligations and the Psychological Contract: A Longitudinal Study," *Academy of Management Journal*, February 1994, pp. 137–152.

63. See, for instance, E. G. Tripp, "Aging Aircraft and Coming Regulations: Political and Media Pressures Have Encouraged the FAA to Expand Its Pursuit of Real and Perceived Problems of Older Aircraft and Their Systems. Operators Will Pay," *Business and Commercial Aviation*, March 2001, pp. 68–75.

64. "A&S Interview: Sully's Tale," *Air & Space Magazine* [www.airspacemag.com], February 18, 2009; A. Altman, "Chesley B. Sullenberger III," *Time* [www.time.com], January 16, 2009; and K. Burke, Pete Donohue, and C. Siemaszko, "US Airways Airplane Crashes in Hudson River—Hero Pilot Chesley Sullenberger III Saves All Aboard," *New York Daily News* [www.nydailynews.com], January 16, 2009.

65. D. Heath and C. Heath, "The Power of Razzle-Dazzle," *Fast Company*, December 2009–January 2010, pp. 69–70.

66. T. Raphael, "It's All in the Cards," *Workforce*, September 2002, p. 18.

67. S. Nassauer, "How Waiters Read Your Table," *Wall Street Journal*, February 22, 2012, pp. D1+.

68. "ASTD's 2013 State of the Industry Report: Workplace Learning," *T&D*, November 2013, pp. 41–44.

69. B. Hall, "The Top Training Priorities for 2003," *Training*, February 2003, p. 40.

70. D. Heath and C. Heath, "The Power of Razzle-Dazzle."

71. J. McGregor, "The Midyear Review's Sudden Impact," *Business Week*, July 6, 2009, pp. 50–52.

72. A. Pace, "The Performance Management Dilemma," *T&D*, July 2011, p. 22.

73. K. Sulkowicz, "Straight Talk at Review Time," *Business Week*, September 10, 2007, p. 16.

74. J. Pfeffer, "Low Grades for Performance Appraisals," *Business Week*, August 3, 2009, p. 68.

75. R. E. Silverman, "Work Reviews Losing Steam," *Wall Street Journal*, December 19, 2011, p. B7.

76. A. Fox, "Upon Further Assessment," *HR Magazine*, August 2013, p. 40.

77. J. D. Glater, "Seasoning Compensation Stew," *New York Times*, March 7, 2001, pp. C1+.

78. M. Korn, "Benefits Matter," *Wall Street Journal*, April 4, 2012, p. B8.

79. This section based on R. I. Henderson, *Compensation Management in a Knowledge-Based World*, 10th ed. (Upper Saddle River, NJ: Prentice Hall, 2006).

80. M. P. Brown, M. C. Sturman, and M. J. Simmering, "Compensation Policy and Organizational Performance: The Efficiency, Operational and Financial Implications of Pay Levels and Pay Structure," *Academy of Management Journal*, December 2003, pp. 752–762; J. D. Shaw, N. P. Gupta, and J. E. Delery, "Pay Dispersion and Workforce Performance: Moderating Effects of Incentives and Interdependence," *Strategic Management Journal*, June 2002, pp. 491–512; E. Montemayor, "Congruence between Pay Policy and Competitive Strategy in High-Performing Firms," *Journal of Management*, vol. 22, no. 6, 1996, pp. 889–908; and L. R. Gomez-Mejia, "Structure and Process of Diversification, Compensation Strategy, and Firm Performance," *Strategic Management Journal*, 13 (1992), pp. 381–397.

81. M. Moskowitz, R. Levering, and C. Tkaczyk, "100 Best Companies to Work For," *Fortune*, February 8, 2010, pp. 75–88.

82. J. D. Shaw, N. Gupta, A. Mitra, and G. E. Ledford, Jr., "Success and Survival of Skill-Based Pay Plans," *Journal of Management,* February 2005, pp. 28–49; C. Lee, K. S. Law, and P. Bobko, "The Importance of Justice Perceptions on Pay Effectiveness: A Two-Year Study of a Skill-Based Pay Plan," *Journal of Management,* vol. 26, no. 6, 1999, pp. 851–873; G. E. Ledford, "Paying for the Skills, Knowledge and Competencies of Knowledge Workers," *Compensation and Benefits Review,* July–August 1995, pp. 55–62; and E. E. Lawler III, G. E. Ledford Jr., and L. Chang, "Who Uses Skill-Based Pay and Why," *Compensation and Benefits Review,* March–April 1993, p. 22.

83. J. D. Shaw, N. Gupta, A. Mitra, and G. E. Ledford Jr., "Success and Survival of Skill-Based Pay Plans."

84. Information from Hewitt Associates Studies: "Aftermath of the Recession on 2009–2010 Compensation Spending," February 2010; "As Fixed Costs Increase, Employers Turn to Variable Pay Programs as Preferred Way to Reward Employees," August 21, 2007; "Hewitt Study Shows Pay-for-Performance Plans Replacing Holiday Bonuses," December 6, 2005; "Salaries Continue to Rise in Asia Pacific, Hewitt Annual Study Reports," November 23, 2005; and "Hewitt Study Shows Base Pay Increases Flat for 2006 with Variable Pay Plans Picking Up the Slack," Hewitt Associates, LLC [www.hewittassociates.com], August 31, 2005.

85. T. J. Erickson, "The Leaders We Need Now," *Harvard Business Review,* May 2010, pp. 63–66.

86. S. Thurm, "Recalculating the Cost of Big Layoffs," *Wall Street Journal,* May 5, 2010, pp. B1+; and J. Pfeffer, "Lay Off the Layoffs," *Newsweek,* February 15, 2010, pp. 32–37.

87. W. F. Cascio, "Use and Management of Downsizing as a Corporate Strategy," *HR Magazine,* June 2010, special insert; D. K. Datta, J. P. Guthrie, D. Basuil, and A. Pandey, "Causes and Effects of Employee Downsizing: A Review and Synthesis," *Journal of Management,* January 2010, pp. 281–348; B. Conaty, "Cutbacks: Don't Neglect the Survivors," *Bloomberg BusinessWeek,* January 11, 2010, p. 68; and P. Korkki, "Accentuating the Positive After a Layoff," *New York Times Online,* August 16, 2009.

88. R. Ceniceros, "Court Finds McDonald's Liable in Employee's Sexual Assault Case," *Workforce Management Online,* November 25, 2009.

89. "Sexual Harassment Charges 2010 - FY 2013," U.S. Equal Employment Opportunity Commission, http://www1.eeoc.gov//eeoc/statistics/enforcement/sexual_harassment_new.cfm?renderforprint=1.

90. B. Braverman, "The High Cost of Sexual Harassment," www.thefiscaltimes.com, August 22, 2013.

91. "Top 25 Workplace Harassment, Bias Settlements," www.insurancejournal.com, October 16, 2012.

92. "Effects of Sexual Harassment," *Stop Violence Against Women* [www.catalyst.org], May 9, 2007; and V. Di Martino, H. Hoel, and C. L. Cooper, "Preventing Violence and Harassment in the Workplace," *European Foundation for the Improvement of Living and Working Conditions,* 2003, p. 39.

93. The Associated Press, "Corruption, Sexual Harassment Charges Cloud Oxford Debating Club Presidential Election," *International Herald Tribune* [www.iht.com], February 6, 2008; G. L. Maatman, Jr., "A Global View of Sexual Harassment: Global Human Resource Strategies," *HR Magazine,* July 2000, pp. 151–156; and W. Hardman and J. Heidelberg, "When Sexual Harassment Is a Foreign Affair," *Personnel Journal,* April 1996, pp. 91–97.

94. "Sexual Harassment," *The U.S. Equal Employment Opportunity Commission* [www.eeoc.gov].

95. Ibid.

96. A. R. Karr, "Companies Crack Down on the Increasing Sexual Harassment by E-Mail," *Wall Street Journal,* September 21, 1999, p. A1; and A. Fisher, "After All This Time, Why Don't People Know What Sexual Harassment Means?" *Fortune,* January 12, 1998, p. 68.

97. See T. S. Bland and S. S. Stalcup, "Managing Harassment," *Human Resource Management,* Spring 2001, pp. 51–61; K. A. Hess and D. R. M. Ehrens, "Sexual Harassment—Affirmative Defense to Employer Liability," *Benefits Quarterly,* Second Quarter 1999, p. 57; J. A. Segal, "The Catch-22s of Remedying Sexual Harassment Complaints," *HR Magazine,* October 1997, pp. 111–117; S. C. Bahls and J. E. Bahls, "Hand-Off Policy," *Entrepreneur,* July 1997, pp. 74–76; J. A. Segal, "Where Are We Now?" *HR Magazine,* October 1996, pp. 69–73; B.

McAfee and D. L. Deadrick, "Teach Employees to Just Say No," *HR Magazine,* February 1996, pp. 86–89; G. D. Block, "Avoiding Liability for Sexual Harassment," *HR Magazine,* April 1995, pp. 91–97; and J. A. Segal, "Stop Making Plaintiffs' Lawyers Rich," *HR Magazine,* April 1995, pp. 31–35. Also, it should be noted here that under the Title VII and the Civil Rights Act of 1991, the maximum award that can be given, under the Federal Act, is $300,000. However, many cases are tried under state laws that permit unlimited punitive damages, such as the $7.1 million that Rena Weeks received in her trial based on California statutes.

98. S. Shellenbarger, "Supreme Court Takes on How Employers Handle Worker Harassment Complaints," *Wall Street Journal,* April 13, 2006, p. D1.

99. J. Yang and A. Gonzalez, "Top Actions Workers Feel Are Grounds for Termination," *USA Today,* May 7, 2012, p. 1B.

100. S. Jayson, "Workplace Romance No Longer Gets the Kiss-Off," *USA Today,* February 9, 2006, p. 9D.

101. J. Yang and V. Salazar, "Would You Date a Co-Worker?" *USA Today,* February 14, 2008, p. 1B.

102. Jayson, "Workplace Romance No Longer Gets the Kiss-off."

103. S. Shellenbarger, "For Office Romance, The Secret's Out," *Wall Street Journal,* February 10, 2010, pp. D1+.

104. C. Boyd, "The Debate Over the Prohibition of Romance in the Workplace," *Journal of Business Ethics,* December 2010, pp. 325–338; R. Mano and Y. Gabriel, "Workplace Romances in Cold and Hot Organizational Climates: The Experience of Israel and Taiwan," *Human Relations,* January 2006, pp. 7–35; J. A. Segal, "Dangerous Liaisons," *HR Magazine,* December 2005, pp. 104–108; "Workplace Romance Can Create Unforeseen Issues for Employers," *HR Focus,* October 2005, p. 2; C. A. Pierce and H. Aguinis, "Legal Standards, Ethical Standards, and Responses to Social-Sexual Conduct at Work," *Journal of Organizational Behavior,* September 2005, pp. 727–732; and C. A. Pierce, B. J. Broberg, J. R. McClure, and H. Aguinis, "Responding to Sexual Harassment Complaints: Effects of a Dissolved Workplace Romance on Decision-Making Standards," *Organizational Behavior and Human Decision Processes,* September 2004, pp. 66–82.

105. J. A. Segal, "Dangerous Liaisons," *HR Magazine,* December 2005, pp. 104–108.

106. E. Zimmerman, "When Cupid Strikes at the Cubicle," *New York Times Online,* April 9, 2010.

107. D. Wilkie, "Workplace Is No Place for Romance," *HR Magazine,* December 2013, p. 13.

108. S. Ali and B. Frankel, "The Work/Life Balancing Act: How 4 Companies Do It," *DiversityInc,* May 18, 2010, pp. 62–68.

109. J. Miller and M. Miller, "Get a Life!" *Fortune,* November 28, 2005, pp. 108–124.

110. L. Vanderkam, "Graduates, You Can Have It All," *USA Today,* May 27, 2010, p. 11A; and M. Elias, "The Family-First Generation," *USA Today,* December 13, 2004, p. 5D.

111. M. Mandel, "The Real Reasons You're Working So Hard...and What You Can Do About It," *BusinessWeek,* October 3, 2005, pp. 60–67.

112. C. Farrell, "The Overworked, Networked Family," *BusinessWeek,* October 3, 2005, p. 68.

113. F. Hansen, "Truths and Myths about Work/Life Balance," *Workforce,* December 2002, pp. 34–39.

114. P. Brough and T. Kalliath, "Work-Family Balance: Theoretical and Empirical Advancements," *Journal of Organizational Behavior,* July 2009, pp. 581–585; E. F. Van Steenbergen and N. Ellemers, "Is Managing the Work-Family Interface Worthwhile? Benefits for Employee Health and Performance," *Journal of Organizational Behavior,* July 2009, pp. 617–642; K. Palmer, "The New Mommy Track," *US News and World Report,* September 3, 2007, pp. 40–45; and J. H. Greenhaus and G. N. Powell, "When Work and Family Are Allies: A Theory of Work-Family Enrichment," *Academy of Management Review,* January 2006, pp. 72–92.

115. Ibid., p. 73.

116. S. Shellenbarger, "What Makes a Company a Great Place to Work Today," *Wall Street Journal,* October 4, 2007, p. D1; and L. B. Hammer, M. B. Neal, J. T. Newsom, K. J. Brockwood, and C. L. Colton, "A Longitudinal Study of the Effects of Dual-Earner Couples' Utilization of Family-Friendly Workplace Supports on Work and Family Outcomes," *Journal of Applied Psychology,* July 2005, pp. 799–810.

117. M. M. Arthur, "Share Price Reactions to Work-Family Initiatives: An Institutional Perspective," *Academy of Management Journal,* August 2003, pp. 497–505.

118. L. B. Hammer et al., "Development and Validation of a Multidimensional Measure of Family Supportive Supervisor Behaviors," *Journal of Management,* August 2009, pp. 837–856; and N. P. Rothbard, T. L. Dumas, and K. W. Phillips, "The Long Arm of the Organization: Work-Family Policies and Employee Preferences for Segmentation," paper presented at the 61st Annual Academy of Management meeting, Washington, DC, August 2001.

119. R. Ceniceros, "Workforce Obesity," *Workforce Management Online,* October 19, 2011; and J. Walsh, "Special Report: Creating a Culture of Wellness Helps Companies Tighten Their Belt," *Workforce Management Online,* April 2011.

120. A. W. Matthews, "Pitting Employees Against Each Other...for Health," *Wall Street Journal,* May 1, 2012, pp. D1+; R. King, "Slimming Down Employees to Cut Costs"; C. Tkaczyk, "Lowering Health-Care Costs," *Fortune,* November 23, 2009, p. 16; and A. W. Matthews, "When All Else Fails: Forcing Workers into Healthy Habits," *Wall Street Journal,* July 8, 2009, pp. D1+.

121. L. Cornwell, "More Companies Penalize Workers with Health Risks," The Associated Press, *Springfield, Missouri News-Leader,* September 10, 2007, p. 10A.

122. B. Pyenson and K. Fitch, "Smoking May Be Hazardous to Your Bottom Line," *Workforce Management Online* [www.workforce.com], December 2007; and L. Cornwell, The Associated Press, "Companies Tack on Fees on Insurance for Smokers," *Springfield, Missouri News-Leader,* February 17, 2006, p. 5B.

123. R. Ceniceros, "Workforce Obesity," J. Walsh, "Special Report: Creating a Culture of Wellness Helps Companies Tighten Their Belt," and M. Scott, "Obesity More Costly to U.S. Companies Than Smoking, Alcoholism," *Workforce Management Online* [www.workforce.com], April 9, 2008.

124. "Obesity Weighs Down Production," *Industry Week,* March 2008, pp. 22–23.

125. J. Appleby, "Companies Step Up Wellness Efforts," *USA Today,* August 1, 2005, pp. 1A+.

126. G. Kranz, "Prognosis Positive: Companies Aim to Get Workers Healthy," *Workforce Management Online* [www.workforce.com], April 15, 2008.

127. M. Conlin, "Hide the Doritos! Here Comes HR," *BusinessWeek,* April 28, 2008, pp. 94–96.

128. J. Fox, "Good Riddance to Pensions," *CNN Money,* January 12, 2006.

129. M. Adams, "Broken Pension System in Crying Need of a Fix," *USA Today,* November 15, 2005, p. 1B+.

130. J. Appleby, "Traditional Pensions Are Almost Gone. Is Employer-Provided Health Insurance Next?" *USA Today,* November 13, 2007, pp. 1A+; S. Kelly, "FedEx, Goodyear Make Big Pension Plan Changes," *Workforce Management Online* [www.workforce.com], March 1, 2007; G. Colvin, "The End of a Dream," *Fortune* [www.cnnmoney.com], June 22, 2006; E. Porter and M. Williams Nash, "Benefits Go the Way of Pensions," *NY Times Online,* February 9, 2006; and J. Fox, "Good Riddance to Pensions."

131. L. Beyer, "The Rise and Fall of Employer-Sponsored Pension Plans," *Workforce Management Online,* February 6, 2012.

132. Based on R. Pyrillis, "Workers Using Medical Marijuana Hold Their Breath, but Employers Worry They'll Take a Hit," *Workforce Management Online,* April 2011; "Puffing Up Over Pot in Workplace," *Workforce Management,* March 2011, p. 41; D. Cadrain, "The Marijuana Exception," *HR Magazine,* November 2010, pp. 40–42; D. Cadrain, "Do Medical Marijuana Laws Protect Usage by Employees?" *HR Magazine,* November 2010, p. 12; A. K. Wiwi and N. P. Crifo, "The Unintended Impact of New Jersey's New Medical Marijuana Law on the Workplace," *Employee Relations Law Journal,* Summer 2010, pp. 33–37; S. Simon, "At Work, A Drug Dilemma," *Wall Street Journal,* August 3, 2010, p. D1; and J. Greenwald, "Medical Marijuana Laws Create Dilemma for Firms," *Business Insurance,* February 15, 2010, pp. 1–20.

133. D. S. Urban, "What to Do About 'Body Art' at Work?" *Workforce Management Online,* March 2010.

134. P. Coy and E. Dwoskin, "Shortchanged: Why Women Get Paid Less Than Men," *Bloomberg BusinessWeek Online,* June 21, 2012.

135. T. Bingham and P. Galagan, "Delivering 'On-Time, Every Time' Knowledge and Skills to a World of Employees," *T&D,* July 2012, pp. 32–37; J. Levitz, "UPS Thinks Outside the Box on Driver Training," *Wall Street Journal,* April 6, 2010, pp. B1+; and K. Kingsbury, "Road to Recovery," *Time,* March 8, 2010, pp. Global 14–16.

136. "Latest Layoffs at Penney Hit Back Office, District Office Workers," Reuters, www.reuters.com, March 7, 2013; K. Bhasin, "JCPenney Is Firing More Store Employees After A 'Secret Broadcast,'" businessinsider.com, March 7, 2013; M. Wilson, "JC Penney's Traffic-Light System Under Fire," www.ragan.com, March 7, 2013; D. Mattioli, "Board's Patience with CEO Wears Thin at J.C. Penney," *Wall Street Journal,* March 6, 2013, p. B1; D. Mattioli, "J.C. Penney's Losses Snowball," *Wall Street Journal,* February 28, 2013, pp. B1+; **S. Clifford, "Chief Talks of Mistakes and Big Losses at J. C. Penney," *New York Times Online,* February 27, 2013**; D. Mattioli, "For Penney's Heralded Boss, the Shine Is Off the Apple," *Wall Street Journal,* February 25, 2013, pp. A1+; and K. Bhasin, "Inside JCPenney: Widespread Fear, Anxiety, and Distrust of Ron Johnson and His New Management Team," businessinsider.com, February 22, 2013.

Managing Your Career *Module*

Managing Your Career *Module*

The main thing to keep in mind if you want to be successful in your career is that YOU are responsible for your career.[1] No one else is going to do it for you, including your employer. That's why we've included this information.

CAREER OPPORTUNITIES in Management

If you've paid any attention to news reports over the last few years, you know about the widespread layoffs both in the United States and worldwide. Merck cut about 11 percent of its workforce. Unisys reduced its workforce by 10 percent. Pfizer Japan Inc. cut its workforce by 5 percent. Kodak eliminated up to 25,000 jobs. So, are management jobs disappearing? You might think so based on these reports. The truth is: The future looks bright! Business administration and management continues to be one of the top 10 most popular college majors, and jobs are likely to be waiting for those graduates!

It's hard to get an exact number of individuals in the United States that are employed as managers because the numbers are aggregated with business and financial operations occupations. According to the U.S. Bureau of Labor Statistics (BLS), almost 30 million individuals are employed in those categories.[2] The BLS estimates an 11 percent growth in executive, administrative, and managerial jobs through the year 2022.[3] The point is that there will be managerial jobs, but these jobs may not be in the organizations or fields that you'd expect. The demand for managers in traditional Fortune 500 organizations, and particularly in the area of traditional manufacturing, is not going to be as strong as the demand for managers in small and medium-sized organizations in the services field, particularly information and health care services. Keep in mind that a good place to land a management position can be a smaller organization.

Finding a Culture That Fits

How can you find a culture that fits?[4] Here are some suggestions.

First, *figure out what suits you*. For instance, do you like working in teams or on your own? Do you like to go out after work with colleagues or go straight home? Are you comfortable in a more formal or a more casual environment? Then, narrow your job search to those kinds of employers.

Once you've gotten through the initial job-screening process and begin interviewing, the real detective work begins, which involves more than investigating the "official" information provided by the employer. *Try to uncover the values that drive the organization.* Ask questions concerning the business's proudest accomplishments or how it responded to past emergencies and crises. Ask, "If I have an idea, how do I make it happen?" Ask if you can talk to someone who's on the "fast track" to

promotions and find out what they're doing and why they're being rewarded. Ask how you'll be evaluated—after all, if you're going to be in the game, shouldn't you know how the score is kept? Also, look for nonverbal clues. What do people have at their desks—family pictures or only work stuff? Are office doors closed or open? Are there doors? How does the physical climate feel? Is it relaxed and casual or more formal? Do people seem to be helping each other as they work? Are the bathrooms dirty, which might indicate a low value placed on anything to do with employees? Look at the material symbols and who seems to have access to them. And finally, during your investigation, *pay particular attention to the specific department or unit where you'd work*. After all, it is the place where you'd spend the majority of your working hours. Can you see yourself being happy there?

Taking Risks

"IYAD-WYAD-YAG-WYAG: If you always do what you've always done, you'll always get what you've always got! So if your life is ever going to improve, you'll have to take chances."—Anonymous[5]

How will you approach your various career moves over the course of your lifetime? Will you want to do what you've always done? Or will you want to take chances, and how comfortable will you be taking chances? Taking career risks doesn't have to be a gamble. Responsible risk taking can make outcomes more predictable. Here are some suggestions for being a responsible, effective risk taker in career decisions. It's important to thoroughly evaluate the risk. Before committing to a career risk, consider what you could lose or who might be hurt. How important are those things or those people to you? Explore whether you can reach your goal in another way, thus making the risk unnecessary. Find out everything you can about what's involved with taking this career risk—the timing; the people involved; the changes it will entail; and the potential gains and losses, both in the short run and the long run. Examine closely your feelings about taking this risk: Are you afraid? Are you ready to act now? Will you know if you have risked more than you can afford to lose? Finally, ensure your employability. The most important thing you can do is ensuring that you have choices by keeping your skills current and continually learning new skills.

As with any decision involving risk, the more information you have available, the better able you are to assess the risk. Then, armed with this information, you can make a more informed decision. Even though you won't be able to eliminate all the negatives associated with taking the risk, you can, at least, know about them.

Reinventing Yourself

Face it. The only sure thing about change is that it is constant. These days, you don't have the luxury of dealing with change only once in a while. No, the workplace seems to change almost continuously. How can you reinvent yourself to deal with the demands of a constantly changing workplace?[6]

Being prepared isn't a credo just for the Boy Scouts; it should be your motto for dealing with a workplace that is constantly changing. Being prepared means taking the initiative and being responsible for your own personal career development. Rather than depending on your organization to provide you with career development and training opportunities, do it yourself. Take advantage of continuing education or graduate courses at local colleges. Sign up for workshops and seminars that can help enhance your skills. Upgrading your skills to keep them current is one of the most important things you can do to reinvent yourself.

It's also important for you to be a positive force when faced with workplace changes. We don't mean you should routinely accept any change that's being implemented. If you think that a proposed change won't work, speak up. Voice your concerns in a constructive manner. Being constructive may mean suggesting an alternative. However, if you feel that the change is beneficial, support it wholeheartedly and enthusiastically.

The changes that organizations make in response to a dynamic environment can be overwhelming and stressful. However, you can take advantage of these changes by reinventing yourself.

Learning to Get Along with Difficult People

We've all been around people who, to put it nicely, are difficult to get along with. These people might be chronic complainers, they might be meddlers who think they know everything about everyone else's job and don't hesitate to tell you so, or they might exhibit any number of other unpleasant interpersonal characteristics. They can make your job as a manager extremely hard and your work day very stressful if you don't know how to deal with them. Being around difficult people tends to bring out the worst in all of us. What can you do? How do you learn to get along with these difficult people?[7]

Getting along with difficult people takes a little bit of patience, planning, and preparation. What you need is an approach that helps you diffuse a lot of the negative aspects of dealing with these individuals. For instance, it helps to write down a detailed description of the person's behavior. Describe what this person does that bothers you. Then, try to understand that behavior. Put yourself in that person's shoes and attempt to see things from his or her perspective. Doing these things initially might help you better understand, predict, and influence behavior.

Unfortunately, trying to understand the person usually isn't enough for getting along. You'll also need some specific strategies for coping with different types of difficult personalities. Here are some of the most common types of difficult people you'll meet and some strategies for dealing with them.

THE HOSTILE, AGGRESSIVE TYPES   With this type, you need to stand up for yourself; give them time to run down; don't worry about being polite, just jump in if you need to; get their attention carefully; get them to sit down; speak from your own point of view; avoid a head-on fight; and be ready to be friendly.

THE COMPLAINERS   With the complainers you need to listen attentively; acknowledge their concerns; be prepared to interrupt their litany of complaints; don't agree, but do acknowledge what they're saying; state facts without comment or apology; and switch them to problem solving.

THE SILENT OR NONRESPONSIVE TYPES   With this type, you need to ask open-ended questions; use the friendly, silent stare; don't fill the silent pauses for them in conversations; comment on what's happening; and help break the tension by making them feel more at ease.

THE KNOW-IT-ALL EXPERTS   The keys to dealing with this type are to be on top of things; listen and acknowledge their comments; question firmly, but don't confront; avoid being a counterexpert; and work with them to channel their energy in positive directions.

What Do I Want from My Job?

Have you ever stopped to think about what you really want from your job?[8] A high salary? Work that challenges you? Autonomy and flexibility? Perhaps the results of

surveys of workers will give you some insights into what you might want from your job. The top reasons that employees took their jobs and stay with their jobs are as follows:

Work–life balance and flexibility	29%
The work itself	27
Compensation offered	26
Coworkers	25
Work culture	13
Training opportunities	5
Advancement opportunities	5

(Total adds up to more than 100% because individuals indicated more than one factor.)

Do any of these characteristics describe what you want from your job? Whether they do or don't, you should spend some time reflecting on what you want your job to provide you. Then, when it's time to do that all-important job search, look for situations that will provide you what you're looking for.

How Can I Have a Successful Career?

Leaving college after graduation to enter the workforce is always a scary step. However, you can make that transition much easier through one "undeniable element: personal accountability."[9] And because you're likely to be the youngest team member, it's especially important that you take responsibility for your actions and behaviors. By taking an active role in managing your career, your work life can be more exciting, enjoyable, satisfying, and rewarding. So, here are some suggestions that will help you on the path to a successful career:

- Understand yourself—your abilities and disabilities; your strengths and weaknesses.
- Protect your personal brand—watch what you share online and in interactions with others, and watch your e-mails.[10]
- Be a team player—focus on knowing your peer group and your organization and on the best ways to work within them.
- Dress appropriately—first impressions count, but so do other impressions that you make every day.
- Network—develop and keep your links to other professionals open and active by participating in professional organizations, staying in touch with classmates and friends, using online networking sites, and so forth.[11]
- Ask for help—if you find yourself facing an issue you're not sure how to handle, ask someone for advice or guidance; seek out a mentor.
- Keep your skills updated—although you might think you know it all, you don't; keep learning about your profession and your industry.
- Set goals and then work hard to achieve them—showing your boss that you're able to set goals and reach them is always impressive.
- Do good work—above all, having a successful career means doing your job well, whatever that job might be.

ENDNOTES

1. S. E. Sullivan and Y. Baruch, "Advances in Career Theory and Research: A Critical Review and Agenda for Future Exploration," *Journal of Management,* December 2009, pp. 1542–1571.
2. "The Employment Situation—July 2012," http://www.bls.gov/news.release/pdf/empsit.pdf, August 3, 2012.
3. "Management and Business and Financial Occupations," *Occupational Outlook Handbook, 2012–13 Edition* [http://www.bls.gov/ooh/management/top-executives.htm].
4. J. Sandberg, "Sometimes an Office Visit Can Feel Like a Visit to a Very Foreign Land," *Wall Street Journal,* October 20, 2005, p. B1; D. Sacks, "Scout's Honor," *Fast Company,* April 2005, p. 94; D. W. Brown, "Searching for Clues," *Black Enterprise,* November 2002, pp. 114–120; L. Bower, "Weigh Values to Decide If Working for 'Beasts' Worthwhile," *Springfield Business Journal,* November 4, 2002, p. 73; S. Shellenbarger, "How to Find Out If You're Going to Hate a New Job Before You Agree to Take It," *Wall Street Journal,* June 13, 2002, p. D1; and M. Boyle, "Just Right," *Fortune,* June 10, 2002, pp. 207–208.
5. S. Caudron, "Some New Rules for the New World of Work," *Business Finance,* October 2001, p. 24; C. Kanchier, *Dare to Change Your Job and Your Life,* 2d ed. (Indianapolis, IN: Jist Publishing, 2000); and S. Hagevik, "Responsible Risk Taking," *Journal of Environmental Health,* November 1999, pp. 29+.
6. A. Feldman, "The Road to Reinvention," *Bloomberg BusinessWeek,* March 8, 2010, pp. 68–70; E. Zimmerman, "Making Yourself Indispensable," *New York Times Online,* February 14, 2010; S. E. Needleman, "Revving a Career While It's in Neutral," *Wall Street Journal,* January 19, 2010, p. D5; and D. Schawbel, "Upping Your Value at Work," *BusinessWeek Online,* December 18, 2009.
7. D. Nishi, "What To Do If Your Boss Is the Problem," *Wall Street Journal,* April 20, 2010, p. D4; M. Weinstein, "Mind Your Manners," *Training,* July–August 2009, pp. 24–29; M. Solomon, *Working with Difficult People* (Upper Saddle River, NJ: Prentice Hall, 2002); M. Gaskill, "Bigger Bullies," *American Way,* August 2001, pp. 92–96; R. Cooper, "Dealing Effectively with Difficult People," *Nursing,* September 1993, pp. 97–100; and R. M. Bramson, *Coping with Difficult People* (Garden City, NY: Anchor Press/Doubleday, 1981).
8. A. Ebron, "All Work and No Play," *Woman's Day,* October 6, 2009, p. 50; and J. Yang and K. Simmons, "Work–Life Balance Tops Pay," *USA Today,* March 13, 2008, p. 1B.
9. D. Hannah, "Just Out of School? Six Ways You Can Get Ahead at Work," *Diversity Inc.,* May 2008, pp. 46–47.
10. S. Lohr, "How Privacy Vanishes Online," *New York Times Online,* March 16, 2010; and A. Bruzzese, "Online Postings Can Sabotage One's Career," Gannett News Service, *Springfield, Missouri, News-Leader,* August 11, 2009, p. 9B; and D. Hannah, "Just Out of School? Six Ways You Can Get Ahead at Work."
11. J. Hempel, "How LinkedIn Will Fire Up Your Career," *Fortune,* April 12, 2010, pp. 74–82; and J. S. Lublin, "A Networking Pro Learns Some New Tricks," *Wall Street Journal,* March 2, 2010, p. D4.

Creating and Managing Teams

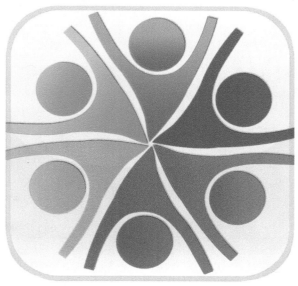

Source: Kev Draws/Shutterstock

A key to success in management and in your career is knowing how to negotiate effectively to maximize outcomes.

Maximizing Outcomes Through Negotiation

A young lawyer was recently asked, "So, what did you learn in three years of law school?" She replied, "Everything is negotiable!"

Lawyers aren't the only people who spend a good part of their time negotiating. Managers negotiate with employees, bosses, colleagues, suppliers, and sometimes even customers. And each of us, in our daily lives, will find ourselves having to negotiate with parents, spouses, children, friends, neighbors, and car salespersons—just to name the obvious.

We know a great deal about what effective negotiators do. Here are some brief suggestions to hone your skills at negotiating:

1. **Do your homework.** Gather as much pertinent information as possible before your negotiation. Know yourself. How do you feel about negotiating? Is it something you're comfortable doing? Do you just want it to be over? Recognize your own negotiating strengths and weaknesses. But also, know who you're negotiating with before you begin. Try to assess their strengths and weaknesses. You can't make good decisions without understanding your and the other person's situation.

2. **Assess goals.** In addition to gauging the personal/people aspects, take the time to assess your own goals and the other party's goals and interests. Know what you want, but also try to anticipate what the other person wants. And...maybe even go one step further by trying to anticipate what the other person thinks you want.

3. **Begin with a positive proposal.** Concessions tend to be reciprocated. So start with something positive. Often, if you expect more, you get more. Your optimism may become a self-fulfilling prophecy.[1]

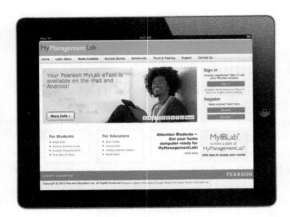

MyManagementLab®

⭐ Improve Your Grade!

When you see this icon, visit
www.mymanagementlab.com for activities that are
applied, personalized, and offer immediate feedback.

Learning Objectives

1 **Define** *groups and the stages of group development.*

2 **Describe** *the major components that determine group performance and satisfaction.*

3 **Define** *teams and best practices influencing team performance.*

- **Know how** to maximize outcomes through effective negotiating.
- **Develop your skill** at coaching team members.

4 **Discuss** *contemporary issues in managing teams.*

---

4. Address problems, not personalities.
Concentrate on the negotiation issues, not on the personal characteristics of your opponent. Don't take the issues or the other person's behavior personally. Don't let the negotiation get sidetracked by personal issues that have nothing to do with what you're negotiating.

5. Pay attention to the interpersonal aspects of the negotiation process. *Negotiating is communicating. Trust is an important part of that communication. Work at building trust by telling the truth, being trustworthy, and honoring your commitments. Also, listen with your ears and your*

eyes. Pay attention to important nonverbal messages, facial expressions, and voice inflections. Listen—really listen—to what the other person is saying verbally and nonverbally.

6. Pay little attention to initial offers. *Initial offers tend to be extreme and idealistic. Treat them as such. Negotiating is a process, not a one-and-done interaction.*

7. Emphasize win-win solutions. *Frame options in terms of your opponent's interests and look for solutions that can allow both you and the person you're negotiating with to declare a victory.*

You've probably had a lot of experience working in groups—class project teams, maybe an athletic team, a fundraising committee, or even a sales team at work. Work teams are one of the realities—and challenges—of managing in today's dynamic global environment. Many organizations have made the move to restructure work around teams rather than individuals. Why? What do these teams look like? And, how can managers build effective teams? We will look at answers to these questions throughout this text. Before we can understand teams, however, we first need to understand some basics about groups and group behavior.

GROUPS and Group Development

L01 Each person in the group had his or her assigned role: The Spotter, The Back Spotter, The Gorilla, and the Big Player. For over 10 years, this group—former MIT students who were members of a secret Black Jack Club—used their extraordinary mathematical abilities, expert training, teamwork, and interpersonal skills to take millions of dollars from some of the major casinos in the United States.[2] Although most groups aren't formed for such dishonest purposes, the success of this group at its task was impressive. Managers would like their groups to be successful at their tasks also. The first step is understanding what a group is and how groups develop.

What Is a Group?

A **group** is defined as two or more interacting and interdependent individuals who come together to achieve specific goals. *Formal groups* are work groups defined by the organization's structure and have designated work assignments and specific tasks directed at accomplishing organizational goals. Exhibit 1 provides some examples. *Informal groups* are social groups. These groups occur naturally in the workplace and tend to form around friendships and common interests. For example, five employees from different departments who regularly eat lunch together are an informal group.

Stages of Group Development

Research shows that groups develop through five stages.[3] As shown in Exhibit 2, these five stages are *forming, storming, norming, performing,* and *adjourning.*

The **forming stage** has two phases. The first occurs as people join the group. In a formal group, people join because of some work assignment. Once they've joined, the second phase begins: defining the group's purpose, structure, and leadership. This phase involves a great deal of uncertainty as members "test the waters" to determine what types of behavior are acceptable. This stage is complete when members begin to think of themselves as part of a group.

The **storming stage** is appropriately named because of the intragroup conflict. There's conflict over who will control the group and what the group needs to be doing. During this stage, a relatively clear hierarchy of leadership and agreement on the group's direction emerge.

The **norming stage** is one in which close relationships develop and the group becomes cohesive. There's now a strong sense of group identity and camaraderie. This stage is complete when the group structure solidifies and the group has assimilated a common set of expectations (or norms) regarding member behavior.

The fourth stage is the **performing stage**. The group structure is in place and accepted by group members. Their energies have moved from getting to know and understand each other to working on the group's task. This is the last stage of development for permanent work groups. However, for temporary groups—project teams, task

group
Two or more interacting and interdependent individuals who come together to achieve specific goals

forming stage
The first stage of group development in which people join the group and then define the group's purpose, structure, and leadership

storming stage
The second stage of group development, characterized by intragroup conflict

norming stage
The third stage of group development, characterized by close relationships and cohesiveness

performing stage
The fourth stage of group development when the group is fully functional and works on group task

Exhibit 1
Examples of Formal Work Groups

- *Command groups*—Groups determined by the organizational chart and composed of individuals who report directly to a given manager.
- *Task groups*—Groups composed of individuals brought together to complete a specific job task; their existence is often temporary because when the task is completed, the group disbands.
- *Cross-functional teams*—Groups that bring together the knowledge and skills of individuals from various work areas or groups whose members have been trained to do each others' jobs.
- *Self-managed teams*—Groups that are essentially independent and that, in addition to their own tasks, take on traditional managerial responsibilities such as hiring, planning and scheduling, and evaluating performance.

Exhibit 2
Stages of Group Development

Stage 1
Forming

Stage 2
Storming

Stage 3
Norming

Stage 4
Performing

Stage 5
Adjourning

forces, or similar groups that have a limited task to do—the final stage is **adjourning**. In this stage, the group prepares to disband. The group focuses its attention on wrapping up activities instead of task performance. Group members react in different ways. Some are upbeat and thrilled about the group's accomplishments. Others may be sad over the loss of camaraderie and friendships.

Many of you have probably experienced these stages as you've worked on a group project for a class. Group members are selected or assigned and then meet for the first time. There's a "feeling out" period to assess what the group is going to do and how it's going to be done. What usually follows is a battle for control: Who's going to be in charge? Once this issue is resolved and a "hierarchy" agreed upon, the group identifies specific work that needs to be done, who's going to do each part, and dates by which the assigned work needs to be completed. General expectations are established. These decisions form the foundation for what you hope will be a coordinated group effort culminating in a project that's been done well. Once the project is complete and turned in, the group breaks up. Of course, some groups don't get much beyond the forming or storming stages. These groups may have serious interpersonal conflicts, turn in disappointing work, and get lower grades.

Does a group become more effective as it progresses through the first four stages? Some researchers say yes, but it's not that simple.[4] That assumption may be generally true, but what makes a group effective is a complex issue. Under some conditions, high levels of conflict are conducive to high levels of group performance. In some situations, groups in the storming stage outperform those in the norming or performing stages. Also, groups don't always proceed sequentially from one stage to the next. Sometimes, groups are storming and performing at the same time. Groups even occasionally regress to previous stages; therefore, don't assume that all groups precisely follow this process or that performing is always the most preferable stage. Think of this model as a general framework that underscores the fact that groups are dynamic entities and managers need to know the stage a group is in so they can understand the problems and issues most likely to surface.

adjourning
The final stage of group development for temporary groups during which group members are concerned with wrapping up activities rather than task performance

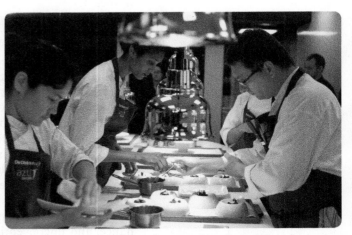

As a permanent work group in the performing stage, chef Andoni Aduriz (right) and his staff prepare a dish in the kitchen of his Mugaritz restaurant in Errenteria, Spain. Aduriz and his team of 35 chefs have a strong sense of group identity and focus their energies on creating elaborate and adventurous dining experiences for their guests.
Source: Vincent West/Reuters Pictures

347

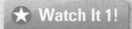 **Watch It 1!** If your professor has assigned this, go to **www.mymanagementlab.com** to watch a video titled: *Rudi's Bakery: Work Teams* and to respond to questions.

WORK **Group Performance and Satisfaction**

LO2 Many people consider them the most successful "group" of our times. Who? The Beatles. "The Beatles were great artists and entertainers, but in many respects they were four ordinary guys who, as a group, found a way to achieve extraordinary artistic and financial success and have a great time together while doing it. Every business team can learn from their story."[5]

Why *are* some groups more successful than others? Why do some groups achieve high levels of performance and high levels of member satisfaction and others do not? The answers are complex, but include variables such as the abilities of the group's members, the size of the group, the level of conflict, and the internal pressures on members to conform to the group's norms. Exhibit 3 presents the major factors that determine group performance and satisfaction.[6] Let's look at each.

External Conditions Imposed on the Group

Work groups are affected by the external conditions imposed on it such as the organization's strategy, authority relationships, formal rules and regulations, availability of resources, employee selection criteria, the performance management system and culture, and the general physical layout of the group's work space. For instance, some groups have modern, high-quality tools and equipment to do their jobs while other groups don't. Or the organization might be pursuing a strategy of lowering costs or improving quality, which will affect what a group does and how it does it.

Group Member Resources

A group's performance potential depends to a large extent on the resources each individual brings to the group. These resources include knowledge, abilities, skills, and personality traits, and they determine what members can do and how effectively they will perform in a group. Interpersonal skills—especially conflict management and resolution, collaborative problem solving, and communication—consistently emerge as important for high performance by work groups.[7]

Personality traits also affect group performance because they strongly influence how the individual will interact with other group members. Research has shown that traits viewed as positive in our culture (such as sociability, self-reliance, and independence) tend to be positively related to group productivity and morale. In contrast, negative personality characteristics, such as authoritarianism, dominance, and unconventionality, tend to be negatively related to group productivity and morale.[8]

Exhibit 3
Group Performance/Satisfaction
Model

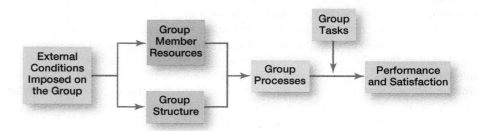

Group Structure

Work groups aren't unorganized crowds. They have an internal structure that shapes members' behavior and influences group performance. The structure defines roles, norms, conformity, status systems, group size, group cohesiveness, and leadership. Let's look at the first six of these aspects of group structure.

ROLES Of course, managers aren't the only individuals in an organization who play various roles. The concept of roles applies to all employees and to their life outside an organization as well. (Think of the various roles you play: student, friend, sibling, employee, spouse or significant other, etc.)

A **role** refers to behavior patterns expected of someone occupying a given position in a social unit. In a group, individuals are expected to do certain things because of their position (role) in the group. These roles are generally oriented toward either getting work done or keeping group members happy.[9] Think about groups you've been in and the roles you played in those groups. Were you continually trying to keep the group focused on getting its work done? If so, you were performing a task accomplishment role. Or were you more concerned that group members had the opportunity to offer ideas and that they were satisfied with the experience? If so, you were performing a group member satisfaction role. Both roles are important to the group's ability to function effectively and efficiently.

A problem arises when individuals play multiple roles and adjust their roles to the group to which they belong at the time. However, the differing expectations of these roles often means that employees face *role conflicts*.

role
Behavior patterns expected of someone occupying a given position in a social unit

NORMS All groups have **norms**—standards or expectations that are accepted and shared by a group's members. Norms dictate things such as work output levels, absenteeism, promptness, and the amount of socializing on the job.

For example, norms dictate the "arrival ritual" among office assistants at Coleman Trust Inc., where the workday begins at 8 A.M. Most employees typically arrive a few minutes before and hang up their coats and put their purses and other personal items on their desk so everyone knows they're "at work." They then go to the break room to get coffee and chat. Anyone who violates this norm by starting work at 8 A.M. is pressured to behave in a way that conforms to the group's standard.

norms
Standards or expectations that are accepted and shared by a group's members

Although a group has its own unique set of norms, common organizational norms focus on effort and performance, dress, and loyalty. The most widespread norms are those related to work effort and performance. Work groups typically provide their members with explicit cues on how hard to work, level of output expected, when to look busy, when it's acceptable to goof off, and the like. These norms are powerful influences on an individual employee's performance. They're so powerful that you can't predict someone's performance based solely on his or her ability and personal motivation. Dress norms frequently dictate what's acceptable to wear to work. If the norm is more formal dress, anyone who dresses casually may face subtle pressure to conform. Finally, loyalty norms will influence whether individuals work late, work on weekends, or move to locations they might not prefer to live.

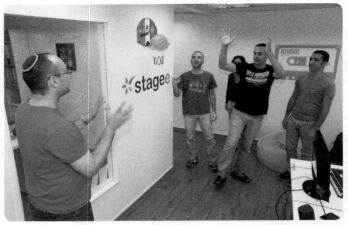

Casual dress, an informal setting, and taking breaks from work to have fun are norms at Stagee, a social networking platform where actors, singers, musicians, dancers, and other entertainers can promote their careers and reach new audiences. High worker output is a performance norm accepted and shared by Stagee's employees as they continue to build their business.
Source: Oren Shalev/PhotoStock-Israel/Alamy

One negative thing about group norms is that being part of a group can increase an individual's antisocial actions. If the norms of the group include tolerating deviant behavior, someone who normally wouldn't engage in such behavior might be more likely to do so. For instance, one study found that those working in a group

Exhibit 4
Examples of Asch's Cards

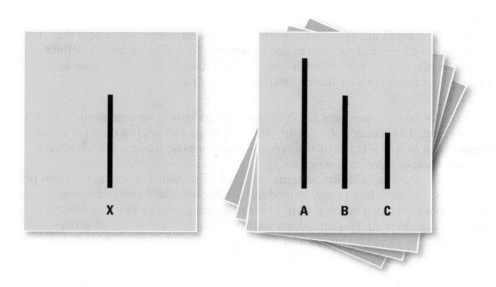

were more likely to lie, cheat, and steal than individuals working alone.[10] Why? Because groups provide anonymity, thus giving individuals—who might otherwise be afraid of getting caught—a false sense of security.

CONFORMITY   Because individuals want to be accepted by groups to which they belong, they're susceptible to pressures to conform. Early experiments done by Solomon Asch demonstrated the impact conformity has on an individual's judgment and attitudes.[11] In these experiments, groups of seven or eight people were asked to compare two cards held up by the experimenter. One card had three lines of different lengths and the other had one line that was equal in length to one of the three lines on the other card (see Exhibit 4). Each group member was to announce aloud which of the three lines matched the single line. Asch wanted to see what would happen if members began to give incorrect answers. Would pressures to conform cause individuals to give wrong answers just to be consistent with the others? The experiment was "fixed" so that all but one of the members (the unsuspecting subject) were told ahead of time to start giving obviously incorrect answers after one or two rounds. Over many experiments and trials, the unsuspecting subject conformed over a third of the time.

Are these conclusions still valid? Research suggests that conformity levels have declined since Asch's studies. However, managers can't ignore conformity because it can still be a powerful force in groups.[12] Group members often want to be seen as one of the group and avoid being visibly different. We find it more pleasant to agree than to be disruptive, even if being disruptive may improve the group's effectiveness. So we conform. But conformity can go too far, especially when an individual's opinion differs significantly from that of others in the group. In such a case, the group often exerts intense pressure on the individual to align his or her opinion to conform to others' opinions, a phenomenon known as **groupthink**. Groupthink seems to occur when group members hold a positive group image they want to protect and when the group perceives a collective threat to this positive image.[13]

STATUS SYSTEMS   Status systems are an important factor in understanding groups. **Status** is a prestige grading, position, or rank within a group. As far back as researchers have been able to trace groups, they have found status hierarchies. Status can be a significant motivator with behavioral consequences, especially when individuals see a disparity between what they perceive their status to be and what others perceive it to be.

Status may be informally conferred by characteristics such as education, age, skill, or experience. Anything can have status value if others in the group evaluate it that way. Of course, just because status is informal doesn't mean it's unimportant or

groupthink
When a group exerts extensive pressure on an individual to align his or her opinion with others' opinions

status
A prestige grading, position, or rank within a group

hard to determine who has it or who does not. Group members have no problem placing people into status categories and usually agree about who has high or low status.

Status is also formally conferred, and it's important for employees to believe the organization's formal status system is congruent—that is, the system shows consistency between the perceived ranking of an individual and the status symbols he or she is given by the organization. For instance, status incongruence would occur when a supervisor earns less than his or her subordinates, a desirable office is occupied by a person in a low-ranking position, or paid country club memberships are provided to division managers but not to vice presidents. Employees expect the "things" an individual receives to be congruent with his or her status. When they're not, employees may question the authority of their managers and may not be motivated by job promotion opportunities.

GROUP SIZE What's an appropriate size for a group? At Amazon, work teams have considerable autonomy to innovate and to investigate their ideas. And Jeff Bezos, founder and CEO, uses a "two-pizza" philosophy; that is, a team should be small enough that it can be fed with two pizzas. This "two-pizza" philosophy usually limits groups to five to seven people depending, of course, on team member appetites.[14]

Group size affects performance and satisfaction, but the effect depends on what the group is supposed to accomplish.[15] Research indicates, for instance, that small groups are faster than larger ones at completing tasks. However, for groups engaged in problem solving, large groups consistently get better results than smaller ones. What do these findings mean in terms of specific numbers? Large groups—those with a dozen or more members—are good for getting diverse input. Thus, if the goal of the group is to find facts, a larger group should be more effective. On the other hand, smaller groups—from five to seven members—are better at doing something productive with those facts.

One important research finding related to group size concerns **social loafing**, which is the tendency for an individual to expend less effort when working collectively than when working individually.[16] Social loafing may occur because people believe others in the group aren't doing their fair share. Thus, they reduce their work efforts in an attempt to make the workload more equivalent. Also, the relationship between an individual's input and the group's output is often unclear. Thus, individuals may become "free riders" and coast on the group's efforts because individuals believe their contribution can't be measured.

social loafing
The tendency for individuals to expend less effort when working collectively than when working individually

group cohesiveness
The degree to which group members are attracted to one another and share the group's goals

The implications of social loafing are significant. When managers use groups, they must find a way to identify individual efforts. If not, group productivity and individual satisfaction may decline.[17]

GROUP COHESIVENESS Cohesiveness is important because it has been found to be related to a group's productivity. Groups in which there's a lot of internal disagreement and lack of cooperation are less effective in completing their tasks than groups in which members generally agree, cooperate, and like each other. Research in this area has focused on **group cohesiveness**, or the degree to which members are attracted to a group and share the group's goals.[18]

Research has generally shown that highly cohesive groups are more effective than less cohesive ones.[19] However, the relationship between cohesiveness and effectiveness is complex. A key moderating variable is the degree to which the group's attitude aligns with its goals or with the goals of the organization.[20] (See Exhibit 5.) The more cohesive the group, the more its members will follow its goals. If the goals are desirable (for instance, high output, quality work, cooperation with individuals outside the group), a cohesive group is more productive than a less cohesive group. But if cohesiveness is high and attitudes are unfavorable, productivity decreases. If cohesiveness is low but goals are

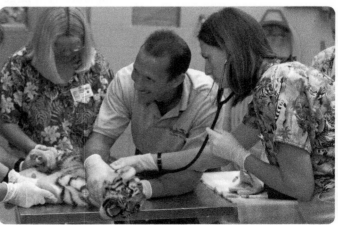

Group cohesiveness is high for these veterinarians at the Detroit Zoo. They are passionate about sharing the zoo's mission of "saving and celebrating wildlife," and they contribute to the zoo's recognition as a leader in animal conservation and welfare. Committed to their work, they cooperate with each other in overseeing the care of wild and exotic animals.
Source: Steve Marcus/Reuters Pictures

Exhibit 5
Group Cohesiveness and
Productivity

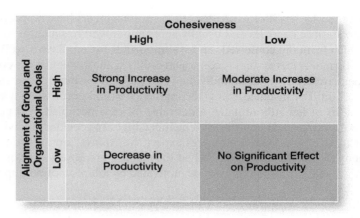

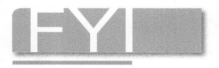

- 25 percent of managers
  say that dealing with issues
  between team coworkers is
  the most challenging aspect of
  managing a team.[21]

supported, productivity increases but not as much as when both cohesiveness and support are high. When cohesiveness is low and goals are not supported, productivity is not significantly affected.

GROUP PROCESSES   The next factor that determines group performance and satisfaction concerns the processes that go on within a work group such as communication, decision making, conflict management, and the like. These processes are important to understanding work groups because they influence group performance and satisfaction positively or negatively. An example of a positive process factor is the synergy of four people on a marketing research team who are able to generate far more ideas as a group than the members could produce individually. However, the group also may have negative process factors such as social loafing, high levels of conflict, or poor communication, which may hinder group effectiveness. We'll look at two important group processes: group decision making and conflict management.

GROUP DECISION MAKING   It's a rare organization that doesn't use committees, task forces, review panels, study teams, or other similar groups to make decisions. Studies show that managers may spend up to 30 hours a week in group meetings.[22] Undoubtedly, a large portion of that time is spent formulating problems, developing solutions, and determining how to implement the solutions. It's possible, in fact, for groups to be assigned any of the eight steps in the decision-making process.

What advantages do group decisions have over individual decisions? One is that groups generate more complete information and knowledge. They bring a diversity of experience and perspectives to the decision process that an individual cannot. In addition, groups generate more diverse alternatives because they have a greater amount and diversity of information. Next, groups increase acceptance of a solution. Group members are reluctant to fight or undermine a decision they helped develop. Finally, groups increase legitimacy. Decisions made by groups may be perceived as more legitimate than decisions made by one person.

Group decisions also have disadvantages. One is that groups almost always take more time to reach a solution than it would take an individual. Another is that a dominant and vocal minority can heavily influence the final decision. In addition, groupthink can undermine critical thinking in the group and harm the quality of the final decision.[23] Finally, in a group, members share responsibility, but the responsibility of any single member is ambiguous.

Determining whether groups are effective at making decisions depends on the criteria used to assess effectiveness.[24] If accuracy, creativity, and degree of acceptance are important, then a group decision may work best. However, if speed and efficiency are important, then an individual decision may be the best. In addition, decision effectiveness is influenced by group size. Although a larger group provides more diverse

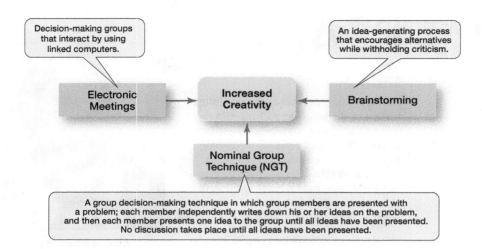

Exhibit 6
Creative Group Decision Making

Decision-making groups that interact by using linked computers.

An idea-generating process that encourages alternatives while withholding criticism.

Electronic Meetings → Increased Creativity ← Brainstorming

Nominal Group Technique (NGT)

A group decision-making technique in which group members are presented with a problem; each member independently writes down his or her ideas on the problem, and then each member presents one idea to the group until all ideas have been presented. No discussion takes place until all ideas have been presented.

representation, it also requires more coordination and time for members to contribute their ideas. Evidence indicates that groups of five, and to a lesser extent seven, are the most effective for making decisions.[25] Having an odd number in the group helps avoid decision deadlocks. Also, these groups are large enough for members to shift roles and withdraw from unfavorable positions but still small enough for quieter members to participate actively in discussions.

What techniques can managers use to help groups make more creative decisions? Exhibit 6 describes three possibilities.

CONFLICT MANAGEMENT   Another important group process is how a group manages conflict. As a group performs its assigned tasks, disagreements inevitably arise. **Conflict** is *perceived* incompatible differences resulting in some form of interference or opposition. Whether the differences are real is irrelevant. If people in a group perceive that differences exist, then there is conflict. Surveys show that managers spend about 25 percent of their time resolving conflicts.[26]

Three different views have evolved regarding conflict.[27] The **traditional view of conflict** argues that conflict must be avoided—that it indicates a problem within the group. Another view, the **human relations view of conflict**, argues that conflict is a natural and inevitable outcome in any group and need not be negative but has potential to be a positive force in contributing to a group's performance. The third and most recent view, the **interactionist view of conflict**, proposes that not only can conflict be a positive force in a group but that some conflict is *absolutely necessary* for a group to perform effectively.

The interactionist view doesn't suggest that all conflicts are good. Some conflicts— **functional conflicts**—are constructive and support the goals of the work group and improve its performance. Other conflicts—**dysfunctional conflicts**—are destructive and prevent a group from achieving its goals. Exhibit 7 on the next page illustrates the challenge facing managers.

When is conflict functional and when is it dysfunctional? Research indicates that you need to look at the *type* of conflict.[28] **Task conflict** relates to the content and goals of the work. **Relationship conflict** focuses on interpersonal relationships. **Process conflict** refers to how the work gets done. Research shows that *relationship* conflicts are almost always dysfunctional because the interpersonal hostilities increase personality clashes and decrease mutual understanding and the tasks don't get done. On the other hand, low levels of process conflict and low-to-moderate levels of task conflict are functional. For *process* conflict to be productive, it must be minimal. Otherwise, intense arguments over who should do what may become dysfunctional and can lead to uncertainty about task assignments, increase the time to complete tasks, and result in members working at cross-purposes. However, a low-to-moderate level of *task* conflict consistently has a positive effect on group performance because it

conflict
Perceived incompatible differences that result in interference or opposition

traditional view of conflict
The view that all conflict is bad and must be avoided

human relations view of conflict
The view that conflict is a natural and inevitable outcome in any group

interactionist view of conflict
The view that some conflict is necessary for a group to perform effectively

functional conflicts
Conflicts that support a group's goals and improve its performance

dysfunctional conflicts
Conflicts that prevent a group from achieving its goals

task conflict
Conflicts over content and goals of the work

relationship conflict
Conflict based on interpersonal relationships

process conflict
Conflict over how work gets done

353

let's get REAL

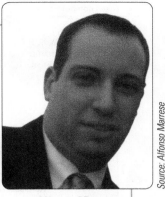

The Scenario:

Fran Waller is the manager of a retail store that's part of a large national chain. Many of her employees are going to school and working. But she also has some full-time employees. A conflict over vacation and holiday work schedules has been building for some time now, and it's creating a very tense atmosphere, which isn't good for customer service. She's got to resolve it NOW.

Alfonso Marrese
Retail Executive

What suggestions would you give Fran for managing this conflict?

In the beginning of the year, when the vacation schedule comes out, the manager should tell all the employees that the vacation schedule is based on tenure. This will help with the arguing of the associates. To handle the issue now, she should talk to the associates that want the same weeks vacation and see if any of them would be willing to switch to a different week and possibly give them a little incentive for switching. Some examples could be giving them an extra weekend off or an extra day of vacation. The same should be done with the holidays; if there are 6 holidays, have each associate work 3. This will help maximize coverage on busy days and provide the best customer service.

Exhibit 7
Conflict and Group Performance

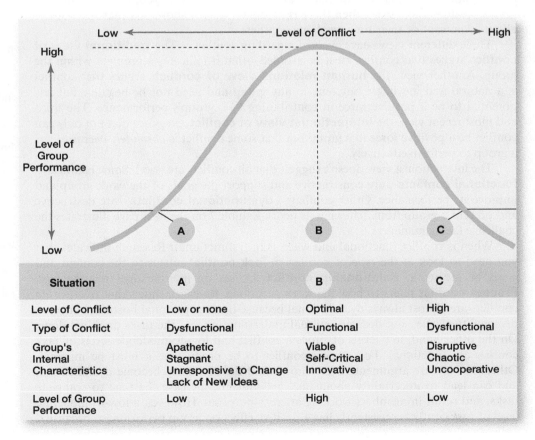

Situation	A	B	C
Level of Conflict	Low or none	Optimal	High
Type of Conflict	Dysfunctional	Functional	Dysfunctional
Group's Internal Characteristics	Apathetic Stagnant Unresponsive to Change Lack of New Ideas	Viable Self-Critical Innovative	Disruptive Chaotic Uncooperative
Level of Group Performance	Low	High	Low

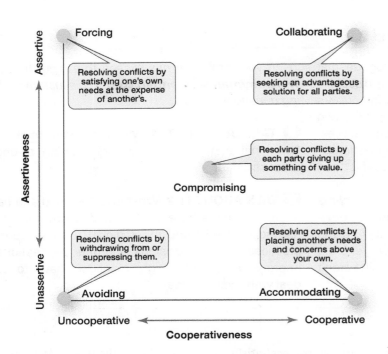

Exhibit 8
Conflict-Management Techniques

Source: K. Thomas, "Conflict and Negotiation Process in Organizations," in M. D. Dunnette and L. J. Hough (eds.), *Handbook of Industrial and Organizational Psychology*, 2 ed. vol. 3 (Palo Alto, CA: Consulting Psychologists Press, 1992), p. 668. Used with permission by Leaetta Hough-Dunnette.

stimulates discussion of ideas that help groups be more innovative.[29] Because we don't yet have a sophisticated measuring instrument for assessing whether conflict levels are optimal, too high, or too low, the manager must try to judge that intelligently.

When group conflict levels are too high, managers can select from five conflict management options: avoidance, accommodation, forcing, compromise, and collaboration.[30] (See Exhibit 8 for a description of these techniques.) Keep in mind that no one option is ideal for every situation. Which approach to use depends on the circumstances.

Have you ever been part of a class group in which all teammates received the same grade, even though some team members didn't fulfill their responsibilities? How did that make you feel? Did it create conflict within the group, and did you feel that the process and outcome were unfair? Recent research also has shown that organizational justice or fairness is an important aspect of managing group conflict.[31] How group members feel about how they're being treated both by each other within the group and by outsiders can affect their work attitudes and behaviors. To promote the sense of fairness, it's important that group leaders build a strong sense of community based on fair and just treatment.

If your professor has assigned this, go to **www.mymanagementlab.com** to complete the Writing Assignment BCOMM 2: Managing Conflict.

★ **Write It 1!**

Group Tasks

At Hackensack University Medical Center in New Jersey, daily reviews of each patient in each nursing unit are conducted in MDRs (multidisciplinary rounds) by teams of nurses, case managers, social workers, and an in-hospital doctor. These teams perform tasks such as prescribing drugs or even recommending a patient be discharged. Employee teams at Lockheed Martin's New York facility custom build complex products such as ground-based radar systems using continuous quality improvement techniques. The six people in the Skinny Improv group in Springfield, Missouri, perform their unique brand of comedy every weekend in a downtown venue.[32] Each of these groups has a different type of task to accomplish.

FUTURE VISION | Conflict 2.0

Successful organizations will come to recognize that functional conflict—in the form of tolerating dissent—makes an organization stronger, not weaker. Tomorrow's organizations will use blogs, social networking sites, and other vehicles to allow employees to question practices, criticize decisions, and offer improvement suggestions.

The historical practice of minimizing conflict and seeking "peace at any price" didn't produce harmony and loyalty. It merely masked employee concerns and frustrations. To maintain competitiveness, organizations will see conflict in a positive light. And the result will be organizations that adapt faster, generate more and better ideas, and have employees who aren't threatened by saying what's on their minds.

If your professor has chosen to assign this, go to **www.mymanagementlab.com** to discuss the following questions.

⭐ **TALK ABOUT IT 1:** What do you think? Will functional conflict make an organization stronger? Discuss.

⭐ **TALK ABOUT IT 2:** What issues—good and bad—might managers have to deal with if employees can use social media and other digital tools to question practices, criticize decisions, and offer suggestions for improvement? What might managers have to do to deal with these issues?

As the group performance/satisfaction model shows, the impact that group processes have on group performance and member satisfaction is modified by the task the group is doing. More specifically, it's the *complexity* and *interdependence* of tasks that influence a group's effectiveness.[33]

Tasks are either simple or complex. Simple tasks are routine and standardized. Complex tasks tend to be novel or nonroutine. It appears that the more complex the task, the more a group benefits from group discussion about alternative work methods. Group members don't need to discuss such alternatives for a simple task, but can rely on standard operating procedures. Similarly, a high degree of interdependence among the tasks that group members must perform means they'll need to interact more. Thus, effective communication and controlled conflict are most relevant to group performance when tasks are complex and interdependent.

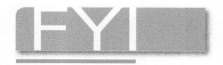

- 50 percent of managers say that their team members collaborate well with other teams.[34]

TURNING Groups into Effective Teams

LO3 When companies like W. L. Gore, Volvo, and Kraft Foods introduced teams into their production processes, it made news because no one else was doing it. Today, it's just the opposite—the organization that *doesn't* use teams would be newsworthy. It's estimated that some 80 percent of *Fortune* 500 companies have at least half of their employees on teams. And 83 percent of respondents in a Center for Creative Leadership study said teams are a key ingredient to organizational success.[35] Without a doubt, team-based work is a core feature of today's organizations. And teams are likely to continue to be popular. Why? Research suggests that teams typically outperform individuals when the tasks being done require multiple skills, judgment, and experience.[36] Organizations are using team-based structures because they've found that teams are more flexible and responsive to changing events than traditional departments or other permanent work groups. Teams have the ability to quickly assemble, deploy, refocus, and disband. In this section, we'll discuss what a work team is, the different types of teams organizations might use, and how to develop and manage work teams.

⭐ **Write It 2!** If your professor has assigned this, go to **www.mymanagementlab.com** to complete the Writing Assignment MGMT 15: Team-Based Structures.

Work Teams	Work Groups
▪ Leadership role is shared	▪ One leader clearly in charge
▪ Accountable to self and team	▪ Accountable only to self
▪ Team creates specific purpose	▪ Purpose is same as broader organizational purpose
▪ Work is done collectively	▪ Work is done individually
▪ Meetings characterized by open-ended discussion and collaborative problem-solving	▪ Meetings characterized by efficiency; no collaboration or open-ended discussion
▪ Performance is measured directly by evaluating collective work output	▪ Performance is measured indirectly according to its influence on others
▪ Work is decided upon and done together	▪ Work is decided upon by group leader and delegated to individual group members
▪ Can be quickly assembled, deployed, refocused, and disbanded	

Exhibit 9
Groups Versus Teams

Sources: J. R. Katzenbach and D. K. Smith, "The Wisdom of Teams," *Harvard Business Review*, July–August 2005, p. 161; A. J. Fazzari and J. B. Mosca, "Partners in Perfection: Human Resources Facilitating Creation and Ongoing Implementation of Self-Managed Manufacturing Teams in a Small Medium Enterprise," *Human Resource Development Quarterly*, Fall 2009, pp. 353–376.

What Is a Work Team?

Most of you are probably familiar with teams, especially if you've watched or participated in organized sports events. Work *teams* differ from work *groups* and have their own unique traits (see Exhibit 9). Work groups interact primarily to share information and to make decisions to help each member do his or her job more efficiently and effectively. There's no need or opportunity for work groups to engage in collective work that requires joint effort. On the other hand, **work teams** are groups whose members work intensely on a specific, common goal using their positive synergy, individual and mutual accountability, and complementary skills. For instance, at the Sparta, Tennessee, facility of Philips Professional Luminaires, a work team came up with a startling innovation. One team member was commenting on the efficient way that Subway restaurants make their sandwiches, with workers lining up all their ingredients in an easy-to-reach, highly adaptable format. The team decided to apply that same flexible principle to their work of producing lighting fixtures and together figured out a way to make that happen.[37]

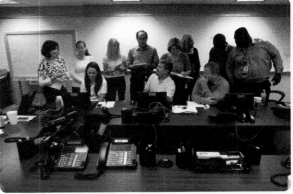

To improve its organizational performance, Florida Power & Light restructured its work processes around high-performing, problem-solving teams. Members of FPL's materials management team shown here collaborate with other company emergency teams in quickly and safely responding to customer power outages caused by accidents and storms.
Source: Bruce R. Bennett/ZUMA Press/Newscom

work teams
Groups whose members work intensely on a specific, common goal using their positive synergy, individual and mutual accountability, and complementary skills

Types of Work Teams

Teams can do a variety of things. They can design products, provide services, negotiate deals, coordinate projects, offer advice, and make decisions.[38] For instance, at Rockwell Automation's facility in North Carolina, teams are used in work process optimization projects. At Sylvania, the New Ventures Group creates cool LED-based products. At Arkansas-based Acxiom Corporation, a team of human resource professionals planned and implemented a cultural change. And every summer weekend at any NASCAR race, you can see work teams in action during drivers' pit stops.[39] The four most common types of work teams are problem-solving teams, self-managed work teams, cross-functional teams, and virtual teams.

When work teams first became popular, most were **problem-solving teams**, teams from the same department or functional area involved in efforts to improve work activities or to solve specific problems. Members share ideas or offer suggestions on how work processes and methods can be improved. However, these teams are rarely given the authority to implement any of their suggested actions.

Although problem-solving teams were helpful, they didn't go far enough in getting employees involved in work-related decisions and processes. This shortcoming led to another type of team, a **self-managed work team**, a formal group of employees who operate without a manager and are responsible for a complete work process or

problem-solving team
A team from the same department or functional area that's involved in efforts to improve work activities or to solve specific problems

self-managed work team
A type of work team that operates without a manager and is responsible for a complete work process or segment

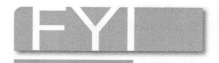

cross-functional team
A work team composed of individuals from various functional specialties

virtual team
A type of work team that uses technology to link physically dispersed members in order to achieve a common goal

segment. A self-managed team is responsible for getting the work done *and* for managing themselves, which usually includes planning and scheduling of work, assigning tasks to members, collective control over the pace of work, making operating decisions, and taking action on problems. For instance, teams at Corning have no shift supervisors and work closely with other manufacturing divisions to solve production-line problems and coordinate deadlines and deliveries. The teams have the authority to make and implement decisions, finish projects, and address problems.[41] Other organizations such as Xerox, Boeing, PepsiCo, and Hewlett-Packard also use self-managed teams. An estimated 30 percent of U.S. employers now use this form of team; among large firms, the number is probably closer to 50 percent.[42] Most organizations that use self-managed teams find them to be effective.[43]

The third type of team is the **cross-functional team**, defined as a work team composed of individuals from various functional specialties. Many organizations use cross-functional teams. For example, ArcelorMittal, the world's biggest steel company, uses cross-functional teams of scientists, plant managers, and salespeople to review and monitor product innovations.[44] The concept of cross-functional teams is even applied in health care. For instance, at Suburban Hospital in Bethesda, Maryland, intensive care unit (ICU) teams composed of a doctor trained in intensive care medicine, a pharmacist, a social worker, a nutritionist, the chief ICU nurse, a respiratory therapist, and a chaplain meet daily with every patient's bedside nurse to discuss and debate the best course of treatment. The hospital credits this team care approach with reducing errors, shortening the amount of time patients spent in ICU, and improving communication between families and the medical staff.[45]

The final type of team is the **virtual team**, a team that uses technology to link physically dispersed members to achieve a common goal. For instance, a virtual team at Boeing-Rocketdyne played a pivotal role in developing a radically new product.[46] Another company, Decision Lens, uses a virtual team environment to generate and evaluate creative ideas.[47] In a virtual team, members collaborate online with tools such as wide-area networks, videoconferencing, fax, e-mail, or Web sites where the team can hold online conferences.[48] Virtual teams can do all the things that other teams can—share information, make decisions, and complete tasks; however, they lack the normal give-and-take of face-to-face discussions. That's why virtual teams tend to be more task-oriented, especially if the team members have never met in person.

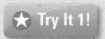

If your professor has assigned this, go to **www.mymanagementlab.com** to complete the Simulation: Virtual Teams and get a better understanding of the challenges of managing virtual teams in organizations.

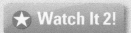

If your professor has assigned this, go to **www.mymanagementlab.com** to watch a video titled: *CH2MHill: Work Teams* and to respond to questions.

Creating Effective Work Teams

As our chapter opener illustrated, teams are not always effective. They don't always achieve high levels of performance. However, research on teams provides insights into the characteristics typically associated with effective teams.[49] These characteristics are listed in Exhibit 10. One element you might notice is missing but think is important to being an effective team is that a team be harmonious and friendly.[50] In fact, friendliness is not a necessary ingredient. Even a grumpy team can be effective if these other team characteristics are present. When a team is productive, has done something good together, and is recognized for its efforts, team members can feel good about their effectiveness.

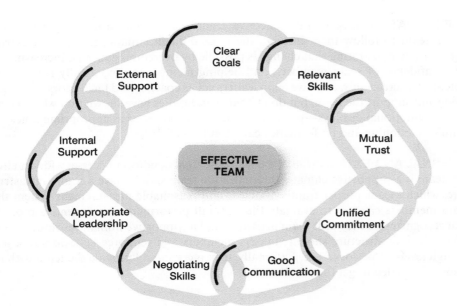

Exhibit 10
Characteristics of Effective Teams

CLEAR GOALS   High-performance teams have a clear understanding of the goal to be achieved. Members are committed to the team's goals, know what they're expected to accomplish, and understand how they will work together to achieve these goals.

RELEVANT SKILLS   Effective teams are composed of competent individuals who have the necessary technical and interpersonal skills to achieve the desired goals while working well together. This last point is important because not everyone who is technically competent has the interpersonal skills to work well as a team member.

MUTUAL TRUST   Effective teams are characterized by high mutual trust among members. That is, members believe in each other's ability, character, and integrity. But as you probably know from personal relationships, trust is fragile. Maintaining this trust requires careful attention by managers.[51]

UNIFIED COMMITMENT   Unified commitment is characterized by dedication to the team's goals and a willingness to expend extraordinary amounts of energy to achieve them. Members of an effective team exhibit intense loyalty and dedication to the team and are willing to do whatever it takes to help their team succeed.

GOOD COMMUNICATION   Not surprisingly, effective teams are characterized by good communication.[53] Members convey messages, verbally and nonverbally, between each other in ways that are readily and clearly understood. Also, feedback helps guide team members and correct misunderstandings. Like a couple who has been together for many years, members of high-performing teams are able to quickly and efficiently share ideas and feelings.

NEGOTIATING SKILLS   Effective teams are continually making adjustments to who does what. This flexibility requires team members to possess negotiating skills. Because problems and relationships regularly change within teams, members need to be able to confront and reconcile differences.

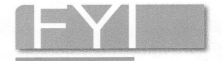

- 72 percent of employees surveyed say that they strongly/moderately trust their coworkers.[52]

Negotiating—If your instructor is using MyManagementLab, log onto **mymanagementlab.com** and test your *negotiating knowledge*. **Be sure to refer back to the chapter opener!**

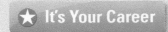

APPROPRIATE LEADERSHIP Effective leaders are important. They can motivate a team to follow them through the most difficult situations. How? By clarifying goals, demonstrating that change is possible by overcoming inertia, increasing the self-confidence of team members, and helping members to more fully realize their potential. Increasingly, effective team leaders act as coaches and facilitators. They help guide and support the team, but don't control it. Studies have shown that when a team leader's emotional displays—positive *and* negative—are used at appropriate times, the team's functioning and performance can be enhanced.[54]

INTERNAL AND EXTERNAL SUPPORT The final condition necessary for an effective team is a supportive climate. Internally, the team should have a sound infrastructure, which means proper training, a clear and reasonable measurement system that team members can use to evaluate their overall performance, an incentive program that recognizes and rewards team activities, and a supportive human resource system. The right infrastructure should support members and reinforce behaviors that lead to high levels of performance. Externally, managers should provide the team with the resources needed to get the job done.

★ **Try It 2!**

If your professor has assigned this, go to **www.mymanagementlab.com** to complete the Simulation: Teams and get a better understanding of the challenges of managing teams in organizations.

let's get REAL

The Scenario:

Barry Murphy is the HR manager at a large agricultural services company. He says, "We've always had an internal recognition program that focused on individual efforts. This recognition provides highly public praise for employees who have exceeded expectations or shown extraordinary effort, plus they get a small monetary incentive. Now, however, since our company is moving to an approach that recognizes team goals rather than individual, how can I make this work?"

What advice would you give Barry?

Barry must meet with his staff and clearly explain the benefits and merits of the company's transition to team-oriented performance objectives. The group goals can be formatted in a similar structure as the individual goals with which everyone was already accustomed. Barry can set up an introductory seminar to get the team motivated and on board with the new program, and then coach each employee to understand their roles in achieving the new team objectives. Challenging, yet attainable, goals combined with proper incentives and recognition can motivate each employee to embrace a team-first outlook.

ToniAnn Petrella-Diaz
Retail Manager

Source: ToniAnn Petrella-Diaz

CURRENT Challenges in Managing Teams

LO4   Few trends have influenced how work gets done in organizations as much as the use of work teams. The shift from working alone to working on teams requires employees to cooperate with others, share information, confront differences, and sublimate personal interests for the greater good of the team. Managers can build effective teams by understanding what influences performance and satisfaction. However, managers also face some current challenges in managing teams, primarily those associated with managing global teams, building team skills, and understanding organizational social networks.

Managing Global Teams

Two characteristics of today's organizations are obvious: they're global and work is increasingly done by teams. These two aspects mean that any manager is likely to have to manage a global team. What do we know about managing global teams? We know there are both drawbacks and benefits in using global teams (see Exhibit 11). Using our group model as a framework, we can see some of the issues associated with managing global teams.

GROUP MEMBER RESOURCES IN GLOBAL TEAMS   In global organizations, understanding the relationship between group performance and group member resources is more challenging because of the unique cultural characteristics represented by members of a global team. In addition to recognizing team members' abilities, skills, knowledge, and personality, managers need to be familiar with and clearly understand the cultural characteristics of the groups and the group members they manage.[55] For instance, is the global team from a culture in which uncertainty avoidance is high? If so, members will not be comfortable dealing with unpredictable and ambiguous tasks. Also, as managers work with global teams, they need to be aware of the potential for stereotyping, which can lead to problems.

GROUP STRUCTURE   Some of the structural areas where we see differences in managing global teams include conformity, status, social loafing, and cohesiveness.

Are conformity findings generalizable across cultures? Research suggests that Asch's findings are culture-bound.[56] For instance, as might be expected, conformity to social norms tends to be higher in collectivistic cultures than in individualistic cultures. Despite this tendency, however, groupthink tends to be less of a problem in global teams because members are less likely to feel pressured to conform to the ideas, conclusions, and decisions of the group.[57]

Also, the importance of status varies between cultures. The French, for example, are extremely status conscious. Also, countries differ on the criteria that confer status. For instance, in Latin America and Asia, status tends to come from family position and formal roles held in organizations. In contrast, while status is important in countries like the United States and Australia, it tends to be less "in your

Drawbacks	Benefits
• Dislike of team members	• Greater diversity of ideas
• Mistrust of team members	• Limited groupthink
• Stereotyping	• Increased attention on understanding others' ideas, perspectives, etc.
• Communication problems	
• Stress and tension	

Exhibit 11
Global Teams

Source: Based on N. Adler, *International Dimensions in Organizational Behavior*, 4th ed. (Cincinnati, OH: South-Western Publishing, 2002), pp. 141–147.

LEADER *making a* DIFFERENCE

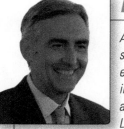

Answering the world's toughest questions is what the some 360,000 employees of Siemens, one of the largest electronics and industrial engineering companies in the world, do.[58] *Former CEO Peter Löscher played an important role in helping those employees do that. Löscher was brought in as CEO after a traumatic time in the company's history, when it was disgraced internationally and paid a $1.6 billion fine for bribery charges. Under his leadership, Löscher turned around the company and returned it to its role of being a leader in the global marketplace. But Löscher didn't do that single-handedly. Employee teams made up of highly dedicated and skilled individuals have been a critical component. For instance, Zhang Wei Ping leads a sales team at Siemens Energy in Shanghai and says the open culture at Siemens is what helps make the company great. "It's like one big family." Löscher also said that trust within a team where "you're no longer just playing individually at your best, but you're also trying to understand what you can do to make the team better" is what he strives for. And that type of culture and atmosphere can be pretty powerful tools in helping make a company strong and competitive in today's world.* What can you learn from this leader making a difference?

face." And it tends to be given based on accomplishments rather than on titles and family history. Managers must understand who and what holds status when interacting with people from a culture different from their own. An American manager who doesn't understand that office size isn't a measure of a Japanese executive's position or who fails to grasp the importance the British place on family genealogy and social class is likely to unintentionally offend others and lessen his or her interpersonal effectiveness.

Social loafing has a Western bias. It's consistent with individualistic cultures, like the United States and Canada, which are dominated by self-interest. It's not consistent with collectivistic societies, in which individuals are motivated by group goals. For instance, in studies comparing employees from the United States with employees from the People's Republic of China and Israel (both collectivistic societies), the Chinese and Israelis showed no propensity to engage in social loafing. In fact, they actually performed better in a group than when working alone.[59]

Cohesiveness is another group structural element where managers may face special challenges. In a cohesive group, members are unified and "act as one." These groups exhibit a great deal of camaraderie, and group identity is high. In global teams, however, cohesiveness is often more difficult to achieve because of higher levels of "mistrust, miscommunication, and stress."[60]

GROUP PROCESSES The processes global teams use to do their work can be particularly challenging for managers. For one thing, communication issues often arise because not all team members may be fluent in the team's working language. This can lead to inaccuracies, misunderstandings, and inefficiencies.[61] However, research also has shown that a multicultural global team is better able to capitalize on the diversity of ideas represented if a wide range of information is used.[62]

Managing conflict in global teams isn't easy, especially when those teams are virtual teams. Conflict can interfere with how information is used by the team. However, research shows that in collectivistic cultures, a collaborative conflict management style can be most effective.[63]

MANAGER'S ROLE Despite the challenges associated with managing global teams, managers can provide the group with an environment in which efficiency and effectiveness are enhanced.[64] First, because communication skills are vital, managers should focus on developing those skills. Also, as we've said earlier, managers must consider cultural differences when deciding what type of global team to use. For instance, evidence suggests that self-managed teams have not fared well in Mexico largely due to that culture's low tolerance of ambiguity and uncertainty and employees' strong respect for hierarchical authority.[65] Finally, it's vital that managers be sensitive to the unique differences of each member of the global team, but it's also important that team members be sensitive to each other.

Building Team Skills

Have you ever participated in a team-building exercise? Such exercises are commonly used to illustrate and develop specific aspects or skills of being on a team. For instance, maybe you've completed *Lost on the Moon* or *Stranded at Sea* or some other written exercise in which you rank-order what items are most important to your survival. Then, you do the same thing with a group—rank-order the most important items. The rank-ordered items are compared against some expert ranking to see how many you got "right." The intent of the exercise is to illustrate how much more effective decisions can be when made as a team. Or maybe you've been part of a trust-building exercise in which you fall back and team members catch you, or an exercise in which your team had to figure out how to get all members across an imaginary river or up a rock wall. Such exercises help team members bond or connect and learn to rely on one another. One of the important tasks managers have is building effective teams.[66] These types of team-building exercises can be an important part of that process. And team-building efforts can work. For example, a research project that looked at star performers with poor team skills who went through two cycles of team-building exercises found that those individuals learned how to collaborate better.[67]

With the emphasis on teams in today's organizations, managers need to recognize that people don't automatically know how to be part of a team or to be an effective team member. Like any behavior, sometimes you have to learn about the skill and then keep practicing and reinforcing it. In building team skills, managers must view their role as more of being a coach and developing team members in order to create more committed, collaborative, and inclusive teams.[68] It's important to recognize that not everyone is a team player or can learn to be a team player. If attempts at team building aren't working, then maybe it's better to put those people in positions where their work is done individually.

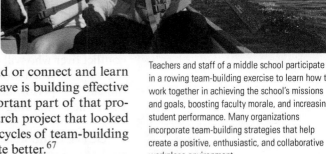

Teachers and staff of a middle school participate in a rowing team-building exercise to learn how to work together in achieving the school's missions and goals, boosting faculty morale, and increasing student performance. Many organizations incorporate team-building strategies that help create a positive, enthusiastic, and collaborative workplace environment.
Source: Gregory Shaver/Associated Press

Understanding Social Networks

We can't leave this text on managing teams without looking at the patterns of informal connections among individuals within groups—that is, at the **social network structure**.[69] What actually happens *within* groups? How *do* group members relate to each other and how does work get done?

Managers need to understand the social networks and social relationships of work groups. Why? Because a group's informal social relationships can help or hinder its effectiveness. For instance, research on social networks has shown that when people need help getting a job done, they'll choose a friendly colleague over someone who may be more capable.[70] Another recent review of team studies showed that teams with high levels of interpersonal interconnectedness actually attained their goals better and were more committed to staying together.[71] Organizations are recognizing the practical benefits of knowing the social networks within teams. For instance, when Ken Loughridge, an IT manager with MWH Global, was transferred from Cheshire, England, to New Zealand, he had a "map" of the informal relationships and connections among company IT employees. This map had been created a few months before using the results of a survey that asked employees who they "consulted most frequently, who they turned to for expertise, and who either boosted or drained their energy levels." Not only did this map help him identify well-connected technical experts, it helped him minimize potential problems when a key manager in the Asia region left the company because Loughridge knew who this person's closest contacts were. Loughridge said, "It's as if you took the top off an ant hill and could see where there's a hive of activity. It really helped me understand who the players were."[72]

social network structure
The patterns of informal connections among individuals within a group

PREPARING FOR: Exams/Quizzes

CHAPTER SUMMARY by Learning Objectives

LO1   **DEFINE groups and the stages of group development.**

A group is two or more interacting and interdependent individuals who come together to achieve specific goals. Formal groups are work groups defined by the organization's structure and have designated work assignments and specific tasks directed at accomplishing organizational goals. Informal groups are social groups.

The forming stage consists of two phases: joining the group and defining the group's purpose, structure, and leadership. The storming stage is one of intragroup conflict over who will control the group and what the group will be doing. The norming stage is when close relationships and cohesiveness develop as norms are determined. The performing stage is when group members begin to work on the group's task. The adjourning stage is when the group prepares to disband.

LO2   **DESCRIBE the major components that determine group performance and satisfaction.**

The major components that determine group performance and satisfaction include external conditions, group member resources, group structure, group processes, and group tasks.

External conditions, such as availability of resources, organizational goals, and other factors, affect work groups. Group member resources (knowledge, skills, abilities, personality traits) can influence what members can do and how effectively they will perform in a group.

Group roles generally involve getting the work done or keeping group members happy. Group norms are powerful influences on a person's performance and dictate things such as work output levels, absenteeism, and promptness. Pressures to conform can heavily influence a person's judgment and attitudes. If carried to extremes, group-think can be a problem. Status systems can be a significant motivator with individual behavioral consequences, especially if incongruence is a factor. What size group is most effective and efficient depends on the task the group is supposed to accomplish. Cohesiveness is related to a group's productivity.

Group decision making and conflict management are important group processes that play a role in performance and satisfaction. If accuracy, creativity, and degree of acceptance are important, a group decision may work best. Relationship conflicts are almost always dysfunctional. Low levels of process conflicts and low-to-moderate levels of task conflicts are functional. Effective communication and controlled conflict are most relevant to group performance when tasks are complex and interdependent.

LO3   **DEFINE teams and best practices influencing team performance.**

Characteristics of work groups include a strong, clearly focused leader; individual accountability; purpose that's the same as the broader organizational mission; individual work product; efficient meetings; effectiveness measured by influence on others; and the ability to discuss, decide, and delegate together. Characteristics of teams include shared leadership roles; individual and mutual accountability; specific team purpose; collective work products; meetings with open-ended discussion and active problem solving; performance measured directly on collective work products; and the ability to discuss, decide, and do real work.

A problem-solving team is one that's focused on improving work activities or solving specific problems. A self-managed work team is responsible for a complete

work process or segment and manages itself. A cross-functional team is composed of individuals from various specialties. A virtual team uses technology to link physically dispersed members in order to achieve a common goal.

The characteristics of an effective team include clear goals, relevant skills, mutual trust, unified commitment, good communication, negotiating skills, appropriate leadership, and internal and external support.

LO4 DISCUSS **contemporary issues in managing teams.**

The challenges of managing global teams can be seen in the group member resources, especially the diverse cultural characteristics; group structure, especially conformity, status, social loafing, and cohesiveness; group processes, especially with communication and managing conflict; and the manager's role in making it all work.

With the emphasis on teams in today's organizations, managers need to recognize that people don't automatically know how to be part of a team or to be an effective team member. Like any behavior, team members have to learn about the skill and then keep practicing and reinforcing it. In building team skills, managers must view their role as more of being a coach and developing others to create more committed, collaborative, and inclusive teams.

Managers need to understand the patterns of informal connections among individuals within groups because those informal social relationships can help or hinder the group's effectiveness.

MyManagementLab

Go to **mymanagementlab.com** to complete the problems marked with this icon ⭐.

⭐ REVIEW AND DISCUSSION QUESTIONS

1. Describe the different types of groups and the five stages of group development.

2. Explain how external conditions and group member resources affect group performance and satisfaction.

3. Discuss how group structure, group processes, and group tasks influence group performance and satisfaction.

4. Compare groups and teams.

5. Describe the four most common types of teams.

6. List the characteristics of effective teams.

7. Explain the role of informal (social) networks in managing teams.

8. How do you think scientific management theorists would react to the increased reliance on teams in organizations? How would behavioral science theorists react?

MyManagementLab

If your professor has assigned these, go to **mymanagementlab.com** for Auto-graded writing questions as well as the following Assisted-graded writing questions:

9. What challenges do managers face in managing global teams? How should those challenges be handled?

10. Why might a manager want to stimulate conflict in a group or team? How could conflict be stimulated?

PREPARING FOR: My Career

⭐ PERSONAL INVENTORY ASSESSMENTS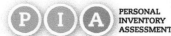

Diagnosing the Need for Team Building

Creating and managing an effective team requires knowing when the team needs some help. Use this PIA to assess teams you're leading or are part of.

⭐ ETHICS DILEMMA

When coworkers work closely on a team project, is there such a thing as TMI (too much information)?[73] At one company, a team that had just finished a major project went out to lunch to celebrate. During lunch, one colleague mentioned that he was training for a 20-mile bike race. In addition to a discussion of his new helmet and Lycra shorts, the person also described shaving his whole body to reduce aerodynamic drag. Later, another team member said, "Why, why, why do we need to go there? This is information about a coworker, not someone I really consider a friend, and now it's forever burned in my brain."

11. What do you think? Why are work colleagues sharing increasingly personal information?

12. How have social media and technology contributed to this type of information disclosure?

13. What are the ethical implications of sharing such personal information in the workplace?

SKILLS EXERCISE Developing Your Coaching Skills

About the Skill

Effective work team managers are increasingly being described as coaches rather than bosses. Just like coaches, they're expected to provide instruction, guidance, advice, and encouragement to help team members improve their job performance.

Steps in Practicing the Skill

- *Analyze ways to improve the team's performance and capabilities.* A coach looks for opportunities for team members to expand their capabilities and improve performance. How? You can use the following behaviors. Observe your team members' behaviors on a day-to-day basis. Ask questions of them: Why do you do a task this way? Can it be improved? What other approaches might be used? Show genuine interest in team members as individuals, not merely as employees. Respect them individually. Listen to each employee.

- *Create a supportive climate.* It's the coach's responsibility to reduce barriers to development and to facilitate a climate that encourages personal performance improvement. How? You can use the following behaviors. Create a climate that contributes to a free and open exchange of ideas. Offer help and assistance. Give guidance and advice when asked. Encourage your team. Be positive and upbeat. Don't use threats. Ask, "What did we learn from this that can help us in the future?" Reduce obstacles. Assure team members that you value their contribution to the team's goals. Take personal responsibility for the outcome, but don't rob team members of their full responsibility. Validate team members' efforts when they succeed. Point to what was missing when they fail. Never blame team members for poor results.

- *Influence team members to change their behavior.* The ultimate test of coaching effectiveness is whether an employee's performance improves. You must encourage ongoing growth and development. How can you do this? Try the following behaviors. Recognize and reward small improvements and treat coaching as a way of helping

employees to continually work toward improvement. Use a collaborative style by allowing team members to participate in identifying and choosing among improvement ideas. Break difficult tasks down into simpler ones. Model the qualities you expect from your team. If you want openness, dedication, commitment, and responsibility from your team members, demonstrate these qualities yourself.

Practicing the Skill

Collaborative efforts are more successful when every member of the group or team contributes a specific role or task toward the completion of the goal. To improve your skill at nurturing team effort, choose two of the following activities and break each one into at least six to eight separate tasks or steps. Be sure to indicate which steps are sequential, and which can be done simultaneously with others. What do you think is the ideal team size for each activity you choose?

a. Making an omelet
b. Washing the car
c. Creating a computerized mailing list
d. Designing an advertising poster
e. Planning a ski trip
f. Restocking a supermarket's produce department

WORKING TOGETHER Team Exercise

Derek Yach, senior vice president for global health policy at PepsiCo, is assembling a team to find alternative snacks for Doritos.[74] These physicians and researchers with doctorate degrees, many of whom have built their reputations at places like the Mayo Clinic, the World Health Organization, and like-minded organizations, are tasked with creating healthier options. Suppose you were put in charge of this elite team. How would you lead it?

Form small groups of three to four individuals. Your team's task is to come up with some suggestions for leading this team. (Hint: Look at Exhibit 10.) Come up with a bulleted list of your ideas. Be prepared to share your ideas with the class.

MY TURN TO BE A MANAGER

- Think of a group to which you belong (or have belonged). Trace its development through the stages of group development as shown in Exhibit 2. How closely did its development parallel the group development model? How might the group development model be used to improve this group's effectiveness?

- Using this same group, write a report describing the following things about this group: types of roles played by whom, group norms, group conformity issues, status system, size of group and how effective/efficient it is, and group cohesiveness.

- Using the same group, describe how decisions are made. Is the process effective? Efficient? Describe what types of conflicts seem to arise most often (relationship, process, or task) and how those conflicts are handled. Add this information to your report on the group's development and structure.

- What traits do you think good team players have? Do some research to answer this question and write up a report detailing your findings using a bulleted list format.

- Select two of the characteristics of effective teams listed in Exhibit 10 and develop a team-building exercise for each characteristic that will help a group improve that characteristic. Be creative. Write a report describing your exercises, and be sure to explain how your exercises will help a group improve or develop that characteristic.

- When working in a group (any group to which you're assigned or to which you belong), pay careful attention to what happens in the group as tasks are completed. How does the group's structure or its processes affect how successful the group is at completing its task?

- Research brainstorming and write a report to your professor explaining what it is and listing suggestions for making it an effective group decision-making tool.

- In your own words, write down three things you learned in this text about being a good manager. Keep a copy of this for future reference.

CASE APPLICATION 1 Far and Wide

A lot of people around the world love to travel. How about you? Have you visited other countries, or do you hope to visit other countries some day? For those who do travel outside their home country, travel advice guides can be quite valuable. Lonely Planet, an Australian company, has set the benchmark for providing accurate, up-to-date travel guides that have accompanied millions of travelers on their journeys worldwide.[75]

Lonely Planet was started by husband-and-wife team Tony and Maureen Wheeler who, in 1971, after Tony finished graduate school in London, decided to embark on an adventurous trip before settling into "real" jobs. They drove through Europe armed with a few maps and sold their car in Afghanistan. From there, they continued their journey using local buses, trains, and boats or by hitchhiking whenever they needed to keep within their daily budget of $6 AUD. Their nine-month journey took them through Pakistan, Kashmir, India, Nepal, Thailand, Malaysia, and Indonesia on their way to their ultimate destination, Australia. The story is they arrived in Sydney on Boxing Day 1971 and had 27 cents left between them. Their plan was to find jobs in Sydney until they had earned enough for plane tickets back to London. However, they found that a lot of people were interested in hearing about their travel experiences. Urged on by friends, they started working on a travel guide titled *Across Asia on the Cheap*. Within a week of the 96-page book's completion and placement in a Sydney bookstore, they had sold 1,500 copies, and the publishing company Lonely Planet was born. They financed their second trip through Asia with profits from the first book and published their second guidebook, *South-East Asia on a Shoestring*. A succession of basic travel guides written by Tony and Maureen produced enough income to cover their own traveling and publishing expenses, but just enough to break even. Their decision to produce a 700-page guidebook to India almost overwhelmed them, but that guidebook was an immediate success, giving Lonely Planet financial stability for the future. Finally, they could afford to hire editors, cartographers, and writers, all of whom worked on a contract basis on individual team projects.

So, how does Lonely Planet produce a product like a guidebook? It's all about teamwork. Commissioning editors (CEs) have a specific geographic area for which they're responsible for commissioning authors of regional content for Lonely Planet's digital and print travel products. CEs research a destination thoroughly to see what travelers are looking for—what's hot and what's not. CEs also get input from specialists and regional experts. Based on this information, the CEs write an author brief. Then, they commission freelance authors who do a lot of pre-trip research before packing their bags. Armed with author briefs, an empty notebook, and a laptop, an author goes on the road doing all the diligent groundwork on location. After concluding their research, the writing of the manuscript begins, which must be completed by a deadline. Once a manuscript is done, it's worked on by CEs and editors at Lonely Planet headquarters to ensure it meets the company's standards of style and quality. Cartographers create new maps from the author's material. The layout designers work with the editors to bring the text, maps, and images together. The design team and image researchers create the cover and photo sections. A proofreader makes sure there are no typographical or layout errors. The book is then sent to a printer, where it's printed, bound, and shipped to bookstores for sale.

From its first simple self-published guidebook, Lonely Planet Publications has grown to become the world's largest independent guidebook publisher. Tony and Maureen realized the business needed a partner that had the necessary resources for future growth, especially in the digital side of the business. They found that partner in BBC Worldwide, which now owns Lonely Planet Publishing.

⭐ **DISCUSSION QUESTIONS**

14. What challenges would there be to creating an effective team in an organization staffed by independent contractors? How could managers deal with these challenges?

15. Why do you think teamwork is crucial to Lonely Planet's business model?

16. Using Exhibit 10, what characteristics of effective teams would be most important to Lonely Planet's guidebook teams? Explain your choices.

CASE APPLICATION 2   737 Teaming Up for Take Off

The Boeing 737, a short- to medium-range twin-engine, narrow-body jet, first rolled off the assembly line in 1967.[76] Here, almost half a century later, it's the best-selling jet airliner in the history of aviation. As airlines replace their aging narrow-body jet fleets, the burden is on Boeing to ramp up production to meet demand and to do so efficiently. As Boeing managers state, "How do you produce more aircraft without expanding the building?" Managing production of the multimillion dollar product—a 737-800 is sold for $84.4 million—means "walking an increasingly fine line between generating cash and stoking an airplane glut." And Boeing is relying on its employee innovation teams to meet the challenge.

Boeing has been using employee-generated ideas since the 1990s, when its manufacturing facility in Renton, Washington, began adopting "lean" manufacturing techniques. Today, employee teams are leaving "few stones unturned." For instance, a member of one team thought of a solution to a problem of stray metal fasteners sometimes puncturing the tires as the airplane advanced down the assembly line. The solution? A canvas wheel cover that hugs the four main landing-gear tires. Another team figured out how to rearrange its work space to make four engines at a time instead of three. Another team of workers in the paint process revamped their work routines and cut 10 minutes to 15 minutes per worker off each job. It took five years for another employee team to perfect a process for installing the plane's landing gear hydraulic tubes, but it eventually paid off.

These employee teams are made up of seven to ten workers with "varying backgrounds"—from mechanics to assembly workers to engineers—and tend to focus on a specific part of a jet, such as the landing gear or the passenger seats or the galleys. These teams may meet as often as once a week. What's the track record of these teams? Today, it takes about 11 days for the final assembly of a 737 jet. That's down from 22 days about a decade ago. The near-term goal is to eventually shave off two more days.

⭐ **DISCUSSION QUESTIONS**

17. What type of team(s) do these employee teams appear to be? Explain.

18. As this story illustrated, sometimes it may take a long time for a team to reach its goal. As a manager, how would you motivate a team to keep on trying?

19. What role do you think a team leader needs to play in this type of setting? Explain.

20. Using Exhibit 10, what characteristics of effective teams would these teams need? Explain.

ENDNOTES

1. E. Brodow, "Ten Tips for Negotiating in 2014," www.brodow.com, 2014.

2. B. Mezrich, *Bringing Down the House: The Inside Story of Six MIT Students Who Took Vegas for Millions* (New York: Free Press, 2002). The 2008 film *21* was a fictional work based loosely on the story.

3. M. F. Maples, "Group Development: Extending Tuckman's Theory," *Journal for Specialists in Group Work*, Fall 1988, pp. 17–23; and B. W. Tuckman and M. C. Jensen, "Stages of Small-Group Development Revisited," *Group and Organizational Studies*, December 1977, pp. 419–427.

4. D. Coutou, interview with J. R. Hackman, "Why Teams Don't Work," *Harvard Business Review*, May 2009, pp. 99–105; M. Kaeter, "Repotting Mature Work Teams," *Training*, April 1994, pp. 54–56; and L. N. Jewell and H. J. Reitz, *Group Effectiveness in Organizations* (Glenview, IL: Scott Foresman, 1981).

5. A. Sobel, "The Beatles Principles," *Strategy & Business*, Spring 2006, p. 42.

6. This model is based on the work of P. S. Goodman, E. Ravlin, and M. Schminke, "Understanding Groups in Organizations," in L. L. Cummings and B. M. Staw (eds.), *Research in Organizational Behavior*, vol. 9 (Greenwich, CT: JAI Press, 1987), pp. 124–128; J. R. Hackman, "The Design of Work Teams," in J. W. Lorsch (ed.), *Handbook of Organizational Behavior* (Upper Saddle River, NJ: Prentice Hall, 1987), pp. 315–342; G. R. Bushe and A. L. Johnson, "Contextual and Internal Variables Affecting Task Group Outcomes in Organizations," *Group and Organization Studies*, December 1989, pp. 462–482; M. A. Campion, C. J. Medsker, and A. C. Higgs, "Relations Between Work Group Characteristics and Effectiveness: Implications for Designing Effective Work Groups," *Personnel Psychology*, Winter 1993, pp. 823–850; D. E. Hyatt and T. M. Ruddy, "An Examination of the Relationship Between Work Group Characteristics, and Performance: Once More into the Breach," *Personnel Psychology*, Autumn 1997, pp. 553–585; and P. E. Tesluk and J. E. Mathieu, "Overcoming Roadblocks to Effectiveness: Incorporating Management of Performance Barriers into Models of Work Group Effectiveness," *Journal of Applied Psychology*, April 1999, pp. 200–217.

7. G. L. Stewart, "A Meta-Analytic Review of Relationships Between Team Design Features and Team Performance," *Journal of Management*, February 2006, pp. 29–54; T. Butler and J. Waldroop, "Understanding 'People' People," *Harvard Business Review*, June 2004, pp. 78–86; J. S. Bunderson, "Team Member Functional Background and Involvement in Management Teams: Direct Effects and the Moderating Role of Power Centralization," *Academy of Management Journal*, August 2003, pp. 458–474; and M. J. Stevens and M. A. Campion, "The Knowledge, Skill, and Ability Requirements for Teamwork: Implications for Human Resource Management," *Journal of Management*, Summer 1994, pp. 503–530.

8. V. U. Druskat and S. B. Wolff, "The Link between Emotions and Team Effectiveness: How Teams Engage Members and Build Effective Task Processes," *Academy of Management Proceedings*, August 1999; D. C. Kinlaw, *Developing Superior Work Teams: Building Quality and the Competitive Edge* (San Diego, CA: Lexington, 1991); and M. E. Shaw, *Contemporary Topics in Social Psychology* (Morristown, NJ: General Learning Press, 1976), pp. 350–351.

9. McMurry, Inc., "The Roles Your People Play," *Managing People at Work*, October 2005, p. 4; G. Prince, "Recognizing Genuine Teamwork," *Supervisory Management*, April 1989, pp. 25–36; R. F. Bales, *SYMOLOG Case Study Kit* (New York: Free Press, 1980); and K. D. Benne and P. Sheats, "Functional Roles of Group Members," *Journal of Social Issues*, vol. 4 (1948), pp. 41–49.

10. A. Erez, H. Elms, and E. Fong, "Lying, Cheating, Stealing: Groups and the Ring of Gyges," paper presented at the Academy of Management annual meeting, Honolulu, HI: August 8, 2005.

11. S. E. Asch, "Effects of Group Pressure upon the Modification and Distortion of Judgments," in H. Guetzkow (ed.), *Groups, Leadership and Men* (Pittsburgh: Carnegie Press, 1951), pp. 177–190; and S. E. Asch, "Studies of Independence and Conformity: A Minority of One Against a Unanimous Majority," *Psychological Monographs: General and Applied*, vol. 70, no. 9, 1956, pp. 1–70.

12. R. Bond and P. B. Smith, "Culture and Conformity: A Meta-Analysis of Studies Using Asch's [1952, 1956] Line Judgment Task," *Psychological Bulletin*, January 1996, pp. 111–137.

13. M. E. Turner and A. R. Pratkanis, "Mitigating Groupthink by Stimulating Constructive Conflict," in C. DeDreu and E. Van deVliert (eds.), *Using Conflict in Organizations* (London: Sage, 1997), pp. 53–71.

14. A. Deutschman, "Inside the Mind of Jeff Bezos," *Fast Company*, August 2004, pp. 50–58.

15. See, for instance, E. J. Thomas and C. F. Fink, "Effects of Group Size," *Psychological Bulletin*, July 1963, pp. 371–384; and M. E. Shaw, *Group Dynamics: The Psychology of Small Group Behavior*, 3rd ed. (New York: McGraw-Hill, 1981).

16. A. Jassawalla, H. Sashittal, and A. Malshe, "Students' Perceptions of Social Loafing: Its Antecedents and Consequences in Undergraduate Business Classroom Teams," *Academy of Management Learning & Education*, March 2009, pp. 42–54; R. C. Liden, S. J. Wayne, R. A. Jaworski, and N. Bennett, "Social Loafing: A Field Investigation," *Journal of Management*, April 2004, pp. 285–304; and D. R. Comer, "A Model of Social Loafing in Real Work Groups," *Human Relations*, June 1995, pp. 647–667.

17. S. G. Harkins and K. Szymanski, "Social Loafing and Group Evaluation," *Journal of Personality and Social Psychology*, December 1989, pp. 934–941.

18. C. R. Evans and K. L. Dion, "Group Cohesion and Performance: A Meta-Analysis," *Small Group Research*, May 1991, pp. 175–186; B. Mullen and C. Copper, "The Relation between Group Cohesiveness and Performance: An Integration," *Psychological Bulletin*, March 1994, pp. 210–227; and P. M. Podsakoff, S. B. MacKenzie, and M. Ahearne, "Moderating Effects of Goal Acceptance on the Relationship between Group Cohesiveness and Productivity," *Journal of Applied Psychology*, December 1997, pp. 974–983.

19. See, for example, L. Berkowitz, "Group Standards, Cohesiveness, and Productivity," *Human Relations*, November 1954, pp. 509–519; and B. Mullen and C. Copper, "The Relation between Group Cohesiveness and Performance: An Integration."

20. S. E. Seashore, *Group Cohesiveness in the Industrial Work Group* (Ann Arbor: University of Michigan, Survey Research Center, 1954).

21. J. Yang and P. Trap, "As a Manager, It's Most Challenging to . . ." *USA Today*, April 19, 2011, p. 1B.

22. C. Shaffran, "Mind Your Meeting: How to Become the Catalyst for Culture Change," *Communication World*, February–March 2003, pp. 26–29.

23. I. L. Janis, *Victims of Groupthink* (Boston: Houghton Mifflin, 1972); R. J. Aldag and S. Riggs Fuller, "Beyond Fiasco: A Reappraisal of the Groupthink Phenomenon and a New Model of Group Decision Processes," *Psychological Bulletin*, May 1993, pp. 533–552; and T. Kameda and S. Sugimori, "Psychological Entrapment in Group Decision Making: An Assigned Decision Rule and a Groupthink Phenomenon," *Journal of Personality and Social Psychology*, August 1993, pp. 282–292.

24. See, for example, L. K. Michaelson, W. E. Watson, and R. H. Black, "A Realistic Test of Individual vs. Group Consensus Decision Making," *Journal of Applied Psychology*, vol. 74, no. 5, 1989, pp. 834–839; R. A. Henry, "Group Judgment Accuracy: Reliability and Validity of Postdiscussion Confidence Judgments," *Organizational Behavior and Human Decision Processes*, October 1993, pp. 11–27; P. W. Paese, M. Bieser, and M. E. Tubbs, "Framing Effects and Choice Shifts in Group Decision Making," *Organizational Behavior and Human Decision Processes*, October 1993, pp. 149–165; N. J. Castellan Jr. (ed.), *Individual and Group Decision Making* (Hillsdale, NJ: Lawrence Erlbaum Associates, 1993); and S. G. Straus and J. E. McGrath, "Does the Medium Matter? The Interaction of Task Type and Technology on Group Performance and Member Reactions," *Journal of Applied Psychology*, February 1994, pp. 87–97.

25. E. J. Thomas and C. F. Fink, "Effects of Group Size," *Psychological Bulletin*, July 1963, pp. 371–384; F. A. Shull, A. L. Delbecq, and L.L.

Cummings, *Organizational Decision Making* (New York: McGraw-Hill, 1970), p. 151; A. P. Hare, *Handbook of Small Group Research* (New York: Free Press, 1976); M. E. Shaw, *Group Dynamics: The Psychology of Small Group Behavior*, 3rd ed. (New York: McGraw-Hill, 1981); and P. Yetton and P. Bottger, "The Relationships Among Group Size, Member Ability, Social Decision Schemes, and Performance," *Organizational Behavior and Human Performance*, October 1983, pp. 145–159.

26. S. Shellenbarger, "Work & Family Mailbox," *Wall Street Journal*, July 17, 2013, p. D2.

27. This section is adapted from S. P. Robbins, *Managing Organizational Conflict: A Nontraditional Approach* (Upper Saddle River, NJ: Prentice Hall, 1974), pp. 11–14. Also, see D. Wagner-Johnson, "Managing Work Team Conflict: Assessment and Preventative Strategies," Center for the Study of Work Teams, University of North Texas [www.workteams.unt.edu/reports], November 3, 2000; and M. Kennedy, "Managing Conflict in Work Teams," Center for the Study of Work Teams, University of North Texas [www.workteams.unt.edu/reports], November 3, 2000.

28. See K. J. Behfar, E. A. Mannix, R. S. Peterson, and W. M. Trochim, "Conflict in Small Groups: The Meaning and Consequences of Process Conflict," *Small Group Research*, April 2011, pp. 127–176; M. A. Korsgaard et al., "A Multilevel View of Intragroup Conflict," *Journal of Management*, December 2008, pp. 1222–1252; C. K. W. DeDreu, "The Virtue and Vice of Workplace Conflict: Food for (Pessimistic) Thought," *Journal of Organizational Behavior*, January 2008, pp. 5–18; K. A. Jehn, "A Multimethod Examination of the Benefits and Detriments of Intragroup Conflict," *Administrative Science Quarterly*, June 1995, pp. 256–282; K. A. Jehn, "A Qualitative Analysis of Conflict Type and Dimensions in Organizational Groups," *Administrative Science Quarterly*, September 1997, pp. 530–557; K. A. Jehn, "Affective and Cognitive Conflict in Work Groups: Increasing Performance Through Value-Based Intragroup Conflict," in C. DeDreu and E. Van deVliert (eds.), *Using Conflict in Organizations* (London: Sage Publications, 1997), pp. 87–100; K. A. Jehn and E. A. Mannix, "The Dynamic Nature of Conflict: A Longitudinal Study of Intragroup Conflict and Group Performance," *Academy of Management Journal*, April 2001, pp. 238–251; C. K. W. DeDreu and A. E. M. Van Vianen, "Managing Relationship Conflict and the Effectiveness of Organizational Teams," *Journal of Organizational Behavior*, May 2001, pp. 309–328; and J. Weiss and J. Hughes, "Want Collaboration? Accept—and Actively Manage—Conflict," *Harvard Business Review*, March 2005, pp. 92–101.

29. C. K. W. DeDreu, "When Too Little or Too Much Hurts: Evidence for a Curvilinear Relationship Between Task Conflict and Innovation in Teams," *Journal of Management*, February 2006, pp. 83–107.

30. A. Somech, H. S. Desivilya, and H. Lidogoster, "Team Conflict Management and Team Effectiveness: The Effects of Task Interdependence and Team Identification," *Journal of Organizational Behavior*, April 2009, pp. 359–378; K. W. Thomas, "Conflict and Negotiation Processes in Organizations," in M. D. Dunnette and L. M. Hough (eds.), *Handbook of Industrial and Organizational Psychology*, 2 ed., vol. 3 (Palo Alto, CA: Consulting Psychologists Press, 1992), pp. 651–717.

31. A. Li and R. Cropanzano, "Fairness at the Group Level: Justice Climate and Intraunit Justice Climate," *Journal of Management*, June 2009, pp. 564–599.

32. K. E. Culp, "Improv Teaches Work Team Building," *Springfield, Missouri News-Leader*, December 9, 2005, p. 5B; T. J. Mullaney and A. Weintraub, "The Tech Guru: Dr. Gerard Burns," *BusinessWeek*, March 28, 2005, p. 84; and J. S. McClenahen, "Lean and Teams: More Than Blips," *Industry Week*, October 2003, p. 63.

33. See, for example, J. R. Hackman and C. G. Morris, "Group Tasks, Group Interaction Process, and Group Performance Effectiveness: A Review and Proposed Integration," in L. Berkowitz (ed.), *Advances in Experimental Social Psychology* (New York: Academic Press, 1975), pp. 45–99; R. Saavedra, P. C. Earley, and L. Van Dyne, "Complex Interdependence in Task-Performing Groups," *Journal of Applied Psychology*, February 1993, pp. 61–72; M. J. Waller, "Multiple-Task Performance in Groups," *Academy of Management Proceedings* on Disk, 1996; and K. A. Jehn, G. B. Northcraft, and M. A. Neale, "Why Differences Make a Difference: A Field Study of Diversity, Conflict,

and Performance in Workgroups," *Administrative Science Quarterly*, December 1999, pp. 741–763.

34. "Smart Pulse," www.smartbrief.com/leadership, November 19, 2013.

35. B. J. West, J. L. Patera, and M. K. Carsten, "Team Level Positivity: Investigating Positive Psychological Capacities and Team Level Outcomes," *Journal of Organizational Behavior*, February 2009, pp. 249–267; T. Purdum, "Teaming, Take 2," *Industry Week*, May 2005, p. 43; and C. Joinson, "Teams at Work," *HRMagazine*, May 1999, p. 30.

36. See, for example, S. A. Mohrman, S. G. Cohen, and A. M. Mohrman, Jr., *Designing Team-Based Organizations* (San Francisco: Jossey-Bass, 1995); P. MacMillan, *The Performance Factor: Unlocking the Secrets of Teamwork* (Nashville, TN: Broadman & Holman, 2001); and E. Salas, C. A. Bowers, and E. Eden (eds.), *Improving Teamwork in Organizations: Applications of Resource Management Training* (Mahwah, NJ: Lawrence Erlbaum, 2002).

37. P. Alpern, "Spreading the Light," *Industry Week*, January 2010, p. 35.

38. See, for instance, J. R. Hollenbeck, B. Beersma, and M. E. Schouten, "Beyond Team Types and Taxonomies: A Dimensional Scaling Conceptualization for Team Description," *Academy of Management Review*, January 2012, p. 85; and E. Sundstrom, K. P. DeMeuse, and D. Futrell, "Work Teams: Applications and Effectiveness," *American Psychologist*, February 1990, pp. 120–133.

39. M. Fitzgerald, "Shine a Light," *Fast Company*, April 2009, pp. 46–48; J. S. McClenahen, "Bearing Necessities," *Industry Week*, October 2004, pp. 63–65; P. J. Kiger, "Acxiom Rebuilds from Scratch," *Workforce*, December 2002, pp. 52–55; and T. Boles, "Viewpoint—Leadership Lessons from NASCAR," *Industry Week* [www.industryweek.com], May 21, 2002.

40. M. B. O'Leary, M. Mortensen, and A. W. Woolley, "Multiple Team Membership: A Theoretical Model of Its Effects on Productivity and Learning for Individuals and Teams," *Academy of Management Review*, July 2011, p. 461.

41. M. Cianni and D. Wanuck, "Individual Growth and Team Enhancement: Moving Toward a New Model of Career Development," *Academy of Management Executive*, February 1997, pp. 105–115.

42. "Teams," *Training*, October 1996, p. 69; and C. Joinson, "Teams at Work," p. 30.

43. G. M. Spreitzer, S. G. Cohen, and G. E. Ledford, Jr., "Developing Effective Self-Managing Work Teams in Service Organizations," *Group & Organization Management*, September 1999, pp. 340–366.

44. "Meet the New Steel," *Fortune*, October 1, 2007, pp. 68–71.

45. J. Appleby and R. Davis, "Teamwork Used to Save Money; Now It Saves Lives," *USA Today* [www.usatoday.com], March 1, 2001.

46. A. Malhotra, A. Majchrzak, R. Carman, and V. Lott, "Radical Innovation without Collocation: A Case Study at Boeing-Rocketdyne," *MIS Quarterly*, June 2001, pp. 229–249.

47. A. Stuart, "Virtual Agreement," *CFO*, November 2007, p. 24.

48. F. Siebdrat, M. Hoegl, and H. Ernst, "How to Manage a Virtual Team," *MIT Sloan Management Review*, Summer 2009, pp. 63–68; A. Malhotra, A. Majchrzak, and B. Rosen, "Leading Virtual Teams," *Academy of Management Perspectives*, February 2007, pp. 60–70; B. L. Kirkman and J. E. Mathieu, "The Dimensions and Antecedents of Team Virtuality," *Journal of Management*, October 2005, pp. 700–718; J. Gordon, "Do Your Virtual Teams Deliver Only Virtual Performance?" *Training*, June 2005, pp. 20–25; L. L. Martins, L. L. Gilson, and M. T. Maynard, "Virtual Teams: What Do We Know and Where Do We Go from Here?" *Journal of Management*, December 2004, pp. 805–835; S. A. Furst, M. Reeves, B. Rosen, and R. S. Blackburn, "Managing the Life Cycle of Virtual Teams," *Academy of Management Executive*, May 2004, pp. 6–20; B. L. Kirkman, B. Rosen, P. E. Tesluk, and C. B. Gibson, "The Impact of Team Empowerment on Virtual Team Performance: The Moderating Role of Face-to-Face Interaction," *Academy of Management Journal*, April 2004, pp. 175–192; F. Keenan and S. E. Ante, "The New Teamwork," *Business Week e.biz*, February 18, 2002, pp. EB12–EB16; and G. Imperato, "Real Tools for Virtual Teams?" *Fast Company*, July 2000, pp. 378–387.

49. B. L. Kirkman, C. B. Gibson, and D. L. Shapiro, "Exporting Teams: Enhancing the Implementation and Effectiveness of Work Teams in Global Affiliates," *Organizational Dynamics*, Summer 2001, pp. 12–29; J. W. Bing and C. M. Bing, "Helping Global Teams Compete," *Train-*

ing & Development, March 2001, pp. 70–71; C. G. Andrews, "Factors That Impact Multi-Cultural Team Performance," Center for the Study of Work Teams, University of North Texas [www.workteams.unt.edu/reports/], November 3, 2000; P. Christopher Earley and E. Mosakowski, "Creating Hybrid Team Cultures: An Empirical Test of Transnational Team Functioning," *Academy of Management Journal,* February 2000, pp. 26–49; J. Tata, "The Cultural Context of Teams: An Integrative Model of National Culture, Work Team Characteristics, and Team Effectiveness," *Academy of Management Proceedings,* 1999; D. I. Jung, K. B. Baik, and J. J. Sosik, "A Longitudinal Investigation of Group Characteristics and Work Group Performance: A Cross-Cultural Comparison," *Academy of Management Proceedings,* 1999; and C. B. Gibson, "They Do What They Believe They Can? Group-Efficacy Beliefs and Group Performance across Tasks and Cultures," *Academy of Management Proceedings,* 1996.

50. D. Coutou, interview with J. R. Hackman, "Why Teams Don't Work."

51. A. C. Costa and N. Anderson, "Measuring Trust in Teams: Development and Validation of a Multifaceted Measure of Formative and Reflective Indicators of Team Trust," *European Journal of Work and Organizational Psychology,* vol. 20, no. 1, 2011, pp. 119–154.

52. "Fast Fact: The Good News About Workplace Trust," *T&D,* October 2012, p. 21.

53. A. Pentland, "The New Science of Building Great Teams," *Harvard Business Review,* April 2012, pp. 60–70.

54. J. C. Santora and M. Esposito, "Do Happy Leaders Make for Better Team Performance," *Academy of Management Perspective,* November 2011, pp. 88–90; G. A. Van Kleef et al., "Searing Sentiment or Cold Calculation? The Effects of Leader Emotional Displays on Team Performance Depend on Followers Epistemic Motivation," *Academy of Management Journal,* June 2009, pp. 562–580.

55. R. Bond and P. B. Smith, "Culture and Conformity: A Meta-Analysis of Studies Using Asch's [1952, 1956] Line Judgment Task," *Psychological Bulletin,* January 1996, pp. 111–137.

56. I. L. Janis, *Groupthink,* 2nd ed. (New York: Houghton Mifflin Company, 1982), p. 175.

57. See P. C. Earley, "Social Loafing and Collectivism: A Comparison of the United States and the People's Republic of China," *Administrative Science Quarterly,* December 1989, pp. 565–581; and P. C. Earley, "East Meets West Meets Mideast: Further Explorations of Collectivistic and Individualistic Work Groups," *Academy of Management Journal,* April 1993, pp. 319–348.

58. Siemens Web site, www.siemens.com/jobs, July 25, 2012; G. Barlett, "Customer Centricity: Siemens' Cultural Centerpiece," *Velocity,* vol. 13, Issue 3, 2011, pp. 17–18; **A. Bryant, "The Trust That Makes a Team Click," *New York Times Online,* July 30, 2011**; H. Struck, D. Fisher, N. Karmali, and G. Epstein, "Urban Outfitter," *Forbes,* May 9, 2011, pp. 80–98; "Siemens Hunts for New Hires as Nation Watches Unemployment Rate," *Forbes.com,* May 5, 2011, p. 62; R. Weiss and B. Kammel, "How Seimens Got Its Geist Back," *Bloomberg BusinessWeek,* January 31, 2011, pp. 18–209; and D. Roberts, "Never Miss a Good Crisis," *Bloomberg BusinessWeek,* October 4, 2010, pp. 79–80.

59. N. J. Adler, *International Dimensions of Organizational Behavior,* 4th ed. (Cincinnati, OH: Southwestern, 2002), p. 142.

60. Ibid., p. 144.

61. K. B. Dahlin, L. R. Weingart, and P. J. Hinds, "Team Diversity and Information Use," *Academy of Management Journal,* December 2005, pp. 1107–1123.

62. Adler, *International Dimensions of Organizational Behavior,* p. 142.

63. P. S. Hempel, Z-X. Zhang, and D. Tjosvold, "Conflict Management Between and Within Teams for Trusting Relationships and Performance in China," *Journal of Organizational Behavior,* January 2009, pp. 41–65; and S. Paul, I. M. Samarah, P. Seetharaman, and P. P. Mykytyn, "An Empirical Investigation of Collaborative Conflict Management Style in Group Support System-Based Global Virtual Teams," *Journal of Management Information Systems,* Winter 2005, pp. 185–222.

64. S. Chang and P. Tharenou, "Competencies Needed for Managing a Multicultural Workgroup," *Asia Pacific Journal of Human Resources* vol. 42, no. 1, 2004, pp. 57–74; and Adler, *International Dimensions of Organizational Behavior,* p. 153.

65. C. E. Nicholls, H. W. Lane, and M. Brehm Brechu, "Taking Self-Managed Teams to Mexico," *Academy of Management Executive,* August 1999, pp. 15–27.

66. M. O'Neil, "Leading the Team," *Supervision,* April 2011, pp. 8-10; and A. Gilley, J. W. Gilley, C. W. McConnell, and A. Veliquette, "The Competencies Used by Effective Managers to Build Teams: An Empirical Study," *Advances in Developing Human Resources,* February 2010, pp. 29–45.

67. B. V. Krishnamurthy, "Use Downtime to Enhance Skills," *Harvard Business Review,* December 2008, pp. 29–30.

68. "Women Leaders: The Hard Truth About Soft Skills," *BusinessWeek Online,* February 17, 2010, p. 8.

69. J. Reingold and J. L. Yang, "The Hidden Workplace: What's Your OQ?" *Fortune,* July 23, 2007, pp. 98–106; and P. Balkundi and D. A. Harrison, "Ties, Leaders, and Time in Teams: Strong Inference About Network Structures' Effects on Team Viability and Performance," *Academy of Management Journal,* February 2006, pp. 49–68.

70. T. Casciaro and M. S. Lobo, "Competent Jerks, Lovable Fools, and the Formation of Social Networks," *Harvard Business Review,* June 2005, pp. 92–99.

71. Balkundi and Harrison, "Ties, Leaders, and Time in Teams: Strong Inference About Network Structures' Effects on Team Viability and Performance."

72. P. Dvorak, "Engineering Firm Charts Ties," *Wall Street Journal,* January 26, 2009, p. B7; and **J. McGregor, "The Office Chart That Really Counts," *Business Week,* February 27, 2006, pp. 48–49.**

73. P. Klaus, "Thank You for Sharing. But Why at the Office? *New York Times Online,* August 18, 2012; and E. Bernstein, "You Did *What?* Spare the Office the Details," *Wall Street Journal,* April 6, 2010, pp. D1+.

74. N. Byrnes, "Pepsi Brings in the Health Police," *Bloomberg BusinessWeek,* January 25, 2010, pp. 50–51.

75. A. Schein, "Lonely Planet Publications," *Hoovers.com,* July 25, 2012; J. Koppisch, "2012 Australian Philanthropists," *Forbes.com,* June 20, 2012, p. 1; N. Denny, "Digital and the Bookshop," *Bookseller,* June 8, 2012, p. 3; M. Costa, "Travel Guru Explores New Routes," *Marketing Week,* April 12, 2012, p. 20; and K. Cuthbertson and R. Haynes, "Duo Came With 27 Cents and Left with $100 Million," *The Herald Sun,* October 2, 2007, p. 11.

76. D. Michaels and J. Ostrower, "Airbus, Boeing Walk a Fine Line on Jetliner Production," *Wall Street Journal,* July 16, 2012, p. B3; D. Kesmodel, "Boeing Teams Speed Up 737 Output," *Wall Street Journal,* February 7, 2012, p. B10; and A. Cohen, "Boeing Sees Demand for Existing, Re-engined 737s," blog on *Seattle Post-Intelligencer Online,* October 26, 2011.

Management Practice: Part 4

Management Practice

A Manager's Dilemma

Management theory suggests that compared to an individual, a diverse group of people will be more creative because team members will bring a variety of ideas, perspectives, and approaches to the group. For an organization like Google, innovation is critical to its success, and teams are a way of life. If management theory about teams is on target, then Google's research and development center in India should excel at innovation. Why? Because there you'll find broad diversity, even though all employees are from India. These Googlers include Indians, Sikhs, Hindus, Muslims, Buddhists, Christians, and Jains. And they speak English, Hindi, Tamil, Bengali, and more of India's 22 officially recognized languages. One skill Google looks for in potential hires is the ability to work as a team member. As Google continues to grow at a rapid pace, new Googlers are continually added to teams.

> Suppose you're a manager at Google's Hyderabad facility. How would you gauge a potential hire's ability to work as a team member, and how would you maintain your team's innovation when new engineers and designers join the group?

Global Sense

Workforce productivity. It's a performance measure that's important to managers and policy makers around the globe. Governments want their labor forces to be productive. Managers want their employees to be productive. Being productive encompasses both efficiency and effectiveness. Efficiency is getting the most output from the least amount of inputs or resources. Or said another way, doing things the right way. Effectiveness was doing those work activities that would result in achieving goals, or doing the right things that would lead to goal achievement. So how does workforce productivity stack up around the world? Here are some of the most recent data on productivity growth rates from the Organization for Economic Cooperation and Development (OECD): Australia, 0.7 percent; Belgium, –1.2 percent; Canada, 0.7 percent; Estonia, –1.7 percent; Greece, –0.9 percent; Ireland, 2.4 percent; Korea, 1.8 percent; Poland, 3.4 percent; Turkey, 2.4 percent; United Kingdom, 1.9 percent; and United States, 0.2 percent. One factor that has a significant effect on workforce productivity rates is the state of the global economy, which is still recovering from the global economic recession. Productivity seems to have spiked through the early part of the downturn, but as the slowdown dragged on, productivity rates for many countries, including the United States, fell. Labor economists suggest that perhaps companies are approaching the limits of how much they can squeeze from the workforce.

Discuss the following questions in light of what you learned:

- *How might workforce productivity be affected by organizational design? Look at the six key elements of organizational design.*
- *What types of adaptive organizational design might be conducive to increasing worker productivity? Which might be detrimental to worker productivity?*
- *How might an organization's human resource management approach affect worker productivity? How could managers use their HR processes to improve worker productivity?*
- *This question is designed to make you think! Are teams more productive than individuals? Discuss and explain.*
- *What's your reaction to the statement by experts that perhaps companies are approaching the limits of how much they can squeeze from the workforce? What are the implications for managers as they make organizing decisions?*

Sources: C. Dougherty, "Workforce Productivity Falls," Wall Street Journal, May 4, 2012, p. A5; "Labour Productivity Growth in the Total Economy," Organization for Economic Cooperation and Development, http://stats.oecd.org/Index.aspx?DatasetCode=PDYGTH, February 2012; and "International Comparisons of Manufacturing Productivity and Unit Labor Cost Trends, 2010," Bureau of Labor Statistics, U.S. Department of Labor, [www.bls.gov], December 1, 2011.

Continuing Case

Starbucks—Organizing

Organizing is an important task of managers. Once the organization's goals and plans are in place, the organizing function sets in motion the process of seeing that those goals and plans are pursued. When managers organize, they're defining what work needs to get done and creating a structure that enables work activities to be completed efficiently and effectively by organizational members hired to do that work. As Starbucks continues its global expansion and pursues innovative strategic initiatives, managers must deal with the realities of continually organizing and reorganizing its work efforts.

Structuring Starbucks

Like many start-up businesses, Starbucks' original founders organized their company around a simple structure based on each person's unique strengths: Zev Siegl became

the retail expert; Jerry Baldwin took over the administrative functions; and Gordon Bowker was the dreamer who called himself "the magic, mystery, and romance man" and recognized from the start that a visit to Starbucks could "evoke a brief escape to a distant world." As Starbucks grew to the point where Jerry recognized that he needed to hire professional and experienced managers, Howard Schultz (now Starbucks' chairman, CEO, and president) joined the company, bringing his skills in sales, marketing, and merchandising. When the original owners eventually sold the company to Schultz, he was able to take the company on the path to becoming what it is today and what it hopes to be in the future.

As Starbucks has expanded, its organizational structure has changed to accommodate that growth. However, the company prides itself on its "lean" corporate structure. Howard Schultz is at the top of the structure and has focused on hiring a team of executives from companies like Nestlé, Procter & Gamble, Corbis, Microsoft, and PepsiCo. Schultz realized how important it was to have an executive team in place that had experience in running divisions or functions of larger companies, and that's what he focused on bringing in to Starbucks. These senior corporate officers include the following: six "C" (chief) officers, seven executive vice presidents, three group presidents, two managing directors, and several "partners." A full description of the team of Starbucks executives and what each is responsible for can be found on the company's Web site.

Although the executive team provides the all-important strategic direction, the "real" work of Starbucks gets done at the company's support center, zone offices, retail stores, and roasting plants. The support center provides support to and assists all other aspects of corporate operations in the areas of accounting, finance, information technology, and sales and supply chain management.

The zone offices oversee the regional operations of the retail stores and provide support in human resource management, facilities management, account management, financial management, and sales management. The essential link between the zone offices and each retail store is the district manager, each of whom oversees 8 to 10 stores, down from the dozen or so stores they used to oversee. Since district managers need to be out working with the stores, most use mobile technology that allows them to spend more time in the stores and still remain connected to their own office. These district managers have been called "the most important in the company" because it's out in the stores that the Starbucks vision and goals are being carried out. Thus, keeping those district managers connected is vital.

In the retail stores, hourly employees (baristas) service customers under the direction of shift supervisors, assistant store managers, and store managers. These managers are responsible for the day-to-day operations of each Starbucks location. One of the organizational challenges

for many store managers has been the company's decision to add more drive-through windows to retail stores, which appears to be a smart, strategic move since the average annual volume at a store with a drive-through window is about 30 percent higher than a store without one. However, a drive-through window often takes up to four people to operate: one to take orders, one to operate the cash register, one to work the espresso machine, and a "floater" who can fill in where needed. And these people have to work rapidly and carefully to get the cars in and out in a timely manner, since the drive-through lane can get congested quickly. Other organizing challenges arise any time the company introduces new products and new, more efficient work approaches.

Finally, without coffee and other beverages and products to sell, there would be no Starbucks. The coffee beans are processed at the company's domestic roasting plants in Washington, Pennsylvania, Nevada, South Carolina, Georgia, and internationally in Amsterdam. There's also a manufacturing plant for Tazo Tea in Oregon, and the company set up a coffee roasting facility with Tata Global Beverages in India. At each manufacturing facility, the production team produces the coffee and other products and the distribution team manages the inventory and distribution of products and equipment to company stores. Because product quality is so essential to Starbucks' success, each person in the manufacturing facilities must be focused on maintaining quality control at every step in the process. The roasting plant in Sandy Run, South Carolina, is a state-of-the art facility that's also an example of the company's commitment to green design. The plant has been awarded LEED® Silver certification for new construction. And the newest plant in Augusta, Georgia, will also be built to LEED® standards. Starbucks also has warehouse/distribution facilities in Georgia, Tennessee, and Washington.

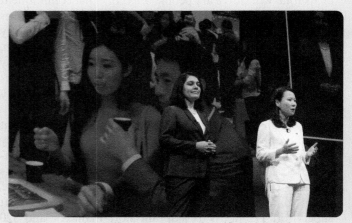

People management is a significant part of the jobs of Avani Davda, left, chief executive officer of Starbucks Tata Limited, the joint-venture company opening Starbucks' stores in India, and Belinda Wong, right, president of Starbucks China. These senior executives are responsible for organizing Starbucks' work force in the two most populous nations in the world with the fastest-growing economies and unique business cultures.
Source: Ted S. Warren/Associated Press

People Management at Starbucks

Starbucks recognizes that what it's been able to accomplish is due to the people it hires. When you have talented and committed people offering their ideas and expertise, success will follow.

Since the beginning, Starbucks has strived to be an employer that nurtured employees and gave them opportunities to grow and be challenged. The company says it is "pro-partner" and has always been committed to providing a flexible and progressive work environment and treating one another with respect and dignity.

As Starbucks continues its expansion both in the United States and internationally, it needs to make sure it has the right number of the right people in the right place at the right time. What kinds of people are "right" for Starbucks? They state they want "people who are adaptable, self-motivated, passionate, creative team players." Starbucks uses a variety of methods to attract potential partners. The company has an interactive and easy-to-use online career center. Job seekers—who must be at least 16—can search and apply online for jobs in the home office (Seattle) support center and in the zone offices, roasting plants, store management, and store hourly (barista) positions in any geographic location. Starbucks also has recruiting events in various locations in the United States throughout the year, which allow job seekers to talk to recruiters and partners face-to-face about working at Starbucks. In addition, job seekers for part-time and full-time hourly positions can also submit an application at any Starbucks store location. The company also has a limited number of internship opportunities for students during the summer.

Starbucks' workplace policies provide for equal employment opportunities and strictly prohibit discrimination. Diversity and inclusion are very important to Starbucks as the following statistics from its U.S. workforce illustrate: 64 percent of its total workforce are women and 33 percent of its total workforce are people of color. That commitment to diversity starts at the top. At one point, senior executives participated in a 360-degree diversity assessment to identify their strengths and needed areas of improvement. Also, an executive diversity learning series, including a full-day diversity immersion exercise, was developed for individuals at the vice-president level and above to build their diversity competencies.

Although diversity training is important to Starbucks, it isn't the only training provided. The company continually invests in training programs and career development initiatives: baristas, who get a "green apron book" that exhorts them to be genuine and considerate, receive 23 hours of initial training; an additional 29 hours of training as shift supervisor; 112 hours as assistant store manager; and 320 hours as store manager. District manager trainees receive 200 hours of training. And every partner takes a class on coffee education, which focuses on Starbucks' passion for coffee and understanding the core product. In addition, the Starbucks corporate support center offers a variety of classes ranging from basic computer skills to conflict resolution to management training. Starbucks' partners aren't "stuck" in their jobs. The company's rapid growth creates tremendous opportunities for promotion and advancement for all store partners. If they desire, they can utilize career counseling, executive coaching, job rotation, mentoring, and leadership development to help them create a career path that meets their needs. One example of the company's training efforts: When oxygen levels in coffee bags were too high in one of the company's roasting plants (which affected product freshness), partners were retrained on procedures and given additional coaching. After the training, the number of bags of coffee placed on "quality hold" declined by 99 percent. Then, on one day in February 2008, Starbucks did something quite unusual—it closed all its U.S. stores for three-and-a-half hours to train and re-train baristas on espresso. A company spokesperson said, "We felt this training was an investment in our baristas and in the Starbucks' experience." The training, dubbed Perfecting the Art of Espresso, was about focusing on the core product, espresso, as well as on the customer experience. Feedback was quite positive. Customers said they appreciated the company taking the time to do the training and felt it had resulted in a better customer experience. The company also embarked on a series of training for partners to find ways to do work more efficiently. A 10-person "lean team" went from region to region encouraging managers and partners to find ways to be more efficient.

One human resource issue that has haunted Starbucks is its position on labor unions. The company takes the position that the fair and respectful "direct employment relationship" it has with its partners— not a third party that acts on behalf of the partners—is the best way to help ensure a great work environment. Starbucks prides itself on how it treats its employees. However, the company did settle a complaint issued by the National Labor Relations Board that contained more than two dozen unfair labor practice allegations brought against the company by the union Industrial Workers of the World. This settlement arose from disputes at three stores in New York City. In 2011, a strike by partners in Chile—which is the only country where the company has a sizable union presence—over low wages led baristas in other countries to call for a "global week of solidarity" in support of the strikers. The Chilean workers eventually abandoned that strike without reaching an agreement with the company. As Starbucks continues to expand globally, it will face challenges in new markets where local labor groups and government requirements honor collective bargaining. And Starbucks realizes it needs to be cautious so that its "we care" image isn't diminished by labor woes.

Discussion Questions

1. What types of departmentalization are being used? Explain your choices. (Hint: In addition to information in the case, you might want to look at the complete list and description of corporate executives on the company's Web site.)

2. Do you think it's a good idea to have a president for the U.S. division and for the other international divisions? What are the advantages of such an arrangement? Disadvantages?

3. What examples of the six organizational structural elements do you see discussed in the case? Describe.

4. Considering the expense associated with having more managers, what are some reasons why you think Starbucks decided to decrease the number of stores each district manager was responsible for, thus increasing the number of managers needed? Other than the expense, can you think of any disadvantages to this decision?

5. Why do you think it was important for Starbucks to keep its mobile workforce "connected?" In addition to the technology used to do this, what other things might the company do to make its adaptive organizational design efficient and effective?

6. Starbucks has said its goal is to open 1,200 new stores globally. In addition, the company has set a financial goal of attaining total net revenue growth of 10 to 13 percent and earnings per share growth between 15 to 20 percent. How will the organizing function contribute to the accomplishment of these goals?

7. Starbucks has said that it wants people who are "adaptable, self-motivated, passionate, and creative team players." How does the company ensure that its hiring and selection process identifies those kinds of people?

8. Select one of the job openings posted on the company's Web site. Do you think the job description and job specification for this job are adequate? Why or why not? What changes might you suggest?

9. Evaluate Starbucks' training efforts. What types of training are available? What other type(s) of training might be necessary? Explain your choices.

10. Pretend that you're a local Starbucks' store manager. You have three new hourly partners (baristas) joining your team. Describe the orientation you would provide these new hires.

11. Which of the company's principles affect the organizing function of management? Explain how the one(s) you chose would affect how Starbucks' managers deal with (a) structural issues; (b) HRM issues; and (c) issues in managing teams. (Hint: The principles can be found on the company's Web site.)

Notes for the Continuing Case

Information from Starbucks Corporation 2013 Annual Report, www.investor.starbucks.com, May 2014; company Web site, www.starbucks.com; Based on Schultz, Howard and Gordon, Joanne, Onward: How Starbucks Fought for Its Life Without Losing Its Soul, © Howard Schultz (New York: Rodale Publishing, 2011); Reuters, M. Moskowitz, R. Levering, O. Akhtar, E. Fry, C. Leahey, and A. VanderMey, "The 100 Best Companies to Work For," Fortune, February 4, 2013, pp. 85+; "Chile Fines, Blacklists Starbucks, Wal-Mart Over Labor Practices," www.reuters.com, August 9, 2012; R. Ahmed, "Tata Setting Up Starbucks Coffee Roasting Facility," online.wsj.com, July 26, 2012; News Release, "Starbucks Spotlights Connection Between Record Performance, Shareholder Value and Company Values at Annual Meeting of Shareholders," news.starbucks.com, March 21, 2012; M. Moskowitz and R. E. Levering, "The 100 Best Companies To Work For," Fortune, February 6, 2012, pp. 117+; J. Jargon, "Baristas Put Pressure on Starbucks," Wall Street Journal, July 26, 2011, p. B3; "Starbucks Finds Ways to Speed Up," Training Online, August 11, 2009; M. Herbst, "Starbucks' Karma Problem," BusinessWeek, January 12, 2009, p. 26; "Fresh Cup of Training," Training Online, May 1, 2008; "Training 135,000 Employees In One Day—Starbucks Closes Store To Do It," www.thecareerrevolution.com, February 27, 2008; K. Maher and J. Adamy," Do Hot Coffee and 'Wobblies' Go Together?" Wall Street Journal, March 21, 2006, pp. B1+; A. Serwer, "Interview with Howard Schultz," Fortune (Europe), March 20, 2006, pp. 35–36; S. Gray, "Fill 'er Up—With Latte," Wall Street Journal, January 6, 2006, pp. A9+; W. Meyers, "Conscience in a Cup of Coffee," US News & World Report, October 31, 2005, pp. 48–50; J. M. Cohn, R. Khurana, and L. Reeves, "Growing Talent as if Your Business Depended on It," Harvard Business Review, October 2005, pp. 62–70; P. B. Nussbaum, R. Berner, and D. Brady, "Get Creative," BusinessWeek, August 1, 2005, pp. 60–68; S. Holmes, "A Bitter Aroma at Starbucks," BusinessWeek, June 6, 2005, p. 13; J. Cummings, "Legislative Grind," Wall Street Journal, April 12, 2005, pp. A1+; "Starbucks: The Next Generation," Fortune, April 4, 2005, p. 20; P. Kafka, "Bean Counter," Forbes, February 28, 2005, pp. 78–80; A. Lustgarten, "A Hot, Steaming Cup of Customer Awareness," Fortune, November 15, 2004, p. 192; and A. Serwer and K. Bonamici, "Hot Starbucks to Go," Fortune, January 26, 2004, pp. 60–74.

Understanding and Managing Individual Behavior

It's Your Career

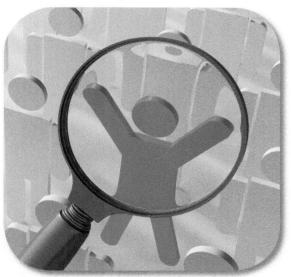

Source: Mooltfilm/Fotolia

A key to success in management and in your career is knowing who you are and how you interact with others.

Self Awareness: You Need to Know Yourself Before You Can Know Others

Do you know your real self? Many of us don't. We work hard to protect, maintain, and enhance our self-concept and the images others have of us. But if you want to maximize your potential, you need to know your weaknesses as well as your strengths. Knowledge of your strengths and weaknesses can help you gain insights into areas you want to change and improve. And it can help you better understand how others see you.

The following identifies five key elements of your personality. Understanding how you rate on these elements is critical to your self-awareness:

Introversion versus Extroversion. *Are you quiet and reserved? Are you shy in new situations? At work, do you prefer quiet for concentration, take care with details, think a lot before you act, and work contentedly alone? If so, you are probably best described as an introvert. In contrast, are you outgoing, sociable, and assertive? At work, do you prefer variety and action; dislike complicated procedures; and are you impatient with long, slow tasks? This characterizes extroverts.*

Thinking versus Feeling. *In making decisions, do you put the emphasis on reason and logic? If so, your preference is for thinking. If you make decisions by emphasizing human values, emotions, and your personal beliefs, then your focus is on feelings.*

Internal Control versus External Control. *Do you believe that you're the master of your own fate? Do you believe you control what happens to you? If so, you have an internal locus of control. If you believe that what happens to you is controlled by outside forces such as luck or chance, you have an external locus of control.*

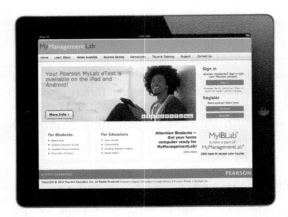

MyManagementLab®

⭐ **Improve Your Grade!**

When you see this icon, visit
www.mymanagementlab.com for activities that are
applied, personalized, and offer immediate feedback.

Learning Objectives

1 *Identify* the focus and goals of individual behavior within organizations.

2 *Explain* the role that attitudes play in job performance.

3 *Describe* different personality theories.

● **Know how** to be more self-aware.

4 *Describe* perception and factors that influence it.

5 *Discuss* learning theories and their relevance in shaping behavior.

● **Develop your skill** at shaping behavior.

6 *Discuss* contemporary issues in organizational behavior.

Organized versus Disorganized. Are you conscientious, responsible, dependable, and consistent? If so, then you'd be organized. Are you easily distracted, unreliable, and have difficulty meeting deadlines and commitments? If so, then you'd be classified as disorganized.

Open to Change versus Comfortable with the Familiar. Finally, do you tend to be creative, curious, and enjoy new experiences? You'd be open to change. If you're better described as someone who is conventional and uncomfortable with change, you'd be described as comfortable with the familiar.

There is no right *personality*. Each side of each dimension has both strengths and weaknesses.

The importance is knowing who you are and where you best fit.

Many of us don't have a good read on who we are. If that's you, here are three suggestions on what you can do to increase your self-awareness:

1. *Seek feedback.* Find individuals you trust and seek their honest feedback.

2. *Reflect.* Review your experiences, situations, and actions to better understand and learn from them.

3. *Keep a journal.* Keep a written, ongoing account that includes comments about personal events and interactions you have with others. Include descriptions of good and bad ways that you handled situations.

Most managers are concerned with the attitudes of their employees and want to attract and retain employees with the right attitudes and personalities. They want people who show up and work hard, get along with coworkers and customers, have good attitudes, and exhibit good work behaviors in other ways. But as you're probably already aware, people don't always behave like that "ideal" employee. They job

hop at the first opportunity or they may post critical comments in blogs. People differ in their behaviors, and even the same person can behave one way one day and a completely different way another day. For instance, haven't you seen family members, friends, or coworkers behave in ways that prompted you to wonder: Why did they do that? In this text, we're going to explore the different aspects of individual behavior so you can better understand "why they did that!"

FOCUS and Goals of Organizational Behavior

behavior
The actions of people

organizational behavior (OB)
The study of the actions of people at work

LO1 Managers need good people skills. The material in this text draws heavily on the field of study that's known as *organizational behavior (OB)*. Although it's concerned with the subject of **behavior**—that is, the actions of people—**organizational behavior** is the study of the actions of people at work.

One of the challenges in understanding organizational behavior is that it addresses issues that aren't obvious. Like an iceberg, OB has a small visible dimension and a much larger hidden portion. (See Exhibit 1.) What we see when we look at an organization is its visible aspects: strategies, goals, policies and procedures, structure, technology, formal authority relationships, and chain of command. But under the surface are other elements that managers need to understand—elements that also influence how employees behave at work. As we'll show, OB provides managers with considerable insights into these important, but hidden, aspects of the organization. For instance, Tony Levitan, founder and former CEO of EGreetings, found out the hard way about the power of behavioral elements. When he tried to "clean up" the company's online greeting-card site for a potential partnership with a large greeting card company, his employees rebelled. He soon realized that he shouldn't have unilaterally made such a major decision without getting input from his staff, and he reversed the move.[1]

Focus of Organizational Behavior

Organizational behavior focuses on three major areas. First, OB looks at *individual behavior*. Based predominantly on contributions from psychologists, this area includes such topics as attitudes, personality, perception, learning, and motivation. Second, OB is concerned with *group behavior*, which includes norms, roles, team building, leadership, and conflict. Our knowledge about groups comes basically from the work of sociologists and social psychologists. Finally, OB also looks at *organizational* aspects including structure, culture, and human resource policies and practices.

Exhibit 1
Organization as Iceberg

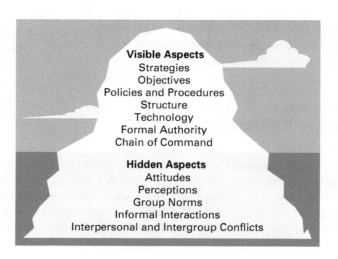

Visible Aspects
Strategies
Objectives
Policies and Procedures
Structure
Technology
Formal Authority
Chain of Command

Hidden Aspects
Attitudes
Perceptions
Group Norms
Informal Interactions
Interpersonal and Intergroup Conflicts

In this text, we'll look at individual behavior.

Goals of Organizational Behavior

The goals of OB are to *explain, predict,* and *influence* behavior. Managers need to be able to *explain* why employees engage in some behaviors rather than others, *predict* how employees will respond to various actions and decisions, and *influence* how employees behave.

What employee behaviors are we specifically concerned with explaining, predicting, and influencing? Six important ones have been identified: employee productivity, absenteeism, turnover, organizational citizenship behavior (OCB), job satisfaction, and workplace misbehavior. **Employee productivity** is a performance measure of both efficiency and effectiveness. Managers want to know what factors will influence the efficiency and effectiveness of employees. **Absenteeism** is the failure to show up for work. It's difficult for work to get done if employees don't show up. Studies have shown that unscheduled absences cost companies around $660 per employee per year and result in the highest net loss of productivity per day.[2] Although absenteeism can't be totally eliminated, excessive levels have a direct and immediate impact on the organization's functioning. **Turnover** is the voluntary and involuntary permanent withdrawal from an organization. It can be a problem because of increased recruiting, selection, and training costs and work disruptions. Just like absenteeism, managers can never eliminate turnover, but it is something they want to minimize, especially among high-performing employees. **Organizational citizenship behavior (OCB)** is discretionary behavior that's not part of an employee's formal job requirements but promotes the effective functioning of the organization.[3] Examples of good OCBs include helping others on one's work team, volunteering for extended job activities, avoiding unnecessary conflicts, and making constructive statements about one's work group and the organization. Organizations need individuals who will do more than their usual job duties, and the evidence indicates that organizations that have such employees outperform those that don't.[4] However, drawbacks of OCB occur when employees experience work overload, stress, and work–family life conflicts.[5] **Job satisfaction** refers to an employee's general attitude toward his or her job. Although job satisfaction is an attitude rather than a behavior, it's an outcome that concerns many managers because satisfied employees are more likely to show up for work, have higher levels of performance, and stay with an organization. **Workplace misbehavior** is any intentional employee behavior that is potentially harmful to the organization or individuals within the organization. Workplace misbehavior shows up in organizations in four ways: deviance, aggression, antisocial behavior, and violence.[6] Such behaviors can range from playing loud music just to irritate coworkers to verbal aggression to sabotaging work, all of which can create havoc in any organization. In the following sections, we'll address how an understanding of four psychological factors—employee attitudes, personality, perception, and learning—can help us predict and explain these employee behaviors.

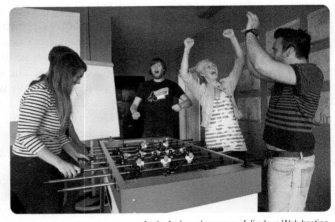

As the feel-good manager of Jimdo, a Web-hosting service in Hamburg, Germany, Magdalena Bethge (raised arms) is charged with creating a positive work environment that will increase employee satisfaction and productivity. She helps employees achieve a work-life balance and organizes ongoing employee feedback sessions, mentoring for new employees, and office get-togethers.
Source: Georg Wendt/Newscom

employee productivity
A performance measure of both efficiency and effectiveness

absenteeism
The failure to show up for work

turnover
The voluntary and involuntary permanent withdrawal from an organization

organizational citizenship behavior (OCB)
Discretionary behavior that is not part of an employee's formal job requirements, but which promotes the effective functioning of the organization

job satisfaction
An employee's general attitude toward his or her job

workplace misbehavior
Any intentional employee behavior that is potentially damaging to the organization or to individuals within the organization

ATTITUDES and Job Performance

L02   **Attitudes** are evaluative statements—favorable or unfavorable—concerning objects, people, or events. They reflect how an individual feels about something. When a person says, "I like my job," he or she is expressing an attitude about work.

An attitude is made up of three components: cognition, affect, and behavior.[7] The **cognitive component** of an attitude refers to the beliefs, opinions, knowledge, or

attitudes
Evaluative statements, either favorable or unfavorable, concerning objects, people, or events

cognitive component
That part of an attitude that's made up of the beliefs, opinions, knowledge, or information held by a person

affective component
That part of an attitude that's the emotional or feeling part

behavioral component
That part of an attitude that refers to an intention to behave in a certain way toward someone or something

information held by a person (for instance, the belief that "discrimination is wrong"). The **affective component** of an attitude is the emotional or feeling part of an attitude. Using our example, this component would be reflected by the statement, "I don't like Pat because he discriminates against minorities." Finally, affect can lead to behavioral outcomes. The **behavioral component** of an attitude refers to an intention to behave in a certain way toward someone or something. To continue our example, I might choose to avoid Pat because of my feelings about him. Understanding that attitudes are made up of three components helps show their complexity. But keep in mind that the term *attitude* usually refers only to the affective component.

Naturally, managers aren't interested in every attitude an employee has. They're especially interested in job-related attitudes. The three most widely known are job satisfaction, job involvement, and organizational commitment. Another concept that's generating widespread interest is employee engagement.[8]

Job Satisfaction

As we know from our earlier definition, job satisfaction refers to a person's general attitude toward his or her job. A person with a high level of job satisfaction has a positive attitude toward his or her job. A person who is dissatisfied has a negative attitude. When people speak of employee attitudes, they usually are referring to job satisfaction.

HOW SATISFIED ARE EMPLOYEES? Studies of U.S. workers over the past 30 years generally indicated that the majority of workers were satisfied with their jobs. A Conference Board study in 1995 found that some 60 percent of Americans were satisfied with their jobs.[9] However, since then the number has been declining. By 2010, that percentage was down to its lowest level, 42.6 percent, but rose slightly in 2011 to 47.2 percent and to 47.3 percent in 2012.[10] Although job satisfaction tends to increase as income increases, only 58 percent of individuals earning more than $50,000 are satisfied with their jobs. For individuals earning less than $15,000, about 45 percent of workers say they are satisfied with their jobs.[11] Even though it's possible that higher pay translates into higher job satisfaction, an alternative explanation for the difference in satisfaction levels is that higher pay reflects different types of jobs. Higher-paying jobs generally require more advanced skills, give jobholders greater responsibilities, are more stimulating and provide more challenges, and allow workers more control. It's more likely that the reports of higher satisfaction among higher-income levels reflect those factors rather than the pay itself. What about job satisfaction levels in other countries? A survey by Kelly Services, a staffing agency, found that 48 percent of global employees were unhappy in their current jobs.[12]

The global recession likely had an impact on global job satisfaction rates. For instance, a study by a British consulting group found that 67 percent of workers surveyed were putting in unpaid overtime. Also, 63 percent said their employers did not appreciate their extra effort, and 57 percent felt that employees were treated like dispensable commodities.[13]

SATISFACTION AND PRODUCTIVITY After the Hawthorne Studies, managers believed that happy workers were productive workers. Because it's not been easy to determine whether job satisfaction caused job productivity or vice versa, some management researchers felt that belief was generally wrong. However, we can say with some certainty that the correlation between satisfaction and productivity is fairly strong.[14] Also, organizations with more satisfied employees tend to be more effective than organizations with fewer satisfied employees.[15]

SATISFACTION AND ABSENTEEISM Although research shows that satisfied employees have lower levels of absenteeism than dissatisfied employees, the correlation isn't strong.[16] It certainly makes sense that dissatisfied employees are more likely to miss work, but other factors affect the relationship. For instance, organizations that

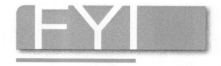

- 22 percent of employees say they've planned to come in to work late or leave work early when they knew their boss was going to be out.[17]

provide liberal sick leave benefits are encouraging all their employees—including those who are highly satisfied—to take "sick" days. Assuming your job has some variety in it, you can find work satisfying and yet still take a "sick" day to enjoy a three-day weekend or to golf on a warm spring day if taking such days results in no penalties.

SATISFACTION AND TURNOVER Research on the relationship between satisfaction and turnover is much stronger. Satisfied employees have lower levels of turnover, while dissatisfied employees have higher levels of turnover.[18] Yet, things such as labor-market conditions, expectations about alternative job opportunities, and length of employment with the organization also affect an employee's decision to leave.[19] Research suggests that the level of satisfaction is less important in predicting turnover for superior performers because the organization typically does everything it can to keep them—pay raises, praise, increased promotion opportunities, and so forth.[20]

JOB SATISFACTION AND CUSTOMER SATISFACTION Is job satisfaction related to positive customer outcomes? For frontline employees who have regular contact with customers, the answer is "yes." Satisfied employees increase customer satisfaction and loyalty.[21] Why? In service organizations, customer retention and defection are highly dependent on how frontline employees deal with customers. Satisfied employees are more likely to be friendly, upbeat, and responsive, which customers appreciate. And because satisfied employees are less likely to leave their jobs, customers are more likely to encounter familiar faces and receive experienced service. These qualities help build customer satisfaction and loyalty. However, the relationship also seems to work in reverse. Dissatisfied customers can increase an employee's job dissatisfaction. Employees who have regular contact with customers report that rude, thoughtless, or unreasonably demanding customers adversely affect their job satisfaction.[22]

A number of companies appear to understand this connection. Service-oriented businesses, such as L.L.Bean, Southwest Airlines, and Starbucks, obsess about pleasing their customers. They also focus on building employee satisfaction—recognizing that satisfied employees will go a long way toward contributing to their goal of having happy customers. These firms seek to hire upbeat and friendly employees, they train employees in customer service, they reward customer service, they provide positive work climates, and they regularly track employee satisfaction through attitude surveys. For instance, at shoe retailer Zappos (now part of Amazon.com), employees are encouraged to "create fun and a little weirdness" and have been given high levels of discretion to make customers satisfied. Zappos even offers a $2,000 bribe to employees to quit the company after training if they're not happy working there.[23]

JOB SATISFACTION AND OCB It seems logical to assume that job satisfaction should be a major determinant of an employee's OCB.[24] Satisfied employees would seem more likely to talk positively about the organization, help others, and go above and beyond normal job expectations. Research suggests a modest overall relationship between job satisfaction and OCB.[25] But that relationship is tempered by perceptions of fairness.[26] Basically, if you don't feel as though your supervisor, organizational procedures, or pay policies are fair, your job satisfaction is likely to suffer significantly. However, when you perceive that these things are fair, you have more trust in your employer and are more willing to voluntarily engage in behaviors that go beyond your formal job requirements. Another factor that influences individual OCB is the type of citizenship behavior a person's work group exhibits. In a work group with low group-level OCB, any individual in that group who engaged in OCB had higher job

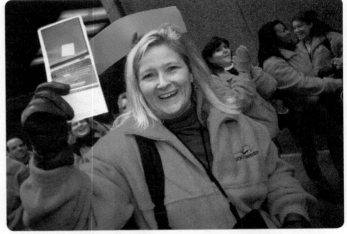

Southwest Airlines marketing employees shown here embody the friendly, fun-loving, upbeat, and helpful behavior that customers appreciate and value. The airline shapes a positive on-the-job attitude by giving employees extensive customer-service training and a supportive work environment and by empowering them to make on-the-spot decisions to satisfy customer needs.
Source: AP Photo/David Zalubowski

performance ratings. One possible explanation may be that the person was trying to find some way to "stand out" from the crowd.[27] No matter why it happens, the point is that OCB can have positive benefits for organizations.

JOB SATISFACTION AND WORKPLACE MISBEHAVIOR When employees are dissatisfied with their jobs, they'll respond somehow. The problem comes from the difficulty in predicting *how* they'll respond. One person might quit. Another might respond by using work time to play computer games. And another might verbally abuse a coworker. If managers want to control the undesirable consequences of job dissatisfaction, they'd be better off attacking the problem—job dissatisfaction—than trying to control the different employee responses. Three other job-related attitudes we need to look at include job involvement, organizational commitment, and employee engagement.

Job Involvement and Organizational Commitment

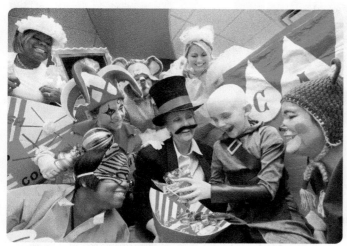

Employee engagement is high at St. Jude Children's Research Hospital, where employees share a deep commitment to the hospital's mission of "finding cures, saving children." Shown here delivering Halloween treats to patients, employees feel their contributions at work are meaningful and make a difference in the lives of young children.
Source: St. Jude Children's Research Hospital/ Associated Press

Job involvement is the degree to which an employee identifies with his or her job, actively participates in it, and considers his or her job performance to be important to his or her self-worth.[28] Employees with a high level of job involvement strongly identify with and really care about the kind of work they do. Their positive attitude leads them to contribute in positive ways to their work. High levels of job involvement have been found to be related to fewer absences, lower resignation rates, and higher employee engagement with their work.[29]

Organizational commitment is the degree to which an employee identifies with a particular organization and its goals and wishes to maintain membership in that organization.[30] Whereas job involvement is identifying with your job, organizational commitment is identifying with your employing organization. Research suggests that organizational commitment also leads to lower levels of both absenteeism and turnover and, in fact, is a better indicator of turnover than job satisfaction.[31] Why? Probably because it's a more global and enduring response to the organization than satisfaction with a particular job.[32] However, organizational commitment is less important as a work-related attitude than it once was. Employees don't generally stay with a single organization for most of their career and the relationship they have with their employer has changed considerably.[33] Although the commitment of *an employee to an organization* may not be as important as it once was, research about **perceived organizational support**—employees' general belief that their organization values their contribution and cares about their well-being— shows that the commitment of *the organization to the employee* can be beneficial. High levels of perceived organizational support lead to increased job satisfaction and lower turnover.[34]

job involvement
The degree to which an employee identifies with his or her job, actively participates in it, and considers his or her job performance to be important to self-worth

organizational commitment
The degree to which an employee identifies with a particular organization and its goals and wishes to maintain membership in that organization

perceived organizational support
Employees' general belief that their organization values their contribution and cares about their well-being

employee engagement
When employees are connected to, satisfied with, and enthusiastic about their jobs

Employee Engagement

A low-level trader employed by Société Générale, a giant French bank, loses billions of dollars through dishonest trades and no one reports suspicious behavior. An internal investigation uncovered evidence that many back-office employees failed to alert their supervisors about the suspicious trades.[35] Employee indifference can have serious consequences.

Managers want their employees to be connected to, satisfied with, and enthusiastic about their jobs. This concept is known as **employee engagement.**[36] Highly engaged employees are passionate about and deeply connected to their work. Disengaged employees have essentially "checked out" and don't care. They

show up for work, but have no energy or passion for it. A global study of more than 12,000 employees found the following factors as contributing to employee engagement: respect, type of work, work-life balance, providing good service to customers, base pay, people you work with, benefits, long-term career potential, learning and development opportunities, flexible work, promotion opportunities, and variable pay/bonuses.[37]

A number of benefits come from having highly engaged employees. First, highly engaged employees are two-and-a-half times more likely to be top performers than their less-engaged coworkers. In addition, companies with highly engaged employees have higher retention rates, which help keep recruiting and training costs low. And both of these outcomes—higher performance and lower costs—contribute to superior financial performance.[38]

Attitudes and Consistency

Have you ever noticed that people change what they say so it doesn't contradict what they do? Perhaps a friend of yours has repeatedly said that she thinks joining a sorority is an important part of college life. But then she goes through rush and doesn't get accepted. All of a sudden, she's saying that sorority life isn't all that great.

Research has generally concluded that people seek consistency among their attitudes *and* between their attitudes and behavior.[39] This tendency means that individuals try to reconcile differing attitudes and align their attitudes and behavior so they appear rational and consistent. When they encounter an inconsistency, individuals will do something to make it consistent by altering the attitudes, altering the behavior, or rationalizing the inconsistency.

For example, a campus recruiter for R&S Information Services who visits college campuses and sells students on the advantages of R&S as a good place to work would experience inconsistency if he personally believed that R&S had poor working conditions and few opportunities for promotion. This recruiter could, over time, find his attitudes toward R&S becoming more positive. He might actually convince himself by continually articulating the merits of working for the company. Another alternative is that the recruiter could become openly negative about R&S and the opportunities within the company for prospective applicants. The original enthusiasm the recruiter might have had would dwindle and might be replaced by outright cynicism toward the company. Finally, the recruiter might acknowledge that R&S is an undesirable place to work but, as a professional, realize that his obligation is to present the positive aspects of working for the company. He might further rationalize that no workplace is perfect and that his job is to present a favorable picture of the company, not to present both sides.

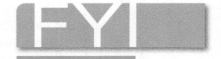

- 79 percent of employees say a sense of humor is important in the workplace.[40]

Cognitive Dissonance Theory

Can we assume from this consistency principle that an individual's behavior can always be predicted if we know his or her attitude on a subject? The answer isn't a simple "yes" or "no." Why? Cognitive dissonance theory.

Cognitive dissonance theory sought to explain the relationship between attitudes and behavior.[41] **Cognitive dissonance** is any incompatibility or inconsistency between attitudes or between behavior and attitudes. The theory argued that inconsistency is uncomfortable and that individuals will try to reduce the discomfort and, thus, the dissonance.

Of course, no one can avoid dissonance. You know you should floss your teeth every day but don't do it. There's an inconsistency between attitude and behavior. How do people cope with cognitive dissonance? The theory proposes that how hard we'll try to reduce dissonance is determined by three things: (1) the *importance* of the factors creating the dissonance, (2) the degree of *influence* the individual believes he or she has over those factors, and (3) the *rewards* that may be involved in dissonance.

cognitive dissonance
Any incompatibility or inconsistency between attitudes or between behavior and attitudes

If the factors creating the dissonance are relatively unimportant, the pressure to correct the inconsistency will be low. However, if those factors are important, individuals may change their behavior, conclude that the dissonant behavior isn't so important, change their attitude, or identify compatible factors that outweigh the dissonant ones.

How much influence individuals believe they have over the factors also affects their reaction to the dissonance. If they perceive the dissonance is something about which they have no choice, they won't be receptive to attitude change or feel a need to be. If, for example, the dissonance-producing behavior was required as a result of a manager's order, the pressure to reduce dissonance would be less than if the behavior had been performed voluntarily. Although dissonance exists, it can be rationalized and justified by the need to follow the manager's orders—that is, the person had no choice or control.

Finally, rewards also influence the degree to which individuals are motivated to reduce dissonance. Coupling high dissonance with high rewards tends to reduce the discomfort by motivating the individual to believe that consistency exists.

Attitude Surveys

attitude surveys
Surveys that elicit responses from employees through questions about how they feel about their jobs, work groups, supervisors, or the organization

Many organizations regularly survey their employees about their attitudes.[42] Exhibit 2 shows an example of an actual attitude survey. Typically, **attitude surveys** present the employee with a set of statements or questions eliciting how they feel about their jobs, work groups, supervisors, or the organization. Ideally, the items will be designed to obtain the specific information that managers desire. An attitude score is achieved by summing up responses to individual questionnaire items. These scores can then be averaged for work groups, departments, divisions, or the organization as a whole. For instance, the Tennessee Valley Authority, the largest U.S. government-run energy company, came up with a "Cultural Health Index" to measure employee attitudes. The organization found business units that scored high on the attitude surveys also were the ones whose performance was high. For poorly performing business units, early signs of potential trouble had shown up in the attitude surveys.[43]

Regularly surveying employee attitudes provides managers with valuable feedback on how employees perceive their working conditions. Policies and practices that managers view as objective and fair may not be seen that way by employees. The use of regular attitude surveys can alert managers to potential problems and employees' intentions early so that action can be taken to prevent repercussions.[44]

Source: Munshi Ahmed/Bloomberg via Getty Images

LEADER making a DIFFERENCE

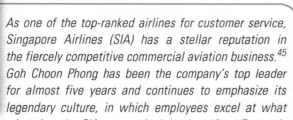

As one of the top-ranked airlines for customer service, Singapore Airlines (SIA) has a stellar reputation in the fiercely competitive commercial aviation business.[45] Goh Choon Phong has been the company's top leader for almost five years and continues to emphasize its legendary culture, in which employees excel at what they do and enjoy what they do. SIA was ranked number 18 on Fortune's The World's Most Admired Companies List in 2014. Passengers appreciate the outstanding customer service provided by the airline's satisfied frontline employees, who have earned a reputation as friendly, upbeat, and responsive. In recruiting flight attendants, the company carefully selects people who are warm, hospitable, and happy to serve others. All employees—from bottom to top—are proud to be part of the SIA family, and over two-thirds of them approve of the CEO. What can you learn from this leader making a difference?

Exhibit 2
Sample Employee Attitude Survey

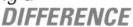

Here are some sample statements from an employee attitude survey:

- I have ample opportunities to use my skills/abilities in my job.
- My manager has a good relationship with my work group.
- My organization provides me professional development opportunities.
- I am told if I'm doing good work or not.
- I feel safe in my work environment.
- My organization is a great place to work.

Implications for Managers

Managers should be interested in their employees' attitudes because they influence behavior. Satisfied and committed employees, for instance, have lower rates of turnover and absenteeism. If managers want to keep resignations and absences down—especially among their more productive employees—they'll want to do things that generate positive job attitudes.

Satisfied employees also perform better on the job. So managers should focus on those factors that have been shown to be conducive to high levels of employee job satisfaction: making work challenging and interesting, providing equitable rewards, creating supportive working conditions, and encouraging supportive colleagues.[46] These factors are likely to help employees be more productive.

Managers should also survey employees about their attitudes. As one study put it, "A sound measurement of overall job attitude is one of the most useful pieces of information an organization can have about its employees."[47]

Finally, managers should know that employees will try to reduce dissonance. If employees are required to do things that appear inconsistent to them or that are at odds with their attitudes, managers should remember that pressure to reduce the dissonance is not as strong when the employee perceives that the dissonance is externally imposed and uncontrollable. It's also decreased if rewards are significant enough to offset the dissonance. So the manager might point to external forces such as competitors, customers, or other factors when explaining the need to perform some work that the individual may have some dissonance about. Or the manager can provide rewards that an individual desires.

PERSONALITY

LO3   "Let's face it, dating is a drag. There was a time when we thought the computer was going to make it all better....But most of us learned the hard way that finding someone who shares our love of film noir and obscure garage bands does not a perfect match make."[48] Using in-depth personality assessment and profiling, Chemistry.com has tried to do something about making the whole dating process better.

Personality. We all have one. Some of us are quiet and passive; others are loud and aggressive. When we describe people using terms such as *quiet, passive, loud, aggressive, ambitious, extroverted, loyal, tense,* or *sociable,* we're describing their personalities. An individual's **personality** is a unique combination of emotional, thought, and behavioral patterns that affect how a person reacts to situations and interacts with others. It's our natural way of doing things and relating to others. Personality is most often described in terms of measurable traits a person exhibits. We're interested in looking at personality because, just like attitudes, it too affects how and why people behave the way they do.

Over the years, researchers have attempted to identify those traits that best describe personality. The two most well-known approaches are the Myers Briggs Type Indicator® (MBTI) and the Big Five Model.

personality
The unique combination of emotional, thought, and behavioral patterns that affect how a person reacts to situations and interacts with others

MBTI®

One popular approach to classifying personality traits is the personality-assessment instrument known as the MBTI®. This 100-question assessment asks people how they usually act or feel in different situations.[49] On the basis of their answers, individuals are classified as exhibiting a preference in four categories: extraversion or introversion (E or I), sensing or intuition (S or N), thinking or feeling (T or F), and judging or perceiving (J or P). These terms are defined as follows:

- *Extraversion (E) versus Introversion (I).* Individuals showing a preference for extraversion are outgoing, social, and assertive. They need a work environment that's varied and action oriented, that lets them be with others, and that gives them

a variety of experiences. Individuals showing a preference for introversion are quiet and shy. They focus on understanding and prefer a work environment that is quiet and concentrated, that lets them be alone, and that gives them a chance to explore in depth a limited set of experiences.

- *Sensing (S) versus Intuition (N).* Sensing types are practical and prefer routine and order. They dislike new problems unless there are standard ways to solve them, have a high need for closure, show patience with routine details, and tend to be good at precise work. On the other hand, intuition types rely on unconscious processes and look at the "big picture." They're individuals who like solving new problems, dislike doing the same thing over and over again, jump to conclusions, are impatient with routine details, and dislike taking time for precision.

- *Thinking (T) versus Feeling (F).* Thinking types use reason and logic to handle problems. They're unemotional and uninterested in people's feelings, like analysis and putting things into logical order, are able to reprimand people and fire them when necessary, may seem hard-hearted, and tend to relate well only to other thinking types. Feeling types rely on their personal values and emotions. They're aware of other people and their feelings, like harmony, need occasional praise, dislike telling people unpleasant things, tend to be sympathetic, and relate well to most people.

- *Judging (J) versus Perceiving (P).* Judging types want control and prefer their world to be ordered and structured. They're good planners, decisive, purposeful, and exacting. They focus on completing a task, make decisions quickly, and want only the information necessary to get a task done. Perceiving types are flexible and spontaneous. They're curious, adaptable, and tolerant. They focus on starting a task, postpone decisions, and want to find out all about the task before starting it.

Combining these preferences provides descriptions of 16 personality types, with every person identified with one of the items in each of the four pairs. Exhibit 3 summarizes two of them. As you can see from these descriptions, each personality type would approach work and relationships differently—neither one better than the other, just different.

More than 2 million people a year take the MBTI® in the United States alone. Some organizations that have used the MBTI® include Apple, AT&T, GE, 3M, hospitals, educational institutions, and even the U.S. Armed Forces. No hard evidence shows that the MBTI® is a valid measure of personality, but that doesn't seem to deter its widespread use.

How could the MBTI® help managers? Proponents believe it's important to know these personality types because they influence the way people interact and solve problems. For instance, if your boss is an intuition type and you're a sensing type, you'll gather information in different ways. An intuitive type prefers gut reactions, whereas a sensor prefers facts. To work well with your boss, you would have to present

Exhibit 3

Examples of MBTI®
Personality Types

Type	Description
I–S–F–P (introversion, sensing, feeling, perceiving)	Sensitive, kind, modest, shy, and quietly friendly. Such people strongly dislike disagreements and will avoid them. They are loyal followers and quite often are relaxed about getting things done.
E–N–T–J (extraversion, intuition, thinking, judging)	Warm, friendly, candid, and decisive; also skilled in anything that requires reasoning and intelligent talk, but may sometimes overestimate what they are capable of doing.

Source: Based on I. Briggs-Myers, *Introduction to Type* (Palo Alto, CA: Consulting Psychologists Press, 1980), pp. 7–8.

more than just facts about a situation and bring out how you feel about it. Also, the MBTI® has been used to help managers better match employees to certain types of jobs.

The Big Five Model

In recent years, research has shown that five basic personality dimensions underlie all others and encompass most of the significant variation in human personality.[50] The five personality traits in the **Big Five Model** are:

1. *Extraversion:* The degree to which someone is sociable, talkative, assertive, and comfortable in relationships with others.
2. *Agreeableness:* The degree to which someone is good-natured, cooperative, and trusting.
3. *Conscientiousness:* The degree to which someone is reliable, responsible, dependable, persistent, and achievement oriented.
4. *Emotional stability:* The degree to which someone is calm, enthusiastic, and secure (positive) or tense, nervous, depressed, and insecure (negative).
5. *Openness to experience:* The degree to which someone has a wide range of interests and is imaginative, fascinated with novelty, artistically sensitive, and intellectual.

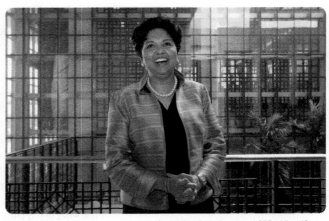

Indra Nooyi, board chairman and CEO of PepsiCo, scores high on all of the personality dimensions of the Big Five Model. She is sociable, agreeable, conscientious, emotionally stable, and open to experiences. These personality traits have contributed to her career success and high job performance in leading PepsiCo to achieve record financial results.
Source: Dario Pignatelli/Bloomberg/Getty Images

The Big Five Model provides more than just a personality framework. Research has shown that important relationships exist between these personality dimensions and job performance. For example, one study examined five categories of occupations: *professionals* (such as engineers, architects, and attorneys), *police, managers, salespeople,* and *semiskilled and skilled employees.*[51] The results showed that conscientiousness predicted job performance for all five occupational groups. Predictions for the other personality dimensions depended on the situation and on the occupational group. For example, extraversion predicted performance in managerial and sales positions—occupations in which high social interaction is necessary. Openness to experience was found to be important in predicting training competency. Ironically, emotional security wasn't positively related to job performance in any of the occupations. Another study that looked at whether the five-factor model could predict managerial performance found it could if 360-degree performance ratings (that is, performance ratings from supervisors, peers, and subordinates) were used.[52] Other studies have shown that employees who score higher in conscientiousness develop higher levels of job knowledge, probably because highly conscientious people learn more. In fact, a review of 138 studies revealed that conscientiousness was rather strongly related to GPA.[53]

Big Five Model
Personality trait model that includes extraversion, agreeableness, conscientiousness, emotional stability, and openness to experience

Additional Personality Insights

Although the traits in the Big Five are highly relevant to understanding behavior, they aren't the only personality traits that can describe someone's personality. Five other personality traits are powerful predictors of behavior in organizations.

1. *Locus of Control.* Some people believe they control their own fate. Others see themselves as pawns, believing that what happens to them in their lives is due to luck or chance. The **locus of control** in the first case is *internal*; these people believe they control their own destiny. The locus of control in the second case is *external*; these people believe their lives are controlled by outside forces.[54] Research indicates that employees who are externals are less satisfied with their jobs, more alienated from the work setting, and less involved in their jobs than those who rate high on internality.[55] A manager might also expect externals to blame a poor performance evaluation on their boss's prejudice, their coworkers, or other events outside their control; internals would explain the same evaluation in terms of their own actions.

locus of control
A personality attribute that measures the degree to which people believe they control their own fate

Machiavellianism
A measure of the degree to which people are pragmatic, maintain emotional distance, and believe that ends justify means

self-esteem
An individual's degree of like or dislike for himself or herself

self-monitoring
A personality trait that measures the ability to adjust behavior to external situational factors

2. *Machiavellianism.* The second characteristic is called **Machiavellianism** (Mach), named after Niccolo Machiavelli, who wrote in the sixteenth century on how to gain and manipulate power. An individual high in Machiavellianism is pragmatic, maintains emotional distance, and believes that ends can justify means.[56] "If it works, use it" is consistent with a high Mach perspective. Do high Machs make good employees? That depends on the type of job and whether you consider ethical factors in evaluating performance. In jobs that require bargaining skills (such as a purchasing manager) or that have substantial rewards for excelling (such as a salesperson working on commission), high Machs are productive.

3. *Self-Esteem.* People differ in the degree to which they like or dislike themselves, a trait called **self-esteem.**[57] Research on self-esteem (SE) offers some interesting behavioral insights. For example, self-esteem is directly related to expectations for success. High SEs believe they possess the ability they need to succeed at work. Individuals with high SEs will take more risks in job selection and are more likely to choose unconventional jobs than people with low SEs.

   The most common finding on self-esteem is that low SEs are more susceptible to external influence than high SEs. Low SEs are dependent on receiving positive evaluations from others. As a result, they're more likely to seek approval from others and are more prone to conform to the beliefs and behaviors of those they respect than high SEs. In managerial positions, low SEs will tend to be concerned with pleasing others and, therefore, will be less likely to take unpopular stands than high SEs. Finally, self-esteem has also been found to be related to job satisfaction. A number of studies confirm that high SEs are more satisfied with their jobs than low SEs.

4. *Self-Monitoring.* Have you ever had the experience of meeting someone new and feeling a natural connection and hitting it off right away? At some time or another, we've all had that experience. That natural ability to "click" with other people may play a significant role in determining career success[58] and is another personality trait called **self-monitoring,** which refers to the ability to adjust behavior to external, situational factors.[59] Individuals high in self-monitoring show considerable adaptability in adjusting their behavior. They're highly sensitive to external cues and can behave differently in different situations. High self-monitors are capable of presenting striking contradictions between their public persona and their private selves. Low self-monitors can't adjust their behavior. They tend to display their true dispositions and attitudes in every situation, and there's high behavioral consistency between who they are and what they do.

   Research on self-monitoring suggests that high self-monitors pay closer attention to the behavior of others and are more flexible than low self-monitors.[60] In addition, high self-monitoring managers tend to be more mobile in their careers, receive more promotions (both internal and cross-organizational), and are more likely to occupy central positions in an organization.[61] The high self-monitor is capable of putting on different "faces" for different audiences, an important trait for managers who must play multiple, or even contradicting, roles.

5. *Risk-Taking.* People differ in their willingness to take chances. Differences in the propensity to assume or to avoid risk have been shown to affect how long it takes managers to make a decision and how much information they require before making their choice. For instance, in one study where managers worked on simulated exercises that required them to make hiring decisions, high risk-taking managers took less time to make decisions and used less information in making their choices than low risk-taking managers.[62] Interestingly, the decision accuracy was the same for the two groups. To maximize organizational effectiveness, managers should try to align employee risk-taking propensity with specific job demands.

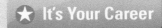

OTHER PERSONALITY TRAITS   A couple of other personality traits deserve mention. The Type A personality describes someone who is continually and aggressively struggling to achieve more and more in less and less time.[63] In the North American culture, the Type A personality is highly valued. Type A individuals subject themselves to continual time pressure and deadlines and have moderate to high levels of stress. They emphasize quantity over quality. On the other hand, a Type B person isn't harried by the desire to achieve more and more. Type Bs don't suffer from a sense of time urgency and are able to relax without guilt.

Another interesting trait that's been studied extensively is the **proactive personality,** which describes people who identify opportunities, show initiative, take action, and persevere until meaningful change occurs. Not surprisingly, research has shown that proactives have many desirable behaviors that organizations want.[64] For instance, they are more likely to be seen as leaders and more likely to act as change agents in organizations; they're more likely to challenge the status quo; they have entrepreneurial abilities; and they're more likely to achieve career success.

Finally, the economic recession prompted a reexamination of **resilience,** an individual's ability to overcome challenges and turn them into opportunities.[65] A study by a global consulting firm showed that it is a key factor in keeping a job: A resilient person is likely to be more adaptable, flexible, and goal-focused. OB researchers also have looked at resilience and other individual characteristics including efficacy, hope, and optimism in a concept called positive psychological capital.[66] These characteristics have been found to be related to higher feelings of well-being and less work stress, which ultimately affect how and why people behave the way they do at work.

proactive personality
A personality trait that describes individuals who are more prone to take actions to influence their environments

resilience
An individual's ability to overcome challenges and turn them into opportunities

Personality Types in Different Cultures

Do personality frameworks, like the Big Five Model, transfer across cultures? Are dimensions like locus of control relevant in all cultures? Let's try to answer these questions.

The five personality factors studied in the Big Five Model appear in almost all cross-cultural studies.[67] These studies include a wide variety of diverse cultures such as China, Israel, Germany, Japan, Spain, Nigeria, Norway, Pakistan, and the United States. Differences are found in the emphasis on dimensions. The Chinese, for example, use the category of conscientiousness more often and use the category of agreeableness less often than do Americans. But a surprisingly high amount of agreement is found, especially among individuals from developed countries. As a case in point, a comprehensive review of studies covering people from the European Community found that conscientiousness was a valid predictor of performance across jobs and occupational groups.[68] Studies in the United States found the same thing.

We know that no personality type is common for a given country. You can, for instance, find high risk takers and low risk takers in almost any culture. Yet a country's culture influences the *dominant* personality characteristics of its people. We can see this effect of national culture by looking at one of the personality traits we just discussed: locus of control.

National cultures differ in terms of the degree to which people believe they control their environment. For instance, North Americans believe they can dominate

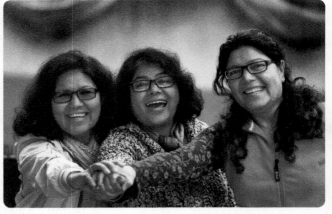

Sisters Lucky, Dicky, and Nicky Chhetri exhibited the personality dimension of conscientiousness in starting 3 Sisters Adventure Trekking Company in Nepal. Persistence and a high achievement drive helped them not only to break into a male-dominated industry but to grow their business by training other women to become guides. Today they run a booming business, with 150 female guides leading some 1,000 trekkers a year.
Source: Niranjan Shrestha/AP Images

let's get REAL

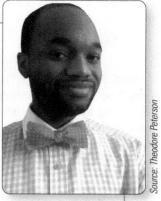

Source: Theodore Peterson

Theodore Peterson
Lead Mentor/
Behavioral Assistant

The Scenario:

"Why can't we all just get along?" wondered Bonnie, as she sat in her office. Today, she had already dealt with an employee who came in nearly every day with a complaint about something another coworker had said or done. Then, on top of that, Bonnie had to soothe over the hurt feelings of another employee who had overheard a conversation in the break room. She thought to herself, "I love being a manager, but there are days when the emotional tension in this place is too much."

What would you tell Bonnie about emotions in the workplace and how to deal with them?

I would tell Bonnie that emotions in the work place are always going to be present and are beyond her control. People will be people. However, don't let the emotions in the work place affect your mood. Unfortunately as a manager, sometimes you have to smile even when you don't feel like doing so. I would recommend Bonnie to find a self-care activity that she can do outside of work, or to take a few minutes during the work day to close the door in her office to take a few deep breaths; or to take a vacation if she has any time available. We all can feel overwhelmed but it's all in how one deals with it that really matters.

their environment; other societies, such as those in Middle Eastern countries, believe life is essentially predetermined. Notice how closely this distinction parallels the concept of internal and external locus of control. On the basis of this particular cultural characteristic, we should expect a larger proportion of internals in the U.S. and Canadian workforces than in the workforces of Saudi Arabia or Iran.

As we have seen throughout this section, personality traits influence employees' behavior. For global managers, understanding how personality traits differ takes on added significance when looking at it from the perspective of national culture.

Emotions and Emotional Intelligence

"Trying to sell wedding gowns to anxious brides-to-be" can be quite a stressful experience for the salesperson, needless to say. To help its employees stay "cheery," David's Bridal, a chain of more than 270 stores, relied on research into joyful emotions. Now, when "faced with an indecisive bride," salespeople have been taught emotional coping techniques and know how to focus on "things that bring them joy."[69]

We can't leave the topic of personality without looking at the important behavioral aspect of emotions. Employees rarely check their feelings at the door to the workplace, nor are they unaffected by things that happen throughout the workday.[70] How we respond emotionally and how we deal with our emotions are typically functions of our personality. **Emotions** are intense feelings directed at someone or something. They're object-specific; that is, emotions are reactions to an object.[71] For instance, when a work colleague criticizes you for the way you spoke to a client, you might become angry at him. That is, you show emotion (anger) toward a specific object (your colleague). Because employees bring an emotional component with them to work every day, managers need to understand the role that emotions play in employee behavior.[72]

emotions
Intense feelings that are directed at someone or something

FUTURE VISION | Increased Reliance on Emotional Intelligence

Whether it goes by the name of emotional intelligence, social intelligence, or something else, the ability to understand yourself and others will be a skill that organizations will seek when hiring employees. In fact, in a survey of critical skills for the workforce in 2020, social intelligence ranked second on a list of the most critical skills.[73] (FYI: the number one skill was sense-making, that is, being able to determine the deeper meaning or significance of what's being expressed.) The ability to get along with others—coworkers, colleagues, team members, bosses, and customers—will be critical to success in most jobs. While more employees are likely to work off-site, there will still be ongoing contact with others. Those employees who have strong technical skills but are weak on emotional intelligence will find it increasingly difficult to find and hold a job.

If your professor has chosen to assign this, go to **www.mymanagementlab.com** *to discuss the following questions.*

⭐ **TALK ABOUT IT 1:** Why do you think the ability to get along with others is so critical?

⭐ **TALK ABOUT IT 2:** How can you develop this ability?

How many emotions are there? Although you could probably name several dozen, research has identified six universal emotions: anger, fear, sadness, happiness, disgust, and surprise.[74] Do these emotions surface in the workplace? Absolutely! I get *angry* after receiving a poor performance appraisal. I *fear* that I could be laid off as a result of a company cutback. I'm *sad* about one of my coworkers leaving to take a new job in another city. I'm *happy* after being selected as employee of the month. I'm *disgusted* with the way my supervisor treats women on our team. And I'm *surprised* to find out that management plans a complete restructuring of the company's retirement program.

People respond differently to identical emotion-provoking stimuli. In some cases, differences can be attributed to a person's personality and because people vary in their ability to express emotions. For instance, you undoubtedly know people who almost never show their feelings. They rarely get angry or show rage. In contrast, you probably also know people who seem to be on an emotional roller coaster. When they're happy, they're ecstatic. When they're sad, they're deeply depressed. And two people can be in the exact same situation—one showing excitement and joy, the other remaining calm.

However, at other times how people respond emotionally is a result of job requirements. Jobs make different demands in terms of what types and how much emotion needs to be displayed. For instance, air traffic controllers, ER nurses, and trial judges are expected to be calm and controlled, even in stressful situations. On the other hand, public-address announcers at sporting events and lawyers in a courtroom must be able to alter their emotional intensity as the need arises.

One area of emotions research with interesting insights into personality is **emotional intelligence (EI),** the ability to notice and to manage emotional cues and information.[76] It's composed of five dimensions:

Self-awareness: The ability to be aware of what you're feeling.

Self-management: The ability to manage one's own emotions and impulses.

Self-motivation: The ability to persist in the face of setbacks and failures.

Empathy: The ability to sense how others are feeling.

Social skills: The ability to handle the emotions of others.

EI has been shown to be positively related to job performance at all levels. For instance, one study looked at the characteristics of Lucent Technologies' engineers who were rated as stars by their peers. The researchers concluded that stars were

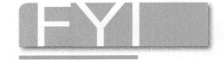

- 49 percent of individuals say they do okay with angry people but that it takes a lot of work on their part.[75]

emotional intelligence (EI)
The ability to notice and to manage emotional cues and information

better at relating to others. That is, it was EI, not academic intelligence, that characterized high performers. A study of Air Force recruiters generated similar findings. Top-performing recruiters exhibited high levels of EI. Despite these findings, EI has been a controversial topic in OB.[77] Supporters say EI has intuitive appeal and predicts important behavior.[78] Critics say that EI is vague, can't be measured, and has questionable validity.[79] One thing we can conclude is that EI appears to be relevant to success in jobs that demand a high degree of social interaction.

Implications for Managers

More than 62 percent of companies are using personality tests when recruiting and hiring.[80] Perhaps the major value in understanding personality differences lies in this area. Managers are likely to have higher-performing and more satisfied employees if consideration is given to matching personalities with jobs. The best-documented personality-job fit theory was developed by psychologist John Holland, who identified six basic personality types.[81] His theory states that an employee's satisfaction with his or her job, as well as his or her likelihood of leaving that job, depends on the degree to which the individual's personality matches the job environment. Exhibit 4 describes the six types, their personality characteristics, and examples of suitable occupations for each.

Holland's theory proposes that satisfaction is highest and turnover lowest when personality and occupation are compatible. Social individuals should be in "people" type jobs, and so forth. The key points of this theory are that (1) intrinsic differences in personality are apparent among individuals; (2) the types of jobs vary; and (3) people in job environments compatible with their personality types should be more satisfied and less likely to resign voluntarily than people in incongruent jobs.

Exhibit 4

Holland's Personality–Job Fit

Source: Based on J. L. Holland, *Making Vocational Choices: A Theory of Vocational Personalities and Work Environments* (Odessa, FL: Psychological Assessment Resources, 1997).

TYPE	PERSONALITY CHARACTERISTICS	SAMPLE OCCUPATIONS
Realistic. Prefers physical activities that require skill, strength, and coordination	Shy, genuine, persistent, stable, conforming, practical	Mechanic, drill press operator, assembly-line worker, farmer
Investigative. Prefers activities involving thinking, organizing, and understanding	Analytical, original, curious, independent	Biologist, economist, mathematician, news reporter
Social. Prefers activities that involve helping and developing others	Sociable, friendly, cooperative, understanding	Social worker, teacher, counselor, clinical psychologist
Conventional. Prefers rule-regulated, orderly, and unambiguous activities	Conforming, efficient, practical, unimaginative, inflexible	Accountant, corporate manager, bank teller, file clerk
Enterprising. Prefers verbal activities that offer opportunities to influence others and attain power	Self-confident, ambitious, energetic, domineering	Lawyer, real estate agent, public relations specialist, small business manager
Artistic. Prefers ambiguous and unsystematic activities that allow creative expression	Imaginative, disorderly, idealistic, emotional, impractical	Painter, musician, writer, interior decorator

In addition, other benefits arise from understanding personality. By recognizing that people approach problem solving, decision making, and job interactions differently, a manager can better understand why an employee is uncomfortable with making quick decisions or why another employee insists on gathering as much information as possible before addressing a problem. Or, for instance, managers can expect that individuals with an external locus of control may be less satisfied with their jobs than internals and that they may be less willing to accept responsibility for their actions.

Finally, being a successful manager and accomplishing goals means working well together with others both inside and outside the organization. In order to work effectively together, you need to understand each other. This understanding comes, at least in part, from an appreciation of personality traits and emotions. Also, one of the skills you have to develop as a manager is learning to fine-tune your emotional reactions according to the situation. In other words, you have to learn to recognize when "you have to smile and when you have to bark."[82]

If your professor has assigned this, go to **www.mymanagementlab.com** to watch a video titled: *CH2MHill: Ability and Personality* and to respond to questions.

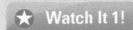

If your professor has assigned this, go to **www.mymanagementlab.com** to watch a video titled: *Rudi's Bakery: Ability and Personality* and to respond to questions.

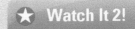

PERCEPTION

LO4 Maybe you've seen this in a Facebook post or on some other online source: AOCRNDICG TO RSCHEEARCH AT CMABRIGDE UINERVTISY, IT DSENO'T MTAETR WAHT OERDR THE LTTERES IN A WROD ARE, THE OLNY IPROAMTNT TIHNG IS TAHT THE FRSIT AND LSAT LTTEER BE IN THE RGHIT PCLAE. TIHS IS BCUSEAE THE HUAMN MNID DEOS NOT RAED ERVEY LTETER BY ISTLEF, BUT THE WROD AS A WLOHE. IF YOU CAN RAED...TIHS, PSOT IT TO YUOR WLAL. OLNY 55% OF PLEPOE CAN.[83] How'd you do in trying to read this? If you were able to make sense out of this jumbled message, that's the perceptual process at work. **Perception** is a process by which we give meaning to our environment by organizing and interpreting sensory impressions. Research on perception consistently demonstrates that individuals may look at the same thing yet perceive it differently. One manager, for instance, can interpret the fact that her assistant regularly takes several days to make important decisions as evidence that the assistant is slow, disorganized, and afraid to make decisions. Another manager with the same assistant might interpret the same tendency as evidence that the assistant is thoughtful, thorough, and deliberate. The first manager would probably evaluate her assistant negatively; the second manager would probably evaluate the person positively. The point is that none of us sees reality. We interpret what we see and call it reality. And, of course, as the example shows, we behave according to our perceptions.

perception
A process by which we give meaning to our environment by organizing and interpreting sensory impressions

Factors That Influence Perception

How do we explain the fact that people can perceive the same thing differently? A number of factors act to shape and sometimes distort perception. These factors are in the *perceiver*, in the *target* being perceived, or in the *situation* in which the perception occurs.

Exhibit 5
What Do You See?

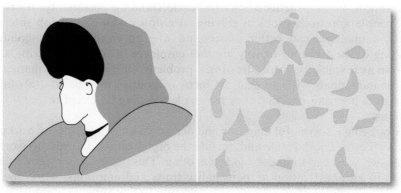

Old woman or young woman?   A knight on a horse?

When a person looks at a target and attempts to interpret what he or she sees, the individual's personal characteristics will heavily influence the interpretation. These personal characteristics include attitudes, personality, motives, interests, experiences, or expectations.

The characteristics of the target being observed can also affect what's perceived. Loud people are more likely than quiet people to be noticed in a group, as are extremely attractive or unattractive individuals. The relationship of a target to its background also influences perception, as does our tendency to group close things and similar things together. You can experience these tendencies by looking at the visual perception examples shown in Exhibit 5. Notice how what you see changes as you look differently at each one.

Finally, the context in which we see objects or events is also important. The time at which an object or event is seen can influence perception, as can location, light, heat, color, and any number of other situational factors.

Attribution Theory

Much of the research on perception is directed at inanimate objects. Managers, however, are concerned with people. Our perceptions of people differ from our perception of inanimate objects because we make inferences about the behaviors of people that we don't make about objects. Objects don't have beliefs, motives, or intentions; people do. The result is that when we observe an individual's behavior, we try to develop explanations of why they behave in certain ways. Our perception and judgment of a person's actions are significantly influenced by the assumptions we make about the person.

Attribution theory was developed to explain how we judge people differently depending on what meaning we attribute to a given behavior.[84] Basically, the theory suggests that when we observe an individual's behavior, we attempt to determine whether it was internally or externally caused. Internally caused behaviors are those believed to be under the personal control of the individual. Externally caused behavior results from outside factors; that is, the person is forced into the behavior by the situation. That determination, however, depends on three factors: distinctiveness, consensus, and consistency.

Distinctiveness refers to whether an individual displays different behaviors in different situations. Is the employee who arrived late today the same person who some employees complain of as being a "goof-off"? What we want to know is whether this behavior is unusual. If it's unusual, the observer is likely to attribute the behavior to external forces, something beyond the control of the person. However, if the behavior isn't unusual, it will probably be judged as internal.

If everyone who's faced with a similar situation responds in the same way, we can say the behavior shows *consensus*. A tardy employee's behavior would meet this criterion if all employees who took the same route to work were also late. From an attribution perspective, if consensus is high, you're likely to give an external attribution to the employee's tardiness; that is, some outside factor—maybe road construction

attribution theory
A theory used to explain how we judge people differently depending on what meaning we attribute to a given behavior

Exhibit 6
Attribution Theory

OBSERVATION	INTERPRETATION	ATTRIBUTION OF CAUSE
Does person behave this way in other situations?	**YES:** Low distinctiveness **NO:** High distinctiveness	Internal attribution External attribution
Do other people behave the same way in similar situations?	**YES:** High consensus **NO:** Low consensus	External attribution Internal attribution
Does person behave this way consistently?	**YES:** High consistency **NO:** Low consistency	Internal attribution External attribution

fundamental attribution error
The tendency to underestimate the influence of external factors and overestimate the influence of internal factors when making judgments about the behavior of others

self-serving bias
The tendency for individuals to attribute their own successes to internal factors while putting the blame for failures on external factors

or a traffic accident—caused the behavior. However, if other employees who come the same way to work made it on time, you would conclude that the cause of the late behavior was internal.

Finally, an observer looks for *consistency* in a person's actions. Does the person engage in the behaviors regularly and consistently? Does the person respond the same way over time? Coming in 10 minutes late for work isn't perceived in the same way if, for one employee, it represents an unusual case (she hasn't been late in months), while for another employee, it's part of a routine pattern (she's late two or three times every week). The more consistent the behavior, the more the observer is inclined to attribute it to internal causes. Exhibit 6 summarizes the key elements of attribution theory.

One interesting finding from attribution theory is that errors or biases distort our attributions. For instance, substantial evidence supports the fact that when we make judgments about the behavior of other people, we have a tendency to *under*estimate the influence of external factors and to *over*estimate the influence of internal or personal factors.[85] This tendency is called the **fundamental attribution error** and can explain why a sales manager may attribute the poor performance of her sales representative to laziness rather than to the innovative product line introduced by a competitor. Another tendency is to attribute our own successes to internal factors, such as ability or effort, while putting the blame for personal failure on external factors, such as luck. This tendency is called the **self-serving bias** and suggests that feedback provided to employees in performance reviews will be distorted by them depending on whether it's positive or negative.

Are these errors or biases that distort attributions universal across different cultures? We can't say for sure, but preliminary evidence indicates cultural differences.[86] For instance, a study of Korean managers found that, contrary to the self-serving bias, they tended to accept responsibility for group failure "because I was not a capable leader" instead of attributing it to group members.[87] Attribution theory was developed largely based on experiments with Americans and Western Europeans. But the Korean study suggests caution in making attribution theory predictions in non-Western societies, especially in countries with strong collectivist traditions.

Shortcuts Used in Judging Others

Perceiving and interpreting people's behavior is a lot of work, so we use shortcuts to make the task more manageable. These techniques can be valuable when they let us make accurate interpretations quickly and provide valid data for making predictions. However, they aren't perfect. They can and do get us into trouble.

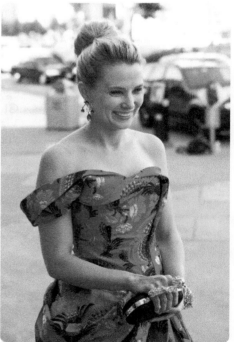

Yahoo CEO Marissa Mayer, shown here arriving at a gala for the San Francisco Opera, is a computer scientist. She challenges the stereotypical view of computer scientists that inaccurately generalizes them as poorly dressed and disorganized white males who have no social skills and no social life and wear thick glasses and pocket protectors. Stereotyping, she believes, may hinder women from pursuing careers in computer science.
Source: Laura Morton/Corbis

assumed similarity
The assumption that others are like oneself

It's easy to judge others if we assume they're similar to us. In **assumed similarity,** or the "like me" effect, the observer's perception of others is influenced more by the observer's own characteristics than by those of the person observed. For example, if you want challenges and responsibility in your job, you'll assume that others want the same. People who assume that others are like them can, of course, be right, but not always.

stereotyping
Judging a person based on a perception of a group to which that person belongs

When we judge someone on the basis of our perception of a group he or she is part of, we're using the shortcut called **stereotyping.** For instance, "Married people are more stable employees than single persons" is an example of stereotyping. To the degree that a stereotype is based on fact, it may produce accurate judgments. However, many stereotypes aren't factual and distort our judgment.[88]

halo effect
A general impression of an individual based on a single characteristic

When we form a general impression about a person on the basis of a single characteristic, such as intelligence, sociability, or appearance, we're influenced by the **halo effect.** This effect frequently occurs when students evaluate their classroom instructor. Students may isolate a single trait such as enthusiasm and allow their entire evaluation to be slanted by the perception of this one trait. An instructor may be quiet, assured, knowledgeable, and highly qualified, but if his classroom teaching style lacks enthusiasm, he might be rated lower on a number of other characteristics.

Implications for Managers

Managers need to recognize that their employees react to perceptions, not to reality. So whether a manager's appraisal of an employee's performance is actually objective and unbiased or whether the organization's wage levels are among the highest in the community is less relevant than what employees perceive them to be. If individuals perceive appraisals to be biased or wage levels as low, they'll behave as if those conditions actually exist. Employees organize and interpret what they see, so the potential for perceptual distortion is always present. The message is clear: Pay close attention to how employees perceive both their jobs and management actions.

LEARNING

L05 When Elvis Andrus was signed by the Texas Rangers, he was excited to learn that the Rangers had signed another shortstop—11-time Gold Glove winner and fellow Venezuelan Omar Vizquel (now retired from baseball). Vizquel's role was clear: to be a mentor to the talented young player. Managers of major league baseball teams "regularly mix savvy veterans with talented young players, hoping tricks of the trade and advice on everything from how to turn a double play to how to avoid trouble in night spots on the road will rub off."[89]

Mentoring is a good example of the last individual behavior concept we're going to look at—learning. Learning is included in our discussion of individual behavior for the obvious reason that almost all behavior is learned. If we want to explain, predict, and influence behavior, we need to understand how people learn.

learning
Any relatively permanent change in behavior that occurs as a result of experience

The psychologists' definition of learning is considerably broader than the average person's view that "it's what we do in school." Learning occurs all the time as we continuously learn from our experiences. A workable definition of **learning** is any relatively permanent change in behavior that occurs as a result of experience. Two learning theories help us understand how and why individual behavior occurs.

Operant Conditioning

operant conditioning
A theory of learning that says behavior is a function of its consequences

Operant conditioning argues that behavior is a function of its consequences. People learn to behave to get something they want or to avoid something they don't want. Operant behavior is voluntary or learned behavior, not reflexive or unlearned behavior. The tendency to repeat learned behavior is influenced by reinforcement or lack of reinforcement that happens as a result of the behavior. Reinforcement strengthens a behavior and increases the likelihood that it will be repeated. Lack of reinforcement weakens a behavior and lessens the likelihood that it will be repeated.

B. F. Skinner's research widely expanded our knowledge of operant conditioning.[90] Behavior is assumed to be determined from without—that is, *learned*—rather than from within—reflexive or unlearned. Skinner argued that people will most likely engage in desired behaviors if they are positively reinforced for doing so, and rewards are most effective if they immediately follow the desired response. In addition, behavior that isn't rewarded or is punished is less likely to be repeated.

You see examples of operant conditioning everywhere. Any situation in which it's either explicitly stated or implicitly suggested that reinforcement (rewards) is contingent on some action on your part is an example of operant conditioning. Your instructor says that if you want a high grade in this course, you must perform well on tests by giving correct answers. A salesperson working on commission knows that earning a sizeable income is contingent on generating high sales in his or her territory. Of course, the linkage between behavior and reinforcement can also work to teach the individual to behave in ways that work against the best interests of the organization. Assume your boss tells you that if you'll work overtime during the next three-week busy season, you'll be compensated for it at the next performance appraisal. Then, when performance appraisal time comes, you are given no positive reinforcements (such as being praised for pitching in and helping out when needed). What will you do the next time your boss asks you to work overtime? You'll probably refuse. Your behavior can be explained by operant conditioning: If a behavior isn't positively reinforced, the probability that the behavior will be repeated declines.

Social Learning

Some 60 percent of the Radio City Rockettes have danced in prior seasons. The veterans help newcomers with "Rockette style"—where to place their hands, how to hold their hands, how to keep up stamina, and so forth.[91]

As the Rockettes are well aware, individuals can also learn by observing what happens to other people and just by being told about something as well as by direct experiences. Much of what we have learned comes from watching others

let's get REAL

The Scenario:

Paul Taylor manages an advertising agency in Sydney. Although he runs his business quite loosely, he has one employee who is chronically late to everything: meetings, appointments, even getting to work.
It's gotten to the point where the other employees are "rumbling" about it. It's time to do something.

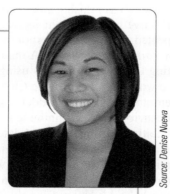

Source: Denise Nueva

Denise Nueva
Art Director

What advice would you give Paul in "shaping" this employee's behavior?

After documenting the tardiness occurrences, Paul should directly address the issue of habitual lateness with his employee. Paul must clearly state his expectation for improved tardiness, such as arriving to work at the scheduled time and being on time to meetings and appointments. Communication is key; asking his employee how s/he can improve, giving suggestions (such as setting calendar reminders/alarms) and requiring an action such as a daily email from the employee when he arrives in the morning may help to shape the employee's behavior.

(models)—parents, teachers, peers, television and movie actors, managers, and so forth. This view that we can learn both through observation and direct experience is called **social learning theory.**

The influence of others is central to the social learning viewpoint. The amount of influence these models have on an individual is determined by four processes:

1. *Attentional processes.* People learn from a model when they recognize and pay attention to its critical features. We're most influenced by models who are attractive, repeatedly available, thought to be important, or seen as similar to us.
2. *Retention processes.* A model's influence will depend on how well the individual remembers the model's action, even after the model is no longer readily available.
3. *Motor reproduction processes.* After a person has seen a new behavior by observing the model, the watching must become doing. This process then demonstrates that the individual can actually do the modeled activities.
4. *Reinforcement processes.* Individuals will be motivated to exhibit the modeled behavior if positive incentives or rewards are provided. Behaviors that are reinforced will be given more attention, learned better, and performed more often.

Shaping: A Managerial Tool

Because learning takes place on the job as well as prior to it, managers are concerned with how they can teach employees to behave in ways that most benefit the organization. Thus, managers will often attempt to "mold" individuals by guiding their learning in graduated steps, through a method called **shaping behavior.**

Consider the situation in which an employee's behavior is significantly different from that sought by a manager. If the manager reinforced the individual only when he or she showed desirable responses, the opportunity for reinforcement might occur too infrequently. Shaping offers a logical approach toward achieving the desired behavior. We shape behavior by systematically reinforcing each successive step that moves the individual closer to the desired behavior. If an employee who has chronically been a half-hour late for work comes in only 20 minutes late, we can reinforce the improvement. Reinforcement would increase as an employee gets closer to the desired behavior.

Four ways to shape behavior include positive reinforcement, negative reinforcement, punishment, and extinction. When a behavior is followed by something pleasant, such as praising an employee for a job well done, it's called *positive reinforcement.* Positive reinforcement increases the likelihood that the desired behavior will be repeated. Rewarding a response by eliminating or withdrawing something unpleasant is *negative reinforcement.* A manager who says, "I won't dock your pay if you start getting to work on time" is using negative reinforcement. The desired behavior (getting to work on time) is being encouraged by the withdrawal of something unpleasant (the employee's pay being docked). On the other hand, *punishment* penalizes undesirable behavior and will eliminate it. Suspending an employee for two days without pay for habitually coming to work late is an example of punishment. Finally, eliminating any reinforcement that's maintaining a behavior is called *extinction.* When a behavior isn't reinforced, it gradually disappears. In meetings, managers who wish to discourage employees from continually asking irrelevant or distracting questions can eliminate this behavior by ignoring those employees when they raise their hands to speak. Soon this behavior should disappear.

Both positive and negative reinforcement result in learning. They strengthen a desired behavior and increase the probability that the desired behavior will be repeated. Both punishment and extinction also result in learning, but do so by weakening an undesired behavior and decreasing its frequency.

Implications for Managers

Employees are going to learn on the job. The only issue is whether managers are going to manage their learning through the rewards they allocate and the examples they set, or allow it to occur haphazardly. If marginal employees are rewarded with pay

social learning theory
A theory of learning that says people can learn through observation and direct experience

shaping behavior
The process of guiding learning in graduated steps using reinforcement or lack of reinforcement

raises and promotions, they will have little reason to change their behavior. In fact, productive employees who see marginal performance rewarded might change their behavior. If managers want behavior A, but reward behavior B, they shouldn't be surprised to find employees learning to engage in behavior B. Similarly, managers should expect that employees will look to them as models. Managers who are consistently late to work, or take two hours for lunch, or help themselves to company office supplies for personal use should expect employees to read the message they are sending and model their behavior accordingly.

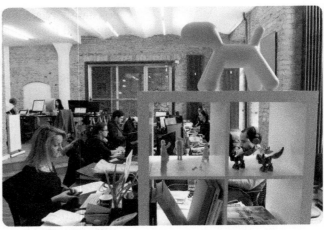

CONTEMPORARY Issues
in Organizational Behavior

LO6 By this point, you're probably well aware of the reasons managers need to understand how and why employees behave the way they do. We conclude this text by looking at two OB issues with a major influence on managers' jobs today.

Fab.com, a shopping portal for design products, understands the attitudes of Gen Y employees and has created a casual and fun environment that appeals to them. Fab offers its tech-savvy employees, like those shown here at their office in Germany, opportunities to develop themselves and their careers in a fast-growing e-commerce firm.
Source: Jens Kalaene/dpa/picture-alliance/ Newscom

Managing Generational Differences

Since 1998, Beloit College in Wisconsin has assembled a Mindset List© that helps identify the experiences that have shaped the lives of incoming freshmen.[92] The authors of the list state that it is an effort to better understand the "experiences that have shaped the lives and formed the mindset of students." Here are some of the observations from the 2017 list (generated in 2013):

- GM refers to "genetically modified" foods, not General Motors.
- Chatting with someone has seldom involved actual talking.
- "Dude" has never had a negative tone.
- They have known only two presidents.
- A tablet is not something you take in the morning.
- GPS means they never needed written directions, just an address.
- Their favorite movies have always been largely, if not totally, computer generated.

What will *this* group of young employees be like when they enter the workforce after graduation? Will they share the characteristics of the earlier members of Gen Y? Let's take a look at how Gen Y is changing the workplace, since by 2025, they'll make up more than 75 percent of the workforce.[93]

They're bright, curious, and eager to learn. But they can also be brash. They wear flip-flops to the office and listen to iPods at their desk. They want to work, but don't want work to be their life. Communicating with them means being concise and being mobile. They get excited about the opportunity to work on exciting or innovative projects, but not so much about job titles. Keeping them engaged in the workplace requires continual feedback and recognition. This is Generation Y, some 70 million of them, many of whom are embarking on their careers, taking their place in an increasingly multigenerational workplace.[94]

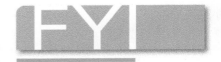

- 80 percent of campus recruiters say that students' way of communicating are too casual for the recruiting process.[95]

JUST WHO IS GEN Y? There's no consensus about the exact timespan that Gen Y comprises, but most definitions include those individuals born from about 1982 to 1997. One thing is for sure—they're bringing new attitudes with them to the workplace. Gen Ys have grown up with an amazing array of experiences and opportunities. And they want their work life to provide that as well. For instance, Stella Kenyi, who is passionately interested in international development, was sent by her employer, the National Rural Electric Cooperative Association, to Yai, Sudan, to survey energy use.[96] At Best Buy's corporate offices, Beth Trippie, a senior scheduling specialist, feels that as long as the results are there, why should it matter how it gets done. She says, "I'm

constantly playing video games, on a call, doing work, and the thing is, all of it gets done, and it gets done well."[97] An assistant account executive from Atlanta described herself and fellow Gen Y'ers as tech-savvy risk takers—individuals who are quite willing to shake up how things currently stand. And from her perspective, appealing work environments are those that offer opportunities to work independently and creatively.[98]

DEALING WITH THE MANAGERIAL CHALLENGES Managing Gen Y workers presents some unique challenges. Conflicts and resentment can arise over issues such as appearance, technology, and management style.

How flexible must an organization be in terms of "appropriate" office attire? It may depend on the type of work being done and the size of the organization. In many organizations, jeans, T-shirts, and flip-flops are acceptable. However, in other settings, employees are expected to dress more conventionally. But even in those more conservative organizations, one possible solution to accommodate the more casual attire preferred by Gen Y is to be more flexible in what's acceptable. For instance, the guideline might be that when the person is not interacting with someone outside the organization, more casual wear (with some restrictions) can be worn.

What about technology? This generation has lived much of their lives with ATMs, DVDs, cell phones, e-mail, texting, laptops, and the Internet. When they don't have information they need, they simply enter a few keystrokes to get it. Having grown up with technology, Gen Ys tend to be totally comfortable with it. They're quite content to meet virtually to solve problems, while bewildered baby boomers expect important problems to be solved with an in-person meeting. Baby boomers complain about Gen Y's inability to focus on one task, while Gen Ys see nothing wrong with multitasking. Again, flexibility from both is the key.

Finally, what about managing Gen Ys? Like the old car advertisement that used to say, "This isn't your father's car," we can say, "This isn't your father's or mother's way of managing." Gen Y employees want bosses who are open minded; experts in their field, even if they aren't tech-savvy; organized; teachers, trainers, and mentors; not authoritarian or paternalistic; respectful of their generation; understanding of their need for work–life balance; providing constant feedback; communicating in vivid and compelling ways; and providing stimulating and novel learning experiences.[99]

Gen Y employees have a lot to offer organizations in terms of their knowledge, passion, and abilities. Mangers, however, have to recognize and understand the behaviors of this group in order to create an environment in which work can be accomplished efficiently, effectively, and without disruptive conflict.

Managing Negative Behavior in the Workplace

Jerry notices the oil is low in his forklift but continues to drive it until it overheats and can't be used. After enduring 11 months of repeated insults and mistreatment from her supervisor, Maria quits her job. An office clerk slams her keyboard and then shouts profanity whenever her computer freezes up. Rudeness, hostility, aggression, and other forms of workplace negativity and incivility have become all too common in today's organizations. In a survey of U.S. employees, 10 percent said they witnessed rudeness daily within their workplaces and 20 percent said they were direct targets of incivility at work at least once a week. In a survey of Canadian workers, 25 percent reported seeing incivility daily, and 50 percent said they were the direct targets at least once per week.[100] Some estimates put the costs of negativity to the U.S. economy at $300 billion a year.[101] Most managers dread having to deal with difficult employees. However, they can't just ignore the problems. So, what can managers do to manage negative behavior in the workplace?

The main thing is to recognize that it's there. Pretending that negative behavior doesn't exist or ignoring such misbehaviors will only confuse employees about what is expected and acceptable behavior. Although some debate among researchers questions whether preventive or responsive actions to negative behaviors are more effective, in reality, both are needed.[102] Preventing negative behaviors by carefully

screening potential employees for certain personality traits and responding immediately and decisively to unacceptable negative behaviors can go a long way toward managing negative workplace behaviors. But it's also important to pay attention to employee attitudes, because negativity will show up there as well. As we said earlier, when employees are dissatisfied with their jobs, they *will* respond somehow.

PREPARING FOR: Exams/Quizzes

CHAPTER SUMMARY by Learning Objectives

LO1

IDENTIFY the focus and goals of individual behavior within organizations.

Just like an iceberg, it's the hidden organizational elements (attitudes, perceptions, norms, etc.) that make understanding individual behavior so challenging.

Organization behavior (OB) focuses on three areas: individual behavior, group behavior, and organizational aspects. The goals of OB are to explain, predict, and influence behavior.

Employee productivity is a performance measure of both efficiency and effectiveness. Absenteeism is the failure to report to work. Turnover is the voluntary and involuntary permanent withdrawal from an organization. Organizational citizenship behavior (OCB) is discretionary behavior that's not part of an employee's formal job requirements, but it promotes the effective functioning of an organization. Job satisfaction is an individual's general attitude toward his or her job. Workplace misbehavior is any intentional employee behavior that is potentially harmful to the organization or individuals within the organization.

LO2

EXPLAIN the role that attitudes play in job performance.

The cognitive component refers to the beliefs, opinions, knowledge, or information held by a person. The affective component is the emotional or feeling part of an attitude. The behavioral component refers to an intention to behave in a certain way toward someone or something.

Job satisfaction refers to a person's general attitude toward his or her job. Job involvement is the degree to which an employee identifies with his or her job, actively participates in it, and considers his or her job performance to be important to his or her self-worth. Organizational commitment is the degree to which an employee identifies with a particular organization and its goals and wishes to maintain membership in that organization. Employee engagement is when employees are connected to, satisfied with, and enthusiastic about their jobs.

Job satisfaction positively influences productivity, lowers absenteeism levels, lowers turnover rates, promotes positive customer satisfaction, moderately promotes OCB, and helps minimize workplace misbehavior.

Individuals try to reconcile attitude and behavior inconsistencies by altering their attitudes, altering their behavior, or rationalizing the inconsistency.

LO3

DESCRIBE different personality theories.

The MBTI measures four dimensions: social interaction, preference for gathering data, preference for decision making, and style of making decisions. The Big Five Model consists of five personality traits: extraversion, agreeableness, conscientiousness, emotional stability, and openness to experience.

The five personality traits that help explain individual behavior in organizations are locus of control, Machiavellianism, self-esteem, self-monitoring, and risk-taking. Other personality traits include Type A/Type B personalities, proactive personality, and resilience.

How a person responds emotionally and how they deal with their emotions is a function of personality. A person who is emotionally intelligent has the ability to notice and to manage emotional cues and information.

LO4 DESCRIBE **perception and factors that influence it.**

Perception is how we give meaning to our environment by organizing and interpreting sensory impressions. Because people behave according to their perceptions, managers need to understand it.

Attribution theory depends on three factors. Distinctiveness is whether an individual displays different behaviors in different situations (that is, is the behavior unusual). Consensus is whether others facing a similar situation respond in the same way. Consistency is when a person engages in behaviors regularly and consistently. Whether these three factors are high or low helps managers determine whether employee behavior is attributed to external or internal causes.

The fundamental attribution error is the tendency to underestimate the influence of external factors and overestimate the influence of internal factors. The self-serving bias is the tendency to attribute our own successes to internal factors and to put the blame for personal failure on external factors.

Three shortcuts used in judging others are assumed similarity, stereotyping, and the halo effect.

LO5 DISCUSS **learning theories and their relevance in shaping behavior.**

Operant conditioning argues that behavior is a function of its consequences. Managers can use it to explain, predict, and influence behavior.

Social learning theory says that individuals learn by observing what happens to other people and by directly experiencing something.

Managers can shape behavior by using positive reinforcement (reinforcing a desired behavior by giving something pleasant), negative reinforcement (reinforcing a desired response by withdrawing something unpleasant), punishment (eliminating undesirable behavior by applying penalties), or extinction (not reinforcing a behavior to eliminate it).

LO6 DISCUSS **contemporary issues in organizational behavior.**

The challenge of managing Gen Y workers is that they bring new attitudes to the workplace. The main challenges are over issues such as appearance, technology, and management style.

Workplace misbehavior can be dealt with by recognizing that it's there; carefully screening potential employees for possible negative tendencies; and most importantly, by paying attention to employee attitudes through surveys about job satisfaction and dissatisfaction.

MyManagementLab

Go to **mymanagementlab.com** to complete the problems marked with this icon ⭐.

⊛ REVIEW AND DISCUSSION QUESTIONS

1. Does the importance of knowledge of OB differ based on a manager's levels in the organization? If so, how? If not, why not? Be specific.

2. Explain why the concept of an organization as an iceberg is important.

3. Define the six important employee behaviors.

4. Describe the three components of an attitude and explain the four job-related attitudes.

5. Contrast the MBTI and the Big Five Model. Describe five other personality traits that help explain individual behavior in organizations.

6. Explain how an understanding of perception can help managers better understand individual behavior. Name three shortcuts used in judging others.

7. Describe the key elements of attribution theory. Discuss the fundamental attribution error and self-serving bias.

8. Describe operant conditioning and how managers can shape behavior.

MyManagementLab

If your professor has assigned these, go to **mymanagementlab.com** for Auto-graded writing questions as well as the following Assisted-graded writing questions:

9. Describe the focus and goals of OB.

10. Explain the challenges facing managers in managing generational differences and negative behavior in the workplace.

PREPARING FOR: My Career

⊛ PERSONAL INVENTORY ASSESSMENTS ⓟⓘⓐ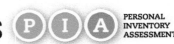

Emotional Intelligence Assessment

How emotionally intelligent are you? This PIA will help you assess your level of emotional intelligence.

⊛ ETHICS DILEMMA

It's been called the "desperation hustle."[103] Employees who want to avoid being laid off want to do whatever they can to look valuable and "irreplaceable." So they clean up their act. Those who might not have paid much attention to their manner of dress now do. Those who were mouthy and argumentative are now quiet and compliant. Those who used to "watch the clock" are now the last to leave. The fear is there, and it's noticeable. Managing employees with that kind of fearful mindset can be a challenge.

11. What ethical issues might arise for both employees and for managers?

12. How could managers approach these circumstances ethically?

SKILLS EXERCISE Developing Your Shaping Behavior Skill

About the Skill

In today's dynamic work environments, learning is continual. But this learning shouldn't be done in isolation or without any guidance. Most employees need to be shown what's expected of them on the job. As a manager, you must teach your employees the behaviors most critical to their, and the organization's, success.

Steps in Practicing the Skill

- *Identify the critical behaviors that have a significant impact on an employee's performance.* Not everything employees do on the job is equally important in terms of performance outcomes. A few critical behaviors may, in fact, account for the majority of one's results. These high-impact behaviors need to be identified.

- *Establish a baseline of performance.* A baseline is obtained by determining the number of times the identified behaviors occur under the employee's present job conditions.

- *Analyze the contributing factors to performance and their consequences.* A number of factors, such as the norms of a group, may be contributing to the baseline performance. Identify these factors and their effect on performance.

- *Develop a shaping strategy.* The change that may occur will entail changing some element of performance—structure, processes, technology, groups, or the task. The purpose of the strategy is to strengthen the desirable behaviors and weaken the undesirable ones.

- *Apply the appropriate strategy.* Once the strategy has been developed, it needs to be implemented. In this step, an intervention occurs.

- *Measure the change that has occurred.* An intervention should produce the desired results in performance behaviors. Evaluate the number of times the identified behaviors now occur. Compare these with the baseline evaluation in step 2.

- *Reinforce desired behaviors.* If an intervention has been successful and the new behaviors are producing the desired results, maintain these behaviors through reinforcement mechanisms.

Practicing the Skill

a. Imagine that your assistant is ideal in all respects but one—he or she is hopeless at taking phone messages for you when you're not in the office. You're often in training sessions and the calls are sales leads you want to follow up, so you have identified taking accurate messages as a high impact behavior for your assistant.

b. Focus on steps 3 and 4, and devise a way to shape your assistant's behavior. Identify some factors that might contribute to his or her failure to take messages—these could range from a heavy workload to a poor understanding of the task's importance (you can rule out insubordination). Then develop a shaping strategy by determining what you can change—the available technology, the task itself, the structure of the job, or some other element of performance.

c. Now plan your intervention and take a brief meeting with your assistant in which you explain the change you expect. Recruit a friend to help you role-play your intervention. Do you think you would succeed in a real situation?

WORKING TOGETHER Team Exercise

You may not like it or want to believe it, but unprofessional dress can be a career-killer.[104] Pretend you're a manager in a large, multinational company. Your company has a dress code policy, but men and women alike "cross the line." One of your female subordinates is the worst offender. Several times, she has come to work dressed in sheer, low-cut, sleeveless blouses with a micro-mini skirt and strappy sandals. How would you change her behavior?

Form small groups of three to four individuals. Your team's task is to come up with a specific plan for changing (shaping) the behavior of any employee who violates the dress code policy. Write this up and be prepared to share your ideas with the class.

MY TURN TO BE A MANAGER

- For one week, pay close attention to how people around you behave, especially those who are close to you (roommates, siblings, significant others, coworkers, etc.). Use what you've learned about attitudes, personality, perception, and learning to understand and explain how

and why they're behaving the way they do. Write your observations and your explanations in a journal.

- Write down three attitudes you have. Identify the cognitive, affective, and behavioral components of those attitudes.

- Survey 15 employees (at your place of work or at some campus office). Be sure to obtain permission before doing this anonymous survey. Ask them what rude or negative behaviors they've seen at work. Compile your findings in a report and be prepared to discuss this in class. If you were the manager in this workplace, how would you handle this behavior?

- If you've never taken a personality or career compatibility test, contact your school's testing center to see if you can take one. Once you get your results, evaluate what they mean for your career choice. Have you chosen a career that "fits" your personality? What are the implications?

- Have you ever heard of the "waiter rule"? A lot of business people think that how you treat service workers says a lot about your character and attitudes. What do you think this means? Do you agree with this idea? Why or why not? How would you be evaluated on the "waiter rule"?

- Like it or not, each of us is continually shaping the behavior of those around us. For one week, keep track of how many times you use positive reinforcement, negative reinforcement, punishment, or extinction to shape behaviors. At the end of the week, which one did you tend to use most? What were you trying to do; that is, what behaviors were you trying to shape? Were your attempts successful? Evaluate. What could you have done differently if you were trying to change someone's behavior?

- Create a job satisfaction survey for a business you're familiar with.

- Now, do a Web search for sample job satisfaction surveys. Find one or two samples. Write a report describing, comparing, and evaluating the examples you found and the survey you created.

- Survey 10 Gen Y'ers. Ask them three questions: (1) What do you think is appropriate office attire? (2) How comfortable are you with using technology, and what types of technology do you rely on most? (3) What do you think the "ideal" boss would be like? Compile your results into a paper that reports your data and summarizes your findings in a bulleted list format.

- In your own words, write down three things you learned in this text about being a good manager. Keep a copy of this for future reference.

CASE APPLICATION 1 Great Place to Work

Have you heard of SAS Institute, Inc.?[105] Maybe, just maybe, you've used a school-based version of their analytical software in a research class. SAS (originally called Statistical Analysis System) is based in Cary, North Carolina, and its analytics and business intelligence software is used by corporations and other customers to analyze operations and forecast trends. For 15 years, SAS has been named to *Fortune's* Best Companies to Work For list. In 2010 and 2011, it was ranked number one; in 2012, it was ranked number three, and in 2013 and 2014, it was ranked number two. One thing that distinguishes SAS is its highly employee-friendly culture.

The good life for employees began over 26 years ago with free M&Ms every Wednesday. Now the sweets have become even sweeter. Today, SAS's almost 13,000 employees enjoy perks such as free onsite health care, subsidized Montessori child care, unlimited sick time, onsite massage, summer camp for employees' children, an enormous fitness and recreation center, car cleaning, soda fountains and snacks in every break room, and others. The SAS dress code is...well, there is no dress code. "Laidback is the unofficial posture here and convenience the motto." To be sure, these benefits help make SAS a desirable place to work. But, the company's commitment to employees goes beyond nice perks. Even in the economic downturn, SAS has refused to lay off employees and has, in fact, even extended its benefits. As SAS's VP of Human Resources says, "SAS's continued success proves our core belief: Happy, healthy employees are more productive."

The masses of programmers who churn out the company's products are paid a competitive wage, but are not offered stock options. SAS is a privately held company so there is no stock. Yet, the extraordinary perks help SAS keep turnover

extraordinarily low: a rate of 3.6 percent versus the industry norm of more than 15 percent. On the survey instrument used to determine those Best Companies, one SAS employee wrote that in his or her opinion, employees continue to work at SAS because the company respects them and cares for them. The company's CEO and cofounder Jim Goodnight would say there's nothing wrong with treating your people well. And it's worked for his company. In 2013, SAS sold over $3 billion of its sophisticated software, and it has never had a year of revenue loss.

⭐ DISCUSSION QUESTIONS

13. What is your impression of this employee-friendly culture? Would this work in other organizations? Why or why not? What would it take to make it work?

14. How might an understanding of organizational behavior help CEO Jim Goodnight lead his company? Be specific. How about first-line company supervisors? Again, be specific.

15. What do you think has contributed to SAS's low turnover? Why is low turnover good for a company?

16. Look back at the statement made by the SAS employee on the Best Companies survey. What does that tell you about the importance of understanding individual behavior?

CASE APPLICATION *2* Employees First

"Employees first." That's the most important and crucial cultural value that HCL Technologies CEO Vineet Nayar believes will take his company into the future.[106] Although most managers think that customers should come first, Nayar's philosophy is that employee satisfaction needs to be the top priority.

As one of the largest companies in India, HCL sells various information technology product services, such as laptop, custom software development, and technology consulting. Luring and keeping top talent is one of the challenges HCL faces. And at its size, it doesn't have the atmosphere of a fun and quirky start-up.

Part of that "employee first" philosophy is a no-layoff policy, which was difficult to uphold during the pressures of the economic downturn. Like its competitors, HCL had excess employees and had suspended raises. But HCL kept its promise and didn't lay off any HCLite (Nayar's name for HCL employees). As business has picked up, however, employees begin looking at competitors' job offers. During the first quarter alone of 2010, HCL lost 22 percent of its workforce. Maybe it's time to monitor and track employee satisfaction.

HCL Technologies is headquartered in the world's largest democracy, so it's quite fitting that the New Delhi–based company is attempting a radical experiment in workplace democracy. CEO Vineet Nayar is committed to creating a company where the job of company leaders is to enable people to find their own destiny by gravitating to their strengths. As we discussed in the chapter opener, one thing that Nayar has done is to pioneer a culture in which employees are first. What has he done to put employees first? Part of the cultural initiative dealt with the organization's structure. HCL inverted its organizational structure and placed more power in the hands of frontline employees, especially those in direct contact with customers and clients. It increased its investment in employee development and improved communication through greater transparency. Employees were encouraged to communicate directly

with Nayar. Through a forum called U&I (You and I), Nayar fielded more than a hundred questions from employees every week. "I threw open the door and invited criticism," he said. However, the signature piece of the company's cultural mission is probably what HCL called "trust pay." In contrast to the industry standard in which the average employee's pay is 30 percent variable, HCL decided to pay higher fixed salaries and reduce the variable component.

Does the unique "employees first" culture at HCL Technologies attract unique employees? Rajeev Sawhney, HCL's European president, would say it does. He uses *Slumdog Millionaire,* the movie that won the Academy Award for Best Picture in 2009, as a parallel. "It (the movie) is a reflection of the Indian race. It shows the adversity that creates the desire in people to reach out and create....With each adversity they face, there is a greater desire to reach out and do something more." Sawhney says that entrepreneurialism is a key value of the HCL culture. "You can still tell an HCL person from a mile off. I think there is a particular DNA for an HCL person. It includes a very high need for achievement and very persuasive skills. HCL people are very energetic; they want to do lots of things and to take risks on behalf of the company."

⭐ DISCUSSION QUESTIONS

17. What is your impression of an "employees first" culture? Would this work in other organizations? Why or why not? What would it take to make it work?

18. How might an understanding of organizational behavior help CEO Vineet Nayar lead his company? Be specific. How about first-line company supervisors? Again, be specific.

19. What aspects of personality do you see in this story about HCL? How have the personality traits of HCL employees contributed to make HCL what it is?

20. Design an employee attitude survey for HCL's employees.

ENDNOTES

1. K. O'Toole, "Cold-Calling Van Horne," *Stanford Business Magazine* [www.gsb.stanford.edu], May 2005; and S. Orenstein, "Feeling Your Way to the Top," *Business 2.0,* June 2004, p. 146.

2. "Unplanned Absence Costs Organizations 8.7 Percent of Payroll, Mercer/Kronos Study" [www.mercer.com], June 28, 2010; and K. M. Kroll, "Absence-Minded," *CFO Human Capital,* 2006, pp. 12–14.

3. K. H. Dekas, T. N. Bauer, B. Welle, J. Kurkoski, and S. Sullivan, "Organizational Citizenship Behavior, Version 2.0: A Review and Qualitative Investigation of OCBs for Knowledge Workers at Google and Beyond," *Academy of Management Perspective,* August 2013, pp. 219–237; D. W. Organ, *Organizational Citizenship Behavior: The Good Soldier Syndrome* (Lexington, MA: Lexington Books, 1988), p. 4. See also J. L. Lavell, D. E. Rupp, and J. Brockner, "Taking a Multifoci Approach to the Study of Justice, Social Exchange, and Citizenship Behavior: The Target Similarity Model," *Journal of Management,* December 2007, pp. 841–866; and J. A. LePine, A. Erez, and D. E. Johnson, "The Nature and Dimensionality of Organizational Citizenship Behavior: A Critical Review and Meta-Analysis," *Journal of Applied Psychology,* February 2002, pp. 52–65.

4. R. Ilies, B. A. Scott, and T. A. Judge, "The Interactive Effects of Personal Traits and Experienced States on Intraindividual Patterns of Citizenship Behavior," *Academy of Management Journal,* June 2006, pp. 561–575; P. Cardona, B. S. Lawrence, and P. M. Bentler, "The Influence of Social and Work Exchange Relationships on Organizational Citizenship Behavior," *Group & Organization Management,* April 2004, pp. 219–247; M. C. Bolino and W. H. Turnley, "Going the Extra Mile: Cultivating and Managing Employee Citizenship Behavior," *Academy*

of Management Executive, August 2003, pp. 60–73; M. C. Bolino, W. H. Turnley, and J. J. Bloodgood, "Citizenship Behavior and the Creation of Social Capital in Organizations," *Academy of Management Review,* October 2002, pp. 505–522; and P. M. Podsakoff, S. B. MacKenzie, J. B. Paine, and D. G. Bachrach, "Organizational Citizenship Behaviors: A Critical Review of the Theoretical and Empirical Literature and Suggestions for Future Research," *Journal of Management,* vol. 26, no. 3, 2000, pp. 543–548.

5. M. C. Bolino and W. H. Turnley, "The Personal Costs of Citizenship Behavior: The Relationship Between Individual Initiative and Role Overload, Job Stress, and Work-Family Conflict," *Journal of Applied Psychology,* July 2005, pp. 740–748.

6. This definition adapted from R. W. Griffin and Y. P. Lopez, "Bad Behavior in Organizations: A Review and Typology for Future Research," *Journal of Management,* December 2005, pp. 988–1005.

7. S. J. Breckler, "Empirical Validation of Affect, Behavior, and Cognition as Distinct Components of Attitude," *Journal of Personality and Social Psychology,* May 1984, pp. 1191–1205; and S. L. Crites Jr., L. R. Fabrigar, and R. E. Petty, "Measuring the Affective and Cognitive Properties of Attitudes: Conceptual and Methodological Issues," *Personality and Social Psychology Bulletin,* December 1994, pp. 619–634.

8. D. R. May, R. L. Gilson, and L. M. Harter, "The Psychological Conditions of Meaningfulness, Safety and Availability and the Engagement of the Human Spirit at Work," *Journal of Occupational and Organizational Psychology,* March 2004, pp. 11–37; R. T. Keller, "Job Involvement and Organizational Commitment as Longitudinal Predictors of Job Performance: A Study of Scientists and Engineers,"

Journal of Applied Psychology, August 1997, pp. 539–545; W. Kahn, "Psychological Conditions of Personal Engagement and Disengagement at Work," *Academy of Management Journal,* December 1990, pp. 692–794; and P. P. Brooke Jr., D. W. Russell, and J. L. Price, "Discriminant Validation of Measures of Job Satisfaction, Job Involvement, and Organizational Commitment," *Journal of Applied Psychology,* May 1988, pp. 139–145.

9. P. Korkki, "With Jobs Few, Most Workers Aren't Satisfied," *New York Times Online,* January 10, 2010.

10. G. Levamon, "The Determinants of Job Satisfaction," https://hcexchange.conference-board.org/blog/post.cfm?post=1927&blogid=1, June 25, 2013; and The Conference Board, "Workers Less Miserable, But Hardly Happy," [www.conference-board.org], June 27, 2012.

11. The Conference Board, "Workers Less Miserable, But Hardly Happy."

12. A. Harjani, "Nearly Half of Global Employees Unhappy in Jobs: Survey," cnbc.com, September 17, 2013.

13. "Overstretched," *The Economist* [www.economist.com], May 20, 2010.

14. T. A. Judge, C. J. Thoresen, J. E. Bono, and G. K. Patton, "The Job Satisfaction-Job Performance Relationship: A Qualitative and Quantitative Review," *Psychological Bulletin,* May 2001, pp. 376–407.

15. J. K. Harter, F. L. Schmidt, and T. L. Hayes, "Business-Unit Level Relationship Between Employee Satisfaction, Employee Engagement, and Business Outcomes: A Meta-Analysis," *Journal of Applied Psychology,* April 2002, pp. 268–279; A. M. Ryan, M. J. Schmit, and R. Johnson, "Attitudes and Effectiveness: Examining Relations at an Organizational Level," *Personnel Psychology,* Winter 1996, pp. 853–882; and C. Ostroff, "The Relationship Between Satisfaction, Attitudes, and Performance: An Organizational Level Analysis," *Journal of Applied Psychology,* December 1992, pp. 963–974.

16. E. A. Locke, "The Nature and Causes of Job Satisfaction," in M. D. Dunnette (ed.), *Handbook of Industrial and Organizational Psychology* (Chicago: Rand McNally, 1976), p. 1331; S. L. McShane, "Job Satisfaction and Absenteeism: A Meta-Analytic Re-Examination," *Canadian Journal of Administrative Science,* June 1984, pp. 61–77; R. D. Hackett and R. M. Guion, "A Reevaluation of the Absenteeism-Job Satisfaction Relationship," *Organizational Behavior and Human Decision Processes,* June 1985, pp. 340–381; K. D. Scott and G. S. Taylor, "An Examination of Conflicting Findings on the Relationship Between Job Satisfaction and Absenteeism: A Meta-Analysis," *Academy of Management Journal,* September 1985, pp. 599–612; R. D. Hackett, "Work Attitudes and Employee Absenteeism: A Synthesis of the Literature," paper presented at the 1988 National Academy of Management Meeting, Anaheim, CA, August 1988; and R. Steel and J. R. Rentsch, "Influence of Cumulation Strategies on the Long-Range Prediction of Absenteeism," *Academy of Management Journal,* December 1995, pp. 1616–1634.

17. J. Yang and S. Ward, "Planned Absenteeism," *USA Today,* April 23, 2014, p. 1B.

18. P. W. Hom and R. W. Griffeth, *Employee Turnover* (Cincinnati, OH: Southwestern, 1995); R. W. Griffith, P. W. Hom, and S. Gaertner, "A Meta-Analysis of Antecedents and Correlates of Employee Turnover: Update, Moderator Tests, and Research Implications for the Next Millennium," *Journal of Management,* vol. 26, no. 3, 2000, p. 479; and P. W. Hom and A. J. Kinicki, "Toward a Greater Understanding of How Dissatisfaction Drives Employee Turnover," *Academy of Management Journal,* October 2001, pp. 975–987.

19. See, for example, J. M. Carsten and P. E. Spector, "Unemployment, Job Satisfaction, and Employee Turnover: A Meta-Analytic Test of the Muchinsky Model," *Journal of Applied Psychology,* August 1987, pp. 374–381; and C. L. Hulin, M. Roznowski, and D. Hachiya, "Alternative Opportunities and Withdrawal Decisions: Empirical and Theoretical Discrepancies and an Integration," *Psychological Bulletin,* July 1985, pp. 233–250.

20. T. A. Wright and D. G. Bonett, "Job Satisfaction and Psychological Well-Being as Nonadditive Predictors of Workplace Turnover," *Journal of Management,* April 2007, pp. 141–160; and D. G. Spencer and R. M. Steers, "Performance as a Moderator of the Job Satisfaction-Turnover Relationship," *Journal of Applied Psychology,* August 1981, pp. 511–514.

21. See, for instance, M. Schulte, C. Ostroff, S. Shmulyian, and A. Kinicki, "Organizational Climate Configurations: Relationships to Collective

Attitudes, Customer Satisfaction, and Financial Performance," *Journal of Applied Psychology,* May 2009, pp. 618–634; S. P. Brown and S. K. Lam, "A Meta-analysis of Relationships Linking Employee Satisfaction to Customer Responses," *Journal of Retailing,* vol. 84, 2008, pp. 243–255; X. Luo and C. Homburg, "Neglected Outcomes of Customer Satisfaction," *Journal of Marketing,* April 2007, pp. 133–149; P. B. Barger and A. A. Grandey, "Service with a Smile and Encounter Satisfaction: Emotional Contagion and Appraisal Mechanisms," *Academy of Management Journal,* December 2006, pp. 1229–1238; C. Homburg and R. M. Stock, "The Link Between Salespeople's Job Satisfaction and Customer Satisfaction in a Business-to-Business Context: A Dyadic Analysis," *Journal of the Academy of Marketing Science,* Spring 2004, pp. 144–158; J. K. Harter, F. L. Schmidt, and T. L. Hayes, "Business-Unit-Level Relationship Between Employee Satisfaction, Employee Engagement, and Business Outcomes: A Meta-Analysis," *Journal of Applied Psychology,* April 2002, pp. 268–279; J. Griffith, "Do Satisfied Employees Satisfy Customers? Support-Services Staff Morale and Satisfaction Among Public School Administrators, Students, and Parents," *Journal of Applied Social Psychology,* August 2001, pp. 1627–1658; D. J. Koys, "The Effects of Employee Satisfaction, Organizational Citizenship Behavior, and Turnover on Organizational Effectiveness: A Unit-Level, Longitudinal Study," *Personnel Psychology,* Spring 2001, pp. 101–114; E. Naumann and D. W. Jackson Jr., "One More Time: How Do You Satisfy Customers?" *Business Horizons,* May–June 1999, pp. 71–76; W. W. Tornow and J. W. Wiley, "Service Quality and Management Practices: A Look at Employee Attitudes, Customer Satisfaction, and Bottom-Line Consequences," *Human Resource Planning,* vol. 4, no. 2, 1991, pp. 105–116; and B. Schneider and D. E. Bowen, "Employee and Customer Perceptions of Service in Banks: Replication and Extension," *Journal of Applied Psychology,* August 1985, pp. 423–433.

22. M. J. Bitner, B. H. Blooms, and L. A. Mohr, "Critical Service Encounters: The Employees' Viewpoint," *Journal of Marketing,* October 1994, pp. 95–106.

23. J. M. O'Brien, "Zappos Knows How to Kick It," *Fortune,* February 2, 2009, pp. 55–60.

24. See T. M. Glomb, D. P. Bhave, A. G. Miner, and M. Wall, "Doing Good, Feeling Good: Examining the Role of Organizational Citizenship Behaviors in Changing Mood," *Personnel Psychology,* Spring 2011, pp. 191–223; L. M. Little, D. L. Nelson, J. C. Wallace, and P. D. Johnson, "Integrating Attachment Style, Vigor at Work, and Extra-Role Performance," *Journal of Organizational Behavior,* April 2011, pp. 464–484; N. P. Podsakoff, P. J. Podsakoff, S. W. Whiting, and P. Hisra, "Effects of Organizational Citizenship Behavior on Selection Decisions in Employment Interviews," *Journal of Applied Psychology,* March 2011, pp. 310–326; J. A. LePine, A. Erez, and D. E. Johnson, "The Nature and Dimensionality of Organizational Citizenship Behavior: A Critical Review and Meta-Analysis," 2002; P. Podsakoff, S. B. Mackenzie, J. B. Paine, and D. G. Bachrach, "Organizational Citizenship Behaviors: A Critical Review of the Theoretical and Empirical Literature and Suggestions for Future Research," *Journal of Management,* May 2000, pp. 513–563; T. S. Bateman and D. W. Organ, "Job Satisfaction and the Good Soldier: The Relationship Between Affect and Employee 'Citizenship,'" *Academy of Management Journal,* December 1983, pp. 587–595.

25. B. J. Hoffman, C. A. Blair, J. P. Maeriac, and D. J. Woehr, "Expanding the Criterion Domain? A Quantitative Review of the OCB Literature," *Journal of Applied Psychology,* vol. 92, no. 2, 2007, pp. 555–566; J. A. LePine, A. Erez, and D. E. Johnson, "The Nature and Dimensionality of Organizational Citizenship Behavior: A Critical Review and Meta-Analysis," 2002; and D. W. Organ and K. Ryan, "A Meta-Analytic Review of Attitudinal and Dispositional Predictors of Organizational Citizenship Behavior," *Personnel Psychology,* Winter 1995, pp. 775–802.

26. N. A. Fassina, D. A. Jones, and K. L. Uggerslev, "Relationship Clean-Up Time: Using Meta-Analysis and Path Analysis to Clarify Relationships Among Job Satisfaction, Perceived Fairness, and Citizenship Behaviors," *Journal of Management,* April 2008, pp. 161–188; M. A. Konovsky and D. W. Organ, "Dispositional and Contextual Determinants of Organizational Citizenship Behavior," *Journal of Organiza-*

tional Behavior, May 1996, pp. 253–266; R. H. Moorman, "Relationship Between Organization Justice and Organizational Citizenship Behaviors: Do Fairness Perceptions Influence Employee Citizenship?" *Journal of Applied Psychology,* December 1991, pp. 845–855; and J. Fahr, P. M. Podsakoff, and D. W. Organ, "Accounting for Organizational Citizenship Behavior: Leader Fairness and Task Scope Versus Satisfaction," *Journal of Management,* December 1990, pp. 705–722.

27. W. H. Bommer, E. C. Dierdorff, and R. S. Rubin, "Does Prevalence Mitigate Relevance? The Moderating Effect of Group-Level OCB on Employee Performance," *Academy of Management Journal,* December 2007, pp. 1481–1494.

28. See, for example, S. Rabinowitz and D. T. Hall, "Organizational Research in Job Involvement," *Psychological Bulletin,* March 1977, pp. 265–288; G. J. Blau, "A Multiple Study Investigation of the Dimensionality of Job Involvement," *Journal of Vocational Behavior,* August 1985, pp. 19–36; and N. A. Jans, "Organizational Factors and Work Involvement," *Organizational Behavior and Human Decision Processes,* June 1985, pp. 382–396.

29. D. A. Harrison, D. A. Newman, and P. L. Roth, "How Important Are Job Attitudes?: Meta-Analytic Comparisons of Integrative Behavioral Outcomes and Time Sequences," *Academy of Management Journal,* April 2006, pp. 305–325; G. J. Blau, "Job Involvement and Organizational Commitment as Interactive Predictors of Tardiness and Absenteeism," *Journal of Management,* Winter 1986, pp. 577–584; and K. Boal and R. Cidambi, "Attitudinal Correlates of Turnover and Absenteeism: A Meta-Analysis," paper presented at the meeting of the American Psychological Association, Toronto, Canada, 1984.

30. G. J. Blau and K. Boal, "Conceptualizing How Job Involvement and Organizational Commitment Affect Turnover and Absenteeism," *Academy of Management Review,* April 1987, p. 290.

31. See, for instance, P. W. Hom, R. Katerberg, and C. L. Hulin, "Comparative Examination of Three Approaches to the Prediction of Turnover," *Journal of Applied Psychology,* June 1979, pp. 280–290; R. T. Mowday, L. W. Porter, and R. M. Steers, *Employee Organization Linkages: The Psychology of Commitment, Absenteeism, and Turnover* (New York: Academic Press, 1982); H. Angle and J. Perry, "Organizational Commitment: Individual and Organizational Influence," *Work and Occupations,* May 1983, pp. 123–145; and J. L. Pierce and R. B. Dunham, "Organizational Commitment: Pre-Employment Propensity and Initial Work Experiences," *Journal of Management,* Spring 1987, pp. 163–178.

32. L. W. Porter, R. M. Steers, R. T. Mowday, and V. Boulian, "Organizational Commitment, Job Satisfaction, and Turnover Among Psychiatric Technicians," *Journal of Applied Psychology,* October 1974, pp. 603–609.

33. D. M. Rousseau, "Organizational Behavior in the New Organizational Era," in J. T. Spence, J. M. Darley, and D. J. Foss (eds.), *Annual Review of Psychology,* vol. 48 (Palo Alto, CA: Annual Reviews, 1997), p. 523.

34. P. Eder and R. Eisenberger, "Perceived Organizational Support: Reducing the Negative Influence of Coworker Withdrawal Behavior," *Journal of Management,* February 2008, pp. 55–68; R. Eisenberger, F. Stinglhamber, C. Vandenberghe, I. L. Sucharski, and L. Rhoades, "Perceived Supervisor Support: Contributions to Perceived Organizational Support and Employee Retention," *Journal of Applied Psychology,* June 2002, pp. 565–573; L. Rhoades and R. Eisenberger, "Perceived Organizational Support: A Review of the Literature," *Journal of Applied Psychology,* August 2002, pp. 698–714; J. L. Kraimer and S. J. Wayne, "An Examination of Perceived Organizational Support as a Multidimensional Construct in the Context of an Expatriate Assignment," *Journal of Management,* vol. 30, no. 2, 2004, pp. 209–237; J. W. Bishop, K. D. Scott, J. G. Goldsby, and R. Cropanzano, "A Construct Validity Study of Commitment and Perceived Support Variables," *Group & Organization Management,* April 2005, pp. 153–180; and J. A-M. Coyle-Shapiro and N. Conway, "Exchange Relationships: Examining Psychological Contracts and Perceived Organizational Support," *Journal of Applied Psychology,* July 2005, pp. 774–781.

35. J. Marquez, "Disengaged Employees Can Spell Trouble at Any Company," *Workforce Management* [www.workforce.com], May 13, 2008.

36. J. Smythe, "Engaging Employees to Drive Performance," *Communication World,* May–June 2008, pp. 20–22; A. B. Bakker and W. B. Schaufeli, "Positive Organizational Behavior: Engaged Employees in Flourishing Organizations," *Journal of Organizational Behavior,* February 2008,

pp. 147–154; U. Aggarwal, S. Datta, and S. Bhargava, "The Relationship Between Human Resource Practices, Psychological Contract, and Employee Engagement—Implications for Managing Talent," *IIMB Management Review,* September 2007, pp. 313–325; M. C. Christian and J. E. Slaughter, "Work Engagement: A Meta-Analytic Review and Directions for Research in an Emerging Area," *AOM Proceedings,* August 2007, pp. 1–6; C. H. Thomas, "A New Measurement Scale for Employee Engagement: Scale Development, Pilot Test, and Replication," *AOM Proceedings,* August 2007, pp. 1–6; A. M. Saks, "Antecedents and Consequences of Employee Engagement," *Journal of Managerial Psychology,* vol. 21, no. 7, 2006, pp. 600–619; and A. Parsley, "Road Map for Employee Engagement," *Management Services,* Spring 2006, pp. 10–11.

37. J. Katz, "The Engagement Dance," *Industry Week,* April 2008, p. 24.

38. "Driving Employee Engagement in a Global Workforce," *Watson Wyatt Worldwide,* 2007–2008, p. 2.

39. A. J. Elliott and P. G. Devine, "On the Motivational Nature of Cognitive Dissonance: Dissonance as Psychological Discomfort," *Journal of Personality and Social Psychology*, September 1994, pp. 382–394.

40. J. Yang and P. Trap, "Is A Sense of Humor Important in the Workplace?" *USA Today,* April 18, 2012, p. 1B.

41. L. Festinger, *A Theory of Cognitive Dissonance* (Stanford, CA: Stanford University Press, 1957); and C. Crossen, "Cognitive Dissonance Became a Milestone in 1950s Psychology," *Wall Street Journal,* December 4, 2006, p. B1.

42. See, for example, S. V. Falletta, "Organizational Intelligence Surveys," *T&D,* June 2008, pp. 52–58; R. Fralicx, P. Foley, H. Friedman, P. Gilberg, D. P. McCauley, and L. F. Parra, "Point of View: Using Employee Surveys to Drive Business Decisions," Mercer Human Resource Consulting, July 1, 2004; L. Simpson, "What's Going on in Your Company? If You Don't Ask, You'll Never Know," *Training,* June 2002, pp. 30–34; and B. Fishel, "A New Perspective: How to Get the Real Story from Attitude Surveys," *Training,* February 1998, pp. 91–94.

43. A. Kover, "And the Survey Says...," *Industry Week,* September 2005, pp. 49–52.

44. See J. Welch and S. Welch, "Employee Polls: A Vote in Favor," *BusinessWeek,* January 28, 2008, p. 90; E. White, "How Surveying Workers Can Pay Off," *Wall Street Journal,* June 18, 2007, p. B3; A. Kover, "And the Survey Says...," R. Fralicx, P. Foley, H. Friedman, P. Gilberg, D. P. McCauley, and L. F. Parra, "Point of View: Using Employee Surveys to Drive Business Decisions"; and S. Shellenbarger, "Companies Are Finding It Really Pays to Be Nice to Employees," *Wall Street Journal,* July 22, 1998, p. B1.

45. Leader Making a Difference box based on Singapore Airlines Reviews, www.glassdoor.com/Reviews/, May 8, 2014; "The World's Most Admired Companies," *Fortune,* February 27, 2014, pp. 123+; "Goh Choon Phong Is Next SIA CEO," [www.asiaone.com.sg], September 3, 2010; L. Heracleous and J. Wirtz, "Singapore Airlines' Balancing Act," *Harvard Business Review,* July–August 2010, pp. 145–149; S. Cendrowski, "Singapore Airlines," *Fortune,* June 14, 2010, p. 22; and S. Govindasamy, "A State of Mind," *Airline Business,* February 2010, pp. 18–21.

46. L. Saari and T. A. Judge, "Employee Attitudes and Job Satisfaction," *Human Resource Management,* Winter 2004, pp. 395–407; and T. A. Judge and A. H. Church, "Job Satisfaction: Research and Practice," in C. L. Cooper and E. A. Locke (eds.), *Industrial and Organizational Psychology: Linking Theory with Practice* (Oxford, UK: Blackwell, 2000).

47. Harrison, Newman, and Roth, "How Important Are Job Attitudes?" pp. 320–321.

48. A. Tugend, "Blinded by Science in the Online Dating Game," *New York Times Online,* July 18, 2009; and Catherine Arnst, "Better Loving Through Chemistry?" *Bloomberg BusinessWeek,* October 23, 2010.

49. I. Briggs-Myers, *Introduction to Type* (Palo Alto, CA: Consulting Psychologists Press, 1980); W. L. Gardner and M. J. Martinko, "Using the Myers-Briggs Type Indicator to Study Managers: A Literature Review and Research Agenda," *Journal of Management,* vol. 22, no. 1, 1996, pp. 45–83; and N. L. Quenk, *Essentials of Myers-Briggs Type Indicator Assessment* (New York: Wiley, 2000).

50. R. D. Meyer, R. S. Dalal, and S. Bonaccio, "A Meta-Analytic Investigation into the Moderating Effects of Situational Strength on the Con-

scientiousness–Performance Relationship," *Journal of Organizational Behavior,* November 2009, pp. 1077–1102; C. G. DeYoung, L. C. Quilty, and J. B. Peterson, "Between Facets and Domains: 10 Aspects of the Big Five," *Journal of Personality and Social Psychology,* November 2007, pp. 880–896; T. A. Judge, D. Heller, and M. K. Mount, "Five-Factor Model of Personality and Job Satisfaction: A Meta-Analysis," *Journal of Applied Psychology,* June 2002, pp. 530–541; G. M. Hurtz and J. J. Donovan, "Personality and Job Performance: The Big Five Revisited," *Journal of Applied Psychology,* December 2000, pp. 869–879; M. K. Mount, M. R. Barrick, and J. P. Strauss, "Validity of Observer Ratings of the Big Five Personality Factors," *Journal of Applied Psychology*, April 1996, pp. 272–280; O. P. John, "The Big Five Factor Taxonomy: Dimensions of Personality in the Natural Language and in Questionnaires," in L. A. Pervin (ed.), *Handbook of Personality Theory and Research* (New York: Guilford Press, 1990), pp. 66–100; and J. M. Digman, "Personality Structure: Emergence of the Five-Factor Model," in M. R. Rosenweig and L. W. Porter (eds.), *Annual Review of Psychology,* vol. 41 (Palo Alto, CA: Annual Review, 1990), pp. 417–440.

51. M. R. Barrick and M. K. Mount, "The Big Five Personality Dimensions and Job Performance: A Meta-Analysis," *Personnel Psychology,* vol. 44, 1991, pp. 1–26; A. J. Vinchur, J. S. Schippmann, F. S. Switzer III, and P. L. Roth, "A Meta-Analytic Review of Predictors of Job Performance for Salespeople," *Journal of Applied Psychology,* August 1998, pp. 586–597; G. M. Hurtz and J. J. Donovan, "Personality and Job Performance Revisited," *Journal of Applied Psychology,* December 2000, pp. 869–879; T. A. Judge and J. E. Bono, "Relationship of Core Self-Evaluations Traits—Self Esteem, Generalized Self-Efficacy, Locus of Control, and Emotional Stability—With Job Satisfaction and Job Performance: A Meta-Analysis," *Journal of Applied Psychology,* February 2001, pp. 80–92; T. A. Judge, D. Heller, and M. K. Mount, "Five-Factor Model of Personality and Job Satisfaction: A Meta-Analysis"; and D. M. Higgins, J. B. Peterson, R. O. Pihl, and A. G. M. Lee, "Prefrontal Cognitive Ability, Intelligence, Big Five Personality, and the Prediction of Advanced Academic and Workplace Performance," *Journal of Personality and Social Psychology,* August 2007, pp. 298–319.

52. I-S. Oh and C. M. Berry, "The Five-Factor Model of Personality and Managerial Performance: Validity Gains Through the Use of 360 Degree Performance Ratings," *Journal of Applied Psychology,* November 2009, pp. 1498–1513.

53. A. E. Poropat, "A Meta-Analysis of the Five-Factor Model of Personality and Academic Performance," *Psychological Bulletin,* vol. 135, no. 2, 2009, pp. 322–338.

54. J. B. Rotter, "Generalized Expectancies for Internal Versus External Control of Reinforcement," *Psychological Monographs* 80, no. 609, 1966.

55. See, for instance, D. W. Organ and C. N. Greene, "Role Ambiguity, Locus of Control, and Work Satisfaction," *Journal of Applied Psychology*, February 1974, pp. 101–102; and T. R. Mitchell, C. M. Smyser, and S. E. Weed, "Locus of Control: Supervision and Work Satisfaction," *Academy of Management Journal*, September 1975, pp. 623–631.

56. S. Weinberg, "Poor, Misunderstood Little Machiavelli," *USA Today,* June 13, 2011, p. 2B; S. R. Kessler, P. E. Spector, W. C. Borman, C. E. Nelson, A. C. Bandelli, and L. J. Penney, "Re-Examining Machiavelli: A Three-Dimensional Model of Machiavellianism in the Workplace," *Journal of Applied Social Psychology,* August 2010, pp. 1868–1896; W. Amelia, "Anatomy of a Classic: Machiavelli's Daring Gift," *Wall Street Journal,* August 30–31, 2008, p. W10; R. G. Vleeming, "Machiavellianism: A Preliminary Review," *Psychological Reports,* February 1979, pp. 295–310; and S. A. Snook, "Love and Fear and the Modern Boss," *Harvard Business Review,* January 2008, pp. 16–17.

57. See J. Brockner, *Self-Esteem at Work: Research, Theory, and Practice* (Lexington, MA: Lexington Books, 1988), chapters 1–4; and N. Branden, *Self-Esteem at Work* (San Francisco: Jossey-Bass, 1998).

58. "Social Studies," *Bloomberg BusinessWeek,* June 14–20, 2010, pp. 72–73.

59. See M. Snyder, *Public Appearances/Private Realities: The Psychology of Self-Monitoring* (New York: W. H. Freeman, 1987); and D. V. Day, D. J. Schleicher, A. L. Unckless, and N. J. Hiller, "Self-Monitoring Personality at Work: A Meta-Analytic Investigation of Construct Validity," *Journal of Applied Psychology,* April 2002, pp. 390–401.

60. Snyder, *Public Appearances/Private Realities*; and J. M. Jenkins, "Self-Monitoring and Turnover: The Impact of Personality on Intent to Leave," *Journal of Organizational Behavior*, January 1993, pp. 83–90.

61. M. Kilduff and D. V. Day, "Do Chameleons Get Ahead? The Effects of Self-Monitoring on Managerial Careers," *Academy of Management Journal,* August 1994, pp. 1047–1060; and A. Mehra, M. Kilduff, and D. J. Brass, "The Social Networks of High and Low Self-Monitors: Implications for Workplace Performance," *Administrative Science Quarterly,* March 2001, pp. 121–146.

62. N. Kogan and M. A. Wallach, "Group Risk Taking as a Function of Members' Anxiety and Defensiveness," *Journal of Personality,* March 1967, pp. 50–63; and J. M. Howell and C. A. Higgins, "Champions of Technological Innovation," *Administrative Science Quarterly*, June 1990, pp. 317–341.

63. M. Friedman and R. H. Rosenman, *Type A Behavior and Your Heart* (New York: Alfred A. Knopf, 1974).

64. S. K. Parker and C. G. Collins, "Taking Stock: Integrating and Differentiating Multiple Proactive Behaviors," *Journal of Management,* May 2010, pp. 633–662; J. D. Kammeyer-Mueller and C. R. Wanberg, "Unwrapping the Organizational Entry Process: Disentangling Multiple Antecedents and Their Pathways to Adjustment," *Journal of Applied Psychology,* October 2003, pp. 779–794; S. E. Seibert, M. L. Kraimer, and J. M. Crant, "What Do Proactive People Do? A Longitudinal Model Linking Proactive Personality and Career Success," *Personnel Psychology,* Winter 2001, pp. 845–874; J. M. Crant, "Proactive Behavior in Organizations," *Journal of Management,* vol. 26, no. 3, 2000, pp. 435–462; J. M. Crant and T. S. Bateman, "Charismatic Leadership Viewed from Above: The Impact of Proactive Personality," *Journal of Organizational Behavior,* February 2000, pp. 63–75; S. E. Seibert, J. M. Crant, and M. L. Kraimer, "Proactive Personality and Career Success," *Journal of Applied Psychology,* June 1999, pp. 416–427; R. C. Becherer and J. G. Maurer, "The Proactive Personality Disposition and Entrepreneurial Behavior Among Small Company Presidents," *Journal of Small Business Management,* January 1999, pp. 28–36; and T. S. Bateman and J. M. Crant, "The Proactive Component of Organizational Behavior: A Measure and Correlates," *Journal of Organizational Behavior,* March 1993, pp. 103–118.

65. "Resilience Key to Keeping Your Job, Accenture Research Finds," Accenture.com, March 5, 2010; J. D. Margolis and P. G. Stoltz, "How to Bounce Back from Adversity," *Harvard Business Review,* January–February, 2010, pp. 86–92; and A. Ollier-Malaterre, "Contributions of Work-Life Resilience Initiatives to the Individual/Organization Relationship," *Human Relations,* January 2010, pp. 41–62.

66. J. B. Avey, F. Luthans, R. M. Smith, and N. F. Palmer, "Impact of Positive Psychological Capital on Employee Well-Being Over Time," *Journal of Occupational Health Psychology,* January 2010, pp. 17–28; and J. B. Avey, F. Luthans, and S. M. Jensen, "Psychological Capital: A Positive Resource for Combating Employee Stress and Turnover," *Human Resource Management,* September–October 2009, pp. 677–693.

67. See, for instance, G. W. M. Ip and M. H. Bond, "Culture, Values, and the Spontaneous Self-Concept," *Asian Journal of Psychology,* vol. 1, 1995, pp. 30–36; J. E. Williams, J. L. Saiz, D. L. FormyDuval, M. L. Munick, E. E. Fogle, A. Adom, A. Haque, F. Neto, and J. Yu, "Cross-Cultural Variation in the Importance of Psychological Characteristics: A Seven-Year Country Study," *International Journal of Psychology,* October 1995, pp. 529–550; V. Benet and N. G. Walker, "The Big Seven Factor Model of Personality Description: Evidence for Its Cross-Cultural Generalizability in a Spanish Sample," *Journal of Personality and Social Psychology,* October 1995, pp. 701–718; R. R. McCrae and P. T. Costa Jr., "Personality Trait Structure as a Human Universal," *American Psychologist,* 1997, pp. 509–516; and M. J. Schmit, J. A. Kihm, and C. Robie, "Development of a Global Measure of Personality," *Personnel Psychology,* Spring 2000, pp. 153–193.

68. J. F. Salgado, "The Five Factor Model of Personality and Job Performance in the European Community," *Journal of Applied Psychology,* February 1997, pp. 30–43. Note: This study covered the original 15-nation European community and did not include the countries that have joined since.

69. J. Zaslow, "Happiness Inc.," *Wall Street Journal,* March 18–19, 2006, p. P1+.

70. N. P. Rothbard and S. L. Wilk, "Waking Up on the Right or Wrong Side of the Bed: Start-of-Workday Mood, Work Events, Employee Affect, and Performance," *Academy of Management Journal,* October 2011, pp. 959–980.

71. N. H. Frijda, "Moods, Emotion Episodes, and Emotions," in M. Lewis and J. M. Havilland (eds.), *Handbook of Emotions* (New York: Guilford Press, 1993), pp. 381–403.

72. T-Y. Kim, D. M. Cable, S-P. Kim, and J. Wang, "Emotional Competence and Work Performance: The Mediating Effect of Proactivity and the Moderating Effect of Job Autonomy," *Journal of Organizational Behavior,* October 2009, pp. 983–1000; J. M. Diefendorff and G. J. Greguras, "Contextualizing Emotional Display Rules: Examining the Roles of Targets and Discrete Emotions in Shaping Display Rule Perceptions," *Journal of Management,* August 2009, pp. 880–898; J. Gooty, M. Gavin, and N. M. Ashkanasy, "Emotions Research in OB: The Challenges That Lie Ahead," *Journal of Organizational Behavior,* August 2009, pp. 833–838; N. M. Ashkanasy and C. S. Daus, "Emotion in the Workplace: The New Challenge for Managers," *Academy of Management Executive,* February 2002, pp. 76–86; and N. M. Ashkanasy, C. E. J. Hartel, and C. S. Daus, "Diversity and Emotions: The New Frontiers in Organizational Behavior Research," *Journal of Management,* vol. 28, no. 3, 2002, pp. 307–338.

73. "Critical Skills for Workforce 2020," *T&D,* September 2011, p. 19.

74. H. M. Weiss and R. Cropanzano, "Affective Events Theory," in B. M. Staw and L. L. Cummings, *Research in Organizational Behavior,* vol. 18 (Greenwich, CT: JAI Press, 1996), pp. 20–22.

75. "How Well Do You Deal with Angry People?" *SmartBrief on Leadership,* www.smartbrief.com/leadership/, October 1, 2013.

76. This section is based on D. Goleman, *Emotional Intelligence* (New York: Bantam, 1995); M. Davies, L. Stankov, and R. D. Roberts, "Emotional Intelligence: In Search of an Elusive Construct," *Journal of Personality and Social Psychology,* October 1998, pp. 989–1015; D. Goleman, *Working with Emotional Intelligence* (New York: Bantam, 1999); R. Bar-On and J. D. A. Parker, eds. *The Handbook of Emotional Intelligence: Theory, Development, Assessment, and Application at Home, School, and in the Workplace* (San Francisco: Jossey-Bass, 2000); and P. J. Jordan, N. M. Ashkanasy, and C. E. J. Hartel, "Emotional Intelligence as a Moderator of Emotional and Behavioral Reactions to Job Insecurity," *Academy of Management Review,* July 2002, pp. 361–372.

77. F. Walter, M. S. Cole, and R. H. Humphrey, "Emotional Intelligence? Sine Qua Non of Leadership or Folderol?" *Academy of Management Perspective,* February 2011, pp. 45–59.

78. E. J. O'Boyle Jr., R. H. Humphrey, J. M. Pollack, T. H. Hawver, and P. A. Story, "The Relation Between Emotional Intelligence and Job Performance: A Meta-Analysis," *Journal of Organizational Behavior Online,* June 2010; R. D. Shaffer and M. A. Shaffer, "Emotional Intelligence Abilities, Personality, and Workplace Performance," *Academy of Management Best Conference Paper—HR,* August 2005; K. S. Law, C. Wong, and L. J. Song, "The Construct and Criterion Validity of Emotional Intelligence and Its Potential Utility for Management Studies," *Journal of Applied Psychology,* August 2004, pp. 483–496; D. L. Van Rooy and C. Viswesvaran, "Emotional Intelligence: A Meta-Analytic Investigation of Predictive Validity and Nomological Net," *Journal of Vocational Behavior,* August 2004, pp. 71–95; P. J. Jordan, N. M. Ashkanasy, and C. E. J. Härtel, "The Case for Emotional Intelligence in Organizational Research," *Academy of Management Review,* April 2003, pp. 195–197; H. A. Elfenbein and N. Ambady, "Predicting Workplace Outcomes from the Ability to Eavesdrop on Feelings," *Journal of Applied Psychology,* October 2002, pp. 963–971; and C. Cherniss, "The Business Case for Emotional Intelligence," Consortium for Research on Emotional Intelligence in Organizations [www.eiconsortium .org], 1999.

79. F. J. Landy, "Some Historical and Scientific Issues Related to Research on Emotional Intelligence," *Journal of Organizational Behavior,* June 2005, pp. 411–424; E. A. Locke, "Why Emotional Intelligence Is an Invalid Concept," *Journal of Organizational Behavior,* June 2005, pp. 425–431; J. M. Conte, "A Review and Critique of Emotional Intelligence Measures," *Journal of Organizational Behavior,* June 2005, pp. 433–440; T. Becker, "Is Emotional Intelligence a Viable Concept?"

Academy of Management Review, April 2003, pp. 192–195; and M. Davies, L. Stankov, and R. D. Roberts, "Emotional Intelligence: In Search of an Elusive Construct," *Journal of Personality and Social Psychology,* October 1998, pp. 989–1015.

80. G. Kranz, "Organizations Look to Get Personal in '07," *Workforce Management* [www.workforce.com], June 19, 2007.

81. J. L. Holland, *Making Vocational Choices: A Theory of Vocational Personalities and Work Environments* (Odessa, FL: Psychological Assessment Resources, 1997).

82. **A. O'Connell, "Smile, Don't Bark in Tough Times," *Harvard Business Review,* November 2009, p. 27;** and G. A. Van Kleef et al., "Searing Sentiment or Cold Calculation? The Effects of Leader Emotional Displays on Team Performance Depend on Follower Epistemic Motivation," *Academy of Management Journal,* June 2009, pp. 562–580.

83. Copyright © 2012 by Matt Davis, Cambridge University. Reprinted with permission.

84. See, for instance, M. J. Martinko (ed.), *Attribution Theory: An Organizational Perspective* (Delray Beach, FL: St. Lucie Press, 1995); and H. H. Kelley, "Attribution in Social Interaction," in E. Jones et al. (eds.), *Attribution: Perceiving the Causes of Behavior* (Morristown, NJ: General Learning Press, 1972).

85. See A. G. Miller and T. Lawson, "The Effect of an Informational Option on the Fundamental Attribution Error," *Personality and Social Psychology Bulletin,* June 1989, pp. 194–204.

86. See, for instance, G. R. Semin, "A Gloss on Attribution Theory," *British Journal of Social and Clinical Psychology,* November 1980, pp. 291–330; and M. W. Morris and K. Peng, "Culture and Cause: American and Chinese Attributions for Social and Physical Events," *Journal of Personality and Social Psychology,* December 1994, pp. 949–971.

87. S. Nam, "Cultural and Managerial Attributions for Group Performance," unpublished doctoral dissertation; University of Oregon. Cited in R. M. Steers, S. J. Bischoff, and L. H. Higgins, "Cross-Cultural Management Research," *Journal of Management Inquiry,* December 1992, pp. 325–326.

88. See, for example, S. T. Fiske, "Social Cognition and Social Perception," *Annual Review of Psychology*, 1993, pp. 155–194; G. N. Powell and Y. Kido, "Managerial Stereotypes in a Global Economy: A Comparative Study of Japanese and American Business Students' Perspectives," *Psychological Reports,* February 1994, pp. 219–226; and J. L. Hilton and W. von Hippel, "Stereotypes," in J. T. Spence, J. M. Darley, and D. J. Foss (eds.), *Annual Review of Psychology,* vol. 47 (Palo Alto, CA: Annual Reviews Inc., 1996), pp. 237–271.

89. P. White, "Baseball Elders Teach Lessons of the Game," *USA Today,* April 14, 2009, p. 1C+.

90. B. F. Skinner, *Contingencies of Reinforcement* (East Norwalk, CT: Appleton-Century-Crofts, 1971).

91. A. Applebaum, "Linear Thinking," *Fast Company,* December 2004, p. 35.

92. "The Mindset List for the Class of 2017," [www.beloit.edu/mindset/2017], May 18, 2014.

93. "Most Common Gen Y Job Titles Today," *T&D,* April 2012, p. 23; and P. Ketter, "Value Proposition? Oh, Yes!" *T&D,* November 2011, p. 10.

94. S. A. Hewlett, L. Sherbin, and K. Sumberg, "How Gen Y & Boomers Will Reshape Your Agenda," *Harvard Business Review,* July–August 2009, pp. 71–76; B. Frankel, "Boomers and Millennials: So Different, Yet So Similar," *Diversity Inc.,* July–August 2009, pp. 20–27; and S. Armour, "Generation Y: They've Arrived at Work with a New Attitude," *USA Today,* p. 2B.

95. J. Yang and P. Trap, "Are Students' Ways of Communicating Too Casual for the Recruiting Process?" *USA Today,* March 29, 2012, p. 1B.

96. N. Ramachandran, "New Paths at Work," *US News & World Report,* March 20, 2006, p. 47.

97. D. Sacks, "Scenes from the Culture Clash," *Fast Company,* January/February 2006, p. 75.

98. S. Armour, "Generation Y: They've Arrived at Work with a New Attitude," p. 2B.

99. J. C. Meister and K. Willyerd, "Mentoring Millennials," *Harvard Business Review,* May 2010, pp. 68–72; P. Trunk, "Motivating Gen Ys in a Downturn," *BusinessWeek Online,* June 9, 2009; S. Armour, "Generation Y: They've Arrived at Work with a New Attitude"; B. Moses,

"The Challenges of Managing Gen Y," *The Globe and Mail,* March 11, 2005, p. C1; and C. A. Martin, *Managing Generation Y* (Amherst, MA: HRD Press, 2001).

100. C. M. Pearson and C. L. Porath, "On the Nature, Consequences, and Remedies of Workplace Incivility: No Time for Nice? Think Again," *Academy of Management Executive,* February 2005, pp. 7–18.

101. J. Robison, "Be Nice: It's Good for Business," *Gallup Brain* [brain.gallup.com], August 12, 2004.

102. D. E. Gibson and R. R. Callister, "Anger in Organizations: Review and Integration," *Journal of Management,* January 2010, pp. 66–93; M. S. Hershcovis and J. Barling, "Towards a Multi-Foci Approach to Workplace Aggression: A Meta-Analytic Review of Outcomes from Different Perpetrators," *Journal of Organizational Behavior,* January 2010, pp. 24–44; S. D. Sidle, "Workplace Incivility: How Should Employees and Managers Respond?" *Academy of Management Perspectives,* November 2009, pp. 88–89; T. G. Reio Jr. and R. Ghosh, "Antecedents and Outcomes of Workplace Incivility: Implications for Human Resource Development Research and Practice," *Human Resource Development Quarterly,* Fall 2009, pp. 237–264; Y. Vardi and E. Weitz, *Misbehavior in Organizations* (Mahwah, NJ: Lawrence Erlbaum Associates, 2004), pp. 246–247.

103. M. Conlin, "Are People in Your Office Acting Oddly?" *BusinessWeek,* April 13, 2009, p. 54; and J. Hoffman, "Working Hard to Look Busy," *New York Times Online,* January 25, 2009.

104. "Unprofessional Dress Can Be a Career-Killer," *Springfield, Missouri, News-Leader,* January 13, 2009, p. 4C.

105. "SAS Institute Review," www.glassdoor.com/reviews/, May 16, 2014; A. Brenoff, "8 Reasons Why Employees Never Want to Leave This Amazing Company," www.huffingtonpost.com, November 18, 2013; M. C. Crowley, "How SAS Became the World's Best Place to Work," www.fastcompany.com/, January 22, 2013; "SAS Ranks No. 2 on 2014 *Fortune* List. Satisfied Customers Are Result of Award-Winning Workplace Culture," SAS Press Release, www.sas.com/, January 16, 2014; R. Karlgaard, "Which CEOs Have the Most Fun?" Forbes.com, February 8, 2012, p. 57; M. Moskowitz and R. Levering, "The 100 Best Companies to Work For," *Fortune,* February 6, 2012, pp. 117+; R. Karlgaard, "Jim Goodnight King of Analytics," *Forbes,* August 22, 2011, p. 28; D. Bracken, "SAS Again Tops Fortune List of Best Places to Work," www.newsobserver.com, January 20, 2011; D. A. Kaplan, "THE Best Company to Work For," *Fortune,* February 8, 2010, pp. 56–64; R. Leung, "Working the Good Life," [www.cbsnews.com/2100-18560_162-550102.html], February 11, 2009; and J. Schu, "Even in Hard Times, SAS Keeps Its Culture Intact," *Workforce,* October 2001, p. 21.

106. R. Mobbs, "The Employee Is Always Right," *In the Black,* April 2011, pp. 12–15; V. Nayar, "Employee Happiness: Zappos vs. HCL," *Bloomberg* BusinessWeek.com, January 5, 2011; G. Hamel, "Extreme Makeover," *Leadership Excellence,* January 2011, pp. 3–4; V. Nayar, "The World in 2036: Vineet Nayar Envisages Bottom-Up Leadership," *Economist,* November 27, 2010, p. 114; V. Nayar, "Employees First, Customers Second," *Chief Learning Officer,* October 2010, pp. 20–23; V. Nayar, "Back to Front," *People Management,* August 12, 2010, pp. 26–29; V. Nayar, "A Maverick CEO Explains How He Persuaded His Team to Leap into the Future," *Harvard Business Review,* June 2010, pp. 110–113; B. Einhorn and K. Gokhale, "Bangalore's Paying Again to Keep the Talent," *Bloomberg BusinessWeek,* May 24, 2010, pp. 14–16; M. Srivastava and S. Hamm, "Using the Slump to Get Bigger in Bangalore," *BusinessWeek,* September 3, 2009, pp. 50–51; and S. Lauchlan, "HCL Embraces Slumdog Effect," *Computer Weekly,* June 23, 2009, p. 8.

Motivating Employees

Motivating Employees

It's Your Career

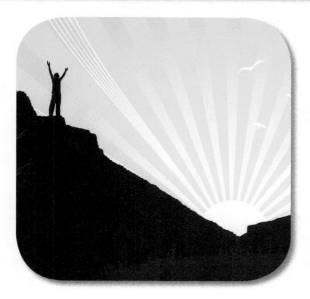

Source: Artplay711/iStock/Getty

A key to success in management and in your career is knowing *what motivates YOU.*

What Motivates You?

What's important to you or excites you in a job? Some say "money." Others might say "challenging work" or "fun co-workers." If you have a solid grounding in and understanding of what motivates you, it can help you make smart career and job choices.

The following is a list of 12 factors that might enter into your decision in selecting a job. Read over the list. Then rank order the items in terms of importance, with 1 being highest in importance and 12 being lowest in importance.

_____ *High pay*

_____ *Good working conditions*

_____ *Friendly and supportive colleagues*

_____ *Flexible working hours*

_____ *Opportunities for growth and new challenges*

_____ *Considerate boss*

_____ *Inclusion in decisions that affect you*

_____ *Fair and equitable treatment*

_____ *Job security*

_____ *Promotion potential*

_____ *Excellent benefits (vacation time; retirement contributions, etc.)*

_____ *Freedom and independence*

Now, compare your list with others in your class. How similar were your preferences? It's rare for lists to be exactly the same. This tells us that people differ in terms of what they value. Second, use these results to better understand what you're looking for in a job.

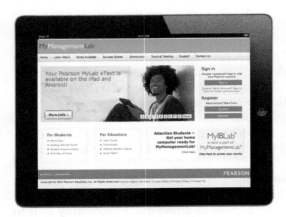

MyManagementLab®

⭐ **Improve Your Grade!**

When you see this icon, visit
www.mymanagementlab.com for activities that are
applied, personalized, and offer immediate feedback.

Learning Objectives

1 **Define** motivation.

2 **Compare** and contrast early theories of motivation.

3 **Compare** and contrast contemporary theories of motivation.

● **Develop your skill** at motivating employees.

4 **Discuss** current issues in motivation.

● **Know how** to identify what motivates you.

Successful managers need to understand that what motivates them personally may have little or no effect on others. Just because *you're* motivated by being part of a cohesive work team, don't assume everyone is. Or just because *you're* motivated by your job doesn't mean that everyone is. Effective managers who get employees to put forth maximum effort know how and why those employees are motivated and tailor motivational practices to satisfy their needs and wants.

WHAT Is Motivation?

L01 Mark Pincus, who founded the social gaming company Zynga, which created the popular game FarmVille, was a perceptive entrepreneur. When Zynga went public, the company was on the cutting edge of the increasing popularity of social gaming. However, two years after its initial public offering of stock, the company faced a dramatically different scenario. The company's performance had faltered and its stock price had tanked. To boost employee morale and help lighten up the mood, Pincus thought it would be a fun prank to hire a half-dozen clowns to swarm company headquarters in San Francisco. However, instead of being a welcome and fun distraction, employees felt terrorized as the unrelenting clowns got into people's faces, disrupted meetings, and generally made an unsettling commotion for days. Company employees were not amused and several were quite upset. The hope of reigniting that playful company spirit didn't have the intended outcome that Pincus (now the former CEO) had imagined.[1]

Would you ever have thought that clowns might be used as a way to motivate someone? Have you *ever even thought about* how to motivate someone? It's an important topic in management, and researchers have long been interested in it.[2] All managers need to be able to motivate their employees, which first requires understanding what motivation is. Let's begin by pointing out what motivation is not. Why? Because

many people incorrectly view motivation as a personal trait; that is, they think some people are motivated and others aren't. Our knowledge of motivation tells us that we can't label people that way because individuals differ in motivational drive and their overall motivation varies from situation to situation. For instance, you're probably more motivated in some classes than in others.

Motivation refers to the process by which a person's efforts are energized, directed, and sustained toward attaining a goal.[3] This definition has three key elements: energy, direction, and persistence.[4]

The *energy* element is a measure of intensity, drive, and vigor. A motivated person puts forth effort and works hard. However, the quality of the effort must be considered as well as its intensity. High levels of effort don't necessarily lead to favorable job performance unless the effort is channeled in a *direction* that benefits the organization. Effort directed toward and consistent with organizational goals is the kind of effort we want from employees. Finally, motivation includes a *persistence* dimension. We want employees to persist in putting forth effort to achieve those goals.

Motivating high levels of employee performance is an important organizational concern, and managers keep looking for answers. For instance, a Gallup poll found that a large majority of U.S. employees—some 70 percent—are not excited about their work.[5] As the researchers stated, "These employees have essentially 'checked out.' They're sleepwalking through their workday, putting time, but not energy or passion, into their work."[6] The number globally is even more disturbing—some 87 percent are not excited about their work.[7] It's no wonder then that both managers and academics want to understand and explain employee motivation.

EARLY Theories of Motivation

L02 We begin by looking at four early motivation theories: *Maslow's hierarchy of needs*, *McGregor's theories X and Y*, *Herzberg's two-factor theory*, and *McClelland's three-needs theory*. Although more valid explanations of motivation have been developed, these early theories are important because they represent the foundation from which contemporary motivation theories were developed and because many practicing managers still use them.

Maslow's Hierarchy of Needs Theory

Having a car to get to work is a necessity for many workers. When two crucial employees of Vurv Technology in Jacksonville, Florida, had trouble getting to work, owner Derek Mercer decided to buy two inexpensive used cars for the employees. One of the employees who got one of the cars said it wasn't the nicest or prettiest car, but it gave him such a sense of relief to know that he had a reliable way to get to work. So when the company needed him to work hard, he was willing to do so.[8] Derek Mercer understands employee needs and their impact on motivation. The first motivation theory we're going to look at addresses employee needs.

The best-known theory of motivation is probably Abraham Maslow's **hierarchy of needs theory**.[9] Maslow was a psychologist who proposed that within every person is a hierarchy of five needs:

1. **Physiological needs**: A person's needs for food, drink, shelter, sex, and other physical requirements.
2. **Safety needs**: A person's needs for security and protection from physical and emotional harm as well as assurance that physical needs will continue to be met.

---

motivation
The process by which a person's efforts are energized, directed, and sustained toward attaining a goal

Motivators for employees of Procter & Gamble's factory in Urlati, Romania, include satisfying their lower-order needs of a salary, a safe job, benefits, and job security. According to Maslow's hierarchy of needs theory, after these needs are met, managers can motivate them by forming work groups and giving them opportunities for socializing to satisfy their needs of friendship and belongingness.
Source: Aga Luczakowska/Bloomberg/Getty Images

hierarchy of needs theory
Maslow's theory that human needs—physiological, safety, social, esteem, and self-actualization—form a sort of hierarchy

physiological needs
A person's needs for food, drink, shelter, sexual satisfaction, and other physical needs

safety needs
A person's needs for security and protection from physical and emotional harm

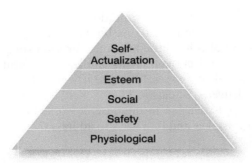

Exhibit 1

Maslow's Hierarchy of Needs

Source: A. H. Maslow, R. D. Frager, and J. Fadiman, *Motivation and Personality*, 3rd Edition, © 1987. Reprinted and electronically reproduced by permission of Pearson Education, Inc., Upper Saddle River, NJ.

3. **Social needs**: A person's needs for affection, belongingness, acceptance, and friendship.
4. **Esteem needs**: A person's needs for internal esteem factors such as self-respect, autonomy, and achievement and external esteem factors such as status, recognition, and attention.
5. **Self-actualization needs**: A person's needs for growth, achieving one's potential, and self-fulfillment; the drive to become what one is capable of becoming.

Maslow argued that each level in the needs hierarchy must be substantially satisfied before the next need becomes dominant. An individual moves up the needs hierarchy from one level to the next. (See Exhibit 1.) In addition, Maslow separated the five needs into higher and lower levels. Physiological and safety needs were considered *lower-order needs*; social, esteem, and self-actualization needs were considered *higher-order needs*. Lower-order needs are predominantly satisfied externally while higher-order needs are satisfied internally.

How does Maslow's theory explain motivation? Managers using Maslow's hierarchy to motivate employees do things to satisfy employees' needs. But the theory also says that once a need is substantially satisfied, an individual is no longer motivated to satisfy that need. Therefore, to motivate someone, you need to understand what need level that person is on in the hierarchy and focus on satisfying needs at or above that level.

Maslow's needs theory was widely recognized during the 1960s and 1970s, especially among practicing managers, probably because it was intuitively logical and easy to understand. But Maslow provided no empirical support for his theory, and several studies that sought to validate it could not.[10]

McGregor's Theory X and Theory Y

Andy Grove, cofounder of Intel Corporation and now a senior advisor to the company, was known for being open with his employees. However, he was also known for his tendency to yell. Intel's current CEO, Paul Otellini, said, "When Andy was yelling at you, it wasn't because he didn't care about you. He was yelling at you because he wanted you to do better."[11] Although managers like Andy Grove want their employees to do better, that approach might not have been the best way to motivate employees, as McGregor's Theory X and Theory Y suggest.

Douglas McGregor is best known for proposing two assumptions about human nature: Theory X and Theory Y.[12] Very simply, **Theory X** is a negative view of people that assumes workers have little ambition, dislike work, want to avoid responsibility, and need to be closely controlled to work effectively. **Theory Y** is a positive view that assumes employees enjoy work, seek out and accept responsibility, and exercise self-direction. McGregor believed that Theory Y assumptions should guide management practice and proposed that participation in decision making, responsible and challenging jobs, and good group relations would maximize employee motivation.

Unfortunately, no evidence confirms that either set of assumptions is valid or that being a Theory Y manager is the only way to motivate employees. For instance,

social needs

A person's needs for affection, belongingness, acceptance, and friendship

esteem needs

A person's needs for internal factors such as self-respect, autonomy, and achievement, and external factors such as status, recognition, and attention

self-actualization needs

A person's need to become what he or she is capable of becoming

Theory X

The assumption that employees dislike work, are lazy, avoid responsibility, and must be coerced to perform

Theory Y

The assumption that employees are creative, enjoy work, seek responsibility, and can exercise self-direction

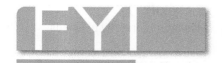

two-factor theory (motivation-hygiene theory)
The motivation theory that intrinsic factors are related to job satisfaction and motivation, whereas extrinsic factors are associated with job dissatisfaction

hygiene factors
Factors that eliminate job dissatisfaction, but don't motivate

motivators
Factors that increase job satisfaction and motivation

Jen-Hsun Huang, founder of Nvidia Corporation, an innovative and successful microchip manufacturer, has been known to use both reassuring hugs and tough love in motivating employees. He also has little tolerance for screw-ups. In one meeting, he supposedly screamed at a project team for its tendency to repeat mistakes. "Do you suck?" he asked the stunned employees. "Because if you suck, just get up and say you suck."[13] His message, delivered in classic Theory X style, was that if you need help, ask for it. It's a harsh approach, but in this case, it worked as employees knew they had to own up to their mistakes and find ways to address them.

Herzberg's Two-Factor Theory

Frederick Herzberg's **two-factor theory** (also called **motivation-hygiene theory**) proposes that intrinsic factors are related to job satisfaction, while extrinsic factors are associated with job dissatisfaction.[15] Herzberg wanted to know when people felt exceptionally good (satisfied) or bad (dissatisfied) about their jobs. (These findings are shown in Exhibit 2.) He concluded that the replies people gave when they felt good about their jobs were significantly different from the replies they gave when they felt badly. Certain characteristics were consistently related to job satisfaction (factors on the left side of the exhibit), and others to job dissatisfaction (factors on the right side). When people felt good about their work, they tended to cite intrinsic factors arising from the job itself such as achievement, recognition, and responsibility. On the other hand, when they were dissatisfied, they tended to cite extrinsic factors arising from the job context such as company policy and administration, supervision, interpersonal relationships, and working conditions.

In addition, Herzberg believed the data suggested that the opposite of satisfaction was not dissatisfaction, as traditionally had been believed. Removing dissatisfying characteristics from a job would not necessarily make that job more satisfying (or motivating). As shown in Exhibit 3, Herzberg proposed that a dual continuum existed: The opposite of "satisfaction" is "no satisfaction," and the opposite of "dissatisfaction" is "no dissatisfaction."

Again, Herzberg believed the factors that led to job satisfaction were separate and distinct from those that led to job dissatisfaction. Therefore, managers who sought to eliminate factors that created job dissatisfaction could keep people from being dissatisfied but not necessarily motivate them. The extrinsic factors that create job dissatisfaction were called **hygiene factors**. When these factors are adequate, people won't be dissatisfied, but they won't be satisfied (or motivated) either. To motivate people, Herzberg suggested emphasizing **motivators**, the intrinsic factors having to do with the job itself.

Herzberg's theory enjoyed wide popularity from the mid-1960s to the early 1980s, despite criticisms of his procedures and methodology. Although some critics said his theory was too simplistic, it has influenced how we currently design jobs, especially when it comes to job enrichment, which we'll discuss at a later point in this text.

Exhibit 2

Herzberg's Two-Factor Theory

Source: Based on F. Herzberg, B. Mausner, and B. B. Snyderman, *The Motivation to Work* (New York: John Wiley, 1959).

Motivators	**Hygiene Factors**
• Achievement	• Supervision
• Recognition	• Company Policy
• Work Itself	• Relationship with Supervisor
• Responsibility	• Working Conditions
• Advancement	• Salary
• Growth	• Relationship with Peers
	• Personal Life
	• Relationship with Subordinates
	• Status
	• Security

| Extremely Satisfied | Neutral | Extremely Dissatisfied |

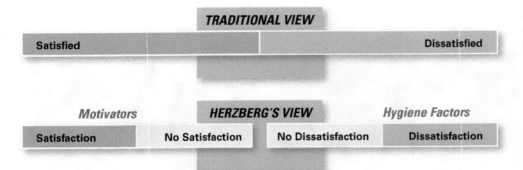

Exhibit 3
Contrasting Views of
Satisfaction–Dissatisfaction

If your professor has assigned this, go to **www.mymanagementlab.com** to watch a video titled: *Rudi's Bakery: Motivation* and to respond to questions.

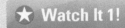

Three-Needs Theory

David McClelland and his associates proposed the **three-needs theory**, which says three acquired (not innate) needs are major motives in work.[16] These three are the **need for achievement (nAch)**, the drive to succeed and excel in relation to a set of standards; the **need for power (nPow)**, the need to make others behave in a way they would not have behaved otherwise; and the **need for affiliation (nAff)**, the desire for friendly and close interpersonal relationships. Of these three needs, the need for achievement has been researched the most.

People with a high need for achievement are striving for personal achievement rather than for the trappings and rewards of success. They have a desire to do something better or more efficiently than it's been done before.[17] They prefer jobs that offer personal responsibility for finding solutions to problems, in which they can receive rapid and unambiguous feedback on their performance in order to tell whether they're improving, and in which they can set moderately challenging goals. High achievers avoid what they perceive to be very easy or very difficult tasks. Also, a high need to achieve doesn't necessarily lead to being a good manager, especially in large organizations. That's because high achievers focus on their *own* accomplishments, while good managers emphasize helping *others* accomplish their goals.[18] McClelland showed that employees can be trained to stimulate their achievement need by being in situations where they have personal responsibility, feedback, and moderate risks.[19]

The other two needs in this theory haven't been researched as extensively as the need for achievement. However, we do know that the best managers tend to be high in the need for power and low in the need for affiliation.[20]

All three of these needs can be measured by using a projective test (known as the Thematic Apperception Test or TAT), in which respondents react to a set of pictures. Each picture is briefly shown to a person who writes a story based on the picture. (See Exhibit 4 on the next page for some examples.) Trained interpreters then determine the individual's levels of nAch, nPow, and nAff from the stories written.

three-needs theory
The motivation theory that says three acquired (not innate) needs—achievement, power, and affiliation—are major motives in work

need for achievement (nAch)
The drive to succeed and excel in relation to a set of standards

need for power (nPow)
The need to make others behave in a way that they would not have behaved otherwise

need for affiliation (nAff)
The desire for friendly and close interpersonal relationships

If your professor has assigned this, go to **www.mymanagementlab.com** to complete the Writing Assignment MGMT 14: Theories of Motivation.

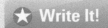

Exhibit 4
TAT Pictures

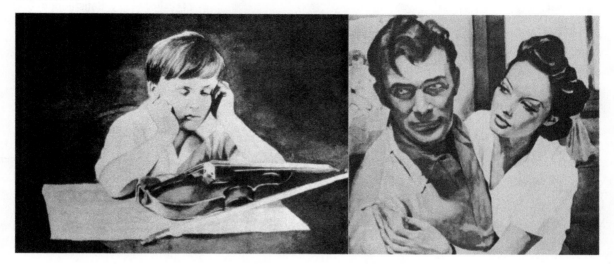

nAch: Indicated by someone in the story wanting to perform or do something better.
nAff: Indicated by someone in the story wanting to be with someone else and enjoy mutual friendship.
nPow: Indicated by someone in the story desiring to have an impact or make an impression on others in the story.

Photo Source: Bill Aron/PhotoEdit

CONTEMPORARY Theories of Motivation

LO3 The theories we look at in this section represent current explanations of employee motivation. Although these theories may not be as well known as those we just discussed, they are supported by research.[21] These contemporary motivation approaches include goal-setting theory, reinforcement theory, job design theory, equity theory, expectancy theory, and high-involvement work practices.

Goal-Setting Theory

At Wyeth's research division, scientists were given challenging new product quotas in an attempt to bring more efficiency to the innovation process, and their bonuses were contingent on meeting those goals.[22] Before a big assignment or major class project presentation, has a teacher ever encouraged you to "Just do your best"? What does that vague statement mean? Would your performance on a class project have been higher had that teacher said you needed to score a 93 percent to keep your A in the class? Research on goal-setting theory addresses these issues, and the findings, as you'll see, are impressive in terms of the effect that goal specificity, challenge, and feedback have on performance.[23]

Research provides substantial support for **goal-setting theory**, which says that specific goals increase performance and that difficult goals, when accepted, result in higher performance than do easy goals. What does goal-setting theory tell us?

First, working toward a goal is a major source of job motivation. Studies on goal setting have demonstrated that specific and challenging goals are superior motivating forces.[24] Such goals produce a higher output than the generalized goal of "do your best." The specificity of the goal itself acts as an internal stimulus. For instance, when a sales rep commits to making eight sales calls daily, this intention gives him a specific goal to try to attain.

It's not a contradiction that goal-setting theory says that motivation is maximized by *difficult* goals, whereas achievement motivation (from three-needs theory) is stimulated by *moderately challenging* goals.[25] First, goal-setting theory deals with people in general, whereas the conclusions on achievement motivation are based on people who

goal-setting theory
The proposition that specific goals increase performance and that difficult goals, when accepted, result in higher performance than do easy goals

have a high nAch. Given that no more than 10 to 20 percent of North Americans are high achievers (a proportion that's likely lower in underdeveloped countries), difficult goals are still recommended for the majority of employees. Second, the conclusions of goal-setting theory apply to those who accept and are committed to the goals. Difficult goals will lead to higher performance *only* if they are accepted.

Next, will employees try harder if they have the opportunity to participate in the setting of goals? Not always. In some cases, participants who actively set goals elicit superior performance; in other cases, individuals performed best when their manager assigned goals. However, participation is probably preferable to assigning goals when employees might resist accepting difficult challenges.[27]

Finally, we know people will do better if they get feedback on how well they're pro-

LEADER *making a* DIFFERENCE

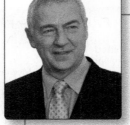

Source: Karl DeBlaker/AP Images

His privately held software company (the world's largest) has made Fortune magazine's list of "Best Companies to Work For" for all 15 years that it's been published.[26] *"He" is Jim Goodnight, CEO and cofounder of Cary, North Carolina–based SAS. Goodnight has always believed in taking care of his employees. His company's approach to giving employees flexibility and perks is "so legendary that even Google uses SAS as a model." Goodnight fashioned SAS's culture around the idea of "trust between our employees and the company." And employees love it! Annual turnover is a low 3.6 percent, and the company is highly profitable. There's something to be said for recognizing that your employees are your most important asset!* What can you learn from this leader making a difference?

gressing toward their goals because feedback helps identify discrepancies between what they have done and what they want to do. But all feedback isn't equally effective. Self-generated feedback—where an employee monitors his or her own progress—has been shown to be a more powerful motivator than feedback coming from someone else.[28]

Three other contingencies besides feedback influence the goal-performance relationship: goal commitment, adequate self-efficacy, and national culture.

First, goal-setting theory assumes an individual is committed to the goal. Commitment is most likely when goals are made public, when the individual has an internal locus of control, and when the goals are self-set rather than assigned.[29]

Next, **self-efficacy** refers to an individual's belief that he or she is capable of performing a task.[30] The higher your self-efficacy, the more confidence you have in your ability to succeed in a task. So, in difficult situations, we find that people with low self-efficacy are likely to reduce their effort or give up altogether, whereas those with high self-efficacy will try harder to master the challenge.[31] In addition, individuals with high self-efficacy seem to respond to negative feedback with increased effort and motivation, whereas those with low self-efficacy are likely to reduce their effort when given negative feedback.[32]

self-efficacy
An individual's belief that he or she is capable of performing a task

Finally, the value of goal-setting theory depends on the national culture. It's well adapted to North American countries because its main ideas align reasonably well with those cultures. It assumes that subordinates will be reasonably independent (not a high score on power distance), that people will seek challenging goals (low in uncertainty avoidance), and that performance is considered important by both managers and subordinates (high in assertiveness). Don't expect goal setting to lead to higher employee performance in countries where the cultural characteristics aren't like this.

Exhibit 5 summarizes the relationships among goals, motivation, and performance. Our overall conclusion is that the intention to work toward hard and specific goals is a powerful motivating force. Under the proper conditions, it can lead to higher performance. However, no evidence indicates that such goals are associated with increased job satisfaction.[33]

Reinforcement Theory

Reinforcement theory says that behavior is a function of its consequences. Those consequences that immediately follow a behavior and increase the probability that the behavior will be repeated are called **reinforcers**.

reinforcement theory
The theory that behavior is a function of its consequences

reinforcers
Consequences immediately following a behavior, which increase the probability that the behavior will be repeated

Exhibit 5
Goal-Setting Theory

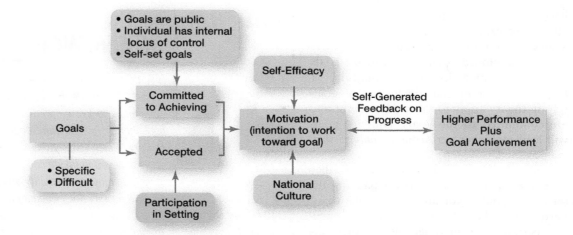

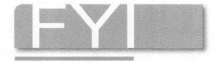

job design
The way tasks are combined to form complete jobs

job scope
The number of different tasks required in a job and the frequency with which those tasks are repeated

job enlargement
The horizontal expansion of a job by increasing job scope

job enrichment
The vertical expansion of a job by adding planning and evaluating responsibilities

Reinforcement theory ignores factors such as goals, expectations, and needs. Instead, it focuses solely on what happens to a person when he or she does something. For instance, Walmart improved its bonus program for hourly employees. Employees who provide outstanding customer service get a cash bonus. And all Walmart hourly full- and part-time store employees are eligible for annual "My$hare" bonuses, which are allocated on store performance and distributed quarterly so that workers are rewarded more frequently.[34] The company's intent: keep the workforce motivated to meet goals by rewarding them when they did, thus reinforcing the behaviors.

Managers use reinforcers to shape behavior, but the concept is also widely believed to explain motivation. According to B. F. Skinner, people will most likely engage in desired behaviors if they are rewarded for doing so. These rewards are most effective if they immediately follow a desired behavior; and behavior that isn't rewarded, or is punished, is less likely to be repeated.[35]

Using reinforcement theory, managers can influence employees' behavior by using positive reinforcers for actions that help the organization achieve its goals. And managers should ignore, not punish, undesirable behavior. Although punishment eliminates undesired behavior faster than nonreinforcement, its effect is often temporary and may have unpleasant side effects, including dysfunctional behavior such as workplace conflicts, absenteeism, and turnover. Although reinforcement is an important influence on work behavior, it isn't the only explanation for differences in employee motivation.[36]

Designing Motivating Jobs

It's not unusual to find shop-floor workers at Cordis LLC's San German, Puerto Rico, facility interacting directly with customers, especially if that employee has special skills or knowledge that could help come up with a solution to a customer's problem.[38] One company executive said, "Our sales guys often encourage this in specific situations because they don't always have all the answers. If by doing this, we can better serve the customers, then we do it." As this example shows, the tasks an employee performs in his or her job are often determined by different factors, such as providing customers what they need—when they need it.

Because managers want to motivate individuals on the job, we need to look at ways to design motivating jobs. If you look closely at what an organization is and how it works, you'll find that it's composed of thousands of tasks. These tasks are, in turn, aggregated into jobs. We use the term **job design** to refer to the way tasks are combined to form complete jobs. The jobs people perform in an organization should not evolve by chance. Managers should design jobs deliberately and thoughtfully to reflect the demands of the changing environment; the organization's technology;

and employees' skills, abilities, and preferences.[39] When jobs are designed like that, employees are motivated to work hard. Let's look at some ways that managers can design motivating jobs.[40]

JOB ENLARGEMENT Job design historically has been to make jobs smaller and more specialized. It's difficult to motivate employees when jobs are like this. An early effort at overcoming the drawbacks of job specialization involved horizontally expanding a job through increasing **job scope**—the number of different tasks required in a job and the frequency with which these tasks are repeated. For instance, a dental hygienist's job could be enlarged so that in addition to cleaning teeth, he or she is pulling patients' files, refiling them when finished, and sanitizing and storing instruments. This type of job design option is called **job enlargement**.

Most job enlargement efforts that focused solely on increasing the number of tasks don't seem to work. As one employee who experienced such a job redesign said, "Before, I had one lousy job. Now, thanks to job enlargement, I have three lousy jobs!" However, research has shown that *knowledge* enlargement activities (expanding the scope of knowledge used in a job) lead to more job satisfaction, enhanced customer service, and fewer errors.[41]

JOB ENRICHMENT Another approach to job design is the vertical expansion of a job by adding planning and evaluating responsibilities—**job enrichment**. Job enrichment increases **job depth**, which is the degree of control employees have over their work. In other words, employees are empowered to assume some of the tasks typically done by their managers. Thus, an enriched job allows workers to do an entire activity with increased freedom, independence, and responsibility. In addition, workers get feedback so they can assess and correct their own performance. For instance, if our dental hygienist had an enriched job, he or she could, in addition to cleaning teeth, schedule appointments (planning) and follow up with clients (evaluating). Although job enrichment may improve the quality of work, employee motivation, and satisfaction, research evidence has been inconclusive as to its usefulness.[42]

JOB CHARACTERISTICS MODEL Even though many organizations implemented job enlargement and job enrichment programs and experienced mixed results, neither approach provided an effective framework for managers to design motivating jobs. But the **job characteristics model (JCM)** does.[43] It identifies five core job dimensions, their interrelationships, and their impact on employee productivity, motivation, and satisfaction. These five core job dimensions are:

1. **Skill variety**, the degree to which a job requires a variety of activities so that an employee can use a number of different skills and talents.
2. **Task identity**, the degree to which a job requires completion of a whole and identifiable piece of work.
3. **Task significance**, the degree to which a job has a substantial impact on the lives or work of other people.
4. **Autonomy**, the degree to which a job provides substantial freedom, independence, and discretion to the individual in scheduling the work and determining the procedures to be used in carrying it out.
5. **Feedback**, the degree to which doing work activities required by a job results in an individual obtaining direct and clear information about the effectiveness of his or her performance.

The JCM is shown in Exhibit 6. Notice how the first three dimensions—skill variety, task identity, and task significance—combine to create meaningful work. In other words, if these three characteristics exist in a job, we can predict that the person will view his or her job as being important, valuable, and worthwhile. Notice, too, that jobs that possess autonomy give the jobholder a feeling of personal

job depth
The degree of control employees have over their work

job characteristics model (JCM)
A framework for analyzing and designing jobs that identifies five primary core job dimensions, their interrelationships, and their impact on outcomes

skill variety
The degree to which a job requires a variety of activities so that an employee can use a number of different skills and talents

task identity
The degree to which a job requires completion of a whole and identifiable piece of work

task significance
The degree to which a job has a substantial impact on the lives or work of other people

autonomy
The degree to which a job provides substantial freedom, independence, and discretion to the individual in scheduling work and determining the procedures to be used in carrying it out

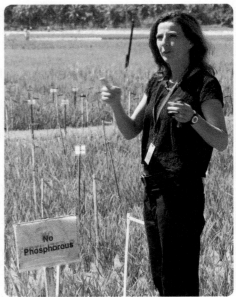

Dr. Sigrid Heuer, a senior scientist at the International Rice Research Institute, leads a multidisciplinary team of scientists whose work scores high in skill variety, task identity, and task significance. The team discovered a gene that increases grain production and helps poor rice farmers grow more rice for sale to poor countries. Meaningful work gives these scientists great motivation and job satisfaction.
Source: Cheryl Ravelo/Reuters Pictures

Exhibit 6
Job Characteristics Model

Source: "Job Characteristics Model," from *Work Redesign*, by J. R. Hackman & G. R. Oldham. Copyright © 1980 by Addison-Wesley (a division of Pearson). Reprinted with permission.

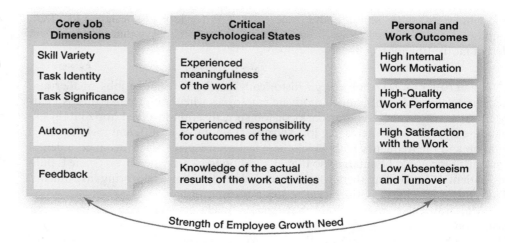

feedback

The degree to which carrying out work activities required by a job results in the individual's obtaining direct and clear information about his or her performance effectiveness

responsibility for the results and that if a job provides feedback, the employee will know how effectively he or she is performing.

The JCM suggests that employees are likely to be motivated when they *learn* (knowledge of results through feedback) that they *personally* (experienced responsibility through autonomy of work) performed well on tasks that they *care about* (experienced meaningfulness through skill variety, task identity, or task significance).[44] The more a job is designed around these three elements, the greater the employee's motivation, performance, and satisfaction and the lower his or her absenteeism and likelihood of resigning. As the model shows, the links between the job dimensions and the outcomes are moderated by the strength of the individual's growth need (the person's desire for self-esteem and self-actualization). Individuals with a high growth need are more likely than low-growth need individuals to experience the critical psychological states and respond positively when their jobs include the core dimensions. This distinction may explain the mixed results with job enrichment: Individuals with low growth need aren't likely to achieve high performance or satisfaction by having their jobs enriched.

The JCM provides specific guidance to managers for job design. These suggestions specify the types of changes most likely to lead to improvement in the five core job dimensions. You'll notice that two suggestions incorporate job enlargement and job enrichment, although the other suggestions involve more than vertical and horizontal expansion of jobs.

1. *Combine tasks.* Put fragmented tasks back together to form a new, larger work module (job enlargement) to increase skill variety and task identity.
2. *Create natural work units.* Design tasks that form an identifiable and meaningful whole to increase employee "ownership" of the work. Encourage employees to view their work as meaningful and important rather than as irrelevant and boring.
3. *Establish client (external or internal) relationships.* Whenever possible, establish direct relationships between workers and their clients to increase skill variety, autonomy, and feedback.
4. *Expand jobs vertically.* Vertical expansion gives employees responsibilities and controls that were formerly reserved for managers, which can increase employee autonomy.
5. *Open feedback channels.* Direct feedback lets employees know how well they're performing their jobs and whether their performance is improving or not.

Research into the JCM continues. For instance, one recent study looked at using job redesign efforts to change job characteristics and improve employee well-being.[45] Another study examined psychological ownership—that is, a personal feeling of "mine-ness" or "our-ness"—and its role in the JCM.[46]

REDESIGNING JOB DESIGN APPROACHES[47]   Although the JCM has proven to be useful, it may not be totally appropriate for today's jobs that are more service and knowledge-oriented. The nature of these jobs has also changed the tasks that employees do in those jobs. Two emerging viewpoints on job design are causing a rethink of the JCM and other standard approaches. Let's take a look at each perspective.

The first perspective, the **relational perspective of work design**, focuses on how people's tasks and jobs are increasingly based on social relationships. In jobs today, employees have more interactions and interdependence with coworkers and others both inside and outside the organization. In doing their job, employees rely more and more on those around them for information, advice, and assistance. So what does this mean for designing motivating jobs? It means that managers need to look at important components of those employee relationships such as access to and level of social support in an organization, types of interactions outside an organization, amount of task interdependence, and interpersonal feedback.

The second perspective, the **proactive perspective of work design**, says that employees are taking the initiative to change how their work is performed. They're much more involved in decisions and actions that affect their work. Important job design factors according to this perspective include autonomy (which *is* part of the JCM), amount of ambiguity and accountability, job complexity, level of stressors, and social or relationship context. Each of these has been shown to influence employee proactive behavior.

One stream of research that's relevant to proactive work design is **high-involvement work practices**, which are designed to elicit greater input or involvement from workers.[48] The level of employee proactivity is believed to increase as employees become more involved in decisions that affect their work. Another term for this approach is employee empowerment.

Equity Theory

Do you ever wonder what kind of grade the person sitting next to you in class makes on a test or on a major class assignment? Most of us do! Being human, we tend to compare ourselves with others. If someone offered you $50,000 a year on your first job after graduating from college, you'd probably jump at the offer and report to work enthusiastic, ready to tackle whatever needed to be done, and certainly satisfied with your pay. How would you react, though, if you found out a month into the job that a coworker—another recent graduate, your age, with comparable grades from a comparable school, and with comparable work experience—was getting $55,000 a year? You'd probably be upset! Even though in absolute terms, $50,000 is a lot of money for a new graduate to make (and you know it!), that suddenly isn't the issue. Now you see the issue as what you believe is *fair*—what is *equitable*. The term *equity* is related to the concept of fairness and equitable treatment compared with others who behave in similar ways. Evidence indicates that employees compare themselves to others and that inequities influence how much effort employees exert.[50]

Equity theory, developed by J. Stacey Adams, proposes that employees compare what they get from a job (outcomes) in relation to what they put into it (inputs), and then they compare their inputs–outcomes ratio with the inputs–outcomes ratios of relevant others (Exhibit 7). If an employee perceives her ratio to be equitable in comparison to those of relevant others, there's no problem. However, if the ratio is inequitable, she views herself as underrewarded or overrewarded. When inequities occur, employees attempt to do something about it.[51] The result might be lower or higher productivity, improved or reduced quality of output, increased absenteeism, or voluntary resignation.

The **referent**—the other persons, systems, or selves individuals compare themselves against in order to assess equity—is an important variable in equity theory.[52] Each of the three referent categories is important. The "persons" category includes other individuals with similar jobs in the same organization but also includes friends,

relational perspective of work design
An approach to job design that focuses on how people's tasks and jobs are increasingly based on social relationships

proactive perspective of work design
An approach to job design in which employees take the initiative to change how their work is performed

high-involvement work practices
Work practices designed to elicit greater input or involvement from workers

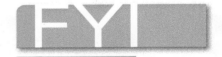

- 92 percent of executives believe that favoritism is used in promotion decisions.[49]

equity theory
The theory that an employee compares his or her job's input–outcomes ratio with that of relevant others and then corrects any inequity

referents
The persons, systems, or selves against which individuals compare themselves to assess equity

Exhibit 7
Equity Theory

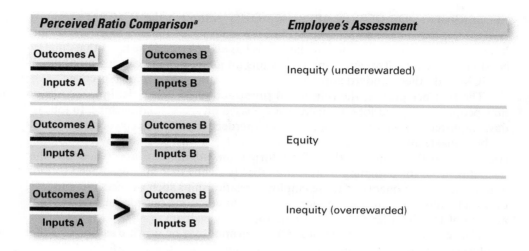

Perceived Ratio Comparison[a]		Employee's Assessment
$\dfrac{\text{Outcomes A}}{\text{Inputs A}} < \dfrac{\text{Outcomes B}}{\text{Inputs B}}$		Inequity (underrewarded)
$\dfrac{\text{Outcomes A}}{\text{Inputs A}} = \dfrac{\text{Outcomes B}}{\text{Inputs B}}$		Equity
$\dfrac{\text{Outcomes A}}{\text{Inputs A}} > \dfrac{\text{Outcomes B}}{\text{Inputs B}}$		Inequity (overrewarded)

distributive justice
Perceived fairness of the amount and allocation of rewards among individuals

procedural justice
Perceived fairness of the process used to determine the distribution of rewards

expectancy theory
The theory that an individual tends to act in a certain way based on the expectation that the act will be followed by a given outcome and on the attractiveness of that outcome to the individual

neighbors, or professional associates. Based on what they hear at work or read about in newspapers or trade journals, employees compare their pay with that of others. The "system" category includes organizational pay policies, procedures, and allocation. The "self" category refers to inputs–outcomes ratios that are unique to the individual. It reflects past personal experiences and contacts and is influenced by criteria such as past jobs or family commitments.

Originally, equity theory focused on **distributive justice**, the perceived fairness of the amount and allocation of rewards among individuals. More recent research has focused on looking at issues of **procedural justice**, the perceived fairness of the process used to determine the distribution of rewards. This research shows that distributive justice has a greater influence on employee satisfaction than procedural justice, while procedural justice tends to affect an employee's organizational commitment, trust in his or her boss, and intention to quit.[53] What are the implications for managers? They should consider openly sharing information on how allocation decisions are made, follow consistent and unbiased procedures, and engage in similar practices to increase the perception of procedural justice. By increasing the perception of procedural justice, employees are likely to view their bosses and the organization as positive even if they're dissatisfied with pay, promotions, and other personal outcomes.

Expectancy Theory

The most comprehensive explanation of how employees are motivated is Victor Vroom's **expectancy theory**.[54] Although the theory has its critics,[55] most research evidence supports it.[56]

Expectancy theory states that an individual tends to act in a certain way based on the expectation that the act will be followed by a given outcome and on the attractiveness of that outcome to the individual. It includes three variables or relationships (see Exhibit 8):

1. *Expectancy* or *effort–performance linkage* is the probability perceived by the individual that exerting a given amount of effort will lead to a certain level of performance.
2. *Instrumentality* or *performance–reward linkage* is the degree to which the individual believes that performing at a particular level is instrumental in attaining the desired outcome.
3. *Valence* or *attractiveness of reward* is the importance an individual places on the potential outcome or reward that can be achieved on the job. Valence considers both the goals and needs of the individual.

This explanation of motivation might sound complicated, but it really isn't. It can be summed up in the questions: How hard do I have to work to achieve a certain

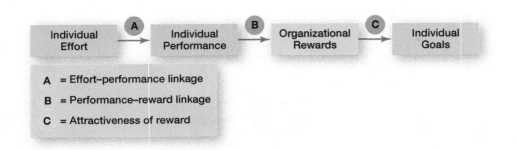

Exhibit 8
Expectancy Model

A = Effort–performance linkage

B = Performance–reward linkage

C = Attractiveness of reward

level of performance, and can I actually achieve that level? What reward will performing at that level of performance get me? How attractive is the reward to me, and does it help me achieve my own personal goals? Whether you are motivated to put forth effort (that is, to work hard) at any given time depends on your goals and your perception of whether a certain level of performance is necessary to attain those goals. Let's look at an example. Your second author had a student many years ago who went to work for IBM as a sales rep. Her favorite work "reward" was having an IBM corporate jet fly into Springfield, Missouri, to pick up her best customers and her and take them for a weekend of golfing at some fun location. But to get that particular "reward," she had to achieve at a certain level of performance, which involved exceeding her sales goals by a specified percentage. How hard she was willing to work (that is, how motivated she was to put forth effort) was dependent on the level of performance that had to be met and the likelihood that if she achieved at that level of performance she would receive that reward. Because she "valued" that reward, she always worked hard to exceed her sales goals. And the performance–reward linkage was clear because her hard work and performance achievements were always rewarded by the company with the reward she valued (access to the corporate jet).

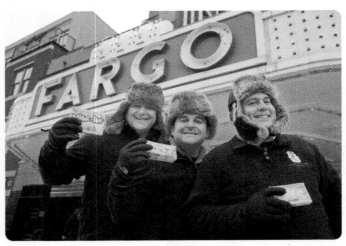

Just Born candy company—makers of Peeps and Mike and Ike brands—uses expectancy theory in motivating employees to achieve annual sales goals. Sales team members shown here expected their efforts would result in winning an all-expense paid trip to Hawaii. But they failed to meet their goal and instead earned jackets and bomber hats and a trip to Fargo, North Dakota.
Source: AP Photo/Ann Arbor Miller

The key to expectancy theory is understanding an individual's goal and the linkage between effort and performance, between performance and rewards, and finally, between rewards and individual goal satisfaction. It emphasizes payoffs, or rewards. As a result, we have to believe that the rewards an organization is offering align with what the individual wants. Expectancy theory recognizes that no universal principle explains what motivates individuals and thus stresses that managers understand why employees view certain outcomes as attractive or unattractive. After all, we want to reward individuals with those things they value positively. Also, expectancy theory emphasizes expected behaviors. Do employees know what is expected of them and how they'll be evaluated? Finally, the theory is concerned with perceptions. Reality is irrelevant. An individual's own perceptions of performance, reward, and goal outcomes—not the outcomes themselves—will determine his or her motivation (level of effort).

Integrating Contemporary Theories of Motivation

Many of the ideas underlying the contemporary motivation theories are complementary, and you'll understand better how to motivate people if you see how the theories fit together.[57] Exhibit 9 presents a model that integrates much of what we know about motivation. Its basic foundation is the expectancy model. Let's work through the model, starting on the left.

The individual effort box has an arrow leading into it. This arrow flows from the individual's goals. Consistent with goal-setting theory, this goals–effort link is meant to illustrate that goals direct behavior. Expectancy theory predicts that an employee will exert a high level of effort if he or she perceives a strong relationship

Exhibit 9

Integrating Contemporary Theories
of Motivation

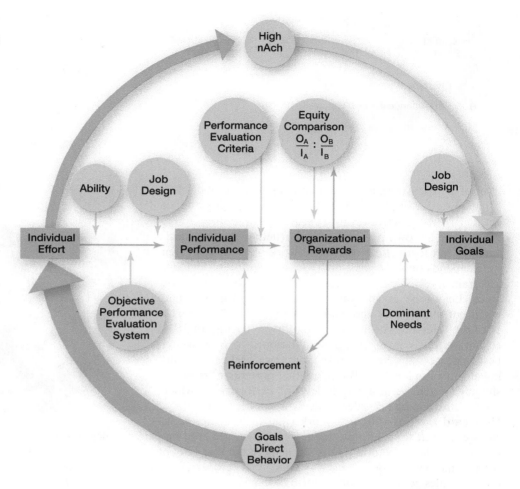

between effort and performance, performance and rewards, and rewards and satisfaction of personal goals. Each of these relationships is in turn influenced by certain factors. You can see from the model that the level of individual performance is determined not only by the level of individual effort but also by the individual's ability to perform and by whether the organization has a fair and objective performance evaluation system. The performance–reward relationship will be strong if the individual perceives that performance (rather than seniority, personal favorites, or some other criterion) is what is rewarded. The final link in expectancy theory is the rewards–goal relationship. The traditional need theories come into play at this point. Motivation would be high to the degree that the rewards an individual received for his or her high performance satisfied the dominant needs consistent with his or her individual goals.

A closer look at the model also shows that it considers the achievement–need, reinforcement, equity, and JCM theories. The high achiever isn't motivated by the organization's assessment of his or her performance or organizational rewards; hence the jump from effort to individual goals for those with a high nAch. Remember that high achievers are internally driven as long as the jobs they're doing provide them with personal responsibility, feedback, and moderate risks. They're not concerned with the effort–performance, performance–reward, or rewards–goals linkages.

Reinforcement theory is seen in the model by recognizing that the organization's rewards reinforce the individual's performance. If managers have designed a reward system that is seen by employees as "paying off" for good performance, the rewards will reinforce and encourage continued good performance. Rewards also play a key part in equity theory. Individuals will compare the rewards (outcomes) they have

let's get REAL

The Scenario:

Sam Grisham is the plant manager at a bathroom vanity manufacturer. When business is brisk, employees have to work overtime to meet customers' demands. Aside from a few people, he has a horrible time getting employees to work overtime. "I practically have to beg for volunteers."

What suggestions do you have for Sam?

As plant manager, I would rotate the overtime for all employees. During busy times, everyone must chip in. I would also suggest implementing mandatory overtime for employees according to seniority in order to keep it fair.

Oscar Valencia
Manufacturing Manager

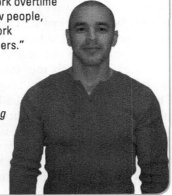

received from the inputs or efforts they made with the inputs–outcomes ratio of relevant others. If inequities exist, the effort expended may be influenced.

Finally, the JCM is seen in this integrative model. Task characteristics (job design) influence job motivation at two places. First, jobs designed around the five job dimensions are likely to lead to higher actual job performance because the individual's motivation will be stimulated by the job itself—that is, they will increase the linkage between effort and performance. Second, jobs designed around the five job dimensions also increase an employee's control over key elements in his or her work. Therefore, jobs that offer autonomy, feedback, and similar task characteristics help to satisfy the individual goals of employees who desire greater control over their work.

If your professor has assigned this, go to **www.mymanagementlab.com** to complete the Simulation: Motivation and get a better understanding of the challenges of knowing how to motivate employees.

CURRENT Issues in Motivation

L04 After Vincent Stevens's church ran an experiment in which 10 members were each given $100 to help their communities, some used it as seed capital to raise thousands more. As a partner in a Bellevue, Washington, accounting firm, he wondered what would happen if he tried the same thing with his employees. To find out, his company launched Caring, Serving, and Giving—a program that lets employees apply for grants of up to $500 to fund community service projects. By empowering employees to use the seed money as they saw fit, they were motivated to make the best use of it. Another benefit was a boost in employee morale.[58]

Understanding and predicting employee motivation is one of the most popular areas in management research. We've introduced you to several motivation theories. However, even the contemporary theories of employee motivation are influenced by some significant workplace issues—motivating in tough economic circumstances, managing cross-cultural challenges, motivating unique groups of workers, and designing appropriate rewards programs.

Motivating in Challenging Economic Circumstances

Zappos, the quirky Las Vegas–based online shoe retailer, has always had a reputation for being a fun place to work.[59] However, during the last economic recession, it, like many companies, had to cut staff—124 employees in total. CEO Tony Hsieh wanted to get out the news fast to lessen the stress for his employees. So he announced the layoff in an e-mail, on his blog, and on his Twitter account. Although some might think these are terrible ways to communicate that kind of news, most employees thanked him for being so open and so honest. The company also took good care of those who were laid off. Laid-off employees with less than two years of service were paid through the end of the year. Longer-tenured employees got four weeks for every year of service. All got six months of continued paid health coverage and, at the request of the employees, got to keep their 40 percent merchandise discount through the Christmas season. Zappos had always been a model of how to nurture employees in good times; now it showed how to treat employees in bad times.

The last economic recession was difficult for many organizations, especially when it came to their employees. Layoffs, tight budgets, minimal or no pay raises, benefit cuts, no bonuses, long hours doing the work of those who had been laid off—this was the reality that many employees faced. As conditions deteriorated, employee confidence, optimism, and job engagement plummeted as well. As you can imagine, it wasn't an easy thing for managers to keep employees motivated under such challenging circumstances.

Managers came to realize that in an uncertain economy, they had to be creative in keeping their employees' efforts energized, directed, and sustained toward achieving goals. They were forced to look at ways to motivate employees that didn't involve money or that were relatively inexpensive.[61] So they relied on actions such as holding meetings with employees to keep the lines of communication open and to get their input on issues; establishing a common goal, such as maintaining excellent customer service, to keep everyone focused; creating a community feel so employees could see that managers cared about them and their work; and giving employees opportunities to continue to learn and grow. And, of course, an encouraging word always went a long way.

Managing Cross-Cultural Motivational Challenges

Scores of employees at Denmark's largest brewer, Carlsberg A/S, walked off their jobs in protest after the company tightened rules on workplace drinking and removed beer coolers from work sites.[62] Now that's a motivational challenge you don't often see in U.S. workplaces!

In today's global business environment, managers can't automatically assume motivational programs that work in one geographic location are going to work in others. Most current motivation theories were developed in the United States by Americans and about Americans.[63] Maybe the most blatant pro-American characteristic in these theories is the strong emphasis on individualism and achievement. For instance, both goal-setting and expectancy theories emphasize goal accomplishment as well as rational and individual thought. Let's look at the motivation theories to see their level of cross-cultural transferability.

Maslow's needs hierarchy argues that people start at the physiological level and then move progressively up the hierarchy in order. This hierarchy, if it has any application at all, aligns with American culture. In countries like Japan, Greece, and Mexico, where uncertainty avoidance characteristics are strong, security needs would be the foundational layer of the needs hierarchy. Countries that score high on nurturing characteristics—Denmark, Sweden, Norway, the Netherlands, and Finland—would have social needs as their foundational level.[64] We would predict, for instance, that group work will be more motivating when the country's culture scores high on the nurturing criterion.

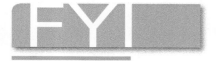

- 48 percent of employees say that a good manager motivates them to stay at their job;
- 46 percent of employees say it's feeling appreciated by a supervisor or employer.[60]

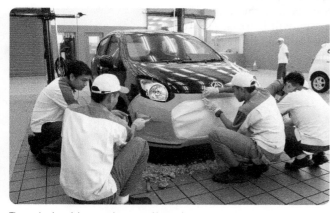

The motivation of these employees working at the research and development facility at the Daihatsu Motor plant near Jakarta, Indonesia, is influenced by their national culture. Indonesia has a strong collectivist culture, where employees are motivated less by receiving individual praise because their culture places a greater emphasis on harmony, belonging, and consensus.
Source: Kyodo/Newscom

Another motivation concept that clearly has an American bias is the achievement need. The view that a high achievement need acts as an internal motivator presupposes two cultural characteristics—a willingness to accept a moderate degree of risk (which excludes countries with strong uncertainty avoidance characteristics) and a concern with performance (which applies almost singularly to countries with strong achievement characteristics). This combination is found in Anglo-American countries such as the United States, Canada, and Great Britain.[65] On the other hand, these characteristics are relatively absent in countries such as Chile and Portugal.

Equity theory has a relatively strong following in the United States, which is not surprising given that U.S.-style reward systems are based on the assumption that workers are highly sensitive to equity in reward allocations. In the United States, equity is meant to closely link pay to performance. However, recent evidence suggests that in collectivist cultures, especially in the former socialist countries of Central and Eastern Europe, employees expect rewards to reflect their individual needs as well as their performance.[66] Moreover, consistent with a legacy of communism and centrally planned economies, employees exhibited a greater "entitlement" attitude—that is, they expected outcomes to be greater than their inputs.[67] These findings suggest that U.S.-style pay practices may need to be modified in some countries in order to be perceived as fair by employees.

Another research study of more than 50,000 employees around the world examined two cultural characteristics from the GLOBE framework—individualism and masculinity—in relation to motivation.[68] The researchers found that in individualistic cultures such as the United States and Canada, individual initiative, individual freedom, and individual achievement are highly valued. In more collective cultures such as Iran, Peru, and China, however, employees may be less interested in receiving individual praise but place a greater emphasis on harmony, belonging, and consensus. They also found that in masculine (achievement/assertive) cultures such as Japan and Slovakia, the focus is on material success. Those work environments are designed to push employees hard and then reward top performers with high earnings. However, in more feminine (nurturing) cultures such as Sweden and the Netherlands, smaller wage gaps among employees are common, and employees are likely to have extensive quality-of-life benefits.

Despite these cross-cultural differences in motivation, some cross-cultural consistencies are evident. In a recent study of employees in 13 countries, the top motivators included (ranked from number one on down): being treated with respect, work-life balance, the type of work done, the quality of people worked with and the quality of the organization's leadership (tied), base pay, working in an environment where good service can be provided to others, long-term career potential, flexible working arrangements, learning and development opportunities and benefits (tied), promotion opportunities, and incentive pay or bonus.[69] And other studies have shown that the desire for interesting work seems important to almost all workers, regardless of their national culture. For instance, employees in Belgium, Britain, Israel, and the United States ranked "interesting work" number one among 11 work goals. It was ranked either second or third in Japan, the Netherlands, and Germany.[70] Similarly, in a study comparing job-preference outcomes among graduate students in the United States, Canada, Australia, and Singapore, growth, achievement, and responsibility were rated the top three and had identical rankings.[71] Both studies suggest some universality to the importance of intrinsic factors identified by Herzberg in his two-factor theory. Another recent study examining workplace motivation trends in Japan also seems to indicate that Herzberg's model is applicable to Japanese employees.[72]

Motivating Unique Groups of Workers

At Deloitte, employees are allowed to "dial up" or "dial down" their job responsibilities to fit their personal and professional goals.[73] The company's program called Mass Career Customization has been a huge hit with its employees! In the first 12 months

after it was rolled out, employee satisfaction with "overall career/life fit" rose by 25 percent. Also, the number of high-performing employees staying with Deloitte increased.

Motivating employees has never been easy! Employees come into organizations with different needs, personalities, skills, abilities, interests, and aptitudes. They have different expectations of their employers and different views of what they think their employer has a right to expect of them. And they vary widely in what they want from their jobs. For instance, some employees get more satisfaction out of their personal interests and pursuits and only want a weekly paycheck—nothing more. They're not interested in making their work more challenging or interesting or in "winning" performance contests. Others derive a great deal of satisfaction in their jobs and are motivated to exert high levels of effort. Given these differences, how can managers do an effective job of motivating the unique groups of employees found in today's workforce? One thing is to understand the motivational requirements of these groups, including diverse employees, professionals, contingent workers, and low-skilled minimum-wage employees.

MOTIVATING A DIVERSE WORKFORCE To maximize motivation among today's workforce, managers need to think in terms of *flexibility*. For instance, studies tell us that men place more importance on having autonomy in their jobs than women. In contrast, the opportunity to learn, convenient and flexible work hours, and good interpersonal relations are more important to women.[74] Having the opportunity to be independent and to be exposed to different experiences is important to Gen Y employees, whereas older workers may be more interested in highly structured work opportunities.[75] Managers need to recognize that what motivates a single mother with two dependent children who's working full time to support her family may be very different from the needs of a single part-time employee or an older employee who is working only to supplement his or her retirement income. A diverse array of rewards is needed to motivate employees with such diverse needs. Many of the work–life balance programs that organizations have implemented are a response to the varied needs of a diverse workforce. In addition, many organizations have developed flexible work arrangements—such as compressed workweeks, flextime, and job sharing—that recognize different needs. Another job alternative is telecommuting. However, keep in mind that not all employees embrace the idea of telecommuting. Some workers relish the informal interactions at work that satisfy their social needs and are a source of new ideas.

FUTURE VISION | Individualized Rewards

Organizations have historically assumed that "one size fits all" when it comes to allocating rewards. Managers typically assumed that everyone wants more money and more vacation time. But as organizations become less bureaucratic and more capable of differentiating rewards, managers will be encouraged to differentiate rewards among employees as well as for individual employees over time.

Organizations control a vast number of potential rewards that employees might find appealing. A partial list would include increased base pay, bonuses, shortened workweeks, extended vacations, paid sabbaticals, flexible work hours, part-time employment, guaranteed job security, increased pension contributions, college tuition reimbursement, personal days off, help in purchasing a home, recognition awards, paid club memberships, and work-from-home options. In the future, most organizations will structure individual reward packages in ways that will maximize employee motivation.

If your professor has chosen to assign this, go to **www.mymanagementlab.com** *to discuss the following questions.*

⭐ **TALK ABOUT IT 1:** What are the positive aspects of having individualized rewards? (Think in terms of employees and managers.)

⭐ **TALK ABOUT IT 2:** What are the negative aspects of having individualized rewards? (Again, think in terms of employees and managers.)

Do flexible work arrangements motivate employees? Although such arrangements might seem highly motivational, both positive and negative relationships have been found. For instance, a recent study that looked at the impact of telecommuting on job satisfaction found that job satisfaction initially increased as the extent of telecommuting increased, but as the number of hours spent telecommuting increased, job satisfaction started to level off, decreased slightly, and then stabilized.[76]

Self-Motivation—If your instructor is using MyManagementLab, log onto **mymanagementlab.com** and test your *self-motivation knowledge*. **Be sure to refer back to the chapter opener!**

⭐ **It's Your Career**

MOTIVATING PROFESSIONALS In contrast to a generation ago, the typical employee today is more likely to be a professional with a college degree than a blue-collar factory worker. What special concerns should managers be aware of when trying to motivate a team of engineers at Intel's India Development Center, software designers at SAS Institute in North Carolina, or a group of consultants at Accenture in Singapore?

Professionals are different from nonprofessionals.[77] They have a strong and long-term commitment to their field of expertise. To keep current in their field, they need to regularly update their knowledge, and because of their commitment to their profession, they rarely define their workweek as 8 A.M. to 5 P.M. five days a week.

What motivates professionals? Money and promotions typically are low on their priority list. Why? They tend to be well paid and enjoy what they do. In contrast, job challenge tends to be ranked high. They like to tackle problems and find solutions. Their chief reward is the work itself. Professionals also value support. They want others to think that what they are working on is important. That may be true for all employees, but professionals tend to be focused on their work as their central life interest, whereas nonprofessionals typically have other interests outside of work that can compensate for needs not met on the job.

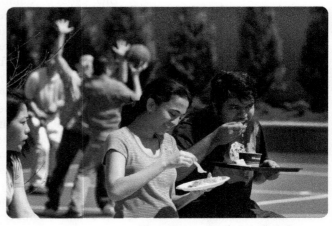

Microsoft managers motivate the firm's diverse work force of more than 100,000 employees by satisfying their differing needs and wants. For young employees in its Entertainment and Devices division, Microsoft built The Commons, a work environment with amenities including sports shops that sell bicycles and snowboards, restaurants, a spa, a soccer field, a basketball court, a post office, and a credit union.
Source: Elaine Thompson/AP Images

MOTIVATING CONTINGENT WORKERS There is an increased number of contingent workers employed by organizations. There's no simple solution for motivating these employees. For that small set of individuals who prefer the freedom of their temporary status, the lack of stability may not be an issue. In addition, temporariness might be preferred by highly compensated physicians, engineers, accountants, or financial planners who don't want the demands of a full-time job. But these individuals are the exceptions. For the most part, temporary employees are not temporary by choice.

What will motivate involuntarily temporary employees? An obvious answer is the opportunity to become a permanent employee. In cases in which permanent employees are selected from a pool of temps, the temps will often work hard in hopes of becoming permanent. A less obvious answer is the opportunity for training. The ability of a temporary employee to find a new job is largely dependent on his or her skills. If an employee sees that the job he or she is doing can help develop marketable skills, then motivation is increased. From an equity standpoint, when temps work alongside permanent employees who earn more and get benefits too for doing the same job, the performance of temps is likely to suffer. Separating such employees or perhaps minimizing interdependence between them might help managers counteract potential problems.[78]

MOTIVATING LOW-SKILLED, MINIMUM-WAGE EMPLOYEES Suppose in your first managerial position after graduating, you're responsible for managing a work group of low-skilled, minimum-wage employees. Offering more pay to these employees for high levels of performance is out of the question: your company just can't afford it. In addition, these employees have limited education and skills. What are your motivational options at this point?

One trap we often fall into is thinking that people are motivated only by money. Although money is important as a motivator, it's not the only reward that people seek and that managers can use. In motivating minimum-wage employees, managers might look at employee recognition programs. Many managers also recognize the power of praise, although these "pats on the back" must be sincere and given for the right reasons.

Designing Appropriate Rewards Programs

Blue Cross of California, one of the nation's largest health insurers, pays bonuses to doctors serving its health maintenance organization members based on patient satisfaction and other quality standards. FedEx's drivers are motivated by a pay system that rewards them for timeliness and how much they deliver.[79] Employee rewards programs play a powerful role in motivating appropriate employee behavior.

OPEN-BOOK MANAGEMENT Within 24 hours after managers of the Heavy Duty Division of Springfield Remanufacturing Company (SRC) gather to discuss a multipage financial document, every plant employee will have seen the same information. If the employees can meet shipment goals, they'll all share in a large year-end bonus.[80] Many organizations of various sizes involve their employees in workplace decisions by opening up the financial statements (the "books"). They share that information so employees will be motivated to make better decisions about their work and better able to understand the implications of what they do, how they do it, and the ultimate impact on the bottom line. This approach is called **open-book management** and many organizations are using it.[81] For instance, at Parrish Medical Center in Titusville, Florida, the CEO struggled with the prospect of massive layoffs, facilities closing, and profits declining. So he turned to "town hall meetings" in which employees received updates on the financial condition of the hospital. He also told his employees it would require their commitment to help find ways to reduce expenses and cut costs.[82] At giant insurance broker Marsh, its employees are taught the ABCs of finance and accounting.[83]

The goal of open-book management is to get employees to think like an owner by seeing the impact their decisions have on financial results. Since many employees don't have the knowledge or background to understand the financials, they have to be taught how to read and understand the organization's financial statements. Once employees have this knowledge, however, managers need to regularly share the numbers with them. By sharing this information, employees begin to see the link between their efforts, level of performance, and operational results.

EMPLOYEE RECOGNITION PROGRAMS **Employee recognition programs** consist of personal attention and expressing interest, approval, and appreciation for a job well done.[84] They can take numerous forms. For instance, Kelly Services introduced a new version of its points-based incentive system to better promote productivity and retention among its employees. The program, called Kelly Kudos, gives employees more choices of awards and allows them to accumulate points over a longer time period. It's working. Participants generate three times more revenue and hours than employees not receiving points.[85] Nichols Foods, a British manufacturer, has a comprehensive recognition program. The main hallway in the production department is hung with "bragging boards" on which the accomplishments of employee teams are noted. Monthly awards are presented to people who have been nominated by peers for extraordinary effort on the job. And monthly award winners are eligible for further

open-book management
A motivational approach in which an organization's financial statements (the "books") are shared with all employees

employee recognition programs
Personal attention and expressing interest, approval, and appreciation for a job well done

recognition at an off-site meeting for all employees.[86] At Wayfair.com, a seller of home furnishings, a recognition wall provides space where anyone in the company can write about anyone else in the company and give them rewards dollars. It's used to recognize someone for something they did for a customer or some other accomplishment.[87] Most managers, however, use a far more informal approach. For example, when Julia Stewart was president of Applebee's restaurants (she's currently the president and CEO of DineEquity, which includes IHOP International and Applebee's Restaurants), she would frequently leave sealed notes on the chairs of employees after everyone had gone home.[88] These notes explained how important Stewart thought the person's work was or how much she appreciated the completion of a project. Stewart also relied heavily on voice mail messages left after office hours to tell employees how appreciative she was for a job well done. And recognition doesn't have to come only from managers. Some 35 percent of companies encourage coworkers to recognize peers for outstanding work efforts.[89] For instance, managers at Yum Brands Inc. (the Kentucky-based parent of food chains Taco Bell, KFC, and Pizza Hut) were looking for ways to reduce employee turnover. They found a successful customer-service program involving peer recognition at KFC restaurants in Australia. Workers there spontaneously rewarded fellow workers with "Champs cards, an acronym for attributes such as cleanliness, hospitality, and accuracy." Yum implemented the program in other restaurants around the world, and credits the peer recognition with reducing hourly employee turnover from 181 percent to 109 percent.[90]

A recent survey of organizations found that 88 percent had some type of program to recognize worker achievements.[91] Another survey found that 12 percent of employees say they receive frequent appreciation for a job well done; 7 percent of employees say their company is excellent at showing appreciation for great work.[92] And do employees think these programs are important? You bet! In a survey conducted a few years ago, a wide range of employees was asked what they considered the most powerful workplace motivator. Their response? Recognition, recognition, and more recognition![93]

Consistent with reinforcement theory, rewarding a behavior with recognition immediately following that behavior is likely to encourage its repetition. And recognition can take many forms. You can personally congratulate an employee in private for a good job. You can send a handwritten note or e-mail message acknowledging something positive that the employee has done. For employees with a strong need for social acceptance, you can publicly recognize accomplishments. To enhance group cohesiveness and motivation, you can celebrate team successes. For instance, you can do something as simple as throw a pizza party to celebrate a team's accomplishments. During the economic recession, managers got quite creative in how they showed employees they were appreciated.[94] For instance, employees at one company got to take home fresh vegetables from the company vegetable garden. In others, managers treated employees who really put forth efforts on a project to a special meal or movie tickets. Also, managers can show employees that no matter his or her role, their contributions matter. Some of these things may seem simple, but they can go a long way in showing employees they're valued.

If your professor has assigned this, go to **www.mymanagementlab.com** to watch a video titled: *CH2MHill: Motivation* and to respond to questions.

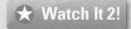

PAY-FOR-PERFORMANCE   Here's a survey statistic that may surprise you: 40 percent of employees see no clear link between performance and pay.[95] So what are the companies where these employees work paying for? They're obviously not clearly communicating performance expectations.[96] **Pay-for-performance programs** are variable compensation plans that pay employees on the basis of some performance measure.[97]

pay-for-performance programs
Variable compensation plans that pay employees on the basis of some performance measure

let's get REAL

The Scenario:

Penny Collins manages an audio supply store in Atlanta. The work hours can be long and work conditions difficult for her three teams of 10 installers. She'd like to implement a recognition program to reward and motivate her employees.

What advice would you give Penny?

My suggestion for a recognition program would be a "hall of fame." A customer service employee should reach out to each individual customer after their installation and post all the best feedback in a conspicuous place where employees gather. This can be an ongoing exercise and at the end of the quarter all of the "hall of famers" will be rewarded with a team bonding group activity. This is an ideal scenario because employees will be motivated AND customers will receive great service.

Katie Pagan
Accounting & HR Manager

Piece-rate pay plans, wage incentive plans, profit-sharing, and lump-sum bonuses are examples. What differentiates these forms of pay from more traditional compensation plans is that instead of paying a person for time on the job, pay is adjusted to reflect some performance measure. These performance measures might include such things as individual productivity, team or work group productivity, departmental productivity, or the overall organization's profit performance.

Pay-for-performance is probably most compatible with expectancy theory. Individuals should perceive a strong relationship between their performance and the rewards they receive for motivation to be maximized. If rewards are allocated only on nonperformance factors—such as seniority, job title, or across-the-board pay raises—then employees are likely to reduce their efforts. From a motivation perspective, making some or all of an employee's pay conditional on some performance measure focuses his or her attention and effort toward that measure, then reinforces the continuation of the effort with a reward. If the employee's team's or organization's performance declines, so does the reward. Thus, there's an incentive to keep efforts and motivation strong.

Pay-for-performance programs are popular. Some 90 percent of employers have some form of variable pay plan.[98] These types of pay plans have also been tried in other countries, such as Canada and Japan. About 30 percent of Canadian companies and 22 percent of Japanese companies have company-wide pay-for-performance plans.[99]

Do pay-for-performance programs work? The jury is still out. For the most part, studies seem to indicate that they do. For instance, one study found companies that used pay-for-performance programs performed better financially than those that did not.[100] Another study showed pay-for-performance programs with outcome-based incentives had a positive impact on sales, customer satisfaction, and profits.[101] In organizations that use work teams, managers should consider group-based performance incentives that will reinforce team effort and commitment. However, others say that linking pay to performance doesn't work.[102] So if a business decides it wants to use pay-for-performance programs, managers need to ensure they're specific about the relationship between an individual's pay and his or her expected level of appropriate performance. Employees must clearly understand exactly how performance—theirs and the organization's—translates into dollars on their paychecks.[103]

PREPARING FOR: Exams/Quizzes

CHAPTER SUMMARY by Learning Objectives

LO1 DEFINE motivation.

Motivation is the process by which a person's efforts are energized, directed, and sustained toward attaining a goal.

The *energy* element is a measure of intensity, drive, or vigor. The high level of effort needs to be *directed* in ways that help the organization achieve its goals. Employees must *persist* in putting forth effort to achieve those goals.

LO2 COMPARE and contrast early theories of motivation.

In Maslow's hierarchy, individuals move up the hierarchy of five needs (physiological, safety, social, esteem, and self-actualization) as needs are substantially satisfied. A need that's substantially satisfied no longer motivates.

A Theory X manager believes people don't like to work or won't seek out responsibility so they have to be threatened and coerced to work. A Theory Y manager assumes people like to work and seek out responsibility, so they will exercise self-motivation and self-direction.

Herzberg's theory proposed that intrinsic factors associated with job satisfaction were what motivated people. Extrinsic factors associated with job dissatisfaction simply kept people from being dissatisfied.

Three-needs theory proposed three acquired needs that are major motives in work: need for achievement, need for affiliation, and need for power.

LO3 COMPARE and contrast contemporary theories of motivation.

Goal-setting theory says that specific goals increase performance, and difficult goals, when accepted, result in higher performance than easy goals. Important points in goal-setting theory include intention to work toward a goal as a major source of job motivation; specific hard goals that produce higher levels of output than generalized goals; participation in setting goals as preferable to assigning goals, but not always; feedback that guides and motivates behavior, especially self-generated feedback; and contingencies that affect goal setting—goal commitment, self-efficacy, and national culture. Reinforcement theory says that behavior is a function of its consequences. To motivate, use positive reinforcers to reinforce desirable behaviors. Ignore undesirable behavior rather than punishing it.

Job enlargement involves horizontally expanding job scope by adding more tasks or increasing how many times the tasks are done. Job enrichment vertically expands job depth by giving employees more control over their work. The job characteristics model says five core job dimensions (skill variety, task identity, task significance, autonomy, and feedback) are used to design motivating jobs. Another job design approach proposed looking at relational aspects and proactive aspects of jobs.

Equity theory focuses on how employees compare their inputs–outcomes ratios to relevant others' ratios. A perception of inequity will cause an employee to do something about it. Procedural justice has a greater influence on employee satisfaction than distributive justice.

Expectancy theory says an individual tends to act in a certain way based on the expectation that the act will be followed by a desired outcome. Expectancy is the effort–performance linkage (how much effort do I need to exert to achieve a certain level of performance?); instrumentality is the performance–reward linkage (achieving at a certain level of performance will get me a specific reward); and valence is the attractiveness of the reward (is it the reward that I want?).

L04 DISCUSS **current issues in motivation.**

Managers must cope with four current motivation issues: motivating in tough economic circumstances, managing cross-cultural challenges, motivating unique groups of workers, and designing appropriate rewards programs.

During tough economic conditions, managers must look for creative ways to keep employees' efforts energized, directed, and sustained toward achieving goals.

Most motivational theories were developed in the United States and have a North American bias. Some theories (Maslow's needs hierarchy, achievement need, and equity theory) don't work well for other cultures. However, the desire for interesting work seems important to all workers, and Herzberg's motivator (intrinsic) factors may be universal.

Managers face challenges in motivating unique groups of workers. A diverse workforce is looking for flexibility. Professionals want job challenge and support and are motivated by the work itself. Contingent workers want the opportunity to become permanent or to receive skills training. Recognition programs and sincere appreciation for work done can be used to motivate low-skilled, minimum-wage workers.

Open-book management is when financial statements (the books) are shared with employees who have been taught what they mean. Employee recognition programs consist of personal attention, approval, and appreciation for a job well done. Pay-for-performance programs are variable compensation plans that pay employees on the basis of some performance measure.

MyManagementLab

Go to **mymanagementlab.com** to complete the problems marked with this icon ⭐.

⭐ REVIEW AND DISCUSSION QUESTIONS

1. What is motivation? Explain the three key elements of motivation.

2. Describe each of the four early theories of motivation.

3. How do goal-setting, reinforcement, and equity theories explain employee motivation?

4. What are the different job design approaches to motivation?

5. Explain the three key linkages in expectancy theory and their role in motivation.

6. What challenges do managers face in motivating today's workforce?

7. Describe open-book management, employee recognition, and pay-for-performance programs.

8. Can an individual be too motivated? Discuss.

MyManagementLab

If your professor has assigned these, go to **mymanagementlab.com** for Auto-graded writing questions as well as the following Assisted-graded writing questions:

9. What economic and cross-cultural challenges do managers face when motivating employees?

10. Most of us have to work for a living, and a job is a central part of our lives. So why do managers have to worry so much about employee motivation issues?

PREPARING FOR: My Career

⭐ PERSONAL INVENTORY ASSESSMENTS 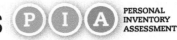 PERSONAL INVENTORY ASSESSMENT

Work Motivation Indicator

How motivated are you? Use this PIA to assess your own level of work motivation.

⭐ ETHICS DILEMMA

Advocates of open-book management point to the advantages of getting employees to think like owners and being motivated to make better decisions about how they do their work once they see how their decisions impact financial results. However, is there such a thing as "too much openness?" At some companies, employees not only have access to company financial details but also to staff performance reviews and individual pay information.[104]

11. What do you think? What are the pros and cons of such an approach?

12. What potential ethical issues do you see here? How might managers address these ethical issues?

SKILLS EXERCISE Developing Your Motivating Employees Skill

About the Skill

Because a simple, all-encompassing set of motivational guidelines is not available, the following suggestions draw on the essence of what we know about motivating employees.

Steps in Practicing the Skill

- *Recognize individual differences.* Almost every contemporary motivation theory recognizes that employees are not homogeneous. They have different needs. They also differ in terms of attitudes, personality, and other important individual variables.

- *Match people to jobs.* A great deal of evidence shows the motivational benefits of carefully matching people to jobs. People who lack the necessary skills to perform successfully will be at a disadvantage.

- *Use goals.* You should ensure that employees have hard, specific goals and feedback on how well they're doing in pursuit of those goals. In many cases, these goals should be participatively set.

- *Ensure goals are perceived as attainable.* Regardless of whether goals are actually attainable, employees who see goals as unattainable will reduce their effort. Be sure, therefore, that employees feel confident that increased efforts can lead to achieving performance goals.

- *Individualize rewards.* Because employees have different needs, what acts as a reinforcer for one may not do so for another. Use your knowledge of employee differences to individualize the rewards over which you have control. Some of the more obvious rewards that you can allocate include pay, promotions, autonomy, and the opportunity to participate in goal setting and decision making.

- *Link rewards to performance.* You need to make rewards contingent on performance. Rewarding factors other than performance will only reinforce the importance of those other factors. Key rewards such as pay increases and promotions should be given for the attainment of employees' specific goals.

- *Check the system for equity.* Employees should perceive that rewards or outcomes are equal to the inputs given. On a simplistic level, experience, ability, effort, and other obvious inputs should explain differences in pay, responsibility, and other obvious outcomes.

- *Don't ignore money.* It's easy to get so caught up in setting goals, creating interesting jobs, and providing opportunities for participation that you forget that money is a major reason why most people work. Thus, the allocation of performance-based wage increases, piece-work bonuses, employee stock ownership plans, and other pay incentives are important in determining employee motivation.

WORKING TOGETHER Team Exercise

Using the chapter-opening *It's Your Career,* break into small groups of three or four and compare your responses. What patterns, if any, did you find? What conclusions can you draw about motivation?

MY TURN TO BE A MANAGER

- A good habit to get into if you don't already do so is goal-setting. Set goals for yourself using the suggestions from goal-setting theory. Write these down and keep them in a notebook. Track your progress toward achieving these goals.

- Describe a task you've done recently for which you exerted a high level of effort. Explain your behavior, using any three of the motivation approaches described in this text.

- Pay attention to times when you're highly motivated and times when you're not as motivated. Write down a description of these. What accounts for the difference in your level of motivation?

- Interview three managers about how they motivate their employees. What have they found that works the best? Write up your findings in a report and be prepared to present it in class.

- Using the job characteristics model, redesign the following jobs to be more motivating: retail store sales associate, utility company meter reader, and checkout cashier at a discount store. In a written report, describe for each job at least two specific actions you would take for each of the five core job dimensions.

- Do some serious thinking about what you want from your job after graduation. Using the chapter-opening *It's Your Career,* make a list of what's important to you. Think about how you will discover whether a particular job will help you get those things.

- Find three different examples of employee recognition programs from organizations with which you're familiar or from articles that you find. Write a report describing your examples and evaluating what you think about the various approaches.

- Find the Web site of Great Place to Work Institute [www.greatplacetowork.com]. What does the Institute say about what makes an organization a great place to work? Next, locate the lists of the Best Companies to Work For. Choose one company from each of the international lists. Now research that company and describe what it does that makes it a great place to work.

- In your own words, write down three things you learned in this text about being a good manager. Keep a copy of this for future reference.

CASE APPLICATION 1 Passion for the Outdoors and for People

At its headquarters in Ventura, California, Patagonia's office space feels more like a national park lodge than the main office of a $400 million retailer.[105] It has a Douglas fir staircase and a portrait of Yosemite's El Capitan. The company's café serves organic food and drinks. There's an infant and toddler child-care room for employees' children. An easy one-block walk from the Pacific Ocean, employees' surfboards are lined up by the cafeteria, ready at a moment's notice to catch some waves. (Current wave reports are noted on a whiteboard in the lobby.) After surfing or jogging or biking, employees can freshen up in the showers in the restrooms. And no one has a private office. If an employee doesn't want to be disturbed, he or she wears headphones. Visitors are evident by the business attire they wear. The company encourages celebrations to boost employee morale. For instance, at the Reno store, the "Fun Patrol" organizes parties throughout the year.

Patagonia has long been recognized as a great workplace for mothers. And it's also earned a reputation for loyal employees, something that many retailers struggle with. Its combined voluntary and involuntary turnover in its retail stores was around 25 percent, while it was only 7 percent at headquarters. (The industry average for retail is around 44 percent.) Patagonia's CEO Casey Sheahan says the company's culture, camaraderie, and way of doing business is very meaningful to employees and they know that "what they do each day is contributing toward a higher purpose—protecting and preserving the areas that most of them love spending time in." Managers are coached to define expectations, communicate deadlines, and then let employees figure out the best way to meet those.

Founded by Yvon Chouinard, Patagonia's first and strongest passion is for the outdoors and the environment. And that attracts employees who are also passionate about those things. But Patagonia's executives do realize that they are first and foremost a business and, even though they're committed to doing the right thing, the company needs to remain profitable to be able to continue to do the things it's passionate about. But that hasn't seemed to be an issue since the recession in the early 1990s, when the company had to make its only large-scale layoffs in its history.

⭐ DISCUSSION QUESTIONS

13. What would it be like to work at Patagonia? (Hint: Go to Patagonia's Web site and find the section on jobs.) What's your assessment of the company's work environment?

14. Using what you've learned from studying the various motivation theories, what does Patagonia's situation tell you about employee motivation?

15. What do you think might be Patagonia's biggest challenge in keeping employees motivated?

16. If you were managing a team of Patagonia employees in the retail stores, how would you keep them motivated?

CASE APPLICATION 2 Best Practices at Best Buy

Do traditional workplaces reward long hours instead of efficient hours? Wouldn't it make more sense to have a workplace in which employees could work however and whenever they wanted to as long as they did their work? Well, that's the approach Best Buy tried.[106] And this radical workplace experiment, which obviously has many implications for employee motivation, was an interesting and enlightening journey for the company.

In 2002, then-CEO Brad Anderson introduced a carefully crafted program called ROWE—Results-Only Work Environment. ROWE was the inspiration of two HRM managers at Best Buy, Cali Ressler and Jody Thompson. These two had been asked to take a flexible work program in effect at corporate headquarters in Minnesota and develop it for implementation throughout the company. Although that flexible work program had had some stunning successes, including high levels of employee engagement and productivity, there was one significant issue. Those involved in the program were perceived to be "not working." And that was a common reaction from managers who didn't really view flexible work employees as actually doing work because they didn't show up at work during the "traditional" hours. The two women set about to change that impression by creating a program in which employees would be evaluated on what they accomplished—their "results only"—not on the amount of hours they spent working.

The first thing to understand about ROWE was that it wasn't about schedules. Instead, it was about changing the work culture of an organization, which is infinitely more difficult than changing schedules. With Anderson's blessing and support, they embarked on this journey to overhaul the company's corporate workplace.

The first step in implementing ROWE was a culture audit at company headquarters, which helped them establish a baseline for how employees perceived their work environment. After four months, the audit was repeated. During this time, Best Buy executives were being educated about ROWE and what it was all about. Obviously, it was important to have their commitment to the program. The second phase involved explaining the ROWE philosophy to all the corporate employees and training managers on how to maintain control in a ROWE workplace. In the third phase, work unit teams were free to figure out how to implement the changes. Each team found a different way to keep the flexibility from spiraling into chaos. For instance, the public relations team got pagers to make sure someone was always available in an emergency. Some employees in the finance department used software that turns voice mail into e-mail files accessible from anywhere, making it easier for them to work at home. Four months after ROWE was implemented, Ressler and Thompson followed up with another culture check to see how everyone was doing.

So what results did Best Buy see with this experiment? Productivity jumped 41 percent, and voluntary turnover fell to 8 percent from 12 percent. They also discovered that when employees' engagement with their jobs increased, average annual sales increased 2 percent. And employees said the freedom changed their lives. ROWE reduced work-family conflict and increased employees' control over their schedules. ROWE employees didn't "count" how many hours they were at work but instead focused on getting their work done, however many or few hours that took. For them, work became "something you do—not a place you go."

Despite the positive aspects of the program, Best Buy's current CEO, Hubert Joly, decided to eliminate the flexible work environment associated with ROWE. Now instead of being able to work whenever and wherever they choose, most corporate staff will be required to work traditional 40-hour weeks in the office. And Ressler and Thompson? Well, they now own their own HR consultancy practice, which promotes the ROWE idea to other companies.

⭐ **DISCUSSION QUESTIONS**

17. Describe the elements of ROWE. What do you think might be the advantages and drawbacks of such a program?

18. Using one or more motivation theories from the chapter, explain why you think ROWE works.

19. What might be the challenges for managers in motivating employees in a program like this?

20. Does this sound like something you would be comfortable with? Why or why not?

21. What's your interpretation of the statement that "Work is something you do, not a place you go"? Do you agree? Why or why not?

ENDNOTES

1. R. Mac, "The Fall of Mark Pincus: From Billionaire to Zynga's Former CEO," www.forbes.com, July 1, 2013; and A. Carr, "Mark Pincus's Clowns Are Still Haunting Zynga," www.fastcompany.com, April 1, 2013.

2. A. Carmeli, B. Ben-Hador, D. A. Waldman, and D. E. Rupp, "How Leaders Cultivate Social Capital and Nurture Employee Vigor: Implications for Job Performance," *Journal of Applied Psychology,* November 2009, pp. 1533–1561.

3. R. M. Steers, R. T. Mowday, and D. L. Shapiro, "The Future of Work Motivation Theory," *Academy of Management Review,* July 2004, pp. 379–387.

4. C. Fritz, C. Fu Lam, and G. M. Spreitzer, "It's the Little Things That Matter: An Examination of Knowledge Workers' Energy Management," *Academy of Management Perspectives,* August 2011, pp. 28–39; A. Carmeli, B. Ben-Hador, D. A. Waldman, and D. E. Rupp, "How Leaders Cultivate Social Capital and Nurture Employee Vigor: Implications for Job Performance," *Journal of Applied Psychology,* November 2009, pp. 1553–1561; and N. Ellemers, D. De Gilder, and S. A. Haslam, "Motivating Individuals and Groups at Work: A Social Identity Perspective on Leadership and Group Performance," *Academy of Management Review,* July 2004, pp. 459–478.

5. Report on State of the American Workplace - 2013, gallup.com, 2013.

6. J. Krueger and E. Killham, "At Work, Feeling Good Matters," *Gallup Management Journal* [http://gmj.gallup.com], December 8, 2005.

7. Report on State of the Global Workplace - 2013, gallup.com, 2013.

8. M. Meece, "Using the Human Touch to Solve Workplace Problems," *New York Times Online,* April 3, 2008.

9. A. Maslow, *Motivation and Personality* (New York: McGraw-Hill, 1954); A. Maslow, D. C. Stephens, and G. Heil, *Maslow on Management* (New York: John Wiley & Sons, 1998); M. L. Ambrose and C. T. Kulik, "Old Friends, New Faces: Motivation Research in the 1990s," *Journal of Management,* vol. 25, no. 3, 1999, pp. 231–292; and "Dialogue," *Academy of Management Review,* October 2000, pp. 696–701.

10. See, for example, D. T. Hall and K. E. Nongaim, "An Examination of Maslow's Need Hierarchy in an Organizational Setting," *Organizational Behavior and Human Performance,* February 1968, pp. 12–35; E. E. Lawler III and J. L. Suttle, "A Causal Correlational Test of the Need Hierarchy Concept," *Organizational Behavior and Human Performance,* April 1972, pp. 265–287; R. M. Creech, "Employee Motivation," *Management Quarterly,* Summer 1995, pp. 33–39; J. Rowan, "Maslow Amended," *Journal of Humanistic Psychology,* Winter 1998, pp. 81–92; J. Rowan, "Ascent and Descent in Maslow's Theory," *Journal of Humanistic Psychology,* Summer 1999, pp. 125–133; and M. L. Ambrose and C. T. Kulik, "Old Friends, New Faces: Motivation Research in the 1990s."

11. E. McGirt, "Intel Risks It All…Again," *Fast Company,* November 2009, pp. 88+.

12. D. McGregor, *The Human Side of Enterprise* (New York: McGraw-Hill, 1960). For an updated description of Theories X and Y, see an annotated edition with commentary of *The Human Side of Enterprise* (McGraw-Hill, 2006); and G. Heil, W. Bennis, and D. C. Stephens, *Douglas McGregor, Revisited: Managing the Human Side of Enterprise* (New York: Wiley, 2000).

13. J. M. O'Brien, "The Next Intel," *Wired,* July 2002, pp. 100–107.

14. "What Motivates Employees?" *T&D,* October 2013, p. 16.

15. F. Herzberg, B. Mausner, and B. Snyderman, *The Motivation to Work* (New York: John Wiley, 1959); F. Herzberg, *The Managerial Choice: To Be Effective or to Be Human,* rev. ed. (Salt Lake City: Olympus, 1982); R. M. Creech, "Employee Motivation"; and M. L. Ambrose and C. T. Kulik, "Old Friends, New Faces: Motivation Research in the 1990s."

16. D. C. McClelland, *The Achieving Society* (New York: Van Nostrand Reinhold, 1961); J. W. Atkinson and J. O. Raynor, *Motivation and Achievement* (Washington, DC: Winston, 1974); D. C. McClelland, *Power: The Inner Experience* (New York: Irvington, 1975); and M. J. Stahl, *Managerial and Technical Motivation: Assessing Needs for Achievement, Power, and Affiliation* (New York: Praeger, 1986).

17. McClelland, *The Achieving Society.*

18. McClelland, *Power;* D. C. McClelland and D. H. Burnham, "Power Is the Great Motivator," *Harvard Business Review,* March–April 1976, pp. 100–110.

19. D. Miron and D. C. McClelland, "The Impact of Achievement Motivation Training on Small Businesses," *California Management Review,* Summer 1979, pp. 13–28.

20. "McClelland: An Advocate of Power," *International Management,* July 1975, pp. 27–29.

21. R. M. Steers, R. T. Mowday, and D. L. Shapiro, "The Future of Work Motivation Theory"; E. A. Locke and G. P. Latham, "What Should We Do About Motivation Theory? Six Recommendations for the Twenty-First Century," *Academy of Management Review,* July 2004, pp. 388–403; and M. L. Ambrose and C. T. Kulik, "Old Friends, New Faces: Motivation Research in the 1990s."

22. A. Barrett, "Cracking the Whip at Wyeth," *BusinessWeek,* February 6, 2006, pp. 70–71.

23. G. P. Latham and E. A. Locke, "Science and Ethics: What Should Count as Evidence Against the Use of Goal Setting?" *Academy of Management Perspective,* August 2009, pp. 88–91; M. L. Ambrose and C. T. Kulik, "Old Friends, New Faces: Motivation Research in the 1990s."

24. J. C. Naylor and D. R. Ilgen, "Goal Setting: A Theoretical Analysis of a Motivational Technique," in B. M. Staw and L. L. Cummings (eds.), *Research in Organizational Behavior,* vol. 6 (Greenwich, CT: JAI Press, 1984), pp. 95–140; A. R. Pell, "Energize Your People," *Managers Magazine,* December 1992, pp. 28–29; E. A. Locke, "Facts and Fallacies About Goal Theory: Reply to Deci," *Psychological Science,* January 1993, pp. 63–64; M. E. Tubbs, "Commitment as a Moderator of the Goal-Performance Relation: A Case for Clearer Construct Definition," *Journal*

of Applied Psychology, February 1993, pp. 86–97; M. P. Collingwood, "Why Don't You Use the Research?" *Management Decision*, May 1993, pp. 48–54; M. E. Tubbs, D. M. Boehne, and J. S. Dahl, "Expectancy, Valence, and Motivational Force Functions in Goal-Setting Research: An Empirical Test," *Journal of Applied Psychology*, June 1993, pp. 361–373; E. A. Locke, "Motivation Through Conscious Goal Setting," *Applied and Preventive Psychology*, vol. 5, 1996, pp. 117–124; M. L. Ambrose and C. T. Kulik, "Old Friends, New Faces: Motivation Research in the 1990s"; E. A. Locke and G. P. Latham, "Building a Practically Useful Theory of Goal Setting and Task Motivation: A 35-Year Odyssey," *American Psychologist*, September 2002, pp. 705–717; Y. Fried and L. H. Slowik, "Enriching Goal-Setting Theory with Time: An Integrated Approach," *Academy of Management Review*, July 2004, pp. 404–422; and G. P. Latham, "The Motivational Benefits of Goal-Setting," *Academy of Management Executive*, November 2004, pp. 126–129.

25. J. B. Miner, *Theories of Organizational Behavior* (Hinsdale, IL: Dryden Press, 1980), p. 65.

26. Leader Making a Difference box based on D. A. Kaplan, "The Best Company to Work For," *Fortune*, February 8, 2010, pp. 56–64; and S. Cooperman, "Goodnight High," *Forbes*, May 5, 2008, pp. 46–48.

27. J. A. Wagner III, "Participation's Effects on Performance and Satisfaction: A Reconsideration of Research and Evidence," *Academy of Management Review*, April 1994, pp. 312–330; J. George-Falvey, "Effects of Task Complexity and Learning Stage on the Relationship Between Participation in Goal Setting and Task Performance," *Academy of Management Proceedings* on Disk, 1996; T. D. Ludwig and E. S. Geller, "Assigned Versus Participative Goal Setting and Response Generalization: Managing Injury Control Among Professional Pizza Deliverers," *Journal of Applied Psychology*, April 1997, pp. 253–261; and S. G. Harkins and M. D. Lowe, "The Effects of Self-Set Goals on Task Performance," *Journal of Applied Social Psychology*, January 2000, pp. 1–40.

28. J. M. Ivancevich and J. T. McMahon, "The Effects of Goal Setting, External Feedback, and Self-Generated Feedback on Outcome Variables: A Field Experiment," *Academy of Management Journal*, June 1982, pp. 359–372; and E. A. Locke, "Motivation Through Conscious Goal Setting."

29. J. R. Hollenbeck, C. R. Williams, and H. J. Klein, "An Empirical Examination of the Antecedents of Commitment to Difficult Goals," *Journal of Applied Psychology*, February 1989, pp. 18–23; see also J. C. Wofford, V. L. Goodwin, and S. Premack, "Meta-Analysis of the Antecedents of Personal Goal Level and of the Antecedents and Consequences of Goal Commitment," *Journal of Management*, September 1992, pp. 595–615; Tubbs, "Commitment as a Moderator of the Goal-Performance Relation"; J. W. Smither, M. London, and R. R. Reilly, "Does Performance Improve Following Multisource Feedback? A Theoretical Model, Meta-Analysis, and Review of Empirical Findings," *Personnel Psychology*, Spring 2005, pp. 171–203.

30. Y. Gong, J-C. Huang, and J-L. Farh, "Employee Learning Orientation, Transformational Leadership, and Employee Creativity: The Mediating Role of Employee Self-Efficacy," *Academy of Management Journal*, August 2009, pp. 765–778; M. E. Gist, "Self-Efficacy: Implications for Organizational Behavior and Human Resource Management," *Academy of Management Review*, July 1987, pp. 472–485; and A. Bandura, *Self-Efficacy: The Exercise of Control* (New York: Freeman, 1997).

31. E. A. Locke, E. Frederick, C. Lee, and P. Bobko, "Effect of Self-Efficacy, Goals, and Task Strategies on Task Performance," *Journal of Applied Psychology*, May 1984, pp. 241–251; M. E. Gist and T. R. Mitchell, "Self-Efficacy: A Theoretical Analysis of Its Determinants and Malleability," *Academy of Management Review*, April 1992, pp. 183–211; A. D. Stajkovic and F. Luthans, "Self-Efficacy and Work-Related Performance: A Meta-Analysis," *Psychological Bulletin*, September 1998, pp. 240–261; and A. Bandura, "Cultivate Self-Efficacy for Personal and Organizational Effectiveness," in E. Locke (ed.), *Handbook of Principles of Organizational Behavior* (Malden, MA: Blackwell, 2004), pp. 120–136.

32. A. Bandura and D. Cervone, "Differential Engagement in Self-Reactive Influences in Cognitively-Based Motivation," *Organizational Behavior and Human Decision Processes*, August 1986, pp. 92–113; and R. Ilies and T. A. Judge, "Goal Regulation Across Time: The Effects

of Feedback and Affect," *Journal of Applied Psychology*, May 2005, pp. 453–467.

33. See J. C. Anderson and C. A. O'Reilly, "Effects of an Organizational Control System on Managerial Satisfaction and Performance," *Human Relations*, June 1981, pp. 491–501; and J. P. Meyer, B. Schacht-Cole, and I. R. Gellatly, "An Examination of the Cognitive Mechanisms by Which Assigned Goals Affect Task Performance and Reactions to Performance," *Journal of Applied Social Psychology*, vol. 18, no. 5, 1988, pp. 390–408.

34. K. Maher and K. Hudson, "Wal-Mart to Sweeten Bonus Plans for Staff," *Wall Street Journal*, March 22, 2007, p. A11; and Reuters, "Wal-Mart Workers to Get New Bonus Plan," CNNMoney.com, March 22, 2007.

35. B. F. Skinner, *Science and Human Behavior* (New York: Free Press, 1953); and Skinner, *Beyond Freedom and Dignity* (New York: Knopf, 1972).

36. The same data, for instance, can be interpreted in either goal-setting or reinforcement terms, as shown in E. A. Locke, "Latham vs. Komaki: A Tale of Two Paradigms," *Journal of Applied Psychology*, February 1980, pp. 16–23. Also, see M. O. Ambrose and C. T. Kulik, "Old Friends, New Faces: Motivation Research in the 1990s."

37. "Few Managers Get Kudos for Helping Develop Employees," *T&D*, August 2012, p. 22.

38. J. Katz, "Cozy Up to Customers," *Industry Week*, January 12, 2010, p. 16.

39. See, for example, A. M. Grant and S. K. Parker, "Redesigning Work Design Theories: The Rise of Relational and Proactive Perspectives," in *The Academy of Management Annals*, J. P. Walsh and A. P. Brief (eds.), 2009, pp. 317–375; R. W. Griffin, "Toward an Integrated Theory of Task Design," in L. L. Cummings and B. M. Staw (eds.), *Research in Organizational Behavior*, vol. 9 (Greenwich, CT: JAI Press, 1987), pp. 79–120; and M. Campion, "Interdisciplinary Approaches to Job Design: A Constructive Replication with Extensions," *Journal of Applied Psychology*, August 1988, pp. 467–481.

40. N. Tasler, "Help Your Best People Do a Better Job," *BusinessWeek Online*, March 26, 2010; S. Caudron, "The De-Jobbing of America," *Industry Week*, September 5, 1994, pp. 31–36; W. Bridges, "The End of the Job," *Fortune*, September 19, 1994, pp. 62–74; and K. H. Hammonds, K. Kelly, and K. Thurston, "Rethinking Work," *BusinessWeek*, October 12, 1994, pp. 75–87.

41. M. A. Campion and C. L. McClelland, "Follow-Up and Extension of the Interdisciplinary Costs and Benefits of Enlarged Jobs," *Journal of Applied Psychology*, June 1993, pp. 339–351; and M. L. Ambrose and C. T. Kulik, "Old Friends, New Faces: Motivation Research in the 1990s."

42. See, for example, J. R. Hackman and G. R. Oldham, *Work Redesign* (Reading, MA: Addison-Wesley, 1980); Miner, *Theories of Organizational Behavior*, pp. 231–266; R. W. Griffin, "Effects of Work Redesign on Employee Perceptions, Attitudes, and Behaviors: A Long-Term Investigation," *Academy of Management Journal*, June 1991, pp. 425–435; J. L. Cotton, *Employee Involvement* (Newbury Park, CA: Sage, 1993), pp. 141–172; and M. L. Ambrose and C. T. Kulik, "Old Friends, New Faces: Motivation Research in the 1990s."

43. J. R. Hackman and G. R. Oldham, "Development of the Job Diagnostic Survey," *Journal of Applied Psychology*, April 1975, pp. 159–170; and J. R. Hackman and G. R. Oldham, "Motivation Through the Design of Work: Test of a Theory," *Organizational Behavior and Human Performance*, August 1976, pp. 250–279.

44. J. R. Hackman, "Work Design," in J. R. Hackman and J. L. Suttle (eds.), *Improving Life at Work* (Glenview, IL: Scott, Foresman, 1977), p. 129; and M. L. Ambrose and C. T. Kulik, "Old Friends, New Faces: Motivation Research in the 1990s."

45. D. J. Holman, C. M. Axtell, C. A. Sprigg, P. Totterdell, and T. D. Wall, "The Mediating Role of Job Characteristics in Job Redesign Interventions: A Serendipitous Quasi-Experiment," *Journal of Organizational Behavior*, January 2010, pp. 84–105.

46. J. L. Pierce, I. Jussila, and A. Cummings, "Psychological Ownership Within the Job Design Context: Revision of the Job Characteristics Model," *Journal of Organizational Behavior*, May 2009, pp. 477–496.

47. A. M. Grant and S. K. Parker, "Redesigning Work Design Theories: The Rise of Relational and Proactive Perspectives."

48. J. Camps and R. Luna-Arocas, "High Involvement Work Practices and Firm Performance," *The International Journal of Human Resource Management,* May 2009, pp. 1056–1077; M. M. Butts, R. J. Vandenberg, D. M. DeJoy, B. S. Schaffer, and M. G. Wilson, "Individual Reactions to High Involvement Work Practices: Investigating the Role of Empowerment and Perceived Organizational Support," *Journal of Occupational Health Psychology,* April 2009, pp. 122–136; P. Boxall and K. Macky, "Research and Theory on High-Performance Work Systems: Progressing the High-Involvement Stream," *Human Resource Management Journal,* vol. 19, no. 1, 2009, pp. 3–23; R. D. Mohr and C. Zoghi, "High-Involvement Work Design and Job Satisfaction," *Industrial and Labor Relations Review,* April 2008, pp. 275–296; and C. D. Zatzick and R. D. Iverson, "High-Involvement Management and Workforce Reduction: Competitive Advantage or Disadvantage?" *Academy of Management Journal,* October 2006, pp. 999–1015.

49. K. Tyler, "Undeserved Promotions," *HR Magazine,* June 2012, p. 79.

50. J. S. Adams, "Inequity in Social Exchanges," in L. Berkowitz (ed.), *Advances in Experimental Social Psychology*, vol. 2 (New York: Academic Press, 1965), pp. 267–300; M. L. Ambrose and C. T. Kulik, "Old Friends, New Faces: Motivation Research in the 1990s"; and T. Menon and L. Thompson, "Envy at Work," *Harvard Business Review,* April 2010, pp. 74–79.

51. See, for example, P. S. Goodman and A. Friedman, "An Examination of Adams' Theory of Inequity," *Administrative Science Quarterly*, September 1971, pp. 271–288; M. R. Carrell, "A Longitudinal Field Assessment of Employee Perceptions of Equitable Treatment," *Organizational Behavior and Human Performance*, February 1978, pp. 108–118; E. Walster, G. W. Walster, and W. G. Scott, *Equity: Theory and Research* (Boston: Allyn & Bacon, 1978); R. G. Lord and J. A. Hohenfeld, "Longitudinal Field Assessment of Equity Effects on the Performance of Major League Baseball Players," *Journal of Applied Psychology*, February 1979, pp. 19–26; J. E. Dittrich and M. R. Carrell, "Organizational Equity Perceptions, Employee Job Satisfaction, and Departmental Absence and Turnover Rates," *Organizational Behavior and Human Performance*, August 1979, pp. 29–40; and J. Greenberg, "Cognitive Reevaluation of Outcomes in Response to Underpayment Inequity," *Academy of Management Journal,* March 1989, pp. 174–184.

52. P. S. Goodman, "An Examination of Referents Used in the Evaluation of Pay," *Organizational Behavior and Human Performance,* October 1974, pp. 170–195; S. Ronen, "Equity Perception in Multiple Comparisons: A Field Study," *Human Relations,* April 1986, pp. 333–346; R. W. Scholl, E. A. Cooper, and J. F. McKenna, "Referent Selection in Determining Equity Perception: Differential Effects on Behavioral and Attitudinal Outcomes," *Personnel Psychology*, Spring 1987, pp. 113–127; and C. T. Kulik and M. L. Ambrose, "Personal and Situational Determinants of Referent Choice," *Academy of Management Review,* April 1992, pp. 212–237.

53. See, for example, R. C. Dailey and D. J. Kirk, "Distributive and Procedural Justice as Antecedents of Job Dissatisfaction and Intent to Turnover," *Human Relations,* March 1992, pp. 305–316; D. B. McFarlin and P. D. Sweeney, "Distributive and Procedural Justice as Predictors of Satisfaction with Personal and Organizational Outcomes," *Academy of Management Journal,* August 1992, pp. 626–637; M. A. Konovsky, "Understanding Procedural Justice and Its Impact on Business Organizations," *Journal of Management,* vol. 26, no. 3, 2000, pp. 489–511; J. A. Colquitt, "Does the Justice of One Interact with the Justice of Many? Reactions to Procedural Justice in Teams," *Journal of Applied Psychology,* August 2004, pp. 633–646; J. Brockner, "Why It's So Hard to Be Fair," *Harvard Business Review,* March 2006, pp. 122–129; and B. M. Wiesenfeld, W. B. Swann Jr., J. Brockner, and C. A. Bartel, "Is More Fairness Always Preferred: Self-Esteem Moderates Reactions to Procedural Justice," *Academy of Management Journal,* October 2007, pp. 1235–1253.

54. V. H. Vroom, *Work and Motivation* (New York: John Wiley, 1964).

55. See, for example, H. G. Heneman III and D. P. Schwab, "Evaluation of Research on Expectancy Theory Prediction of Employee Performance," *Psychological Bulletin*, July 1972, pp. 1–9; and L. Reinharth and M. Wahba, "Expectancy Theory as a Predictor of Work Motivation, Effort Expenditure, and Job Performance," *Academy of Management Journal*, September 1975, pp. 502–537.

56. See, for example, V. H. Vroom, "Organizational Choice: A Study of Pre- and Postdecision Processes," *Organizational Behavior and Human Performance*, April 1966, pp. 212–225; L. W. Porter and E. E. Lawler III, *Managerial Attitudes and Performance* (Homewood, IL: Richard D. Irwin, 1968); W. Van Eerde and H. Thierry, "Vroom's Expectancy Models and Work-Related Criteria: A Meta-Analysis," *Journal of Applied Psychology*, October 1996, pp. 575–586; and M. L. Ambrose and C. T. Kulik, "Old Friends, New Faces: Motivation Research in the 1990s."

57. See, for instance, M. Siegall, "The Simplistic Five: An Integrative Framework for Teaching Motivation," *The Organizational Behavior Teaching Review*, vol. 12, no. 4, 1987–1988, pp. 141–43.

58. I. Mount, "Building a Community—and Staff Loyalty," CNNMoney.com, June 5, 2009.

59. J. M. O'Brien, "Zappos Know How to Kick It," *Fortune,* February 2, 2009, pp. 54–60.

60. "What Motivates U.S. Employees to Stay at Their Jobs?" *T&D,* April 2013, p. 16.

61. T. Barber, "Inspire Your Employees Now," *Bloomberg BusinessWeek Online,* May 18, 2010; D. Mattioli, "CEOs Welcome Recovery to Look After Staff," *Wall Street Journal,* April 5, 2010, p. B5; J. Sullivan, "How Do We Keep People Motivated Following Layoffs?" *Workforce Management Online,* March 2010; S. Crabtree, "How to Bolster Employees' Confidence," *The Gallup Management Journal Online,* February 25, 2010; S. E. Needleman, "Business Owners Try to Motivate Employees," *Wall Street Journal,* January 14, 2010, p. B5; H. Mintzberg, "Rebuilding Companies as Communities," *Harvard Business Review,* July–August 2009, pp. 140–143; and R. Luss, "Engaging Employees Through Periods of Layoffs," *Towers Watson* [www.towerswatson.com], March 3, 2009.

62. J. W. Miller and D. Kesmodel, "Drinking on the Job Comes to a Head at Carlsberg," *Wall Street Journal,* April 10–11, 2010, pp. A1+; and Associated Press, "Carlsberg Workers Balk at Loss of On-the-Job Beer," *Wall Street Journal,* April 9, 2010, p. B2.

63. N. J. Adler with A. Gundersen, *International Dimensions of Organizational Behavior*, 5th ed. (Cincinnati, OH: South-Western College Pub., 2008).

64. G. Hofstede, "Motivation, Leadership and Organization: Do American Theories Apply Abroad?" *Organizational Dynamics,* Summer 1980, p. 55.

65. Ibid.

66. J. K. Giacobbe-Miller, D. J. Miller, and V. I. Victorov, "A Comparison of Russian and U.S. Pay Allocation Decisions, Distributive Justice Judgments and Productivity Under Different Payment Conditions," *Personnel Psychology,* Spring 1998, pp. 137–163.

67. S. L. Mueller and L. D. Clarke, "Political-Economic Context and Sensitivity to Equity: Differences Between the United States and the Transition Economies of Central and Eastern Europe," *Academy of Management Journal,* June 1998, pp. 319–329.

68. S. D. Sidle, "Building a Committed Global Workforce: Does What Employees Want Depend on Culture?" *Academy of Management Perspective,* February 2009, pp. 79–80; and G. A. Gelade, P. Dobson, and K. Auer, "Individualism, Masculinity, and the Sources of Organizational Commitment," *Journal of Cross-Cultural Psychology,* vol. 39, no. 5, 2008, pp. 599–617.

69. P. Brotherton, "Employee Loyalty Slipping Worldwide; Respect, Work-Life Balance Are Top Engagers," *T&D,* February 2012, p. 24.

70. I. Harpaz, "The Importance of Work Goals: An International Perspective," *Journal of International Business Studies,* First Quarter 1990, pp. 75–93.

71. G. E. Popp, H. J. Davis, and T. T. Herbert, "An International Study of Intrinsic Motivation Composition," *Management International Review,* January 1986, pp. 28–35.

72. R. W. Brislin, B. MacNab, R. Worthley, F. Kabigting Jr., and B. Zukis, "Evolving Perceptions of Japanese Workplace Motivation: An Employee-Manager Comparison," *International Journal of Cross-Cultural Management,* April 2005, pp. 87–104.

73. J. T. Marquez, "Tailor-Made Careers," *Workforce Management Online,* January 2010.

74. J. R. Billings and D. L. Sharpe, "Factors Influencing Flextime Usage Among Employed Married Women," *Consumer Interests Annual,*

1999, pp. 89–94; and I. Harpaz, "The Importance of Work Goals: An International Perspective," *Journal of International Business Studies,* First Quarter 1990, pp. 75–93.

75. N. Ramachandran, "New Paths at Work," *US News & World Report,* March 20, 2006, p. 47; S. Armour, "Generation Y: They've Arrived at Work with a New Attitude," *USA Today,* November 6, 2005, pp. B1+; and R. Kanfer and P. L. Ackerman, "Aging, Adult Development, and Work Motivation," *Academy of Management Review,* July 2004, pp. 440–458.

76. T. D. Golden and J. F. Veiga, "The Impact of Extent of Telecommuting on Job Satisfaction: Resolving Inconsistent Findings," *Journal of Management,* April 2005, pp. 301–318.

77. See, for instance, M. Alpert, "The Care and Feeding of Engineers," *Fortune,* September 21, 1992, pp. 86–95; G. Poole, "How to Manage Your Nerds," *Forbes ASAP,* December 1994, pp. 132–136; T. J. Allen and R. Katz, "Managing Technical Professionals and Organizations: Improving and Sustaining the Performance of Organizations, Project Teams, and Individual Contributors," *Sloan Management Review,* Summer 2002, pp. S4–S5; and S. R. Barley and G. Kunda, "Contracting: A New Form of Professional Practice," *Academy of Management Perspectives,* February 2006, pp. 45–66.

78. J. P. Broschak and A. Davis-Blake, "Mixing Standard Work and Nonstandard Deals: The Consequences of Heterogeneity in Employment Arrangements," *Academy of Management Journal,* April 2006, pp. 371–393; M. L. Kraimer, S. J. Wayne, R. C. Liden, and R. T. Sparrowe, "The Role of Job Security in Understanding the Relationship Between Employees' Perceptions of Temporary Workers and Employees' Performance," *Journal of Applied Psychology,* March 2005, pp. 389–398; and C. E. Connelly and D. G. Gallagher, "Emerging Trends in Contingent Work Research," *Journal of Management,* November 2004, pp. 959–983.

79. C. Haddad, "FedEx: Gaining on the Ground," *BusinessWeek,* December 16, 2002, pp. 126–128; and L. Landro, "To Get Doctors to Do Better, Health Plans Try Cash Bonuses," *Wall Street Journal,* September 17, 2004, pp. A1+.

80. K. E. Culp, "Playing Field Widens for Stack's Great Game," *Springfield, Missouri, News-Leader,* January 9, 2005, pp. 1A+.

81. D. Meinert, "An Open Book," *HR Magazine,* April 2013, pp. 43–46; K. Berman and J. Knight, "What Your Employees Don't Know Will Hurt You," *Wall Street Journal,* February 27, 2012, p. R4; J. Case, "The Open-Book Revolution," *Inc.,* June 1995, pp. 26–50; J. P. Schuster, J. Carpenter, and M. P. Kane, *The Power of Open-Book Management* (New York: John Wiley, 1996); J. Case, "Opening the Books," *Harvard Business Review,* March–April 1997, pp. 118–127; and D. Drickhamer, "Open Books to Elevate Performance," *Industry Week,* November 2002, p. 16.

82. J. Ruhlman and C. Siegman, "Boosting Engagement While Cutting Costs," *The Gallup Management Journal Online,* June 18, 2009.

83. D. McCann, "No Employee Left Behind," *CFO,* April 2012, p. 29.

84. P. Lencioni, "The No-Cost Way to Motivate," *BusinessWeek,* October 5, 2009, p. 84; and F. Luthans and A. D. Stajkovic, "Provide Recognition for Performance Improvement," in E. A. Locke (ed.), *Principles of Organizational Behavior* (Oxford, England: Blackwell, 2000), pp. 166–180.

85. C. Huff, "Recognition That Resonates," *Workforce Management Online,* April 1, 2008.

86. D. Drickhamer, "Best Plant Winners: Nichols Foods Ltd.," *Industry Week,* October 1, 2001, pp. 17–19.

87. A. Bryant, "A Wall of Honor That's Built by Your Colleagues," *New York Times Online,* June 30, 2012.

88. M. Littman, "Best Bosses Tell All," *Working Woman,* October 2000, p. 54; and Hoover's Online [www.hoovers.com], June 20, 2003.

89. E. White, "Praise from Peers Goes a Long Way," *Wall Street Journal,* December 19, 2005.

90. Ibid.

91. S. Ladika, "Companies Recognizing Importance of Recognition," *Workforce,* December 2013, pp. 52–56.

92. K. Piombino, "Infographic: Only 12% of Workers Get Frequent Appreciation," www.hrcommunication.com, January 4, 2013.

93. Cited in S. Caudron, "The Top 20 Ways to Motivate Employees," *Industry Week,* April 3, 1995, pp. 15–16. See also B. Nelson, "Try Praise," *Inc.,* September 1996, p. 115; and J. Wiscombe, "Rewards Get Results," *Workforce,* April 2002, pp. 42–48.

94. R. Flandez, "Vegetable Gardens Help Morale Grow," *Wall Street Journal Online,* August 18, 2009; "Pay Raise Alternatives = Motivated Employees," *Training,* July/August 2009, p. 11; D. Koeppel, "Strange Brew: Beer and Office Democracy," CNNMoney.com, June 9, 2009; and B. Brim and T. Simon, "Strengths on the Factory Floor," *The Gallup Management Journal Online,* March 10, 2009.

95. V. M. Barret, "Fight the Jerks," *Forbes,* July 2, 2007, pp. 52–54.

96. E. White, "The Best vs. the Rest," *Wall Street Journal,* January 30, 2006, pp. B1+.

97. R. K. Abbott, "Performance-Based Flex: A Tool for Managing Total Compensation Costs," *Compensation and Benefits Review,* March–April 1993, pp. 18–21; J. R. Schuster and P. K. Zingheim, "The New Variable Pay: Key Design Issues," *Compensation and Benefits Review,* March–April 1993, pp. 27–34; C. R. Williams and L. P. Livingstone, "Another Look at the Relationship Between Performance and Voluntary Turnover," *Academy of Management Journal,* April 1994, pp. 269–298; A. M. Dickinson and K. L. Gillette, "A Comparison of the Effects of Two Individual Monetary Incentive Systems on Productivity: Piece Rate Pay Versus Base Pay Plus Incentives," *Journal of Organizational Behavior Management,* Spring 1994, pp. 3–82; and C. B. Cadsby, F. Song, and F. Tapon, "Sorting and Incentive Effects of Pay for Performance: An Experimental Investigation," *Academy of Management Journal,* April 2007, pp. 387–405.

98. J. B. Kelleher, "90 Percent of Employers Tie Workers' Pay to Company Performance," www.huffingtonpost.com, September 1, 2013.

99. "More Than 20 Percent of Japanese Firms Use Pay Systems Based on Performance," *Manpower Argus,* May 1998, p. 7; and E. Beauchesne, "Pay Bonuses Improve Productivity, Study Shows," *Vancouver Sun,* September 13, 2002, p. D5.

100. H. Rheem, "Performance Management Programs," *Harvard Business Review,* September–October 1996, pp. 8–9; G. Sprinkle, "The Effect of Incentive Contracts on Learning and Performance," *Accounting Review,* July 2000, pp. 299–326; and "Do Incentive Awards Work?" *HRFocus,* October 2000, pp. 1–3.

101. R. D. Banker, S. Y. Lee, G. Potter, and D. Srinivasan, "Contextual Analysis of Performance Impacts on Outcome-Based Incentive Compensation," *Academy of Management Journal,* August 1996, pp. 920–948.

102. B. S. Frey and M. Osterloh, "Stop Typing Pay to Performance," *Harvard Business Review,* January–February 2012, pp. 51–52.

103. T. Reason, "Why Bonus Plans Fail," *CFO,* January 2003, p. 53; and "Has Pay For Performance Had Its Day?" *The McKinsey Quarterly,* no. 4, 2002, accessed on Forbes Web site [www.forbes.com].

104. L. Weber and R. E. Silverman, "Workers Share Their Salary Secrets," *Wall Street Journal,* April 17, 2013, pp. B1+; R. E. Silverman, "Psst…This Is What Your Co-Worker Is Paid," *Wall Street Journal,* January 30, 2013, p. B6; and R. E. Silverman, "My Colleague, My Paymaster," *Wall Street Journal,* April 4, 2012, pp. B1+.

105. "Patagonia CEO & President Casey Sheahan Talks Business, Conservation & Compassion," offyonder.com, February 13, 2012; T. Henneman, "Patagonia Fills Payroll with People Who Are Passionate," www.workforce.com, November 4, 2011; M. Hanel, "Surf's Up at Patagonia," *Bloomberg BusinessWeek,* September 5–11, 2011, pp. 88–89; J. Wang, "Patagonia, from the Ground Up," *Entrepreneur,* June 2010, pp. 26–32; and J. Laabs, "Mixing Business with Pleasure," *Workforce,* March 2000, pp. 80–85.

106. M. Valcour, "The End of 'Results Only' at Best Buy Is Bad News," http://blogs.hbr.org/2013/03/goodbye-to-flexible-work-at-be/, March 8, 2013; C. Ressler, "Welcome to the Past: Best Buy Embraces Last Century Management Practices," http://info.gorowe.com/blog/bid/327538/Welcome-to-the-Past-Best-Buy-Embraces-Last-Century-Management-Practices, March 5, 2013; M. Nisen, "The Creators of Best Buy's Flexible Work Program Are Furious That It's Getting Dropped," www.businessinsider.com, March 5, 2013; S. Miller, "Study: Flexible Schedule Reduce Conflict, Lower Turnover," www.shrm.org, April 13, 2011; K. M. Butler, "We Can ROWE Our Way to a Better

Work Environment," EBN.BenefitNews.com, April 1, 2011, p. 8; P. Moen, E. L. Kelly, and R. Hill, "Does Enhancing Work-Time Control and Flexibility Reduce Turnover? A Naturally Occurring Experiment," *Social Problems,* February 2011, pp. 69–98; M. Conlin, "Is Optimism a Competitive Advantage?" *BusinessWeek,* August 24 & 31, 2009, pp. 52–53; "New ROLE," *Training,* June 2009, p. 4; C. Ressler and J.

Thompson, *Why Work Sucks and How to Fix It* (New York: Penguin Group, 2008); J. Marquez, "Changing a Company's Culture, Not Just Its Schedules, Pays Off," *Workforce Management Online,* November 17, 2008; S. Brown, "Results Should Matter, Not Just Working Late," *USA Today,* June 16, 2008, p. 4B; and J. Thottam, "Reworking Work," *Time,* July 25, 2005, pp. 50–55.

Being an Effective Leader

It's Your Career

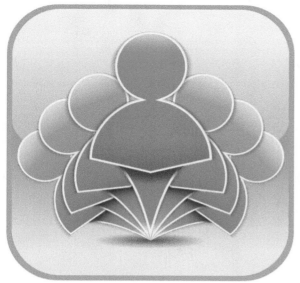

Source: Aleksandr Bryliaev/Shutterstock

A key to success in management and in your career is knowing *how to step into a leadership position.*

I'm a Leader: Now What?

You've been promoted to a supervisory position. Or you've been asked to head up a temporary task force. Or your team asks you to lead them on a new project. What now?

Sometime during your work career, you're likely to be asked to step up and take a leadership position. As a leader, you'll want a team that's motivated, committed, engaged, and ready to give their best. Here are some suggestions to help you successfully make that transition to being an effective leader:

1. Assess the leadership situation by looking at these three variables: *(a) Assess the individual capabilities of your group members. How competent and capable is each member? What does each bring to the team/group? (b) Assess the willingness and motivation of your group members. How motivated are the members toward the group's goals? (c) Determine how much power you have to reward or punish group members. All things being equal, it helps to have influence over factors such as hiring, firing, discipline, and salary increases. Assessing these three variables will give you important insights into what type of leadership style will be most effective in your new situation.*

2. Build trust. *Trust is so critically important. People tend to not follow those they don't trust. Start earning your team members' trust by telling them the truth and keeping your promises. (Look in the chapter for more information on how to build trust.)*

3. Be consistent. *Set clear priorities and follow them consistently and daily. If employees see you changing direction or behaving randomly, they'll lose confidence in your ability to lead them.*

4. Engage your team members. *Leaders are successful when they have the buy-in and commitment of their people. Be deliberate in establishing*

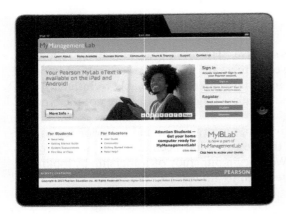

MyManagementLab®

⭐ Improve Your Grade!

When you see this icon, visit **www.mymanagementlab.com** for activities that are applied, personalized, and offer immediate feedback.

Learning Objectives

1 **Define** *leader and leadership.*

2 **Compare** *and contrast early theories of leadership.*

3 **Describe** *the three major contingency theories of leadership.*

- **Develop your skill** at choosing an effective leadership style.

4 **Describe** *contemporary views of leadership.*

5 **Discuss** *contemporary issues affecting leadership.*

- **Know how** to prepare for an effective transition to a leadership position.

---

relationships. Expecting your team members to be open to your leading them simply because of your credentials or experience isn't realistic. Talk with them about your vision, goals, and tasks. Let them know you have the organization's interests and their interests in mind.

5. Don't distance yourself from those you're leading. *Being arrogant or distant can disengage your*

team members. They need to know you are there for them and want to see them succeed.

6. Be adaptable. *Leading others isn't a one-size-fits-all scenario. Adapt your leadership approach to what the situation calls for. Sometimes you have to be more direct; sometimes more personable. This is a skill that you'll continue to develop as you're faced with leading different individuals and in different situations.*

If someone asked you to name a great leader, who would you name? Many individuals point to the late Steve Jobs of Apple as a great leader. And he does provide a fascinating example of the "whats" and "hows" of leadership. His leadership approach and style is totally not what you'd read about in most books on leadership. And how he led Apple probably wouldn't work in all situations, if any others. But leadership *is* needed in *all* organizations. Why? Because it's the leaders in organizations who make things happen.

WHO Are Leaders and What is Leadership?

LO1 Let's begin by clarifying who leaders are and what leadership is. Our definition of a **leader** is someone who can influence others and who has managerial authority. **Leadership** is a process of leading a group and influencing that group to achieve its goals. It's what leaders do.

Are all managers leaders? Because leading is one of the four management functions, yes, ideally, all managers *should* be leaders. Thus, we're going to study leaders

leader
Someone who can influence others and who has managerial authority

leadership
A process of influencing a group to achieve goals

and leadership from a managerial perspective.[1] However, even though we're looking at these from a managerial perspective, we're aware that groups often have informal leaders who emerge. Although these informal leaders may be able to influence others, they have not been the focus of most leadership research and are not the types of leaders we're studying in this text.

Leaders and leadership, like motivation, are organizational behavior topics that have been researched a lot. Most of that research has been aimed at answering the question: *What is an effective leader?* We'll begin our study of leadership by looking at some early leadership theories that attempted to answer that question.

EARLY Leadership Theories

LO2 People have been interested in leadership since they started coming together in groups to accomplish goals. However, it wasn't until the early part of the twentieth century that researchers actually began to study leadership. These early leadership theories focused on the *leader* (leadership trait theories) and how the *leader interacted* with his or her group members (leadership behavior theories).

Leadership Trait Theories

Researchers at the University of Cambridge in England recently reported that men with longer ring fingers, compared to their index fingers, tended to be more successful in the frantic high-frequency trading in the London financial district.[2] What does a study of the finger lengths of financial traders have to do with trait theories of leadership? Well, that's also what leadership trait theories have attempted to do—identify certain traits that all leaders have.

Leadership research in the 1920s and 1930s focused on isolating leader traits—that is, characteristics—that would differentiate leaders from nonleaders. Some of the traits studied included physical stature, appearance, social class, emotional stability, fluency of speech, and sociability. Despite the best efforts of researchers, it proved impossible to identify a set of traits that would *always* differentiate a leader (the person) from a nonleader. Maybe it was a bit optimistic to think that a set of consistent and unique traits would apply universally to all effective leaders, no matter whether they were in charge of Mondelez International (formerly Kraft Foods), the Moscow Ballet, the country of France, a local collegiate chapter of Alpha Chi Omega, Ted's Malibu Surf Shop, or Oxford University. However, later attempts to identify traits consistently associated with *leadership* (the process of leading, not the person) were more successful. The eight traits shown to be associated with effective leadership are described briefly in Exhibit 1.[3]

Researchers eventually recognized that traits alone were not sufficient for identifying effective leaders since explanations based solely on traits ignored the interactions of leaders and their group members as well as situational factors. Possessing the appropriate traits only made it more likely that an individual would be an effective leader. Therefore, leadership research from the late 1940s to the mid-1960s concentrated on the preferred behavioral styles that leaders demonstrated. Researchers wondered whether something unique in what effective leaders *did*—in other words, in their *behavior*—was the key.

Leadership Behavior Theories

Bill Watkins, former CEO of disk drive manufacturer Seagate Technology, once responded when asked how he handled his board of directors, "You never ask board members what they think. You tell them what you're going to do" (Jeffery M. O'Brien, Senior Editor, *Fortune* magazine, November 30, 2006). In contrast, Joe Lee, CEO of Darden Restaurants during the aftermath of 9/11, was focused on only two things that morning: his Darden people who were traveling and his company's Muslim

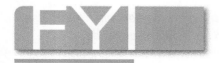

Exhibit 1

Eight Traits Associated with Leadership

Sources: Based on S. A. Kirkpatrick and E. A. Locke, "Leadership: Do Traits Really Matter?" *Academy of Management Executive,* May 1991, pp. 48–60; T. A. Judge, J. E. Bono, R. Ilies, and M. W. Gerhardt, "Personality and Leadership: A Qualitative and Quantitative Review," *Journal of Applied Psychology,* August 2002, pp. 765–780; and R. L. Schaumberg and F. J. Flynn, "Uneasy Lies the Head That Wears the Crown: The Link Between Guilt Proneness and Leadership," *Journal of Personality and Social Psychology,* August 2012, pp. 327–342.

1. *Drive.* Leaders exhibit a high effort level. They have a relatively high desire for achievement, they are ambitious, they have a lot of energy, they are tirelessly persistent in their activities, and they show initiative.

2. *Desire to lead.* Leaders have a strong desire to influence and lead others. They demonstrate the willingness to take responsibility.

3. *Honesty and integrity.* Leaders build trusting relationships with followers by being truthful or nondeceitful and by showing high consistency between word and deed.

4. *Self-confidence.* Followers look to leaders for an absence of self-doubt. Leaders, therefore, need to show self-confidence in order to convince followers of the rightness of their goals and decisions.

5. *Intelligence.* Leaders need to be intelligent enough to gather, synthesize, and interpret large amounts of information, and they need to be able to create visions, solve problems, and make correct decisions.

6. *Job-relevant knowledge.* Effective leaders have a high degree of knowledge about the company, industry, and technical matters. In-depth knowledge allows leaders to make well-informed decisions and to understand the implications of those decisions.

7. *Extraversion.* Leaders are energetic, lively people. They are sociable, assertive, and rarely silent or withdrawn.

8. *Proneness to guilt.* Guilt proneness is positively related to leadership effectiveness because it produces a strong sense of responsibility for others.

colleagues.[5] These two leaders of successful companies, as you can see, behaved in two very different ways. What do we know about leader behavior and how can it help us in our understanding of what an effective leader is?

Researchers hoped that the **behavioral theories** approach would provide more definitive answers about the nature of leadership than did the trait theories.[6] The four main leader behavior studies are summarized in Exhibit 2.

UNIVERSITY OF IOWA STUDIES The University of Iowa studies explored three leadership styles to find which was the most effective.[7] The **autocratic style** described a leader who dictated work methods, made unilateral decisions, and limited employee participation. The **democratic style** described a leader who involved employees in decision making, delegated authority, and used feedback as an opportunity for coaching employees. Finally, the **laissez-faire style** leader let the group make decisions and complete the work in whatever way it saw fit. The researchers' results seemed to indicate that the democratic style contributed to both good quantity and quality of work. Had the answer to the question of the most effective leadership style been found? Unfortunately, it wasn't that simple. Later studies of the autocratic and democratic styles showed mixed results. For instance, the democratic style sometimes produced higher performance levels than the autocratic style, but at other times, it didn't. However, more consistent results were found when a measure of employee satisfaction was used. Group members were more satisfied under a democratic leader than under an autocratic one.[8]

Now leaders had a dilemma! Should they focus on achieving higher performance or on achieving higher member satisfaction? This recognition of the dual nature of a leader's behavior—that is, focus on the task and focus on the people—was also a key characteristic of the other behavioral studies.

THE OHIO STATE STUDIES The Ohio State studies identified two important dimensions of leader behavior.[9] Beginning with a list of more than 1,000 behavioral dimensions, the researchers eventually narrowed it down to just two that accounted for most of the leadership behavior described by group members. The first was called **initiating structure**, which referred to the extent to which a leader defined his or her role and the roles of group members in attaining goals. It included behaviors that

behavioral theories
Leadership theories that identify behaviors that differentiate effective leaders from ineffective leaders

autocratic style
A leader who dictates work methods, makes unilateral decisions, and limits employee participation

democratic style
A leader who involves employees in decision making, delegates authority, and uses feedback as an opportunity for coaching employees

laissez-faire style
A leader who lets the group make decisions and complete the work in whatever way it sees fit

initiating structure
The extent to which a leader defines his or her role and the roles of group members in attaining goals

Exhibit 2
Behavioral Theories of Leadership

	Behavioral Dimension	**Conclusion**
University of Iowa	*Democratic style:* involving subordinates, delegating authority, and encouraging participation	Democratic style of leadership was most effective, although later studies showed mixed results.
	Autocratic style: dictating work methods, centralizing decision making, and limiting participation	
	Laissez-faire style: giving group freedom to make decisions and complete work	
Ohio State	*Consideration:* being considerate of followers' ideas and feelings	High–high leader (high in consideration and high in initiating structure) achieved high subordinate performance and satisfaction, but not in all situations
	Initiating structure: structuring work and work relationships to meet job goals	
University of Michigan	*Employee oriented:* emphasized interpersonal relationships and taking care of employees' needs	Employee-oriented leaders were associated with high group productivity and higher job satisfaction.
	Production oriented: emphasized technical or task aspects of job	
Managerial Grid	*Concern for people:* measured leader's concern for subordinates on a scale of 1 to 9 (low to high)	Leaders performed best with a 9,9 style (high concern for production and high concern for people).
	Concern for production: measured leader's concern for getting job done on a scale of 1 to 9 (low to high)	

consideration
The extent to which a leader has work relationships characterized by mutual trust and respect for group members' ideas and feelings

high–high leader
A leader high in both initiating structure and consideration behaviors

involved attempts to organize work, work relationships, and goals. The second was called **consideration**, which was defined as the extent to which a leader had work relationships characterized by mutual trust and respect for group members' ideas and feelings. A leader who was high in consideration helped group members with personal problems, was friendly and approachable, and treated all group members as equals. He or she showed concern for (was considerate of) his or her followers' comfort, well-being, status, and satisfaction. Research found that a leader who was high in both initiating structure and consideration (a **high–high leader**) sometimes achieved high group task performance and high group member satisfaction, but not always.

UNIVERSITY OF MICHIGAN STUDIES Leadership studies conducted at the University of Michigan at about the same time as those done at Ohio State also hoped to identify behavioral characteristics of leaders that were related to performance effectiveness. The Michigan group also came up with two dimensions of leadership behavior, which they labeled employee oriented and production oriented.[10] Leaders

who were *employee oriented* were described as emphasizing interpersonal relationships. The *production-oriented* leaders, in contrast, tended to emphasize the task aspects of the job. Unlike the other studies, the Michigan researchers concluded that leaders who were employee oriented were able to get high group productivity and high group member satisfaction.

THE MANAGERIAL GRID   The behavioral dimensions from these early leadership studies provided the basis for the development of a two-dimensional grid for appraising leadership styles. This **managerial grid** used the behavioral dimensions "concern for people" (the vertical part of the grid) and "concern for production" (the horizontal part of the grid) and evaluated a leader's use of these behaviors, ranking them on a scale from 1 (low) to 9 (high).[11] Although the grid had 81 potential categories into which a leader's behavioral style might fall, only five styles were named: impoverished management (1,1 or low concern for production, low concern for people), task management (9,1 or high concern for production, low concern for people), middle-of-the-road management (5,5 or medium concern for production, medium concern for people), country club management (1,9 or low concern for production, high concern for people), and team management (9,9 or high concern for production, high concern for people). Of these five styles, the researchers concluded that managers performed best when using a 9,9 style. Unfortunately, the grid offered no answers to the question of what made a manager an effective leader; it only provided a framework for conceptualizing leadership style. In fact, little substantive evidence supports the conclusion that a 9,9 style is most effective in all situations.[12]

Leadership researchers were discovering that predicting leadership success involved something more complex than isolating a few leader traits or preferable behaviors. They began looking at situational influences; specifically, which leadership styles might be suitable in different situations and what these different situations might be.

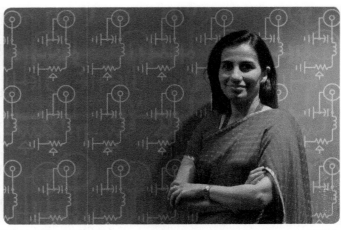

Chanda Kochhar, the managing director and CEO of ICICI Bank in India, is an employee-oriented leader whose compassionate and nurturing behavior towards subordinates in helping them realize their full potential results in high group member satisfaction and productivity. Under her leadership, ICICI Bank has grown to become the largest private retail bank in India.
Source: Vivek Prakash/Reuters Pictures

managerial grid
A two-dimensional grid for appraising leadership styles

CONTINGENCY Theories of Leadership

L03   "The corporate world is filled with stories of leaders who failed to achieve greatness because they failed to understand the context they were working in."[13] In this section, we examine three contingency theories—Fiedler, Hersey-Blanchard, and path-goal. Each looks at defining leadership style and the situation, and attempts to answer the *if-then* contingencies (that is, *if* this is the context or situation, *then* this is the best leadership style to use).

The Fiedler Model

The first comprehensive contingency model for leadership was developed by Fred Fiedler.[14] The **Fiedler contingency model** proposed that effective group performance depended on properly matching the leader's style and the amount of control and influence in the situation. The model was based on the premise that a certain leadership style would be most effective in different types of situations. The keys were to (1) define those leadership styles and the different types of situations, and then (2) identify the appropriate combinations of style and situation.

Fiedler proposed that a key factor in leadership success was an individual's basic leadership style, either task oriented or relationship oriented. To measure a leader's style, Fiedler developed the **least-preferred coworker (LPC) questionnaire**. This questionnaire contained 18 pairs of contrasting adjectives—for example, pleasant–unpleasant, cold–warm, boring–interesting, or friendly–unfriendly. Respondents were asked to think of all the coworkers they had ever had and to describe that one person they *least enjoyed* working with by rating him or her on a scale of 1 to 8 for each of

Fiedler contingency model
A leadership theory proposing that effective group performance depends on the proper match between a leader's style and the degree to which the situation allows the leader to control and influence

least-preferred coworker (LPC) questionnaire
A questionnaire that measures whether a leader is task or relationship oriented

the 18 sets of adjectives (the 8 always described the positive adjective out of the pair and the 1 always described the negative adjective out of the pair).

If the leader described the least preferred coworker in relatively positive terms (in other words, a "high" LPC score—a score of 64 or above), then the respondent was primarily interested in good personal relations with coworkers, and the style would be described as *relationship oriented*. In contrast, if you saw the least preferred coworker in relatively unfavorable terms (a low LPC score—a score of 57 or below), you were primarily interested in productivity and getting the job done; thus, your style would be labeled as *task oriented*. Fiedler did acknowledge that a small number of people might fall in between these two extremes and not have a cut-and-dried leadership style. One other important point is that Fiedler assumed a person's leadership style was fixed regardless of the situation. In other words, if you were a relationship-oriented leader, you'd always be one, and the same for task-oriented.

After an individual's leadership style had been assessed through the LPC, it was time to evaluate the situation in order to be able to match the leader with the situation. Fiedler's research uncovered three contingency dimensions that defined the key situational factors in leader effectiveness.

- **Leader–member relations:** the degree of confidence, trust, and respect employees have for their leader; rated as either good or poor.
- **Task structure:** the degree to which job assignments are formalized and structured; rated as either high or low.
- **Position power:** the degree of influence a leader has over activities such as hiring, firing, discipline, promotions, and salary increases; rated as either strong or weak.

Each leadership situation was evaluated in terms of these three contingency variables, which, when combined, produced eight possible situations that were either favorable or unfavorable for the leader. (See the bottom of the chart in Exhibit 3.) Situations I, II, and III were classified as highly favorable for the leader. Situations IV, V, and VI were moderately favorable for the leader. And situations VII and VIII were described as highly unfavorable for the leader.

Once Fiedler had described the leader variables and the situational variables, he had everything he needed to define the specific contingencies for leadership effectiveness. To do so, he studied 1,200 groups where he compared relationship-oriented

leader–member relations
One of Fiedler's situational contingencies that describes the degree of confidence, trust, and respect employees have for their leader

task structure
One of Fiedler's situational contingencies that describes the degree to which job assignments are formalized and structured

position power
One of Fiedler's situational contingencies that describes the degree of influence a leader has over activities such as hiring, firing, discipline, promotions, and salary increases

Exhibit 3
The Fiedler Model

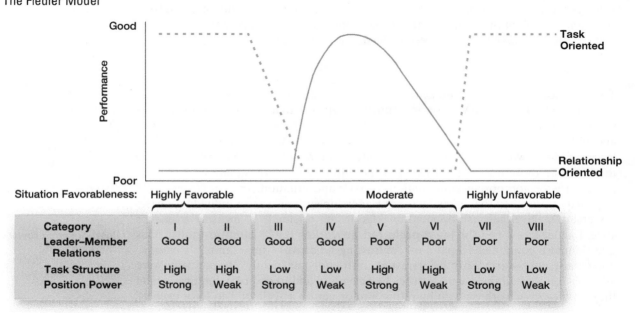

Category	I	II	III	IV	V	VI	VII	VIII
Leader–Member Relations	Good	Good	Good	Good	Poor	Poor	Poor	Poor
Task Structure	High	High	Low	Low	High	High	Low	Low
Position Power	Strong	Weak	Strong	Weak	Strong	Weak	Strong	Weak

versus task-oriented leadership styles in each of the eight situational categories. He concluded that task-oriented leaders performed better in very favorable situations and in very unfavorable situations. (See the top of Exhibit 3, where performance is shown on the vertical axis and situation favorableness is shown on the horizontal axis.) On the other hand, relationship-oriented leaders performed better in moderately favorable situations.

Because Fiedler treated an individual's leadership style as fixed, only two ways could improve leader effectiveness. First, you could bring in a new leader whose style better fit the situation. For instance, if the group situation was highly unfavorable but was led by a relationship-oriented leader, the group's performance could be improved by replacing that person with a task-oriented leader. The second alternative was to change the situation to fit the leader. This could be done by restructuring tasks; by increasing or decreasing the power that the leader had over factors such as salary increases, promotions, and disciplinary actions; or by improving the leader–member relations.

Research testing the overall validity of Fiedler's model has shown considerable evidence to support the model.[15] However, his theory wasn't without criticisms. The major one is that it's probably unrealistic to assume that a person can't change his or her leadership style to fit the situation. Effective leaders can, and do, change their styles. Another is that the LPC wasn't very practical. Finally, the situation variables were difficult to assess.[16] Despite its shortcomings, the Fiedler model showed that effective leadership style needed to reflect situational factors.

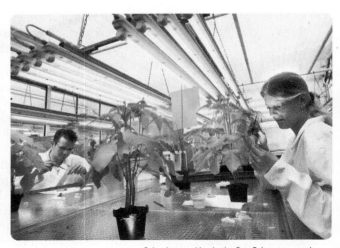

Scientists working in the CropScience research laboratory of Bayer AG, a German chemical and pharmaceutical firm, have a high level of follower readiness. Responsible and experienced, they are willing and able to complete their tasks under leadership that gives them freedom to make and implement decisions, a relationship consistent with Hersey and Blanchard's situational theory.
Source: Bayer AG/AP Images

Hersey and Blanchard's Situational Leadership Theory

Paul Hersey and Ken Blanchard developed a leadership theory that has gained a strong following among management development specialists.[17] This model, called **situational leadership theory (SLT)**, is a contingency theory that focuses on followers' readiness. Before we proceed, two points need clarification: why a leadership theory focuses on the followers and what is meant by the term *readiness*.

The emphasis on the followers in leadership effectiveness reflects the reality that it *is* the followers who accept or reject the leader. Regardless of what the leader does, the group's effectiveness depends on the actions of the followers. This important dimension has been overlooked or underemphasized in most leadership theories. And **readiness**, as defined by Hersey and Blanchard, refers to the extent to which people have the ability and willingness to accomplish a specific task.

SLT uses the same two leadership dimensions that Fiedler identified: task and relationship behaviors. However, Hersey and Blanchard go a step further by considering each as either high or low and then combining them into four specific leadership styles described as follows:

- *Telling* (high task–low relationship): The leader defines roles and tells people what, how, when, and where to do various tasks.
- *Selling* (high task–high relationship): The leader provides both directive and supportive behavior.
- *Participating* (low task–high relationship): The leader and followers share in decision making; the main role of the leader is facilitating and communicating.
- *Delegating* (low task–low relationship): The leader provides little direction or support.

The final component in the model is the four stages of follower readiness:

- *R1:* People are both *unable and unwilling* to take responsibility for doing something. Followers aren't competent or confident.
- *R2:* People are *unable but willing* to do the necessary job tasks. Followers are motivated but lack the appropriate skills.

situational leadership theory (SLT)
A leadership contingency theory that focuses on followers' readiness

readiness
The extent to which people have the ability and willingness to accomplish a specific task

- *R3:* People are *able but unwilling* to do what the leader wants. Followers are competent, but don't want to do something.
- *R4:* People are both *able and willing* to do what is asked of them.

SLT essentially views the leader–follower relationship as like that of a parent and a child. Just as a parent needs to relinquish control when a child becomes more mature and responsible, so too should leaders. As followers reach higher levels of readiness, the leader responds not only by decreasing control over their activities but also decreasing relationship behaviors. The SLT says if followers are at R1 (*unable* and *unwilling* to do a task), the leader needs to use the telling style and give clear and specific directions; if followers are at R2 (*unable* and *willing*), the leader needs to use the selling style and display high task orientation to compensate for the followers' lack of ability and high relationship orientation to get followers to "buy into" the leader's desires; if followers are at R3 (*able* and *unwilling*), the leader needs to use the participating style to gain their support; and if employees are at R4 (both *able* and *willing*), the leader doesn't need to do much and should use the delegating style.

SLT has intuitive appeal. It acknowledges the importance of followers and builds on the logic that leaders can compensate for ability and motivational limitations in their followers. However, research efforts to test and support the theory generally have been disappointing.[18] Possible explanations include internal inconsistencies in the model as well as problems with research methodology. Despite its appeal and wide popularity, we have to be cautious about any enthusiastic endorsement of SLT.

Path-Goal Model

Another approach to understanding leadership is **path-goal theory**, which states that the leader's job is to assist followers in attaining their goals and to provide direction or support needed to ensure that their goals are compatible with the goals of the group or organization. Developed by Robert House, path-goal theory takes key elements from the expectancy theory of motivation.[20] The term *path-goal* is derived from the belief that effective leaders remove the roadblocks and pitfalls so that followers have a clearer path to help them get from where they are to the achievement of their work goals.

House identified four leadership behaviors:

- *Directive leader:* Lets subordinates know what's expected of them, schedules work to be done, and gives specific guidance on how to accomplish tasks.
- *Supportive leader:* Shows concern for the needs of followers and is friendly.
- *Participative leader:* Consults with group members and uses their suggestions before making a decision.
- *Achievement oriented leader:* Sets challenging goals and expects followers to perform at their highest level.

In contrast to Fiedler's view that a leader couldn't change his or her behavior, House assumed that leaders are flexible and can display any or all of these leadership styles depending on the situation.

As Exhibit 4 illustrates, path-goal theory proposes two situational or contingency variables that moderate the leadership behavior–outcome relationship: those in the *environment* that are outside the control of the follower (factors including task structure, formal authority system, and the work group) and those that are part of the personal characteristics of the *follower* (including locus of control, experience, and perceived ability). Environmental factors determine the type of leader behavior required if subordinate outcomes are to be maximized; personal characteristics of the follower determine how the environment and leader behavior are interpreted. The theory proposes that a leader's behavior won't be effective if it's redundant with what

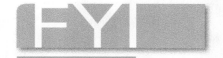

path-goal theory
A leadership theory that says the leader's job is to assist followers in attaining their goals and to provide direction or support needed to ensure that their goals are compatible with the goals of the group or organization

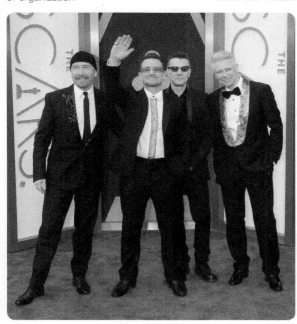

Bono (waving), U2's leader, lead singer, and lyricist, uses the supportive and participative approaches of the path-goal theory. He includes band members in decision making, believing that their input is necessary to achieve excellence. And he supports them by expressing his appreciation for their talents in contributing to U2's success and in achieving the band's goal of improving the world through its music and influence.
Source: Gregg DeGuire/WireImage/Getty Images

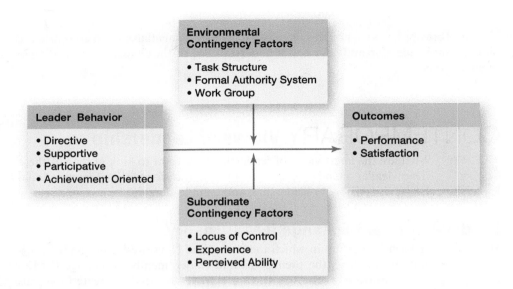

Exhibit 4
Path-Goal Model

the environmental structure is providing or is incongruent with follower characteristics. For example, some predictions from path-goal theory are:

- Directive leadership leads to greater satisfaction when tasks are ambiguous or stressful than when they are highly structured and well laid out. The followers aren't sure what to do, so the leader needs to give them some direction.
- Supportive leadership results in high employee performance and satisfaction when subordinates are performing structured tasks. In this situation, the leader only needs to support followers, not tell them what to do.
- Directive leadership is likely to be perceived as redundant among subordinates with high perceived ability or with considerable experience. These followers are quite capable, so they don't need a leader to tell them what to do.
- The clearer and more bureaucratic the formal authority relationships, the more leaders should exhibit supportive behavior and deemphasize directive behavior. The organizational situation has provided the structure as far as what is expected of followers, so the leader's role is simply to support.
- Directive leadership will lead to higher employee satisfaction when there is substantive conflict within a work group. In this situation, the followers need a leader who will take charge.
- Subordinates with an internal locus of control will be more satisfied with a participative style. Because these followers believe they control what happens to them, they prefer to participate in decisions.
- Subordinates with an external locus of control will be more satisfied with a directive style. These followers believe that what happens to them is a result of the external environment, so they would prefer a leader who tells them what to do.
- Achievement-oriented leadership will increase subordinates' expectancies that effort will lead to high performance when tasks are ambiguously structured. By setting challenging goals, followers know what the expectations are.

Testing path-goal theory has not been easy. A review of the research suggests mixed support.[21] To summarize the model, however, an employee's performance and satisfaction are likely to be positively influenced when the leader chooses a leadership style that compensates for shortcomings in either the employee or the work setting. However, if the leader spends time explaining tasks that are already clear or when the employee has the ability and experience to handle them without interference, the employee is likely to see such directive behavior as redundant or even insulting.

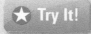 If your professor has assigned this, go to **www.mymanagementlab.com** to complete the Simulation: Leadership and get a better understanding of the challenges of leading in organizations.

CONTEMPORARY Views of Leadership

LO4 What are the latest views of leadership? We want to look at four of these views: leader–member exchange theory, transformational-transactional leadership, charismatic-visionary leadership, and team leadership.

Leader–Member Exchange (LMX) Theory

Have you ever been in a group in which the leader had "favorites" who made up his or her in-group? If so, that's the premise behind leader–member exchange (LMX) theory.[22] **Leader–member exchange theory (LMX)** says leaders create in-groups and out-groups and those in the in-group will have higher performance ratings, less turnover, and greater job satisfaction.

LMX theory suggests that early on in the relationship between a leader and a given follower, a leader will implicitly categorize a follower as an "in" or as an "out." That relationship tends to remain fairly stable over time. Leaders also encourage LMX by rewarding those employees with whom they want a closer linkage and punishing those with whom they do not.[24] For the LMX relationship to remain intact, however, both the leader and the follower must "invest" in the relationship.

It's not exactly clear how a leader chooses who falls into each category, but evidence shows that in-group members have demographic, attitude, personality, and even gender similarities with the leader or they have a higher level of competence than out-group members.[25] The leader does the choosing, but the follower's characteristics drive the decision.

Research on LMX has been generally supportive. It appears that leaders do differentiate among followers; that these disparities are not random; and followers with in-group status will have higher performance ratings, engage in more helping or "citizenship" behaviors at work, and report greater satisfaction with their boss.[26] A recent LMX study found that leaders who establish a supportive relationship with key subordinates by providing emotional and other kinds of support generate organizational commitment on the part of these employees, which leads to increases in employee performance.[27] This probably shouldn't be surprising since leaders invest their time and other resources in those whom they expect to perform best.

Transformational-Transactional Leadership

Many early leadership theories viewed leaders as **transactional leaders**; that is, leaders who lead primarily by using social exchanges (or transactions). Transactional leaders guide or motivate followers to work toward established goals by exchanging rewards for their productivity.[29] But another type of leader—a **transformational leader**—stimulates and inspires (transforms) followers to achieve extraordinary outcomes. Examples include

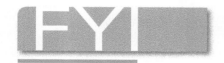

leader–member exchange theory (LMX)
The leadership theory that says leaders create in-groups and out-groups and those in the in-group will have higher performance ratings, less turnover, and greater job satisfaction

transactional leaders
Leaders who lead primarily by using social exchanges (or transactions)

transformational leaders
Leaders who stimulate and inspire (transform) followers to achieve extraordinary outcomes

LEADER making a DIFFERENCE

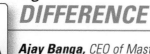

Ajay Banga, CEO of MasterCard, has had well-rounded leadership experiences. Born in India, Banga honed his leadership skills at Nestlé and PepsiCo before moving to Citigroup to head up its Asia-Pacific division. Citigroup was a challenging situation as he found a vast banking group where product groups worked well alone but did not coordinate or work with each other. Banga undertook the painful process of breaking down the internal barriers and rejoining them again in a unified, coordinated structure. When he was offered a position at MasterCard as president and chief operating officer, Banga jumped at the chance. Now as CEO, Banga is the company's cheerleader, shaking up the company's low-key corporate culture with hugs and fist bumps in the hallways. One analyst describes him as "energetic, open, and engaging."[28] What can you learn from this leader making a difference?

Source: Keith Bedford / Reuters Pictures

Jim Goodnight of SAS Institute and Andrea Jung of Avon. They pay attention to the concerns and developmental needs of individual followers; they change followers' awareness of issues by helping those followers look at old problems in new ways; and they are able to excite, arouse, and inspire followers to exert extra effort to achieve group goals.

Transactional and transformational leadership shouldn't be viewed as opposing approaches to getting things done.[30] Transformational leadership develops from transactional leadership. Transformational leadership produces levels of employee effort and performance that go beyond what would occur with a transactional approach alone. Moreover, transformational leadership is more than charisma because the transformational leader attempts to instill in followers the ability to question not only established views but those views held by the leader.[31]

The evidence supporting the superiority of transformational leadership over transactional leadership is overwhelmingly impressive. For instance, studies that looked at managers in different settings, including the military and business, found that transformational leaders were evaluated as more effective, higher performers, more promotable than their transactional counterparts, and more interpersonally sensitive.[32] In addition, evidence indicates that transformational leadership is strongly correlated with lower turnover rates and higher levels of productivity, employee satisfaction, creativity, goal attainment, follower well-being, and corporate entrepreneurship, especially in start-up firms.[33]

Charismatic-Visionary Leadership

Jeff Bezos, founder and CEO of Amazon.com, is a person who exudes energy, enthusiasm, and drive.[34] He's fun-loving (his legendary laugh has been described as a flock of Canadian geese on nitrous oxide), but he has pursued his vision for Amazon with serious intensity and has demonstrated an ability to inspire his employees through the ups and downs of a rapidly growing company. Bezos is what we call a **charismatic leader**—that is, an enthusiastic, self-confident leader whose personality and actions influence people to behave in certain ways.

Several authors have attempted to identify personal characteristics of the charismatic leader.[35] The most comprehensive analysis identified five such characteristics: they have a vision, the ability to articulate that vision, a willingness to take risks to achieve that vision, a sensitivity to both environmental constraints and follower needs, and behaviors that are out of the ordinary.[36]

An increasing body of evidence shows impressive correlations between charismatic leadership and high performance and satisfaction among followers.[37] Although one study found that charismatic CEOs had no impact on subsequent organizational performance, charisma is still believed to be a desirable leadership quality.[38]

If charisma is desirable, can people learn to be charismatic leaders? Or are charismatic leaders born with their qualities? Although a small number of experts still think that charisma can't be learned, most believe that individuals can be trained to exhibit charismatic behaviors.[39] For example, researchers have succeeded in teaching undergraduate students to "be" charismatic. How? They were taught to articulate a far-reaching goal, communicate high performance expectations, exhibit confidence in the ability of subordinates to meet those expectations, and empathize with the needs of their subordinates; they learned to project a powerful, confident, and dynamic presence; and they practiced using a captivating and engaging voice tone. The researchers also trained the student leaders to use charismatic nonverbal behaviors, including leaning toward the follower when communicating, maintaining direct eye contact, and having a relaxed posture and animated facial expressions. In groups with these "trained" charismatic leaders, members had higher task performance, higher task adjustment, and better adjustment to the leader and to the group than did group members who worked in groups led by noncharismatic leaders.

One last thing we should say about charismatic leadership is that it may not always be necessary to achieve high levels of employee performance. It may be most

charismatic leader
An enthusiastic, self-confident leader whose personality and actions influence people to behave in certain ways

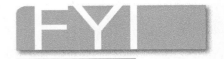

- A 60 percent increase in leadership ratings is what executives saw after they had been trained in charismatic tactics.[40]

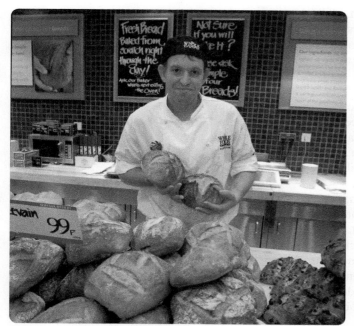

This team leader of the bakery department at a Whole Foods Market store serves as a coach in training and motivating team members to maintain good relationships with each other and vendors and to achieve team goals for sales, growth, and productivity. Leading his 13-member team requires enthusiasm, good communication skills, and working well with others.
Source: Daily Mail/Rex/Alamy

visionary leadership
The ability to create and articulate a realistic, credible, and attractive vision of the future that improves upon the present situation

appropriate when the follower's task has an ideological purpose or when the environment involves a high degree of stress and uncertainty.[41] This distinction may explain why, when charismatic leaders surface, it's more likely to be in politics, religion, or wartime, or when a business firm is starting up or facing a survival crisis. For example, Martin Luther King Jr. used his charisma to bring about social equality through nonviolent means, and Steve Jobs achieved unwavering loyalty and commitment from Apple's technical staff in the early 1980s by articulating a vision of personal computers that would dramatically change the way people lived.

Although the term *vision* is often linked with charismatic leadership, **visionary leadership** is different; it's the ability to create and articulate a realistic, credible, and attractive vision of the future that improves on the present situation.[42] This vision, if properly selected and implemented, is so energizing that it "in effect jump-starts the future by calling forth the skills, talents, and resources to make it happen."[43]

An organization's vision should offer clear and compelling imagery that taps into people's emotions and inspires enthusiasm to pursue the organization's goals. It should be able to generate possibilities that are inspirational and unique and offer new ways of doing things that are clearly better for the organization and its members. Visions that are clearly articulated and have powerful imagery are easily grasped and accepted. For instance, Michael Dell (Dell Computer) created a vision of a business that sells and delivers customized PCs directly to customers in less than a week. The late Mary Kay Ash's vision of women as entrepreneurs selling products that improved their self-image gave impetus to her cosmetics company, Mary Kay Cosmetics.

Team Leadership

Because leadership is increasingly taking place within a team context and more organizations are using work teams, the role of the leader in guiding team members has become increasingly important. The role of team leader *is* different from the traditional leadership role, as J. D. Bryant, a supervisor at Texas Instruments' Forest Lane plant in Dallas, discovered. One day he was contentedly overseeing a staff of 15 circuit board assemblers. The next day, he was told that the company was going to use employee teams and he was to become a "facilitator." He said, "I'm supposed to teach the teams everything I know and then let them make their own decisions." Confused about his new role, he admitted, "There was no clear plan on what I was supposed to do."[44] What *is* involved in being a team leader?

Many leaders are not equipped to handle the change to employee teams. As one consultant noted, "Even the most capable managers have trouble making the transition because all the command-and-control type things they were encouraged to do before are no longer appropriate. There's no reason to have any skill or sense of this."[45] This same consultant estimated that "probably 15 percent of managers are natural team leaders; another 15 percent could never lead a team because it runs counter to their personality—that is, they're unable to sublimate their dominating style for the good of the team. Then there's that huge group in the middle: Team leadership doesn't come naturally to them, but they can learn it."[46]

The challenge for many managers is learning how to become an effective team leader. They have to learn skills such as patiently sharing information, being able to trust others and to give up authority, and understanding when to intervene. And effective team leaders have mastered the difficult balancing act of knowing when to leave their teams alone and when to get involved. New team leaders may try to retain too much control at a time when team members need more autonomy, or they may abandon their teams at times when the teams need support and help.[47]

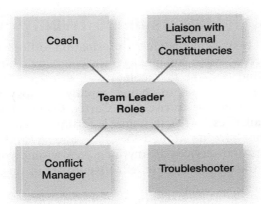

Exhibit 5
Team Leadership Roles

One study looking at organizations that reorganized themselves around employee teams found certain common responsibilities of all leaders. These leader responsibilities included coaching, facilitating, handling disciplinary problems, reviewing team and individual performance, training, and communication.[48] However, a more meaningful way to describe the team leader's job is to focus on two priorities: (1) managing the team's external boundary and (2) facilitating the team process.[49] These priorities entail four specific leadership roles, which are identified in Exhibit 5.

If your professor has assigned this, go to **www.mymanagementlab.com** to watch a video titled: *CH2MHill: Power and Political Behavior* and to respond to questions.

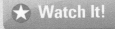

let's get REAL

The Scenario:

Linda Bustamante owns a thriving company that manufactures scented potpourris and other products. She's getting ready to expand her sales team again and wants to promote one of the current sales reps to team leader. This is a big step, and Linda desperately wants that person to succeed because it would take a load off her shoulders.

What advice could Linda give her newly appointed team leader?

Linda will need to have a long conversation with the new team leader about his/her strengths and why they have earned this position. It will be important to let them know that she has confidence in their ability to do the job and do it well. At the same time, it's important to gently note some challenges that the team leader may face. Linda will need to tailor the 'challenge discussion' to her employee's weaknesses.

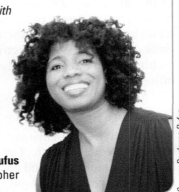

Prudence Rufus
Business Owner/Photographer

LEADERSHIP Issues in the Twenty-First Century

L05 It's not easy being a chief information officer (CIO) today. The person responsible for managing a company's information technology activities will find that the task comes with a lot of external and internal pressures. Technology continues to change rapidly—almost daily, it sometimes seems. Business costs continue to rise. Rob Carter, CIO of FedEx, is on the hot seat facing such challenges.[50] He's responsible for all the computer and communication systems that provide around-the-clock and around-the-globe support for FedEx's products and services. If anything goes wrong, you know who takes the heat. However, Carter has been an effective leader in this seemingly chaotic environment.

Leading effectively in today's environment is likely to involve such challenging circumstances for many leaders. In addition, twenty-first-century leaders do face some important leadership issues. In this section, we look at these issues that include managing power, developing trust, empowering employees, leading across cultures, and becoming an effective leader.

Managing Power

Where do leaders get their power—that is, their right and capacity to influence work actions or decisions? Five sources of leader power have been identified: legitimate, coercive, reward, expert, and referent.[51]

Legitimate power and authority are the same. Legitimate power represents the power a leader has as a result of his or her position in the organization. Although people in positions of authority are also likely to have reward and coercive power, legitimate power is broader than the power to coerce and reward.

Coercive power is the power a leader has to punish or control. Followers react to this power out of fear of the negative results that might occur if they don't comply. Managers typically have some coercive power, such as being able to suspend or demote employees or to assign them work they find unpleasant or undesirable.

Reward power is the power to give positive rewards. A reward can be anything a person values such as money, favorable performance appraisals, promotions, interesting work assignments, friendly colleagues, and preferred work shifts or sales territories.

Expert power is power based on expertise, special skills, or knowledge. If an employee has skills, knowledge, or expertise that's critical to a work group, that person's expert power is enhanced.

Finally, **referent power** is the power that arises because of a person's desirable resources or personal traits. If I admire you and want to be associated with you, you can exercise power over me because I want to please you. Referent power develops out of admiration of another and a desire to be like that person.

Most effective leaders rely on several different forms of power to affect the behavior and performance of their followers. For example, the commanding officer of one of Australia's state-of-the-art submarines, the HMAS *Sheean,* employs different types of power in managing his crew and equipment. He gives orders to the crew (legitimate), praises them (reward), and disciplines those who commit infractions (coercive). As an effective leader, he also strives to have expert power (based on his expertise and knowledge) and referent power (based on his being admired) to influence his crew.

Developing Trust

In today's uncertain environment, an important consideration for leaders is building trust and credibility, both of which can be extremely fragile. Before we can discuss ways leaders can build trust and credibility, we have to know what trust and credibility are and why they're so important.

legitimate power
The power a leader has as a result of his or her position in the organization

coercive power
The power a leader has to punish or control

reward power
The power a leader has to give positive rewards

expert power
Power that's based on expertise, special skills, or knowledge

referent power
Power that arises because of a person's desirable resources or personal traits

let's get REAL

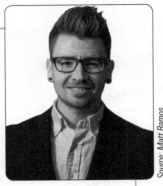

Source: Matt Ramos

Matt Ramos
Director of Marketing

The Scenario:

Adhita Chopra is stumped. Three months ago, he was assigned to lead a team of phone app designers, and although no one has come out and said anything directly, he feels like his team doesn't trust him. They have been withholding information and communicating only selectively when asked questions. And they have persistently questioned the team's goals and strategies and even Adhita's actions and decisions. How can he build trust with his team?

What advice would you give Adhita?

Trust in the workplace is always a tricky subject. I've seen a similar situation unfold once before. If Adhita feels this, but hasn't heard it directly, he's probably right. Earning trust at work comes down to 3 things: being good at what you do, being passionate about your work and the people around you, and the ability to listen and follow through. Adhita should make sure he's producing top notch work and set up weekly one-on-one meetings with the team. Hard work and careful listening will see Adhita through this.

The main component of credibility is honesty. Surveys show that honesty is consistently singled out as the number one characteristic of admired leaders. "Honesty is absolutely essential to leadership. If people are going to follow someone willingly, whether it be into battle or into the boardroom, they first want to assure themselves that the person is worthy of their trust."[52] In addition to being honest, credible leaders are competent and inspiring. They are personally able to effectively communicate their confidence and enthusiasm. Thus, followers judge a leader's **credibility** in terms of his or her honesty, competence, and ability to inspire.

Trust is closely entwined with the concept of credibility and, in fact, the terms are often used interchangeably. **Trust** is defined as the belief in the integrity, character, and ability of a leader. Followers who trust a leader are willing to be vulnerable to the leader's actions because they are confident that their rights and interests will not be abused.[53] Research has identified five dimensions that make up the concept of trust:[54]

- *Integrity:* honesty and truthfulness
- *Competence:* technical and interpersonal knowledge and skills
- *Consistency:* reliability, predictability, and good judgment in handling situations
- *Loyalty:* willingness to protect a person, physically and emotionally
- *Openness:* willingness to share ideas and information freely

Of these five dimensions, integrity seems to be the most critical when someone assesses another's trustworthiness.[55] Both integrity and competence were seen in our earlier discussion of leadership traits found to be consistently associated with leadership. Workplace changes have reinforced why such leadership qualities are important. For instance, the trends toward empowerment and self-managed work teams have reduced many of the traditional control mechanisms used to monitor employees. If a work team is free to schedule its own work, evaluate its own performance, and even make its own hiring decisions, trust becomes critical. Employees have to trust managers to treat them fairly, and managers have to trust employees to conscientiously fulfill their responsibilities.

credibility
The degree to which followers perceive someone as honest, competent, and able to inspire

trust
The belief in the integrity, character, and ability of a leader

Exhibit 6
Building Trust

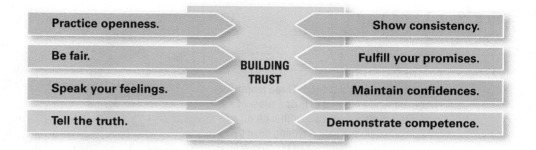

Practice openness.	BUILDING TRUST	Show consistency.
Be fair.		Fulfill your promises.
Speak your feelings.		Maintain confidences.
Tell the truth.		Demonstrate competence.

Also, leaders have to increasingly lead others who may not be in their immediate work group or may even be physically separated—members of cross-functional or virtual teams, individuals who work for suppliers or customers, and perhaps even people who represent other organizations through strategic alliances. These situations don't allow leaders the luxury of falling back on their formal positions for influence. Many of these relationships, in fact, are fluid and fleeting. So the ability to quickly develop trust and sustain that trust is crucial to the success of the relationship.

Why is it important that followers trust their leaders? Research has shown that trust in leadership is significantly related to positive job outcomes including job performance, organizational citizenship behavior, job satisfaction, and organizational commitment.[56] Given the importance of trust to effective leadership, how can leaders build trust? Exhibit 6 lists some suggestions.[57]

Now, more than ever, managerial and leadership effectiveness depends on the ability to gain the trust of followers.[58] Downsizing, financial challenges, and the increased use of temporary employees have undermined employees' trust in their leaders and shaken the confidence of investors, suppliers, and customers. Today's leaders are faced with the challenge of rebuilding and restoring trust with employees and with other important organizational stakeholders.

Empowering Employees

Employees at DuPont's facility in Uberaba, Brazil, planted trees to commemorate the site's 10th anniversary. Although they had several things to celebrate, one of the most important was the fact that since production began, the facility has had zero environmental incidents and no recordable safety violations. The primary reason for this achievement was the company's implementation of STOP (Safety Training Observation Program)—a program in which empowered employees were responsible for observing one another, correcting improper procedures, and encouraging safe procedures.[59]

As we've described in different places throughout the text, managers are increasingly leading by empowering their employees. As we've said before, empowerment involves increasing the decision-making discretion of workers. Millions of individual employees and employee teams are making the key operating decisions that directly affect their work. They're developing budgets, scheduling workloads, controlling inventories, solving quality problems, and engaging in similar activities that until very recently were viewed exclusively as part of the manager's job.[60] For instance, at The Container Store, any employee who gets a customer request has permission to take care of it. Garret Boone, chairman emeritus, says, "Everybody we hire, we hire as a leader. Anybody in our store can take an action that you might think of typically being a manager's action."[61]

One reason more companies are empowering employees is the need for quick decisions by those people who are most knowledgeable about the issues—often those at lower organizational levels. If organizations want to successfully compete in a dynamic global economy, employees have to be able to make decisions and implement changes quickly. Another reason is that organizational downsizings left many

managers with larger spans of control. In order to cope with the increased work demands, managers had to empower their people. Although empowerment is not a universal answer, it can be beneficial when employees have the knowledge, skills, and experience to do their jobs competently.

Leading Across Cultures

"In the United States, leaders are expected to look great, sound great, and be inspiring. In other countries—not so much."[62] In this global economy, how can managers account for cross-cultural differences as they lead?

One general conclusion that surfaces from leadership research is that effective leaders do not use a single style. They adjust their style to the situation. Although not mentioned explicitly, national culture is certainly an important situational variable in determining which leadership style will be most effective. What works in China isn't likely to be effective in France or Canada. For instance, one study of Asian leadership styles revealed that Asian managers preferred leaders who were competent decision makers, effective communicators, and supportive of employees.[63]

National culture affects leadership style because it influences how followers will respond. Leaders can't (and shouldn't) just choose their styles randomly. They're constrained by the cultural conditions their followers have come to expect. Exhibit 7 provides some findings from selected examples of cross-cultural leadership studies. Because most leadership theories were developed in the United States, they have an American bias. They emphasize follower responsibilities rather than rights; assume self-gratification rather than commitment to duty or altruistic motivation; assume centrality of work and democratic value orientation; and stress rationality rather than spirituality, religion, or superstition.[64] However, the GLOBE research program is the most extensive and comprehensive cross-cultural study of leadership ever undertaken. The GLOBE study found that leadership has some universal aspects. Specifically, a number of elements of transformational leadership appear to be associated with effective leadership regardless of what country the leader is in.[65] These elements include vision, foresight, providing encouragement, trustworthiness, dynamism, positiveness, and proactiveness. The results led two members of the GLOBE team to conclude that "effective business leaders in

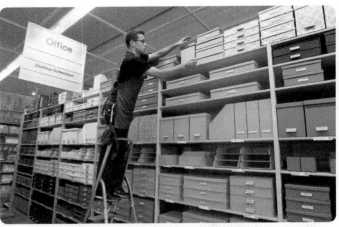

Managers of The Container Store provide goals for employees, give them extensive training, and then let them use what CEO Kip Tindell calls their "creative genius" to solve problems. Encouraged to take ownership in their jobs and to make decisions based on company guidelines, empowered employees feel they are respected and valued contributors to their store's team.
Source: © James Borchuck/Tampa Bay Times/ ZUMAPRESS.com/Alamy Live News

---

- Korean leaders are expected to be paternalistic toward employees.
- Arab leaders who show kindness or generosity without being asked to do so are seen by other Arabs as weak.
- Japanese leaders are expected to be humble and speak frequently.
- Scandinavian and Dutch leaders who single out individuals with public praise are likely to embarrass, not energize, those individuals.
- Effective leaders in Malaysia are expected to show compassion while using more of an autocratic than a participative style.
- Effective German leaders are characterized by high performance orientation, low compassion, low self-protection, low team orientation, high autonomy, and high participation.

Exhibit 7
Cross-Cultural Leadership

Sources: Based on J. C. Kennedy, "Leadership in Malaysia: Traditional Values, International Outlook," *Academy of Management Executive,* August 2002, pp. 15–17; F. C. Brodbeck, M. Frese, and M. Javidan, "Leadership Made in Germany: Low on Compassion, High on Performance," *Academy of Management Executive,* February 2002, pp. 16–29; M. F. Peterson and J. G. Hunt, "International Perspectives on International Leadership," *Leadership Quarterly,* Fall 1997, pp. 203–231; R. J. House and R. N. Aditya, "The Social Scientific Study of Leadership: Quo Vadis?" *Journal of Management,* vol. 23, no. 3, 1997, p. 463; and R. J. House, "Leadership in the Twenty-First Century," in A. Howard (ed.), *The Changing Nature of Work* (San Francisco: Jossey-Bass, 1995), p. 442.

FUTURE VISION | **Flexible Leadership**

As organizations become flatter (that is, fewer hierarchical levels) and more globally and technologically interconnected, old leadership models will become outdated. Although the three elements of leadership—the leader, the followers, and the situation—will still be part of the whole leadership equation, how these three elements interact to successfully accomplish a team's mission and goals is changing. Successful leaders in tomorrow's workplaces will need to be more like chameleons, adapting to complex and dynamic environments. Under these circumstances, leaders can do three things: (1) share responsibility and accountability by empowering employees; recognize that "leading" can come from anywhere and everywhere and that sometimes the best approach may be to step out of the way and let someone else take charge; (2) keep calm and stay focused in the midst of the fast pace and the uncertainty; when

faced with such conditions, focus on the most important tasks at hand and present a confident demeanor when others may be panicking or at a loss as to what to do; and (3) be a leader who listens, encourages participation, recognizes that others' needs are as important as your own, encourages and supports collaboration in achieving common goals—that is, a leader who puts people first. After all, without people, leaders are nothing.

If your professor has chosen to assign this, go to **www.mymanagementlab.com** *to discuss the following questions.*

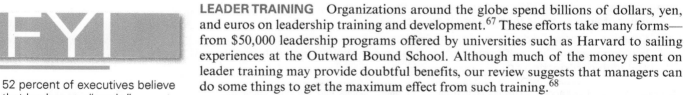 **TALK ABOUT IT 1:** Why are old leadership models becoming outdated?

TALK ABOUT IT 2: Without people, leaders are nothing. What does this mean?

any country are expected by their subordinates to provide a powerful and proactive vision to guide the company into the future, strong motivational skills to stimulate all employees to fulfill the vision, and excellent planning skills to assist in implementing the vision."[66] Some people suggest that the universal appeal of these transformational leader characteristics is due to the pressures toward common technologies and management practices as a result of global competitiveness and multinational influences.

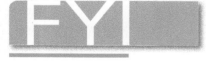 **It's Your Career**

Leadership Transition—If your instructor is using MyManagementLab, log onto mymanagementlab.com and test your *leadership transition knowledge*. **Be sure to refer back to the chapter opener!**

Becoming an Effective Leader

Organizations need effective leaders. Two issues pertinent to becoming an effective leader are leader training and recognizing that sometimes being an effective leader means *not* leading. Let's take a look at these issues.

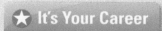

LEADER TRAINING Organizations around the globe spend billions of dollars, yen, and euros on leadership training and development.[67] These efforts take many forms—from $50,000 leadership programs offered by universities such as Harvard to sailing experiences at the Outward Bound School. Although much of the money spent on leader training may provide doubtful benefits, our review suggests that managers can do some things to get the maximum effect from such training.[68]

First, let's recognize the obvious. Some people don't have what it takes to be a leader. Period. For instance, evidence indicates that leadership training is more likely to be successful with individuals who are high self-monitors than with low self-monitors. Such individuals have the flexibility to change their behavior as different situations may require. In addition, organizations may find that individuals with

- 52 percent of executives believe that leaders are "made."
- 19 percent believe they are born.
- 29 percent believe they're equally born and "made."[69]

higher levels of a trait called motivation to lead are more receptive to leadership development opportunities.[70]

What kinds of things can individuals learn that might be related to being a more effective leader? It may be a bit optimistic to think that "vision-creation" can be taught, but implementation skills can be taught. People can be trained to develop "an understanding about content themes critical to effective visions."[71] We can also teach skills such as trust-building and mentoring. And leaders can be taught situational analysis skills. They can learn how to evaluate situations, how to modify situations to make them fit better with their style, and how to assess which leader behaviors might be most effective in given situations.

SUBSTITUTES FOR LEADERSHIP Despite the belief that some leadership style will always be effective regardless of the situation, leadership may not always be important! Research indicates that, in some situations, any behaviors a leader exhibits are irrelevant. In other words, certain individual, job, and organizational variables can act as "substitutes for leadership," negating the influence of the leader.[72]

For instance, follower characteristics such as experience, training, professional orientation, or need for independence can neutralize the effect of leadership. These characteristics can replace the employee's need for a leader's support or ability to create structure and reduce task ambiguity. Similarly, jobs that are inherently unambiguous and routine or intrinsically satisfying may place fewer demands on leaders. Finally, such organizational characteristics as explicit formalized goals, rigid rules and procedures, or cohesive work groups can substitute for formal leadership.

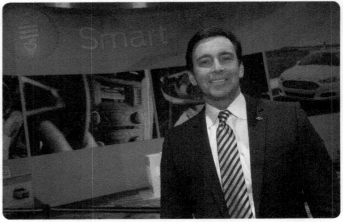

Global executive leadership programs at Ford Motor Company develop effective leaders such as Mark Fields, a 25-year Ford employee who has been elected as the company's new CEO and president. Ford offers a wide range of leadership development programs for employees at all levels that focus on fostering functional and technical excellence, risk taking, decision making, managing change, and entrepreneurial thinking.
Source: Paul Warner/Getty Images Entertainment/Getty Images

PREPARING FOR: Exams/Quizzes

CHAPTER SUMMARY by Learning Objectives

LO1

DEFINE **leader and leadership.**

A leader is someone who can influence others and who has managerial authority. Leadership is a process of leading a group and influencing that group to achieve its goals. Managers should be leaders because leading is one of the four management functions.

LO2

COMPARE **and contrast early theories of leadership.**

Early attempts to define leader traits were unsuccessful, although later attempts found eight traits associated with leadership.

The University of Iowa studies explored three leadership styles. The only conclusion was that group members were more satisfied under a democratic leader than under an autocratic one. The Ohio State studies identified two dimensions of leader behavior—initiating structure and consideration. A leader high in both those dimensions at times achieved high group task performance and high group member satisfaction, but not always. The University of Michigan studies looked at employee-oriented leaders and production-oriented leaders. They concluded that leaders who were employee oriented could get high group productivity and high group member satisfaction. The Managerial Grid looked at leaders' concern for production and concern for people and identified five leader styles. Although it suggested that a leader who was high in concern for production and high in concern for people was the best, there was no substantive evidence for that conclusion.

As the behavioral studies showed, a leader's behavior has a dual nature: a focus on the task and a focus on the people.

L03 · DESCRIBE the three major contingency theories of leadership.

Fiedler's model attempted to define the best style to use in particular situations. He measured leader style—relationship oriented or task oriented—using the least-preferred coworker questionnaire. Fiedler also assumed a leader's style was fixed. He measured three contingency dimensions: leader–member relations, task structure, and position power. The model suggests that task-oriented leaders performed best in very favorable and very unfavorable situations, and relationship-oriented leaders performed best in moderately favorable situations.

Hersey and Blanchard's situational leadership theory focused on followers' readiness. They identified four leadership styles: telling (high task–low relationship), selling (high task–high relationship), participating (low task–high relationship), and delegating (low task–low relationship). They also identified four stages of readiness: unable and unwilling (use telling style), unable but willing (use selling style), able but unwilling (use participative style), and able and willing (use delegating style).

The path-goal model developed by Robert House identified four leadership behaviors: directive, supportive, participative, and achievement-oriented. He assumed that a leader can and should be able to use any of these styles. The two situational contingency variables were found in the environment and in the follower. Essentially the path-goal model says that a leader should provide direction and support as needed; that is, structure the path so the followers can achieve goals.

L04 · DESCRIBE contemporary views of leadership.

Leader–member exchange theory (LMX) says that leaders create in-groups and out-groups and those in the in-group will have higher performance ratings, less turnover, and greater job satisfaction.

A transactional leader exchanges rewards for productivity where a transformational leader stimulates and inspires followers to achieve goals.

A charismatic leader is an enthusiastic and self-confident leader whose personality and actions influence people to behave in certain ways. People can learn to be charismatic. A visionary leader is able to create and articulate a realistic, credible, and attractive vision of the future.

A team leader has two priorities: manage the team's external boundary and facilitate the team process. Four leader roles are involved: liaison with external constituencies, troubleshooter, conflict manager, and coach.

L05 · DISCUSS contemporary issues affecting leadership.

The five sources of a leader's power are legitimate (authority or position), coercive (punish or control), reward (give positive rewards), expert (special expertise, skills, or knowledge), and referent (desirable resources or traits).

Today's leaders face the issues of managing power, developing trust, empowering employees, leading across cultures, and becoming an effective leader.

MyManagementLab

Go to **mymanagementlab.com** to complete the problems marked with this icon ⭐.

⭐ REVIEW AND DISCUSSION QUESTIONS

1. What does each of the four behavioral leadership theories say about leadership?
2. Explain Fiedler's contingency model of leadership.
3. How do situational leadership theory and path-goal theory each explain leadership?
4. What is leader–member exchange theory, and what does it say about leadership?
5. Differentiate between transactional and transformational leaders and between charismatic and visionary leaders.

6. What are the five sources of a leader's power?
7. Do you think most managers in real life use a contingency approach to increase their leadership effectiveness? Explain.
8. Do the followers make a difference in whether a leader is effective? Discuss.

MyManagementLab

If your professor has assigned these, go to **mymanagementlab.com** for Auto-graded writing questions as well as the following Assisted-graded writing questions:

9. Define leader and leadership and explain why managers should be leaders.
10. What issues do today's leaders face?

PREPARING FOR: My Career

⭐ PERSONAL INVENTORY ASSESSMENTS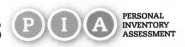

Leadership Style Inventory

What's your leadership style? Take this PIA and find out!

⭐ ETHICS DILEMMA

Have you ever watched the show *Undercover Boss?* It features a company's "boss" working undercover in his or her own company to find out how the organization really works. Typically, the executive works undercover for a week, and then the employees the leader has worked with are summoned to company headquarters and either rewarded or punished for their actions. Bosses from organizations ranging from Waste Management and White Castle to NASCAR and Family Dollar have participated.

11. What do you think? Is it ethical for a leader to go undercover in his or her organization? Why or why not?
12. What ethical issues could arise? How could managers deal with those issues?

SKILLS EXERCISE Developing Your Choosing an Effective Leadership Style Skill

About the Skill

Effective leaders are skillful at helping the groups they lead be successful as the group goes through various stages of development. No leadership style is consistently effective. Situational factors, including follower characteristics, must be taken into consideration in the selection of an effective leadership style. The key situational factors that determine leadership effectiveness include stage of group development, task structure, position power, leader–member relations, the work group, employee characteristics, organizational culture, and national culture.

Steps in Practicing the Skill

You can choose an effective leadership style if you use the following six suggestions.

- *Determine the stage in which your group or team is operating: forming, storming, norming, or performing.* Because each team stage involves specific and different issues and behaviors, it's important to know in which stage your team is. *Forming* is the first stage of group development, during which people join a group and then help define the group's purpose, structure, and leadership. *Storming* is the second stage, characterized by intragroup conflict. *Norming* is the third stage, characterized by close relationships and cohesiveness. *Performing* is the fourth stage, when the group is fully functional.

- *If your team is in the forming stage, you want to exhibit certain leader behaviors.* These include making certain that all team members are introduced to one another, answering member questions, working to establish a foundation of trust and openness, modeling the behaviors you expect from the team members, and clarifying the team's goals, procedures, and expectations.

- *If your team is in the storming stage, you want to exhibit certain leader behaviors.* These behaviors include identifying sources of conflict and adopting a mediator role, encouraging a win-win philosophy, restating the team's vision and its core values and goals, encouraging open discussion, encouraging an analysis of team processes in order to identify ways to improve, enhancing team cohesion and commitment, and providing recognition to individual team members as well as the team.

- *If your team is in the norming stage, you want to exhibit certain leader behaviors.* These behaviors include clarifying the team's goals and expectations, providing performance feedback to individual team members and the team, encouraging the team to articulate a vision for the future, and finding ways to publicly and openly communicate the team's vision.

- *If your team is in the performing stage, you want to exhibit certain leader behaviors.* These behaviors include providing regular and ongoing performance feedback, fostering innovation and innovative behavior, encouraging the team to capitalize on its strengths, celebrating achievements (large and small), and providing the team whatever support it needs to continue doing its work.

- *Monitor the group for changes in behavior and adjust your leadership style accordingly.* Because a group is not a static entity, it will go through up periods and down periods. You should adjust your leadership style to the needs of the situation. If the group appears to need more direction from you, provide it. If it appears to be functioning at a high level on its own, provide whatever support is necessary to keep it functioning at that level.

Practicing the Skill

The following suggestions are activities you can do to practice the behaviors in choosing an effective leadership style.

1. Think of a group or team to which you currently belong or of which you have been a part. What type of leadership style did the leader of this group appear to exhibit? Give some specific examples of the types of leadership behaviors he or she used. Evaluate the leadership style. Was it appropriate for the group? Why or why not? What would you have done differently? Why?

2. Observe a sports team (either college or professional) that you consider extremely successful and one that you would consider not successful. What leadership styles appear to be used in these team situations? Give some specific examples of the types of leadership behaviors you observe. How would you evaluate the leadership style? Was it appropriate for the team? Why or why not? To what degree do you think leadership style influenced the team's outcomes?

WORKING TOGETHER Team Exercise

Everybody's probably had at least one experience with a *bad boss.* But what *is* a bad boss? And more importantly, what can you do in such a situation?

Break into small groups of three to four other class members. Come up with a bulleted list of characteristics and behaviors you believe a bad boss would have or exhibit. Then, come up with another bulleted list of what you can do if you find yourself in a situation with a bad boss. Be realistic about your suggestions; that is, don't suggest tampering with the person's coffee or slashing the person's tires!

MY TURN TO BE A MANAGER

- Think of the different organizations to which you belong. Note the different styles of leadership used by the leaders in these organizations. Write a paper describing these individual's style of leading (no names, please) and evaluate the styles being used.

- Write down three people you consider effective leaders. Make a bulleted list of the characteristics these individuals exhibit that you think make them effective leaders.

- Think about the times you have had to lead. Describe your own personal leadership style. What could you do to improve your leadership style? Come up with an action plan of steps you can take. Put all this information into a brief paper.

- Managers say that increasingly they must use influence to get things done. Do some research on the art of persuasion. Make a bulleted list of suggestions you find on how to improve your skills at influencing others.

- Here's a list of leadership skills. Choose two and develop a training exercise that will help develop or improve that skill: building employee communities; building teams; coaching and motivating others; communicating with impact, confidence, and energy; leading by example; leading change; making decisions; providing direction and focus; and valuing diversity.

- Select one of the topics in the section on leadership issues in the twenty-first century. Do some additional research on the topic, and put your findings in a bulleted list that you are prepared to share in class. Be sure to cite your sources.

- Interview three managers about what they think it takes to be a good leader. Write up your findings in a report and be prepared to present it in class.

- In your own words, write down three things you learned in this text about being a good manager. Keep a copy of this for future reference.

CASE APPLICATION 1   Growing Leaders

How important are excellent leaders to organizations? If you were to ask the recently-retired 3M CEO George Buckley, he'd say extremely important.[73] But he'd also say that excellent leaders don't just pop up out of nowhere. A company has to cultivate leaders who have the skills and abilities to help it survive and thrive. And like a successful baseball team with strong performance statistics that has a player development plan in place, 3M has its own farm system. Except its farm system is designed to develop company leaders.

3M's leadership development program is so effective that it has been one of the "Top 20 Companies for Leadership" in three of the last four years and ranks as one of the top 25 companies for grooming leadership talent according to Hay Consulting Group and *Fortune* magazine. What is 3M's leadership program all about? About 10 years ago, the company's former CEO (Jim McNerney, who is now Boeing's CEO) and his top team spent 18 months developing a new leadership model for the company. After numerous brainstorming sessions and much heated debate, the group finally agreed on six "leadership attributes" they believed were essential for the company to become skilled at executing strategy and being accountable. Those six attributes included the ability to "chart the course; energize and inspire others; demonstrate ethics, integrity, and compliance; deliver results; raise the bar; and innovate resourcefully." And under Buckley's guidance and continued under the leadership of newly appointed CEO Inge Thulin, the company is continuing and reinforcing its pursuit of leadership excellence with these six attributes.

When asked about his views on leadership, Buckley said he believes leaders differ from managers. He believes the key to developing leaders is to focus on those things that can be developed—like strategic thinking. Buckley also believes leaders should not be promoted up and through the organization too quickly. They need time to experience failures and what it takes to rebuild.

Finally, when asked about his own leadership style, Buckley said he believed the best way for him to succeed as a leader was to surround himself with people who were better than him. But doing that takes a great deal of emotional self-confidence, an attribute that is vital to being a great leader. When you have people working for you who are excellent at what they do, you respect them. When you respect them, you build trust. That type of leadership approach worked well for Buckley, as illustrated by 3M's number 18 ranking on *Fortune's* most admired global companies list for 2012.

⭐ DISCUSSION QUESTIONS

13. What do you think about Buckley's statement that leaders and managers differ? Do you agree? Why or why not?

14. What leadership models/theories/issues do you see in this case? List and describe.

15. Take each of the six leadership attributes that the company feels is important. Explain what you think each one involves. Then discuss how those attributes might be developed and measured.

16. What did this case teach you about leadership?

CASE APPLICATION **2** # Serving Up Leaders

Thirty-five million dollars. Five thousand live coffee plants. One thousand lighting instruments. One hundred twenty speakers. Twenty-one projection screens. These are just a few of the "numbers" describing the spectacle known as the Starbucks Leadership Lab.[74] For three days in the fall of 2012, some 9,600 Starbucks store managers trekked to a conference center in Houston to be immersed in an massive interactive experience. While there, these managers were steeped in the Starbucks brand.

The Leadership Lab was part leadership training and part trade show. The company's store managers were given a behind-the-scenes look and introduced up close and personal to what makes Starbucks go. From an exhibit featuring live coffee shrubs to a drying patio where they could get hands-on experience raking through coffee beans to an enormous exhibit of used shoes with customer experiences noted on cards (sort of a "walk in my shoes" theme). Most of these experiences were designed to be instructive for the store managers. However, in addition, the store managers—who are on the "firing line" day in and day out—had the opportunity to interact with top managers of the company's roasting process, blend development, and customer service functions. Managers also were encouraged to share what they had learned from the Leadership Lab by stopping at a station lined with laptops.

The lights, the music, and the dramatic presentation were all designed to immerse the store managers in the Starbucks brand and culture. The goal was to "mobilize its employees to become brand evangelists." And since presentation is a significant component of what the Starbucks experience is built on—the sights, the sounds, the smells—the entire presentation at the Leadership Lab was well thought out and intentional.

⭐ DISCUSSION QUESTIONS

17. Describe the leadership lessons you think Starbucks Leadership Lab provided store managers.

18. What role do you think an organization's culture plays in how its leaders lead? Relate this to the story told above.

19. Using the behavioral theories as a guideline, what do you think would be more important to a Starbucks store manager: focus on task, focus on people, or both? Explain.

20. How might a Starbucks store manager use situational leadership theory? Path-goal theory? Transformational leadership?

ENDNOTES

1. Most leadership research has focused on the actions and responsibilities of managers and extrapolated the results to leaders and leadership in general.
2. "Study: Long Finger Equals Success," *Springfield, Missouri, News-Leader,* January 13, 2009, p. 4B.
3. See R. L. Schaumberg and F. J. Flynn, "Uneasy Lies the Head That Wears the Crown: The Link Between Guilt Proneness and Leadership," *Journal of Personality and Social Psychology,* August 2012, pp. 327–342; D. S. Derue, J. D. Nahrgang, N. Wellman, and S. E. Humphrey, "Trait and Behavioral Theories of Leadership: An Integration and Meta-Analytic Test of Their Relative Validity," *Personnel Psychology,* Spring 2011, pp. 7–52; T. A. Judge, J. E. Bono, R. Ilies, and M. W. Gerhardt, "Personality and Leadership: A Qualitative and Quantitative Review," *Journal of Applied Psychology,* August 2002, pp. 765–780; and S. A. Kirkpatrick and E. A. Locke, "Leadership: Do Traits Matter?" *Academy of Management Executive,* May 1991, pp. 48–60.
4. R. Working, "Executive Qualities Differ by Gender, Study Finds," www.hrcommunication.com, March 8, 2013.
5. "Ensemble Acting in Business," *New York Times Online,* June 7, 2009; and J. M. O'Brien, "Ousted Seagate CEO Provocative to the End," CNNMoney.com, January 13, 2009.
6. D. S. Derue, J. D. Nahrgang, N. Wellman, and S. E. Humphrey, "Trait and Behavioral Theories of Leadership: An Integration and Meta-Analytic Test of Their Relative Validity."
7. K. Lewin and R. Lippitt, "An Experimental Approach to the Study of Autocracy and Democracy: A Preliminary Note," *Sociometry,* vol. 1, 1938, pp. 292–300; K. Lewin, "Field Theory and Experiment in Social Psychology: Concepts and Methods," *American Journal of Sociology,* vol. 44, 1939, pp. 868–896; K. Lewin, L. Lippitt, and R. K. White, "Patterns of Aggressive Behavior in Experimentally Created Social Climates," *Journal of Social Psychology,* vol. 10, 1939, pp. 271–301; and L. Lippitt, "An Experimental Study of the Effect of Democratic and Authoritarian Group Atmospheres," *University of Iowa Studies in Child Welfare,* vol. 16, 1940, pp. 43–95.
8. B. M. Bass, *Stogdill's Handbook of Leadership* (New York: Free Press, 1981), pp. 289–299.
9. R. M. Stogdill and A. E. Coons (eds.), *Leader Behavior: Its Description and Measurement,* Research Monograph no. 88 (Columbus: Ohio State University, Bureau of Business Research, 1951). For an updated literature review of Ohio State research, see S. Kerr, C. A. Schriesheim, C. J. Murphy, and R. M. Stogdill, "Toward a Contingency Theory of Leadership Based upon the Consideration and Initiating Structure Literature," *Organizational Behavior and Human Performance,* August 1974, pp. 62–82; and B. M. Fisher, "Consideration and Initiating Structure and Their Relationships with Leader Effectiveness: A Meta-Analysis," in F. Hoy (ed.), *Proceedings* of the 48th Annual Academy of Management Conference, Anaheim, California, 1988, pp. 201–205.
10. R. Kahn and D. Katz, "Leadership Practices in Relation to Productivity and Morale," in D. Cartwright and A. Zander (eds.), *Group Dynamics: Research and Theory,* 2d ed. (Elmsford, NY: Row, Paterson, 1960).
11. R. R. Blake and J. S. Mouton, *The Managerial Grid III* (Houston: Gulf Publishing, 1984).
12. L. L. Larson, J. G. Hunt, and R. N. Osborn, "The Great Hi-Hi Leader Behavior Myth: A Lesson from Occam's Razor," *Academy of Management Journal,* December 1976, pp. 628–641; and P. C. Nystrom, "Managers and the Hi-Hi Leader Myth," *Academy of Management Journal,* June 1978, pp. 325–331.
13. W. G. Bennis, "The Seven Ages of the Leader," *Harvard Business Review,* January 2004, p. 52.
14. F. E. Fiedler, *A Theory of Leadership Effectiveness* (New York: McGraw-Hill, 1967).
15. R. Ayman, M. M. Chemers, and F. Fiedler, "The Contingency Model of Leadership Effectiveness: Its Levels of Analysis," *Leadership Quarterly,* Summer 1995, pp. 147–167; C. A. Schriesheim, B. J. Tepper, and L. A. Tetrault, "Least Preferred Coworker Score, Situational Control, and Leadership Effectiveness: A Meta-Analysis of Contingency Model Performance Predictions," *Journal of Applied Psychology,* August 1994, pp. 561–573; and L. H. Peters, D. D. Hartke, and J. T. Pholmann, "Fiedler's Contingency Theory of Leadership: An Application of the Meta-Analysis Procedures of Schmidt and Hunter," *Psychological Bulletin,* March 1985, pp. 274–285.
16. See E. H. Schein, *Organizational Psychology,* 3rd ed. (Upper Saddle River, NJ: Prentice Hall, 1980), pp. 116–117; and B. Kabanoff, "A Critique of Leader Match and Its Implications for Leadership Research," *Personnel Psychology,* Winter 1981, pp. 749–764.
17. P. Hersey and K. Blanchard, "So You Want to Know Your Leadership Style?" *Training and Development Journal,* February 1974, pp. 1–15; and P. Hersey and K. H. Blanchard, *Management of Organizational Behavior: Leading Human Resources,* 8th ed. (Englewood Cliffs, NJ: Prentice Hall, 2001).
18. See, for instance, E. G. Ralph, "Developing Managers' Effectiveness: A Model with Potential," *Journal of Management Inquiry,* June 2004, pp. 152–163; C. L. Graeff, "Evolution of Situational Leadership Theory: A Critical Review," *Leadership Quarterly,* vol. 8, no. 2, 1997, pp. 153–170; and C. F. Fernandez and R. P. Vecchio, "Situational Leadership Theory Revisited: A Test of an Across-Jobs Perspective," *Leadership Quarterly,* vol. 8, no. 1, 1997, pp. 67–84.
19. Smart Pulse, "How Willing Are You to Step Outside Your Leadership Style 'Comfort Zone' and Try New Techniques?" www.smartbrief.com/leadership/, December 10, 2013.
20. R. J. House, "A Path-Goal Theory of Leader Effectiveness," *Administrative Science Quarterly,* September 1971, pp. 321–338; R. J. House and T. R. Mitchell, "Path-Goal Theory of Leadership," *Journal of Contemporary Business,* Autumn 1974, p. 86; and R. J. House, "Path-Goal Theory of Leadership: Lessons, Legacy, and a Reformulated Theory," *Leadership Quarterly,* Fall 1996, pp. 323–352.
21. M. L. Dixon and L. K. Hart, "The Impact of Path-Goal Leadership Styles on Work Group Effectiveness and Turnover Intention," *Journal of Managerial Issues,* Spring 2010, pp. 52–69; J. C. Wofford and L. Z. Liska, "Path-Goal Theories of Leadership: A Meta-Analysis," *Jour-*

nal of Management, Winter 1993, pp. 857–876; and A. Sagie and M. Koslowsky, "Organizational Attitudes and Behaviors as a Function of Participation in Strategic and Tactical Change Decisions: An Application of Path-Goal Theory," *Journal of Organizational Behavior*, January 1994, pp. 37–47.

22. R. M. Dienesch and R. C. Liden, "Leader–Member Exchange Model of Leadership: A Critique and Further Development," *Academy of Management Review,* July 1986, pp. 618–634; G. B. Graen and M. Uhl-Bien, "Relationship-Based Approach to Leadership: Development of Leader–Member Exchange (LMX) Theory of Leadership Over 25 Years: Applying a Multi-Domain Perspective," *Leadership Quarterly,* Summer 1995, pp. 219–247; R. C. Liden, R. T. Sparrowe, and S. J. Wayne, "Leader–Member Exchange Theory: The Past and Potential for the Future," in G. R. Ferris (ed.), *Research in Personnel and Human Resource Management,* vol. 15 (Greenwich, CT: JAI Press, 1997), pp. 47–119; and C. P. Schriesheim, S. L. Castro, X. Zhou, and F. J. Yammarino, "The Folly of Theorizing 'A' but Testing 'B': A Selective Level-of-Analysis Review of the Field and a Detailed Leader–Member Exchange Illustration," *Leadership Quarterly,* Winter 2001, pp. 515–551.

23. P. Drexler, "The Upside of Favoritism," *Wall Street Journal,* June 8–9, 2013, p. C3.

24. R. C. Liden and G. Graen, "Generalizability of the Vertical Dyad Linkage Model of Leadership," *Academy of Management Journal,* September 1980, pp. 451–465; R. C. Liden, S. J. Wayne, and D. Stilwell, "A Longitudinal Study of the Early Development of Leader–Member Exchanges," *Journal of Applied Psychology,* August 1993, pp. 662–674; S. J. Wayne, L. J. Shore, W. H. Bommer, and L. E. Tetrick, "The Role of Fair Treatment and Rewards in Perceptions of Organizational Support and Leader–Member Exchange," *Journal of Applied Psychology,* June 2002, pp. 590–598; and S. S. Masterson, K. Lewis, and B. M. Goldman, "Integrating Justice and Social Exchange: The Differing Effects of Fair Procedures and Treatment on Work Relationships," *Academy of Management Journal,* August 2000, pp. 738–748.

25. D. Duchon, S. G. Green, and T. D. Taber, "Vertical Dyad Linkage: A Longitudinal Assessment of Antecedents, Measures, and Consequences," *Journal of Applied Psychology,* February 1986, pp. 56–60; R. C. Liden, S. J. Wayne, and D. Stilwell, "A Longitudinal Study of the Early Development of Leader–Member Exchanges"; M. Uhl-Bien, "Relationship Development as a Key Ingredient for Leadership Development," in S. E. Murphy and R. E. Riggio (eds.), *Future of Leadership Development* (Mahwah, NJ: Lawrence Erlbaum, 2003), pp. 129–147; R. Vecchio and D. M. Brazil, "Leadership and Sex-Similarity: A Comparison in a Military Setting," *Personnel Psychology,* vol. 60, 2007, pp. 303–335; and V. L. Goodwin, W. M. Bowler, and J. L. Whittington, "A Social Network Perspective on LMX Relationships: Accounting for the Instrumental Value of Leader and Follower Networks," *Journal of Management,* August 2009, pp. 954–980.

26. See, for instance, C. R. Gerstner and D. V. Day, "Meta-Analytic Review of Leader–Member Exchange Theory: Correlates and Construct Issues," *Journal of Applied Psychology,* December 1997, pp. 827–844; R. Ilies, J. D. Nahrgang, and F. P. Morgeson, "Leader–Member Exchange and Citizenship Behaviors: A Meta-analysis," *Journal of Applied Psychology,* January 2007, pp. 269–277; Z. Chen, W. Lam, and J. A. Zhong, "Leader–Member Exchange and Member Performance: A New Look at Individual-Level Negative Feedback-Seeking Behavior and Team-Level Empowerment Culture," *Journal of Applied Psychology,* January 2007, pp. 202–212; and Z. Zhang, M. Wang, and J. Shi, "Leader-Follower Congruence in Proactive Personality and Work Outcomes: The Mediating Role of Leader-Member Exchange," *Academy of Management Journal,* February 2012, pp. 111–130.

27. R. Eisenberger, G. Karagonlar, F. Stinglhamber, P. Neves, T. Becker, M. Gonzalez-Morales, and M. Steiger-Mueller, "Leader-Member Exchange and Affective Organizational Commitment: The Contribution of Supervisor's Organizational Embodiment," *Journal of Applied Psychology,* vol. 95, 2010, pp. 1085–1103.

28. Leader Making a Difference box based on D. Roberts, "Dynamic Duos," *Fortune,* June 11, 2012, pp. 24–25; R. Sidel, "Banga to Be MasterCard's Protector," *Wall Street Journal,* May 29–30, 2010, pp. B1+; A. Saha-Bubna and M. Jarzemsky, "MasterCard President Is Named CEO," *Wall Street Journal,* April 13, 2010, p. C3; "Why Banga Quit Citi," *Euromoney,* July 2009, p. 41; and E. Wilson, "Banga Demolishes Citi's Asia-Pac Silos," *Euromoney,* May 2009, p. 49.

29. B. M. Bass and R. E. Riggio, *Transformational Leadership,* 2d ed. (Mahwah, NJ: Lawrence Erlbaum Associates, Inc., 2006), p. 3.

30. B. M. Bass, "Leadership: Good, Better, Best," *Organizational Dynamics,* Winter 1985, pp. 26–40; and J. Seltzer and B. M. Bass, "Transformational Leadership: Beyond Initiation and Consideration," *Journal of Management,* December 1990, pp. 693–703.

31. B. J. Avolio and B. M. Bass, "Transformational Leadership, Charisma, and Beyond." Working paper, School of Management, State University of New York, Binghamton, 1985, p. 14.

32. B. J. Hoffman, B. H. Bynum, R. F. Piccolo, and A. W. Sutton, "Person-Organization Value Congruence: How Transformational Leaders Influence Work Group Effectiveness," *Academy of Management Journal,* August 2011, pp. 779–796; G. Wang, In-Sue Oh, S. H. Courtright, and A. E. Colbert, "Transformational Leadership and Performance Across Criteria and Levels: A Meta-Analytic Review of 25 Years of Research," *Group & Organization Management,* 36, no. 2, 2011, pp. 223–270; M. Tims, A. B. Bakker, and D. Xanthopoulou, "Do Transformational Leaders Enhance Their Followers' Daily Work Engagement?" *The Leadership Quarterly,* February 2011, pp. 121–131; S. J. Peterson and F. O. Walumba, "CEO Positive Psychological Traits, Transformational Leadership, and Firm Performance in High-Technology Start-up and Established Firms," *Journal of Management,* April 2009, pp. 348–368; R. S. Rubin, D. C. Munz, and W. H. Bommer, "Leading from Within: The Effects of Emotion Recognition and Personality on Transformational Leadership Behavior," *Academy of Management Journal,* October 2005, pp. 845–858; T. A. Judge and J. E. Bono, "Five-Factor Model of Personality and Transformational Leadership," *Journal of Applied Psychology,* October 2000, pp. 751–765; B. M. Bass and B. J. Avolio, "Developing Transformational Leadership: 1992 and Beyond," *Journal of European Industrial Training,* January 1990, p. 23; and J. J. Hater and B. M. Bass, "Supervisors' Evaluation and Subordinates' Perceptions of Transformational and Transactional Leadership," *Journal of Applied Psychology,* November 1988, pp. 695–702.

33. Y. Ling, Z. Simsek, M. H. Lubatkin, and J. F. Veiga, "Transformational Leadership's Role in Promoting Corporate Entrepreneurship: Examining the CEO-TMT Interface," *Academy of Management Journal,* June 2008, pp. 557–576; A. E. Colbert, A. L. Kristof-Brown, B. H. Bradley, and M. R. Barrick, "CEO Transformational Leadership: The Role of Goal Importance Congruence in Top Management Teams," *Academy of Management Journal,* February 2008, pp. 81–96; R. F. Piccolo and J. A. Colquitt, "Transformational Leadership and Job Behaviors: The Mediating Role of Core Job Characteristics," *Academy of Management Journal,* April 2006, pp. 327–340; O. Epitropaki and R. Martin, "From Ideal to Real: A Longitudinal Study of the Role of Implicit Leadership Theories on Leader–Member Exchanges and Employee Outcomes," *Journal of Applied Psychology,* July 2005, pp. 659–676; J. E. Bono and T. A. Judge, "Self-Concordance at Work: Toward Understanding the Motivational Effects of Transformational Leaders," *Academy of Management Journal,* October 2003, pp. 554–571; T. Dvir, D. Eden, B. J. Avolio, and B. Shamir, "Impact of Transformational Leadership on Follower Development and Performance: A Field Experiment," *Academy of Management Journal,* August 2002, pp. 735–744; N. Sivasubramaniam, W. D. Murry, B. J. Avolio, and D. I. Jung, "A Longitudinal Model of the Effects of Team Leadership and Group Potency on Group Performance," *Group and Organization Management,* March 2002, pp. 66–96; J. M. Howell and B. J. Avolio, "Transformational Leadership, Transactional Leadership, Locus of Control, and Support for Innovation: Key Predictors of Consolidated-Business-Unit Performance," *Journal of Applied Psychology,* December 1993, pp. 891–911; R. T. Keller, "Transformational Leadership and the Performance of Research and Development Project Groups," *Journal of Management,* September 1992, pp. 489–501; and Bass and Avolio, "Developing Transformational Leadership."

34. F. Vogelstein, "Mighty Amazon," *Fortune,* May 26, 2003, pp. 60–74.

35. F. Walter and H. Bruch, "An Affective Events Model of Charismatic Leadership Behavior: A Review, Theoretical Integration, and Research

Agenda," *Journal of Management,* December 2009, pp. 1428–1452; A. Pentland, "We Can Measure the Power of Charisma," *Harvard Business Review,* January–February 2010, pp. 34–35; J. M. Crant and T. S. Bateman, "Charismatic Leadership Viewed from Above: The Impact of Proactive Personality," *Journal of Organizational Behavior,* February 2000, pp. 63–75; G. Yukl and J. M. Howell, "Organizational and Contextual Influences on the Emergence and Effectiveness of Charismatic Leadership," *Leadership Quarterly,* Summer 1999, pp. 257–283; and J. A. Conger and R. N. Kanungo, "Behavioral Dimensions of Charismatic Leadership," in J. A. Conger, R. N. Kanungo et al., *Charismatic Leadership* (San Francisco: Jossey-Bass, 1988), pp. 78–97.

36. J. A. Conger and R. N. Kanungo, *Charismatic Leadership in Organizations* (Thousand Oaks, CA: Sage, 1998).

37. F. Walter and H. Bruch, "An Affective Events Model of Charismatic Leadership Behavior: A Review, Theoretical Investigation, and Research Agenda," *Journal of Management,* December 2009, pp. 1428–1452; K. S. Groves, "Linking Leader Skills, Follower Attitudes, and Contextual Variables via an Integrated Model of Charismatic Leadership," *Journal of Management,* April 2005, pp. 255–277; J. J. Sosik, " The Role of Personal Values in the Charismatic Leadership of Corporate Managers: A Model and Preliminary Field Study," *Leadership Quarterly,* April 2005, pp. 221–244; A. H. B. deHoogh, D. N. den Hartog, P. L. Koopman, H. Thierry, P. T. van den Berg, J. G. van der Weide, and C. P. M. Wilderom, "Leader Motives, Charismatic Leadership, and Subordinates' Work Attitudes in the Profit and Voluntary Sector," *Leadership Quarterly,* February 2005, pp. 17–38; J. M. Howell and B. Shamir, "The Role of Followers in the Charismatic Leadership Process: Relationships and Their Consequences," *Academy of Management Review,* January 2005, pp. 96–112; J. Paul, D. L. Costley, J. P. Howell, P. W. Dorfman, and D. Trafimow, "The Effects of Charismatic Leadership on Followers' Self-Concept Accessibility," *Journal of Applied Social Psychology,* September 2001, pp. 1821–1844; J. A. Conger, R. N. Kanungo, and S. T. Menon, "Charismatic Leadership and Follower Effects," *Journal of Organizational Behavior,* vol. 21, 2000, pp. 747–767; R. W. Rowden, "The Relationship Between Charismatic Leadership Behaviors and Organizational Commitment," *Leadership & Organization Development Journal,* January 2000, pp. 30–35; G. P. Shea and C. M. Howell, "Charismatic Leadership and Task Feedback: A Laboratory Study of Their Effects on Self-Efficacy," *Leadership Quarterly,* Fall 1999, pp. 375–396; S. A. Kirkpatrick and E. A. Locke, "Direct and Indirect Effects of Three Core Charismatic Leadership Components on Performance and Attitudes," *Journal of Applied Psychology,* February 1996, pp. 36–51; D. A. Waldman, B. M. Bass, and F. J. Yammarino, "Adding to Contingent-Reward Behavior: The Augmenting Effect of Charismatic Leadership," *Group & Organization Studies,* December 1990, pp. 381–394; and R. J. House, J. Woycke, and E. M. Fodor, "Charismatic and Noncharismatic Leaders: Differences in Behavior and Effectiveness," in Conger and Kanungo, *Charismatic Leadership,* pp. 103–104.

38. B. R. Agle, N. J. Nagarajan, J. A. Sonnenfeld, and D. Srinivasan, "Does CEO Charisma Matter? An Empirical Analysis of the Relationships Among Organizational Performance, Environmental Uncertainty, and Top Management Team Perceptions of CEO Charisma," *Academy of Management Journal,* February 2006, pp. 161–174.

39. J. Antonakis, M. Fenley, and S. Liechti, "Learning Charisma," *Harvard Business Review,* June 2012, pp. 127–130; J. Antonakis, M. Fenley, and S. Liechti, "Can Charisma Be Taught? Tests of Two Interventions," *Academy of Management Learning & Education,* September 2011, pp. 374–396; R. Birchfield, "Creating Charismatic Leaders," *Management,* June 2000, pp. 30–31; S. Caudron, "Growing Charisma," *Industry Week,* May 4, 1998, pp. 54–55; and J. A. Conger and R. N. Kanungo, "Training Charismatic Leadership: A Risky and Critical Task," in Conger and Kanungo, *Charismatic Leadership,* pp. 309–323.

40. J. Antonakis et.al., "Learning Charisma."

41. J. G. Hunt, K. B. Boal, and G. E. Dodge, "The Effects of Visionary and Crisis-Responsive Charisma on Followers: An Experimental Examination," *Leadership Quarterly,* Fall 1999, pp. 423–448; R. J. House and R. N. Aditya, "The Social Scientific Study of Leadership: Quo Vadis?" *Journal of Management,* vol. 23, no. 3, 1997, pp. 316–323; and R. J. House, "A 1976 Theory of Charismatic Leadership."

42. This definition is based on M. Sashkin, "The Visionary Leader," in Conger and Kanungo et al., *Charismatic Leadership,* pp. 124–125; B. Nanus, *Visionary Leadership* (San Francisco: Jossey-Bass, 1992), p. 8; N. H. Snyder and M. Graves, "Leadership and Vision," *Business Horizons,* January–February 1994, p. 1; and J. R. Lucas, "Anatomy of a Vision Statement," *Management Review,* February 1998, pp. 22–26.

43. B. Nanus, *Visionary Leadership* (San Francisco: Jossey-Bass, 1992), p. 8.

44. S. Caminiti, "What Team Leaders Need to Know," *Fortune,* February 20, 1995, pp. 93–100.

45. Ibid., p. 93.

46. Ibid., p. 100.

47. S. B. Sitkin and J. R. Hackman, "Developing Team Leadership: An Interview with Coach Mike Krzyzewski," *Academy of Management Learning and Education,* September 2011, pp. 494–501; and N. Steckler and N. Fondas, "Building Team Leader Effectiveness: A Diagnostic Tool," *Organizational Dynamics,* Winter 1995, p. 20.

48. R. S. Wellins, W. C. Byham, and G. R. Dixon, *Inside Teams* (San Francisco: Jossey-Bass, 1994), p. 318.

49. Steckler and Fondas, "Building Team Leader Effectiveness," p. 21.

50. P. High, "FedEx's Rob Carter on What It Takes to Be a Board-Level CEO," www.forbes.com, March 10, 2014; and G. Colvin, "The FedEx Edge," *Fortune,* April 3, 2006, pp. 77–84.

51. See J. R. P. French Jr. and B. Raven, "The Bases of Social Power," in D. Cartwright and A. F. Zander (eds.), *Group Dynamics: Research and Theory* (New York: Harper & Row, 1960), pp. 607–623; P. M. Podsakoff and C. A. Schriesheim, "Field Studies of French and Raven's Bases of Power: Critique, Reanalysis, and Suggestions for Future Research," *Psychological Bulletin,* May 1985, pp. 387–411; R. K. Shukla, "Influence of Power Bases in Organizational Decision Making: A Contingency Model," *Decision Sciences,* July 1982, pp. 450–470; D. E. Frost and A. J. Stahelski, "The Systematic Measurement of French and Raven's Bases of Social Power in Workgroups," *Journal of Applied Social Psychology,* April 1988, pp. 375–389; and T. R. Hinkin and C. A. Schriesheim, "Development and Application of New Scales to Measure the French and Raven (1959) Bases of Social Power," *Journal of Applied Psychology,* August 1989, pp. 561–567.

52. J. M. Kouzes and B. Z. Posner, *Credibility: How Leaders Gain and Lose It, and Why People Demand It* (San Francisco: Jossey-Bass, 1993), p. 14.

53. Based on F. D. Schoorman, R. C. Mayer, and J. H. Davis, "An Integrative Model of Organizational Trust: Past, Present, and Future," *Academy of Management Review,* April 2007, pp. 344–354; G. M. Spreitzer and A. K. Mishra, "Giving up Control Without Losing Control," *Group & Organization Management,* June 1999, pp. 155–187; R. C. Mayer, J. H. Davis, and F. D. Schoorman, "An Integrative Model of Organizational Trust," *Academy of Management Review,* July 1995, p. 712; and L. T. Hosmer, "Trust: The Connecting Link Between Organizational Theory and Philosophical Ethics," *Academy of Management Review,* April 1995, p. 393.

54. P. L. Schindler and C. C. Thomas, "The Structure of Interpersonal Trust in the Workplace," *Psychological Reports,* October 1993, pp. 563–573.

55. H. H. Tan and C. S. F. Tan, "Toward the Differentiation of Trust in Supervisor and Trust in Organization," *Genetic, Social, and General Psychology Monographs,* May 2000, pp. 241–260.

56. H. H. Brower, S. W. Lester, M. A. Korsgaard, and B. R. Dineen, "A Closer Look at Trust Between Managers and Subordinates: Understanding the Effects of Both Trusting and Being Trusted on Subordinate Outcomes," *Journal of Management,* April 2009, pp. 327–347; R. C. Mayer and M. B. Gavin, "Trust in Management and Performance: Who Minds the Shop While the Employees Watch the Boss?" *Academy of Management Journal,* October 2005, pp. 874–888; and K. T. Dirks and D. L. Ferrin, "Trust in Leadership: Meta-Analytic Findings and Implications for Research and Practice," *Journal of Applied Psychology,* August 2002, pp. 611–628.

57. See, for example, Dirks and Ferrin, "Trust in Leadership: Meta-Analytic Findings and Implications for Research and Practice"; J. K. Butler Jr., "Toward Understanding and Measuring Conditions of Trust: Evolution of a Conditions of Trust Inventory," *Journal of Man-*

agement, September 1991, pp. 643–663; and F. Bartolome, "Nobody Trusts the Boss Completely—Now What?" *Harvard Business Review*, March–April 1989, pp. 135–142.

58. P. H. Kim, K. T. Dirks, and C. D. Cooper, "The Repair of Trust: A Dynamic Bilateral Perspective and Multilevel Conceptualization," *Academy of Management Review*, July 2009, pp. 401–422; R. Zemke, "The Confidence Crisis," *Training*, June 2004, pp. 22–30; J. A. Byrne, "Restoring Trust in Corporate America," *BusinessWeek*, June 24, 2002, pp. 30–35; S. Armour, "Employees' New Motto: Trust No One," *USA Today*, February 5, 2002, p. 1B; J. Scott, "Once Bitten, Twice Shy: A World of Eroding Trust," *New York Times*, April 21, 2002, p. WK5; J. Brockner, P. A. Siegel, J. P. Daly, T. Tyler, and C. Martin, "When Trust Matters: The Moderating Effect of Outcome Favorability," *Administrative Science Quarterly*, September 1997, p. 558; and J. Brockner, P. A. Siegel, J. P. Daly, T. Tyler, and C. Martin, "When Trust Matters: The Moderating Effect of Outcome Favorability," *Administrative Science Quarterly*, September 1997, p. 558.

59. T. Vinas, "DuPont: Safety Starts at the Top," *Industry Week*, July 2002, p. 55.

60. A. Srivastava, K. M. Bartol, and E. A. Locke, "Empowering Leadership in Management Teams: Effects on Knowledge Sharing, Efficacy, and Performance," *Academy of Management Journal*, December 2006, pp. 1239–1251; P. K. Mills and G. R. Ungson, "Reassessing the Limits of Structural Empowerment: Organizational Constitution and Trust as Controls," *Academy of Management Review*, January 2003, pp. 143–153; W. A. Rudolph and M. Sashkin, "Can Organizational Empowerment Work in Multinational Settings?" *Academy of Management Executive*, February 2002, pp. 102–115; C. Gomez and B. Rosen, "The Leader–Member Link Between Managerial Trust and Employee Empowerment," *Group & Organization Management*, March 2001, pp. 53–69; C. Robert and T. M. Probst, "Empowerment and Continuous Improvement in the United States, Mexico, Poland, and India," *Journal of Applied Psychology*, October 2000, pp. 643–658; R. C. Herrenkohl, G. T. Judson, and J. A. Heffner, "Defining and Measuring Employee Empowerment," *Journal of Applied Behavioral Science*, September 1999, p. 373; R. C. Ford and M. D. Fottler, "Empowerment: A Matter of Degree," *Academy of Management Executive*, August 1995, pp. 21–31; and W. A. Rudolph, "Navigating the Journey to Empowerment," *Organizational Dynamics*, Spring 1995, pp. 19–32.

61. T. A. Stewart, "Just Think: No Permission Needed," *Fortune*, January 8, 2001, pp. 190–192.

62. M. Elliott, "Who Needs Charisma?" *Time*, July 20, 2009, pp. 35–38.

63. F. W. Swierczek, "Leadership and Culture: Comparing Asian Managers," *Leadership & Organization Development Journal*, December 1991, pp. 3–10.

64. House, "Leadership in the Twenty-First Century," p. 443; M. F. Peterson and J. G. Hunt, "International Perspectives on International Leadership," *Leadership Quarterly*, Fall 1997, pp. 203–231; and J. R. Schermerhorn and M. H. Bond, "Cross-Cultural Leadership in Collectivism and High Power Distance Settings," *Leadership & Organization Development Journal*, vol. 18, issue 4/5, 1997, pp. 187–193.

65. R. J. House, P. J. Hanges, S. A. Ruiz-Quintanilla, P. W. Dorfman et al., "Culture Specific and Cross-Culturally Generalizable Implicit Leadership Theories: Are the Attributes of Charismatic/Transformational Leadership Universally Endorsed?" *Leadership Quarterly*, Summer 1999, pp. 219–256; and D. E. Carl and M. Javidan, "Universality of Charismatic Leadership: A Multi-Nation Study," paper presented at

the National Academy of Management Conference, Washington, DC, August 2001.

66. D. E. Carl and M. Javidan, "Universality of Charismatic Leadership: A Multi-Nation Study," paper presented at the National Academy of Management Conference, Washington, DC, August 2001.

67. See, for instance, R. Lofthouse, "Herding the Cats," *EuroBusiness*, February 2001, pp. 64–65; and M. Delahoussaye, "Leadership in the 21st Century," *Training*, September 2001, pp. 60–72.

68. See, for example, D. S. DeRue and N. Wellman, "Developing Leaders via Experience: The Role of Developmental Challenge, Learning Organization, and Feedback Availability," *Journal of Applied Psychology*, July 2009, pp. 859–875; A. A. Vicere, "Executive Education: The Leading Edge," *Organizational Dynamics*, Autumn 1996, pp. 67–81; J. Barling, T. Weber, and E. K. Kelloway, "Effects of Transformational Leadership Training on Attitudinal and Financial Outcomes: A Field Experiment," *Journal of Applied Psychology*, December 1996, pp. 827–832; and D. V. Day, "Leadership Development: A Review in Context," *Leadership Quarterly*, Winter 2000, pp. 581–613.

69. P. Brotherton, "Leadership: Nature or Nurture?" *T&D*, February 2013, p. 25.

70. K. Y. Chan and F. Drasgow, "Toward a Theory of Individual Differences and Leadership: Understanding the Motivation to Lead," *Journal of Applied Psychology*, June 2001, pp. 481–498.

71. M. Sashkin, "The Visionary Leader," in J. A. Conger, R. N. Kanungo et al. (eds.), *Charismatic Leadership* (San Francisco: Jossey-Bass, 1988), p. 150.

72. S. Kerr and J. M. Jermier, "Substitutes for Leadership: Their Meaning and Measurement," *Organizational Behavior and Human Performance*, December 1978, pp. 375–403; J. P. Howell, P. W. Dorfman, and S. Kerr, "Leadership and Substitutes for Leadership," *Journal of Applied Behavioral Science* 22, no. 1, 1986, pp. 29–46; J. P. Howell, D. E. Bowen, P. W. Dorfman, S. Kerr, and P. M. Podsakoff, "Substitutes for Leadership: Effective Alternatives to Ineffective Leadership," *Organizational Dynamics*, Summer 1990, pp. 21–38; and P. M. Podsakoff, B. P. Niehoff, S. B. MacKenzie, and M. L. Williams, "Do Substitutes for Leadership Really Substitute for Leadership? An Empirical Examination of Kerr and Jermier's Situational Leadership Model," *Organizational Behavior and Human Decision Processes*, February 1993, pp. 1–44.

73. S. Adams, "The World's Best Companies for Leadership," Forbes.com, May 2, 2012; J. R. Hagerty and J. S. Lublin, "3M Taps 33-Year Veteran and Operating Chief as CEO," *Wall Street Journal*, February 9, 2012, p. B3; R. M. Murphy, "How Do Great Companies Groom Talent?" [management.fortune.cnn.com], November 3, 2011; J. R. Hagerty and B. Tita, "3M Works on Succession Plan," *Wall Street Journal*, December 21, 2010, p. B2; A. Bernasek, "World's Most Admired Companies," *Fortune*, March 22, 2010, pp. 121+; "Selected Results from Best Companies for Leadership Survey," *Bloomberg BusinessWeek Online*, February 16, 2010; J. Kerr and R. Albright, "Finding and Cultivating Finishers," *Leadership Excellence*, July 2009, p. 20; **D. Jones, "3M CEO Emphasizes Importance of Leaders," *USA Today*, May 18, 2009, p. 4B**; G. Colvin, "World's Most Admired Companies 2009," *Fortune*, March 16, 2009, pp. 75+; and M. C. Mankins and R. Steele, "Turning Great Strategy into Great Performance," *Harvard Business Review*, July–August 2005, pp. 64–72.

74. S. Kessler, "Take a Peek Inside Starbucks's $35 Million Leadership Lab," fastcompany.com, March 6, 2013; L. Sinclair, "Fast Company Goes Inside Starbucks' Leadership Lab," sprudge.com, November 5, 2012; and J. Jennings, "Successful Reinventors," *Leadership Excellence*, August 2012, p. 13.

Management Practice: Part 5

Management Practice

A Manager's Dilemma

How would you feel as a new employee if your boss asked you to do something and you had to admit that you didn't know how to do it? Most of us would probably feel pretty inadequate and incompetent. Now imagine how strange and uncomfortable it would be if, after experiencing such an incident, you went home with the boss because you were roommates and have been friends since fourth grade. That's the situation faced by John, Glen, and Kurt. John and Kurt are employees at a software company that their friend Glen and four others started. The business now has 39 employees, and the "friends" are finding out that mixing work and friendships can be tricky! At home, they're equals. They share a three-bedroom condo and divide up housework and other chores. However, at work, equality is out the door. Glen is John's boss and Kurt's boss is another company manager. Recently, the company moved into a new workspace. As part of the four-person management team, Glen has a corner office with windows. However, John was assigned a cubicle and is annoyed at Glen for not standing up for him when offices were assigned. But John didn't complain because he didn't want to get an office only because of his friendship with Glen. Another problem brewing is that the roommates compete to outlast one another at working late. Kurt's boss is afraid that he's going to burn out. Other awkward moments arise whenever the company's performance is discussed. When Glen wants to get something off his chest about work matters, he has to stop himself. And then there's the "elephant in the room." If the software company is ever bought out by a larger company, Glen (and his three partners) stand to profit dramatically, thereby creating some interesting emotional issues for the roommates. Although it might seem easy to say the solution is to move, real estate is too expensive and, besides that, these guys are good friends.

Put yourself in Glen's shoes. Using what you've learned about individual behavior, communication, employee motivation, and leadership, how would you handle this situation?

Global Sense

As you discovered in this part of the text, employee engagement is an important focus for managers. Managers want their employees to be connected to, satisfied with, and enthusiastic about their jobs; that is, to be engaged. Why is employee engagement so important? The level of employee engagement serves as an indicator of organizational health and ultimately business results—success or failure. The latest available data (2013) on global employee engagement levels showed that only 13 percent of employees (surveyed from 142 countries) were engaged in their jobs; 63 percent were not engaged, and 24 percent were actively disengaged (*The State of the Global Workplace: Employee Engagement Insights for Business Leaders Worldwide,* Gallup Organization, http://www.gallup.com/strategicconsulting/164735/state-global-workplace.aspx, accessed August 15, 2014). That is, only 13 percent of employees worldwide say they're passionate about and deeply connected to their work. The region of East Asia showed the lowest proportion of engaged employees at six percent. The global regions of Australia and New Zealand and the United States and Canada showed the highest levels of employee engagement at around 24 percent. And the highest level of active disengagement of employees in the MENA region—Middle East and North Africa.

So what can managers do to get and keep employees engaged? Some important efforts include providing opportunities for career advancement, offering recognition, and having a good organization reputation.

Discuss the following questions in light of what you learned.

- *What role do you think external factors such as the global economic downturn or a country's culture play in levels of employee engagement? Discuss.*
- *What role does an organization's motivational programs play in whether an employee is engaged or not? Discuss.*
- *How might a manager's leadership style affect an employee's level of engagement? Discuss.*
- *Look at what we discussed about managerial communication. What could a manager do in the way he or she communicates to affect an employee's level of engagement?*
- *You're a manager of a workplace that has different "generations." How will you approach engaging your employees? Do you think Gen Y employees are going to be more difficult to "engage"? Discuss.*

Sources: The State of the Global Workplace: Employee Engagement Insights for Business Leaders Worldwide, *Gallup Organization, http://www.gallup.com/strategicconsulting/164735/state-global-workplace.aspx, accessed August 15, 2014;* M. Wilson, "Study: Employee Engagement Ticking Up, But It's Not All Good News," [www.hrcommunication.com], June 18, 2012; "2012 Trends in Global Employee Engagement," www.aon.com, June 17, 2012; K. Gurchiek, "Engagement Erosion Plagues Employers Worldwide," HR Magazine, *June 2012, p. 17; and* T. Maylett and J. Nielsen, "There Is No Cookie-Cutter Approach to Engagement," T&D, *April 2012, pp. 54–59.*

Continuing Case
Starbucks—Leading

Once people are hired or brought into organizations, managers must oversee and coordinate their work so that organizational goals can be pursued and achieved. This is the leading function of management. And it's an important one! However, it also can be quite challenging. Managing people successfully means understanding their attitudes, behaviors, personalities, individual and team work efforts, motivation, conflicts, and so forth. That's not an easy thing to do. In fact, understanding how people behave and why they do the things they do is downright difficult at times. Starbucks has worked hard to create a workplace environment in which employees (partners) are *encouraged to* and *want to* put forth their best efforts. Howard Schultz says he believes that people everywhere have the same desire—to be respected, valued, and appreciated.

Starbucks—Focus on Individuals

Even with some 200,000 full- and part-time partners around the world, one thing that's been important to Howard Schultz from day one is the relationship he has with employees. Schultz is an ardent proponent of a people-first approach and recognizes that the success of Starbucks is due to its partners (employees). And one way Starbucks demonstrates the concern it has for the relationship with its partners is through an attitude survey that gives partners an opportunity to voice their opinions about their experiences. It also measures overall satisfaction and engagement—the degree to which partners are connected to the company. It's been an effective way for Starbucks to show that it cares about what its employees think.

For example, a partner view survey was conducted in early 2010 with partners in the United States and Canada and in the international regional support centers in Europe/Middle East/Africa, Asia Pacific and Latin America, at Starbucks Coffee Trading Company in Switzerland, at Starbucks Coffee Agronomy Company in Costa Rica, and at the coffee roasting facility in Amsterdam. At the end of the survey, Howard Schultz thanked partners for taking the survey. He also acknowledged that the previous year and a half had been difficult (it was the time of Schultz transitioning back into the CEO position) and that partners had been asked to do a lot during that time. The tough and emotional decisions to be made and the company's financial crisis weren't easy for any of them—from the top to the bottom of the organization. But, Schultz also reiterated that his number-one commitment was to the company's partners and reinventing the partner experience at Starbucks. Although results aren't publicly available, it's likely that managers heard the good and the bad stuff that partners experienced and were feeling. It was a good barometer for gauging employee attitudes after a difficult time of transition and transformation for the company. Earlier partner surveys have provided relevant and important clues to employee attitudes. For instance, in a survey from 2005, well over half (64 percent) of partners responded to the survey—much higher than the number of respondents to the previous survey in 2003, in which the partner response rate was only 46 percent. Responses to questions about partner satisfaction and partner engagement were extremely positive: 87 percent of partners said they were satisfied or very satisfied, and 73 percent said they were engaged with the company. (The numbers in 2003 were 82 percent satisfied and 73 percent engaged.) In addition, partners specifically said they "Know what is expected of them at work; believe someone at work cares about them; and work for managers who promote work/life balance." But partners also identified some areas where they felt improvements were needed. These included "Celebrate successes more; provide more effective coaching and feedback; and improve communication with partners" (Corporate Social Responsibility, Starbucks Fiscal 2005 Annual Report, "Beyond the Cup," p. 65 [http://globalassets.starbucks.com/assets/64d30f4e24724986a9e9823901567867.pdf]). And Starbucks' managers try to address any concerns raised in these surveys or concerns expressed in other ways. In another review published by Glassdoor.com, Starbucks employees gave the company 3.7 stars out of 5 and 88 percent approved of CEO Howard Schultz.

Every organization needs employees who will be able to do their jobs efficiently and effectively. Starbucks states that it wants employees who are "adaptable, self-motivated, passionate, creative team players" (Corporate Social

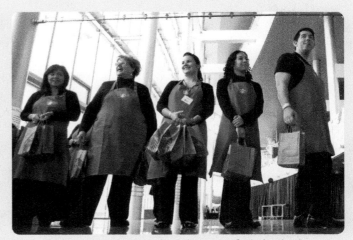

Knowing that its people are the heart and soul of its success, Starbucks values its employees and has created an environment that motivates them to work efficiently and effectively, rewards their accomplishments, and gives them training opportunities and generous benefits. The baristas shown here handing out gift bags to shareholders at an annual meeting represent Starbucks' "ideal" employee who is adaptable, self-motivated, passionate, and a creative team player.
Source: Elaine Thompson/Associated Press

Responsibility, Starbucks Fiscal 2005 Annual Report, "Beyond the Cup," p. 65 [http://globalassets.starbucks.com/assets/64d30f4e24724986a9e9823901567867.pdf]). As you can see, this "ideal" Starbucks partner should have individual strengths and should be able to work as part of a team. In the retail store setting, especially, individuals must work together as a team to provide the experience that customers expect when they walk into a Starbucks. If that doesn't happen, the company's ability to pursue its mission and goals is likely to be affected.

Communication at Starbucks

Keeping organizational communication flowing in all directions is important to Starbucks. And that commitment starts at the top. Howard Schultz tries to visit at least 30 to 40 stores a week. Not only does this give him an upfront view of what's happening out in the field, it gives partners a chance to talk with the top guy in the company. The CEO also likes to "get out in the field" by visiting the stores and roasting facilities. For instance, when Starbucks was first moving into the China market, Schultz spent time in Beijing with more than 1,200 Starbucks partners and their parents and family members. The event recognized the special role Chinese families play and highlighted Starbucks' commitment to its partners. Despite these efforts by the top executives, partners have indicated on past employee surveys that communication needed improvement. Managers listened and made some changes.

An initial endeavor was the creation of an internal video newsletter that conveyed information to partners about company news and announcements. Another change was the implementation of an internal communication audit that asks randomly selected partners for feedback on how to make company communication more effective. In addition, partners can voice concerns about actions or decisions where they believe the company is not operating in a manner consistent with the guiding principles to the Mission Review team, a group formed in 1991 and consisting of company managers and partners. The concept worked so well in North America that many of Starbucks' international units have provided similar communication forums to their partners.

Starbucks—Motivating Employees

A story from Howard Schultz's childhood provides some clues into what has shaped his philosophy about how to treat people. Schultz's father worked hard at various blue-collar jobs. However, when he didn't work, he didn't get paid. When his father broke his ankle when Howard was seven years old, the family "had no income, no health insurance, no worker's compensation, nothing to fall back on." The image of his father with his leg in a cast unable to work left a lasting impression on the young Schultz. Many years later, when his father died of lung cancer, "he had no savings, no pension, and more important, he

had never attained fulfillment and dignity from work he found meaningful." The sad realities of the types of work environments his father endured had a powerful effect on Howard, and he vowed that if he were "ever in a position where I could make a difference, I wouldn't leave people behind" (Based On: Schultz, Howard and Gordon, Joanne, *Onward: How Starbucks Fought For Its Life Without Losing Its Soul*, © Howard Schultz (New York: Rodale Publishing, 2011). And those personal experiences have shaped the way that Starbucks cares for its partners—the relationships and commitments the company has with each and every employee. In fact, during the recent economic recession, Schultz was contacted by an institutional shareholder about trimming the health insurance for part-time employees. Schultz's reply? There's no way that benefit at Starbucks is being cut.

One of the best reflections of how Starbucks treats its eligible part- and full-time partners is its Total Pay package, which includes competitive base pay, bonuses, a comprehensive health plan, paid time-off plans, stock options, a savings program, and partner perks (which includes a pound of coffee each week). Although specific benefits differ between regions and countries, all Starbucks international partners share the "Total Pay" philosophy. For instance, in Malaysia and Thailand, partners are provided extensive training opportunities to further their careers in addition to health insurance, paid vacation, sick leave, and other benefits. In Turkey, the "Total Pay" package for Starbucks' partners includes transportation subsidies and access to a company doctor who provides free treatment.

Partner (employee) recognition is important to Starbucks. The company has several formal recognition programs in place that partners can use as tools to encourage, reward, and inspire one another. These programs range from formal company awards to informal special acknowledgments given by coworkers. One tool—developed in response to suggestions on the partner survey—is an on-the-spot recognition card that celebrates partner and team successes.

To assist partners who are facing particularly difficult circumstances (such as natural disaster, fire, illness), the company has a CUP (Caring Unites Partners) fund that provides financial support. After Hurricanes Katrina and Rita in 2005, more than 300 partners from the Gulf Coast region received more than $225,000 in assistance from the CUP fund. In China, Starbucks has set aside RMB1 million (about $158,000 in today's currency exchange) for the Starbucks China CUP fund to be used to provide financial assistance to partners in times of significant or immediate needs. This is the type of caring and compassion that Howard Schultz vowed to provide after seeing his father not able to work and have an income because of a broken ankle.

In 2013, Starbucks again was named one of *Fortune* magazine's 100 Best Companies to Work For—the fifteenth time since 1998 that Starbucks has received this recognition. Although being recognized as a great company to

work for is commendable, Starbucks has seen its ranking drop. In 2008, it was ranked number 7; in 2009, number 24; in 2010, number 93; and in 2011, number 98. However, in 2012, its ranking rose to number 73, but it fell to number 94 in 2013, and did not make the list in 2014. Like many companies, Starbucks had to make some tough strategic decisions during one of the toughest economic periods faced recently. Despite the challenges, it's a testament to Starbucks' treatment of its partners that it made the top 100 list for 15 years straight. However, there may be some underlying employee issues to address after failing to be cited as one of the 100 Best Companies to Work For in the most recent survey.

Starbucks—Fostering Leadership

Not surprisingly, Howard Schultz has some definite views about leading and leadership. He says being a great leader involves finding a balance between celebrating what's made a company successful in the past and knowing when to not continue following the status quo. He also said being a great leader means identifying a path your organization needs to follow and then creating enough confidence in your people so they follow that path and don't "veer off course because it's an easier route to go" (W. Meyers, "Conscience In a Cup of Coffee," *US News & World Report*, October 31, 2005, pp. 48–50). He also said leaders, particularly of growing companies, need to stay true to those values and principles that have guided how their business is done and not let those values be compromised by ambitions of growth.

Since 1982, Howard Schultz has led Starbucks in a way that has allowed the company to successfully grow and meet and exceed its goals *and* to do so ethically and responsibly. From the creation of the company's Guiding Principles to the various innovative strategic initiatives, Schultz has never veered from his belief about what Starbucks, the company, could be and should be. In 2011, *Fortune* named Howard Schultz the Businessperson of the Year.

Unlike many companies, Starbucks and Howard Schultz have taken their leadership succession responsibilities seriously. In 2000 when Schultz was still CEO, he decided to move into the chairman's position. His replacement, Orin Smith (president and chief operating officer of Starbucks Coffee U.S.), had been "groomed" to take over the CEO position. Smith made it a top priority to plan his own succession. First, he established an exit date—in 2005 at age 62. Then he monitored the leadership skills development of his top executives. Two years into the job, Smith recognized that the internal candidates most likely to replace him would still be too "unseasoned" to assume the CEO position by his stated exit date. At that point, the decision was made to look externally for a promising successor. That's when Jim Donald was hired from Pathmark, a regional grocery chain, where he was chairman, president, and CEO. For three years, Donald was immersed in Starbucks' business as president of the largest division, the North American unit, before assuming the CEO position in 2005, as planned. In early 2008, Jim Donald stepped down from the CEO position, and Howard Schultz once again assumed the position. At that time, Schultz realized his job was to step up as a leader to transform and revitalize Starbucks.

Starbucks also recognizes the importance of having individuals with excellent leadership skills throughout the company. In addition to the leadership development training for upper-level managers, Starbucks offers a program called Learning to Lead for hourly employees (baristas) to develop leadership skills. This training program also covers store operations and effective management practices. In addition, Starbucks offers to managers at all organizational levels additional training courses on coaching and providing feedback to help managers improve their people skills.

Discussion Questions

1. Do the overwhelmingly positive results from the 2005 partner survey surprise you? Why or why not? Do you think giving employees an opportunity to express their opinions in something like an attitude survey is beneficial? Why or why not?

2. How might the results of the partner survey affect the way a local store manager does his or her job? How about a district manager? How about the president of global development? Do you think there are differences in the impact of employee surveys on how managers at different organizational levels lead? Why or why not?

3. As Starbucks continues to expand globally, what factors might affect partner responses on a partner view survey? What are the implications for managers?

4. Look at the description of the types of people Starbucks seeks. What individual behavior issues might arise in managing these types of people? (Think in terms of attitudes, personality, etc.) What work team issues might arise? (Think in terms of what makes teams successful. Hint: Can a person be self-motivated and passionate *and* be a good team player?)

5. Discuss the "ideal" Starbucks employee in terms of the various personality trait theories.

6. Describe in your own words the workplace environment Starbucks has tried to create. What impact might such an environment have on motivating employees?

7. Using the Job Characteristics Model, redesign a part-time hourly worker's job to be more motivating. Do the same with a store manager's job.

8. Does Starbucks "care" too much for its partners? Can a company ever treat its employees too well? Why or why not?

9. Howard Schultz says, "We all want the same thing as people—to be respected and valued as employees and appreciated as customers." Does the company respect and value its partners (employees)? Explain. What do you think this implies for its employee relationships?

10. Former CEO Jim Donald once said, "Spending money to put people first is smart money." Do you agree or disagree? Why?

11. If you were an executive, would you be concerned about the drastic drop in ranking on the list of best companies to work for and not being ranked in the most current list? Why or why not? What actions might you take?

12. Give some examples of the types of communication taking place at Starbucks.

13. Suppose you're a Starbucks store manager in Birmingham, Alabama. How do you find out what's going on in the company? How might you communicate your concerns or issues?

14. Describe Howard Schultz's leadership style. Would his approach be appropriate in other types of organizations? Why or why not?

15. Do you agree that leadership succession planning is important? Why or why not?

16. What is Starbucks doing "right" with respect to the leading function? Are they doing anything "wrong?" Explain.

17. Which of the company's principles (see Web site) influence the leading function of management? Explain how the one(s) you chose would affect how Starbucks' managers deal with (a) individual behavior issues; (b) communication issues; (c) motivational techniques; and (d) leadership styles or approaches.

Notes for the Continuing Case

Information from Starbucks Corporation 2013 Annual Report, www.investor.starbucks.com, May 2014; company Web site, www.starbucks.com; Glassdoor Company Review, "Starbucks," http://www.glassdoor.com/Overview/Working-at-Starbucks-EI_IE2202.11,20.htm, May 12, 2014; News Release, "Starbucks Strengthens Commitment to Being the Employer of Choice in China," news.starbucks.com, April 18, 2012; J. Certner, "Starbucks: For Infusing a Steady Stream of New Ideas to Revive Its Business," *Fast Company,* March 2012, pp. 112+; D. A. Kaplan, "Strong Coffee," *Fortune,* December 12, 2011, pp. 100+; "Howard Schultz, On Getting A Second Shot," *Inc.,* April 2011, pp. 52–54; C. Cain Miller, "A Changed Starbucks. A Changed CEO," *New York Times Online,* March 12, 2011; "Howard Schultz Promises Partners a Better Starbucks Experience in the Future," *StarbucksMelody.com,* www.starbucksmelody.com/2010/03/06/howard-schultz-promises-partners-a-better-starbucks-experience-in-the-future/, March 6, 2010; M. Moskowitz, R. Levering, and C. Tkaczyk, "The List: 100 Best Companies to Work For," *Fortune,* February 8, 2010, pp. 75+; Starbucks Ad, *USA Today,* May 19, 2009, p. 9A; Interview with Jim Donald, *Smart Money,* May 2006, pp. 31–32; A. Serwer, "Interview with Howard Schultz," *Fortune (Europe),* March 20, 2006, pp. 35–36; W. Meyers, "Conscience in a Cup of Coffee," *US News & World Report,* October 31, 2005, pp. 48–50; J. M. Cohn, R. Khurana, and L. Reeves, "Growing Talent as If Your Business Depended on It," *Harvard Business Review,* October 2005, pp. 62–70; Interview with Jim Donald, *Fortune,* April 4, 2005, p. 30; P. Kafka, "Bean Counter," *Forbes,* February 28, 2005, pp. 78–80; S. Gray, "Starbucks' CEO Announces Plan to Retire in March," *Wall Street Journal,* October 13, 2004, p. A6; and A. Serwer and K. Bonamici, "Hot Starbucks to Go," *Fortune,* January 26, 2004, pp. 60–74.

Monitoring and Controlling

From Chapter 18 of *Management*, Thirteenth Edition. Stephen P. Robbins and Mary Coulter. Copyright © 2016 by Pearson Education, Inc. All rights reserved.

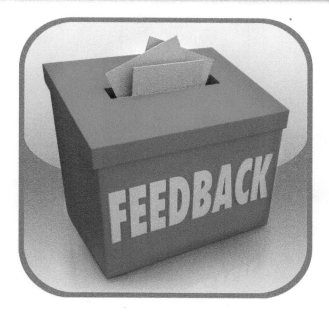

Source: iQoncept/Shutterstock

A key to success in management and in your career is knowing *how to be effective at giving feedback.*

How to Be a Pro at Giving Feedback

Everyone needs feedback! If you want people to do their best, they need to know what they're doing well and what they can do better. That's why providing feedback is such an important skill to have. But being effective at giving feedback is tricky! That's why we often see managers either (a) not wanting to give feedback or (b) giving feedback in such a way that it doesn't result in anything positive.

You can feel more comfortable with and be more effective at providing feedback if you use the following specific suggestions:[1]

1. Be straightforward by focusing on specific behaviors. *Feedback should be specific rather than general. Avoid such statements as "You have a bad attitude" or "I'm really impressed with the good job you did." They're vague and although they provide information, they don't tell the recipient enough to correct the "bad attitude" or on what basis you concluded that a "good job" had been done so the person knows what behaviors to repeat or to avoid.*

2. Be realistic. *Focus your feedback on what can be changed. When people get comments on things over which they have no control, it can be frustrating.*

3. Keep feedback impersonal. *Feedback, particularly the negative kind, should be descriptive rather than judgmental or evaluative. No matter how upset you are, keep the feedback focused on job-related behaviors and never criticize someone personally because of an inappropriate action.*

Keep feedback goal oriented. Feedback should not be given primarily to "blow off steam" or "unload" on another person. If you have to say something negative, make sure it's directed toward the recipient's goals. Ask yourself whom the feedback is supposed to help. If the answer is you, bite your tongue

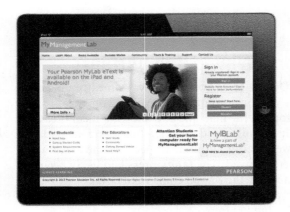

Learning Objectives

1 **Explain** *the nature and importance of control.*

2 **Describe** *the three steps in the control process.*

3 **Explain** *how organizational and employee performance are measured.*

   ● **Know how** to be effective at giving feedback.

4 **Describe** *tools used to measure organizational performance.*

5 **Discuss** *contemporary issues in control.*

   ● **Develop your skill** at dealing with difficult people.

---

and hold the comment. Such feedback undermines your credibility and lessens the meaning and influence of future feedback.

   4. ***Know when to give feedback—make it well timed.*** *Feedback is most meaningful to a recipient when there's a very short interval between his or her behavior and the receipt of feedback about that behavior. Moreover, if you're particularly concerned with changing behavior, delays in providing feedback on the undesirable actions lessen the likelihood that the feedback will be effective in bringing about the desired change. Of course, making feedback prompt merely for the sake of promptness can backfire if you have insufficient information, if you're angry,*

or if you're otherwise emotionally upset. In such instances, "well timed" could mean "somewhat delayed."

   5. ***Ensure understanding.*** *Make sure your feedback is concise and complete so that the recipient clearly and fully understands the communication. It may help to have the recipient rephrase the content of your feedback to find out whether it fully captured the meaning you intended.*

   6. ***Watch your body language, tone of voice, and facial expressions.*** *Your body language and tone of voice can speak louder than words. Think about what you want to communicate and make sure your body language supports that message.*

Things don't always go as planned. That's why controlling is so important! Controlling is the final step in the management process. Managers must monitor whether goals that were established as part of the planning process are being accomplished efficiently and effectively as planned. That's what they do when they control. Appropriate controls can help managers look for specific performance gaps and areas for improvement. And that's what we're going to look at in this text—the control process, the types of controls that managers can use, and contemporary issues in control.

WHAT Is Controlling and Why Is It Important?

LO1
- A press operator at the Denver Mint noticed a flaw—an extra up leaf or an extra down leaf—on Wisconsin state quarters being pressed at one of his five press machines. He stopped the machine and left for a meal break. When he returned, he saw the machine running and assumed that someone had changed the die in the machine. However, after a routine inspection, the machine operator realized the die had not been changed. The faulty press had likely been running for over an hour and thousands of the flawed coins were now commingled with unblemished quarters. As many as 50,000 of the faulty coins entered circulation, setting off a coin collector buying frenzy.[2]
- After an above-ground radioactive release at a nuclear waste storage vault in New Mexico, a report blamed managers who failed to "understand and control the risks."[3]
- Security lapses, including unlocked doors and defective airflow, at a federal Center for Disease Control lab in Atlanta generated serious concerns.[4]
- After a number of negatively publicized incidents on its cruise ships, Carnival Corporation accelerated its schedule of maintenance and other renovations.[5]
- A technical error on Walmart's Web site led to certain products showing unbelievably low prices (for instance, a treadmill for $33). The error was not the result of hacking, but an internal glitch, and was quickly corrected.[6]
- For more than a century, the venerable *New York Times* had an error on its front page every single day. Somehow, back in 1898, the issue number was inflated by 500. The paper did correct the error once it was discovered in 1999.[7]
- Clothing return fraud costs U.S. retailers almost $9 billion annually. To combat this, many high-end retailers have started placing large black plastic tags in highly visible places on dresses and other pricey clothing items.[8]
- No fast-food chain wants its employees doing gross stuff behind the scenes, but social media photos and videos of a Taco Bell employee licking a stack of taco shells, a Wendy's employee bending down under a Frosty machine with mouth wide open gobbling the treat, and a Domino's Pizza employee performing vulgar and unsanitary actions while preparing food have all shown up online.[9]

Yikes! Can you see why controlling is such an important managerial function?

controlling
Management function that involves monitoring, comparing, and correcting work performance

What is **controlling**? It's the process of monitoring, comparing, and correcting work performance. All managers should control even if their units are performing as planned because they can't really know that unless they've evaluated what activities have been done and compared actual performance against the desired standard.[10] Effective controls ensure that activities are completed in ways that lead to the attainment of goals. Whether controls are effective, then, is determined by how well they help employees and managers achieve their goals.[11]

In David Lee Roth's autobiography (yes, *that* David Lee Roth, the former front man for Van Halen), he tells the story of how he had a clause (article 126) in his touring contract asking for a bowl of M&Ms backstage, but no brown ones.[12] Now, you might think that is just typical demanding rock star behavior, but instead it was a well-planned effort by Roth to see whether the venue management had paid attention. With the technical complexity of his show, he figured if they couldn't get the M&Ms right, he needed to demand a line check of the entire production to ensure that no technical errors would occur during a performance. Now that's how managers should use control!

Why is control so important? Planning can be done, an organizational structure created to facilitate efficient achievement of goals, and employees motivated through effective leadership. But there's no assurance that activities are going as planned and that the goals employees and managers are working toward are, in fact, being attained. Control is important, therefore, because it's the only way that managers know whether organizational goals are being met and, if not, the reasons why. The value of the control function can be seen in three specific areas: planning, empowering employees, and protecting the workplace.

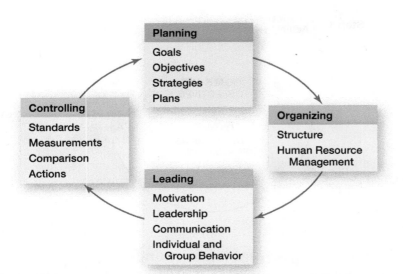

Exhibit 1
Planning-Controlling Link

Goals provide specific direction to employees and managers, as the foundation of planning. However, just stating goals or having employees accept goals doesn't guarantee that the necessary actions to accomplish those goals have been taken. As the old saying goes, "The best-laid plans often go awry." The effective manager follows up to ensure that what employees are supposed to do is, in fact, being done and goals are being achieved. Controlling provides a critical link back to planning. (See Exhibit 1.) If managers didn't control, they'd have no way of knowing whether their goals and plans were being achieved and what future actions to take.

The second reason controlling is important is because of employee empowerment. Many managers are reluctant to empower their employees because they fear something will go wrong for which they would be held responsible. But an effective control system can provide information and feedback on employee performance and minimize the chance of potential problems.

The final reason why managers control is to protect the organization and its assets.[13] Today's environment brings heightened threats from natural disasters, financial scandals, workplace violence, global supply chain disruptions, security breaches, and even possible terrorist attacks. Managers must protect organizational assets in the event that any of these things should happen. Comprehensive controls and back-up plans will help assure minimal work disruptions.

THE Control Process

L02 Zebra. That's the name of a company with an RFID sensor tracking product called MotionWorks that Nascar's Michael Waltrip Racing pit crew is clamoring over, although it's not yet been approved for use in races. This RFID sensing technology will allow pit crews to track in real-time what they've only been able to do with videos and stopwatches. By controlling every movement and action, the team hopes to maximize speed in pit stops and prevent penalties. It would allow them to measure their performance in ways not available before.[14] What a great example of managers using the control process to address issues both leading to and resolving problems and trying to be more efficient and effective.

The **control process** is a three-step process of measuring actual performance, comparing actual performance against a standard, and taking managerial action to correct deviations or to address inadequate standards. (See Exhibit 2.) The control process assumes that performance standards already exist, and they do. They're the specific goals created during the planning process.

control process
A three-step process of measuring actual performance, comparing actual performance against a standard, and taking managerial action to correct deviations or inadequate standards

Exhibit 2
The Control Process

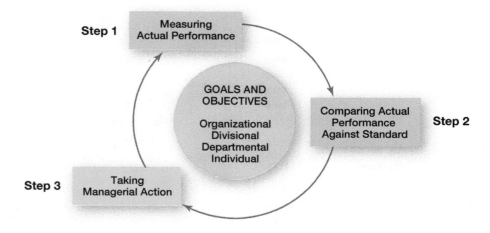

Step 1: Measuring Actual Performance

To determine what actual performance is, a manager must first get information about it. Thus, the first step in control is measuring.

HOW WE MEASURE   Four approaches used by managers to measure and report actual performance are personal observations, statistical reports, oral reports, and written reports. Exhibit 3 summarizes the advantages and drawbacks of each approach. Most managers use a combination of these approaches.

WHAT WE MEASURE   At Office Depot, customer service was measured by metrics—such as the cleanliness of bathrooms—that didn't drive sales. The company's president is trying to address this by identifying what measures are most important and then retraining the staff on achieving those measures.[15] Yes, what is measured is probably more critical to the control process than how it's measured. Why? Because selecting the wrong criteria can create serious problems. Besides, *what* is measured often determines what employees will do.[16] What control criteria might managers use?

Some control criteria can be used for any management situation. For instance, all managers deal with people, so criteria such as employee satisfaction or turnover and absenteeism rates can be measured. Keeping costs within budget is also a fairly common control measure. Other control criteria should recognize the different activities that managers supervise. For instance, a manager at a pizza delivery location might use measures such as number of pizzas delivered per day, average delivery time for

Exhibit 3
Sources of Information for Measuring Performance

	Benefits	Drawbacks
Personal Observations	• Get firsthand knowledge • Information isn't filtered • Intensive coverage of work activities	• Subject to personal biases • Time-consuming • Obtrusive
Statistical Reports	• Easy to visualize • Effective for showing relationships	• Provide limited information • Ignore subjective factors
Oral Reports	• Fast way to get information • Allow for verbal and nonverbal feedback	• Information is filtered • Information can't be documented
Written Reports	• Comprehensive • Formal • Easy to file and retrieve	• Take more time to prepare

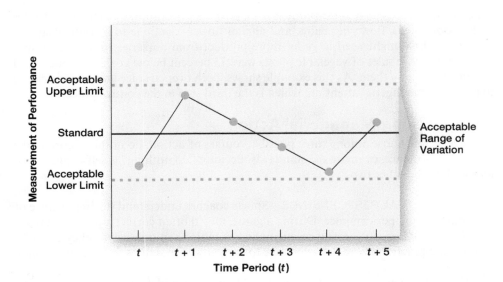

Exhibit 4
Acceptable Range of Variation

phone orders versus online orders, or number of coupons redeemed. A manager in a governmental agency might use applications typed per day, client requests completed per hour, or average time to process paperwork.

Most work activities can be expressed in quantifiable terms. However, managers should use subjective measures when necessary. Although such measures may have limitations, they're better than having no standards at all and doing no controlling.

Step 2: Comparing Actual Performance Against the Standard

The comparing step determines the variation between actual performance and the standard. Although some variation in performance can be expected in all activities, it's critical to determine an acceptable **range of variation** (see Exhibit 4). Deviations outside this range need attention. Let's work through an example.

Chris Tanner is a sales manager for Green Earth Gardening Supply, a distributor of specialty plants and seeds in the Pacific Northwest. Chris prepares a report during the first week of each month that describes sales for the previous month, classified by product line. Exhibit 5 displays both the sales goals (standard) and actual sales figures for the month of June. After looking at the numbers, should Chris be concerned? Sales were a bit higher than originally targeted, but does that mean there were no significant deviations? That depends on what Chris thinks is *significant*; that is, outside the acceptable range of variation. Even though overall performance was

range of variation
The acceptable parameters of variance between actual performance and the standard

Product	Standard	Actual	Over (Under)
Vegetable plants	1,075	913	(162)
Perennial flowers	630	634	4
Annual flowers	800	912	112
Herbs	160	140	(20)
Flowering bulbs	170	286	116
Flowering bushes	225	220	(5)
Heirloom seeds	540	672	132
Total	3,600	3,777	177

Exhibit 5
Green Earth Gardening Supply—
June Sales

generally quite favorable, some product lines need closer scrutiny. For instance, if sales of heirloom seeds, flowering bulbs, and annual flowers continue to be over what was expected, Chris might need to order more product from nurseries to meet customer demand. Because sales of vegetable plants were 15 percent below goal, Chris may need to run a special on them. As this example shows, both overvariance and undervariance may require managerial attention, which is the third step in the control process.

Step 3: Taking Managerial Action

Managers can choose among three possible courses of action: do nothing, correct the actual performance, or revise the standards. Because "do nothing" is self-explanatory, let's look at the other two.

CORRECT ACTUAL PERFORMANCE   Sports coaches understand the importance of correcting actual performance. During a game, they'll often correct a player's actions. But if the problem is recurring or encompasses more than one player, they'll devote time during practice before the next game to correcting the actions.[17] That's what managers need to do as well.

Depending on what the problem is, a manager could take different corrective actions. For instance, if unsatisfactory work is the reason for performance variations, the manager could correct it by things such as training programs, disciplinary action, changes in compensation practices, and so forth. One decision a manager must make is whether to take **immediate corrective action**, which corrects problems at once to get performance back on track, or to use **basic corrective action**, which looks at how and why performance deviated before correcting the source of deviation. It's not unusual for managers to rationalize that they don't have time to find the source of a problem (basic corrective action) and continue to perpetually "put out fires" with immediate corrective action. Effective managers analyze deviations and, if the benefits justify it, take the time to pinpoint and correct the causes of variance.

REVISE THE STANDARD   It's possible that the variance was a result of an unrealistic standard—too low or too high a goal. In that situation, the standard needs the corrective action, not the performance. If performance consistently exceeds the goal, then a manager should look at whether the goal is too easy and needs to be raised. On the other hand, managers must be cautious about revising a standard downward. It's natural to blame the goal when an employee or a team falls short. For instance, students who get a low score on a test often attack the grade cut-off standards as too high. Rather than accept the fact that their performance was inadequate, they will argue that the standards are unreasonable. Likewise, salespeople who don't meet their monthly quota often want to blame what they think is an unrealistic quota. The point is that when performance isn't up to par, don't immediately blame the goal or standard. If you believe the standard is realistic, fair, and achievable, tell employees that you expect future work to improve, and then take the necessary corrective action to help make that happen.

Managerial Decisions in Controlling

Exhibit 6 summarizes the decisions a manager makes in controlling. The standards are goals developed during the planning process. These goals provide the basis for the control process, which involves measuring actual performance and comparing it against the standard. Depending on the results, a manager's decision is to do nothing, correct the performance, or revise the standard.

immediate corrective action
Corrective action that corrects problems at once to get performance back on track

basic corrective action
Corrective action that looks at how and why performance deviated before correcting the source of deviation

⭐ **Watch It 1!**   If your professor has assigned this, go to **www.mymanagementlab.com** to watch a video titled: *CH2MHill: Foundations of Control* and to respond to questions.

Exhibit 6
Managerial Decisions in the Control Process

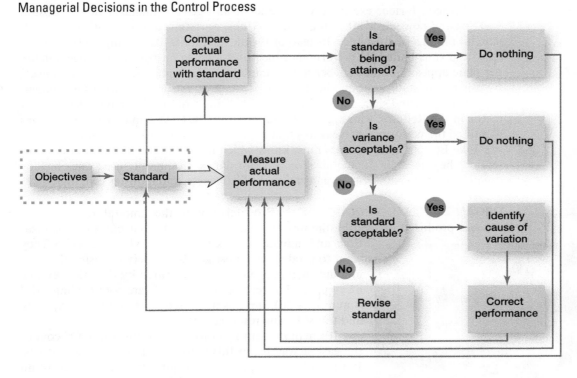

CONTROLLING for Organizational and Employee Performance

LO3 Cost efficiency. The length of time customers are kept on hold. Customer satisfaction with service provided. These are just a few of the important performance indicators that executives in the intensely competitive call-center service industry measure. To make good decisions, managers in this industry want and need this type of information so they can manage organizational and employee performance. Managers in all types of businesses are responsible for managing organizational and employee performance.

What Is Organizational Performance?

When you hear the word *performance,* what do you think of? A summer evening concert by a local community orchestra? An Olympic athlete striving for the finish line in a close race? A Southwest Airlines ramp agent in Ft. Myers, Florida, loading passengers as efficiently as possible in order to meet the company's 20-minute gate turnaround goal? **Performance** is all of these things. It's the end result of an activity. And whether that activity is hours of intense practice before a concert or race or whether it's carrying out job responsibilities as efficiently and effectively as possible, performance is what results from that activity.

Managers are concerned with **organizational performance**—the accumulated results of all the organization's work activities. It's a multifaceted concept, but managers need to understand the factors that contribute to organizational performance. After all, it's unlikely that they want (or intend) to manage their way to mediocre performance. They *want* their organizations, work units, or work groups to achieve high levels of performance.

performance
The end result of an activity

organizational performance
The accumulated results of all the organization's work activities

499

Measures of Organizational Performance

Theo Epstein, former executive vice president and general manager of the Boston Red Sox and now president of the Chicago Cubs, uses some unusual statistics to evaluate his players' performance. Instead of the old standards like batting average, home runs, and runs batted in, performance measures include on-base percentage, pitches per plate appearance, at-bats per home run, and on-base plus slugging percentage.[18] By using these statistics to predict future performance, Epstein identified some potential star players and signed them for a fraction of the cost of a big-name player, a key factor in the Red Sox winning the World Series in 2004. As a manager, Epstein has identified the performance measures that are most important to his decisions.

Like Epstein, all managers must know which measures will give them the information they need about organizational performance. Commonly used ones include organizational productivity, organizational effectiveness, and industry rankings.

productivity
The amount of goods or services produced divided by the inputs needed to generate that output

organizational effectiveness
A measure of how appropriate organizational goals are and how well those goals are being met

ORGANIZATIONAL PRODUCTIVITY **Productivity** is the amount of goods or services produced divided by the inputs needed to generate that output. Organizations and individual work units want to be productive. They want to produce the most goods and services using the least amount of inputs. Output is measured by the sales revenue an organization receives when goods are sold (selling price × number sold). Input is measured by the costs of acquiring and transforming resources into outputs.

It's management's job to increase this ratio. Of course, the easiest way to do this is to raise prices of the outputs. But in today's competitive environment, that may not be an option. The only other option, then, is to decrease the inputs side. How? By being more efficient in performing work and thus decreasing the organization's expenses.

ORGANIZATIONAL EFFECTIVENESS **Organizational effectiveness** is a measure of how appropriate organizational goals are and how well those goals are met. That's the bottom line for managers, and it's what guides managerial decisions in designing strategies and work activities and in coordinating the work of employees.

INDUSTRY AND COMPANY RANKINGS Rankings are a popular way for managers to measure their organization's performance. And there's not a shortage of these rankings, as Exhibit 7 shows. Rankings are determined by specific performance measures, which are different for each list. For instance, *Fortune's* Best Companies to

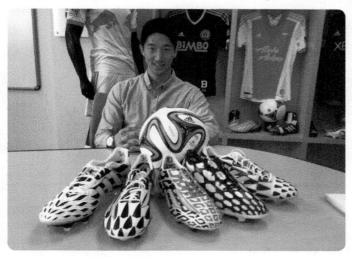

Peter Hong, merchandise manager for Adidas, display's the firm's Battle Pack soccer boots and Brazuca soccer ball. According to a global survey of 200,000 business students, Adidas ranks in the top 50 list of the world's most attractive employers. This ranking of Adidas as an ideal employer is one way that the firm's managers can measure their organization's performance.
Source: Anne Peterson/Associated Press

Exhibit 7
Popular Industry and Company Rankings

Fortune (www.fortune.com)	*IndustryWeek* (www.industryweek.com)
Fortune 500	*IndustryWeek* 1000
Global 500	*IndustryWeek* U.S. 500
World's Most Admired Companies	50 Best Manufacturers
100 Best Companies to Work For	*IndustryWeek* Best Plants
100 Fastest-Growing Companies	
Forbes (www.forbes.com)	**Customer Satisfaction Indexes**
World's Biggest Public Companies	American Customer Satisfaction Index— University of Michigan Business School
	Customer Satisfaction Measurement Association

Work For are chosen by answers given by thousands of randomly selected employees on a questionnaire called "The Great Place to Work® Trust Index®" and on materials filled out by thousands of company managers, including a corporate culture audit created by the Great Place to Work Institute. These rankings give managers (and others) an indicator of how well their company performs in comparison to others.

Controlling for Employee Performance

Since managers manage employees, they also have to be concerned about controlling for employee performance; that is, making sure employees' work efforts are of the quantity and quality needed to accomplish organizational goals. How do managers do that? By following the control process: measure actual performance; compare that performance to standard (or expectations); and take action, if needed. It's particularly important for managers to deliver effective performance feedback and to be prepared, if needed, to use **disciplinary actions**—actions taken by a manager to enforce the organization's work standards and regulations.[19] Let's look first at effective performance feedback.

disciplinary actions
Actions taken by a manager to enforce the organization's work standards and regulations

DELIVERING EFFECTIVE PERFORMANCE FEEDBACK Throughout the semester, do you keep track of all your scores on homework, exams, and papers? If you do, why do you like to know that information? For most of us, it's because we like to know where we stand in terms of where we'd like to be and what we'd like to accomplish in our work. We like to know how we're doing. Managers need to provide their employees with feedback so that the employees know where they stand in terms of their work. When giving performance feedback, both parties need to feel heard, understood, and respected. And if done that way, positive outcomes can result. "In a productive performance discussion, organizations have the opportunity to reinforce company values, strengthen workplace culture, and achieve strategic goals."[21] Sometimes, however, performance feedback doesn't work. An employee's performance may continue to be an issue. Under those circumstances, disciplinary actions may be necessary to address the problems.

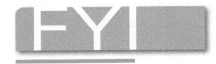

- 73 percent of managers say they deliver difficult feedback well although they struggle with it sometimes and it doesn't always go perfectly.[20]

Providing Good Feedback—If your instructor is using MyManagementLab, log onto **mymanagementlab.com** and test your *providing good feedback knowledge.* **Be sure to refer back to the chapter opener!**

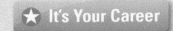

USING DISCIPLINARY ACTIONS Fortunately, most employees do their jobs well and never need formal correction. Yet, sometimes it is needed. Exhibit 8 lists some common types of work discipline problems and examples of each. In those

PROBLEM TYPE	EXAMPLES OF EACH
Attendance	Absenteeism, tardiness, abuse of sick leave
On-the-Job Behaviors	Insubordination, failure to use safety devices, alcohol or drug abuse
Dishonesty	Theft, lying to supervisors, falsifying information on employment application or on other organizational forms
Outside Activities	Criminal activities, unauthorized strike activities, working for a competing organization (if no-compete clause is part of employment)

Exhibit 8
Types of Discipline Problems and Examples of Each

let's get REAL

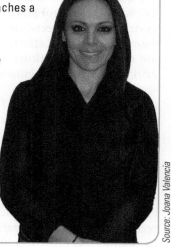

The Scenario:

Maddy Long supervises a team of data specialists. One of her team members doesn't like to be told what to do, even though that's part of Maddy's responsibility as the manager—to outline the work that has to be done each week. Some of the other team members are starting to complain among themselves. Maddy knows she needs to address this problem before it reaches a crisis stage.

What should Maddy do now?

Maddy needs to address this sooner rather than later in order to avoid bad habits from her team members. She needs to tell them that although she trusts them completely and is not trying to micromanage them, there are tasks that need to be done and she is responsible for seeing that everyone is sharing the workload. In order to be an efficient team, there needs to be control of the workload and as the team supervisor, this is her job.

Joana Valencia
Senior Project Manager

Source: Joana Valencia

circumstances, it's important for a manager to know what the organization's policies are on discipline. Is there a process for dealing with unsatisfactory job performance? Do warnings need to be given when performance is inadequate? What happens if, after the warnings, performance or the troublesome behavior doesn't improve? Disciplinary actions are never easy or pleasant; however, discipline can be used to both control and correct employee performance, and managers must know how to discipline. (See the end-of-chapter Skill Application on Disciplining Employees Effectively for more suggestions.)

TOOLS for Measuring Organizational Performance

LO4 • Missoni-loving fashionistas scrambling to buy the high-end Italian designer's clothes at Target crashed the company's Web site. Target executives admitted being unprepared for online shoppers' demand for the items.
• When someone typed the word "bailout" into a Domino's promo code window and found it was good for a free medium pizza, the news spread like wildfire across the Web. Domino's ended up having to give away thousands of free pizzas.
• A simple mistyped Web address by a Google employee caused all search results worldwide during a 55-minute period to warn, "This site may be harmful to your computer," even though it wasn't.[22]

What kinds of tools could managers at these companies have used for monitoring and measuring performance?

All managers need appropriate tools for monitoring and measuring organizational performance. Before describing some specific types of control tools, let's look at the concept of feedforward, concurrent, and feedback control.

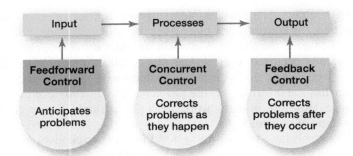

Exhibit 9
Types of Control

Feedforward/Concurrent/Feedback Controls

Managers can implement controls *before* an activity begins, *during* the time the activity is going on, and *after* the activity has been completed. The first type is called feedforward control; the second, concurrent control; and the last, feedback control (see Exhibit 9).

FEEDFORWARD CONTROL The most desirable type of control—**feedforward control**—prevents problems because it takes place before the actual activity.[23] For instance, hospital emergency rooms are looking to prevent mistakes such as an 18-year-old with fever and chills being sent home from the emergency room with Tylenol and later dying of sepsis, a blood infection; or a 42-year-old woman with chest pains being discharged, only to suffer a heart attack two hours later. Medical experts know that a serious ailment can look a lot like something else in the hubbub and chaos of the ER. So that's why many are setting protocols and oversights in place to prevent these kinds of mistakes.[24] When McDonald's opened its first restaurant in Moscow, it sent company quality control experts to help Russian farmers learn techniques for growing high-quality potatoes and to help bakers learn processes for baking high-quality breads. Why? McDonald's demands consistent product quality no matter the geographical location. They want a cheeseburger in Moscow to taste like one in Omaha. Still another example of feedforward control is the scheduled preventive maintenance programs on aircraft done by the major airlines. These programs are designed to detect and hopefully to prevent structural damage that might lead to an accident.

The key to feedforward controls is taking managerial action *before* a problem occurs. That way, problems can be prevented rather than having to correct them after any damage (poor-quality products, lost customers, lost revenue, etc.) has already been done. However, these controls require timely and accurate information that isn't always easy to get. Thus, managers frequently end up using the other two types of control.

CONCURRENT CONTROL **Concurrent control**, as its name implies, takes place while a work activity is in progress. For instance, Nicholas Fox is director of business product management at Google. He and his team keep a watchful eye on one of Google's most profitable businesses—online ads. They watch "the number of searches and clicks, the rate at which users click on ads, the revenue this generates—everything is tracked hour by hour, compared with the data from a week earlier and charted."[25] If they see something that's not working particularly well, they fine-tune it.

The best-known form of concurrent control is direct supervision. Another term for it is **management by walking around**, which is when a manager is in the work area interacting directly with employees. For example, Nvidia's CEO, Jen-Hsun Huang, tore down his cubicle and replaced it with a conference table so he's available to employees at all times to discuss what's going on.[26] Even GE's CEO, Jeff Immelt, spends a large portion of his workweek on the road talking to employees and visiting the company's numerous locations.[27] All managers can benefit from using concurrent control, but especially first-line managers, because they can correct problems before they become too costly.

feedforward control
Control that takes place before a work activity is done

concurrent control
Control that takes place while a work activity is in progress

management by walking around
A term used to describe when a manager is out in the work area interacting directly with employees

503

feedback control
Control that takes place after a work activity is done

FEEDBACK CONTROL   The most popular type of control relies on feedback. In **feedback control**, the control takes place *after* the activity is done. For instance, the Denver Mint discovered the flawed Wisconsin quarters using feedback control. The damage had already occurred, even though the organization corrected the problem once it was discovered. And that's the major problem with this type of control. By the time a manager has the information, the problems have already occurred, leading to waste or damage. However, in many work areas (for example, financial), feedback is the only viable type of control.

Feedback controls have two advantages.[28] First, feedback gives managers meaningful information on how effective their planning efforts were. Feedback that shows little variance between standard and actual performance indicates that the planning was generally on target. If the deviation is significant, a manager can use that information to formulate new plans. Second, feedback can enhance motivation. People want to know how well they're doing and feedback provides that information. Now, let's look at some specific control tools that managers can use.

Financial Controls

Every business wants to earn a profit. To achieve this goal, managers need financial controls. For instance, they might analyze quarterly income statements for excessive expenses. They might also calculate financial ratios to ensure that sufficient cash is available to pay ongoing expenses, that debt levels haven't become too high, or that assets are used productively.

Managers might use traditional financial measures such as ratio analysis and budget analysis. Exhibit 10 summarizes some of the most popular financial ratios. Liquidity ratios measure an organization's ability to meet its current debt obligations. Leverage ratios examine the organization's use of debt to finance its assets and whether it's able to meet the interest payments on the debt. Activity ratios assess how efficiently a company uses its assets. Finally, profitability ratios measure how efficiently and effectively the company uses its assets to generate profits. These ratios are calculated using selected information from the organization's two primary financial statements (the balance sheet and the income statement), which are then expressed as

let's get REAL

The Scenario:

Lily Wong manages a product testing lab. Although her team works normal hours (8 to 5), there are times when the product testers need to work after hours or even on the weekend. She doesn't have a supervisor there when these associates are working but is wondering whether she needs to.

What would you suggest to Lily?

Lily needs to start training a few of her key associates to become lead associates. When the supervisor or manager is not around, the lead associate can oversee the project. By doing this, she can have a group of associates work on the weekend with the lead to get more of the projects done. You always need a supervisor around. While the associates are working, the lead will keep them focused and will keep the project going.

Alfonso Marrese
Retail Executive

Source: Alfonso Marrese

Objective	Ratio	Calculation	Meaning
Liquidity	Current ratio	$\dfrac{\text{Current assets}}{\text{Current liabilities}}$	Tests the organization's ability to meet short-term obligations
	Acid test	$\dfrac{\text{Current assets less inventories}}{\text{Current liabilities}}$	Tests liquidity more accurately when inventories turn over slowly or are difficult to sell
Leverage	Debt to assets	$\dfrac{\text{Total debt}}{\text{Total assets}}$	The higher the ratio, the more leveraged the organization
	Times interest earned	$\dfrac{\text{Profits before interest and taxes}}{\text{Total interest charges}}$	Measures how many times the organization is able to meet its interest expenses
Activity	Inventory turnover	$\dfrac{\text{Sales}}{\text{Inventory}}$	The higher the ratio, the more efficiently inventory assets are used
	Total asset turnover	$\dfrac{\text{Sales}}{\text{Total assets}}$	The fewer assets used to achieve a given level of sales, the more efficiently management uses the organization's total assets
Profitability	Profit margin on sales	$\dfrac{\text{Net profit after taxes}}{\text{Total sales}}$	Identifies the profits that are generated
	Return on investment	$\dfrac{\text{Net profit after taxes}}{\text{Total assets}}$	Measures the efficiency of assets to generate profits

Exhibit 10
Popular Financial Ratios

a percentage or ratio. Because you've probably studied these ratios in other accounting or finance courses, or will in the near future, we aren't going to elaborate on how they're calculated. We mention them here to remind you that managers use such ratios as internal control tools.

Budgets are planning and control tools. When a budget is formulated, it's a planning tool, because it indicates which work activities are important and what and how much resources should be allocated to those activities. But budgets are also used for controlling, because they provide managers with quantitative standards against which to measure and compare resource consumption. If deviations are significant enough to require action, the manager examines what has happened and tries to uncover why. With this information, necessary action can be taken. For example, if you use a personal budget for monitoring and controlling your monthly expenses, you might find that one month your miscellaneous expenses were higher than you had budgeted for. At that point, you might cut back spending in another area or work extra hours to get more income.

Information Controls

During the most critical—and worst possible—time period for retailers, Target Corporation found that cybercriminals caused an enormous data breach in late 2013. Six months after the attack, Target executives were still trying to fix the mess. Cyberattackers from China targeted Google and 34 other companies in an attempt to steal information. A large criminal theft of credit card data—account information belonging to millions of people—happened to Heartland Payment Systems, a

payments processor. American Express found its Web site under attack, one of several and powerful attacks on American financial institutions. An ex-worker at Goldman Sachs stole "black box" computer programs that Goldman uses to make lucrative, rapid-fire trades in the financial markets. Even the U.S. government is getting serious about controlling information. Financial-market sensitive data (think Consumer Price Index, housing starts, inflation numbers, gas prices, corn yields, etc.) will be guarded as a precaution against anyone who might want to take advantage of an accidental or covert leak to get an insider's edge in the financial markets.[29] Talk about the need for information controls! Managers deal with information controls in two ways: (1) as a tool to help them control other organizational activities and (2) as an organizational area they need to control.

HOW IS INFORMATION USED IN CONTROLLING?   Managers need the right information at the right time and in the right amount to monitor and measure organizational activities and performance.

In measuring actual performance, managers need information about what is happening within their area of responsibility and about the standards in order to be able to compare actual performance with the standards. They also rely on information to help them determine if deviations are acceptable. Finally, they rely on information to help them develop appropriate courses of action. Information *is* important! Most of the information tools managers use come from the organization's management information system.

management information system (MIS)
A system used to provide management with needed information on a regular basis

A **management information system (MIS)** is a system used to provide managers with needed information on a regular basis. In theory, this system can be manual or computer-based, although most organizations have moved to computer-supported applications. The term *system* in MIS implies order, arrangement, and purpose. Further, an MIS focuses specifically on providing managers with *information* (processed and analyzed data), not merely *data* (raw, unanalyzed facts). A library provides a good analogy. Although it can contain millions of volumes, a library doesn't do you any good if you can't find what you want quickly. That's why librarians spend a great deal of time cataloging a library's collections and ensuring that materials are returned to their proper locations. Organizations today are like well-stocked libraries. The issue is not a lack of data; instead, the issue is whether an organization has the ability to process that data so that the right information is available to the right person when he or she needs it. An MIS collects data and turns them into relevant information for managers to use.

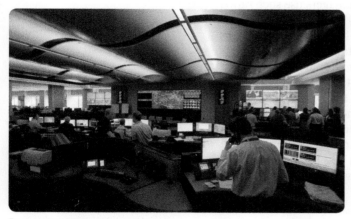

The goal of United Airlines Network Operations Center is to get the right information to the right people at the right time so managers can make decisions that provide safe and efficient travel. In monitoring and measuring the airline's real-time activities and performance, employees plan flights, forecast weather, route aircraft, coordinate with air traffic controllers, and monitor geopolitical conditions.
Source: Kiichiro Sato/Associated Press

CONTROLLING INFORMATION   Using pictures of a cute kitty attached to e-mails or as a link, companies are using "ethical hackers" to demonstrate how easily employees can put company data at risk by clicking on them.[30] Although these cute kitties are simulated attacks, it seems that every week, there's another news story about actual information security breaches. A survey shows that 60 percent of companies had a network security breach in the past year.[31] Because information is critically important to everything an organization does, managers must have comprehensive and secure controls in place to protect that information. Such controls can range from data encryption to system firewalls to data back-ups, and other techniques as well.[32] Problems can lurk in places that an organization might not even have considered, like blogs, search engines, and Twitter accounts. Sensitive, defamatory, confidential, or embarrassing organizational information has found its way into search engine results. For instance, detailed monthly expenses and employee salaries on the National Speleological Society's Web site turned up in a Google search.[33] Equipment such as tablet and laptop computers, smartphones, and even RFID (radio-frequency identification)

tags are vulnerable to viruses and hacking. Needless to say, information controls should be monitored regularly to ensure that all possible precautions are in place to protect important information.

Balanced Scorecard

The **balanced scorecard** approach is a way to evaluate organizational performance from more than just the financial perspective.[35] A balanced scorecard typically looks at four areas that contribute to a company's performance: financial, customer, internal processes, and people/innovation/growth assets. According to this approach, managers should develop goals in each of the four areas and then measure whether the goals are being met.

Although a balanced scorecard makes sense, managers will tend to focus on areas that drive their organization's success and use scorecards that reflect those strategies.[36] For example, if strategies are customer-centered, then the customer area is likely to get more attention than the other three areas. Yet, you can't focus on measuring only one performance area because others are affected as well. For instance, at IBM Global Services in Houston, managers developed a scorecard around an overriding strategy of customer satisfaction. However, the other areas (financial, internal processes, and people/innovation/growth) support that central strategy. The division manager described it as follows, "The internal processes part of our business is directly related to responding to our customers in a timely manner, and the learning and innovation aspect is critical for us since what we're selling our customers above all is our expertise. Of course, how successful we are with those things will affect our financial component."[37]

Benchmarking of Best Practices

The Cleveland Clinic is world renowned for delivering high-quality health care, with a top-ranked heart program that attracts patients from around the world. But what you may not realize is that it's also a model of cost-effective health care.[38] It could serve as a model for other health care organizations looking to be more effective and efficient.

Managers in such diverse industries as health care, education, and financial services are discovering what manufacturers have long recognized—the benefits of **benchmarking**, which is the search for the best practices among competitors or noncompetitors that lead to their superior performance. Benchmarking should identify various **benchmarks**, the standards of excellence against which to measure and compare. For instance, the American Medical Association developed more than 100 standard measures of performance to improve medical care. Carlos Ghosn, CEO of Nissan, benchmarked Walmart operations in purchasing, transportation, and logistics.[39] Target Corporation benchmarked Amazon by mimicking its online offerings including recurring diaper delivery, free shipping, and member discounts.[40] At its most basic, benchmarking means learning from others. As a tool for monitoring and measuring organizational performance, benchmarking can be used to identify specific performance gaps and potential areas of improvement. But best practices aren't just found externally.

Sometimes those best practices can be found inside the organization and just need to be shared. One fertile area for finding good performance improvement ideas is an

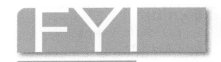
balanced scorecard
A performance measurement tool that looks at more than just the financial perspective

benchmarking
The search for the best practices among competitors or noncompetitors that lead to their superior performance

benchmark
The standard of excellence against which to measure and compare

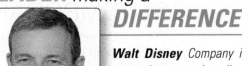

LEADER making a
DIFFERENCE

Source: Stewart Cook/ Associated Press

Walt Disney *Company is one of the world's largest entertainment and media companies and has had a long record of success.[41] When Bob Iger was named CEO in 2005, analysts believed that the Disney brand had become outdated. The perception was that there were too many Disney products in the marketplace lacking the quality people expected. Iger decided to address that perception with what he called the Disney Difference. What is the Disney Difference? It's taking the content created company-wide and spreading it out over many different markets and in many different forms. The company's new, obsessive focus on product quality led it to a number-seven ranking in* Fortune's *Most Admired list for 2014. What can you learn from this leader making a difference?*

Exhibit 11
Suggestions for Internal Benchmarking

1. *Connect best practices to strategies and goals.* The organization's strategies and goals should dictate what types of best practices might be most valuable to others in the organization.

2. *Identify best practices throughout the organization.* Organizations must have a way to find out what practices have been successful in different work areas and units.

3. *Develop best practices reward and recognition systems.* Individuals must be given an incentive to share their knowledge. The reward system should be built into the organization's culture.

4. *Communicate best practices throughout the organization.* Once best practices have been identified, that information needs to be shared with others in the organization.

5. *Create a best practices knowledge-sharing system.* There needs to be a formal mechanism for organizational members to continue sharing their ideas and best practices.

6. *Nurture best practices on an ongoing basis.* Create an organizational culture that reinforces a "we can learn from everyone" attitude and emphasizes sharing information.

Source: Based on "Extracting Diamonds in the Rough," by Tad Leahy, from *Business Finance*, August 2000.

employee suggestion box. Research shows that best practices frequently already exist within an organization but usually go unidentified and unnoticed.[42] In today's environment, organizations seeking high performance levels can't afford to ignore such potentially valuable information. For example, Ameren Corporation's power plant managers used internal benchmarking to help identify performance gaps and opportunities.[43] Exhibit 11 provides some suggestions for internal benchmarking.

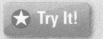 **Try It!**

If your professor has assigned this, go to **www.mymanagementlab.com** to complete the Simulation: Controlling and get a better understanding of the challenges of monitoring and controlling in organizations.

CONTEMPORARY Issues in Control

L05 The employees of Integrated Information Systems Inc. didn't think twice about exchanging digital music over a dedicated office server they had set up. Like office betting on college and pro sports, it was technically illegal, but harmless, or so they thought. But after the company had to pay a $1 million settlement to the Recording Industry Association of America, managers wished they had controlled the situation better.[44] Control is an important managerial function. We're going to look at four control issues that managers face today: cross-cultural differences, workplace concerns, customer interactions, and corporate governance.

Adjusting Controls for Cross-Cultural Differences and Global Turmoil

The concepts of control that we've been discussing are appropriate for an organization whose work units are not geographically separated or culturally distinct. But control techniques can be quite different for different countries. The differences are primarily in the measurement and corrective action steps of the control process. In a global corporation, managers of foreign operations tend to be less controlled by the

home office, if for no other reason than the distance keeping managers from being able to observe work directly. Because distance creates a tendency to formalize controls, such organizations often rely on extensive formal reports for control, most of which are communicated electronically.

Technology's impact on control is also seen when comparing technologically advanced nations with less technologically advanced countries. Managers in countries where technology is more advanced often use indirect control devices such as computer-generated reports and analyses in addition to standardized rules and direct supervision to ensure that work activities are going as planned. In less technologically advanced countries, however, managers tend to use more direct supervision and highly centralized decision making for control.

Managers in foreign countries also need to be aware of constraints on investigating complaints and corrective actions they can take. Some countries' laws prohibit closing facilities, laying off employees, taking money out of the country, or bringing in a new management team from outside the country.

Another challenge for global managers in collecting data for measurement and comparison is comparability. For instance, a company that manufactures apparel in Cambodia might produce the same products at a facility in Scotland. However, the Cambodian facility might be more labor intensive than its Scottish counterpart to take advantage of lower labor costs in Cambodia. This difference makes it hard to compare, for instance, labor costs per unit.

Finally, global organizations need to have controls in place for protecting their workers and other assets during times of global turmoil and disasters. For instance, when the earthquake/tsunami hit Japan in March 2011, companies scrambled to activate their disaster management plans. In the volatile Middle East, many companies have had to evacuate workers during times of crisis. The best time to be prepared is before an emergency occurs, and many organizations are doing just that, so that if a crisis occurs, employees and other organizational assets are protected as best as possible.

Workplace Concerns

The month-long World Cup games are a big drain on global productivity. A survey by the Chartered Management Institute says that in the United Kingdom, productivity losses could total just under 1 billion pounds ($1.45 billion). In the United States, March Madness also leads to a drop in productivity—estimated at $1.8 billion during the first week of the tournament—as employees fill out their brackets and survey the message boards and blogs.[45]

Today's workplaces present considerable control challenges for managers. From monitoring employees' computer usage at work to protecting the workplace against disgruntled employees intent on doing harm, managers need controls to ensure that work can be done efficiently and effectively, as planned.

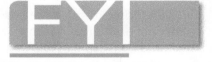

• 31 percent of employees say they shop online while at work.[46]

WORKPLACE PRIVACY If you work, do you think you have a right to privacy at your job? What can your employer find out about you and your work? You might be surprised at the answers! Employers can (and do), among other things, read your e-mail (even those marked "personal" or "confidential"), tap your telephone, monitor your work by computer, store and review computer files, monitor you in an employee bathroom or dressing room, and track your whereabouts in a company vehicle. And these actions aren't that uncommon. In fact, some 26 percent of companies have fired an employee for e-mail misuse; 26 percent have fired workers for misusing the Internet; 6 percent have fired employees for inappropriate cell phone use; 4 percent have fired someone for instant messaging misuse; and 3 percent have fired someone for inappropriate text messaging.[47]

Why do managers feel they need to monitor what employees are doing? A big reason is that employees are hired to work, not to surf the Web checking stock prices, watching online videos, playing fantasy baseball, or shopping for presents for family or

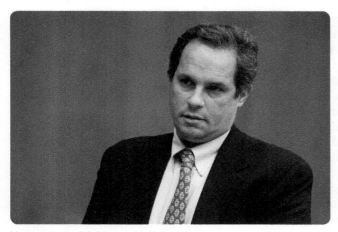

Most organizational theft is committed by employees such as Thomas Rica, former Ridgewood, New Jersey, public works inspector who pleaded guilty to stealing $460,000 in quarters from the village's parking meter collection room over two years and depositing it in his personal bank account. To deter future theft, village officials adopted tighter internal security controls.
Source: Mitsu Yasukawa/Associated Press

friends. Recreational on-the-job Web surfing is thought to cost billions of dollars in lost work productivity annually. In fact, a survey of U.S. employers said that 87 percent of employees look at non-work-related Web sites while at work and more than half engage in personal Web site surfing every day.[48] Watching online videos has become an increasingly serious problem not only because of the time being wasted by employees but also because it clogs already-strained corporate computer networks.[49] All this nonwork adds up to significant costs to businesses.

Another reason why managers monitor employee e-mail and computer usage is that they don't want to risk being sued for creating a hostile workplace environment because of offensive messages or an inappropriate image displayed on a coworker's computer screen. Concerns about racial or sexual harassment are one reason companies might want to monitor or keep back-up copies of all e-mail. Electronic records can help establish what actually happened so managers can react quickly.[50]

Finally, managers want to ensure that company secrets aren't being leaked.[51] In addition to typical e-mail and computer usage, companies are monitoring instant messaging and banning camera phones in the office. Managers need to be certain that employees are not, even inadvertently, passing information on to others who could use that information to harm the company.

Because of the potentially serious costs and given the fact that many jobs now entail computers, many companies have workplace monitoring policies. Such policies should control employee behavior in a nondemeaning way, and employees should be informed about those policies.[52]

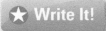 **Write It!**

If your professor has assigned this, go to **www.mymanagementlab.com** to complete the Writing Assignment MGMT 3: Technology

FUTURE VISION | Wearable Technology: Eyes (and Ears) Checking Up on You

Yes, technological advances make the process of managing an organization much easier, but they also provide employers a means of sophisticated employee monitoring.[53] For instance, employees may be asked to wear sensors that measure when and how they're the most productive. Other companies are using biometric technology (such as a facial recognition device) to keep track of when an employee checks in and leaves work. Most of this monitoring is designed to enhance worker productivity, but it could be, and has been, a source of concern over worker privacy. As wearable technology becomes more commonplace, these advantages bring with them difficult questions regarding what managers have the right to know about employees and how far they can go in controlling employee behavior.

Although such monitoring and controlling may appear unjust or unfair, nothing in our legal system prevents employers from engaging in these practices. Rather, the law is based on the premise that if employees don't like the rules, they have the option of quitting. Managers, too, typically defend their actions in terms of ensuring quality, productivity, and proper employee behavior.

If your professor has chosen to assign this, go to **www.mymanagementlab.com** *to discuss the following questions.*

⭐ **TALK ABOUT IT 1:** When does management's need for information about employee performance cross over the line and interfere with a worker's right to privacy?

⭐ **TALK ABOUT IT 2:** Is any action by management acceptable as long as employees are notified ahead of time that they will be monitored? Discuss.

EMPLOYEE THEFT At the Saks flagship store in Manhattan, a 23-year-old sales clerk was caught ringing up $130,000 in false merchandise returns and putting the money onto a gift card.[54] And such practices have occurred at other retailers as well.

Would you be surprised to find that up to 85 percent of all organizational theft and fraud is committed by employees, not outsiders?[55] And it's a costly problem—estimated to be around $4,500 per worker per year.[56]

Employee theft is defined as any unauthorized taking of company property by employees for their personal use.[57] It can range from embezzlement to fraudulent filing of expense reports to removing equipment, parts, software, or office supplies from company premises. Although retail businesses have long faced serious potential losses from employee theft, loose financial controls at start-ups and small companies and the ready availability of information technology have made employee stealing an escalating problem in all kinds and sizes of organizations. Managers need to educate themselves about this control issue and be prepared to deal with it.[58]

Why do employees steal? The answer depends on whom you ask.[59] Experts in various fields—industrial security, criminology, clinical psychology—have different perspectives. The industrial security people propose that people steal because the opportunity presents itself through lax controls and favorable circumstances. Criminologists say it's because people have financial-based pressures (such as personal financial problems) or vice-based pressures (such as gambling debts). And the clinical psychologists suggest that people steal because they can rationalize whatever they're doing as being correct and appropriate behavior ("everyone does it," "they had it coming," "this company makes enough money and they'll never miss anything this small," "I deserve this for all that I put up with," and so forth).[60] Although each approach provides compelling insights into employee theft and has been instrumental in attempts to deter it, unfortunately, employees continue to steal. What can managers do?

The concept of feedforward, concurrent, and feedback control is useful for identifying measures to deter or reduce employee theft.[61] Exhibit 12 summarizes several possible managerial actions.

employee theft
Any unauthorized taking of company property by employees for their personal use

FEEDFORWARD	CONCURRENT	FEEDBACK
Use careful prehiring screening.	Treat employees with respect and dignity.	Make sure employees know when theft or fraud has occurred—not naming names but letting people know this is not acceptable.
Establish specific policies defining theft and fraud and discipline procedures.	Openly communicate the costs of stealing.	Use the services of professional investigators.
Involve employees in writing policies.	Let employees know on a regular basis about their successes in preventing theft and fraud.	Redesign control measures.
Educate and train employees about the policies.	Use video surveillance equipment if conditions warrant.	Evaluate your organization's culture and the relationships of managers and employees.
Have a professional review of your internal security controls.	Install "lock-out" options on computers, telephones, and e-mail. Use corporate hotlines for reporting incidences. Set a good example.	

Exhibit 12
Controlling Employee Theft

Sources: Based on A. H. Bell and D. M. Smith, "Protecting the Company Against Theft and Fraud," *Workforce Management Online,* December 3, 2000; J. D. Hansen, "To Catch a Thief," *Journal of Accountancy,* March 2000, pp. 43–46; and J. Greenberg, "The Cognitive Geometry of Employee Theft," in S. B. Bacharach, A. O'Leary-Kelly, J. M. Collins, and R. W. Griffin (eds.), *Dysfunctional Behavior in Organizations: Nonviolent and Deviant Behavior* (Stamford, CT: JAI Press, 1998), pp. 147–193.

Workplace Violence

In April 2014, an individual who worked as a baggage handler opened fire at a FedEx facility near Atlanta injuring six employees. In August 2010, a driver about to lose his job at Hartford Distributors in Hartford, Connecticut, opened fire killing eight other employees and himself. In July 2010, a former employee at a solar products manufacturer in Albuquerque, New Mexico, walked into the business and opened fire killing two people and wounding four others. On November 6, 2009, in Orlando, Florida, an engineer who had been dismissed from his job for poor performance returned and shot and killed one person while wounding five others. This incident happened only one day after an army psychiatrist went on a shooting rampage at Fort Hood army post killing 13 and wounding 27.[62] These are just a few of the deadly workplace attacks in recent years. Is workplace violence really an issue for managers? Yes. Despite these examples, thankfully the number of workplace shootings has decreased.[63] However, the U.S. National Institute of Occupational Safety and Health still says that each year, some 2 million American workers are victims of some form of workplace violence. In an average week, one employee is killed and at least 25 are seriously injured in violent assaults by current or former coworkers. And according to a Department of Labor survey, 58 percent of firms reported that managers received verbal threats from workers.[64] Anger, rage, and violence in the workplace are intimidating to coworkers and adversely affect their productivity. The annual cost to U.S. businesses is estimated to be between $20 billion and $35 billion.[65] And office rage isn't a uniquely American problem. A survey of aggressive behavior in Britain's workplaces found that 18 percent of managers say they have personally experienced harassment or verbal bullying, and 9 percent claim to have experienced physical attacks.[66]

What factors are believed to contribute to workplace violence? Undoubtedly, employee stress caused by an uncertain economic environment, job uncertainties, declining value of retirement accounts, long hours, information overload, other daily interruptions, unrealistic deadlines, and uncaring managers play a role. Even office layout designs with small cubicles where employees work amid the noise and commotion from those around them have been cited as contributing to the problem.[67] Other experts have described dangerously dysfunctional work environments characterized by the following as primary contributors to the problem:[68]

- Employee work driven by TNC (time, numbers, and crises).
- Rapid and unpredictable change where instability and uncertainty plague employees.
- Destructive communication style where managers communicate in an excessively aggressive, condescending, explosive, or passive-aggressive style; excessive workplace teasing or scapegoating.
- Authoritarian leadership with a rigid, militaristic mindset of managers versus employees; employees aren't allowed to challenge ideas, participate in decision making, or engage in team-building efforts.
- Defensive attitude where little or no performance feedback is given; only numbers count; and yelling, intimidation, or avoidance is the preferred way of handling conflict.
- Double standards in terms of policies, procedures, and training opportunities for managers and employees.
- Unresolved grievances because the organization provides no mechanisms or only adversarial ones for resolving them; dysfunctional individuals may be protected or ignored because of long-standing rules, union contract provisions, or reluctance to take care of problems.
- Emotionally troubled employees and no attempt by managers to get help for these people.
- Repetitive, boring work with no chance for doing something else or for new people coming in.

- Faulty or unsafe equipment or deficient training, which keeps employees from being able to work efficiently or effectively.
- Hazardous work environment in terms of temperature, air quality, repetitive motions, overcrowded spaces, noise levels, excessive overtime, and so forth. To minimize costs, no additional employees are hired when workload becomes excessive, leading to potentially dangerous work expectations and conditions.
- Culture of violence that has a history of individual violence or abuse; violent or explosive role models; or tolerance of on-the-job alcohol or drug abuse.

Reading through this list, you surely hope that workplaces where you'll spend your professional life won't be like this. However, the competitive demands of succeeding in a 24/7 global economy put pressure on organizations and employees in many ways.

What can managers do to deter or reduce possible workplace violence? Once again, the concept of feedforward, concurrent, and feedback control can help identify actions that managers can take.[69] Exhibit 13 summarizes several suggestions.

Controlling Customer Interactions

Every month, every local branch of Enterprise Rent-a-Car conducts telephone surveys with customers.[70] Each branch earns a ranking based on the percentage of its customers who say they were "completely satisfied" with their last Enterprise experience—a level of satisfaction referred to as "top box." Top box performance is important to Enterprise because completely satisfied customers are far more likely

Feedforward	Concurrent	Feedback
Use MBWA (managing by walking around) to identify potential problems; observe how employees treat and interact with each other.	Ensure management commitment to functional, not dysfunctional, work environments.	Communicate openly about incidences and what's being done.
Provide employee assistance programs (EAPs) to help employees with behavioral problems.	Allow employees or work groups to "grieve" during periods of major organizational change.	Investigate incidents and take appropriate action.
Enforce organizational policy that any workplace rage, aggression, or violence will not be tolerated.	Be a good role model in how you treat others.	Review company policies and change, if necessary.
Use careful prehiring screening.	Use corporate hotlines or some other mechanism for reporting and investigating incidents.	
Never ignore threats.	Use quick and decisive intervention.	
Train employees about how to avoid danger if situation arises.	Get expert professional assistance if violence erupts.	
Clearly communicate policies to employees.	Provide necessary equipment or procedures for dealing with violent situations (cell phones, alarm system, code names or phrases, and so forth).	

Exhibit 13
Controlling Workplace Violence

Sources: Based on M. Gorkin, "Five Strategies and Structures for Reducing Workplace Violence," *Workforce Management Online,* December 3, 2000; "Investigating Workplace Violence: Where Do You Start? *Workforce Management Online,* December 3, 2000; "Ten Tips on Recognizing and Minimizing Violence," *Workforce Management Online,* December 3, 2000; and "Points to Cover in a Workplace Violence Policy," *Workforce Management Online,* December 3, 2000.

to be repeat customers. By using this service quality index measure, employees' careers and financial aspirations are linked with the organizational goal of providing consistently superior service to each and every customer. Managers at Enterprise Rent-a-Car understand the connection between employees and customers and the importance of controlling these customer interactions.

There's probably no better area to see the link between planning and controlling than in customer service. If a company proclaims customer service as one of its goals, it quickly and clearly becomes apparent whether that goal is being achieved by seeing how satisfied customers are with their service! How can managers control the interactions between the goal and the outcome when it comes to customers? The concept of a service profit chain can help.[71]

service profit chain
The service sequence from employees to customers to profit

A **service profit chain** is the service sequence from employees to customers to profit. According to this concept, the company's strategy and service delivery system influence how employees deal with customers; that is, how productive they are in providing service and the quality of that service. The level of employee service productivity and service quality influences customer perceptions of service value. When service value is high, it has a positive impact on customer satisfaction, which leads to customer loyalty. And customer loyalty improves organizational revenue growth and profitability.

What does this concept mean for managers? Managers who want to control customer interactions should work to create long-term and mutually beneficial relationships among the company, employees, and customers. How? By creating a work environment that enables employees to deliver high levels of quality service and which makes them feel they're capable of delivering top-quality service. In such a service climate, employees are motivated to deliver superior service. Employee efforts to satisfy customers, coupled with the service value provided by the organization, improve customer satisfaction. And when customers receive high service value, they're loyal and return, which ultimately improves the company's growth and profitability.

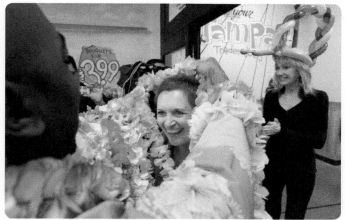

To celebrate a new store opening in Florida, a Trader Joe's employee welcomes customers with leis. Courteous, cheerful, well-informed, and helpful employees make Trader Joe's a place where people love to shop. Employees are important to Trader Joe's service profit chain as they provide high-quality service that leads to high customer satisfaction and loyalty and results in revenue growth and profitability.
Source: © Daniel Wallace/Tampa Bay Times/ ZUMAPRESS.com/Alamy Live News

There's no better example of this concept in action than Southwest Airlines, which is the most consistently profitable U.S. airline (the year 2013 marked 41 straight years of profitability). Its customers are fiercely loyal because the company's operating strategy (hiring, training, rewards and recognition, teamwork, and so forth) is built around customer service. Employees consistently deliver outstanding service value to customers. And Southwest's customers reward the company by coming back. It's through efficiently and effectively controlling these customer interactions that companies like Southwest and Enterprise have succeeded.

★ **Watch It 2!**   If your professor has assigned this, go to **www.mymanagementlab.com** to watch a video titled: *Zane's Cycles: Foundations of Control* and to respond to questions.

Corporate Governance

Although Andrew Fastow—Enron's former chief financial officer who pled guilty to wire and securities fraud—had an engaging and persuasive personality, that still didn't explain why Enron's board of directors failed to raise even minimal concerns about management's questionable accounting practices. The board even allowed Fastow to set up off-balance-sheet partnerships for his own profit at the expense of Enron's shareholders.

Corporate governance, the system used to govern a corporation so that the interests of corporate owners are protected, failed abysmally at Enron, as it has at many companies caught in financial scandals. In the aftermath of these scandals, corporate governance has been reformed. Two areas where reform has taken place are the role of boards of directors and financial reporting. Such reforms aren't limited to U.S. corporations; corporate governance problems are global.[72] Some 75 percent of senior executives at U.S. and Western European corporations expect their boards of directors to take a more active role.[73]

corporate governance
The system used to govern a corporation so that the interests of corporate owners are protected

THE ROLE OF BOARDS OF DIRECTORS The original purpose of a board of directors was to have a group, independent from management, looking out for the interests of shareholders who were not involved in the day-to-day management of the organization. However, it didn't always work that way. Board members often enjoyed a cozy relationship with managers in which each took care of the other.

This type of "quid pro quo" arrangement has changed. The Sarbanes-Oxley Act puts greater demands on board members of publicly traded companies in the United States to do what they were empowered and expected to do.[74] To help boards do this better, the Business Roundtable developed a document outlining principles of corporate governance. (See [http://businessroundtable.org/sites/default/files/BRT_Principles_of_Corporate_Governance_-2012_Formatted_Final.pdf] for a list and discussion of these principles.)

FINANCIAL REPORTING AND THE AUDIT COMMITTEE In addition to expanding the role of boards of directors, the Sarbanes-Oxley Act also called for more disclosure and transparency of corporate financial information. In fact, senior managers in the United States are now required to certify their companies' financial results. Such changes have led to better information—that is, information that is more accurate and reflective of a company's financial condition.

PREPARING FOR: Exams/Quizzes

CHAPTER SUMMARY by Learning Objectives

LO1 EXPLAIN the nature and importance of control.

Controlling is the process of monitoring, comparing, and correcting work performance. As the final step in the management process, controlling provides the link back to planning. If managers didn't control, they'd have no way of knowing whether goals were being met.

Control is important because (1) it's the only way to know if goals are being met, and if not, why; (2) it provides information and feedback so managers feel comfortable empowering employees; and (3) it helps protect an organization and its assets.

LO2 DESCRIBE the three steps in the control process.

The three steps in the control process are measuring, comparing, and taking action. Measuring involves deciding how to measure actual performance and what to measure. Comparing involves looking at the variation between actual performance and the standard (goal). Deviations outside an acceptable range of variation need attention.

Taking action can involve doing nothing, correcting the actual performance, or revising the standards. Doing nothing is self-explanatory. Correcting the actual performance can involve different corrective actions, which can either be immediate or basic. Standards can be revised by either raising or lowering them.

LO3 EXPLAIN **how organizational and employee performance are measured.**

Organizational performance is the accumulated results of all the organization's work activities. Three frequently used organizational performance measures include (1) productivity, the output of goods or services produced divided by the inputs needed to generate that output; (2) effectiveness, a measure of how appropriate organizational goals are and how well those goals are being met; and (3) industry and company rankings compiled by various business publications.

Employee performance is controlled through effective performance feedback and through disciplinary actions, when needed.

LO4 DESCRIBE **tools used to measure organizational performance.**

Feedforward controls take place before a work activity is done. Concurrent controls take place while a work activity is being done. Feedback controls take place after a work activity is done.

Financial controls that managers can use include financial ratios (liquidity, leverage, activity, and profitability) and budgets. One information control managers can use is an MIS, which provides managers with needed information on a regular basis. Others include comprehensive and secure controls such as data encryption, system firewalls, data back-ups, and so forth that protect the organization's information.

Balanced scorecards provide a way to evaluate an organization's performance in four different areas rather than just from the financial perspective. Benchmarking provides control by finding the best practices among competitors or noncompetitors and from inside the organization itself.

LO5 DISCUSS **contemporary issues in control.**

Adjusting controls for cross-cultural differences may be needed primarily in the areas of measuring and taking corrective actions.

Workplace concerns include workplace privacy, employee theft, and workplace violence. For each of these issues, managers need to have policies in place to control inappropriate actions and ensure that work is getting done efficiently and effectively.

Control is important to customer interactions because employee service productivity and service quality influences customer perceptions of service value. Organizations want long-term and mutually beneficial relationships among their employees and customers.

Corporate governance is the system used to govern a corporation so that the interests of corporate owners are protected.

MyManagementLab

Go to **mymanagementlab.com** to complete the problems marked with this icon ⭐.

⭐ REVIEW AND DISCUSSION QUESTIONS

1. What are the three steps in the control process? Describe in detail.

2. What is organizational performance?

3. Contrast feedforward, concurrent, and feedback controls.

4. Discuss the various types of tools used to monitor and measure organizational performance.

5. What workplace concerns do managers have to deal with? How might those concerns be controlled?

6. Why is control important to customer interactions?

7. The white-water rapids view of change refers to situations in which unpredictable change is normal and expected, and managing it is a continual process. Do you think it's possible to establish and maintain effective standards and controls in this type of environment? Discuss.

8. "Every individual employee in an organization plays a role in controlling work activities." Do you agree with this statement, or do you think control is something that only managers are responsible for? Explain.

MyManagementLab

If your professor has assigned these, go to **mymanagementlab.com** for Auto-graded writing questions as well as the following Assisted-graded writing questions:

9. Why is control important to customer interactions?

10. What are some work activities in which the acceptable range of variation might be higher than average? What about lower than average? (Hint: Think in terms of the output from the work activities, whom it might affect, and how it might affect them.)

PREPARING FOR: My Career

⭐ PERSONAL INVENTORY ASSESSMENTS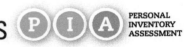

Workplace Discipline Indicator

Disciplining. It's usually not a manager's favorite thing to do. But it is important. Take this PIA and discover how you prefer to discipline employees.

⭐ ETHICS DILEMMA

"The restaurant industry faces a sobering image mess: how to convince consumers it will stop accidentally serving alcohol drinks to toddlers."[75] In separate incidents, a 10-year-old boy was accidently served a drink with rum in it; a toddler was served alcoholic sangria instead of orange juice; and a toddler was served a margarita.

11. Other than the obvious, what problems do you see here, especially as it relates to control?

12. How would you handle this? How could organizations make sure they're addressing work controls ethically?

SKILLS EXERCISE Dealing with Difficult People

About the Skill
Almost all managers will, at one time or another, have to deal with people who are difficult. There is no shortage of characteristics that can make someone difficult to work with. Some examples include people being short-tempered, demanding, abusive, angry, defensive, complaining, intimidating, aggressive, narcissistic, arrogant, and rigid. Successful managers have learned how to cope with difficult people.

Steps in Practicing the Skill
No single approach is always effective in dealing with difficult people.[76] However, we can offer several suggestions that are likely to lessen the angst these people create in your

life and may have some influence in reducing their difficult behavior.

- Don't let your emotions rule. Our first response to a difficult person is often emotional. We get angry. We show frustration. We want to lash out at them or "get even" when we think they've insulted or demeaned us. This response is not likely to reduce your angst and may escalate the other person's negative behavior. So fight your natural tendencies and keep your cool. Stay rational and thoughtful. At worst, while this approach may not improve the situation, it is also unlikely to encourage and escalate the undesirable behavior.

- Attempt to limit contact. If possible, try to limit your contact with the difficult person. Avoid places where they hang out and limit nonrequired interactions. Also, use communication channels—like e-mail and text messaging—that minimize face-to-face contact and verbal intonations.

- Try polite confrontation. If you can't avoid the difficult person, consider standing up to them in a civil but firm manner. Let them know that you're aware of their behavior, that you find it unacceptable, and that you won't tolerate it. For people who are unaware of the effect their actions have on you, confrontation might awaken them to altering their behavior. For those who are acting purposefully, taking a clear stand might make them think twice about the consequences of their actions.

- Practice positive reinforcement. We know that positive reinforcement is a powerful tool for changing behavior. Rather than criticizing undesirable behavior, try reinforcing desirable behaviors with compliments or other positive comments. This focus will tend to weaken and reduce the exhibiting of the undesirable behaviors.

- Recruit fellow victims and witnesses. Finally, we know strength lies in numbers. If you can get others who are also offended by the difficult person to support your case, several positive things can happen. First, it's likely to lessen your frustrations because others will be confirming your perception and can offer support. Second, people in the organization with authority to reprimand are more likely to act when complaints are coming from multiple

sources. And third, the difficult person is more likely to feel pressure to change when a group is speaking out against his or her specific behaviors than if the complaint is coming from a single source.

Based on N. Pelusi, "Dealing with Difficult People," *Psychology Today*, September–October 2006, pp. 68–69; and R. I. Sutton, *The No Asshole Rule: Building a Civilized Workplace and Surviving One That Isn't* (New York: Business Plus, 2007).

Practicing the Skill

Read through the following scenario and discuss how you would handle it:

Your career has progressed even faster than you thought possible. After graduating from college with an accounting degree, you passed your CPA exam and worked three years for a major accounting firm. Then you joined General Electric in their finance department. Two employers and four jobs later, you have just been hired by a Fortune 100 mining company as their vice president for finance. What you didn't expect in the new job was having to deal with Mark Hundley.

Mark is the vice president of company operations. He has been with the company for eight years. Your first impression of Mark was that he was a "know-it-all." He was quick to put you down and acted as if he was your superior rather than an equal. Based on comments you've heard around the offices, it seems you are not alone. Other executives all seemed to agree that Mark is a brilliant engineer and operations manager but very difficult to work with. Specific comments you've heard include "an abrasive attitude"; "talks down to people"; "arrogant"; "thinks everyone is stupid"; and "poor listener."

In your short time in the new job, you've already had several run-ins with Mark. You've even talked to your boss, the company president, about him. The president's response wasn't surprising: "Mark isn't easy to deal with. But no one knows this company's operations like he does. If he ever leaves, I don't know how we'd replace him. But, that said, he gives me a lot of grief. Sometimes he makes me feel like I work for him rather than the other way around." What could you do to improve your ability to work with Mark?

WORKING TOGETHER Team Exercise

Research says that up to 80 percent of U.S. teens have worked for pay at some time during high school.[77] As the number of employed teens has risen, so has the likelihood of their getting hurt on the job. How can organizations keep teen workers safe?

Form small groups of three to four students. Come up with some ideas about things an organization could do to keep its teen workers safe. Put your ideas in a bulleted list format and be prepared to share those ideas with the class.

MY TURN TO BE A MANAGER

- You have a major class project due in a month. Identify some performance measures you could use to help determine whether the project is going as planned and will be completed efficiently (on time) and effectively (with high quality).

- How could you use the concept of control in your personal life? Be specific. (Think in terms of feedforward, concurrent, and feedback controls as well as specific controls for the different aspects of your life—school, work, family relationships, friends, hobbies, etc.)

- Survey 30 people as to whether they have experienced office rage. Ask them specifically whether they have experienced any of the following: yelling or other verbal abuse from a coworker, yelling at coworkers themselves, crying over work-related issues, seeing someone purposely damaging machines or furniture, seeing physical violence in the workplace, or striking a coworker. Compile your findings in a table. Are you surprised at the results? Be prepared to present these in class.

- Pretend you're the manager of a customer call center for timeshare vacations. What types of control measures would you use to see how efficient and effective an employee is? How about measures for evaluating the entire call center?

- Disciplining employees is one of the least favorite tasks of managers, but it is something that all managers have to do. Survey three managers about their experiences with employee discipline. What types of employee actions have caused the need for disciplinary action? What disciplinary actions have they used? What do they think is the most difficult thing to do when disciplining employees? What suggestions do they have for disciplining employees?

- Research "The Great Package Race." Write a paper describing what it is and how it's a good example of organizational control.

- In your own words, write down three things you learned in this text about being a good manager. Keep a copy of this for future reference.

CASE APPLICATION 1 Top Secret

"Prisons are easier to enter than Visa's top-secret Operations Center East (OCE), its biggest, newest and most advanced U.S. data center."[78] And Rick Knight, Visa's head of global operations and engineering, is responsible for its security and functioning. Why all the precautions? Because Visa acknowledges that (1) hackers are increasingly savvy, (2) data is an increasingly desirable black-market commodity, and (3) the best way to keep itself safe is with an information network in a fortress that instantly responds to threats.

Every day, Visa processes some 150 million retail electronic payments from around the globe. (Its current record for processing transactions is 300.7 million on December 23, 2011.) And every day, Visa's system connects up to 2 billion debit and credit cards, millions of acceptance locations, 1.9 million ATMs, and 15,000 financial institutions. So what seems to us a simple swipe of a card or keying in our card numbers on an online transaction actually triggers a robust set of activities including the basic sales transaction processing, risk management, and information-based services. That's why OCE's 130 workers have two jobs: "Keep hackers out and keep the network up, no matter what." And that's why Visa doesn't reveal the location of OCE— on the eastern seaboard is as specific as the description gets.

Beneath the road leading to the OCE, hydraulic posts can rise up fast enough to stop a car going 50 miles per hour. And a car won't be able to go that fast or it will miss a "vicious hairpin turn" and drive off into a drainage pond. Back in medieval

days, that would have been known as the castle moat, which was also designed as protection. There are also hundreds of security cameras and a superb security team of former military personnel. If you're lucky enough to be invited as a guest to OCE (which few people are), you'll have your photo taken and right index fingerprint encoded on a badge. Then you're locked into a "mantrap portal" where you put your badge on a reader that makes sure you are you, and then put it on another reader with your finger on a fingerprint detector. If you make it through, you're clear to enter the network operations center. With a wall of screens in front of them, each employee sits at a desk with four monitors. In a room behind the main center, three security über-experts keep an eye on things. "Knight says about 60 incidents a day warrant attention."

Although hackers are a primary concern, Knight also worries about network capacity. Right now, maximum capacity is currently at 24,000 transactions per second. "At some point, over that 24,000-message limit, 'the network doesn't stop processing one message. It stops processing all of them,' Knight says." So far, on its busiest day, OCE hit 11,613 messages processed. OCE is described as a "Tier-4" center, which is a certification from a data center organization. To achieve that certification, every (and yes, we mean every) mainframe, air conditioner, and battery has a backup.

⭐ DISCUSSION QUESTIONS

13. Is Visa being overly cautious? Why or why not? Why is this level of controls necessary?

14. Which controls would be more important to Visa: feedforward, concurrent, or feedback? Explain.

15. What other managerial controls might be useful to the company?

16. What could other organizations learn from Visa's approach?

CASE APPLICATION 2 Deepwater in Deep Trouble

When all is said and done, it's likely to be one of the worst environmental disasters, if not the worst, in U.S. history.[79] British Petroleum's (BP) Deepwater Horizon offshore rig in the Gulf of Mexico exploded in a ball of flames on April 20, 2010, killing 11 employees. This initial tragedy set in motion frantic efforts to stop the flow of oil, followed by a long and arduous cleanup process. Although the impacts of the explosion and oil spill were felt most intensely by businesses and residents along the coast and by coastal wildlife, those of us inland who watched the disaster unfold were also stunned and dismayed by what we saw happening. What led to this disaster, and what should BP do to minimize the likelihood of it ever happening again?

One thing that has come to light in the disaster investigation is that it's no surprise that something like this happened. After Hurricane Dennis blew through in July 2005, a passing ship was shocked to see BP's new massive $1 billion Thunder Horse oil platform "listing precariously to one side, looking for all the world as if it were about to sink." Thunder Horse "was meant to be the company's crowning glory, the embodiment of its bold gamble to outpace its competitors in finding and exploiting the vast reserves of oil beneath the waters of the gulf." But the problems with this rig soon became evident. A valve installed backwards caused it to flood during the hurricane even before any oil had been pumped. Other problems included a welding job so shoddy that it left underwater pipelines brittle and full of cracks. "The problems

at Thunder Horse were not an anomaly, but a warning that BP was taking too many risks and cutting corners in pursuit of growth and profits."

Then came the tragic explosion on the Deepwater Horizon. Before the rig exploded, there were strong warning signs that something was terribly wrong with the oil well. Among the red flags were several equipment readings suggesting that gas was bubbling into the well, a potential sign of an impending blowout. Those red flags were ignored. Other decisions made in the 24 hours before the explosion included a critical decision to replace heavy mud in the pipe rising from the seabed with seawater, again possibly increasing the risk of an explosion. Internal BP documents also show evidence of serious problems and safety concerns with Deepwater. Those problems involved the well casing and blowout preventer. One BP senior drilling engineer warned, "This would certainly be a worst-case scenario."

The federal panel charged with investigating the spill examined 20 "anomalies in the well's behavior and the crew's response." The panel is also investigating in particular why "rig workers missed telltale signs that the well was close to an uncontrolled blowout." The panel's final report blamed both BP and its contractors for the failures that led to the explosion on the Deepwater Horizon. Many of those failings stemmed from shortcuts to save time and money. However, the report also faulted the government for lax oversight of the companies.

⭐ DISCUSSION QUESTIONS

17. What type(s) of control—feedforward, concurrent, or feedback—do you think would have been most useful in this situation? Explain your choice(s).

18. Using Exhibit 2, explain what BP could have done better.

19. Why do you think company employees ignored the red flags? How could such behavior be changed in the future?

20. What could other organizations learn from BP's mistakes?

ENDNOTES

1. Based on A. Tugend, "You've Been Doing a Fantastic Job. Just One Thing...," *New York Times Online,* April 5, 2013; C. R. Mill, "Feedback: The Art of Giving and Receiving Help," in L. Porter and C. R. Mill (eds.), *The Reading Book for Human Relations Training* (Bethel, ME: NTL Institute for Applied Behavioral Science, 1976), pp. 18–19; and S. Bishop, *The Complete Feedback Skills Training Book* (Aldershot, UK: Gower Publishing, 2000).

2. B. Hagenbaugh, "State Quarters Extra Leaf Grew out of Lunch Break," *USA Today,* January 20, 2006, p. 1B.

3. J. R. Emshwiller, "Managers Blamed in Nuclear Leak," *Wall Street Journal,* April 25, 2014, p. A6.

4. A. Young, "Security Lapses Found at CDC Bioterror Lab in Atlanta," *USA Today,* June 28, 2012, p. 5A.

5. M. Murphy and S. Chaudhuri, "Carnival to Step up Maintenance After Mishaps," *Wall Street Journal,* March 16–17, 2013, p. B3.

6. E. A. Harris, "Error Creates Deals Too Good to Be True on Walmart's Site," *New York Times Online,* November 6, 2013.

7. R. J. Rosen, "The *New York Times* Had a Mistake on Its Front Page Every Day for More Than a Century," www.theatlantic.com, January 16, 2014.

8. C. Timberlake, R. Dudley, and C. Burritt, "Don't Even Think About Returning This Dress," *Bloomberg BusinessWeek,* September 30–October 6, 2013, pp. 29–31.

9. B. Horovitz, "Gross Photo with Wendy's Frosty Is Latest to Go Viral," *USA Today,* June 14, 2013, p. 2B; and S. Clifford, "Video Prank at Domino's Taints Brand," *New York Times Online,* April 16, 2009.

10. K. A. Merchant, "The Control Function of Management," *Sloan Management Review,* Summer 1982, pp. 43–55.

11. E. Flamholtz, "Organizational Control Systems Managerial Tool," *California Management Review,* Winter 1979, p. 55.

12. S. D. Levitt and S. J. Dubner, "Traponomics," *Wall Street Journal,* May 10–11, 2014; and D. Heath and C. Heath, "The Telltale Brown M&M," *Fast Company,* March 2010, pp. 36–38.

13. T. Vinas and J. Jusko, "5 Threats That Could Sink Your Company," *Industry Week,* September 2004, pp. 52–61; "Workplace Security: How Vulnerable Are You?" Special section in *Wall Street Journal,* September 29, 2003, pp. R1–R8; P. Magnusson, "Your Jitters Are Their Lifeblood," *BusinessWeek,* April 14, 2003, p. 41; and T. Purdum, "Preparing for the Worst," *Industry Week,* January 2003, pp. 53–55.

14. M. Hartigan, "Why Nascar Is Putting RFID Sensors on Every Person in the Pit," www.fastcolabs.com, May 23, 2014.

15. K. Peters, "Office Depot's President on How 'Mystery Shopping' Helped Spark a Turnaround," *Harvard Business Review,* November 2011, pp. 47–50.

16. S. Kerr, "On the Folly of Rewarding A, While Hoping for B," *Academy of Management Journal,* December 1975, pp. 769–783.

17. D. Heath and C. Heath, "Watch the Game Film," *Fast Company,* June 2010, pp. 52–54.

18. M. Starr, "State-of-the-Art Stats," *Newsweek,* March 24, 2003, pp. 47–49.

19. A. H. Jordan and P. G. Audia, "Self-Enhancement and Learning from Performance Feedback," *Academy of Management Review,* April 2012, pp. 211–231; D. Busser, "Delivering Effective Performance Feedback," *T&D,* April 2012, pp. 32–34; and "U.S. Employees Desire More Sources of Feedback for Performance Reviews," *T&D,* February 2012, p. 18.

20. "How Well Do You Deliver Difficult Feedback?" smartbrief.com/leadership, October 22, 2013.

21. D. Busser, "Delivering Effective Performance Feedback."

22. S. Clifford, "Demand at Target for Fashion Line Crashes Web Site," *New York Times Online*, September 13, 2011; "Domino's Delivered Free Pizzas," *Springfield, Missouri, News-Leader*, April 3, 2009, p. 3B; and L. Robbins, "Goggle Error Sends Warning Worldwide," *New York Times Online*, February 1, 2009.

23. H. Koontz and R. W. Bradspies, "Managing Through Feedforward Control," *Business Horizons*, June 1972, pp. 25–36.

24. L. Landro, "Hospitals Overhaul ERs to Reduce Mistakes," *Wall Street Journal*, May 10, 2011, p. D3.

25. M. Helft, "The Human Hands Behind the Google Money Machine," *New York Times Online*, June 2, 2008.

26. B. Caulfield, "Shoot to Kill," *Forbes*, January 7, 2008, pp. 92–96.

27. T. Laseter and L. Laseter, "See for Yourself," *Strategy+Business* [www.strategy-business.com], November 29, 2007.

28. W. H. Newman, *Constructive Control: Design and Use of Control Systems* (Upper Saddle River, NJ: Prentice Hall, 1975), p. 33.

29. E. A. Harris, "After Data Breach, Target Plans to Issue More Secure Chip-and-Pin Cards," *New York Times Online*, April 29, 2014; N. Perlroth and D. E. Sanger, "Cyberattacks Seem Meant to Destroy, Not Just Disrupt," *New York Times Online*, March 28, 2013; J. H. Cushman Jr., "U.S. Tightens Security for Economic Data," *New York Times Online*, July 16, 2012; B. Worthen, "Private Sector Keeps Mum on Cyber Attacks," *Wall Street Journal*, January 19, 2010, p. B4; G. Bowley, "Ex-Worker Said to Steal Goldman Code," *New York Times Online*, July 7, 2009; and R. King, "Lessons from the Data Breach at Heartland," *BusinessWeek Online*, July 6, 2009.

30. G. A. Fowler, "You Won't Believe How Adorable This Kitty Is! Click for More!" *Wall Street Journal*, March 27, 2013, pp. A1+.

31. B. Acohido, "To Be a Hacker, You'd Better Be Sneaky," *USA Today*, February 28, 2013, p. 2B.

32. B. Grow, K. Epstein, and C-C. Tschang, "The New E-Spionage Threat," *BusinessWeek*, April 21, 2008, pp. 32–41; S. Leibs, "Firewall of Silence," *CFO*, April 2008, pp. 31–35; J. Pereira, "How Credit-Card Data Went out Wireless Door," *Wall Street Journal*, May 4, 2007, pp. A1+; and B. Stone, "Firms Fret as Office E-Mail Jumps Security Walls," *New York Times Online*, January 11, 2007.

33. D. Whelan, "Google Me Not," *Forbes*, August 16, 2004, pp. 102–104.

34. O. Kharif, "Google Glass Invades the Workplace," *Bloomberg BusinessWeek*, September 23, 2013, pp. 34–35.

35. K. Hendricks, M. Hora, L. Menor, and C. Wiedman, "Adoption of the Balance Scorecard: A Contingency Variables Analysis," *Canadian Journal of Administrative Sciences*, June 2012, pp. 124–138; E. R. Iselin, J. Sands, and L. Mia, "Multi-Perspective Performance Reporting Systems, Continuous Improvement Systems, and Organizational Performance," *Journal of General Management*, Spring 2011, pp. 19–36; T. L. Albright, C. M. Burgess, A. R. Hibbets, and M. L. Roberts, "Four Steps to Simplify Multimeasure Performance Evaluations Using the Balanced Scorecard," *Journal of Corporate Accounting & Finance*, July–August 2010, pp. 63–68; H. Sundin, M. Granlund, and D. A. Brown, "Balancing Multiple Competing Objectives with a Balanced Scorecard," *European Accounting Review*, vol. 19, no. 2, 2010, pp. 203–246; R. S. Kaplan and D. P. Norton, "How to Implement a New Strategy Without Disrupting Your Organization," *Harvard Business Review*, March 2006, pp. 100–109; L. Bassi and D. McMurrer, "Developing Measurement Systems for Managers in the Knowledge Era," *Organizational Dynamics*, May 2005, pp. 185–196; G. M. J. DeKoning, "Making the Balanced Scorecard Work (Part 2)," *Gallup Brain* [brain.gallup.com], August 12, 2004; G. J. J. DeKoning, "Making the Balanced Scorecard Work (Part 1)," *Gallup Brain* [brain.gallup.com], July 8, 2004; K. Graham, "Balanced Scorecard," *New Zealand Management*, March 2003, pp. 32–34; K. Ellis, "A Ticket to Ride: Balanced Scorecard," *Training*, April 2001, p. 50; and T. Leahy, "Tailoring the Balanced Scorecard," *Business Finance*, August 2000, pp. 53–56.

36. T. Leahy, "Tailoring the Balanced Scorecard."

37. Ibid.

38. V. Fuhrmans, "Replicating Cleveland Clinic's Success Poses Major Challenges," *Wall Street Journal*, July 23, 2009, p. A4.

39. R. Pear, "A.M.A. to Develop Measure of Quality of Medical Care," *New York Times Online*, February 21, 2006; and A. Taylor III, "Double Duty," *Fortune*, March 7, 2005, pp. 104–110.

40. P. Ziobro, "Target Fills Its Cart with Amazon Ideas," *Wall Street Journal*, November 12, 2013, pp. B1+.

41. Leader Making a Difference box based on S. M. Mehta and C. Fairchild, "The World's Most Admired Companies," *Fortune*, March 17, 2014, pp. 123+; J. Reingold and M. Adamo, "The Fun King," *Fortune*, May 21, 2012, pp. 166–174; P. Sanders, "Disney Angles for Cash, Loyalty," *Wall Street Journal*, March 11, 2009, p. B4; and R. Siklos, "Bob Iger Rocks Disney," *CNN Online* [www.cnnmoney.com], January 5, 2009.

42. S. Minter, "How Good Is Your Benchmarking?" *Industry Week*, October 2009, pp. 24–26; and T. Leahy, "Extracting Diamonds in the Rough," *Business Finance*, August 2000, pp. 33–37.

43. B. Bruzina, B. Jessop, R. Plourde, B. Whitlock, and L. Rubin, "Ameren Embraces Benchmarking as a Core Business Strategy," *Power Engineering*, November 2002, pp. 121–124.

44. J. Yaukey and C. L. Romero, "Arizona Firm Pays Big for Workers' Digital Downloads," *Associated Press, Springfield, Missouri, News-Leader*, May 6, 2002, p. 6B.

45. L.Petrecca, "Office Madness," *USA Today*, March 15, 2012, pp. 1A+; D. Mattioli and J. Espinoza, "World Cup Poses Challenge to Bosses," *Wall Street Journal*, June 14, 2010, p. B9; "March Madness Leads to Drop in Productivity," *Delaware County Daily Times Online*, March 16, 2010; and "March Madness at Work Raises Questions of Priorities, Productivity," *FoxSports Online*, March 15, 2010.

46. A. R. Carey and P. Trap, "U.S. Workers Who Shop While on the Clock," *USA Today*, December 2, 2013, p. 1A.

47. L. Petrecca, "Feel Like Someone's Watching? You're Right," *USA Today*, March 17, 2010, pp. 1B+.

48. S. Armour, "Companies Keep an Eye on Workers' Internet Use," *USA Today*, February 21, 2006, p. 2B.

49. B. White, "The New Workplace Rules: No Video-Watching," *Wall Street Journal*, March 4, 2008, pp. B1+.

50. P-W. Tam, E. White, N. Wingfield, and K. Maher, "Snooping E-Mail by Software Is Now a Workplace Norm," *Wall Street Journal*, March 9, 2005, pp. B1+; D. Hawkins, "Lawsuits Spur Rise in Employee Monitoring," *U.S. News & World Report*, August 13, 2001, p. 53; and L. Guernsey, "You've Got Inappropriate Mail," *New York Times*, April 5, 2000, pp. C1+.

51. S. Armour, "More Companies Keep Track of Workers' E-Mail," *USA Today*, June 13, 2005, p. 4B; and E. Bott, "Are You Safe? Privacy Special Report," *PC Computing*, March 2000, pp. 87–88.

52. B. Acohido, "An Invitation to Crime," *USA Today*, March 4, 2010, pp. A1+; W. P. Smith and F. Tabak, "Monitoring Employee E-mails: Is There Any Room for Privacy?" *Academy of Management Perspectives*, November 2009, pp. 33–38; and S. Boehle, "They're Watching You," *Training*, September 2008, pp. 23–29.

53. Future Vision box based on S. E. Ante and L. Weber, "Memo to Workers: The Boss Is Watching," *Wall Street Journal*, October 23, 2013, pp. B1+; V. Giang, "Employees Tracked with 'Productivity' Sensors," jobs.aol.com, March 18, 2013; S. F. Gale, "Employers Turn to Biometric Technology to Track Attendance," www.workforce.com, March 5, 2013; C. A. Ciocchetti, "The Eavesdropping Employer: A Twenty-First-Century Framework for Employee Monitoring," *American Business Law Journal*, Summer 2011, pp. 285–369; and G. M. Amsler, H. M. Findley, and E. Ingram, "Performance Monitoring: Guidance for the Modern Workplace," *Supervision*, January 2011, pp. 16–22; T. Harbert, "When IT Is Asked to Spy"; D. Searcey, "Employers Watching Workers Online Spurs Privacy Debate," *Wall Street Journal*, April 23, 2009, p. A13; D. Darlin, "Software That Monitors Your Work, Wherever You Are," *New York Times Online*, April 12, 2009; S. Boehle, "They're Watching You," *Training*, September 2008, pp. 23+; S. Shellenbarger, "Work at Home? Your Employer May Be Watching You," *Wall Street Journal*, July 30, 2008, p. D1+; J. Jusko, "A Watchful Eye," *Industry Week*, May 7, 2001, p. 9; "Big Brother Boss," *U.S. News and World Report*, April 30, 2001, p. 12; and L. Guernsey, "You've Got Inappropriate E-Mail," *New York Times*, April 5, 2000, pp. C1+.

54. S. Greenhouse, "Shoplifters? Studies Say Keep an Eye on Workers," *New York Times Online*, December 30, 2009.

55. A. M. Bell and D. M. Smith, "Theft and Fraud May Be an Inside Job," *Workforce Online* [www.workforce.com], December 3, 2000.

56. C. C. Verschoor, "New Evidence of Benefits from Effective Ethics Systems," *Strategic Finance,* May 2003, pp. 20–21; and E. Krell, "Will Forensic Accounting Go Mainstream?" *Business Finance,* October 2002, pp. 30–34.

57. J. Greenberg, "The STEAL Motive: Managing the Social Determinants of Employee Theft," in R. Giacalone and J. Greenberg (eds.), *Antisocial Behavior in Organizations* (Newbury Park, CA: Sage, 1997), pp. 85–108.

58. B. E. Litzky, K. A. Eddleston, and D. L. Kidder, "The Good, the Bad, and the Misguided: How Managers Inadvertently Encourage Deviant Behaviors," *Academy of Management Perspective,* February 2006, pp. 91–103; "Crime Spree," *BusinessWeek,* September 9, 2002, p. 8; B. P. Niehoff and R. J. Paul, "Causes of Employee Theft and Strategies That HR Managers Can Use for Prevention," *Human Resource Management,* Spring 2000, pp. 51–64; and G. Winter, "Taking at the Office Reaches New Heights: Employee Larceny Is Bigger and Bolder," *New York Times,* July 12, 2000, pp. C1+.

59. This section is based on J. Greenberg, *Behavior in Organizations: Understanding and Managing the Human Side of Work,* 8th ed. (Upper Saddle River, NJ: Prentice Hall, 2003), pp. 329–330.

60. A. H. Bell and D. M. Smith, "Why Some Employees Bite the Hand That Feeds Them," *Workforce Management Online,* December 3, 2000.

61. B. E. Litzky et al., "The Good, the Bad, and the Misguided"; A. H. Bell and D. M. Smith, "Protecting the Company Against Theft and Fraud," *Workforce Management Online,* December 3, 2000; J. D. Hansen, "To Catch a Thief," *Journal of Accountancy,* March 2000, pp. 43–46; and J. Greenberg, "The Cognitive Geometry of Employee Theft," in *Dysfunctional Behavior in Organizations: Nonviolent and Deviant Behavior* (Stamford, CT: JAI Press, 1998), pp. 147–193.

62. L. Copeland and D. Stanglin, "'Rambo' Gunman Injures 6 at FedEx Facility," *USA Today Online,* April 29, 2014; R. Rivera and L. Robbins, "Troubles Preceded Connecticut Workplace Killing," *New York Times Online,* August 3, 2010; J. Griffin, "Workplace Violence News" [www.workplaceviolencenews.com], July 16, 2010; and J. Smerd, "Workplace Shootings in Florida, Texas Again Put Focus on Violence on the Job," *Workforce Management Online,* November 6, 2009.

63. "Workplace Homicides from Shootings," U.S. Bureau of Labor Statistics, http://www.bls.gov/iif/oshwc/cfoi/osar0016.htm, January 2013.

64. J. McCafferty, "Verbal Chills," *CFO,* June 2005, p. 17; S. Armour, "Managers Not Prepared for Workplace Violence," July 15, 2004, pp. 1B+; and "Workplace Violence," OSHA Fact Sheet, U.S. Department of Labor, Occupational Safety and Health Administration, 2002.

65. "Ten Tips on Recognizing and Minimizing Violence," *Workforce Management Online,* December 3, 2000.

66. "Bullying Bosses Cause Work Rage Rise," *Management Issues News* [www.management-issues.com], January 28, 2003.

67. R. McNatt, "Desk Rage," *BusinessWeek,* November 27, 2000, p. 12.

68. M. Gorkin, "Key Components of a Dangerously Dysfunctional Work Environment," *Workforce Management Online,* December 3, 2000.

69. "Ten Tips on Recognizing and Minimizing Violence"; M. Gorkin, "Five Strategies and Structures for Reducing Workplace Violence"; "Investigating Workplace Violence: Where Do You Start?"; and "Points to Cover in a Workplace Violence Policy," all articles from *Workforce Management Online,* December 3, 2000.

70. A. Taylor, "Enterprise Asks What Customer's Thinking and Acts," *USA Today,* May 22, 2006, p. 6B; and A. Taylor, "Driving Customer Satisfaction," *Harvard Business Review,* July 2002, pp. 24–25.

71. S. D. Pugh, J. Dietz, J. W. Wiley, and S. M. Brooks, "Driving Service Effectiveness Through Employee–Customer Linkages," *Academy of Management Executive,* November 2002, pp. 73–84; J. L. Heskett, W. E. Sasser, and L. A. Schlesinger, *The Service Profit Chain* (New York: Free Press, 1997); and J. L. Heskett, T. O. Jones, G. W. Loveman, W. E. Sasser Jr., and L. A. Schlesinger, "Putting the Service Profit Chain to Work," *Harvard Business Review,* March–April 1994, pp. 164–170.

72. T. Buck and A. Shahrim, "The Translation of Corporate Governance Changes Across National Cultures: The Case of Germany," *Journal of International Business Studies,* January 2005, pp. 42–61; and "A Revolution Where Everyone Wins: Worldwide Movement to Improve Corporate-Governance Standards," *BusinessWeek,* May 19, 2003, p. 72.

73. J. S. McClenahen, "Executives Expect More Board Input," *Industry Week,* October 2002, p. 12.

74. D. Salierno, "Boards Face Increased Responsibility," *Internal Auditor,* June 2003, pp. 14–15.

75. "Restaurant Serves Rum Drink to Boy, 10," www.wishtv.com, April 20, 2012; B. Horovitz, "Restaurants Reel After Babies Get Booze," *USA Today,* April 15, 2011, p. 1B; "Toddler Given Sangria at Restaurant," www.wishtv.com, April 14, 2011; and A. Hillaker, "Applebee's Serves Alcohol to 15-month-old Child Instead of Apple Juice," MiNBCnews.com, April 11, 2011.

76. N. Pelusi, "Dealing with Difficult People," *Psychology Today,* September–October 2006, pp. 68–69; and R. I. Sutton, *The No Asshole Rule: Building a Civilized Workplace and Surviving One That Isn't* (New York: Business Plus, 2007).

77. A. Andors, "Keeping Teen Workers Safe," *HR Magazine,* June 2010, pp. 76–80.

78. J. Swartz, "Visa Stores Data Like Gold: In Its Own Fort Knox," *USA Today,* March 26, 2012, p. 4B; M. Fitzgerald, "Visa Is Ready for Anything," FastCompany.com, November 2011, pp. 54–58; and "Visa Launches New Operating System, Data Center," *CardLine,* November 20, 2009, p. 37.

79. P. Elkind and D. Whitford, "An Accident Waiting to Happen," *Fortune,* February 7, 2011, pp. 105–132; G. Chazan, "BP's Safety Drive Faces Rough Road," *Wall Street Journal,* February 1, 2011, pp. A1+; C. Hausman, "Report Says Lack of Oversight Contributed to the Gulf Spill Disaster," *Ethics Newsline Online,* January 11, 2011; B. Casselman, "Supervisor Says Flaw Was Found in Key Safety Device," *Wall Street Journal,* July 21, 2010, pp. A6; R. Gold, "Rig's Final Hours Probed," *Wall Street Journal,* July 19, 2010, pp. A1+; **S. Lyall, "In BP's Record, a History of Boldness and Costly Blunders," *New York Times Online,* July 12, 2010**; B. Casselman and R. Gold, "Unusual Decisions Set Stage for BP Disaster," *Wall Street Journal,* May 27, 2010, pp. A1+; H. Fountain and T. Zeller Jr., "Panel Suggests Signs of Trouble Before Rig Explosion," *New York Times Online,* May 25, 2010; and R. Gold and N. King Jr., "The Gulf Oil Spill: Red Flags Were Ignored Aboard Doomed Rig," *Wall Street Journal,* May 13, 2010, p. A6.

Managing Operations *Module*

Using millions of parts as small as rivets and as large as five-story buildings, employees at Hyundai Heavy Industries Inc. build as many as 30 ships at one time.[1] And the "factory" stretches for miles over land and sea. "It's an environment that is too large and complex to be able to keep track of the movement in parts and inventory in real time." Hwang See-young, chief information officer at Hyundai Heavy, knew that production efficiency was limited without real-time data. The solution? High-speed wireless networks that employees can access at anytime and anywhere with notebook computers.

With the new technology, data fly around the shipyard complex at 4 megabits per second. Radio sensors track the movements of parts from fabrication shops to the dry dock and onto a ship being constructed. Also, workers on a ship can access plans using notebook computers or handheld phones. They're also able to hold two-way video conversations with ship designers in the office over a mile away. Eventually, they hope to establish communication capabilities with workers inside a ship that is below ground or at sea level. Now, however, Hyundai Heavy wants to implement the technology in its other construction divisions. Suppose you were in charge of doing this. What would you do?

As the world's largest maker of ships, Hyundai hopes its new technology helps it reduce expenses and streamline production, an important consideration in today's environment. You've probably never given much thought to how organizations "produce" the goods and services that you buy or use. But it's an important process. Without it, you wouldn't have a car to drive or McDonald's fries to snack on, or even a hiking trail in a local park to enjoy. Organizations need to have well-thought-out and well-designed operating systems, organizational control systems, and quality programs to survive in today's increasingly competitive global environment. And it's the manager's job to manage those systems and programs.

THE Role of Operations Management

What is **operations management**? The term refers to the transformation process that converts resources into finished goods and services. Exhibit 1 portrays this process in a simplified fashion. The system takes in inputs—people, technology, capital, equipment, materials, and information—and transforms them through various processes, procedures, work activities, and so forth into finished goods and services. Because every unit in an organization produces something, managers need to be familiar with operations management concepts in order to achieve goals efficiently and effectively.

Operations management is important to organizations and managers for three reasons: (1) it encompasses both services and manufacturing; (2) it's important in effectively and efficiently managing productivity; and (3) it plays a strategic role in an organization's competitive success.

Services and Manufacturing

With a menu that offers more than 200 items, The Cheesecake Factory restaurants rely on a finely tuned production system. One food-service consultant says, "They've evolved with this highly complex menu combined with a highly efficient kitchen."[2]

Every organization produces something. Unfortunately, this fact is often overlooked except in obvious cases such as in the manufacturing of cars, cell phones, or lawnmowers. After all, **manufacturing organizations** produce physical goods. It's easy to see the operations management (transformation) process at work in these types of organizations because raw materials are turned into recognizable physical products. But the transformation process isn't as readily evident in **service organizations** that produce nonphysical outputs in the form of services. For instance, hospitals provide medical and health care services that help people manage their personal health, airlines provide transportation services that move people from one location to another, a cruise line provides a vacation and entertainment service, military forces provide defense capabilities, and the list goes on. These service organizations also transform inputs into outputs, although the transformation process isn't as easily recognizable as that in manufacturing organizations. Take a university, for example. University administrators bring together inputs—professors, books, academic journals, technology materials, computers, classrooms, and similar resources—to transform "unenlightened" students into educated and skilled individuals who are capable of making contributions to society.

The reason we're making this point is that the U.S. economy, and to a large extent the global economy, is dominated by the creation and sale of services. Most of the world's developed countries are predominantly service economies. In the United States, for instance, almost 80 percent of all economic activity is services, and in the European Union it's over 72 percent. In lesser-developed countries, the services sector is less important. For instance, in Nigeria, it accounts for only 26 percent of economic activity; in Laos, only 21 percent; and in Vietnam, about 31 percent.[3]

Managing Productivity

One jetliner has roughly 4 million parts. Efficiently assembling such a finely engineered product requires intense focus. Boeing and Airbus, the two major global manufacturers, have copied techniques from Toyota. However, not every technique can be copied

operations management
The transformation process that converts resources into finished goods and services

manufacturing organizations
Organizations that produce physical goods

service organizations
Organizations that produce nonphysical products in the form of services

Exhibit 1
The Operations System

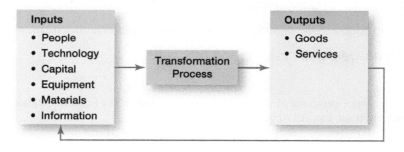

because airlines demand more customization than do car buyers and significantly more rigid safety regulations apply to jetliners than to cars.[4] At the Evans Findings Company in East Providence, Rhode Island, which makes the tiny cutting devices on dental-floss containers, one production shift each day is run without people.[5] The company's goal is to do as much as possible with no labor. And it's not because they don't care about their employees. Instead, like many U.S. manufacturers, Evans needed to raise productivity in order to survive, especially against low-cost competitors. So they turned to "lights-out" manufacturing where machines are designed to be so reliable that they make flawless parts on their own, without people operating them.

Although most organizations don't make products that have 4 million parts and most organizations can't function without people, improving productivity has become a major goal in virtually every organization. For countries, high productivity can lead to economic growth and development. Employees can receive higher wages and company profits can increase without causing inflation. For individual organizations, increased productivity gives them a more competitive cost structure and the ability to offer more competitive prices.

Over the past decade, U.S. businesses have made dramatic improvements to increase their efficiency. For example, at Latex Foam International's state-of-the-art digital facility in Shelton, Connecticut, engineers monitor all of the factory's operations. The facility boosted capacity by 50 percent in a smaller space but with a 30 percent efficiency gain.[6] And it's not just in manufacturing that companies are pursuing productivity gains. Pella Corporation's purchasing office improved productivity by reducing purchase order entry times anywhere from 50 percent to 86 percent, decreasing voucher processing by 27 percent, and eliminating 14 financial systems. Its information technology department slashed e-mail traffic in half and implemented work design improvements for heavy PC users such as call center users. The human resources department cut the time to process benefit enrollment by 156.5 days. And the finance department now takes 2 days instead of 6 to do its end-of-month closeout.[7]

Organizations that hope to succeed globally are looking for ways to improve productivity. For example, McDonald's Corporation drastically reduced the time it takes to cook its french fries—65 seconds as compared to the 210 seconds it once took, saving time and other resources.[8] The Canadian Imperial Bank of Commerce, based in Toronto, automated its purchasing function, saving several million dollars annually.[9] And Skoda, the Czech car company that's a subsidiary of Germany's Volkswagen AG, improved its productivity through an intensive restructuring of its manufacturing process.[10]

Productivity is a composite of people and operations variables. To improve productivity, managers must focus on both. The late W. Edwards Deming, a renowned quality expert, believed that managers, not workers, were the primary source of increased productivity. Some of his suggestions for managers included planning for the long-term future, never being complacent about product quality, understanding whether problems were confined to particular parts of the production process or stemmed from the overall process itself, training workers for the job they're being asked to perform, raising the quality of line supervisors, requiring workers to do quality work, and so forth.[11] As you can see, Deming understood the interplay between people and operations. High productivity can't come solely from good "people management." The truly effective organization will maximize productivity by successfully integrating people into the overall operations system. For instance, at Simplex Nails Manufacturing in Americus, Georgia, employees were an integral part of the company's much-needed turnaround effort.[12] Some production workers were redeployed on a plant-wide cleanup and organization effort, which freed up floor space. The company's sales force was retrained and refocused to sell what customers wanted rather than what was in inventory. The results were dramatic. Inventory was reduced by more than 50 percent, the plant had 20 percent more floor space, orders were more consistent, and employee morale improved. Here's a company that recognized the important interplay between people and the operations system.

Strategic Role of Operations Management

Modern manufacturing originated over 100 years ago in the United States, primarily in Detroit's automobile factories. The success that U.S. manufacturers experienced during World War II led manufacturing executives to believe that troublesome production problems had been conquered. These executives focused, instead, on improving other functional areas, such as finance and marketing, and paid little attention to manufacturing.

However, as U.S. executives neglected production, managers in Japan, Germany, and other countries took the opportunity to develop modern, computer-based, and technologically advanced facilities that fully integrated manufacturing operations into strategic planning decisions. The competition's success realigned world manufacturing leadership. U.S. manufacturers soon discovered that foreign goods were made not only less expensively but also with better quality. Finally, by the late 1970s, U.S. executives recognized they were facing a true crisis and responded. They invested heavily in improving manufacturing technology, increased the corporate authority and visibility of manufacturing executives, and began incorporating existing and future production requirements into the organization's overall strategic plan. Today, successful organizations recognize the crucial role that operations management plays as part of the overall organizational strategy to establish and maintain global leadership.[13]

The strategic role that operations management plays in successful organizational performance can be seen clearly as more organizations move toward managing their operations from a value chain perspective, which we're going to discuss next.

WHAT Is Value Chain Management and Why Is It Important?

It's 11 P.M., and you're reading a text message from your parents saying they want to buy you a laptop for your birthday this year and to order it. You log on to Dell's Web site and configure your dream machine. You hit the order button and, not long after, your dream computer is delivered to your front door, built to your exact specifications, ready to set up and use immediately to type that management assignment due tomorrow. Or consider Siemens AG's Computed Tomography manufacturing plant in Forchheim, Germany, which has established partnerships with about 30 suppliers. These suppliers are partners in the truest sense, as they share responsibility with the plant for overall process performance. This arrangement has allowed Siemens to eliminate all inventory warehousing and has streamlined the number of times paper changes hands to order parts from 18 to one. At the Timken's plant in Canton, Ohio, electronic purchase orders are sent across the street to an adjacent "Supplier City," where many of its key suppliers have set up shop. The process takes milliseconds and costs less than 50 cents per purchase order. And when Black & Decker extended its line of handheld tools to include a glue gun, it totally outsourced the entire design and production to the leading glue gun manufacturer. Why? Because they understood that glue guns don't require motors, which was what Black & Decker did best.[14]

As these examples show, closely integrated work activities among many different players are possible. How? The answer lies in value chain management. The concepts of value chain management have transformed operations management strategies and turned organizations around the world into finely tuned models of efficiency and effectiveness, strategically positioned to exploit competitive opportunities.

WHAT Is Value Chain Management?

Every organization needs customers if it's going to survive and prosper. Even a not-for-profit organization must have "customers" who use its services or purchase its products. Customers want some type of value from the goods and services they

purchase or use, and these customers decide what has value. Organizations must provide that value to attract and keep customers. **Value** is defined as the performance characteristics, features, and attributes and any other aspects of goods and services for which customers are willing to give up resources (usually money). For example, when you purchase Rihanna's new CD at Best Buy, a new pair of Australian sheepskin Ugg boots online at Zappos, a Wendy's bacon cheeseburger at the drive-through location on campus, or a haircut from your local hair salon, you're exchanging (giving up) money in return for the value you need or desire from these products—providing music during your evening study time, keeping your feet warm *and* fashionable during winter's cold weather, alleviating the lunchtime hunger pangs quickly since your next class starts in 15 minutes, or looking professionally groomed for the job interview you've got next week.

How *is* value provided to customers? Through transforming raw materials and other resources into some product or service that end users need or desire when, where, and how they want it. However, that seemingly simple act of turning varied resources into something that customers value and are willing to pay for involves a vast array of interrelated work activities performed by different participants (suppliers, manufacturers, and even customers)—that is, it involves the value chain. The **value chain** is the entire series of organizational work activities that add value at each step from raw materials to finished product. In its entirety, the value chain can encompass the supplier's suppliers to the customer's customer.[15]

Value chain management is the process of managing the sequence of activities and information along the entire value chain. In contrast to supply chain management, which is *internally* oriented and focuses on efficient flow of incoming materials (resources) to the organization, value chain management is *externally* oriented and focuses on both incoming materials and outgoing products and services. Although supply chain management is efficiency oriented (its goal is to reduce costs and make the organization more productive), value chain management is effectiveness oriented and aims to create the highest value for customers.[16]

Goal of Value Chain Management

Who has the power in the value chain? Is it the suppliers providing needed resources and materials? After all, they have the ability to dictate prices and quality. Is it the manufacturer who assembles those resources into a valuable product or service? Their contribution in creating a product or service is quite obvious. Is it the distributor that makes sure the product or service is available where and when the customer needs it? Actually, it's none of these! In value chain management, ultimately customers are the ones with power.[17] They're the ones who define what value is and how it's created and provided. Using value chain management, managers hope to find that unique combination that offers customers solutions to truly meet their unique needs incredibly fast and at a price that can't be matched by competitors.

With these factors in mind then, the goal of value chain management is to create a value chain strategy that meets and exceeds customers' needs and desires and allows for full and seamless integration among all members of the chain. A good value chain involves a sequence of participants working together as a team, each adding some component of value—such as faster assembly, more accurate information, better customer response and service, and so forth—to the overall process.[18] The better the collaboration among the various chain participants, the better the customer solutions. When value is created for customers and their needs and desires are satisfied, everyone along the chain benefits. For example, at Johnson Controls Inc., managing the value chain started first with improved relationships with internal suppliers, then expanded out to external suppliers and customers. As the company's experience with value chain management improved, so did its connection with its customers, which ultimately paid off for all its value chain partners.[19]

value
The performance characteristics, features, and attributes, and any other aspects of goods and services for which customers are willing to give up resources

value chain
The entire series of organizational work activities that add value at each step from raw materials to finished product

value chain management
The process of managing the sequence of activities and information along the entire value chain

Benefits of Value Chain Management

Collaborating with external and internal partners in creating and managing a successful value chain strategy requires significant investments in time, energy, and other resources, and a serious commitment by all chain partners. Given these demands, why would managers ever choose to implement value chain management? A survey of manufacturers noted four primary benefits of value chain management: improved procurement, improved logistics, improved product development, and enhanced customer order management.[20]

MANAGING Operations Using Value Chain Management

Even though it's the world's largest retailer, Walmart still looks for ways to more effectively and efficiently manage its value chain. Its current efforts involve taking over U.S. transportation services from suppliers in an effort to reduce the cost of transporting goods. The goal: "to handle suppliers' deliveries in instances where Walmart can do the same job for less, then use those savings to reduce prices in stores." Walmart believes it has the size and scale to allow it to ship most products more efficiently than the companies that produce the goods.[21]

Even if you're Walmart, managing an organization from a value chain perspective isn't easy. Approaches to giving customers what they want that may have worked in the past are likely no longer efficient or effective. Today's dynamic competitive environment demands new solutions from global organizations. Understanding how and why value is determined by the marketplace has led some organizations to experiment with a new business model. For example, IKEA transformed itself from a small Swedish mail-order furniture operation into one of the world's largest furniture retailers by reinventing the value chain in that industry. The company offers customers well-designed products at substantially lower prices in return for their willingness to take on certain key tasks traditionally done by manufacturers and retailers—assembling furniture and getting it home.[22] The company's creation of a new business model and willingness to abandon old methods and processes has worked well.

Value Chain Strategy

Exhibit 2 shows the six main requirements of a successful value chain strategy: coordination and collaboration, technology investment, organizational processes, leadership, employees, and organizational culture and attitudes.

COORDINATION AND COLLABORATION For the value chain to achieve its goal of meeting and exceeding customers' needs and desires, collaborative relationships

Exhibit 2
Value Chain Strategy Requirement

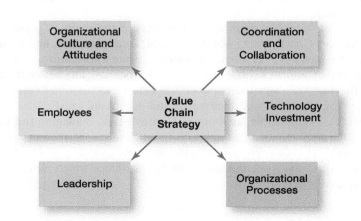

among all chain participants must exist.[23] Each partner must identify things he or she may not value but that customers do. Sharing information and being flexible as far as who in the value chain does what are important steps in building coordination and collaboration. This sharing of information and analysis requires more open communication among the various value chain partners. For example, Kraft Foods believes that better communication with customers and with suppliers has facilitated timely delivery of goods and services.[24]

TECHNOLOGY INVESTMENT   Successful value chain management isn't possible without a significant investment in information technology. The payoff from this investment, however, is that information technology can be used to restructure the value chain to better serve end users. For example, each year the Houston-based food distributor Sysco ships 21.5 million tons of produce, meats, prepared meals, and other food-related products to restaurants, cafeterias, and sports stadiums. To get all that food safely to the right place at the right time, Sysco relies on a complex web of software, databases, scanning systems, and robotics.[25]

ORGANIZATIONAL PROCESSES   At Pactiv Corporation, which manufactures consumer and food-service packaging, the company relied on a planning process that included three-year breakthrough goals, which were then translated into one-year goals, annual improvement priorities, and measurable targets. This disciplined approach to planning has helped the company grow and achieve its goals.[26]

Value chain management radically changes **organizational processes**—that is, the ways that organizational work is done. When managers decide to manage operations using value chain management, old processes are no longer appropriate. All organizational processes must be critically evaluated from beginning to end to see where value is being added. Non-value-adding activities should be eliminated. Questions such as "Where can internal knowledge be leveraged to improve the flow of material and information?" "How can we better configure our product to satisfy both customers and suppliers?" "How can the flow of material and information be improved?" and "How can we improve customer service?" should be asked for each and every process. For example, when managers at Deere and Company implemented value chain management, a thorough process evaluation revealed that work activities needed to be better synchronized and interrelationships between multiple links in the value chain better managed. They changed numerous work processes division-wide in order to realize greater value.[27]

Three important conclusions can be made about organizational processes. First, better demand forecasting is necessary *and* possible because of closer ties with customers and suppliers. For example, in an effort to make sure that Listerine was on the store shelves when customers wanted it (known in the retail industry as *product replenishment rates*), Walmart and Pfizer's Consumer Healthcare Group collaborated on improving product demand forecast information. Through their mutual efforts, the partners boosted Walmart's sales of Listerine, an excellent outcome for both supplier and retailer. Customers also benefited because they were able to purchase the product when and where they wanted it.

Second, selected functions may need to be done collaboratively with other partners in the value chain. This collaboration may even extend to sharing employees. For instance, Saint-Gobain Performance Plastics places its own employees in customer sites and brings in employees of suppliers and customers to work on its premises.[28]

Finally, new measures are needed for evaluating performance of various activities along the value chain. Because the goal in value chain management is meeting and exceeding customers' needs and desires, managers need a better picture of how well this value is being created and delivered to customers. For example, when Nestlé USA implemented value chain management, it redesigned its metrics system to focus on one consistent set of measurements—including, for instance, accuracy of demand forecasts

organizational processes
The ways that organizational work is done

and production plans, on-time delivery, and customer-service levels—that allowed them to more quickly identify problem areas and take actions to resolve them.[29]

LEADERSHIP Successful value chain management isn't possible without strong and committed leadership. From top organizational levels to lower levels, managers must support, facilitate, and promote the implementation and ongoing practice of value chain management. Managers must seriously commit to identifying what value is, how that value can best be provided, and how successful those efforts have been. A culture where all efforts are focused on delivering superb customer value isn't possible without a serious commitment on the part of the organization's leaders.

Also, it's important that managers outline expectations for what's involved in the organization's pursuit of value chain management. Ideally, managers start with a vision or mission statement that expresses the organization's commitment to identifying, capturing, and providing the highest possible value to customers. For instance, when American Standard began using value chain management, the CEO held dozens of meetings across the United States to explain the new competitive environment and why the company needed to create better working relationships with its value chain partners in order to better serve the needs of its customers.[30]

Then, managers should clarify expectations regarding each employee's role in the value chain. But clear expectations aren't just important for internal partners. Being clear about expectations also extends to external partners. For example, managers at American Standard identified clear requirements for suppliers and were prepared to drop any that couldn't meet them, and did so. The upside, though, was that those suppliers who met the expectations benefited from more business and American Standard had partners willing to work with them in delivering better value to customers.

EMPLOYEES/HUMAN RESOURCES When new employees at the Thermo Fisher Scientific plant in Marietta, Ohio, have work-related questions, they can consult with a member of the facility's "Tree of Knowledge." The "tree" is actually a bulletin board with pictures of employees who have worked at the plant for decades.[31]

We know from our discussions of management theories throughout this text that employees are an organization's most important resource. Without employees, no products are produced and no services are delivered—in fact, no organized efforts in the pursuit of common goals would be possible. So not surprisingly, employees play an important role in value chain management. The three main human resource requirements for value chain management are flexible approaches to job design, an effective hiring process, and ongoing training.

Flexibility is the key to job design in value chain management. Traditional functional job roles—such as marketing, sales, accounts payable, customer service, and so forth—won't work. Instead, jobs must be designed around work processes that create and provide value to customers. It takes flexible jobs and flexible employees. For instance, at Nordson Corporation's facility in Swainsboro, Georgia, workers are trained to do several different tasks, which isn't all that uncommon in many manufacturing plants. What's unique about this facility is that even salaried employees are expected to spend four hours every month building products on the shop floor.[32]

In a value chain organization, employees may be assigned to work teams that tackle a given process and may be asked to do different things on different days depending on need. In such an environment, where customer value is best delivered through collaborative relationships that may change as customer needs change and where processes or job descriptions are not standardized, an employee's ability to be flexible is critical. Therefore, the organization's hiring process must be designed to identify those employees who have the ability to learn and adapt.

Finally, the need for flexibility also requires a significant investment in continual and ongoing employee training. Whether that training involves learning how to use information technology software, how to improve the flow of materials throughout

the chain, how to identify activities that add value, how to make better decisions faster, or how to improve any other number of potential work activities, managers must see to it that employees have the knowledge and tools they need to do their jobs efficiently and effectively.

ORGANIZATIONAL CULTURE AND ATTITUDES The last requirement for value chain management is having a supportive organizational culture and attitudes. From our extensive description of value chain management, you could probably guess the type of organizational culture that's going to support its successful implementation! Those cultural attitudes include sharing, collaborating, openness, flexibility, mutual respect, and trust. These attitudes encompass not only the internal partners in the value chain, but extend to external partners as well.

Obstacles to Value Chain Management

As desirable as these benefits may be, managers must tackle several obstacles in managing the value chain, including organizational barriers, cultural attitudes, required capabilities, and people (see Exhibit 3).

ORGANIZATIONAL BARRIERS At General Cable's manufacturing facility in Manchester, New Hampshire, one of the most interesting challenges faced by managers and employees in maintaining its world-class competitiveness is the 23 different nationalities that speak 12 languages besides English. Multiple languages make getting new messages out about anything that comes up especially tricky. But they've made it work using visual cues throughout the plant.[33]

Organizational barriers are among the most difficult obstacles to handle. These barriers include refusal or reluctance to share information, reluctance to shake up the status quo, and security issues. Without shared information, close coordination and collaboration is impossible. And the reluctance or refusal of employees to shake up the status quo can impede efforts toward value chain management and prevent its successful implementation. Finally, because value chain management relies heavily on a substantial information technology infrastructure, system security and Internet security breaches are issues that need to be addressed.

CULTURAL ATTITUDES Unsupportive cultural attitudes—especially trust and control—also can be obstacles to value chain management. The trust issue is a critical one, both lack of trust and too much trust. To be effective, partners in a value chain must trust each other. A mutual respect for, and honesty about, each partner's activities all along the chain is essential. When that trust doesn't exist, the partners will be reluctant to share information, capabilities, and processes. But too much trust also can be a problem. Just about any organization is vulnerable to theft of **intellectual property**—that is, proprietary information that's critical to an organization's efficient and effective functioning and competitiveness. You need to be able to trust your value chain partners so your organization's valuable assets aren't compromised.[34] Another cultural attitude that can be an obstacle is the belief that

intellectual property
Proprietary information that's critical to an organization's efficient and effective functioning and competitiveness

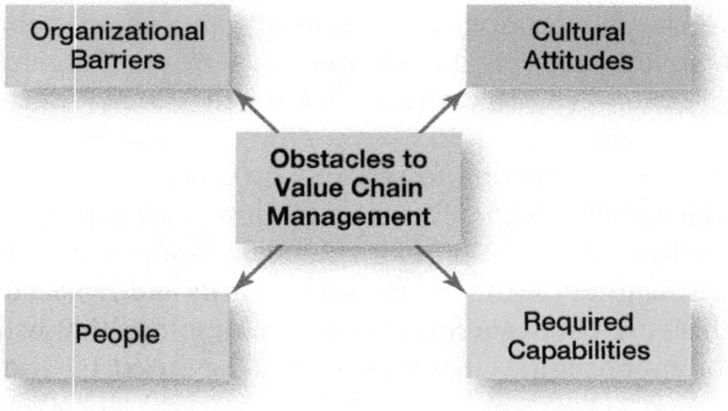

Exhibit 3
Obstacles to Value Chain Management

when an organization collaborates with external and internal partners, it no longer controls its own destiny. However, this lack of control just isn't the case. Even with the intense collaboration that's important to value chain management, organizations still control critical decisions such as what customers value, how much value they desire, and what distribution channels are important.[35]

REQUIRED CAPABILITIES We know from our earlier discussion of requirements for the successful implementation of value chain management that value chain partners need numerous capabilities. Several of these capabilities—coordination and collaboration, the ability to configure products to satisfy customers and suppliers, and the ability to educate internal and external partners—aren't easy, but they're essential to capturing and exploiting the value chain. Many of the companies we've described throughout this section endured critical, and oftentimes difficult, self-evaluations of their capabilities and processes in order to become more effective and efficient at managing their value chains.

PEOPLE The final obstacles to successful value chain management can be an organization's people. Without their unwavering commitment to do whatever it takes, value chain management won't be successful. If employees refuse to be flexible in their work—how and with whom they work—collaboration and cooperation throughout the value chain will be hard to achieve.

In addition, value chain management takes an incredible amount of time and energy on the part of an organization's employees. Managers must motivate those high levels of effort from employees, which is not an easy thing to do.

Finally, a major human resource problem is the lack of experienced managers who can lead value chain management initiatives. It's not that widespread, so there aren't a lot of managers who've done it successfully. However, progressive organizations see the benefits to be gained from value chain management and pursue it despite obstacles.

CURRENT Issues in Managing Operations

Rowe Furniture had an audacious goal: make a sofa in 10 days. It wanted to "become as efficient at making furniture as Toyota is at making cars." Reaching that goal, however, required revamping its operations management process to exploit technology *and* maintain quality.[36] Rowe's actions illustrate three of today's most important operations management issues: technology, quality, and mass customization and lean organizations.

Technology's Role in Operations Management

Global positioning systems (GPS) are changing a number of enterprises from shipping to shopping, from health care to law enforcement, and even farming.[37] Like many other technologies, GPS was invented for military use to track weapons and personnel as they moved. Now GPS is being used to track shipping fleets, revitalize consumer products such as watches or photos, and monitor parolees or sex offenders.

As we know from our previous discussion of value chain management, today's competitive marketplace has put tremendous pressure on organizations to deliver products and services that customers value in a timely manner. Smart companies are looking at ways to harness technology to improve operations management. Many fast-food companies are competing to see who can provide faster and better service to drive-through customers. With drive-through now representing a huge portion of sales, faster and better delivery can be a significant competitive edge. For instance, Wendy's has added awnings to some of its menu boards and replaced some of the text with pictures. Others use confirmation screens, a technology that helped McDonald's boost accuracy by more than 11 percent. Technology used by two national chains

tells managers how much food they need to prepare by counting vehicles in the drive-through line and factoring in demand for current promotional and popular staple items. Even Domino's is using a new point-of-sale system to attract customers and streamline online orders.[38]

Although an organization's production activities are driven by the recognition that the customer is king, managers still need to be more responsive. For instance, operations managers need systems that can reveal available capacity, status of orders, and product quality while products are in the process of being manufactured, not just after the fact. To connect more closely with customers, production must be synchronized across the enterprise. To avoid bottlenecks and slowdowns, the production function must be a full partner in the entire business system.

What's making such extensive collaboration possible is technology. Technology is also allowing organizations to control costs particularly in the areas of predictive maintenance, remote diagnostics, and utility cost savings. For instance, new Internet-compatible equipment contains embedded Web servers that can communicate pro-actively—that is, if a piece of equipment breaks or reaches certain preset parameters indicating that it's about to break, it asks for help. But technology can do more than sound an alarm or light up an indicator button. For instance, some devices have the ability to initiate e-mail or signal a pager at a supplier, the maintenance department, or contractor describing the specific problem and requesting parts and service. How much is such e-enabled maintenance control worth? It can be worth quite a lot if it prevents equipment breakdowns and subsequent production downtime.

Managers who understand the power of technology to contribute to more effective and efficient performance know that managing operations is more than the traditional view of simply producing the product. Instead, the emphasis is on working together with all the organization's business functions to find solutions to customers' business problems. Even service providers understand the power of technology for these tasks. For example, Southwest Airlines upgraded its cockpit software, enabling its pilots (who have been extensively trained) to fly precise satellite-based navigation approaches to airports, thus saving fuel, reducing delays, and cutting noise.[39]

Quality Initiatives

Quality problems are expensive. For example, even though Apple has had phenomenal success with its iPod, the batteries in the first three versions died after 4 hours instead of lasting the up-to-12 hours that buyers expected. Apple's settlement with consumers cost close to $100 million. At Schering-Plough, problems with inhalers and other pharmaceuticals were traced to chronic quality control shortcomings, for which the company eventually paid a $500 million fine. And the auto industry paid $14.5 billion to cover the cost of warranty and repair work in one year.[40]

Many experts believe that organizations unable to produce high-quality products won't be able to compete successfully in the global marketplace. What is quality? When you consider a product or service to have quality, what does that mean? Does it mean that the product doesn't break or quit working—that is, that it's reliable? Does it mean that the service is delivered in a way that you intended? Does it mean that the product does what it's supposed to do? Or does quality mean something else? We're going to define **quality** as the ability of a product or service to reliably do what it's supposed to do and to satisfy customer expectations.

quality
The ability of a product or service to reliably do what it's supposed to do and to satisfy customer expectations

How is quality achieved? That's an issue managers must address. A good way to look at quality initiatives is with the management functions—planning, organizing, leading, and controlling—that need to take place.

PLANNING FOR QUALITY Managers must have quality improvement goals and strategies and plans to achieve those goals. Goals can help focus everyone's attention toward some objective quality standard. For instance, Caterpillar's goal is to apply quality improvement techniques to help cut costs.[41] Although this goal is specific and

challenging, managers and employees are partnering together to pursue well-designed strategies to achieve the goals, and are confident they can do so.

ORGANIZING AND LEADING FOR QUALITY Because quality improvement initiatives are carried out by organizational employees, it's important for managers to look at how they can best organize and lead them. For instance, at the Moosejaw, Saskatchewan, plant of General Cable Corporation, every employee participates in continual quality assurance training. In addition, the plant manager believes wholeheartedly in giving employees the information they need to do their jobs better. He says, "Giving people who are running the machines the information is just paramount. You can set up your cellular structure, you can cross-train your people, you can use lean tools, but if you don't give people information to drive improvement, there's no enthusiasm." Needless to say, this company shares production data and financial performance measures with all employees.[42]

Organizations with extensive and successful quality improvement programs tend to rely on two important people approaches: cross-functional work teams, and self-directed or empowered work teams. Because achieving product quality is something that all employees from upper to lower levels must participate in, it's not surprising that quality-driven organizations rely on well-trained, flexible, and empowered employees.

CONTROLLING FOR QUALITY Quality improvement initiatives aren't possible without having some way to monitor and evaluate their progress. Whether it involves standards for inventory control, defect rate, raw materials procurement, or other operations management areas, controlling for quality is important. For instance, at the Northrup Grumman Corporation plant in Rolling Meadows, Illinois, several quality controls have been implemented, such as automated testing and IT that integrates product design and manufacturing and tracks process quality improvements. Also, employees are empowered to make accept/reject decisions about products throughout the manufacturing process. The plant manager explains, "This approach helps build quality into the product rather than trying to inspect quality into the product." But one of the most important things they do is "go to war" with their customers—soldiers preparing for war or in live combat situations. Again, the plant manager says, "What discriminates us is that we believe if we can understand our customer's mission as well as they do, we can help them be more effective. We don't wait for our customer to ask us to do something. We find out what our customer is trying to do and then we develop solutions."[43]

These types of quality improvement success stories aren't just limited to U.S. operations. For example, at a Delphi assembly plant in Matamoros, Mexico, employees worked hard to improve quality and made significant strides. Their customer rejection rate on shipped products is now 10 ppm (parts per million), down from 3,000 ppm—an improvement of almost 300 percent.[44] Quality initiatives at several Australian companies, including Alcoa of Australia, Wormald Security, and Carlton and United Breweries, have led to significant quality improvements.[45] And at Valeo Klimasystemme GmbH of Bad Rodach, Germany, assembly teams build different climate-control systems for high-end German cars including Mercedes and BMW. Quality initiatives by Valeo's employee teams have led to significant improvements in various quality standards.[46]

Quality Goals

To publicly demonstrate their quality commitment, many organizations worldwide have pursued challenging quality goals—the two best-known being ISO 9000 and Six Sigma.

ISO 9000 **ISO 9000** is a series of international quality management standards established by the International Organization for Standardization (www.iso.org), which set uniform guidelines for processes to ensure that products conform to customer requirements. These standards cover everything from contract review to product design to

ISO 9000
A series of international quality management standards that set uniform guidelines for processes to ensure products conform to customer requirements

product delivery. The ISO 9000 standards have become the internationally recognized standard for evaluating and comparing companies in the global marketplace. In fact, this type of certification can be a prerequisite for doing business globally. Achieving ISO 9000 certification provides proof that a quality operations system is in place.

As of 2012, more than 1 million certifications had been awarded to organizations in 175 countries. Almost 40,000 U.S. businesses are ISO 9000 certified. Over 200,000 Chinese firms have received certification.[47]

SIX SIGMA Motorola popularized the use of stringent quality standards more than 30 years ago through a trademarked quality improvement program called Six Sigma.[48] Very simply, **Six Sigma** is a quality program designed to reduce defects to help lower costs, save time, and improve customer satisfaction. It's based on the statistical standard that establishes a goal of no more than 3.4 defects per million units or procedures. What does the name mean? Sigma is the Greek letter that statisticians use to define a standard deviation from a bell curve. The higher the sigma, the fewer the deviations from the norm—that is, the fewer the defects. At One Sigma, two-thirds of whatever is being measured falls within the curve. Two Sigma covers about 95 percent. At Six Sigma, you're about as close to defect-free as you can get.[49] It's an ambitious quality goal! Although it is an extremely high standard to achieve, many quality-driven businesses are using it and benefiting from it. For instance, General Electric estimates that it has saved billions in costs since 1995, according to company executives.[50] Other well-known companies pursuing Six Sigma include ITT Industries, Dow Chemical, 3M Company, American Express, Sony Corporation, Nokia Corporation, and Johnson & Johnson. Although manufacturers seem to make up the bulk of Six Sigma users, service companies such as financial institutions, retailers, and health care organizations are beginning to apply it. What impact can Six Sigma have? Let's look at an example.

It used to take Wellmark Blue Cross & Blue Shield, a managed-care health care company, 65 days or more to add a new doctor to its medical plans. Now, thanks to Six Sigma, the company discovered that half the processes they used were redundant. With those unnecessary steps gone, the job now gets done in 30 days or less and with reduced staff. The company also has been able to reduce its administrative expenses by $3 million per year, an amount passed on to consumers through lower health care premiums.[51]

Although it's important for managers to recognize that many positive benefits come from reaching Six Sigma or obtaining ISO 9000 certification, the key benefit comes from the quality improvement journey itself. In other words, the goal of quality certification should be having work processes and an operations system in place that enable organizations to meet customers' needs and employees to perform their jobs in a consistently high-quality way.

Six Sigma
A quality program designed to reduce defects and help lower costs, save time, and improve customer satisfaction

Mass Customization and Lean Organization

The term *mass customization* seems an oxymoron. However, the design-to-order concept is becoming an important operations management issue for today's managers. **Mass customization** provides consumers with a product when, where, and how they want it.[52] Companies as diverse as BMW, Ford, Levi Strauss, Wells Fargo, Mattel, and Dell are adopting mass customization to maintain or attain a competitive advantage. Mass customization requires flexible manufacturing techniques and continual customer dialogue.[53] Technology plays an important role in both.

With flexible manufacturing, companies have the ability to quickly readjust assembly lines to make products to order. Using technology such as computer-controlled factory equipment, intranets, industrial robots, barcode scanners, digital printers, and logistics software, companies can manufacture, assemble, and ship customized products with customized packaging to customers in incredibly short timeframes. Dell is a good example of a company that uses flexible manufacturing techniques and technology to custom-build computers to customers' specifications.

mass customization
Providing customers with a product when, where, and how they want it

Technology also is important in the continual dialogue with customers. Using extensive databases, companies can keep track of customers' likes and dislikes. And the Internet has made it possible for companies to have ongoing dialogues with customers to learn about and respond to their exact preferences. For instance, on Amazon's Web site, customers are greeted by name and can get personalized recommendations of books and other products. The ability to customize products to a customer's desires and specifications starts an important relationship between the organization and the customer. If the customer likes the product and it provides value, he or she is more likely to be a repeat customer.

An intense focus on customers is also important in order to be a **lean organization**, which is an organization that understands what customers want, identifies customer value by analyzing all activities required to produce products, and then optimizes the entire process from the customer's perspective.[54] Lean organizations drive out all activities that do not add value in customers' eyes. For instance, companies like United Parcel Service, LVMH Moet Hennessy Louis Vuitton, and Harley-Davidson have pursued lean operations. "Lean operations adopt a philosophy of minimizing waste by striving for perfection through continuous learning, creativity, and teamwork."[55] As more manufacturers and service organizations adopt lean principles, they must realize that it's a never-ending journey toward being efficient and effective.

lean organization
An organization that understands what customers want, identifies customer value by analyzing all activities required to produce products, and then optimizes the entire process from the customer's perspective

MyManagementLab

Go to **mymanagementlab.com** to complete the problems marked with
this icon ⭐.

⭐ REVIEW AND DISCUSSION QUESTIONS

1. What is operations management?

2. Do you think that manufacturing or service organizations have the greater need for operations management? Explain.

3. What is a value chain and what is value chain management? What is the goal of value chain management? What are the benefits of value chain management?

4. What is required for successful value chain management? What obstacles exist to successful value chain management?

5. How could you use value chain management in your everyday life?

6. How does technology play a role in manufacturing?

7. What are ISO 9000 and Six Sigma?

8. Describe lean management and explain why it's important.

9. How might operations management apply to other managerial functions besides control?

10. Which is more critical to success in organizations: continuous improvement or quality control? Support your position.

ENDNOTES

1. K. Baxter, "Seoul Showcases Its Talent," *MEED: Middle East Economic Digest,* May 14, 2010, pp. 13–24; E. Ramstad, "High-Speed Wireless Transforms a Shipyard," *Wall Street Journal,* March 16, 2010, p. B6; and Datamonitor, "Company Profile: Hyundai Heavy Industries Co., Ltd." [www.datamonitor.com], November 27, 2009.

2. D. McGinn, "Faster Food," *Newsweek,* April 19, 2004, pp. E20–E22.

3. *World Factbook 2014,* available online at [https://www.cia.gov/library/publications/the-world-factbook/].

4. D. Michaels and J. L. Lunsford, "Streamlined Plane Making," *Wall Street Journal,* April 1, 2005, pp. B1+.

5. T. Aeppel, "Workers Not Included," *Wall Street Journal,* November 19, 2002, pp. B1+.

6. A. Aston and M. Arndt, "The Flexible Factory," *BusinessWeek,* May 5, 2003, pp. 90–91.

7. P. Panchak, "Pella Drives Lean Throughout the Enterprise," *Industry Week,* June 2003, pp. 74–77.

8. J. Ordonez, "McDonald's to Cut the Cooking Time of Its French Fries," *Wall Street Journal,* May 19, 2000, p. B2.

9. C. Fredman, "The Devil in the Details," *Executive Edge,* April–May 1999, pp. 36–39.

10. Information from [http://new.skoda-auto.com/Documents/AnnualReports/skoda_auto_annual_report_2007_%20EN_FINAL.pdf], July 8, 2008; and T. Mudd, "The Last Laugh," *Industry Week,* September 18, 2000, pp. 38–44.

11. W. E. Deming, "Improvement of Quality and Productivity Through Action by Management," *National Productivity Review,* Winter 1981–1982, pp. 12–22.

12. T. Vinas, "Little Things Mean a Lot," *Industry Week,* November 2002, p. 55.

13. "The Future of Manufacturing 2009," *Industry Week,* November 2009, pp. 25–31; T. D. Kuczmarski, "Remanufacturing America's Factory Sector," *BusinessWeek Online,* September 9, 2009; P. Panchak, "Shaping the Future of Manufacturing," *Industry Week,* January 2005, pp. 38–44; M. Hammer, "Deep Change: How Operational Innovation Can Transform Your Company," *Harvard Business Re-*

view, April 2004, pp. 84–94; S. Levy, "The Connected Company," *Newsweek,* April 28, 2003, pp. 40–48; and J. Teresko, "Plant Floor Strategy," *Industry Week,* July 2002, pp. 26–32.

14. T. Laseter, K. Ramdas, and D. Swerdlow, "The Supply Side of Design and Development," *Strategy+Business,* Summer 2003, p. 23; J. Jusko, "Not All Dollars and Cents," *Industry Week,* April 2002, p. 58; and D. Drickhamer, "Medical Marvel," *Industry Week,* March 2002, pp. 47–49.

15. J. H. Sheridan, "Managing the Value Chain," *Industry Week* [www.industryweek.com], September 6, 1999, pp. 1–4.

16. Ibid., p. 3.

17. J. Teresko, "Forward, March!" *Industry Week,* July 2004, pp. 43–48; D. Sharma, C. Lucier, and R. Molloy, "From Solutions to Symbiosis: Blending with Your Customers," *Strategy+Business,* Second Quarter 2002, pp. 38–48; and S. Leibs, "Getting Ready: Your Suppliers," *Industry Week* [www.industryweek.com], September 6, 1999.

18. D. Bartholomew, "The Infrastructure," *Industry Week* [www.industryweek.com], September 6, 1999, p. 1.

19. T. Stevens, "Integrated Product Development," *Industry Week,* June 2002, pp. 21–28.

20. T. Vinas, "A Map of the World: IW Value-Chain Survey," *Industry Week,* September 2005, pp. 27–34.

21. C. Burritt, C. Wolf, and M. Boyle, "Why Wal-Mart Wants to Take the Driver's Seat," *Bloomberg BusinessWeek,* May 31–June 6, 2010, pp. 17–18.

22. R. Normann and R. Ramirez, "From Value Chain to Value Constellation," *Harvard Business Review on Managing the Value Chain* (Boston, MA: Harvard Business School Press, 2000), pp. 185–219.

23. "Collaboration Is the Key to Reducing Costs," *Industry Week,* October 2009, p. 35; J. Teresko, "The Tough Get Going," *Industry Week,* March 2005, pp. 25–32; D. M. Lambert and A. M. Knemeyer, "We're in This Together," *Harvard Business Review,* December 2004, pp. 114–122; and V. G. Narayanan and A. Raman, "Aligning Incentives in Supply Chains," *Harvard Business Review,* November 2004, pp. 94–102.

24. D. Drickhamer, "Looking for Value," *Industry Week,* December 2002, pp. 41–43.
25. J. L. Yang, "Veggie Tales," *Fortune,* June 8, 2009, pp. 25–30.
26. J. Jusko, "Focus. Discipline. Results," *Industry Week,* June 2010, pp. 16–17.
27. J. H. Sheridan, "Managing the Value Chain," p. 3.
28. S. Leibs, "Getting Ready: Your Customers," *Industry Week* [www.industryweek.com], September 6, 1999, p. 1.
29. G. Taninecz, "Forging the Chain," *Industry Week,* May 15, 2000, pp. 40–46.
30. S. Leibs, "Getting Ready: Your Customers."
31. J. Katz, "Empowering the Workforce," *Industry Week,* January 2009, p. 43.
32. D. Blanchard, "In the Rotation," *Industry Week,* January 2009, p. 42.
33. N. Zubko, "Mindful of the Surroundings," *Industry Week,* January 2009, p. 38.
34. "Top Security Threats and Management Issues Facing Corporate America: 2003 Survey of *Fortune* 1000 Companies," ASIS International and Pinkerton [www.asisonline.org].
35. J. H. Sheridan, "Managing the Value Chain," p. 4.
36. R. Russell and B. W. Taylor, *Operations Management,* 5th ed. (New York: Wiley, 2005); C. Liu-Lien Tan, "U.S. Response: Speedier Delivery," *Wall Street Journal,* November 18, 2004, pp. D1+; and C. Salter, "When Couches Fly," *Fast Company,* July 2004, pp. 80–81.
37. D. Joseph, "The GPS Revolution: Location, Location, Location," *BusinessWeek Online,* May 27, 2009.
38. J. Jargon, "Domino's IT Staff Delivers Slick Site, Ordering System," *Wall Street Journal,* November 24, 2009, p. B5; and S. Anderson, The Associated Press, "Restaurants Gear Up for Window Wars," *Springfield, Missouri, News-Leader,* January 27, 2006, p. 5B.
39. S. McCartney, "A Radical Cockpit Upgrade Southwest Fliers Will Feel," *Wall Street Journal,* April 1, 2010, p. D1.
40. D. Bartholomew, "Quality Takes a Beating," *Industry Week,* March 2006, pp. 46–54; J. Carey and M. Arndt, "Making Pills the Smart Way," *BusinessWeek,* May 3, 2004, pp. 102–103; and A. Barrett, "Schering's Dr. Feelbetter?" *BusinessWeek,* June 23, 2003, pp. 55–56.
41. T. Vinas, "Six Sigma Rescue," *Industry Week,* March 2004, p. 12.
42. J. S. McClenahen, "Prairie Home Companion," *Industry Week,* October 2005, pp. 45–46.
43. T. Vinas, "Zeroing In on the Customer," *Industry Week,* October 2004, pp. 61–62.
44. W. Royal, "Spotlight Shines on Maquiladora," *Industry Week,* October 16, 2000, pp. 91–92.
45. See B. Whitford and R. Andrew (eds.), *The Pursuit of Quality* (Perth: Beaumont Publishing, 1994).
46. D. Drickhamer, "Road to Excellence," *Industry Week,* October 16, 2000, pp. 117–118.
47. J. Heizer and B. Render, *Operations Management,* 10th ed. (Upper Saddle River, NJ: Prentice Hall, 2011), p. 193.
48. G. Hasek, "Merger Marries Quality Efforts," *Industry Week,* August 21, 2000, pp. 89–92.
49. M. Arndt, "Quality Isn't Just for Widgets," *BusinessWeek,* July 22, 2002, pp. 72–73.
50. E. White, "Rethinking the Quality Improvement Program," *Wall Street Journal,* September 19, 2005, p. B3.
51. M. Arndt, "Quality Isn't Just for Widgets."
52. S. McMurray, "Ford's F-150: Have It Your Way," *Business 2.0,* March 2004, pp. 53–55; "Made-to-Fit Clothes Are on the Way," *USA Today,* July 2002, pp. 8–9; and L. Elliott, "Mass Customization Comes a Step Closer," *Design News,* February 18, 2002, p. 21.
53. E. Schonfeld, "The Customized, Digitized, Have-It-Your-Way Economy," *Fortune,* October 28, 1998, pp. 114–120.
54. Heizer and Render, *Operations Management,* p. 636; and S. Minter, "Measuring the Success of Lean," *Industry Week,* February 2010, pp. 32–35.
55. Heizer and Render, *Operations Management,* p. 636.

Management Practice: Part 6

Management Practice

A Manager's Dilemma

Vancouver, Canada–based Lululemon Athletica Inc. is a well-known manufacturer of yoga and athletic apparel, which is sold in over 250 stores, mostly in North America but also in Australia and New Zealand. Lululemon has built a loyal, almost obsessive/cult-like, customer base. One customer commented that, "Once you go Lululemon, you never go back" (H. Malcom, "Lulu's No Downward Dog," *USA Today*, March 20, 2013, p. 1B+). Others have credited the company's apparel as the reason they started—or continued to—exercise. Retail experts portray the brand positioning to be as much about selling a way of life as selling cute and colorful yoga pants. Customers can take a free yoga class at the stores and be assisted by cheery, knowledgeable employees. All seemed to be well and good, even fantastic, in Lululemon's world. Then, a batch of too-sheer stretchy pants—one of the company's core products—happened. This problem was the company's fourth quality-control issue in the span of a year. And for a company that built a billion-dollar business selling premium yoga gear at high prices, this particular problem was a costly stumble. The company responded by recalling the batch of sheer, too-revealing black yoga pants and commenting that, "This event is not the result of changing manufacturers or quality of ingredients" ("Black luon pants shortage expected," Lululemon Athletica, Press Release March 18, 2003). The recall of its top-selling pants proved to be expensive and embarrassing to the company, which had long hyped itself as a premium brand.

Pretend you're part of the management team. Using what you've learned about monitoring and controlling, what five things would you suggest the team focus on? Think carefully about your suggestions to the team.

Global Sense

This is a story about the global economy. It's about markets, politics, and public opinion. And as jobs—especially white-collar and professional jobs—continue to be outsourced and offshored, the story hits closer and closer to home. Although the terms *offshoring* and *outsourcing* are often used interchangeably, they do mean different things. **Offshoring** is relocating business processes (production and services) from one country to another. **Outsourcing** is moving noncore activities from being done internally to being done externally by an entity that specializes in that activity.

One of the realities of a global economy is that to be competitive, strategic decision makers must look for the best places to do business. If a car can be made more cheaply in Mexico, maybe it should be. If a telephone inquiry can be processed more cheaply in India or the Philippines, maybe it should be. And if programming code can be written more cheaply in China or Russia, maybe it should be. Almost any professional job that can be done outside the organization is up for grabs. There's nothing political or philosophical about the reason for shipping jobs elsewhere. The bottom line is that it can save companies money. But there's a price to be paid in terms of angry and anxious employees. So, are offshoring and outsourcing bad?

Critics say "yes." It's affecting jobs once considered "safe" across a wider range of professional work activities. And the offshoring and outsourcing have taken place at a breathtaking pace. What this means is that the careers college students are preparing for probably won't sustain them in the long run. This structural change in the U.S. economy also means that the workforce is likely to face frequent career changes and downward pressures on wages.

Proponents say "no." Their argument is based on viewing economic development as a ladder with every country trying to climb to the next rung. And it's foolish to think that in the United States we've reached the top of the ladder and there's nowhere else to go. Although people fear that educated U.S. workers will face the same fate as blue-collar workers whose jobs shifted to lower-cost countries, the truth is that the United States currently still has a competitive advantage in innovation; although, as discussed earlier, that may be in jeopardy. The biggest danger to U.S. workers isn't overseas competition; it's worrying too much about other countries climbing up the economic ladder and not worrying enough about finding that next higher rung.

Finally, economic forces at work in the latest global recession that led to rapidly rising labor rates in those geographic areas where costs had been low, coupled with higher materials and shipping costs and attractive tax incentives from various U.S. states, may combine to lure back U.S. firms.

Who's right? We probably can't answer that question just yet. Only time will tell. However, we do know that what we're seeing with offshoring and outsourcing is another example of why decision makers need to be aware of the context within which their organizations are doing business.

Discuss the following questions in light of what you learned:

• *How are offshoring and outsourcing similar? How are they different?*

- *What arguments do critics use to say offshoring and outsourcing are bad?*
- *What arguments do proponents use to say offshoring and outsourcing are not bad?*
- *How does the decision to offshore and outsource affect monitoring and controlling activities?*
- *Is it just manufacturers that deal with these decisions/issues? Discuss.*

Sources: D. Searcey, "Judges Turn to Outsourcing as Cases Get More Complex," Wall Street Journal, September 30, 2013; A. Fisher, "Got a Back-Office Job? It May Be Headed Overseas," management.fortune.cnn.com, September 12, 2013; S. Cendrowski, "Can Outsourcing Be Improved? Fortune, June 10, 2013, pp. 14–17; A. Fox, "America Inc.," HR Magazine, May 2013, pp. 44–48; K. O'Sullivan, "Practiced, But Not Perfect," CFO, March 2013, pp. 52–53; J. Bussey, "Will Costs Drive Firms Home?" Wall Street Journal, May 5, 2011, pp. B1+; D. Wessel, "Big U.S. Firms Shift Hiring Abroad," Wall Street Journal, April 19, 2011, pp. B1+; P. Engardio, M. Arndt, and D. Foust, "The Future of Outsourcing," BusinessWeek, January 30, 2006, pp. 50–58; J. Thottam, "Is Your Job Going Abroad?" Time, March 1, 2004, pp. 26–36; L. D. Tyson, "Outsourcing: Who's Safe Anymore?" BusinessWeek, February 23, 2004, p. 26; A. Fisher, "Think Globally, Save Your Job Locally," Fortune, February 23, 2004, p. 60; "The New Job Migration," The Economist, February 21, 2004, p. 11; O. Thomas, "The Outsourcing Solution," Business 2.0, September 2003, pp. 159–160; and K. Madigan and M. J. Mandel, "Outsourcing Jobs: Is It Bad?" BusinessWeek, August 25, 2003, pp. 36–38.

Starbucks—Controlling

Once managers have established goals and plans and organized and structured to pursue those goals, the manager's job isn't done. Quite the opposite! Managers must now monitor work activities to make sure they're being done as planned and correct any significant deviations. At Starbucks, managers control various functions, activities, processes, and procedures to ensure that desired performance standards are achieved at all organizational levels.

Controlling the Coffee Experience

Why has Starbucks been so successful? Although many factors have contributed to its success, one significant factor is its ability to provide customers with a unique product of the highest quality delivered with exceptional service. Everything that each Starbucks partner does, from top level to bottom level, contributes to the company's ability to do that efficiently and effectively. And managers need controls in place to help monitor and evaluate what's being done and how it's being done. Starbucks' managers use different types of controls to ensure that the company meets its goals. These controls include transactions controls, security controls, employee controls, and organizational performance controls.

A legal recruiter stops by Starbucks on her way to her office in downtown Chicago and orders her daily Caffè Mocha tall. A construction site supervisor pulls into the drive-through line at the Starbucks store in Rancho Cucamonga, California, for a cinnamon chip scone and Tazo tea. It's 11 P.M. and, needing a break from studying for her next-day's management exam, a student heads to the local Starbucks for a tasty treat—a Raspberry Pomegranate Starbucks Refresher. Now she's ready again to tackle that chapter material on managerial controls.

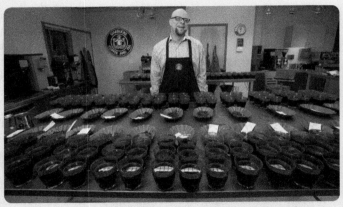

Scott McMartin, Starbucks' director of global coffee advocacy, poses in the cupping room at company headquarters where quality control tastings take place daily. Starbuck's coffee buyers, tasters, and quality control team members taste an average 1,000 cups per day as part of Starbucks' stringent control activities to meet its goal of providing customers with a unique product of the highest quality.
Source: Marcus Donner/Reuters

Every week, an average 60 million transactions take place at a Starbucks store. The average dollar sale per transaction is $7.01. These transactions between partners (employees) and customers—the exchange of products for money—are the major source of sales revenue for Starbucks. Measuring and evaluating the efficiency and effectiveness of these transactions for both walk-in customers and customers at drive-through windows is important. As Starbucks has been doing walk-in transactions for a number of years, numerous procedures and processes are in place to make those transactions go smoothly. However, as Starbucks adds more drive-through windows, the focus of the transaction is on being fast as well as on quality—a different metric than for walk-in transactions. When a customer walks into a store and orders, he can step aside while the order is being prepared; that's not possible in a drive-through line. Recognizing these limitations, the company is taking steps to improve its drive-through service. For instance, digital timers are placed where employees can easily see them to measure service times; order confirmation screens are used to help keep accuracy rates high; and additional pastry racks have been conveniently located by the drive-through windows.

Security is also an important issue for Starbucks. Keeping company assets (such as people, equipment, products, financial information, and so forth) safe and secure requires security controls. The company is committed to providing all partners with a clean, safe, and healthy work environment. All partners share the responsibility to follow all safety rules and practices; to cooperate with officials who enforce those rules and practices; to take necessary steps to protect ourselves and other partners; to attend required safety training; and to report immediately all accidents, injuries, and unsafe practices or conditions. When hired, each partner is provided with a manual that covers

safety, security, and health standards and is trained on the requirements outlined in the manual. In addition, managers receive ongoing training about these issues and are expected to keep employees trained and up-to-date on any changes. And at any time, any partner can contact the Partner & Asset Protection Department for information and advice.

One security area that has been particularly important to Starbucks has been with its gift cards, in which it does an enormous volume of business. With gift cards, there are lots of opportunities for an unethical employee to "steal" from the company. The company's director of compliance has said that detecting such fraud can be difficult because it's often not apparent from an operations standpoint. However, Starbucks uses transactional data analysis technology to detect multiple card redemptions in a single day and has identified other "telltale" activities that pinpoint possible fraud. When the company's technology detects transaction activity outside the norm, Starbucks' corporate staff is alerted and a panel of company experts reviews the data. Investigators have found individuals at stores who confess to stealing as much as $42,000. When smaller exceptions are noted, the individuals are sent letters asking them to explain what's going on. Employees who have been so "notified" often quit.

Starbucks' part-time and full-time hourly partners are the primary—and most important—source of contact between the company and the customer, and exemplary customer service is a top priority at Starbucks. Partners are encouraged to strive to make every customer's experience pleasant and fulfilling and to treat customers with respect and dignity. What kinds of employee controls does Starbucks use to ensure that this happens? Partners are trained in and are required to follow all proper procedures relating to the storage, handling, preparation, and service of Starbucks' products. In addition, partners are told to notify their managers immediately if they see anything that suggests a product may pose a danger to the health or safety of themselves or of customers. Partners also are taught the warning signs associated with possible workplace violence and how to reduce their vulnerability if faced with a potentially violent situation. In either circumstance where product or partner safety and security are threatened, store managers have been trained as far as the appropriate steps to take if such a situation occurs.

The final types of control that are important to Starbucks' managers are the organizational performance and financial controls. Starbucks uses the typical financial control measures, but also looks at growth in sales at stores open at least one year as a performance standard. One continual challenge is trying to control store operating costs. There's a fine balance the company has to achieve between keeping costs low and keeping quality high. However, there are steps the company has taken to control costs. For instance, new thinner garbage bags will save the company half a million dollars a year.

In addition to the typical financial measures, corporate governance procedures and guidelines are an important part of Starbucks' financial controls, as they are at any public corporation that's covered by Sarbanes-Oxley legislation. The company has identified guidelines for its board of directors with respect to responsibilities, processes, procedures, and expectations.

Starbucks' Value Chain: From Bean to Cup

The steaming cup of coffee placed in a customer's hand at any Starbucks store location starts as coffee beans (berries) plucked from fields of coffee plants. From harvest to storage to roasting to retail to cup, Starbucks understands the important role each participant in its value chain plays.

Starbucks offers a selection of coffees from around the world, and its coffee buyers personally travel to the coffee-growing regions of Latin America, Africa/Arabia, and Asia/Pacific in order to select and purchase the highest-quality *arabica* beans. Once the beans arrive at any one of the five roasting facilities in the United States and three global facilities, Starbucks' master professional roasters take over. These individuals know coffee and do their "magic" in creating the company's rich signature roast coffee in a process that brings balance to all of its flavor attributes. There are many potential challenges to "transforming" the raw material into the quality product and experience that customers have come to expect at Starbucks. Weather, shipping and logistics, technology, political instability, and so forth all could potentially impact what Starbucks is in business to do.

One issue of great importance to Starbucks is environmental protection. Starbucks has taken actions throughout its entire supply chain to minimize its "environmental footprint." For instance, suppliers are asked to sign a code of conduct that deals with certain expectations in business standards and practices. Even company stores are focused on the environmental impact of their store operations. For instance, partners at stores around the world have found innovative ways to reuse coffee grounds. In Japan, for example, a team of Starbucks partners realized that coffee grounds could be used as an ingredient to make paper. A local printing company uses this paper to print the official Starbucks Japan newsletter. In Bahrain, partners dry coffee grounds in the sun, package them, and give them to customers as fertilizer for house plants.

Discussion Questions

1. What companies might be good benchmarks for Starbucks? Why? What companies might want to benchmark Starbucks? Why?
2. Describe how the following Starbucks managers might use forecasting, budgeting, and scheduling (be specific): (a) a retail store manager; (b) a regional marketing manager; (c) the manager for global development; and (d) the CEO.

3. What control criteria might be useful to a retail store manager? To a barista at one of Starbucks's walk-in-only retail stores? How about for a store that has a drive-through?

4. What types of feedforward, concurrent, and feedback controls does Starbucks use? Are there others that might be important to use? If so, describe.

5. What "red flags" might indicate significant deviations from standard for (a) an hourly partner; (b) a store manager; (c) a district manager; (d) the executive vice president of finance; and (e) the CEO? Are there any similarities? Why or why not?

6. Evaluate the control measures Starbucks is using with its gift cards from the standpoint of the three steps in the control process.

7. Using the company's most current financial statements, calculate the following financial ratios: current, debt to assets, inventory turnover, total asset turnover, profit margin on sales, and return on investment. What do these ratios tell managers?

8. Would you describe Starbucks' production/operations technology in its retail stores as unit, mass, or process? How about in its roasting plants?

9. Can Starbucks manage the uncertainties in its value chain? If so, how? If not, why not?

10. Go to the company's Web site [www.starbucks.com]. Find the information on the company's environmental activities from bean to cup. Select one of the steps in the chain (or your professor may assign you one). Describe and evaluate what environmental actions it's taking. How might these affect the planning, organizing, and controlling taking place in these areas?

11. Look at the company's mission and guiding principles on its Web site. How might these affect the way Starbucks controls? How do the ways Starbucks controls contribute to the attainment or pursuit of these?

Notes for the Continuing Case

Information from Starbucks Corporation 2013 Annual Report, www.investor.starbucks.com, May, 2014; Company Web site, www.starbucks.com; C. Cain Miller, "Starbucks and Square to Team Up," *New York Times Online*, August 8, 2012; Starbucks Corporation 2011 Annual Report, www.investor.starbucks.com, August 6, 2012; Starbucks News Release, "Starbucks Reports Record Third Quarter Results," www.investor.starbucks.com, July 26, 2012; R. Ahmed, "Tata Setting Up Starbucks Coffee Roasting Facility," www.online.wsj.com, July 26, 2012; B. Horovitz, "Starbucks Rolling Out Pop with Pep," *USA Today*, March 22, 2012, p. 1B; Starbucks News Release, "Starbucks Spotlights Connection Between Record Performance, Shareholder Value, and Company Values at Annual Meeting of Shareholders," news.starbucks.com, March 21, 2012; D. A. Kaplan, "Strong Coffee," *Fortune*, December 12, 2011, pp. 100–116; J. A. Cooke, ed., "From Bean to Cup: How Starbucks Transformed Its Supply Chain," www.supplychainquarterly.com, Quarter 4, 2010; R. Ruggless, "Starbucks Exec: Security from Employee Theft Important When Implementing Gift Card Strategies," *Nation's Restaurant News*, December 12, 2005, p. 24; and R. Ruggless, "Transaction Monitoring Boosts Safety, Perks Up Coffee Chain Profits," *Nation's Restaurant News*, November 28, 2005, p. 35.

Index

Work, 3-27, 30, 32-42, 48, 52, 55, 57, 63-64, 67, 69,
    72, 74-76, 80-81, 84-87, 89-91, 93-95,
    97-99, 102-104, 106-108, 110-111, 117, 121,
    124, 126, 128-130, 132, 134-137, 139-140,
    142, 144, 148-153, 155-156, 158-163, 165,
    167-174, 176-179, 183-184, 186-205,
    208-209, 211, 213, 216, 219-220, 222-223,
    226, 228, 231, 235, 239-240, 244-248,
    250-257, 259-264, 266-269, 272-281,
    283-290, 292-298, 301-308, 311, 313-324,
    326-327, 329-335, 338-342, 345-349,
    351-372, 374-377, 380-399, 401-405,
    408-416, 418-431, 433-451, 454-455,
    457-458, 462-464, 466, 468-471, 473, 476,
    479-482, 484-489, 494-505, 508-510,
    512-519, 522-523, 526-529, 531-537,
    542-543
    attitudes toward, 172, 176, 387
Work councils, 307
work products, 364
Work schedules, 354
Work specialization, 161, 246-248, 256, 261-262, 273,
    276
Work teams, 7, 35, 91, 195, 274, 278, 289, 322, 345,
    348, 351, 356-358, 361, 370-372, 440, 466,
    469, 532, 536
    Cross-functional, 274, 289, 357-358, 536
    global, 195, 278, 289, 345, 361, 371-372
    types of, 356-357, 440, 536
Work unit orientation, 315
Workers, 7, 15, 18-19, 23, 26, 30-34, 41, 63, 84, 87,
    99-100, 104, 106, 121, 125, 139, 141-142,
    150, 152, 155, 170-172, 174, 176-177, 232,
    238, 240, 246-247, 254, 257-258, 272,
    277-278, 285-286, 289, 293, 296-298,
    304-305, 307-308, 310, 314, 319-323, 325,
    332, 334-335, 341, 355, 357-358, 369, 376,
    384, 404, 406, 409, 411-413, 418, 420-421,
    426-429, 433, 435-437, 439, 442, 447-450,
    470, 509, 512, 518-519, 521-523, 525, 527,
    532, 539, 542
    skilled, 84, 247, 285, 304, 308, 436, 442
    unskilled, 247
Workers' compensation, 125
workforce, 4, 6, 12, 14, 26-27, 72, 74, 85, 106-108,
    140-142, 146, 172, 174, 176, 180, 191, 205,
    253, 268, 273, 281, 284-286, 289, 293,
    296-298, 302, 304, 307-310, 313, 319, 323,
    332-335, 338, 341, 371, 374, 376-377, 395,
    403, 410, 413, 415-416, 426, 436, 442,
    449-451, 511, 513, 522-523, 540, 542
    diversity in, 180
    women in, 74, 307
Workforce Management, 26-27, 108, 140, 172, 174,
    281, 296-297, 332-335, 413, 415, 449-451,
    511, 513, 523
Workforce reduction, 449
Work-life balance, 170, 307, 320, 323, 332, 341-342,
    383, 387, 404, 435-436, 449
    cultural differences in, 435
workplace, 1-2, 4-27, 36, 42-43, 74, 84-85, 97-101,
    108, 117, 121, 125, 134-135, 142, 145, 148,
    153, 155, 157, 170-174, 176-180, 193, 208,
    259, 269, 272-273, 276, 283-286, 289, 293,
    296, 306-307, 319-320, 322-324, 326-328,
    333-335, 339, 346, 363, 366, 371-372, 376,
    383, 386-387, 394-395, 403-407, 409-410,
    412-416, 426, 433-435, 438-439, 445-447,
    449, 469, 481, 485-486, 488, 494-495, 501,
    508-510, 512-513, 516-519, 521-523, 544
    changing, 4-6, 13-14, 20, 43, 135, 142, 148, 155,
        319, 333, 339, 403, 412, 426, 446, 518
Workplace discrimination, 14
Workplace environment, 4, 179, 363, 486, 488, 510
Workplace incivility, 416
Workplace misbehavior, 383, 386, 405-406
Workplace spirituality, 97-98, 100-101, 108
    characteristics of, 98, 100
Workplace violence, 495, 512-513, 516, 523, 544
World, 2-5, 8, 13, 16-17, 21, 26, 32, 37, 41, 48, 56, 59,
    62-65, 67, 69, 72, 74-76, 82-86, 94, 97,
    105-107, 111-113, 115-118, 121, 123, 127,
    129, 131-134, 136-138, 140-142, 145,
    147-148, 151, 154, 160, 169-172, 174,
    176-177, 179, 181, 187, 189, 193-195, 197,
    204-205, 208-210, 215, 218, 220, 231,
    233-236, 238-240, 245, 259, 268, 273,
    276-277, 279-280, 283-284, 296-297, 302,
    307, 309-311, 329-330, 332-335, 342, 358,

362, 367-368, 370, 374-377, 388, 390, 410,
    413, 415-416, 425, 435, 439, 450, 459, 462,
    482, 486, 488-489, 500, 507, 509, 520, 522,
    525-526, 528, 530, 533, 539, 542, 544
World Economic Forum, 72, 84, 118
World economy, 83
World Factbook, 26, 539
World Health Organization, 367
World War, 37, 528
Written essays, 326
Written reports, 496
Written tests, 326
WWW, 3, 7-9, 15, 18, 26-27, 47, 54, 57, 60, 63, 67,
    71-72, 74, 76-77, 81, 85, 94-95, 98, 106,
    111, 113, 115, 117-118, 121, 124, 129-131,
    136, 139-142, 145-146, 160-162, 171-174,
    176-177, 179-181, 185, 193, 195-196,
    204-205, 209, 211, 213-214, 219, 221, 224,
    234-236, 240-241, 245, 257, 259, 268, 273,
    277, 287-288, 296-298, 301, 305, 309, 312,
    316, 319, 324, 329, 331-335, 342, 345, 348,
    355-356, 358, 360, 370-372, 374, 377, 381,
    395, 397, 411-413, 415-416, 419, 423, 433,
    436, 439, 444, 447, 449-450, 455, 464, 467,
    472, 479, 481, 485, 489, 493, 498, 500, 508,
    510, 514, 521-523, 536, 539-540, 545

X
Xers, 308

Y
Yen, 268, 472
YouTube, 105, 151, 216
Yuan, 174

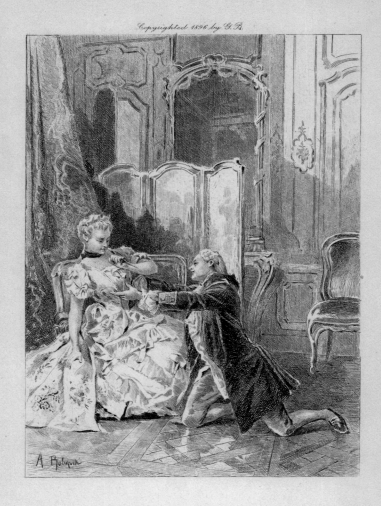

LA ZAMBINELLA AND SARRASINE

———

"'If you approach,' she said, 'I shall be forced to plunge this weapon in your heart. Go! You would despise me. I have conceived too much respect for your character to deliver myself thus. I do not wish to destroy the sentiment which you have for me.'

"'Ah! ah!' said Sarrasine, 'it is a bad way to extinguish a passion by exciting it.'

The *Edition Définitive* of the *Comédie
Humaine* by HONORÉ DE BALZAC,
now for the first time completely translated
into English.

*THE HOUSE OF NUCINGEN. THE SECRETS OF
LA PRINCESSE DE CADIGNAN. SARRASINE.
FACINO CANE. A MAN OF BUSINESS. THE
INVOLUNTARY COMEDIANS. IN ONE
VOLUME. TRANSLATED BY WILLIAM
WALTON, AND ILLUSTRATED
WITH FOUR ETCHINGS.*

PHILADELPHIA: PRINTED FOR SUBSCRIBERS
ONLY BY GEORGE BARRIE & SON.

THE HOUSE OF NUCINGEN

Is it not to you, Madame, whose lofty and upright intelligence is as a treasure for all your friends, to you, who are at once for me an entire public and the most indulgent of sisters, that I should dedicate this work? Deign to accept it in testimony of a friendship of which I am proud. You and some other souls, fine as your own, will comprehend my design in reading *The House of Nucingen* coupled with *César Birotteau*. In this contrast, is there not an entire social lesson?

DE BALZAC.

THE HOUSE OF NUCINGEN

*

You are acquainted with the thinness of the partitions which separate the little apartments, the *cabinets particuliers*, in the most elegant restaurants in Paris. In that of Véry, for instance, the largest room is cut in two by a partition which is removed and restored at will. This scene is not laid there, but in a good locality, which it is not convenient for me to designate. There were two of us. I will say, then, like the Prudhomme of Henry Monnier: "I would not wish to compromise her." We were lingering over the delicacies of a dinner, admirable in many respects, in a little apartment, in which we were conversing in low tones, having due regard for the lack of thickness of partition. We had progressed as far as the roast without having had any neighbors in the apartment adjoining ours, in which we heard only the crackling of the fire. Eight o'clock sounded. There was a great noise of feet, the sound of words exchanged, the waiters brought candles. It was demonstrated to us that the neighboring apartment was occupied. In recognizing the voices, I knew what sort of personages were these

occupants. They were four of the most enterprising
cormorants sprung from the foam which tops the
incessantly renewed waves of the present generation; good-natured youths, whose support is prob-
lematical, who are not known to possess either
incomes or estates, and yet who live well. These
clever *condottieri* of modern industry, which has
become the cruelest of wars, leave all the worries to
their creditors, keep all the pleasures for themselves,
and have no other care than that of their apparel.
Moreover, bold enough to smoke, like Jean Bart,
their cigar over a barrel of powder, perhaps in order
not to fail in their particular rôle; greater scoffers,
even, than the smaller newspapers, scoffers that
would not hesitate to ridicule themselves; perspi-
cacious and incredulous, inquirers into the affairs
of others, avaricious and prodigal, envious of others,
but satisfied with themselves; profound politicians
at moments, analyzing all, guessing at everything,
they had not yet been able to shine in the world in
which they wished to display themselves. One
only of the four had succeeded, but only to the foot
of the ladder. It is nothing to have money, and a
parvenu only knows what is deficient in him after
six months of flatteries. Not much of a talker, cold,
affectedly grave, without wit, this parvenu, whose
name was Andoche Finot, had had heart enough to
prostrate himself on his stomach before those who
could serve him, and wit enough to be insolent to
those of whom he had no need. Like one of the
grotesque figures of the ballet of "Gustave," he was

marquis behind and a villain in front. This industrial prelate kept a train-bearer, Émile Blondet, editor of a newspaper, a man of a good deal of ingenuity, but ill-regulated, bright, capable, lazy, knowing himself exploited, but permitting himself to be so; perfidious, as he was good, by impulses; one of those men whom you like and for whom you have no respect. Sharp as a soubrette of comedy, incapable of refusing his pen to any one who asked it and his heart to anyone who borrowed it, Émile is the most attractive of these girl-men of whom the most fanciful of our wits has said: "I like them better in satin slippers than in boots." The third man, named Couture, supported himself by speculations. He grafted one enterprise upon another; the success of one covered the failure of the other. Thus he maintained himself on the surface, sustained by the nervous strength of his activity, by sharp and audacious strokes. He swam about here and there, seeking in the immense sea of Parisian affairs an islet sufficiently contestable for him to lodge himself thereon. Evidently, he was not in his place. As to the last, the most malicious of the four, his name alone will suffice: Bixiou! Alas, it was no longer the Bixiou of 1825, but the one of 1836, the misanthropical buffoon, with his mad fancy and biting wit, a poor devil exasperated at having expended so much wit in pure loss, furious at not having picked up his lucky find in the last revolution, giving a kick to each one like a true Pierrot of the Funambules, having the

knowledge of his own epoch and of its scandalous
adventures on the tips of his fingers, ornamenting
them with his own droll inventions, leaping on
everybody's shoulders like a clown and endeavoring to leave a mark there like an executioner.

After having satisfied the first cravings of gour-
mandizing, our neighbors arrived at the station in
which we were in our dinner, at the dessert; and,
thanks to our silence, they thought themselves alone.
With the smoke of the cigars, with the aid of
the champagne, interspersed with the gastronomical
pleasures of the dessert, they fell into familiar conversation. Characterized by that icy spirit which
stiffens the most elastic sentiments, arrests the
most generous inspirations, and gives to laughter
something cutting, this talking, full of the bitter
irony which changes gaiety into sneering, betrayed
the exhaustion of souls delivered over entirely to
themselves, without any other aim than the satisfaction of egotism, a fruit of the peace in which we
dwell. That pamphlet against man which Diderot
did not dare to publish, *le Neveu de Rameau,* that
book, which reveals everything in order to show
the wounds, is alone comparable to this pamphlet
uttered without any after-thought, in which the language does not even respect that which the thinker
is still discussing, in which nothing is constructed
save with ruins, in which everything is denied, in
which nothing is admired save that which skepti-
cism adopts,—the omnipotence, the omniscience, the
all-congruity of money. After having taken stray

shots in the circle of acquaintances, back-biting now began to massacre intimate friends. One indication will suffice to explain the desire which I had to remain and to listen to the moment when Bixiou began to speak, as will be seen. We then heard one of those terrible improvisations which secured for this artist his reputation among a certain number of blasé spirits; and though often interrupted, commenced and recommenced, it was stenographed in my memory. Opinions and form, everything was outside of all literary conditions. But this is what it was,—a pot-pourri of sinister things which paint our time, of which should be recounted none but similar histories, and I leave the responsibility, moreover, to the principal narrator. The pantomime, the gestures, in harmony with the frequent changes of the voice by which Bixiou depicted the various personages brought on to the scene, must have been perfect, for his three auditors uttered from time to time approving exclamations and satisfied interjections.

"And Rastignac refused you?" said Blondet to Finot.

"Flatly."

"But did you threaten him with the papers?" asked Bixiou.

"He just laughed," answered Finot.

"Rastignac is the direct heir of the late De Marsay; he makes his way in politics as in the world," said Blondet.

"But how did he make his fortune?" asked

Couture. "He was in 1819, with the illustrious
Bianchon, in a miserable boarding-house of the Latin
Quarter; his family dined on scraps and drank raw
wine, so as to send him a hundred francs a month;
the estate of his father was not worth a thousand
écus; he had two sisters and a brother on his hands,
and now—"

"Now, he has an income of forty thousand
francs," resumed Finot; "each of his sisters is
richly dowered, married in the nobility, and he has
left the usufruct of his estate to his mother—"

"In 1827," said Blondet, "I saw him still without a sou."

"Oh! in 1827!" said Bixiou.

"Well," resumed Finot, "to-day we see him in a
fair way to become a minister, peer of France, and
everything that he could wish! Three years ago
he got rid of Delphine comfortably; he will only
marry under good conditions, and he can marry
some young girl of noble rank, he can!—The scamp
has had the good sense to attach himself to a rich
woman."

"My friends, give him credit for favorable circumstances," said Blondet; "he fell into the hands
of a clever man when he escaped from the clutches
of poverty."

"You know Nucingen well," said Bixiou; "in
the early days, Delphine and Rastignac found him
good; a wife seemed to be for him in his house, a
plaything, an ornament. And this is what, for me,
makes this man so remarkable and decided,—

Nucingen does not hesitate to say that his wife is the representation of his fortune, an indispensable *thing*, but one of secondary value in the life at high pressure of men in politics and the great financiers. He said, before me, that Bonaparte was as stupid as a bourgeois in his first relations with Joséphine, and that, after having had the courage to take her for a stepping-stone, he was ridiculous in being willing to make a companion of her."

"Every man of superior qualities should have concerning women the opinions of the Orient," said Blondet.

"The baron melted the Oriental and Occidental doctrines together into a charming Parisian doctrine. He held De Marsay in horror, as he was not manageable, but Rastignac pleased him a great deal and he exploited him without Rastignac's having the least idea of it: he put on him all the charge of his household. Rastignac took on his back all the whims of Delphine, he drove her to the Bois, he accompanied her to the theatre. This great little man of politics of to-day for a long time passed his life in reading and writing pretty notes. In the commencement of things, Eugène was scolded for trifles; he was lively with Delphine when she was gay, he was melancholy when she was sad; he supported the weight of all her headaches, of her confidences; he gave her all his time, his hours, his precious youth, to fill up the emptiness of the idleness of this Parisian woman. Delphine and he held great consultations over the adornments which were

most becoming to her, he sustained all the fire of
her anger and the broadsides of her poutings; during which time, in compensation, she made herself
charming for the baron. The baron, for his part,
laughed in his sleeve; then, when he saw Rastignac
bending under the weight of his duties, he assumed
the air of suspecting something and reunited the two
lovers by a common fear.''

"I can understand that a rich woman could have
made Rastignac live, and live honorably; but
where did he get his fortune?'' asked Couture.
"A fortune as considerable as his is to-day has
to be found somewhere, and no one has ever
accused him of having invented a good piece of
business?''

"He inherited,'' said Finot.

"Of whom?'' said Blondet.

"Of imbeciles whom he met,'' answered Couture.

"He did not take it all, my little loves,'' said
Bixiou:—

> "—Dispense with your unwonted fear;
> The age with fraud holds compact dear.''

"I will relate to you the origin of his fortune. In
the first place, let us pay homage to talent! Our
friend is not a scamp, as Finot says, but a gentleman who knows the game, who is acquainted with
the cards, and whom the gallery respects. Rastignac
has all the wit which it is necessary to have at a
given moment, like a military man who only stakes
his courage at ninety days, three signatures and an

endorsement. He may seem heedless, scatter-brained, without connection in his ideas, without constancy in his projects, without any fixed opinion; but, if there should present itself a serious affair, a combination to follow, he will not scatter himself, like Blondet, whom you see, and who goes off into discussions for the account of his neighbor. Rastignac concentrates himself, gathers himself up, studies the point at which he must charge, and he charges furiously. With the valor of Murat, he drives in the squares, the shareholders, the founders, and the whole shop; when the charge has made its hole, he returns to his soft and careless life, he becomes again the man of the *Midi*, the voluptuous, the sayer of nothings, the unoccupied Rastignac, who can lie abed till mid-day because he did not go to bed at the moment of the crisis.''

"All this is very well, but let us get to his fortune," said Finot.

"Bixiou will only give us one charge," added Blondet. "The fortune of Rastignac, it is Delphine de Nucingen, a remarkable woman, and one who joins audacity to foresight."

"Has she borrowed money of you?" asked Bixiou. A general laugh broke out.

"You are mistaken about her," said Couture to Blondet; "her wit consists in saying more or less piquant words, in loving Rastignac with a wearying fidelity, in obeying him blindly, a woman altogether Italian."

"Money apart," said Andoche Finot, sharply.

"Come, come," resumed Bixiou, in a wheedling voice, "after what we have just said, will you still dare to reproach this poor Rastignac with having lived at the expense of the house of Nucingen, with having been set up in his house neither more nor less than was La Torpille formerly by our friend des Lupeaulx? You will fall into the vulgarity of the Rue Saint-Denis. To begin with, speaking abstractly, as Royer-Collard says, the question may bring up 'the criticism of pure reason;' while as to that of impure reason—"

"Now he is off," said Finot to Blondet.

"But," cried Blondet, "he is right. The question is very ancient; it was the great word in the famous duel to death between La Châtaigneraie and Jarnac. Jarnac was accused of being on good terms with his mother-in-law, who furnished the pomp of the too-much loved son-in-law. When a fact is so true, it should not be uttered. Through his devotion for the king, Henri II., who had permitted himself this evil speaking, La Châtaigneraie took it on his own account; hence this duel, which has enriched the French language with the expression *coup de jarnac.*"

"Ah! if the expression comes from so far back, it is then noble?" said Finot.

"You might be ignorant of that in your character of a former proprietor of newspapers and reviews," said Blondet.

"There are women," resumed Bixiou, gravely, "there are also men, who can saw their existence in

two, and only give away a part of it—observe that I phrase my opinion after the humanitarian formula—. For those men, all material interest is outside of the sentiments; they give their life, their time, their honor, to a woman, and consider that it is not good style to spend between them that silk paper on which is engraved: 'The law punishes the counterfeiter with death.' Reciprocally, these individuals accept nothing from a woman. Yes, everything becomes dishonoring if there is a community of interest as there is a community of souls. This doctrine is confessed; it is rarely applied."

"Well," said Blondet, "what punctiliousness! The Maréchal de Richelieu, who was versed in the science of gallantry, granted a pension of a thousand louis to Madame de la Popelinière, after the adventure of the chimney plaque. Agnes Sorel brought quite naïvely to the king, Charles VII., her fortune, and the king took it. Jacques Cœur contributed to the support of the French crown, which allowed him to do so, and was as ungrateful as a woman."

"Monsieur," said Bixiou, "that love which does not consist of an indissoluble friendship seems to me a momentary libertinism. What is an entire abandonment in which something is reserved? Between these two doctrines, thus opposed and as profoundly immoral one as the other, there is no possible conciliation. According to my ideas, those who fear a complete liaison doubtless fear that it may come to an end, and then, adieu illusion! Passion

which does not believe itself eternal is hideous.
—This is from Fénelon direct.—Thus, those who
know the world, the observers, the people *comme
il faut,* the men well-gloved and well-cravated, who
do not blush to marry a woman for her fortune, they
proclaim as indispensable a complete separation of
interests and of sentiments.   The others are the
fools who love, who believe themselves alone in the
world with their mistress! For them, millions are
but mud; the glove, the camelia, worn by the idol
is worth the millions. If you never find among
them any traces of the base metal dissipated, you
will find the remains of flowers hidden in pretty
cedar-boxes.   They are not to be distinguished one
from the other.   For them, there is no longer any
I. THOU, that is their incarnate Word.   What
would you have! Would you hinder this secret
malady of the heart? There are idiots who love
without any kind of calculation, and there are sages
who calculate in loving."

"Bixiou seems to me sublime," cried Blondet.
"What does Finot say about it?"

"Everywhere else," replied Finot, settling his
cravat, "I would say like the gentleman; but, here,
I think—"

"Like the infamous badly disposed persons with
whom you have the honor of being," interrupted
Bixiou.

"Faith, yes," said Finot.

"And you?" said Bixiou to Couture.

"Imbecilities," cried Couture. "A woman who

does not make of her body a stepping-stone to enable the man she distinguishes to arrive at his aim, is a woman who has a heart for no one but herself."

"And you, Blondet?"

"I—I practice."

"Well," resumed Bixiou, in his most biting voice, "Rastignac was not of your opinion. To take and not to give is horrible and even somewhat light; but to take in order to have the right to imitate the Lord, in returning an hundred-fold, is a chivalrous act. Thus thought Rastignac. Rastignac was profoundly humiliated at his community of interests with Delphine de Nucingen. I can speak of his regrets; I have seen him with tears in his eyes, deploring his position. Yes, he wept of it veritably—after supper! Well, according to us—"

"Ah! now you are ridiculing us," said Finot.

"Not the least in the world. It concerns Rastignac, whose mortification would be, according to you, a proof of his corruption; for he then loved Delphine much less. But what would you have! the poor boy had this thorn in his heart. He is a gentleman profoundly depraved, as you see, and we are virtuous artists. Then, Rastignac wished to enrich Delphine, he poor, she rich! Would you believe it?—he succeeded. Rastignac, who would have combated like Jarnac, went over from that time to the opinion of Henri II., in virtue of his fine saying: 'There is no absolute virtue, but there are circumstances.' This is connected with the history of his fortune."

2

"You would do well to go on with your story instead of enticing us to calumniate ourselves," said Blondet, with a gracious good-fellowship.

"Ah! ah! my little one," said Bixiou to him, giving him the baptism of a little tap on the occiput, "you will pick yourself up again in the champagne."

"Oh! by the holy name of the stockholder," said Couture, "tell us your story!"

"I am within a notch of it," answered Bixiou; "but, with your oath, you have brought me to the dénouement."

"There are, then, stockholders in the history?" asked Finot.

"Multo-rich as yours," answered Bixiou.

"It seems to me," said Finot in a stiff voice, "that you owe some consideration to a good lad with whom you find occasionally a note of five hundred—"

"Waiter!" cried Bixiou.

"What are you going to ask of the waiter?" said Blondet to him.

"Five hundred francs, to return them to Finot, in order that I may disengage my tongue and tear up my receipt."

"Tell your story," resumed Finot, feigning to laugh.

"You are all witnesses," said Bixiou, "that I do not belong to this impertinent who thinks that my silence is only worth five hundred francs! You will never be minister if you do not know how to gauge

consciences. Well, yes," he said, in a cajoling voice, "my good Finot, I will tell the history without any personalities, and we will be quits."

"He is going to demonstrate to us," said Couture, smiling, "that Nucingen made the fortune of Rastignac."

"You are not so far from it as you think," resumed Bixiou. "You do not know what Nucingen is, financially speaking."

"You do not even know," said Blondet, "one thing about his beginnings?"

"I have only known him in his own house," said Bixiou, "but we might have seen each other in other times on the highway."

"The prosperity of the house of Nucingen is one of the most extraordinary phenomena of our epoch," resumed Blondet. "In 1804, Nucingen was but little known; the bankers of that day would have trembled to have known that there were on the market a hundred thousand écus of his acceptances. This grand financier was conscious of his inferiority. How to make himself known? He suspended payment. Good! His name, restricted to Strasbourg and to the Quartier Poissonnière, resounded in all the exchanges! He indemnified all his creditors with non-interest bearing securities and resumed payment; immediately his papers circulated throughout France. By an unheard-of chance, the stocks came up again, resumed their value, paid dividends. Nucingen was very much sought after. The year 1815 arrived, my hero consolidates his capital, buys

funds before the Battle of Waterloo, suspends payment at the moment of the crisis, liquidates with shares in the mines of Wortschin which he had procured at twenty per cent less than the value at which he had put them out himself! yes, Messieurs! He took from Grandet a hundred and fifty thousand bottles of champagne to cover himself, foreseeing the failure of this virtuous father of the present Comte d'Aubrion, and as many from Duberghe in Bordeaux wines. These three hundred thousand bottles *accepted*, accepted, my dear fellow, at thirty sous, he caused the allies to drink at six francs, at the Palais-Royal, from 1817 to 1819. The paper of the house of Nucingen and his name became European. This illustrious baron had lifted himself out of the abyss in which others would have sunk. Twice his liquidation had produced immense advantages to his creditors: he wished to get the best of them, impossible! He passed for the most honest man in the world. At the third suspension, the paper of the house of Nucingen was circulating in Asia, in Mexico, in Australia, among the savages. Ouvrard is the only one who had found out this Alsatian, the son of some Jew converted through ambition: 'When Nucingen lets go of his gold,' said he, 'you may believe that he is seizing diamonds!'"

"His ally, Du Tillet, is well worthy of him," said Finot. "You must know that Du Tillet is a man who, as far as birth went, had only that which is absolutely indispensable for existence, and that

this beggar, who had not a liard in 1814, has become what you see; but what none of us—I am not speaking of you, Couture,—has been able to do, he has had friends instead of having enemies. In short, he so well hid his antecedents, that it was necessary to search the sewers to find him, no later than 1814, clerk in a perfumer's shop in the Rue Saint-Honoré."

"Ta, ta, ta!" resumed Bixiou, "never compare Nucingen to a little timid gambler like Du Tillet, a jackal who succeeds through his sense of smell, who scents the carcass and arrives the first to get the best bone. Besides, look at the two men,—one of them has the sharp look of cats, he is thin, lank; the other is cubical, he is fat, he is heavy as a sack, immovable as a diplomat. Nucingen has a thick hand and the look of a lynx, which never becomes animated; his profundity is not before, but behind: he is impenetrable, he is never seen to come, while the sharpness of Du Tillet resembles, as Napoléon said of someone, I have forgotten whom, 'cotton spun too fine, it breaks.'"

"I do not see in Nucingen any other advantage over Du Tillet than that of having the good sense to understand that a financier should be no more than a baron, whilst Du Tillet wishes to have himself made a count in Italy," said Blondet.

"Blondet,—a word, my child," said Couture. "In the first place, Nucingen has ventured to say that he has only the semblance of an honest man; then, to know him well, it is necessary to deal

with him. With him the bank is a very small department,—there is the furnishing of government supplies, the wines, the wools, the indigoes, in short, all that might be made to contribute to any gain whatsoever. His genius embraces everything. This elephant of finance would sell deputies to the minister, and the Greeks to the Turks. For him, commerce is, as Cousin would say, the totality of varieties, the unity of specialties. Banking, considered in this light, thus becomes a whole political system; it requires a powerful head and carries a man whose metal is well tempered to lift himself above the laws of probity, in which he finds himself cramped."

"You are right, my son," said Blondet. "But we alone, we comprehend what it is thus to have war carried into the monetary world. The banker is a conqueror who sacrifices masses to arrive at hidden results, his soldiers are the interests of individuals. He has his stratagems to combine, his ambuscades to prepare, his partisans to send out, his cities to take. The greater number of these men are so close to politics that they end by going into it, and there losing their fortunes. The house of Necker was thus destroyed, the famous Samuel Bernard was there almost ruined. In every century there may be found a banker with a colossal fortune who leaves neither fortune nor successor. The brothers Pâris, who contributed to bring down Law, and Law himself, besides whom all those who float stock companies are pigmies; Bouret, Beaujon,

all have disappeared without leaving a family to
represent them.   Like Saturn, the bank devours its
own children.   In order to subsist, the banker
should become a noble, found a dynasty like the
money-lenders of Charles V., the Fuggers, created
princes of Babenhausen, and who still exist—in the
Almanach de Gotha.   The bank seeks nobility
through an instinct of self-preservation, and without
knowing it, perhaps.   Jacques Cœur founded a
great noble house, that of Noirmoutier, extinct under
Louis XIII.   What energy in that man, ruined for
having made a legitimate king!   He died prince of
an island in the Archipelago, where he built a magnificent cathedral."

"Ah! if you are going to give a course of history,
we will get away from present time, when the
throne is devoid of the right of conferring nobility,
when barons and counts are made behind closed
doors.   What a pity!" said Finot.

"You regret the *savonnette à vilain*,"* said Bixiou; "you are right.   I return to our subject.   Do
you know Beaudenord?   No, no, no!   Good.   See
how everything passes away!   That poor boy was
the flower of dandyism ten years ago.   But he has
been so completely absorbed that you no longer
know him any more than Finot knew, just now, the
origin of the *coup de jarnac*—it is for the sake of the
phrase and not in order to tease you that I say that,
Finot!—In truth, he belonged to the Faubourg

---

*A proverbial expression in allusion to such posts or offices as were
purchased with a view to nobility.

Saint-Germain.   Well, Beaudenord is the first
pigeon that I am going to put on the stage for you.
In the first place, he called himself Godefroid de
Beaudenord.   Neither Finot, nor Blondet, nor
Couture, nor I, none of us, will despise such an advantage.   The youth did not suffer in his self-
love in hearing his domestics called when coming
out of a ball, while thirty pretty women, hooded
and flanked by their husbands and their adorers,
were waiting for their carriages.   Then he was in
the enjoyment of all the members which God has
given to man,—whole and entire, neither film on
the eye, nor false wigs, nor false calves; his legs
were neither knock-kneed nor bowed; knees not
too prominent, spinal column straight, figure slender, hand white and handsome, hair black; complexion neither pink, like that of a grocer's ap-
prentice, nor too brown, like that of a Calabrais.
Finally, the essential thing! Beaudenord was not
a too-pretty man, as are those of our friend who
have the air of making a business of their beauty,
of not having any other affair; but let us not dwell
on that subject; we have said it, it is infamous!
He was a good shot with a pistol, a very good eques-
trian; he had fought for a punctilio, and had not
killed his adversary.   Do you know that, to portray that which constitutes an entire happiness,
pure without alloy, in the nineteenth century, in
Paris, and the happiness of a young man of twenty-
six, it is necessary to enter into the infinitely
little things of life?   The boot-maker had quite

compassed the foot of Beaudenord and shod him well, his tailor loved to array him. Godefroid did not get fat, did not gasconnade, did not Norman-ade, he spoke purely and correctly, and tied his cravat exceedingly well, like Finot. A cousin by marriage of the Marquis d'Aiglemont, his guardian—he was orphaned of both father and mother, another happiness!—he could go, and did go, among the bankers, without the Faubourg Saint-Germain reproaching him with frequenting them, for, fortunately, a young man has the right to make pleasure his only law, to go wherever there is amusement, and to flee the sombre corners in which chagrin flourishes. Finally, he had been vaccinated—you understand me, Blondet—. Despite all these virtues, he might have been able to find himself very unhappy. Eh! eh! happiness has the misfortune of appearing to signify something absolute; an appearance which leads so many simpletons to ask: 'What is happiness?' A woman of much wit said: 'Happiness is where one puts it.'"

"She proclaimed a sad truth," said Blondet.

"And a moral one," added Finot.

"Arch-moral! HAPPINESS, like VIRTUE, like EVIL, expresses something relative," replied Blondet. "Thus, La Fontaine hoped that, in course of time, the damned would become accustomed to their situation, and would finish by being, in Hell, just like fish in the water."

"The grocers know all La Fontaine's sayings!" said Bixiou.

"The happiness of a man of twenty-six who lives at Paris is not the happiness of a man of twenty-six who lives at Blois," said Blondet, without hearing the interruption. "Those who start from this to rail against the instability of opinions are either knaves or ignoramuses. Modern medicine, of which the finest title to glory is in having, between 1799 and 1837, passed from the state of conjecture to the state of a positive science, and that, through the influence of the great analytical school of Paris, it has demonstrated that, in a certain period of time, man is completely renewed—"

"After the manner of Jeannot's knife, and you think him always the same," resumed Bixiou. "There are, then, several lozenges in this harlequin costume that we denominate happiness; well, the costume of my Godefroid had neither rents nor spots. A young man of twenty-six, who would be happy in love, that is to say, loved, not because of the flower of his youth, not for his wit, not for his appearance, but irresistibly, not even because of love in himself, but even when this love shall be abstract, to return to the phrase of Royer-Collard, this aforesaid young man may well not have even a liard in the purse which the loving object has embroidered for him, he may owe his rent to his landlord, his boots to the boot-maker already named, his clothes to the tailor, who may finish, like France, by becoming alienated. In short, he may be poor! Poverty spoils the happiness of the young man who does not partake of our transcendental opinions on

the community of interests. I know of nothing more wearying than to be morally very happy and materially very unhappy. Is it not to have one leg frozen, as mine is, by the draught that comes through that door, and the other grilled by the hot coals of the fire? I trust that I make myself understood. Is there an echo in the pocket of your waistcoat, Blondet? Between ourselves, let us leave the heart, it spoils the wit. We will proceed. Godefroid de Beaudenord had, then, the esteem of his haberdashers, for his haberdashers received, with sufficient regularity, their payments. The woman of a good deal of wit already cited, and who cannot be named, because, thanks to her lack of heart, she lives—"

"Who is it?"

"The Marquise d'Espard! She said that a young man should live in an entresol, have in his domicile nothing which smelt of housekeeping, neither cook nor kitchen, be served by an old domestic, and make no pretension to stability. According to her, any other establishment would be in bad taste. Godefroid de Beaudenord, faithful to this programme, lodged on the Quay Malaquais, in an entresol; nevertheless, he had been obliged to have a little resemblance to married people by putting in his chamber a bed, which, however, was so narrow that it made but little difference. An Englishwoman who might have happened to enter his lodging, would have been able to find nothing *improper* there. Finot, you will explain to yourself the great

law of the *improper* which rules England! But, since we are united by a note of one thousand, I am going to give you an idea. I have been in England, I have"—in a low tone in Blondet's ear: "I give him wit for more than two thousand francs.— In England, Finot, you become extremely well acquainted with a woman, at night, at a ball or elsewhere; you meet her the next morning in the street, and you appear to recognize her: *improper!* You find at dinner, under the black coat of your neighbor on your left, a charming man, witty, no haughtiness, an easy freedom; he has nothing of the English; following the ancient laws of French society, so flexible, so courteous, you speak to him: *improper!* You accost a pretty woman at a ball to ask her to dance: *improper!* You warm up, you discuss, you laugh, you expand your heart, your soul, your spirit in your conversation; you express in it feeling; you play when you are at play, you talk in talking and you eat in eating: *improper! improper! improper!* One of the most spiritual and most profound men of this epoch, Stendhal, has very well characterized the *improper* in saying that there is a certain lord of Great Britain who, when alone, dares not cross his legs before his own fire, for fear of being *improper.* An English lady, were she of the furious sect of the *saints*—double-dyed Protestants who would let all their family die of hunger rather than be *improper*—would not be *improper* in making the devil of an ado in her bed-chamber, and would consider herself lost if she received a friend

in this same chamber.   Thanks to the *improper*,
some day London and all its inhabitants will be
found petrified.''

"When one thinks that there are in France simpletons who wish to import here the solemn stupidities which the English commit at home with
that fine complacency which you see in them," said
Blondet, "it is enough to make anyone shudder who
has seen England and who thinks of the graceful
and charming French manners.   In his later years,
Walter Scott, who did not dare to paint women as
they are, for fear of being *improper*, repented of having drawn the charming figure of Effie in the Prison
of Edinburgh.''

"Would you like to know how not to be *improper*
in England?" said Bixiou to Finot.

"Well?" said Finot.

"Go to the Tuileries and see a species of fireman
in marble entitled Themistocles by the statuary,
and endeavor to walk like the statue of the commander; you will never be *improper*. It was by
a rigorous application of the great law of the
improper that the happiness of Godefroid was completed. This is the story: He had a tiger, and
not a groom, as those people who know nothing
about the world write.   His tiger was a little Irish-
man, named Paddy, Joby, Toby—at will—, three
feet high, twenty inches wide, with the face of a
weasel, nerves of steel, made by gin, active as a
squirrel, managing a landau with a skill which was
never found in default, neither in London nor in

Paris; the eye of a lizard, fine as mine, mounting a
horse like the old Franconi, hair as blond as that
of a Virgin by Rubens, pink cheeks, dissembling as
a prince, learned as a retired lawyer, aged ten
years, in short a true flower of perversity, swearing and playing, loving jam and punch, insulting as
a newspaper, bold and pilfering as a gamin of
Paris. He had been the honor and the profit of a
celebrated English lord, for whom he had gained
seven hundred thousand francs on the race-course.
The lord prized very highly this infant: his tiger
was a curiosity, no one in London had a tiger so
little. Mounted on a race horse, Joby looked like
a falcon. Well, the lord dismissed Toby, not for
gluttony, nor for theft, nor for murder, nor for
criminal conversation, nor for failure in style, nor
for insolence to milady, nor for having made holes
in the pocket of milady's first maid, nor for having
been bribed by milord's adversaries at the races,
nor for having amused himself on Sunday, in short,
for no reproachable act. Toby might have done all
these things, he might even have spoken to milord
without being questioned, milord would again have
pardoned this domestic crime. Milord would have
endured a great many things for Toby, so much
milord was attached to him. His tiger could handle
a two-wheeled carriage, tandem, mounted in the
saddle of the rear horse, his legs not reaching below
the shafts, having the appearance in fact of one of
those heads of cherubs which the Italian painters
scatter around the Eternal Father. An English

journalist made a delicious description of this little angel. He found him too pretty for a tiger; he offered to bet that Paddy was a tamed tigress. The description threatened to envenom and to become in the highest degree *improper*. The superlative of the *improper* leads to the gallows. Milord was much praised for his circumspection by milady. Toby could not find any other situation, after having his civil status thus contested in the Britannic Zoölogy. At this period Godefroid was flourishing at the French embassy in London, where he heard of the adventure of Toby, Joby, Paddy. Godefroid took possession of the tiger, whom he found weeping beside a pot of jam, for the infant had already lost the guineas with which milord had gilded his misfortune. On his return, Godefroid de Beaudenord then imported amongst us the most charming tiger of England; he was known by his tiger as Couture attracts attention by his waistcoats. Thus he entered with facility into the confederation of the club called to-day De Grammont. He did not disturb any ambition after having renounced the diplomatic career; he had not a dangerous spirit, he was well received by everybody. We others, we would be offended in our self-love if we encountered only smiling faces. We are pleased to see the bitter grimace of the envious. Godefroid did not love to be hated. Everyone to his taste! Let us get to the solid facts, to the material life. His apartment, in which I have discussed more than one déjeuner, recommended itself by a mysterious dressing-room, well ornamented,

full of comfortable things, with a fire-place, with a bath-tub; opening on a little stairway, folding-doors that made no noise, easy locks, discreet hinges, windows of ground glass with impassable curtains. If the chamber offered and should have offered the very finest disorder that the most exacting water-color painter could have desired, if everything in it exhaled the Bohemian charm of the life of an elegant young man, the dressing-room was like a sanctuary,—white, clean, well-ordered, warm, no draughts, a carpet made for alighting on in naked feet, in one's chemise, affrighted. There could be found the signature of the young man, a real beau and one who knows life! for there during several minutes he may reveal himself either imbecile or great in those little details of existence which betray character. The marquise already cited, no, it was the Marquise de Rochefide, issued furious from this dressing-room and never returned there; she found in it nothing *improper*. Godefroid had there a little cupboard full—"

"Of night-shirts?" said Finot.

"Come now, there you are, you gross Turcaret! —I shall never be able to make anything of him!— Not at all,—of cakes, of fruit, of pretty little flasks of Malaga wine, of Lunel, a little refection à la Louis XIV., all that could amuse delicate and well-educated stomachs, the stomachs of sixteen quarterings. A malicious old domestic, very strong in the veterinary art, looked after the horses and waited on Godefroid, for he had been in the service of the late

Monsieur Beaudenord, and had for Godefroid an
inveterate affection, that malady of the heart which
the savings banks have ended, by curing, for all
servants. All material happiness reposes on figures.
You, to whom Parisian life is known even to its
exostosis, you will understand that he required about
seventeen thousand francs of income, for he had
seventeen francs of imposts and a thousand écus of
fancies. Well, my dear infants, the day on which
he attained his majority the Marquis d'Aiglemont
presented him with the accounts of his stewardship,
such as we should not be able to render to our
nephews, and handed to him his statement of eighteen thousand francs of income from investments in
the public funds, the remnants of the paternal opulence, somewhat mauled by the great Republican
reduction and riddled by the arrears of the Empire.
This virtuous guardian put into his pupil's hands
some thirty thousand francs of savings placed in
the house of Nucingen, saying to him, with all the
courtesy of a grand seigneur and the easy freedom
of a soldier of the Empire, that he had saved this
sum for his youthful follies. 'If you will listen to
me, Godefroid,' he added, 'instead of expending this
sottishly, like so many others, practice some useful
follies, accept a post as attaché to the embassy at
Turin, from there go to Naples, from Naples to London, and for your money you will be amused,
instructed. Later, if you wish to adopt a career,
you will have lost neither your time nor your
money.' The late D'Aiglemont quite deserved his

3

reputation; no one will be able to say as much of us."

"A young man who starts life at twenty-one with eighteen thousand francs of income is a young man ruined," said Couture.

"If he is not avaricious, or very superior," said Blondet.

"Godefroid sojourned awhile in the four capitals of Italy," resumed Bixiou. "He saw Germany and England, a little of St. Petersburg, traversed Holland; but he separated himself from the aforesaid thirty thousand francs by living as if he had thirty thousand francs of income. He found everywhere 'the best part of the fowl, jellied meats,' and 'the wines of France,' heard French spoken everywhere, in fact he was not able to get out of Paris. He would have been quite willing to have depraved his heart, to have put it in a cuirass, to have lost his illusions, to have learned to hear everything without blushing, to talk without saying anything, to penetrate the secret interests of the powers.—Bah! it was scarcely worth his while to furnish himself with four languages, that is to say, to provide himself with four words for one idea. He returned widowed of several very tedious dowagers, called *good fortunes,* abroad, timid and scarcely formed, a good fellow, full of confidence, incapable of speaking evil of those who did him the honor to admit him to their houses, having too much good faith to be a diplomat, in short, what we call an honest fellow."

"In short, a *brat* who held his eighteen thousand francs of income for the first investment that should come along," said Couture.

"This devil of a Couture is so much in the habit of anticipating his dividends that he anticipates the dénouement of my history. Where was I? At Beaudenord's return. When he was installed in the Quay Malaquais, he found that a thousand francs above his needs were insufficient for his box at the Italiens and at the Opera. When he lost twenty-five or thirty louis at play in betting, naturally he paid; then, he spent them when he won, which always happens to us if we are stupid enough to allow ourselves to take to betting. Beaudenord, cramped in his eighteen thousand francs of income, felt the necessity of creating that which we call to-day *funds for running expenses*. He was quite resolved *not to get himself in too deep*. He went to consult his guardian: 'My dear child,' said D'Aiglemont to him, 'Rentes are at par, sell your Rentes; I have sold mine and those of my wife. Nucingen has all my capital, and gives me for it six per cent; do like me, you will have one per cent the more, and this one per cent will permit you to be perfectly comfortable.' In three days our Godefroid was quite comfortable. His revenues were in a state of perfect equilibrium with his superfluousness, his material happiness was complete. If it were possible to interrogate all the young people of Paris with one glance, as it appears will be done at the time of the last judgment for the billions of

generations which have splashed about on all the
worlds, as National Guards or as savages, and to
demand of them if the happiness of a young man
of twenty-six did not consist in being able to go
out on horseback, in a tilbury, or in a cabriolet
with a tiger as big as your fist, fresh and rosy as
Toby, Joby, Paddy; to have in the evening for
twelve francs a very convenient coupé to hire; to
show oneself elegantly gotten up according to the
laws of apparel which regulate eight o'clock, noon,
four o'clock, and the evening; to be well received
in all the embassies, and to gather there the ephem-
eral flowers of cosmopolitan and superficial friendships; to be of a supportable beauty, and to carry
well one's name, one's coat and one's head; to live
in a charming little entresol arranged as I have told
you was the entresol of the Quay Malaquais; to be
able to invite your friends to accompany you to the
Rocher de Cancale without having to previously interrogate one's pocket, and not to be arrested in
every reasonable movement by this word, 'but how
about the money?' to be able to renew the pink
tufts which ornament the ears of one's three thor-
oughbred horses, and to have always a new lining
to one's hat? Everybody, ourselves, superior persons, all would reply that this happiness is incomplete, that it is the Madeleine without an altar, that
it is necessary to love and be loved, or to love without being loved, or to be loved without loving, or to
be able to love through thick and thin. We will
arrive at the moral happiness. When, in January,

1823, he found himself comfortably settled in all his
enjoyments, after having established his footing in
all the different Parisian societies in which it pleased
him to go, he felt the necessity of putting himself
under the shelter of a parasol, of being able to complain to some woman *comme il faut*, of not having
to chew the stem of a rose bought for ten sous from
Madame Prévost, after the fashion of the little young
people who cluck in the corridors of the Opera
House, like pullets in a chicken-house. In short, he
resolved to carry all his sentiments, his ideas, his
affections to a woman, *a woman!* LA PHAMME! Ah!
—He conceived at first the absurd idea of having
an unhappy passion, he hovered for some time
around his charming cousin, Madame d'Aiglemont,
without perceiving that a diplomatist had already
danced the waltz of 'Faust' with her. The year '25
passed in essays, in researches, in useless flirta-
tions. The loving object demanded did not present
itself. Passions are extremely rare. At this epoch,
there were set up as many barricades in manners as
in the streets! Verily, my brethren, I say to you
the *improper* is overcoming us! As we have been
reproached with imitating the method of the painters of portraits, of the auctioneers and of the
dressmakers, I will not make you undergo the description of the person in whom Godefroid recognized his female. Aged nineteen years; stature one
metre fifty centimetres; blond hair, eyebrows *idem*,
eyes blue, forehead medium, nose arched, mouth
small, chin short and high, visage oval; particular

indications, none. Such was the passport of the loved object. Do not be more hard to please than the police, than Messieurs the mayors of all the towns and communes of France, than the gendarmes and other constituted authorities. Moreover, this is the block of the Venus de Medici, word of honor. The first time that Godefroid went to the house of Madame de Nucingen, who had invited him to one of those balls by which she acquired, at a reasonable price, a certain reputation, he perceived there, in a quadrille, the person to love and was astonished by this figure of a metre and fifty centimetres. These blond locks flowed in rippling cascades on a little head ingenuous and fresh as that of a naiad who had put her nose out of the crystalline window of her stream to see the flowers of Spring.—This is our new style, phrases which spin themselves out as our macaroni did just now.—The *idem* of the eyebrows, without offence to the prefecture of police, might have demanded six verses from the amiable Parny; that playful poet would have compared them very agreeably to Cupid's bow, observing that the dart was below, but a dart without force, a blunted dart, for there reigns there still to-day the sheep-like softness which the chimney-panels attribute to Mademoiselle de la Vallière, at the moment when she bore witness to her tenderness before God, through lack of being able to bear witness before a notary. You know the effect of these blond locks and blue eyes, in combination with a dance, soft, voluptuous, and decent? Such a young

person does not strike you at first audaciously to
the heart, like those brunettes who by their glance
have the air of saying to you, like Spanish beggars:
'Your purse or your life! Five francs or I scorn
you.' These insolent beauties—and somewhat dangerous!—may be able to please many men; but
according to me, the blond who has the happiness
of appearing excessively tender and yielding, without losing her right of remonstrance, of teasing, of
immoderate discourses, of unfounded jealousy and
all that which renders woman adorable, will be
always more certain of marriage than the ardent
brunette. Wood is dear. Isaure, white as an
Alsatian—she had first seen the day at Strasbourg
and spoke German with a very agreeable little
French accent—, danced marvelously. Her feet,
which the police employé had not mentioned and
which, however, might find their place under the
rubric *particular indications*, were remarkable for
their smallness, for that peculiar action which the
old masters denominated *flic flac*, and comparable to
the agreeable recitative of Mademoiselle Mars, for all
Muses are sisters, the dancer and the poet alike
have their feet on the earth. The feet of Isaure
conversed with a clearness, a precision, a lightness,
a rapidity of excellent augury for the things of the
heart. 'She has the *flic flac*,' was the supreme
eulogy of Marcel, the only dancing-master who has
merited the title of great. He was called the great
Marcel, like the great Frederick, and of the times of
Frederick.''

"Did he compose ballets?" asked Finot.

"Yes, something like 'The Four Elements,' 'Gallant Europe.'"

"What a period," said Finot; "like the times in which the grand seigneurs dressed the danseuses."

"*Improper!*" resumed Bixiou. "Isaure did not raise herself on her toes, she remained upon the earth, she balanced herself without shaking, neither more nor less voluptuously than a young person should balance herself. Marcel said, with profound philosophy, that each state had its peculiar dance, —a married woman should dance in a different fashion from a young person, a limb of the law otherwise than a financier, and a military man otherwise than a page; he went so far as to pretend that a foot soldier should dance in a different way than a cavalryman: and from this he set out to analyze the whole of society. All these fine shades are quite out of our line."

"Ah!" said Blondet, "you put your finger on a great misfortune. If Marcel had been comprehended, the French Revolution would never have taken place."

"Godefroid," resumed Bixiou, "had not had the advantage of traversing Europe without observing foreign dances closely. Without that profound knowledge of choregraphy, which is qualified as futile, perhaps he would not have loved this young person; but of the three hundred guests who crowded the handsome salons of the Rue Saint-Lazare, he was the only one to comprehend the

unpublished love which is betrayed by a talkative
dance. There were many who noticed the manner
of Isaure d'Aldrigger; but, in that century in which
everyone cries: 'Slide, do not bear on!' one said:
'there is a young girl who dances famously well'
—this was a notary's clerk—; another, 'there is a
young person who dances ravishingly'—this was a
lady in a turban—; the third, a woman of thirty:
'there is a young person who does not dance badly!'
Let us return to the great Marcel, and say, parody-
ing his most famous saying: 'how many things in a
forward-two!' "

"And let us get on a little faster!" said Blondet.
"You are sentimentalizing."

"Isaure," resumed Bixiou, who looked at Blondet
askance, "had a simple dress of white crêpe ornamented with green ribbons, a camelia in her hair,
a camelia at her waist, another camelia at the bottom of her dress, and a camelia—"

"Oh! come on; here are the three hundred goats
of Sancho!"

"It is like all literature, my dear fellow. 'Clar-
issa' is a masterpiece, there are fourteen volumes,
and the dullest vaudevillist will recount it to you
in an act. So long as I amuse you, of what do you
complain? This toilet had a delicious effect. Do
you not love camelias? would you like to have
dahlias? No. Well, then, a chestnut, here!" said
Bixiou, who doubtless threw a chestnut at Blondet,
for we heard the noise on a plate.

"Go on, I was wrong; continue!" said Blondet.

"I resume," said Bixiou. "'Would it not be nice to marry?' said Rastignac to Beaudenord, indicating to him the little one with the white camelias, pure and without a leaf missing. Rastignac was one of the intimate friends of Godefroid. 'Eh! well, I was thinking of it,' replied Godefroid in his ear. 'I was saying to myself that, instead of trembling at each moment in his happiness, of only being able to utter occasionally a word in an inattentive ear, of looking, at the Italiens, to see if there were a red or a white flower in a coiffure, if there were at the Bois a gloved hand on the panel of a carriage, as is done at Milan, on the Corso; that instead of stealing a mouthful of sweetness behind a door, like a lackey who finishes a bottle; of using all his intelligence to give and to receive a letter, like a postman; that instead of receiving infinite tendernesses in two lines, of having five volumes in folio to read to-day, to-morrow a pamphlet of two pages, which is fatiguing; that instead of dragging one's self along the ruts and behind the hedges, it would be much better to give one's self up to the adorable passion envied by Jean-Jacques Rousseau, to love quite honestly a young person like Isaure, with the intention of making her his wife if, during the exchange of feelings, the hearts should come to an agreement, in short, to be Werther happy!'—'That is just as absurd as anything else,' said Rastignac, without laughing. 'In your place, perhaps, I would throw myself into the infinite delights of this asceticism; it is new, original and not costly. Your Mona Lisa

is sweet and soft, but simple as ballet music, I fore-
warn you.' The manner in which Rastignac uttered
this last phrase suggested to Beaudenord that his
friend had some interest in disenchanting him, and
he believed him his rival in his quality of a former
diplomat. The professions that have failed often color
a whole lifetime. Godefroid became so enamored
of Mademoiselle Isaure d'Aldrigger, that Rastignac
went in search of a tall girl who was conversing in
the card-room, and whispered to her: 'Malvina,
your sister has just caught in her net a fish that
weighs eighteen thousand francs of income; he has
a name, a certain place in the world and very good
style; watch over them; if they should spin out the
perfect love, have a care to be Isaure's confidante in
order that she may not reply a single word which
you have not corrected.' Toward two o'clock in
the morning the valet de chambre came to say to a
little Alpine shepherdess, forty years old, coquettish as the Zerlina of the opera of 'Don Juan,' and
under whose charge was Isaure: 'the carriage of
Madame la Baronne is at the door.' Godefroid then
saw his beauty of the German ballad conducting her
fantastic mother into the salon of departure, where
these two ladies were followed by Malvina. Godefroid, who pretended—the infant!—to be going to see
in what pot of jam Joby had lost himself, had the
happiness of perceiving Isaure and Malvina envel-
oping their sprightly mamma in her pelisse, rendering her all those little cares of the toilet required for
a nocturnal journey in Paris. The two sisters

examined him out of the corners of their eyes like
well-trained cats, who watch a mouse without
appearing to pay any attention to it. He experienced a certain satisfaction in seeing the style, the
appearance, the manners, of the big Alsatian in
livery, very well gloved, who brought the comfortable furred slippers to his three mistresses. Never
were two sisters more unlike than were Isaure and
Malvina. The elder, tall and brunette, Isaure petite
and blonde; this one with fine and delicate features;
the other much more vigorous and pronounced;
Isaure was the woman who rules by her lack of
strength and whom a lyceum student would have
felt himself called upon to protect; Malvina was the
woman of '*Avez-vous vu dans Barcelone?*' By the
side of her sister, Isaure had the effect of a miniature in contrast with a portrait in oil. 'She is rich!'
said Godefroid to Rastignac returning to the
ball.—'Who?'—'That young person.'—'Ah! Isaure
d'Aldrigger! Why, yes. The mother is a widow;
her husband had employed Nucingen in his offices
at Strasbourg. Should you like to see her again,
turn off a compliment to Madame de Restaud, who
gives a ball the day after to-morrow; the Baronne
d'Aldrigger and her two daughters will be there;
you will get an invitation!' For three days, in the
camera obscura of his brain, Godefroid saw *his*
Isaure and the white camelias, and the little movements of her head, just as when, after having long
contemplated an object brilliantly lighted, we see it
again when our eyes are shut, in a smaller form,

radiant and colored, sparkling in the midst of the obscurity.''

"Bixiou, you are falling into phenomena; pull your picture together more!" said Couture.

"Here you are!" resumed Bixiou, assuming doubtless, the attitude of a waiter, "here, messieurs, is your picture! Attention, Finot! you will have to pull at your mouth as a cab-driver does at that of his old horse! Madame Théodora-Marguerite-Wilhelmine Adolphus—of the house of Adolphus & Co., Mannheim—widow of the Baron d'Aldrigger, was not a good, fat German woman, compact and deliberate, fair-skinned, with a face gilded like the froth of a pot of beer, enriched with all the patriarchal virtues which Germany possesses, romantically speaking. Her cheeks were still fresh, colored on the cheek-bones like those of a Nuremburg doll, very sprightly corkscrew curls at her temples, enticing eyes, not a single white hair, a slender figure whose pretensions were set forth by tight-fitting dresses. She had on the forehead and on the temples some involuntary wrinkles which she would have very willingly, like Ninon, banished to her heels; but the wrinkles persisted in designing their zigzags in the most visible localities. The outline of her nose was drooping a little and the end reddening, which was all the more embarrassing that the nose thus came into harmony with the color of the cheeks. In her quality of sole heiress, spoiled by her parents, spoiled by her husband, spoiled by the city of Strasbourg, and always spoiled by her

two daughters, who adored her, the baroness favored pink, wore short skirts, and the bow at the point of the corset which defined her figure. When a Parisian saw this baroness passing on the Boulevard, he smiled; he condemned her without admitting, as the jury always does, the extenuating circumstances in a fratricide! The scoffer is always a superficial being and consequently a cruel one; the knave never takes into account that for which society is responsible in the absurdity at which he laughs, for nature only made beasts; we owe the dolt to the social state.''

"That which I find so fine in Bixiou," said Blondet, "is that he is complete; when he is not railing at others, he is laughing at himself."

"Blondet, I will be even with you for that," said Bixiou, in a shrewd tone. "If this baroness was giddy, careless, egotistical, incapable of reflection, the responsibility of her defects all fell upon the house of Adolphus & Co., of Mannheim, on the blind love of the Baron d'Aldrigger. Soft as a lamb, this baroness had a tender heart, easy to move, but, unluckily the emotion was of short duration and consequently was often renewed. When the baron died, this shepherdess all but followed him, so violent and real was her grief; but—the next day, at déjeuner, she was served with French peas, which she loved, and these delicious *petits pois* calmed the crisis. She was so blindly loved by her two daughters, by her servants, that all the household was happy at a circumstance which

enabled them to prevent her from seeing the dolorous spectacle of the funeral. Isaure and Malvina hid their tears from this adored mother, and occupied her in selecting her mourning, in ordering it whilst the *Requiem* was sung. When a coffin is placed under that great catafalque black and white, spotted with wax drippings, which served for three thousand corpses of well-to-do people before being renewed, according to the estimate of a philosophic undertaker's man whom I consulted on this point, between two glasses of *petit blanc;* when the inferior clergy, very indifferent, bawl the *Dies iræ,* when the superior clergy, equally indifferent, sing the Office, do you know what the friends in mourning, seated or standing about in the church, say to each other?—Here is your picture.—Well, would you like to see? 'How much do you think Papa d'Aldrigger left?' said Desroches to Taillefer, who gave us, before his death, the very finest orgie known—"

"Was Desroches an attorney at that time?"

"He was admitted in 1822," said Couture. "And it was a good deal for the son of a poor employé who had never had more than eighteen hundred francs, and whose mother conducted an establishment for the sale of stamped paper. But he worked hard from 1818 to 1822. Entered as a fourth clerk in the office of Derville, he was second clerk in 1819!"

"Desroches?"

"Yes," said Bixiou. "Desroches rolled along,

like us, on the dung-hills of favoritism. Tired of
wearing coats too small and sleeves too short, he ate
up his fee in despair and secured a bare title.   An
attorney without a sou, without any clients, without any other friends than us, he had to pay the
interest on a commission and on his securities.''

"He looked to me then like a tiger from the Jardin
des Plantes,'' said Couture.   "Thin, with reddish
hair, his eyes the color of Spanish tobacco, a harsh
skin, a cold and phlegmatic air, but harsh for the
widow, merciless for the orphan, a hard worker, the
terror of his clerks, who did not dare to waste their
time, learned, shrewd, two-sided, with a honeyed
elocution, never excited, hateful after the manner
of a judicial man.''

"And there was some good in him,'' cried Finot;
"he was devoted to his friends, and his first care
was to take Godeschal, the brother of Mariette, for
head clerk.''

"At Paris,'' said Blondet, "advocates are of only
two kinds,—there is the advocate who is an honest
man, who keeps within the terms of the law, pushes
his suits, does not run after business, neglects nothing, gives his clients good advice, comes to an
agreement with them on all doubtful points, a Derville, in short.   Then, there is the starveling advocate, for whom everything is good, provided only
that his fees are assured; who would bring into
action not the mountains, he would sell them, but the
planets; who would interest himself in the triumph
of a rascal over an honest man if by chance the

honest man did not have the best case. When one of these advocates has done a trick, after the manner of Master Gonin, a little too strong, the Chamber compels him to sell out. Desroches, our friend Desroches, understood this trade, so badly managed by the sorry fellows; he took charge of the cases of those persons who feared to lose them; he threw himself eagerly into chicanery like a man determined to get out of his poverty. He was right; he followed his trade very honestly. He found protectors in men of political affairs by straightening out their embarrassed transactions, as in the case of our dear des Lupeaulx, whose position was so compromised. It required all this to get him into a good position, for Desroches had commenced by being very badly considered by the court, he who rectified with so much trouble the errors of his clients!—Well, Bixiou, to return—. How did Desroches come to be in the church?"

" 'D'Aldrigger left seven or eight hundred thousand francs!" answered Taillefer to Desroches. 'Ah, bah! there is only one person who knows what *their* fortune is,' said Werbrust, a friend of the deceased.—'Who?'—'That big scamp of a Nucingen; he will go to the cemetery; d'Aldrigger was his patron, and through gratitude he will appraise the property of the worthy man.' 'His widow will find a very great difference!' 'What do you mean?' 'But d'Aldrigger loved his wife so much! Don't laugh, people are looking at us.' 'Well, here is Du Tillet; he is very late; he gets here in time to hear

4

the epistle.' 'He will doubtless marry the elder.'
'Is it possible?' said Desroches. 'He is more than
ever engaged with Madame Roguin.' 'He! Engaged?—you do not know him.' 'Do you know the
position of Nucingen and of Du Tillet?' asked Desroches. 'Here it is,' said Taillefer,—'Nucingen is
a man to eat up the capital of his former patron and
to give it back to him.' 'Heu! Heu!' said Werbrust. 'It is devilishly damp in the churches, heu!
heu!' 'How give it up again?'—'Well, Nucingen
knows that Du Tillet has a great fortune, he wants
to marry him to Malvina; but Du Tillet mistrusts
Nucingen. For those who watch the play, this
game is amusing.' 'How,' said Werbrust, 'is she
already old enough to marry? How fast we grow
old!' 'Malvina d'Aldrigger is more than twenty,
my dear fellow. The goodman d'Aldrigger was
married in 1800! He gave us some very good fêtes
at Strasbourg on the occasion of his marriage and
at the birth of Malvina. That was in 1801, at the
Peace of Amiens, and we are now in 1823, Papa
Werbrust. In those times, everything was Ossi-
anized! he named his daughter Malvina. Six years
later, under the Empire, there was for some time a
fury for chivalric things, it was all *Partant pour la
Syrie,*—a heap of foolishnesses. He named his
second daughter Isaure; she is seventeen. There
are two marriageable girls!' 'Those women will
not have a sou in ten years,' said Werbrust, confi-
dentially, to Desroches. 'There is,' replied Taillefer, 'the valet de chambre of d'Aldrigger, that old

fellow who bellows at the back of the church; he
has seen the two demoiselles brought up; he is capable of doing everything to preserve them their
property.' The chanters: *Dies iræ!* The children
of the choir: *Dies illa!* Taillefer: 'Adieu, Werbrust; when I hear the *Dies iræ, it* reminds me too
strongly of my poor son.' 'I am going too, it is too
damp here,' said Werbrust.—*In favilla.*—The beggars at the door: 'A few pennies, my dear gentlemen!' The beadle: 'Pan! Pan! *for the needs of
the church.*' The chanters: '*Amen!*' A friend:
'What did he die of?' An inquisitive joker: 'Of
a broken blood-vessel in the heel.' A passer-by:
'Do you know who is the personage who has died?'
A relative: 'The President de Montesquieu.' The
sacristan to the beggars: 'Get away from here;
they have given to us for you. Don't ask any
more!'"

"What *verve!*" said Couture.

—In fact, it seemed to us that we heard everything
that happened in the church. Bixiou imitated
everything, even to the noise of those who went
away with the body, by a shuffling of his feet on
the floor.—

"There are poets, romancers, writers, who say a
great many pretty things about Parisian manners,"
resumed Bixiou, "but this is the truth about funer-
als. Of a hundred persons who render the last
duties to a poor devil of a dead man, ninety-nine talk
of business and of pleasure openly in the church.
In order to see some poor little real grief, it requires

impossible circumstances. Further! is there a grief without selfishness?—"

"Heu! Heu!" said Blondet. "There is nothing in the world less respected than death, perhaps because there is nothing less respectable?"—

"It is so common!" resumed Bixiou. "When the service was over, Nucingen and Du Tillet accompanied the body to the cemetery. The old valet de chambre followed on foot. The coachman drove the carriage behind that of the clergy. 'Vel, my gude vrent,' said Nucingen to Du Tillet, as they turned the corner of the Boulevard, 'dis is a gude zhance to marry Malvina; you vil be de prodecdor ov dat boor vamily veeping, you vould haf a family, a home; you vould find a house alretty vurnished, und Malvina for zure is a real dresure.' "

"It is just like hearing him speak, that old Robert Macaire of a Nucingen!" said Finot.

" 'A charming young woman,' " said Ferdinand du Tillet, with enthusiasm, and without exciting himself,' " resumed Bixiou.

"It is all of Du Tillet in one word!" cried Couture.

" 'She might seem ugly to those who do not know her, but, I am sure of it, she has a fine soul,' said Du Tillet. 'And a hart, dat is de best ov it, my tear vellow; zhe vould haf tefotion und indelligence. In our tog ov a drade, you nefer know who vil life und who vil tie; it is a great habbiness do be able do drust in the hart of your vife. I vould sed off Telvine, who, you know, brought me more dan

a million, against Malvina, who has nod so gread a
dod.' 'But how much has she?' 'I do nod know
schust,' said the Baron de Nucingen, 'but zhe has
somedings.' 'She has a mother who likes to wear
pink!' said Du Tillet. This speech put an end to
the attempts of Nucingen. After dinner, the baron
informed Wilhelmine Adolphus that there remained
in his keeping scarcely four hundred thousand
francs. The daughter of the Adolphuses of Mannheim, reduced to twenty-four thousand francs of
income, lost herself in calculations which bewildered her. 'What!' said she to Malvina, 'what! I
have always had six thousand francs for us to spend
at the dressmakers! but where did your father get
the money? We shall have nothing at all with
twenty-four thousand francs; we shall starve. Ah!
if my father should see me thus reduced he would
die of it, if he were not already dead! Poor
Wilhelmine!' And she wept. Malvina, not knowing how to console her mother, represented to
her that she was still young and pretty; that pink
was still becoming to her; that she would go to the
Opera, to the Bouffons in the box of Madame de
Nucingen. She lulled her mother to sleep in dreams
of fêtes, of balls, of music, of beautiful toilets and
of success, a dream which commenced under the curtains of a bed in blue silk, in an elegant chamber,
adjoining that in which had expired, two nights previously, Monsieur Jean-Baptiste Baron d'Aldrigger, whose history may be given in three words.
During his life-time, this respectable Alsatian,

a banker at Strasbourg, had acquired a fortune of
about three millions.   In 1800, at the age of thirty-
six, at the climax of a fortune made during the Revolution, he had married, through ambition and by
inclination, the heiress of all the Adolphuses of
Mannheim, a young girl adored by a whole family,
and naturally she received the ancestral fortune in
the space of ten years.   D'Aldrigger was then made
a baron by His Majesty, the Emperor and King, for
his fortune doubled itself.   But he had a passion for
the great man who had given him his title; therefore, between 1814 and 1815, he was ruined for
having taken seriously the sun of Austerlitz.   The
honest Alsatian did not suspend payment, did not
satisfy his creditors with values which he considered doubtful; he paid everything over the counter,
retired from the bank and deserved the description
of his former head clerk, Nucingen: 'Honest man,
but a fool!' Everything included, there remained to
him five hundred thousand francs and obligations
due under the Empire, which no longer existed. 'See
vat it is to haf beliefed too much in Nappolion,'
said he, when he saw the result of his liquidation.   When one has been one of the first citizens,
what a descent to be one of the lesser ones!—The
banker of Alsace did as do all the ruined provin-
cials,—he came to Paris, he there wore courageously
tri-colored suspenders on which were embroidered
the imperial eagles, and he concentrated himself in
Bonapartist society.   He placed all his funds in the
hand of the Baron de Nucingen, who gave him

eight per cent for everything, accepting his imperial claims at sixty per cent only of loss, which
was the cause of d'Aldrigger's clasping the hand of
Nucingen and saying to him: 'I vas very zure to
vind a hart in an Elzacien!' Nucingen secured
payment in full from our friend, des Lupeaulx.
Though much shorn, the Alsatian still had a working revenue of forty-four thousand francs. His
chagrin was complicated with the *spleen* which
affects those who are accustomed to live in the midst
of affairs when they are separated from them. The
banker gave himself for a duty the task of sacrificing himself, noble heart! to his wife, whose fortune
had been made away with, and which she had
allowed to be taken with the indifference of a young
woman to whom monetary affairs were entirely unknown. The Baroness d'Aldrigger, then, was able
to find again the pleasures to which she had been
accustomed, the void which had been caused by the
loss of the society of Strasbourg was filled by the
pleasures of Paris. The house of Nucingen held
then, as it still holds, the supremacy in financial
society, and the clever baron made it a point of
honor to treat well the honest baron. This fine
virtue did good service in the Salon Nucingen.
Each winter curtailed the capital of d'Aldrigger;
but he did not dare to make the least reproach to
the pearl of the Adolphuses; his tenderness was the
most ingenuous and the most unintelligent that there
is in this world. An honest man, but stupid! He
died asking himself: 'What will become of them

without me?' And during a moment in which he
was alone with his old valet de chambre, Wirth, the
good man, between two suffocations, commended
to him his wife and his two daughters, as if this
Caleb of Alsace was the only reasonable being that
there was in the house. Three years later, in
1826, Isaure was twenty years old and Malvina was
not yet married. In going out into the world, Malvina had ended by becoming convinced of the super-
ficiality of all its relations, of the extent to which
everything there is examined, defined. Like the
greater number of young women said to be *well
brought-up,* Malvina was ignorant of the mechanism
of life, of the importance of a fortune, the difficulty
of acquiring the smallest amount of money, the price
of things. Thus, during these six years, every
enlightenment had been to her like a wound. The
four hundred thousand francs left by the late d'Aldrigger in the house of Nucingen were carried to
the credit of the baroness, for the estate of her husband was indebted to her in the sum of twelve
hundred thousand francs; and in times of need, the
shepherdess of the Alps drew from it as from an
inexhaustible treasury. At the moment in which
our pigeon was advancing toward his turtle-dove,
Nucingen, knowing the character of his ancient
patroness, felt himself obliged to explain to Malvina
the financial situation in which the widow was
placed,—he had no more than three hundred thous-
and francs in his hands, the twenty-four thousand
francs of income were, therefore, reduced to eighteen

thousand. Wirth had maintained the status during three years! After the banker's revelation, the horses were disposed of, the carriages sold and the coachman dispensed with by Malvina, without her mother's knowledge. The furniture of the hotel, which had been in use for ten years, could not be renewed, but everything had faded in the same time. For those who love harmony, this was only a semi-misfortune. The baroness, this flower so well preserved, had taken the aspect of a rose, cold and shriveled which remains alone on the bush in the middle of November. I who speak to you, I have seen this opulence vanishing by shades, by demitones! It was frightful, on my honor! That was my last grief. After it I said to myself: 'It is idiotic to take so much interest in others!' While I was an employé, I was stupid enough to interest myself in all the houses in which I dined, I defended them in case of scandal. I did not calumniate them, I—Oh! I was an infant! When her daughter had explained to her her position, the ci-devant pearl exclaimed: 'My poor children! Who will then make my gowns! I cannot then have any more new bonnets, nor receive, nor go out in society!'— In what way do you think love can be recognized in a man?" said Bixiou, interrupting himself; "it concerns us to know if Beaudenord was really in love with this little blond."

"He neglects his affairs," replied Couture.

"He puts on three shirts in one day," said Finot.

"A preliminary question," said Blondet,—"a superior man, can he and should he be in love?"

"My friends," resumed Bixiou, with a sentimental air, "beware, as you would of a venomous beast, of the man who, feeling himself taken with love for a woman, snaps his fingers or throws away his cigar, saying: 'Bah! there are others in the world!' But the government may employ this citizen in the Ministry of Foreign Affairs. Blondet, I'd have you note that this Godefroid had quit the diplomatic career."

"Well, he has been absorbed; love offers fools their only chance of growing," replied Blondet.

"Blondet, Blondet, why are we, then, so poor?" cried Bixiou.

"And why is Finot so rich?" replied Blondet; "I will tell you; come, my boy, we will understand each other. Just see, there is Finot, who pours out my wine as if I had carried up his fire-wood for him. But toward the end of the dinner you should *sip* your wine.—Well, then?"

"As you say, the absorbed Godefroid became very well acquainted with the tall Malvina, the fair baroness and the little danseuse. Ah! he fell into a state of servantism of the most detailed and the most astringent character.   These remnants of a cadaverous opulence did not frighten him. Ah, bah! he became accustomed by degrees to all these rags. The green lampas of the salon, with its white ornaments, never appeared to this youth worn or old, nor spotted, nor in need of being renewed.   The

curtains, the tea-table, the Chinese ornaments on
the chimney-piece, the rococo glass chandelier, the
carpet in imitation Cashmere worn threadbare, the
piano, the little flowered table service, the napkins
fringed and also open-worked in the Spanish style,
the Persian salon, which opened into the bed-chamber, in blue, of the baroness, with its accessories,
everything to him was saintly and sacred. Women
who are commonplace, and in whom beauty shines,
so as to throw into the shade wit, the heart and
the soul, alone can inspire such complete forgetfulness, for a spiritual woman never abuses her advantages; it is necessary to be petite and foolish thus
to carry a man away. Beaudenord, he told me so
himself, loved the old and solemn Wirth! This old
fellow respected his future master as a Catholic
believer respects the Eucharist. This honest
Wirth was a German Gaspard, one of those beer-
drinkers who conceal their shrewdness in their
good-nature, as a cardinal of the Middle Ages his
poniard in his sleeve. Wirth, seeing a husband for
Isaure, surrounded Godefroid with the ambages and
flowery circumlocutions of his Alsatian good-nature,
the most binding of all adhesive things. Madame
d'Aldrigger was profoundly *improper*, she found love
the most natural thing in the world. When Isaure
and Malvina went out together to the Tuileries or to
the Champs-Élysées, where they would meet the
young people of their society, the mother would say
to them: 'Amuse yourselves, my dear daughters.'
Their friends, the only persons who could speak

evil of the two sisters, defended them; for the great
liberty which reigned in the salon of the d'Aldriggers rendered it an unique locality in Paris.   With
a fortune of millions, it would have been difficult to
have obtained such evenings, in which everything
was discussed with spirit, in which a careful partic-
ularity was not required, in which every one was
at his ease, even to the extent of asking for supper.
The two sisters wrote to whomsoever they pleased,
received peacefully their letters by their mother's
side, without the idea ever occurring to the baroness
to make any inquiries.   This adorable mother gave
to her daughters all the benefits of her egoism, the
most amiable passion in the world, in this respect
that the egoists, not wishing to be interfered with,
interfere with no one, and do not in the least embarrass the life of those who surround them with
the brambles of good advice, with the thorns of
remonstrance, nor with the wasp-like teasing which
are permitted those excessive friendships which
wish to know everything, to control everything.—"

"You go to my heart," said Blondet.   "But, my
dear fellow, you are not telling your story, you are
hoaxing—"

"Blondet, if you were not drunk, you would give
me pain!   Of us four, he is the only man who is
seriously literary!   For his sake, I am doing you
the honor to treat you as epicures, I am distilling
to you my history, and he criticises me!   My
friends, the greatest evidence of mental sterility
is the heaping up of fact.   The sublime comedy of

the *Misanthrope* proves that art consists in building a palace on the point of a needle. The myth of my idea is in the wand of the fairy which can make of the plain of Sablons an Interlaken, in ten seconds—the time to empty this glass!—Would you have me make a recital to you that should go like a cannon-ball, a report of the general-in-chief? We are conversing, we are laughing, this newspaper man, bibliophobe fasting, wishes, when he is drunk, that I should give to my language the sottish attraction of a book—he pretends to weep.— Woe to the French imagination, the needles of its pleasantry are to be blunted! *Dies iræ.* Weep, Candide, and long live the *Critique de la raison pure!* the *Symbolique*, and the systems in five compact volumes, printed by the Germans, who have not known at Paris since 1750, to put it neatly, the diamonds of our national intelligence. Blondet conducts the funeral train of its suicide, he who utters in his journal the last words of all the great men who have died for us without saying anything."

"Go your own gait," said Finot.

"I wish to explain to you in what consists the happiness of a man who is not a shareholder—this is a politeness to Couture!—Well, do you not see now at what price Godefroid procured the greatest happiness that a young man could dream of!—He studied Isaure to be sure of being comprehended!— Those things which comprehend each other should be similar. Now, there are only like each other two things, nothingness and the infinite; nothingness

is stupidity, genius is the infinite. These two lovers wrote to each other the most stupid letters in the world, sending them on paper perfumed with the words then in the fashion: 'Angel! Æolian harp! with thee I shall be complete! There is a heart in my manly chest! Feeble woman! poor me!' all the frippery of a modern heart. Godefroid scarcely remained ten minutes in a salon, he talked with women without any pretension, and they found him very witty. He was of those who have no other wit than that which is lent them. In short, you may judge of his absorption,—Joby, his horses, his carriages, became secondary things in his existence. He was only happy when ensconced in her comfortable sofa before the baroness, at the corner of that chimney-piece in verd-antique, occupied in watching Isaure, in drinking tea while conversing with a little group of friends who came every evening, between eleven o'clock and midnight, to Rue Joubert, and where one could always have a game of bouillotte without fear:—I always won. When Isaure had put out her pretty little foot, shod with a black satin slipper and when Godefroid had looked at it for a long time, he remained after all the others and said to Isaure: 'Give me thy shoe'—Isaure raised her foot, rested it on a chair, took off her shoe, gave it to him, throwing upon him a look, one of those looks—in short, you understand! Godefroid ended by discovering a great mystery in Malvina. When Du Tillet knocked at the door, the lively red which colored the cheeks of Malvina said: 'Ferdinand!'

when looking at this tiger with two paws, the eyes of
the poor girl lit up like a brazier on which a current
of air is turned; she betrayed an infinite pleasure
when Ferdinand took her aside to tell her something
by a console or at the window. How very rare
and beautiful it is, a woman enough in love to become candid and to permit her heart to be read!
Mon Dieu, it is as scarce in Paris as is in the Indies
the flower that sings. Notwithstanding this friendship, commenced the day on which the d'Aldriggers appeared at the Nucingens, Ferdinand did not
marry Malvina. Our ferocious friend, Du Tillet had
not seemed jealous of the assiduous court which
Desroches paid to Malvina, for, to finish paying for
his practice charges with a dot which appeared to
be not less than fifty thousand écus, he had feigned
love, he, a man of the law! Although profoundly
humiliated by the indifference of Du Tillet, Malvina
loved him too much to shut the door on him. In this
young woman, all soul, all sentiment, all expansion,
sometimes pride yielded to love, sometimes offended
love permitted pride to triumph. Calm and cold,
our friend Ferdinand accepted this tenderness, he
inhaled it with the tranquil satisfaction of a tiger
licking the blood which stains its paws; he came to
get fresh proofs of it; he did not allow two days to
pass without presenting himself in the Rue Joubert.
The scamp possessed at this time about eighteen
hundred thousand francs; the question of fortune
should have been a secondary one in his eyes, and
he had resisted not only Malvina, but the Barons of

Nucingen and of Rastignac, who, both of them, had made him do seventy-five leagues a day, with four francs to the guides, the postilion in advance, and with no clew! in the labyrinths of their shrewdness. Godefroid could not restrain himself from speaking to his future sister-in-law of the unfortunate situation in which she was placed between a banker and an advocate. 'You wish to sermonize me on the subject of Ferdinand, to know the secret which is between us,' she said frankly. 'Dear Godefroid, do not speak of it again. The birth of Ferdinand, his antecedents, his fortune, count for nothing; therefore you may believe in something extraordinary.' Nevertheless, a few days later, Malvina took Beaudenord aside and said to him: 'I do not think Monsieur Desroches is an honest man—such is the instinct of love!—he would like to marry me, and is paying court to a grocer's daughter. I should much like to know if I am a make-shift, if marriage is for him only an affair of money!' Despite his great intelligence Desroches could not make out Du Tillet, and he feared to see him marry Malvina. Thus the youth had managed a retreat; his position was intolerable; he gained with difficulty, all expenses paid, the interest of his debt. Women never understand anything of these situations. For them, the heart is always a millionaire!"

"But, as neither Desroches nor Du Tillet married Malvina," said Finot, "explain to us Ferdinand's secret."

"The secret, here it is," replied Bixiou. "General rule: A young person who has once given her slipper, if she should refuse it for ten years, is never married by him to whom—"

"Nonsense!" said Blondet, interrupting, "one loves also because one has loved. The secret, here it is. General rule: Do not marry as a sergeant, when you can become Duc de Dantzick and Marshal of France. Thus, see what an alliance Du Tillet did make! He married one of the daughters of the Comte de Granville, one of the oldest families of the French magistracy."

"The mother of Desroches had a friend," resumed Bixiou, "the wife of a druggist, which druggist had retired swollen with a fortune. These druggists have very absurd ideas,—in order to give his daughter a good education he had put her in a boarding-school!—This Matifat counted on marrying his daughter well, by virtue of two hundred thousand francs, in good and sound money which did not smell of drugs."

"The Matifat of Florine?" said Blondet.

"Well, yes, Lousteau's, ours, in short! These Matifats, then lost to us, had taken a house in the Rue du Cherche-Midi, the most opposite quarter to the Rue des Lombards, in which they had made their fortune. As for myself, I cultivated them, the Matifats! During my time in the ministerial galleys, in which I was locked up eight hours every day among dunces of twenty-two carats, I saw some originals which convinced me that shadows have

5

their asperities, and that in the greatest flatness one may encounter angles! Yes, my dear fellow, one bourgeois is to another as Raphaël is to Natoire. The widow Desroches had brought about with all her influence this marriage to her son, notwithstanding the enormous obstacle presented by a certain Cochin, a son of the sleeping-partner of the Matifats, a young man employed in the Ministry of Finance. In the eyes of Monsieur and Madame Matifat, the standing of an advocate appeared, as they expressed it, to offer guarantees for the happiness of a wife. Desroches lent himself to his mother's plans in order to have a certain choice. He accordingly kept on good terms with the druggist of the Rue du Cherche-Midi. To be able to understand another species of happiness, it would be necessary to describe for you these two trades-people, male and female, enjoying a little garden, lodged in a fine ground-floor, amusing themselves with watching a little fountain, thin and long as a spike, which played perpetually and sprang from a little round table in freestone, in the middle of a basin six feet in diameter; rising early to see if the flowers in their garden had grown, unemployed and unquiet, dressing for the sake of dressing, boring themselves at the theatre, and forever between Paris and Luzarches, where they had a country-house, and where I have dined. Blondet, one day when they wished me to do something for them, I related to them a story from nine o'clock in the evening to midnight, an adventure of episodes. I

had arrived at the introduction of my twenty-ninth
personage—the serial novels stole it from me !—when
Father Matifat, who, in his character as head of the
house, had kept up a good appearance, fell to snoring
like the others, after having been winking for five
minutes. The next day everybody complimented
me on the ending of my story. These grocers had
for society Monsieur and Madame Cochin, Adolphe
Cochin, Madame Desroches, a little Popinot, a druggist exercising his profession, who brought them
the news of the Rue des Lombards—a man of your
acquaintance, Finot.—Madame Matifat, who loved
the arts, bought lithographs, chromo-lithographs,
colored designs, everything that was of the cheap-
est. The Sieur Matifat interested himself in
watching new enterprises and in endeavoring to
speculate with some funds in order to experience
some emotion—Florine had cured him of the styles
of the Regency.—A single word will enable you to
comprehend the profundity of my Matifat. The
good man bade his nieces good-night in these words :
'Go thou to bed, my nieces !' He was afraid, he
said, to hurt their feelings by saying *you* to them.
Their daughter was a young person without any
manners, with the appearance of a waiting-maid
in a good house, playing a sonata indifferently well,
with a pretty English hand-writing, knowing French
and orthography, in short, a complete bourgeois education. She was sufficiently impatient to be married,
in order to be able to leave the paternal mansion, in
which she was as much bored as a naval officer

during a night-watch; it must be said that the watch here lasted the whole day. Desroches or Cochin's son, a notary or a Garde du Corps, an imitation English lord, any husband would do for her. As she evidently knew nothing of life, I took pity on her; I wished to reveal to her its great mystery. Bah! the Matifats shut their door on me: the bourgeois and I, we shall never comprehend each other."

"She married General Gouraud," said Finot.

"In forty-eight hours, Godefroid de Beaudenord, the ex-diplomat, had taken the measure of the Matifats and their intriguing corruption," resumed Bixiou. "As it happened, Rastignac was present in the house of the light baroness, talking, at a corner of the fire, while Godefroid made his report to Malvina. Some words reached his ear, he guessed at the subject under discussion, especially because of the bitterly satisfied air of Malvina. Rastignac remained there until two o'clock in the morning,—and people said that he was egotistical! Beaudenord left when the baroness went to bed. 'Dear child,' said Rastignac to Malvina, in a good-humored and paternal tone, when they were alone, 'remember that a poor fellow heavy with sleep has kept himself awake with tea until two o'clock in the morning in order to be able to say to you solemnly: *Get married.* Do not raise any difficulties, do not concern yourself with feelings, do not think of the ignoble calculations of men who have one foot here and one foot at the Matifats, reflect on nothing: get married! For a girl to get married, that is to impose herself on a

man who engages to support her in a position more
or less happy, but in which the material question
is assured.   I know the world: young girls, mam-
mas and grandmothers are all hypocrites in making
so much ado about feelings when it is a question of
marriage.   No one thinks of any other thing than
being well-established.   When her daughter is well
married, a mother says that she has done an excellent thing.'   And Rastignac proceeded to develop to
her his theory upon marriage, which, according to
him, is a commercial society instituted to support
life.   'I do not ask your secret,' said he, in conclusion, to Malvina, 'I know it.   Men talk about everything among themselves, just as you do when you
go out after dinner.   Well, then, this is my last
word: Get married.   If you do not get married,
remember that I begged you here, this evening, to
get married!'   Rastignac spoke with a certain
accent which commanded, not attention, but reflection.   His insistence was of a nature to surprise.
Malvina was so much struck with it in her keenest
intelligence, which Rastignac wished to reach, that
she was still thinking of it the next day, and un-
availingly sought to discover the reason for this
advice.''

"I do not see in all these peg-tops which you set
off, anything which resembles the origin of Rastignac's fortune, and you take us for the Matifats
multiplied by six bottles of champagne!'' cried
Couture.

"We are there," replied Bixiou.   "You have

followed the course of all the little streams which have made the forty thousand francs of income which so many people envy! Rastignac then held in his hands the thread of all these existences."

"Desroches, the Matifats, Beaudenord, the d'Aldriggers, d'Aiglemont?"

"And of a hundred others!—" said Bixiou.

"Well, now, how?" cried Finot. "I know a good many things, and I do not see the answer to this enigma."

"Blondet has described to you briefly the first two liquidations of Nucingen, here is the third in detail," resumed Bixiou. "At the Peace of 1815, Nucingen had comprehended that which we only understand to-day,—that money is a power only when it is in disproportionate quantities. He was secretly jealous of the brothers Rothschild. He possessed five millions, he wished to have ten! With ten millions he would know how to gain thirty, and with five he would only have fifteen. He had therefore resolved to bring about a third liquidation! This great man consequenty planned to pay his creditors with fictitious values while keeping their money. On the exchanges, an operation of this kind does not present itself in quite such a mathematical expression. A liquidation of this kind consists in giving a little pâté for a golden louis to big children, who, like the little children formerly, preferred the pâté to the coin, without knowing that for the coin they could have two hundred pâtés."

"What is it you are saying to us, Bixiou?" cried

Couture, "but nothing is more fair, there is not a week goes by nowadays without some one presenting pâtés to the public and demanding a louis for each. But is the public forced to give its money? has it not the right to inform itself?"

"You would like it better if compelled to buy its shares of stock," said Blondet.

"No," said Finot, "or where would be our smartness?"

"That is very good for Finot," said Bixiou.

"Who gave him that idea?" asked Couture.

"In short," resumed Bixiou, "Nucingen had had on two occasions the happinesses of giving, without intending it, a pâté which came to possess more value than he had received. This unlucky good fortune had caused him remorse. Happiness such as this, ends by killing a man. He waited during ten years for an occasion in which he would not deceive himself, in which to create values that should have the appearance of being worth something and which—"

"But," said Couture, "with this explanation of banking, no commerce is possible. More than one honest banker has persuaded, under the approval of a loyal government, the most able treasurers to accept funds which in the course of time have become depreciated. You have seen better than that! Have there not been issued, always with the advice, with the support of governments, securities with which to pay the interest of certain funds, in order to maintain their circulation and to enable

them to be disposed of? These operations have more or less analogy with liquidation in the manner of Nucingen."

"In small affairs," said Blondet, "the transaction might appear singular; but on a great scale it is high financiering. There are certain arbitrary acts which are criminal between individuals, but which amount to nothing when they are expanded through any multitude whatever, like a drop of Prussic acid which becomes harmless in a tub of water. You kill a man and you are guillotined. But, with any governmental conviction whatever, you kill five hundred men, the political crime is respected. You take five thousand francs from my writing-desk, you go to the galleys. But, with the pimento of a profit to make, skilfully put in the mouths of a thousand purse-holders, you force them to take the stocks of I-know-not-what republic or monarchy in default, issued, as Couture says, to pay the interest of these same stocks,—no one can complain. These are the true principles of the age of gold in which we live!"

"The setting in operation of so vast a machine," resumed Bixiou, "required a great many punchinellos. In the first place, the house of Nucingen had knowingly, and with design, employed its five millions in an American enterprise, the profits of which had been calculated in such a manner as to come in too late. They had been put out of the way with premeditation. Every liquidation should be justified. The bank possessed in individual funds

and in values issued about six millions. Among the individual funds were the three hundred thousand francs of the Baroness d'Aldrigger, the four hundred thousand of Beaudenord, a million belonging to d'Aiglemont, three hundred thousand francs to Matifat, a half million to Charles Grandet, the hus-band of Mademoiselle d'Aubrion, etc. If he had created himself some industrial enterprise with the shares of which he proposed to satisfy his creditors by means of manœuvres more or less skilful, Nucingen might have been suspected, but he went about it with much more adroitness: he caused it to be created by another!—that machine destined to play the part which the Mississippi did in the system of Law. The peculiar quality of Nucingen is to make the most able negotiators serve his projects without communiating his own to them. Nucingen accordingly let slip before Du Tillet a suggestion of this pyramidal and victorious scheme of getting up an enterprise by subscription with a capital sufficiently large to pay very heavy interest to the shareholders at first. If tried for the first time, at a period when there was an abundance of credulous capital, this combination should bring about a rise in the shares, and consequently a bene-fit for the banker who issued them. Remember that this was in 1826. Although struck with this idea, fruitful as ingenious, Du Tillet naturally reflected that, if the enterprise did not succeed, there would be some blame laid somewhere. Therefore, he would suggest putting forward some visible

director for this commercial machine. You know to-day the secret of the house of Claparon, founded by Du Tillet, one of his finest inventions!—"

"Yes," said Blondet, "the responsible financial editor, the agent that prepares the way, the scape-goat; but, to-day, we are more clever, we put out: 'Address the Management of the thing, such a street, such a number,' where the public will find employés in green caps, pretty as bailiff's men."

"Nucingen had supported the house of Charles Claparon with all his credit," resumed Bixiou. "A million of the paper of Claparon could be issued without any fear on some exchanges. Du Tillet proposed, therefore, to bring the house of Claparon forward. Adopted. In 1825, the shareholder was not spoiled in industrial enterprises. The funds destined to provide for *running expenses* were un-known! The directors did not undertake to ever issue their interest-bearing shares; they deposited nothing in the Bank of France, they guaranteed nothing. The shareholder could not expect to have the workings of the company explained to him when informed that he was fortunate in not having more than a thousand, or more than five hundred, or even two hundred and fifty francs demanded of him! It was not published that the experience *in ære publico* would only endure for seven years, five years or even three years, and that therefore the dénouement would not have to be long waited for. It was the infancy of the art! There had not even been called in the publicity of those gigantic announcements by

which imaginations are now stimulated, by demanding money from everyone—"

"This happens when no one wishes to subscribe,"
said Couture.

"In short, the competition in this sort of enterprises did not exist," resumed Bixiou. "The
manufacturers of papier-maché, of printed calicoes,
the rollers of zinc, the theatres, the newspapers,
did not throw themselves in like dogs of the chase
at 'the death' of the expiring shareholder. The
fine affairs by subscription, as Couture says, so
ingenuously published, supported by the reports of
experts—the princes of science!—were then trans-
acted shamefacedly in the silence and in the obscurity of the Bourse. The monetary lynxes executed,
financially speaking, the air of the Calumny of
the *Barber of Seville*. They went *piano, piano*,
proceeding by light cancans, on the good qualities
of the enterprise, spoken from ear to ear. They did
not exploit the patient, the shareholder, only at his
house, at the Bourse, or in society, by that rumor
skilfully created, and which increased to the *tutti* of
a number of four figures—"

"But, since we are among ourselves and can say
anything, I return to our subject," said Couture.

"You are a goldsmith, Monsieur Josse!" said
Finot.

"Finot will remain classical, constitutional, and
bewigged," said Blondet.

"Yes, I am a goldsmith," resumed Couture, "seeing that Cérizet has been condemned by the police

tribunals.   I maintain that the new method is infinitely less treacherous, more honest, less assassinating, than the old one.   The publicity allows of reflection and examination.   If any stockholder is gullible, he comes to it deliberately; he has not been made to purchase 'a pig in a poke.' Industry—"

"Ah! now we are coming to industry!" cried Bixiou.

"Industry would profit by it," said Couture, without paying any attention to the interruption. "Every government that interferes with commerce and does not leave it unrestricted, undertakes a costly folly; it brings about either the *maximum* or the monopoly.   To my thinking, nothing is more conformable to the principles of the liberty of commerce than the societies of shareholders!   To meddle with them, is to answer for both capital and profits, which is stupid.   In every transaction, the profits are in proportion to the risks!   What matters it to the state the manner in which is brought about the free circulation of money, provided that it be kept in perpetual activity?   What matter who is rich, who is poor, if there is always the same quantity of taxable wealth?   Moreover, for the last twenty years the societies of shareholders, stock-companies, premiums under all possible forms, have been in use in the most commercial country in the world, in England, where everything is disputed, where Parliament hatches out a thousand or twelve hundred laws each session, and

where a member of either House has never risen to
speak against the method—"

"Curative for full coffers, and a vegetarian one!"
said Bixiou; "carrots!" *

"Come now!" said Couture, excitedly. "You
have ten thousand francs, you take ten shares of a
thousand each in ten different enterprises. You are
robbed nine times—this is not so! the public is
wiser than any one person! but I make the suppo-
sition—one enterprise alone succeeds—by chance!—
agreed!—it has not been made expressly!—oh, go
ahead! talk nonsense!—Well, the *punter* who is
wise enough thus to divide up his forces will find a
superb investment, as did those who took the shares
of the mines of Wortschin. Messieurs, let us admit
among ourselves that the people who cry out are the
hypocrites in despair at having neither the conception of an enterprise, nor the power to proclaim it,
nor the skill to exploit it. The proof will not long
be waited for. In a little while you will see the
aristocracy, the people of the Court, the ministeri-
alists, descending in solid columns into business
speculations, and reaching out hands more grasping
and finding more tortuous ideas than ours, without
having our superiority. What a head it requires
to set on foot a good enterprise at an epoch in
which the avidity of the shareholder is equal to that
of the inventor! What a great magnetizer must be
the man who creates a Claparon, who finds new
expedients! Do you know the moral of all this?

* Carotte, a trick for obtaining money by skill or deception.

Our time is no better than we are! We live in an epoch of avidity in which no one concerns himself about the value of a thing, provided he can make something on it and pass it on to his neighbor; and it is passed on to the neighbor because the avidity of the shareholder, who hopes for a profit, is equal to that of the founder who proposed one to him!"

"Isn't he fine, Couture, isn't he fine!" said Bixiou to Blondet; "he is going to ask that statues be erected to him, as to a benefactor of humanity."

"It will be necessary to bring him to conclude that the money of fools is, by right divine, the patrimony of clever men," said Blondet.

"Messieurs," resumed Couture, "let us laugh here in return for the seriousness which we preserve elsewhere, when we hear uttered the respectable stupidities which consecrate the laws made without forethought."

"He is right. What a time, Messieurs," said Blondet, "is that in which as soon as the fire of intelligence appears it is quickly extinguished by the application of a circumstantial law! The legislators, nearly all of them come from little arrondissements where they have made their social studies in the newspapers, put the fire in the engine. When the engine blows up, then there are tears and grindings of teeth! A time in which the only laws made are fiscal and penal! The true word of all that happens, do you wish to know it! *There is no longer any religion in the state!* "

"Ah!" said Bixiou, "bravo, Blondet! you have

put your finger on the tender spot of France,—the code of fiscal laws, which has taken more conquests from our country than all the vexations of war. In the ministry where I served seven years at the galleys, yoked with the bourgeois, there was an employé, a man of talent, who had resolved to change the entire financial system—ah! well, we very soon dismissed him. France had been too happy, she would have amused herself by reconquering Europe, and we acted in the interest of the repose of nations. I killed Rabourdin by a caricature!"—See *The Civil Service*.

"When I said *religion*, I did not mean to say a stupid Capuchin's sermon; I understand the word in a grand political sense," resumed Blondet.

"Explain yourself," said Finot.

"In this way," continued Blondet. "There has been much talk of the affairs at Lyons, of the Republic cannonaded in the streets; no one has told the truth. The Republic took possession of the riot just as an insurgent grasps a gun. The real truth, I will give it to you, both absurd and profound. The commerce of Lyons is a commerce without any soul, which does not manufacture a yard of silk unless it is ordered and unless the payment is sure. When the orders cease, the workman dies of hunger; he earns with difficulty enough to live on when he works. The galley slaves are happier than he. After the Revolution of July, the misery reached such a point that the CANUTS* hoisted the flag,

* Canut, operative in the silk factories of Lyons.

'Bread or death!' one of those proclamations which
the government should study; it was produced by the
dearness of living at Lyons. Lyons wished to build
theatres and to become a capital, hence came sense-
less octroi duties. The Republicans scented this
revolt in the cause of bread, and they organized the
Canuts, who fought in two parties. Lyons has had
its three days, but everything has returned to order
and the Canut into his hole. The Canut, honest up
to this period, returning in the woven stuff the silk
which was weighed out to him in hanks, has turned
his honesty out of the door, believing that the merchant had victimized him, and has put oil on his
fingers,—he has returned weight for weight, but he
had sold oil represented as silk, and the trade in
French silks has been infested with 'loaded silks,'
which may bring about the destruction of Lyons
and that of a branch of the commerce of France.
The manufacturers and the government, instead of
suppressing the cause of the evil, have, like certain
physicians, driven in the disease by a violent
topical remedy. There should have been sent to
Lyons a skilful man, one of those who are called
immoral, an Abbé Terray, but the situation was
looked at only from the military point of view!
The troubles, therefore, have produced gros-grain at
forty sous the aune. This gros-grain, it can be
said, is sold to-day, and the manufacturers have
doubtless invented I know not what system of veri-
fication. This method of manufacture without forethought is naturally established in a country in

which RICHARD LENOIR, one of the greatest citizens which France ever had, had ruined himself by giving employment to six thousand workmen without any orders, by supporting them, and had found ministers stupid enough to let him succumb to the revolution which 1814 brought about in the price of stuffs. This is the only case in which a merchant has merited a statue. Well, this man is to-day the object of the subscription to which there are no subscribers, whilst a million has been raised for the children of General Foy. Lyons is consistent; it knows France; it is without any religious sentiment. The story of Richard Lenoir is one of those faults which Fouché found to be worse than a crime."

"If in the manner in which affairs present themselves," resumed Couture, going back to the point where he was before the interruption, "there is a tinge of charlatanism, a word which has become dishonoring and set astride the partition-wall between the just and the unjust, I demand where commences, or where finishes, charlatanism, what is charlatanism? Have the kindness to tell me who is not a charlatan? Come, now, let us have a little good faith, the rarest social ingredient! That commerce which should consist in going to seek at night that which could be sold in the day would be nonsense. A seller of matches has the instinct of monopoly. To monopolize merchandise is the idea of the shop-keeper of the Rue Saint-Denis, *called* the most virtuous, as of the speculator *called* the most shameless. When the stores are full, there

6

is a necessity to sell. To sell, it is necessary to *excite* the customer, hence the sign of the Middle Ages and the advertisement of to-day! Between calling in the customers and forcing them to enter, to purchase, I do not see the difference of a hair! It may happen, it should happen, it often does happen, that merchants get caught with damaged merchandise, for the seller is incessantly cheating the buyer. Well, consult the most honest people in Paris, the distinguished merchants, in short,—they will all relate to you triumphantly the trick which they have invented to get rid of their merchandise when it has been sold to them in a damaged condition. The famous House of Minard commenced by sales of this description. The Rue Saint-Denis will only sell you a dress of loaded silk; it has no other. The most virtuous merchant will repeat to you with the most candid air this phrase of the most brazen dishonesty: 'You get out of a bad bargain the best way you can.' Blondet has shown you the affair of Lyons in its causes and in its consequences; for my part, I will get to the application of my theory by an anecdote. A workman in wool, ambitious and overloaded with children by a wife too much loved, believes in the Republic. My fine fellow bought a lot of red wool and made these caps in knitted wool which you may have seen on the heads of all the gamins of Paris, and you will know why. The Republic was overcome. After the affair of Saint-Merri, the caps were unsalable. When a workman finds himself in his

household with a wife, children and ten thousand red woolen caps which no hatter on any shore wants, there come into his head as many ideas as would present themselves to a banker loaded with ten millions of shares to place in an enterprise which he mistrusts. Do you know what he did, this workman, this Law of the Faubourgs, this Nucingen of caps? He hunted up a dandy of the taverns, one of those fellows who are the despair of the police sergeants in the Bals Champêtres of the barriers, and requested him to play the part of an American captain trading in colonial goods, stopping at the Hôtel Meurice, to go and *inquire for* ten thousand red woolen caps at the establishment of a rich hatter who had still one of them in his stock. The hatter foresaw a large transaction in America, he hastened to the workman and eagerly took possession of all the caps, cash down. You understand, —no more American captain, but a great many caps. To attack commercial liberty because of these inconveniences, would be to attack justice under the pretext that there are delinquencies which it does not punish, or to accuse society of being badly organized because of the misfortunes to which it gives rise! From caps and the Rue Saint-Denis to shares of stock and the Bank of France, draw your own conclusions!"

"Couture, a crown!" said Blondet, placing on his head his twisted napkin. "I go farther, Messieurs. If there be a vice in the actual theory, whose is the fault? that of the law! the law considered in its

entire system, legislation! of those great men of the arrondissements whom the provinces send puffed up with moral ideas, ideas indispensable in the conduct of life, at least to combat by the side of justice, but stupid as soon as they prevent a man from lifting himself to the height at which the legislator should maintain himself. Though the laws may forbid to the passions such or such a development—gambling, the lottery, the Ninons of the barriers, whatever you like,—they will never extirpate the passions. To kill the passions, that would be to kill society, which, if it does not engender them, at least develops them. Thus, if you fetter with restrictions the desire to gamble which lurks at the bottom of every heart, that of the young girl, that of the man of the provinces, as in that of a diplomat, for all the world sighs for a fortune *gratis*, gambling will then display itself in other spheres. You suppress the lottery stupidly; the cooks will not the less steal from their masters, they will carry their thefts to the savings-bank, and the stake is for them two hundred and fifty francs instead of being forty sous, for the shares in industrial enterprises, the stock-companies, become the lottery, the play without the green carpet, but with an invisible rake and with a calculated success for the bank. The gambling places are closed, the lottery no longer exists, behold France much more moral, exclaim the imbeciles, as if they had suppressed the *punters!* Gambling still goes on, only the benefit no longer accrues to the state, which replaces a tax paid with pleasure

by a vexatious tax, without diminishing the number of suicides, for the gambler does not die, but only his victim! I do not say anything about funds invested abroad, lost to France, nor of the lotteries of Frankfort, against the hawking about of which the Convention proclaimed the death penalty, and to which the *procureurs-syndics* themselves were addicted! Here you may see the sense of the silly philanthropy of our legislator. The encouragement given to the savings-bank is a gross political stupidity. Suppose any distrust whatever about the conduct of affairs, the government would have created *la queue* de l'argent* as they created during the Revolution, *la queue du pain.* So many savings-banks, so many riots. If, in a corner, three street boys set up a solitary flag, you will have a revolution. But this danger, however great it may be, seems to me less to be feared than that of the demoralization of the people. A savings-bank is the inoculation of all the vices engendered by interest, to those whom neither education nor reflection restrain in their tacitly criminal combinations. And there you have the effects of philanthropy. A great politician should be a blackguard in the abstract; without which societies are badly conducted. A politician who is an honest man is a steam-engine which has feelings, or a pilot who makes love while at the helm,—the vessel founders. A prime minister who takes a hundred millions and who renders France great and happy, is he not

---

* *Queue,* a long line of people waiting to be served.

to be preferred to a minister who has to be buried
at the expense of the state, but who had ruined his
country? Between Richelieu, Mazarin, Potemkin,
all three of them possessed at certain epochs three
hundred millions, and the virtuous Robert Lindet,
who did not know enough to make anything either
from the assignats, nor from the national property,
or the virtuous imbeciles who ruined Louis XVI.,
would you hesitate? Go on with your story,
Bixiou."

"I will not explain to you," resumed Bixiou,
"the nature of the enterprise invented by the financial genius of Nucingen, it would be all the more
inconvenient, as it is still existing to-day; its shares
are quoted on the Bourse; the combinations were
so real, the object of the enterprise so permanent,
that, created with a nominal capital of a thousand
francs, established by royal ordinance, fallen to
three hundred francs, they went up again to seven
hundred, and will arrive at par after having traversed the storms of the years '27, '30 and '32. The
financial crisis of 1827 made them shrink, the Revolution of July brought them down, but the enterprise is sound at bottom—Nucingen would not know
how to invent a bad affair—In short, as several
first-class banking houses have participated in it,
it would not be parliamentary to enter more into
details. The nominal capital was fixed at ten millions, the real capital seven, three millions were to
go to the originators and to the bankers who had
charge of the issuing of the shares. Everything

was calculated so as to cause in the first six months
each share to gain two hundred francs by the distribution of a fictitious dividend.   Hence, twenty
per cent on ten millions.   The interest of Du
Tillet amounted to five hundred thousand francs.
In the financial vocabulary this gain is called the
glutton's part!   Nucingen proposed to operate, with
his millions made from a quire of pink paper, with
the aid of a lithographic stone, some nice little
marketable shares, preciously preserved in his
cabinet.   The real shares would go to help establish the enterprise, to buy a magnificent hôtel
and commence operations.   Nucingen found still
other shares in I-know-not-what mines of silver-
bearing lead ore, in oil wells and in two canals,
interest-bearing shares issued to aid in the presentation of these four enterprises in full activity,
equipped in a superior manner and flourishing,
thanks to the dividend drawn on the capital.
Nucingen could count upon an *agio* if the shares
went up, but the baron left this out of his calculations; he allowed it to remain at its par value,
on the market, in order to attract the fish!
He had thus massed his funds, as Napoléon massed
his troops, in order to be able to liquidate during
the crisis which was revealing itself and which rev-
olutionized, in '26 and '27, the European markets.
If he had had his Prince de Wagram, he would have
been able to say, as did Napoléon on the heights of
Santon : 'Examine the locality well; on such a day,
at such an hour, there will funds be scattered!'

But in whom could he confide? Du Tillet did not
suspect his involuntary complicity. His first two
liquidations had demonstrated to our puissant baron
the necessity of attaching to himself a man who
could serve him as a piston to act on the creditor.
Nucingen had no nephew, did not dare to take a
confidant; he required a devoted man, an intelligent
Claparon, gifted with good manners, a veritable
diplomat, a man worthy of being a minister and
worthy of him. Such connections are not formed in
a day nor in a year. Rastignac had been so well
twisted up by the baron, that, like the Prince of
the Peace, who was loved as much by the king as by
the queen of Spain, he believed he had conquered
in Nucingen an invaluable dupe. After having
laughed at a man whose capacity was long unknown
to him, he had finished by vowing to him a grave
and serious worship in recognizing in him the
strength which he thought he alone possessed.
From the date of his début in Paris, Rastignac had
been led to despise society in its entirety. From
1820, he had thought, like the baron, that there
were only apparently honest men, and he regarded
the world as the reunion of all corruptions and of all
dishonesties. If he admitted exceptions, he condemned the mass; he did not believe in any virtue,
but in certain circumstances in which man is virtuous. This science was the result of a moment; it
was acquired at the top of Père-Lachaise, the day
on which he conducted there the funeral of a poor,
honest man, the father of his Delphine, who had

died the dupe of our society, of the truest feelings,
and abandoned by his daughters and by his sons-
in-law. He resolved to get the better of all this
world, and to maintain himself in a fine costume of
virtue, of probity, of beautiful manners. Egotism
armed this young noble cap-a-pie. When he met
Nucingen clothed with the same armor, he esteemed
him as, in the Middle Ages, in the tournament, a
knight in damascene steel from the feet to the head,
mounted on a war horse, would esteem his adversary
caparisoned and mounted like himself. But he
softened for a while in the delights of Capua. The
friendship of a woman like the Baroness de Nucingen is of a nature to banish all egotism. After having been deceived a first time in her affections by
meeting a piece of Birmingham mechanism, such
as was the late De Marsay, Delphine naturally felt
for a man young and full of the religious sentiment
of the provinces, an attachment without bounds.
This tenderness reacted on Rastignac. When
Nucingen had passed over to his wife's friend the
harness which every exploiter puts on his exploitee,
which happened precisely at the moment when he
was meditating his third liquidation, he confided to
him his position, presenting to him, as an obligation
growing out of his intimacy, as a reparation, the
rôle of accomplice to take up and to play. The
baron thought it dangerous to initiate his conjugal
collaborator into his plan. Rastignac feared a misfortune, and the baron let him believe that he might
save the shop. But, when a skein has so many

threads, there are sure to be knots.   Rastignac
trembled for the fortune of Delphine; he stipulated
for the independence of the baroness, requiring a
separation of property, swearing to himself to join
his account with hers and triple her fortune.   As
Eugène did not speak for himself, Nucingen begged
him to accept, in case of complete success, twenty-
five shares of a thousand francs each in the mines
of silver-bearing lead ore, which Rastignac took so
as not to offend him!   Nucingen taught Rastignac
his tunes the evening before the day in which our
friend advised Malvina to get married.   At the
sight of the hundred happy families who came and
went in Paris tranquil in the possession of their fortunes, the Godefroid de Beaudenords, the d'Aldriggers, the d'Aiglemonts, etc., Rastignac was seized
with a shiver like a young general who for the first
time contemplates an army before the battle.   The
poor little Isaure and Godefroid, playing at love, did
they not represent Acis and Galatea under the rock
which the great Polyphemus is about to tumble on
them?—"

"This monkey of a Bixiou," said Blondet, "he
has almost a talent."

"Ah! I am not sentimentalizing, then, any
more?" said Bixiou, enjoying his success, and
looking at his surprised auditors.—"During two
months," he resumed, after this interruption,
"Godefroid gave himself up to all the little happinesses of a man who is about to marry.   He
resembles at this period those birds who make their

nests in springtime, come and go, pick up straws, carry them in their beaks, and line the domicile of their eggs. The future husband of Isaure had taken in the Rue de la Planche a little hôtel for a thousand écus, commodious, suitable, neither too large nor too small. He went every morning to see the workmen working and to inspect the painting. He had introduced comfort there, the only good thing that there is in England,—a heater to maintain an equal temperature in the house; furniture well chosen, neither too brilliant nor too elegant; colors fresh and pleasant to the eye, interior and exterior blinds to all the windows; silverware, new carriages. He had arranged the stable, the harness-house, the carriage-house, where Toby, Joby, Paddy agitated himself, fidgeting about like a marmot unchained, and apparently delighted to know that there would be women in the household and a *lady!* This passion of the man who sets up housekeeping, who selects clocks, who comes into the house of his betrothed with his pockets full of samples of stuffs, consults her on the furnishing of the bed-chamber, who goes, comes, trots, when he goes, comes, and trots animated by love, is one of those things which most rejoice an honest heart, and especially the furnishers. And, as nothing pleases the world more than the marriage of a pretty young man of twenty-seven with a charming girl of twenty who dances well, Godefroid, embarrassed by the bridegroom's gifts, invited Rastignac and Madame de Nucingen to déjeuner, in order to consult them on this capital affair.

He had the excellent idea of inviting his cousin d'Aiglemont and his wife, as well as Madame de Sérizy. Fashionable women like very well these little occasional dissipations in bachelor apartments, they like to breakfast there."

"It is their way of playing truant," said Blondet.

"Every one had to go and see in the Rue de la Planche the little hôtel of the future married pair," resumed Bixiou. "The women are for these little expeditions just like ogres for fresh flesh, they freshen up their own present with this young joy which has not yet begun to pall through enjoyment. The table was laid in the little salon, which, for the interment of this bachelor life, was adorned like a show horse in a cavalcade. The déjeuner had been selected so as to offer a variety of those pretty little dishes which the women love to eat, to craunch, to suck, in the mornings, a time of the day in which they have a frightful appetite, which they do not wish to admit, for it seems that they compromise themselves in saying: 'I am hungry!' 'And why are you all alone?' said Godefroid, seeing Rastignac arrive. 'Madame de Nucingen is indisposed, I will tell you all about it,' replied Rastignac, who had the appearance of a man much disturbed. 'Some disagreement?' cried Godefroid. 'No,' said Rastignac. At four o'clock, when the ladies had all flown away to the Bois de Boulogne, Rastignac remained in the salon, looking in a melancholy manner through the window at Toby, Joby, Paddy, who was posted audaciously before the horse harnessed to the

tilbury, the arms folded like Napoléon; he could not keep him in check otherwise than by his clear, shrill voice, and the horse feared Joby, Toby. 'Well, what is the matter with you, my dear friend?' said Godefroid to Rastignac. 'You are sombre, disquieted; your gayety is not spontaneous. It is incomplete happiness which vexes your soul. It is, in fact, very unfortunate not to be married at the Mayor's office and at the church to the woman you love.' 'Have you courage, my dear fellow, to hear what I have to say to you, and will you know how to recognize to what a degree it is necessary to be attached to some one in order to commit the indiscretion of which I am about to be culpable?' said Rastignac to him in that tone which resembled a stroke of a whip. 'What?' said Godefroid, turning pale. 'I was grieved at your joy, and I have not the heart, in seeing all these preparations, this happiness in flower, to keep such a secret.' 'Tell me in three words.' 'Swear to me on your honor that you will be in this as silent as the tomb.' 'As the tomb.' 'That, if one of your nearest friends is interested in this secret, he shall not know it.' 'He shall not.' 'Well, Nucingen has gone off last night to Brussels; it will be necessary to go into bankruptcy if liquidation cannot be effected. Delphine has petitioned this very morning at the Palais for the separation of her property. You may yet save your fortune.' 'How?' said Godefroid, feeling an icy blood in his veins. 'Write simply to the Baron de Nucingen a letter antedated fifteen days, in which

you will give him the order to employ all your
funds in shares—and he named to him the Claparon
Company—You will have two weeks, a month,
three months, perhaps, to sell them above the present price; they will rise still higher.' 'But
d'Aiglemont, who breakfasted with us, d'Aiglemont, who has a million invested with Nucingen!'
'Listen, I do not know if there are enough of these
shares to cover him, and then I am not his friend.
I cannot betray the secrets of Nucingen; you
must not speak to him about it. If you say one
word, you will answer to me for the consequences.'
Godefroid remained for ten minutes perfectly
motionless. 'Do you accept, yes or no?' said Rastignac to him, pitilessly. Godefroid took pen and
ink, he wrote and signed the letter which Rastignac
dictated to him. 'My poor cousin!' he cried. 'Each
one for himself,' said Rastignac. 'And one saved
from the game,' he added, in leaving Godefroid.
While Rastignac was manœuvering in Paris, this
was the state of affairs on the Bourse. I have a
friend from the provinces, a stupid, who asked me,
when passing the Bourse, between four and five
o'clock, the reason for this assemblage of eager
talkers, who came and went, what they could be
saying to each other, and why they were thus going
about after the final settlement of the price of the
public funds. 'My friend,' I said to him, 'they
have eaten, they are digesting; during digestion, they gossip about their neighbors; without
that, no commercial security in Paris.' There

enterprises are launched, and there is such and such a man, Palma, for example, whose authority is like that of Sinard at the Royal Academy of Sciences. He says: 'Let there be speculation,' and speculation there is.''

"What a man, Messieurs," said Blondet, "is this Jew, who possesses an education not of the Universities, but universal. In him, the universality does not exclude profundity; what he knows, he knows all the way to the bottom; his genius is intuitive in business; he is the great referendary of the lynxes who rule the Exchange of Paris, and who do not undertake an enterprise until Palma has examined it. He is grave, he listens, he studies, he reflects, and says to his interlocutor, who, seeing his attention, believes him secured: 'That does not interest me.' That which seems to me to be the most extraordinary, is, that after having been for ten years the associate of Werbrust, there have never arisen any differences between them.''

"That only happens between those who are very strong or very weak; all those who are between these two extremes quarrel and speedily separate enemies," said Couture.

"You understand," said Bixiou, "that Nucingen had knowingly and with a skilful hand thrown under the columns of the Bourse a little shell which exploded about four o'clock. 'Do you know of a grave piece of news?' said Du Tillet to Werbrust, drawing him into a corner. 'Nucingen is in Brussels, his wife has presented to the court a petition for

her separation of property.' 'Are you his accomplice in a liquidation?' said Werbrust, smiling. 'No nonsense, Werbrust,' said Du Tillet; 'you know the people who have his paper; listen to me, we have an affair to arrange. The shares of our new company earn twenty per cent, they will gain twenty-five at the end of the quarter; you know why. There will be a magnificent dividend.' 'You are sly,' said Werbrust, 'go on, go your way; you are a devil whose claws are long and pointed, and you plunge them in butter.' 'But let me tell you, or we will not have time in which to operate. I found my idea when I heard the news, and I have positively seen Madame de Nucingen in tears; she has fears for her fortune.' 'Poor little thing!' said Werbrust, with an ironical air. 'Well?' resumed this old Alsatian Jew, interrogating Du Tillet, who was silent. 'Well, there are in my office a thousand shares of a thousand francs which Nucingen delivered to me to put on the market, do you understand?' 'Good!' 'We will buy at ten, at twenty per cent discount, paper of the House of Nucingen for a million, we will gain a fine premium on this million, for we will be creditors and debtors, there will be uncertainty! But we must act carefully; the holders might believe that we are manœuvering in the interests of Nucingen.' Werbrust now comprehended the thing to be done and grasped Du Tillet's hand, throwing upon him the look of a woman who is playing a trick on her neighbor. 'Well, have you heard the news?' said Martin Falleix to them. 'The House of Nucingen

has suspended!' 'Bah!' replied Werbrust; 'Do
not noise that about, let the people who hold his
paper attend to their affairs.' 'Do you know the
cause of the disaster ?—' said Claparon, intervening.
'You, you know nothing,' said Du Tillet to him;
'there will not be the least disaster, there will be
payment in full. Nucingen will resume and will
find all the funds he requires in my hands. I know
the cause of the suspension,—he has put all his
capital in Mexican investments, which repay him
in metals, in Spanish cannon so ridiculously cast
that there is gold in them, bells, church silver,
all the débris of the Spanish monarchy in the
Indies. The return of these values is delayed.
The dear baron is cramped, that is all.' 'That is
true,' said Werbrust, 'I take his paper at twenty
per cent discount. The news circulated thencefor-
ward with the rapidity of fire under a stack of
straw. The most contradictory things were said.
But there was so much confidence in the House of
Nucingen, always because of the two preceding
liquidations, that everybody kept its paper. 'It is
necessary that Palma give us a lift,' said Werbrust.
Palma was the oracle of the Kellers, who were gorged
with Nucingen securities. A word of alarm from
him would suffice. Werbrust persuaded Palma to
sound this tocsin. The next day, alarm pervaded
the Bourse. The Kellers, advised by Palma, disposed of their securities at ten per cent rebate, and
were accepted as authority at the Bourse; they
were known to be very shrewd. Taillefer then

7

disposed of three hundred thousand francs at twenty per cent, Martin Falleix two hundred thousand at fifteen per cent. Gigonnet guessed the trick! He encouraged the panic in order to be able to procure the Nucingen paper so as to gain some two or three per cent, by selling it to Werbrust. He perceived, in a corner of the Bourse the poor Matifat, who had three hundred thousand francs in the hands of Nucingen. The druggist, pale and ghastly, did not see without a shudder the terrible Gigonnet, the discounter of his ancient quarter, coming to him to terrify him. 'That is bad, the crisis is at hand. Nucingen is making an arrangement! but that does not concern you, Father Matifat; you have retired from business.' 'Well, you are mistaken, Gigonnet, I am caught with three hundred thousand francs with which I wished to operate in Spanish funds.' 'They are saved; the Spanish funds would have entirely devoured you, whilst I will give you something like fifty per cent for your account with Nucingen.' 'I had rather see the liquidation,' replied Matifat; 'a banker has never given less than fifty per cent. Ah, if it were only a question of ten per cent loss,' said the former druggist. 'Well, will you have it at fifteen?' said Gigonnet. 'You seem to me very eager,' said Matifat. 'Good-evening,' said Gigonnet. 'Will you have it at twelve?' 'Agreed,' said Gigonnet. Two millions were bought up that evening and balanced at Nucingen's by Du Tillet, for the account of these three fortunate associates, who, the next day,

received their premium. The old, pretty and little Baroness d'Aldrigger was breakfasting with her two daughters and Godefroid, when Rastignac came with a diplomatic air and engaged the conversation on the financial crisis. The Baron de Nucingen had a lively affection for the d'Aldrigger family; he had arranged in case of misfortune to cover the account of the baroness with his most valuable securities, shares in the mines of silver-bearing lead ore; but, for the security of the baroness, she should request him to employ her funds in this manner. 'That poor Nucingen,' said the baroness. 'And what has happened to him, then?' 'He is in Belgium; his wife has demanded a separation of her property; but he has gone to find other resources among the bankers.' *Mon Dieu,* that reminds me of my poor husband! Dear Monsieur de Rastignac, how badly this must make you feel, you who are so attached to that house.' 'Provided that all the outsiders are protected, his friends will be recompensed later. He will get out of it; he is a clever man.' 'An honest man, above all,' cried the baroness. At the end of a month the liquidation of the liabilities of the House of Nucingen had been accomplished, without any other process than letters by which each one requested the employment of his money in certain designated securities, and without any other formalities on the part of the banking-houses than the transfer of the Nucingen securities to those stocks which were preferred. Whilst Du Tillet, Werbrust, Claparon, Gigonnet

and some others, who thought themselves clever, brought back from abroad the paper of the House of Nucingen with one per cent premium, for they made a further profit in exchanging it against rising stocks, the rumor was still more widely spread on the Paris Exchange that no one had longer anything to fear. There was much talk about Nucingen. He was examined, he was judged; means were found to calumniate him! His luxury, his enterprises! When a man carries on so, he will sink himself, etc. In the midst of all this *tutti*, some persons were much astonished to receive letters from Geneva, Basle, from Milan, from Naples, from Genoa, from Marseilles, from London, in which their correspondents announced, not without astonishment, that they were offered one per cent premium on Nucingen's paper, of whose failure they were advised. 'Something is going on,' said the financial lynxes. The courts had pronounced separation of property between Nucingen and his wife. The affair became still more complicated,—the newspapers announced the return of Monsieur le Baron de Nucingen, who had just concluded a negotiation with a well-known Belgium manufacturer for the operation of some ancient coal mines, then in difficulties, the pits of the forests of Bossut. The Baron reappeared on the Bourse, without even taking the trouble to deny the injurious rumors which had been in circulation concerning him. He disdained to claim reparation through the newspapers; he purchased for two millions a magnificent property at the gates of Paris.

Six weeks later the journals of Bordeaux announced
the arrival of two vessels, consigned to the House
of Nucingen, with cargoes of metals of the value
of seven millions. Palma, Werbrust and Du
Tillet comprehended that the operation was completed, but they were the only ones who comprehended it. These scholars studied the theatrical
arrangement of this financial *puff*, recognized that
it had been prepared eleven months previously,
and proclaimed Nucingen the greatest European
financier. Rastignac comprehended nothing of it,
but he had gained thereby four hundred thousand
francs which Nucingen had allowed him to shear
from the Parisian lambs, and with which he had
provided dots for his two sisters. D'Aiglemont,
notified by his cousin Beaudenord, had come to
entreat Rastignac to accept ten per cent of his million if he would obtain for him the employment of
the million in shares of a canal which was yet to be
made, for Nucingen had so well involved the government in this affair that the concessionaires of
the canal were interested in not having it completed. Charles Grandet had implored Delphine's
lover to permit him to exchange his money for
shares. In short, Rastignac had played, during
ten days, the rôle of Law, supplicated by the prettiest duchesses to give them shares, and to-day
the scamp may have forty thousand francs of
income, the origin of which might be traced to
the shares in the mines of the silver-bearing lead
ore."

"If everybody made money, who then lost?" said Finot.

"Conclusion," resumed Bixiou. "Allured by the pseudo-dividend which they had received some months after the exchange of their money for shares, the Marquis d'Aiglemont and Beaudenord kept theirs—I give you these to represent all the others—They had three per cent more than their capitals; they chanted the praises of Nucingen, and defended him at the very moment when he was suspected of suspending payment. Godefroid married his dear Isaure, and received a hundred thousand francs in shares in the mines. On the occasion of this marriage, the Nucingens gave a ball, the magnificence of which surpassed anything that can be conceived of it. Delphine offered to the young wife a charming set of rubies. Isaure danced, no longer as a young girl, but as a happy wife. The litttle baroness was more than ever shepherdess of the Alps. Malvina, the woman of *Avez-vous vu dans Barcelone?* heard, in the midst of the ball, Du Tillet dryly counselling her to become Madame Desroches. Desroches, excited by the Nucingens, by Rastignac, undertook to treat of pecuniary affairs; but, at the first words concerning mining stocks given in dowry, he broke off and returned to the Matifats. In the Rue du Cherche-Midi the lawyer found the damned canal shares with which Gigonnet had stuffed Matifat, instead of giving him money. So you see Desroches finding Nucingen's rake upon the two dots on which he had fixed his attention! The catastrophes were not

delayed. The Claparon Company was engaged in too many affairs, there was a choking up; it ceased to pay interest and to declare dividends, although its operations were excellent. This misfortune happened in combination with the events of 1827. In 1829, Claparon was too well known to be the man of straw of these two colossi, and he fell from his pedestal to the earth. From twelve hundred and fifty francs, the shares fell to four hundred francs, although their intrinsic value was six hundred. Nucingen, who knew their real value, bought them in. The little Baroness d'Aldrigger had sold her shares in the mines which brought in nothing, and Godefroid sold his wife's for the same reason. Like the baroness, Beaudenord had exchanged his mining stock for shares of the Claparon Company. Their debts forced them to sell on a declining market. Of that which represented to them seven hundred thousand francs, they had two hundred and thirty thousand francs. They took their losses, and the remnant was prudently placed in the three per cents at seventy-five. Godefroid, that happy youth, without care, who had only to enjoy life, saw himself charged with a little wife stupid as a goose, incapable of supporting misfortune, for, at the end of six months, he perceived a transformation in the object so lightly loved; and, moreover, he was saddled with a mother-in-law without means who dreamed of toilets. The two families were living together in order to exist. Godefroid was obliged to call upon all his former influential connections,

now chilled, to secure a situation of a thousand écus
at the Ministry of Finance.   His friends?—at the
watering places.   His relatives?—astonished, promising: *'What, my dear fellow, but count upon me!
Poor boy!'*   Clean forgotten a quarter of an hour afterwards, Beaudenord was indebted for his situation
to the influence of Nucingen and of Vandenesse.
These persons, so estimable and so unfortunate,
live to-day in the Rue du Mont-Thabor, on the
third floor above the entresol.   The pearl of the
daughter of the Adolphuses, Malvina, has nothing; she gives piano-lessons in order not to be
a charge on her brother-in-law.   Dark, tall, thin,
dry, she resembles a mummy escaped from the
museum of Passalacqua running about on foot
through Paris.   In 1830, Beaudenord lost his situation, and his wife presented him with a fourth
child.   Eight masters and two servants—Wirth and
his wife—! money: eight thousand francs of income.
The mines pay to-day such considerable dividends,
that the thousand francs' share is worth a thousand
francs of income.   Rastignac and Madame de Nucingen have purchased the stocks sold by Godefroid and
by the baroness.   Nucingen was made peer of France
by the Revolution of July, and Grand Officer of the
Legion of Honor.   Although he has not liquidated
since 1830, he has, it is said, sixteen to eighteen
millions.   Foreseeing the Ordinance of July, he
sold all his funds and replaced them courageously
when the three per cents were at forty-five; he caused
it to be believed at the Château that this was

IN THE RUE DE RIVOLI

"*The little old woman had a green capote lined with pink, a flowered dress, a mantilla; in short, she was still, and more than ever, shepherdess of the Alps, for she no more comprehended the causes of her misfortune than the causes of her opulence. She was leaning on the poor Malvina, that model of heroic devotion, who had the air of being the old mother, while the baroness had that of being the young daughter; and Wirth followed them with an umbrella.*"

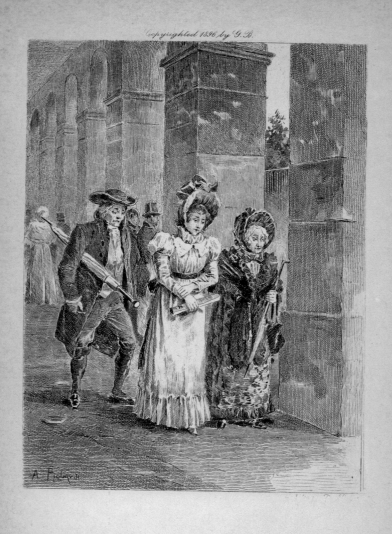

A. Foligno

through loyalty, and he has in this period gobbled up, in concert with Du Tillet, three millions from that great rogue of a Philippe Bridau! Recently, passing through the Rue de Rivoli on his way to the Bois de Boulogne, our baron perceived under the arcades the Baroness d'Aldrigger. The little old woman had a green capote lined with pink, a flowered dress, a mantilla; in short, she was still, and more than ever, shepherdess of the Alps, for she no more comprehended the causes of her misfortune than the causes of her opulence. She was leaning on the poor Malvina, that model of heroic devotion, who had the air of being the old mother, while the baroness had that of being the young daughter; and Wirth followed them with an umbrella. 'Dere are zome beebles,' said the baron to Monsieur Cointet, a minister, with whom he was walking, 'whose vortunes it was imbossible for me to make. De vlurry of high brincibles is over, dake dis boor Peautenord pack.' Beaudenord returned to the finances through the care of Nucingen, whom the d'Aldriggers praise as a hero of friendship, for he always invites the little shepherdess of the Alps and her daughters to his balls. It is impossible to anyone, no matter whom, in the world to demonstrate how this man has, three times and without breaking the law, wished to rob the public enriched by him, despite him. Nobody had any reproaches for him. Whoever would say that this great banking is often throat-cutting would utter the basest calumny. If stocks rise and fall, if values

augment and decrease, this flux and reflux is produced by some movement mutual, atmospheric,
brought about by the influence of the moon, and the
great Arago is culpable in not giving any scientific
theory for this important phenomenon. The only
result of all this is a pecuniary verity which I have
never seen written anywhere—"

"Which one?"

"The debtor is stronger than the creditor."

"Oh!" said Blondet, "for myself, I see in what
we have said the paraphrase of a saying of Montesquieu, in which he has concentrated all the
Ésprit des lois."

"What?" said Finot.

"Laws are spiders' webs through which the big
flies pass and in which the little ones are caught."

"What do you want to arrive at?" said Finot to
Blondet.

"An absolute government, the only one in which
enterprises of the wits against the law can be
repressed! Yes, the arbitrary power rescues the
people in coming to the aid of justice, for the right
of pardon has no reverse,—the king, who may pardon the fraudulent bankrupt, restores nothing to the
plundered victim.   Legality kills modern society."

"Make the electors comprehend that!" said
Bixiou.

"There is some one who has taken charge of it."

"Who?"

"Time.   As the bishop of Léon said: 'If liberty
is ancient, royalty is eternal;' every nation of

sound mind will return to it under one form or another."

"Look out, there is someone on the other side," said Finot, hearing us go out.

"There is always some one on the other side," replied Bixiou, who was probably by this time well wine-seasoned.

Paris, November, 1837.

THE SECRETS OF
LA PRINCESSE DE CADIGNAN

TO THEOPHILE GAUTIER

LA PRINCESSE DE CADIGNAN

*

After the disasters of the Revolution of July, which destroyed more than one of the aristocratic fortunes sustained by the Court, Madame la Princesse de Cadignan had the cleverness to lay to the account of the current political events the complete ruin due to her extravagances. The prince had left France with the royal family, leaving the princess in Paris, inviolable through his absence,—for the debts, for the satisfaction of which the sale of the salable property could not suffice, weighed on him only. The revenues of the entail had been seized. In short, the affairs of this great family were in as evil a state as those of the elder branch of the Bourbons. This woman, so well known under her first name of the Duchesse de Maufrigneuse, then decided wisely to live in profound retirement,—she wished to be forgotten. Paris was carried away by a current of events so bewildering that very shortly the Duchesse de Maufrigneuse, buried in the Princesse de Cadignan—a change of name unknown to the greater number of the new actors in society brought on the stage by the Revolution of July— became like a stranger.

8 (113)

In France, the title of duke precedes all others, even that of prince, although in heraldic thesis, free from sophism, titles signify absolutely nothing and there should be perfect equality among gentlemen. This admirable equality was formerly carefully maintained by the Royal House of France; and, in our day, it still is, at least nominally, by the care which the kings take to give the simple title of count to their children. It was in virtue of this system that Francis I. eclipsed the splendor of the titles which the pompous Charles V. gave himself by signing a reply to him: "François, Seigneur de Vanves." Louis XI. did better still, by marrying his daughter to an untitled gentleman, Pierre de Beaujeu. The feudal system was so well broken up by Louis XIV. that the title of duke became in his reign the highest honor of the aristocracy, and the one the most envied. Nevertheless, there are two or three families in France of which the princedom, formerly richly possessed, is put before that of the duchy. The House of Cadignan, which possesses the title of Duc de Maufrigneuse for its eldest son, while all the others are entitled simply Chevaliers de Cadignan, is one of these exceptional families. As was formerly the case with two princes of the House of Rohan, the princes de Cadignan were entitled to a throne amongst them; they were entitled to have pages and gentlemen in their service. This explanation is necessary, as much to avoid the foolish criticisms of those who know nothing as to declare the important things of a world which, it is said, is

departing, and which so many people promote without comprehending it.   The Cadignans bore *d'or with five fusils sable coupled and placed fesse*, with the word "MEMINI" for device, and the closed crown, without supporters or mantling.   To-day, the great number of foreigners who throng to Paris, and an almost general ignorance of the science of heraldry, tend to bring the title of prince into fashion.   There are no real princes excepting those who have landed possessions and who are entitled "Highness."   The disdain of the French nobility for the title of prince and the reasons which induced Louis XIV. to give supremacy to the title of duke, have operated to prevent in France claims to the title of Highness for the few princes who exist in this nation, those of Napoléon excepted.   This is the reason why the Princes de Cadignan found themselves in an inferior position, nominally speaking, to the other Continental princes.

The princess was protected by that society called "of the Faubourg Saint-Germain" through a respectful discretion due to her name, which is one of those always honored; to her misfortunes, which were not discussed, and to her beauty, the only thing which she had preserved of her lost opulence.   The world, of which she was the ornament, was thankful to her for having taken, as it were, the veil in cloistering herself in her own house.   This good taste was for her, more than for any other woman, an immense sacrifice.   The great events are always so keenly felt in France, that the princess regained

by her retirement all that she might have lost in
public opinion in the middle of her splendors. She
saw only one of her ancient friends, the Marquise
d'Espard; she went neither to the grand social
reunions nor to the festivities. The princess and
the marchioness visited each other in the early
morning, and, as it were, secretly. When the princess came to dine with her friend, the marchioness
closed her doors. Madame d'Espard was admirably
considerate for the princess; she changed her box at
the Italiens, and left the front row for a box on
the ground floor, so that Madame de Cadignan could
go to the theatre without being seen, and depart
incognito. Very few women would have been
capable of a delicacy which deprived them of the
pleasure of dragging in their suite a fallen former
rival, of proclaiming themselves her benefactress.
The princess, being thus able to dispense with the
ruinous extravagance of toilets, went privately in
the carriage of the marchioness, which she would
not have accepted publicly. No one has ever
known the reasons which induced Madame d'Espard
to act thus with the Princesse de Cadignan; but
her conduct was sublime, and permitted for a long
time a multitude of little things which, seen singly,
seem to be but sillinesses, but which, taken altogether, attain the gigantic. In 1832, the snows of
three years had drifted over the adventures of the
Duchesse de Maufrigneuse, and had so nearly
covered them that serious efforts of the memory
were required to recall the grave circumstances of

her previous life. Of this queen, adored by so many
courtiers, and whose light adventures might have
furnished material for several romances, there still
remained a delightfully handsome woman, thirty-
six years of age, but authorized to claim no more
than thirty, although she was the mother of the Duc
Georges de Maufrigneuse, a young man of nineteen, handsome as Antinous, poor as Job, who was
entitled to the utmost success and whom his mother
wished, before all, to make a rich marriage. Perhaps
in this project might be found a secret of the intimacy which she preserved with the marchioness,
whose salon enjoyed the reputation of being the
first in Paris, and in which she might some day
choose, among the heiresses, a wife for Georges.
The princess foresaw five years yet to pass between
the present moment and the epoch of her son's marriage; solitary and deserted years, for, in order to
secure a good marriage, it would be necessary that
her conduct should be marked with prudence.

The princess lived in the Rue de Miromesnil in a
little hôtel, on the ground floor, at a moderate rent.
She had brought thither a part of the remnants of
her magnificence. Her elegance of the *grande dame*
might still be felt there. She was still surrounded
there by those things which announce a superior
existence. On her chimney-piece might be seen a
magnificent miniature, the portrait of Charles X.,
by Madame de Mirbel, under which were engraved
these words: *"Presented by the king;"* and, as a
companion, the portrait of MADAME, which was so

peculiarly excellent in her case.   On a table was a
resplendent album of the utmost costliness, which
not one of the bourgeois who enthrone themselves in
our industrial society, so shifting and uncertain,
would dare to display.   This audacity portrayed the
woman admirably.   The album contained a number
of portraits among which might be recognized some
thirty intimate friends whom the world had called
her lovers.   This number was a calumny; but, if
we were to say ten, perhaps that might be somewhat near it, as said the Marquise d'Espard, with
good honest scandal.   The portraits of Maxime de
Trailles, of De Marsay, of Rastignac, of the Marquis
d'Esgrignon, of General de Montriveau, of the two
Marquises, de Ronquerolles and d'Ajuda-Pinto, of the
Prince Galathionne, of the young Ducs de Grandlieu,
de Rhétoré, of the handsome Lucien de Rubempré,
of the young Vicomte de Sérizy, had, moreover,
been rendered with the greatest and most flattering
skill by the most celebrated artists.   As the princess no longer received more than two or three persons of this collection, she alluded to this book
pleasantly as "the collection of her errors."   Misfortune had made of this woman a good mother.
During the fifteen years of the Restoration she had
amused herself too constantly to think of her son;
but, when taking refuge in obscurity, this illustrious egotist reflected that the maternal sentiment
pushed to its extreme development might become
for her past life an absolution, confirmed by all right-
thinking people, who pardon everything to an

excellent mother. She loved her son all the more
that she no longer had any other thing to love.
Georges de Maufrigneuse is, moreover, one of those
children who might flatter all a mother's vanities;
and thus the princess made for him all kinds of sacrifices: she maintained for Georges a stable and a carriage-house, over which he lived in a little entresol
on the street, consisting of three apartments, beauti-
fully furnished; she had imposed upon herself some
privations that he might have a saddle-horse, a horse
for his cabriolet, and a small servant. She herself
kept no longer anything but her femme de chambre,
and, for cook, one of her former kitchen-maids. The
duke's tiger had at this period a somewhat exacting
service. Toby, the former tiger of the late Beaudenord—for such was the pleasant jest of the gay
world on this ruined dandy—this young tiger, who
at twenty-five was everywhere thought to be only
fourteen years old, was expected to take care of the
horses, clean the cabriolet or the tilbury, follow his
master, keep the apartments in order and be present
in the antechamber of the princess to announce her
guest if, by chance, she was receiving the visit of
some personage. When we reflect on that which
was, under the Restoration, the beautiful Duchesse
de Maufrigneuse, one of the queens of Paris, a
splendid queen, whose luxurious existence would
have been worthy of one of the richest women of
the world of London, there was something inde-
scribably touching to see her in a little shell of the
Rue de Miromesnil, a few steps only from her

immense hôtel, which no fortune was able to maintain and which the hammer of the speculators has now demolished. The woman who could scarcely be served comfortably by thirty servants, who possessed the finest reception apartments in Paris, the most charming little apartments, who gave in them such admirable fêtes, now lived in a suite of five rooms,—an antechamber, a dining-room, a salon, a bed-chamber, and a dressing-room, with two women for her only servants.

"Ah! she is admirable for her son," said that fine gossip, the Marquise d'Espard, "and admirable without affectation; she is happy. One would never have thought this woman, so light, capable of resolutions followed so persistently; and our good Archbishop has encouraged her, has shown the greatest consideration for her, and has persuaded the old Comtesse de Cinq-Cygne to pay her a visit."

Let us admit it, moreover, it is necessary to have been a queen to know how to abdicate and to descend nobly from an elevated position which, however, is never entirely lost. Those only who are conscious in themselves of being nothing manifest their regrets in thus falling, or murmur continually, and go back in imagination to a past which will never return, feeling sure, as they do, that they can never attain it a second time. Compelled to abandon the rare flowers in the midst of which she had been accustomed to live, and which so well set off her person, for it was impossible not to compare her to a

flower, the princess had skilfully chosen her ground-floor apartment,—she there had the enjoyment of a pretty little garden full of shrubs and bushes, and of which the turf, always green, enlivened her peaceful retreat. She might have had at this period about twelve thousand francs of income. This modest revenue was composed of an annual stipend donated by the old Duchesse de Navarreins, paternal aunt of the young duke, which would be continued to the day of his marriage, and of another stipend sent by the Duchesse d'Uxelles, from her estate, where she was economizing as the old duchesses know how to economize, for, compared with them, Harpagon was only a scholar. The prince lived abroad, constantly at the orders of his exiled masters, sharing their evil fortune and serving them with a disinterested devotion, the most intelligent perhaps of all those who surrounded them. The position of the Prince de Cadignan still protected his wife at Paris. It was in the apartments of the princess that the mar-shal to whom we owe the conquest of Africa had, at the period of the attempt of MADAME in La Ven-dée, conferences with the principal chiefs of the Légitimistes,—so complete was the obscurity of the princess, so little did her poverty excite the sus-picion of the actual government! In seeing the approach of the terrible failure of love, that age of forty years, beyond which there is so little for a woman, the princess had thrown herself into the kingdom of philosophy. She read, she who had, for sixteen years, manifested the greatest horror for

serious things.   Literature and politics are to-day
that which formerly devotion was for women, the
last refuge of their pretensions.   In the elegant circles of society, it was said that Diane would wish
to write a book.   Since the period when, from a
charming, from a beautiful woman, the princess had
passed into a clever woman, before she should pass
away altogether, she had made of a reception under
her roof a supreme honor which distinguished pro-
digiously the favored person.   Under cover of these
occupations she could deceive one of her first lovers,
De Marsay, the most influential personage in bourgeois politics, put into power July, 1830; she
received him sometimes in the evenings, while the
marshal and several Légitimistes were discussing,
with lowered voices, in her bed-chamber, the conquest of the kingdom, which could not be brought
about without the aid of ideas, the only element of
success which the conspirators forgot.   It was a
charming vengeance of a pretty woman, thus to
trick a Prime Minister by making him serve as a
screen for a conspiracy against his own government.
This adventure, worthy of the best days of the
Fronde, furnished a text for the most ingenious letter
in the world, in which the princess rendered an
account of the negotiations to MADAME.   The Duc
de Maufrigneuse went to La Vendée and was able to
return secretly, without being compromised, but not
without having shared the perils of MADAME, who,
unfortunately, sent him back when everything
appeared lost.   Perhaps the enthusiastic vigilance

of this young man might have baffled the treason. However great may have been the errors of the Duchesse de Maufrigneuse in the eyes of the bourgeois world, the conduct of her son has certainly effaced them in the eyes of the aristocratic world. There was something of nobility and of grandeur in thus risking the only son and the heir of an historical house.   There are those, reputed clever, who repair the errors of private life by political services, and reciprocally; but no sordid calculations entered into the actions of the Princesse de Cadignan. Perhaps there were none, either, in any of those who thus contributed.   Events count for at least half in these misconceptions.

On one of the first fine days of the month of May, 1833, the Marquise d'Espard and the princess were slowly promenading, it could not be called walking, in the only garden alley which surrounded the turf of the little enclosure, about two o'clock in the afternoon, in the declining sunlight.   The rays reflected by the walls made a warm atmosphere in this little space perfumed by the flowers, a present from the marchioness.

"We will soon lose De Marsay," said Madame d'Espard to the princess, "and with him will go your last hope of fortune for the Duc de Maufrigneuse; for, since you have tricked him so prettily, this great politician has again found his affection for you."

"My son will never yield to the younger branch," replied the princess, "should he die of hunger, should

I have to work for him.   But Berthe de Cinq-Cygne
does not hate him."

"Children," said Madame d'Espard, "have not
the same engagements as their fathers—"

"Do not speak of it," said the princess.   "It will
be well enough, if I cannot bring the Marquise de
Cinq-Cygne to reason, to marry my son to some
blacksmith's daughter, as did that little d'Esgrignon!"

"Did you love him?" asked the marchioness.

"No," replied the princess gravely.   "The
naïvete of d'Esgrignon was a species of departmental dulness of which I became aware a little too
late, or a little too early, if you prefer."

"And De Marsay?"

"De Marsay played with me as if I were a doll.
I was so young! We never fall in love with the
men who constitute themselves our instructors; they
ruffle too much our little vanities."

"And that little miserable who hanged himself?"

"Lucien? That was an Antinous and a great
poet. I very sincerely loved him. I might have become happy.   But he loved a young girl, and I
yielded him to Madame de Sérizy—.   If he had loved
me, would I have yielded him?"

"What a fantastical thing! you to come in conflict with an Esther!"

"She was more beautiful than I," said the princess.   "Here are now nearly three years which I
have passed in a complete solitude," she resumed
after a pause; "well, this calm has had in it nothing

painful.   To you alone, I would dare to say that
here I have found myself happy.   I was weary of
adoration, fatigued without pleasure, moved super-
ficially without ever having my heart touched by
emotion.   I have found all the men whom I have
known, little, mean, superficial; not one of them has
ever caused me the slightest surprise; they were
without innocence, without grandeur, without delicacy.   I would have liked to have met someone
who would have seemed imposing to me."

"Would you be, then, like me, my dear?" asked
the marchioness; "would you have never encountered love in endeavoring to love?"

"Never," replied the princess, interrupting the
marchioness, and laying her hand on her arm.

Both of them went and seated themselves on a
rustic wooden bench, under a bush of flowering
jessamine.   Both of them had uttered one of those
words so solemn for women of their age.

"Like you," resumed the princess, "perhaps I
have been more loved than are other women; but
through so many adventures, I feel it, I have not
known happiness.   I have committed many follies,
but they all had an object, and the object recoiled
in proportion as I advanced!   In my heart grown
old, I am conscious of an innocence which has not
yet been touched.   Yes, under so much experience
still lies a first love which might be abused; just
as, notwithstanding so much wear and fatigue, I
still feel myself young and handsome.   We can love
without being happy, we can be happy and not love;

but to love and to have happiness, to bring together these two immense human enjoyments, that is
a prodigy.   This prodigy has not been accomplished
by me."

"Nor by me," said Madame d'Espard.

"I am pursued in my retreat by a frightful
regret,—I have amused myself, but I have never
loved."

"What an incredible secret!" cried the marchioness.

"Ah! my dear," replied the princess, "these
secrets, we can only confide them to ourselves: no
one in Paris would believe us."

"And," resumed the marchioness, "if we had not
both of us passed the age of thirty-six, we should
not, perhaps, make this avowal to ourselves—"

"Yes, when we are young we have some very
stupid fatuities!" said the princess.   "We resemble at times those poor young people who play with
a tooth-pick to make believe that they have dined
well."

"In short, here we are," replied Madame d'Espard,
with a coquettish grace, making a charming gesture
of sapient innocence, "and we are, it seems to me,
still enough alive to take a revenge."

"When you told me, the other day, that Béatrix
had gone off with Conti, I thought about it all
night long," resumed the princess, after a pause.
"One must be very happy to sacrifice thus one's
position, one's future, and renounce the world
forever!"

"She is a little fool," said Madame d'Espard, gravely. "Mademoiselle de Touches was enchanted to be rid of Conti. Béatrix did not comprehend how much this abandonment, made by a superior woman, who has not for a single moment defended her pretended happiness, revealed the nothingness of Conti."

"She will then be unhappy?"

"She is so already," replied Madame d'Espard. "Of what good is it to leave your husband? In a woman, is not this an avowal of want of power?"

"Thus you believe that Madame de Rochefide was not influenced by the desire to enjoy in peace a real happiness, that happiness the enjoyment of which, for us two, is still a dream?"

"No; she mimicked Madame de Beauséant and Madame de Langeais, who, it may be said between us, in a century less vulgar than ours, would have been, like you, moreover, figures as great as those of the La Vallières, of the Montespans, of the Dianes de Poitiers, of the Duchesses d'Étampes and de Châteauroux."

"Oh! without the king, my dear. Ah! I would like to be able to evoke those women and ask them if—"

"But," said the marchioness, interrupting the princess, "it is not necessary to make the dead speak; we know some living women who are happy. There are more than twenty times that I have had lately, intimate conversations on such matters with the Comtesse de Montcornet, who, for

the last fifteen years, has been the happiest
woman in the world with that little Émile Blondet,
—not one infidelity, not one wandering thought;
they are to-day as on the very first day; but we
have always been interfered with, interrupted at
the most interesting moment.   These long attachments, like those of Rastignac and of Madame de
Nucingen, of Madame de Camps, your cousin, for
her Octave, have a secret, and this secret we are
ignorant of, my dear.   The world does us the extreme honor to take us for profligates worthy of
the Court of the Regent, and we are as innocent as
two little school-girls.''

"I should be still happy in that innocence,"
cried the princess, jestingly; "but ours is worse,
there is in it something humiliating.   What would
you have!   We will offer this mortification to
God in expiation of our fruitless researches; for,
my dear, it is not probable that we shall find, in the
late autumn, the fine flower which we have missed
during the spring and the summer.''

"That is not the question," resumed the marchioness after a pause full of retrospective medita-
tions.   "We are still handsome enough to inspire
a passion; but we shall never convince anyone of
our innocence and of our virtue.''

"If it were a lie, it would be soon enough ornamented with commentaries, served up with pretty
preparations which would make it believable and
devoured like a delicious fruit; but to make a truth
believed!   Ah! the greatest men have perished in

that attempt," added the princess, with one of those fine smiles which the brush of Leonardo da Vinci alone could render.

"The simpletons love well enough sometimes," said the marchioness.

"But," observed the princess, "for this, the simpletons themselves would not have sufficient credulity."

"You are right," said the marchioness, laughing. "But it is neither a fool nor even a man of talent that we should seek for. To solve such a problem will require a man of genius. Genius alone has the faith of childhood, the religion of love, and willingly lets its eyes be bandaged. Look at Canalis and the Duchesse de Chaulieu. If, you and I, we have met with men of genius, they were perhaps too far from us, too much occupied, and we were too frivolous, too much carried away, too much taken up with other things."

"Ah, I would very much like, however, not to quit this world without having known the pleasures of a true love," cried the princess.

"It is nothing to inspire it only," said Madame d'Espard; "it is a question of experiencing it. I see many women who are only the pretext of a passion, instead of being at once the cause and the effect of it."

"The last passion which I inspired was a saintly and beautiful thing," said the princess; "it had a future. Fortune sent to me this time that man of genius who is due to us, and who is so difficult to

9

take, for there are more pretty women than gen·
iuses.   But the devil interfered in the adventure."

"Tell me that, my dear; that is entirely new to
me."

"I only became aware of this fine passion in the
middle of the winter of 1829.   Every Friday, at the
Opera, I saw in the orchestra seats a young man of
about thirty years of age, who came there for my
sake, always in the same seat, looking at me with
eyes of fire, but often saddened by the distance
which he found between us, or perhaps also by the
impossibility of succeeding."

"Poor boy! When one is in love, one becomes
very stupid," said the marchioness.

"Between each act he slipped into the corridor,"
resumed the princess, smiling at the friendly
epigram with which the marchioness had interrupted her; "then, once or twice, to see me or
to make himself seen, he showed his nose at the
glass of a box opposite mine.   If I received a visit,
I perceived him flattened in my doorway; he could
then throw me a furtive glance; he had ended by
knowing by sight the persons of my society; he followed them when they came toward my box, in
order to have the benefit of the opening of my door.
The poor youth doubtless soon learned who I was,
for he knew by sight Monsieur de Maufrigneuse and
my father-in-law.   I found, after that, my mysterious unknown at the Italiens, in a seat in which he
could admire me, directly opposite, in a simple
ecstasy:—it was very pretty.   When coming out of

the Opera, as out of the Bouffons, I saw him planted
in the crowd, motionless on his two legs,—he was
elbowed, but he was not moved.   His eyes became
less brilliant when he perceived me leaning on the
arm of some favorite.   All this time, not a word,
not a letter, not a demonstration.   You must admit
that it was in good taste.   Sometimes, on returning
home in the morning, I found my man seated on
one of the sides of my porte-cochère.   This loving
one had very fine eyes, a thick and long beard
cut fan-shaped, an imperial, a mustache and
whiskers; you could only see two white cheeks and
a handsome forehead; in short, a veritable antique
head.   The prince, as you know, defended the
Tuileries on the side of the quays during the days
of July.   He returned in the evening to Saint-Cloud
when everything was lost.   'My dear,' he said to
me, 'I just escaped being killed about four o'clock.
I was aimed at by one of the insurgents, when a
young man with a long beard, whom I think I have
seen at the Italiens and who led the attack, turned
aside the barrel of the musket.'   The ball struck
I know not what man, a quartermaster in the regiment, and who was within two steps of my husband.   This young man must then have been a
Republican.   In 1831, when I came back to live here,
I encountered him leaning against the wall of this
house; he seemed joyful because of my disasters,
which, perhaps it seemed to him, would bring us
nearer; but, since the affair of Saint-Merri I have
no longer seen him: he perished in it.   The evening

of the funeral of General Lamarque, I went out on foot with my son, and my Republican followed us, sometimes behind, sometimes before us, from the Madeleine to the Passage des Panoramas, where I was going."

"Is that all?" said the marchioness.

"All," replied the princess. "Ah! the morning of the taking of Saint-Merri, a street boy wished to speak to me and handed me a letter, written on common paper, signed with the name of the unknown."

"Show it to me," said the marchioness.

"No, my dear. This love was too great and too holy in this man's heart for me to violate his secret. This letter, short and terrible, still moves me to the heart when I think of it. This dead man causes me more emotion than all the living ones whom I have distinguished, he returns again into my thoughts."

"His name?" asked the marchioness.

"Oh, a very common name, Michel Chrestien."

"You have done very well to tell it to me," replied Madame d'Espard, quickly, "I have often heard him spoken of. This Michel Chrestien was the friend of a celebrated man whom you have already wished to see, of Daniel d'Arthez, who comes once or twice a winter to my house. This Chrestien, who was really killed at Saint-Merri, did not lack for friends. I have heard it said that he was one of those great politicians to whom, as to De Marsay, it is only needful that the foot-ball of circumstances should come their way for them to become all at once what they should be."

"It is better, then, that he should be dead," said the princess, with a melancholy air under which she concealed her thoughts.

"Would you like to meet d'Arthez some evening at my house?" asked the marchioness; "you could talk of your apparition."

"Willingly, my dear."

Some days after this conversation, Blondet and Rastignac, who knew d'Arthez, promised Madame d'Espard to induce him to come and dine with her. This promise would without doubt have been imprudent were it not for the name of the princess, the meeting with whom could not be indifferent to this great writer.

Daniel d'Arthez, one of those rare men, who in our day, unite a fine character to a fine talent, had already obtained, not all the popularity which his works should have procured him, but a respectful esteem to which chosen souls could add nothing. His reputation would certainly increase still more, but it had already attained its full development in the eyes of connoisseurs,—he is of those authors who, sooner or later, find their true place, and retain it. A poor gentleman, he had comprehended his epoch in requiring everything from a personal illustration. He had combated for a long period in the Parisian arena, against the will of a rich uncle, who, through a contradiction which vanity endeavors to justify, after having left him a prey to the greatest poverty, had bequeathed to the celebrated man the fortune pitilessly refused to the

unknown writer.   This sudden change had changed
nothing in the manners of Daniel d'Arthez: he continued his labors with a simplicity worthy of antique
times, and imposed new ones on himself by accepting a seat in the Chamber of Deputies, where he
took a place on the Right.   Since his attainment
to fame he had gone out sometimes into society.
One of his old friends, a great physician, Horace
Bianchon, had made him acquainted with the Baron
de Rastignac, Under-Secretary of State to a minister, and friend of De Marsay.   These two men of
politics had with sufficient nobility lent their aid to
Daniel, Horace and some intimate friends of Michel
Chrestien, who wished to withdraw the body of this
Republican from the church of Saint-Merri and render it funeral honors.   Gratitude for a service
which contrasted so strongly with the administrative rigors displayed at this period in which political passions were so freely unchained, had bound, as
it were, d'Arthez to Rastignac.   The Under-Secretary of State and the illustrious minister were too
skilful not to profit by this circumstance; they
thus gained over some friends of Michel Chrestien,
who, moreover, did not share his opinions, and who
henceforth attached themselves to the new government.   One of them, Léon Giraud, appointed at
first Maître des Requêtes, became Councillor of
State.   The existence of Daniel d'Arthez is entirely
consecrated to work, he only sees society in occasional glimpses; it is for him like a dream.   His
house is a convent, in which he leads the life of a

Benedictine,—the same sobriety in the regimen, the same regularity in the occupations. His friends know that up to the present time woman has only been for him an accident always dreaded, he has observed her too much not to fear her; but, by dint of studying her, he has ended by no longer knowing her, resembling in this those profound tacticians who will always be beaten on unforeseen ground where their scientific axioms are modified and contradicted. He has remained the most candid child, while showing himself the most learned observer. This contrast, apparently impossible, is easily explicable for those who are able to measure the depth which separates the faculties from the feelings: one proceeds from the head and the other from the heart. One can be a great man and a wicked one, as one can be a fool and a sublime lover. D'Arthez is one of those privileged beings in whom the finesse of the intellect, the wide extent of the qualities of the brain, exclude neither the strength nor the grandeur of feeling. He is, by a rare privilege, a man of action and a man of reflection, both at once. His private life is noble and pure. If he had carefully avoided love up to this time, he knew himself well; he knew in advance what would be the empire of a passion over him. During a long period, the heavy labors by which he prepared the solid ground of his glorious works, and the cold of poverty, had been a marvelous preservative. When he had attained to ease, he had the most vulgar and the most incomprehensible liaison with a woman

sufficiently attractive, but who belonged to the lower
orders, without any instruction, without manners,
and carefully concealed from all observation.
Michel Chrestien conceded to men of genius the
power to transform the most massive creatures into
sylphids, the stupid ones into women of wit, the
peasant women into marchionesses: the more a
woman was accomplished, the more she lost in their
eyes; for, according to him, their imagination had no
part to play in this business. According to him also,
love, the simple craving of the senses in inferior
beings, was, in the superior beings, the most immense and the most attaching of all moral creations.
In order to justify d'Arthez, he fell back upon the
example given by Raphaël and the Fornarina.   He
might have offered himself as a model in this
respect, he who saw an angel in the Duchesse
de Maufrigneuse.   The curious whim of d'Arthez
might, moreover, be justified in various ways,—perhaps he had promptly and at once despaired of ever
encountering here below a woman who would
respond in any degree to that delightful chimera
which every man of intelligence creates for himself;
perhaps he was possessed of a heart too sensitive,
too delicate, to be yielded up to a woman of the
world; perhaps he thought it better to give to nature
her due merely and to keep his illusions intact by
cultivating his ideal; perhaps he had put aside love
as something incompatible with his work, with the
regularity of a monastic life in which passion would
have disarranged everything.   For the last few

months d'Arthez had been the object of the jests of
Blondet and of Rastignac, who reproached him with
knowing neither the world nor women. According
to them, his works were sufficiently numerous and
carried sufficiently far for him to permit himself
some distractions,—he had a fine fortune and he
lived like a poor scholar; he enjoyed nothing,
neither his gold nor his glory; he was ignorant of
the exquisite pleasure of that noble and delicate
passion which certain women well-born and well-
educated inspire in others or feel themselves; was
it not unworthy of himself to have never known
anything but the grossness of love? Love, reduced
to that which nature makes of it, was in their eyes
the most sottish thing in the world. One of the
glories of society, is to have created *the woman*
where nature had made a female; to have created
the perpetuity of desire where nature had thought
only of the perpetuity of the species; to have, in
short, invented love, the very finest human religion. D'Arthez knew nothing of the charming
delicacies of language, nothing of those proofs of
affection incessantly given by soul and spirit, nothing of those desires ennobled by manners, nothing
of those angelic forms lent to the grossest things by
refined and charming women. He was, perhaps,
acquainted with the woman, but he was ignorant of
the divinity. It requires an extraordinary art, very
many beautiful toilets of the body and of the soul in
a woman to secure true love. Finally, in lauding
the delightful depravations of the thought which

constitute the Parisian coquetry, these two cor-
ruptors pitied d'Arthez, whose diet was simple and
wholesome, and without any seasoning, for never
having tasted the delicacies of the finest Parisian
cooking, and they greatly stimulated his curiosity.
Doctor Bianchon, in whom d'Arthez confided, was
aware that this curiosity had been finally aroused.
The long liaison of this great writer with a common
woman, far from becoming satisfactory through
habit, had now become to him insupportable; but he
was restrained from breaking away by the excessive
timidity which takes possession of all solitary men.

"How," said Rastignac, "when one bears *party
per bend dexter gules and or to a bezant and a torteau
from one to the other,* why not make this old Picard
shield glitter on a carriage panel? You have thirty
thousand francs of income and the products of
your pen; you have justified your motto, which
makes the pun so much desired by our ancestors:
ARS, THE*Saurusque virtus* and you do not promenade yourself in the Bois de Boulogne! We are in
a century in which virtue should show itself."

"If you read your works to that species of gross
Laforêt who makes your delights, I would pardon
you for keeping her," said Blondet. "But, my
dear fellow, if you are reduced to dry bread in material things, with respect to the spiritual you have
not even bread—"

This little friendly warfare had been going on
between Daniel and his friends for several months
when Madame d'Espard asked Rastignac and Blondet

to persuade d'Arthez to come and dine with her, saying to them that the Princesse de Cadignan had a very great desire to meet this celebrated man. These species of curiosity are, for certain women, what the magic lantern is for children, a pleasure for the eyes, a poor enough one, moreover, and full of disenchantments. The greater the curiosity and interest which a clever and distinguished man excites at a distance, the less satisfactory he is when brought near; the more brilliant he has been dreamed to be, the sooner he tarnishes. In this connection, the disappointed curiosity often goes to the extreme of injustice. Neither Blondet nor Rastignac could deceive d'Arthez, but they said to him laughingly that it would offer him the most seductive opportunity to clean up his heart and to become acquainted with the supreme delights which the love of a great Parisian lady might give. The princess was positively enamored of him; he had nothing to fear, he had everything to gain in this interview; it would be impossible for him to descend from the pedestal on which Madame de Cadignan had placed him. Neither Blondet nor Rastignac saw any impropriety in imputing this love to the princess; she could support this calumny, she had given rise to enough stories in the past. One and the other, they set to work to recount to d'Arthez the adventures of the Duchesse de Maufrigneuse,—her first indiscretions with De Marsay, her second inconsistency with d'Ajuda, whom she had turned away from his wife, thus avenging

Madame de Beauséant; her third liaison with the
young d'Esgrignon, who had accompanied her into
Italy and had horribly compromised himself for her;
then how she had been unhappy with a celebrated
ambassador, happy with a Russian general; how
she had been the Egeria of two Ministers of Foreign
Affairs, etc.   D'Arthez informed them that he knew
more concerning her than they could tell him,
through their poor friend, Michel Chrestien, who
had adored her in secret for four years, and had
almost gone mad over it.

"I often went with my friend," said Daniel, "to
the Italiens, to the Opera.   The unhappy man ran
with me through the streets, going as fast as the
horses, and admiring the princess through the windows of her coupé.   It was to this love that the
Prince de Cadignan owed his life; Michel prevented
a gamin who would have killed him."

"Well, then, you will have a subject all ready,"
said Blondet, smiling.   "There is the woman that
you require; she will only be cruel through delicacy,
and will initiate you very graciously into the
mysteries of elegance; but, beware, she has devoured
many fortunes!   The beautiful Diane is one of those
dissipators who do not cost a centime, and for whom
millions are expended.   Give yourself, body and
soul; but keep your money in your own hands, like
the old man in Girodet's 'Deluge.'"

According to this conversation, the princess had
all the profundity of an abyss, the grace of a queen,
the corruption of a diplomat, the mystery of an

initiation, the danger of a siren. These two men of
wit, incapable of foreseeing the dénouement of this
pleasantry, had finished by making of Diane
d'Uxelles the most monstrous Parisian woman, the
most skilful coquette, the most intoxicating courtesan in the world. Although they might have been
right, the woman whom they treated so lightly was
saintly and sacred for d'Arthez, whose curiosity had
no need of being excited; he consented to come
immediately, and the two friends wished nothing
better of him.

Madame d'Espard went to see the princess as soon
as she had a reply.

"My dear, do you feel yourself in the way to be
beautiful, coquettish?" she said to her; "come and
dine with me in a few days; I will serve up to you
d'Arthez. Our man of genius is of a nature the
wildest; he fears women, and has never loved. You
can prepare your theme on those lines. He is
excessively intelligent, with a simplicity which gets
the better of you by depriving you of all suspicion.
His penetration, all retrospective, acts after the
stroke and deranges all calculations. You have
surprised him to-day, to-morrow he will be no longer
dupe in anything."

"Ah!" said the princess, "if I were only thirty,
I would amuse myself greatly! That which has
always failed me up to the present time has been a
man of wit to play with. I have only had partners
and never adversaries. Love was only a game instead of being a combat."

"Dear princess, admit that I am very generous, for, as you know, all well-regulated charity—"

The two women looked at each other laughingly and clasped each other's hands with friendship. Certainly, they knew important secrets of each other, not even excepting love affairs, and little service rendered; for, to have sincere and durable friendships between women, it is necessary that they should have been united by some little crimes. When two female friends are about to kill each other, and may be seen, poisoned dagger in hand, they offer a touching spectacle of a harmony which is only destroyed at the moment when one of them has, inadvertently, dropped her weapon. Therefore, a week later, there was in the house of the marchioness one of those evenings called *des petits jours,* reserved for intimate friends, to which no one comes without a verbal invitation, and during which the door is closed. This entertainment was given for five persons,—Emile Blondet and Madame de Montcornet, Daniel d'Arthez, Rastignac, and the Princesse de Cadignan. Including the mistress of the house, there were as many men as women. Never did fortune permit of more skilful preparations than these for the meeting of d'Arthez and Madame de Cadignan. The princess still enjoys to-day the reputation of being one of the most skilful women in all matters of the toilet, which is, for women, the first of all arts. She wore a gown of blue velvet with large white flowing sleeves, the bodice showing, in guimpe cf tulle

slightly gathered and bordered with blue, rising to within four finger breadths of the neck and covering the shoulders, as may be seen in some of Raphaël's portraits. Her maid had dressed her hair with some white heather skilfully arranged in the ripples of her blond tresses, one of those aids to beauty to which she owed her celebrity. Certainly Diane did not seem to be twenty-five years old. Four years of solitude and repose had restored the clearness to her skin. Are there not, moreover, moments in which the desire to please gives an increase of beauty to women? The will is not without influence on the variations of the countenance. If violent emotions have the power of yellowing the white tints in people of a sanguine temperament, or a melancholy one, of turning lymphatic countenances greenish, should there not be given to desire, to joy, to hope, the quality of clearing the skin, of illuminating the glance with a lively light, of animating beauty by a vivid illumination like that of a fine morning? The fairness of the princess, so celebrated, had taken a ripened tint which lent to her an august air. In this moment of her life, animated by so many self-reflections and by serious thoughts, her pensive and sublime forehead was in admirable accord with the slow and majestic glance of her blue eyes. It would have been impossible for the most skilful physiognomist to have discovered calculation and decision under this most unusual delicacy of feature. There are women's faces which deceive all science and vanquish observation

by their calm and by their fineness; it would
be necessary to be able to examine them when the
passions are speaking, which is difficult; or when
they have spoken, which serves for nothing,—then,
the woman is old and no longer dissimulates. The
princess is one of those impenetrable women; she
is able to make herself whatever she wishes to be,
—playful, infantile, hopelessly innocent; or shrewd,
serious and profound to a disquieting extent. She
came to the house of the marchioness with the
intention of being a woman sweet and simple, to
whom life was known by its deceptions only, a
woman full of spirit and sentiment and calumniated, but resigned; in short, an angel martyred.
She arrived early, so that she might be found posed
on a little sofa, at the corner of the fire, near to
Madame d'Espard, as she would wish to be seen, in
one of those attitudes in which science is carefully
concealed under an appearance of exquisite naturalness, one of those poses studied, thought out, which
bring into relief that beautiful serpentine line,
which, starting from the feet, mounts gracefully to
the hips and continues by admirable curves to the
shoulders, offering to the regard all the profile of the
body. A woman nude would be less dangerous
than in a robe thus knowingly displayed, which
covers everything and reveals everything at the
same time. By a refinement which very few women
would have invented, Diane, to the great stupefaction of the marchioness, was accompanied by the
Duc de Maufrigneuse. After a moment of reflection,

Madame d'Espard grasped the hand of the princess with an air of intelligence:

"I understand you! In compelling d'Arthez to accept all the difficulties at the first outset, you will not have them to overcome later."

The Comtesse de Montcornet came with Blondet. Rastignac brought d'Arthez. The princess did not pay to the celebrated man any of those compliments with which the vulgar overwhelmed him; but she displayed those little attentions full of grace and of respect which seemed as though they might be the last limit of her concessions. She was doubtless thus with the King of France, with the princes. She seemed happy to see this great man and pleased with having sought him. Persons of good taste, like the princess, are distinguished above all by their manner of listening, by an affability without mockery, which is to politeness what practice is to virtue. When the celebrated man spoke, she had an attentive air a thousand times more flattering than the most skilful compliments. This mutual introduction was performed without any emphasis, and gracefully, by the marchioness. At dinner, d'Arthez was placed near the princess, who, far from imitating the little exaggerations of dieting which are permitted by affectation, ate with a very good appetite, and made it a point to show herself as a natural woman, without any strange fashions. Between two services, she profited by a moment during which the conversation became general to speak to d'Arthez aside.

10

"The secret of the pleasure which I have procured myself in meeting you," she said, "is the desire of learning something of an unfortunate friend of yours, Monsieur, who died for another cause than ours, to whom I am under great obligation, without having been able to recognize them and to acquit myself of them. The Prince de Cadignan has shared my regrets. I have learned that you were one of the best friends of this poor youth. Your mutual friendship, pure and unaltered, was a title to my consideration. You will not, then, find it extraordinary that I have wished to know all that you could tell me of this being who is so dear to you. Though I am attached to the exiled family, and held to entertain monarchical opinions, I am not of the number of those who believe it to be impossible to be at once Republican and noble of heart. The Monarchy and the Republic are the only two forms of government which do not suppress elevated sentiments."

"Michel Chrestien was an angel, Madame," replied Daniel, in a voice of emotion. "I do not know, among the heroes of antiquity, a man who was superior to him. Avoid entertaining for one of these Republicans those narrow ideas which would set up again the Convention and the pretty ways of the Committee of Public Safety; no. Michel dreamed of the Swiss Federation applied to the whole of Europe. Let us admit it, between ourselves, after the admirable government of one only, which, I believe, is more peculiarly adapted

to our country, the system of Michel is the suppression of war in the Old World and its reconstruction on bases other than those of conquest which formerly feudalized it. The Republicans were, in this respect, the nearest to his idea; this is why he lent them his aid in July and at Saint-Merri. Although entirely divided in opinion, we remained closely united."

"It is the finest eulogy of your two characters," said Madame de Cadignan, timidly.

"In the last four years of his life," resumed Daniel, "he confided to me only his love for you, and this confidence knit still tighter the already strong bonds of our fraternal friendship. He alone, Madame, would have loved you as you should be loved. How many times have I not endured the rain in accompanying your carriage to your house, in contending in speed with your horses, so as to keep at the same point on a parallel line in order to see you,—to admire you!"

"But, Monsieur," said the princess, "I am going to hold myself bound to indemnify you."

"Why is Michel not here?" replied Daniel, with an accent full of melancholy.

"He would perhaps have not loved me long," said the princess, shaking her head with a sorrowful movement. "The Republicans are even more absolute in their ideas than we other absolutists, who sin by indulgence. He doubtless dreamed of me as perfect; he would have been cruelly undeceived. We are pursued, we women, by as many calumnies

as you have to endure in a literary life, and we are not able to defend ourselves, neither by glory, nor by our works. We are not believed to be that which we really are, but that which we are said to be. There are those who would have very soon covered up for him the unknown woman which is in me under the false portrait of the imaginary woman, which is the true one for the world. He would have believed me unworthy of the noble sentiments which he entertained for me, incapable of comprehending them."

Here, the princess shook her head, agitating her beautiful blond tresses crowned with heather, by a sublime gesture. That which she expressed of desolating doubts, of hidden miseries, is unspeakable. Daniel comprehended everything, and looked at the princess with a lively emotion.

"However, the day on which I saw him again, long after the revolt of July," she resumed, "I was on the point of yielding to the desire which I felt, to take him by the hand, to grasp it before all the world, under the peristyle of the Théâtre-Italien, in giving him my bouquet. I thought that this testimony of gratitude would be misinterpreted, like so many other noble things which to-day pass for the follies of Madame de Maufrigneuse, and which I could never explain, for there is only my son and God who will ever know me."

These words, breathed into the listener's ear in such a manner as to be unheard by all the other guests, and with an accent worthy of the most skilful

comedienne, should have gone direct to the heart; and they did attain to that of d'Arthez. It did not concern the celebrated writer; this woman sought to reëstablish herself in the favor of a dead man. She might have been slandered, she wished to know if nothing had tarnished her in the eyes of him who loved her. Had he died with all his illusions?

"Michel," replied d'Arthez, "was one of those men who love absolutely, and who, if they choose badly, know how to suffer for it without ever renouncing her whom they have elected."

"Was I, then, loved in this manner?—" she cried, with an air of exalted beatitude.

"Yes, Madame."

"I, then, made his happiness?"

"During four years."

"A woman never learns such a thing as this without experiencing a proud satisfaction," she said, turning her gentle and noble countenance towards d'Arthez with a movement full of modest confusion.

One of the most knowing manœuvres of these comediennes is to veil their manners when the words are too expressive, and to make the eyes speak when the discourse is restrained. These skilful dissonances, slipped into the music of their love, false or true, bring about invincible seductions.

"Is it not," she resumed, lowering her voice still more, and after assuring herself of having produced the desired effect, "is it not to have accomplished

her destiny to have rendered happy, and without crime, a great man?"

"Did he not write it to you?"

"Yes; but I wished to be very sure of it, for, believe me, Monsieur, in setting me so high, he did not deceive himself."

Women know how to give to their words a peculiar saintliness; they communicate to them I know not what of vibration which extends the sense of their ideas and lends them profundity; if, later, their charmed auditor no longer recalls what they have said, the object has been completely attained, which is the proper quality of eloquence. The princess might at this moment have worn the diadem of France, her forehead would not have been more imposing than it was under the beautiful diadem of her tresses elevated in coils like a tower, and ornamented with the pretty heather. This woman seemed to walk on the flood of calumny, like the Saviour on the waves of the Lake of Tiberius, enveloped in the winding-sheet of this love, like an angel in his nimbus. There was nothing in it which suggested either the necessity of being thus, or the desire to appear grand or loving,—it was all simple and calm. A living man could never have rendered to the princess the services which she obtained of this dead one. D'Arthez, a solitary worker, to whom the practices of the world were unknown, and whom study had enveloped with its protecting veils, was the dupe of this accent and of these words. He was under the charm of these

exquisite manners; he admired this perfect beauty,
ripened by unhappiness, restored in retirement; he
adored the union, so rare, of a fine intelligence and
a beautiful soul.   Finally, he wished to obtain for
himself the heritage of Michel Chrestien.   The
commencement of this passion was, as it is among
most profound thinkers, an idea.   In seeing the
princess, in studying the shape of her head, the
disposition of her so gentle features, her figure, her
foot, her hands so finely modeled, so much more
closely than he had been able to do while accompanying his friend in his foolish courses through the
street, he remarked the surprising phenomenon of
the moral second sight which the man exalted by
love finds in himself.   With what lucidity had not
Michel Chrestien read this heart, this soul, lit up
by the fires of love?   The Federalist had then been
divined, he also! he would have doubtless been
happy.   The princess had thus in the eyes of
d'Arthez a great charm, she was surrounded by an
aureole of poesy.   During the dinner, the writer
recalled to himself the despairing confidences of the
Republican and his hopes when he thought himself
loved; the beautiful poem which a true feeling
inspires had been sung for him alone because of this
woman.   Unknowingly, Daniel was to profit by
these preparations due to chance.   It is but seldom
that a man passes without remorse from the position
of a confidant to that of a rival, and d'Arthez could
now do so without crime.   In a moment he perceived the enormous differences which exist between

superior women, these flowers of the great world, and vulgar women, whom he knew, however, as yet, by but one specimen; he was then assailed by the most accessible sides, the most tender, of his soul and of his genius.   Instigated by his simplicity, by the impetuosity of his ideas, to take possession of this woman, he found himself restrained by the world and by the barrier which the manner, let us say the word, which the majesty, of the princess put between herself and him.   Thus, for this man, not accustomed to respect that which he loved, there was here something, I know not what, of irritating, a charm all the more great, that he was forced to conceal its effects upon himself and to guard his attempts without betraying himself.   The con-versation, which related to Michel Chrestien through the dinner to the dessert, furnished an admirable pretext to Daniel, as to the princess, for conversing with lowered voices,—love, sympathy, divination; for her to pose as a woman misunder-stood, calumniated; for him to slip his feet into the shoes of the dead Republican.   Perhaps this ingen-uous man was surprised to find himself regretting his friend so little.   At the moment when the mar-vels of the dessert were resplendent on the table, in the light of the candelabra, under the shelter of the bouquets of natural flowers which separated the guests by a brilliant hedge, richly colored with fruits and with sweetmeats, the princess was pleased to bring to a close this succession of confidences by a delicious word, accompanied by one of those glances

by the aid of which blond women seem to be
brunettes, and in which she expressed finely this
idea that Daniel and Michel were two twin souls.
D'Arthez from this moment threw himself into the
general conversation, bringing to it an infantile joy
and a little fatuous air worthy of a scholar. The
princess took in the simplest manner his arm to
return into the little salon of the marchioness. In
traversing the grand salon, she walked slowly; and,
when she was separated from the marchioness, to
whom Blondet had given his arm, by a sufficiently
considerable interval, she halted d'Arthez.

"I do not desire to be inaccessible to the friend of
that poor Republican," she said to him. "And,
although I have made a law for myself to receive no
one, you alone of all the world should be able to
enter my house. Do not think that this is a favor.
A favor is always something for strangers only, and
it seems to me that we are old friends,—I would
wish to see in you the brother of Michel."

D'Arthez could only press the arm of the princess,
he found nothing to reply. When the coffee was
served, Diane de Cadignan enveloped herself, by a
coquettish movement, in a large shawl and rose.
Blondet and Rastignac were men too high in the
world of politics and too much accustomed to the
ways of society to utter the slightest bourgeois exclamation and endeavor to retain the princess; but
Madame d'Espard caused her friend to seat herself
again by taking her by the hand and saying in her
ear:

"Wait till the domestics have dined; the carriage is not ready."

And she made a sign to the valet de chambre, who carried away the coffee service. Madame de Montcornet understood that the princess and Madame d'Espard had something to say to each other, and engrossed the attention of d'Arthez, Rastignac and Blondet, whom she amused by one of those extravagant paradoxical attacks of which the Parisian women have such a marvelous understanding.

"Well," said the marchioness to Diane, "what do you make of him?"

"Why, he is an adorable child; he is just out of his swaddling-clothes. Truly, this time again, there will be, as always, a triumph without any contest."

"It is desperately discouraging," said Madame d'Espard, "but there is one resource."

"How?"

"Let me become your rival."

"As you like," replied the princess; "I have made up my mind. Genius is in a certain manner a being of the brain, I do not know what will touch its heart; we will talk about it later."

Hearing this last word, the meaning of which was impenetrable, Madame d'Espard took part in the general conversation and appeared neither hurt as to the "As you like," nor curious to know what this interview would lead to. The princess remained about an hour seated on the little sofa near the fire, in the attitude, full of nonchalance and abandonment, which Guérin has given to Didon,

listening with all the attention of one absorbed, and looking at Daniel from time to time, without disguising an admiration which, nevertheless, did not exceed due bounds. She made her escape when the carriage was announced, after having exchanged a clasp of the hand with the marchioness and an inclination of the head with Madame de Montcornet.

The evening came to a termination without further reference to the princess. The species of exaltation experienced by d'Arthez was taken advantage of by the others, and he displayed all the treasures of his mind. Certainly he had in Rastignac and in Blondet two acolytes of the first quality in regard to finesse of wit and extended intelligence. As for the two ladies, they have long been known as among the most spirituelle of the higher society. This was then a halt in an oasis, an enjoyment rare and perfectly appreciated by these personages habitually possessed by the "Beware" of the world, of the salons and of political life. There are those who have the privilege of being among men, as it were, the beneficent stars whose light illumines all minds, whose rays warm all hearts. D'Arthez was one of those fine souls. A writer, who elevates himself to his height, acquires the habit of reflecting on all things, and forgets sometimes in the world that it is not necessary to say everything; it is impossible for him to have the restraint of those who live in it continually; but, as his flights are nearly always marked by a quality of originality, no one could complain of him. This savor so rare among talents,

this youthfulness full of simplicity, which rendered
d'Arthez so nobly original, made of this evening
something delightful. He went away with the
Baron de Rastignac, who, in conducting him to his
own house, naturally spoke of the princess, asking
him what he had thought of her.

"Michel was right to love her," replied d'Arthez;
"she is an extraordinary woman."

"Very truly extraordinary," replied Rastignac, in
a tone of raillery. "By your accent, I see that you
love her already; you will be in her house before
three days, and I am too old an habitué of Paris not
to know what will come to pass between you. Well,
my dear Daniel, I entreat you to not allow your
personal interests to become involved in the least
confusion. Love the princess if you feel love for
her in your heart; but think of your fortune. She
has never taken nor demanded two farthings from
any one whatever, she is far too much a d'Uxelles
and Cadignan for that; but, from my certain knowledge, outside her own fortune, which was very
considerable, she has dissipated several millions.
How? why? by what means? no one knows; she
does not know herself. I have seen her make away
with, thirteen years ago, the fortune of a charming
young man and that of an old notary in twenty
months."

"Thirteen years ago!" said d'Arthez; "why, how
old is she?"

"You did not then see," replied Rastignac, laughing, "at the table her son, the Duc de Maufrigneuse,

a young man of nineteen? Now, nineteen and
seventeen make—"

"Thirty-six!" cried the author, in surprise; "I
would have given her twenty years."

"She would have accepted them," said Rastignac; "but you need not worry on that subject,
she will never be more than twenty for you. You are
about to enter into the most fantastic world.—Goodnight, here you are at home," said the baron, seeing
his carriage enter the Rue de Bellefond, in which
d'Arthez lived in a pretty house of his own; "we
will see each other during the week at Mademoiselle
des Touches."

D'Arthez allowed love to penetrate into his heart
after the manner of Uncle Toby, without making
the least resistance; he proceeded by adoration
without criticism, by pure admiration. The princess,
this beautiful creature, one of the most remarkable
creatures of this monstrous Paris, in which everything is possible in good as in evil, became—however common the misfortune of the times has rendered this word,—the angel dreamed of. In order
to thoroughly comprehend the sudden transformation
of this illustrious author, it would be necessary to
know all that solitude and constant labor leave of
innocence in the heart; all that love, reduced to mere
need and become tedious by the side of an ignoble
woman, develops of desires and of fancies, how
much it excites regrets and gives birth to divine
sentiment in the very highest regions of the soul.
D'Arthez was indeed the child, the collegian whom

the tact of the princess had suddenly recognized.
An almost similar illumination had taken place in
the beautiful Diane.   She had then, at last, encountered that superior man whom all women desire, if
only to amuse themselves with him; that puissance
to which they consent to obey were it only for the
pleasure of mastering it; she had found, in short,
the great qualities of intelligence united to the simplicity of the heart, to a newness of passion; then
she saw, by an unheard-of good fortune, all these
riches contained in a form which pleased her.
D'Arthez seemed to her handsome, perhaps he was.
Although he had arrived at the serious age of man,
at thirty-eight years, he had preserved a flower of
youth due to the sober and chaste life which he had
led, and, like studious men, like men of the state,
he had acquired a reasonable *embonpoint.*   While
very young he had offered a slight resemblance to
General Bonaparte.   This resemblance was still
visible, as much so as a man with black eyes, with
thick brown hair, can resemble this sovereign with
blue eyes, with chestnut locks; but all that there
had been formerly of ardent and noble ambition in
the eyes of d'Arthez had been, as it were, made
tender by success.   The thoughts with which his
forehead had been burdened had flowered, the hollow
lines of his face had been filled out.   A happy
comfort had spread its golden tones where in
his youth poverty had mingled the yellowish tints
of the temperaments whose forces were banded together in order to sustain the crushing and continuous

combat. If you observe with care the fine faces
of the antique philosophers, you will perceive
in them always the deviations from the perfect type
of the human countenance to which each physiognomy owes its originality, rectified by the habit of
meditation, by the constant calm indispensable to
intellectual labor.   The most unquiet countenances,
like that of Socrates, become finally of a serenity
almost divine.   To this noble simplicity which
adorned his majestic head, d'Arthez joined a
candid expression, the naturalness of children,
and a touching benevolence.   He had not that
politeness, always with a touch of falseness, by
which, in this world, those persons the best educated
and the most amiable assume qualities which are
often lacking to them, and which leave seriously
wounded those who recognize that they have been
duped.   He might fail to come up to the requirement of some of the worldly laws in consequence of
his isolation; but, as he never offended, this sort of
perfume of wildness rendered still more gracious the
affability peculiar to men of great talent, who know
how to leave their superiority at home in order to
let themselves down to the social level, in order to,
like Henry IV., lend their backs to the children and
their wit to the simpletons.

In returning home, the princess did not debate
with herself, any more than d'Arthez had defended
himself against the charm which she had thrown
over him.   Everything was now said for her: she
loved with her science and with her ignorance.   If

she interrogated herself, it was to ask herself if she merited so great a happiness, and what she had done that Heaven had sent her such an angel. She wished to be worthy of this love, to perpetuate it, to appropriate it to herself forever, and to finish softly her life of a pretty woman in that paradise of which she caught glimpses. As for resistance, for quibbling with herself, for coquetting, she did not even think of it. She was thinking of a very different thing! She had comprehended the grandeur of men of genius, she had divined that they do not submit superior women to ordinary laws. Thus, by one of those rapid perceptions peculiar to these great feminine spirits, she had promised herself to be yielding at the very first desire. From the knowledge which she had gained, in one interview only, of the character of d'Arthez, she had suspected that this desire would not be soon enough expressed not to leave her the time in which to make of herself that which she wished, that which she should be in the eyes of this sublime lover.

Here commences one of those unknown comedies played, in the interior tribunal of the conscience, between two beings, of which one will be the dupe of the other, and which push back the boundaries of perversity, one of those black and comic dramas, compared with which that of *Tartuffe* is a bagatelle; but which are not of the scenic world, and which, that everything in them may be extraordinary, are natural, conceivable and justified by necessity, a horrible drama which should be named

the seamy side of vice. The princess commenced
by sending for the works of d'Arthez. She had not
read the first word of them; and, nevertheless, she
had sustained twenty minutes of eulogistic discussion with him, without *quid pro quo!* She read
them all. Then she wished to compare his books
with the best which contemporary literature had
produced. She had an indigestion of the mind the
day on which d'Arthez came to see her. Expecting
this visit, she had every day made a superior toilet,
one of those toilets which express an idea and cause
it to be accepted by the eyes, without knowing
how or why. She offered to the regard a harmonious combination of gray colors, a sort of half-mourn-
ing, a grace full of abandonment, the vestments
of a woman who no longer held to life but by
a few natural ties, her child perhaps, and who was
weary. She bore witness to an elegant disgust
which, however, would not go as far as suicide; she
would complete her term in the terrestrial bagnio.
She received d'Arthez like a woman who is waiting for him, and as if he had already been a hundred times in her house; she did him the honor to
treat him like an old acquaintance; she put him at
his ease by a single gesture indicating to him a sofa
on which to be seated, while she finished the letter
already commenced. The conversation began in
the commonest manner,—the weather, the ministry, the illness of De Marsay, the hopes of the
Legitimistes. D'Arthez was an Absolutist, the princess could not ignore the opinions of a man seated

11

in the Chamber among the fifteen or twenty persons
who represented the Legitimiste party; she found
an opportunity to relate to him how she had tricked
De Marsay; then, by a transition which was furnished her by the devotion of the Prince de Cadignan to the royal family and MADAME, she drew
the attention of d'Arthez to the prince.

"He has at least in his favor the love he bears
his masters and his devotion to them," said she.
"His public character consoles me for all the suffering which his private character has caused me.—
For," she went on, leaving the prince lightly aside,
"have you not remarked, you who know all, that
men have two characters,—they have one for their
household, for their wives, for their private life, and
which is the true one; there, no more mask, no
more dissimulation, they do not give themselves the
trouble to pretend, they are what they are, and are
often horrible; then the world, others, the salons,
the Court, the sovereign, politics, see them grand,
noble, generous, in a costume embroidered with
virtues, adorned with beautiful language, full of
exquisite qualities.   What a horrible pleasantry!
And people are surprised sometimes at the smile of
certain women, at their air of superiority with their
husbands, at their indifference!—"

She let her hand fall on the arm of her chair,
without finishing her sentence, but this gesture completed her speech admirably.   As she saw d'Arthez
occupied in studying her flexible figure, so well disposed in the depths of her cushioned arm-chair,

occupied with the fall of her skirts, and with
a pretty little gather which relieved the stiffness of
her corsage, one of those hardihoods of the toilet
which are only possible for figures sufficiently
slender to lose nothing by them, she resumed the
sequence of her thoughts as if she were speaking to
herself:

"I will not continue. You have ended, you
writers, by rendering very ridiculous the women
who pretend to be misunderstood, who are unfortunately married, who make themselves dramatic,
interesting, which seems to me to the last degree
bourgeois. One yields, and everything is said, or
one resists and you are amused. In both cases,
silence should be kept. It is true that I have neither
known how to yield altogether nor to resist altogether; but perhaps this is a still greater reason to
keep silence. What foolishness it is in women to
complain! If they have not been the strongest,
they have been wanting in wit, in tact, in finesse;
they deserve their fate. Are they not the queens
in France? They play with you as they wish,
when they wish, and as much as they wish."

She made her perfume flask dance with a marvelous movement of feminine impertinence and of
mocking gayety.

"I have often heard miserable little specimens
regret that they were women, wished that they were
men; I have always looked at them with pity," she
said, continuing. "If I had to choose, I should still
prefer to be a woman. A fine pleasure it is to owe

one's triumphs to strength, to all the powers which
are given you by the laws made by you! But,
when we see you at our feet, uttering and doing
sillinesses, is it not then an intoxicating happiness
to feel in one's self the weakness which triumphs?
When we succeed, we are obliged to keep silent,
under pain of losing our empire. Beaten, women
are still obliged to keep silent through pride. The
silence of the slave frightens the master."

This cackling was chirruped in a voice so softly
mocking, so delicate, with such coquettish movements of the head, that d'Arthez, to whom this
species of woman was totally unknown, remained exactly like the partridge charmed by the hunting dog.

"I pray you, Madame," said he, finally, "explain
to me how a man has been able to make you suffer,
and you may be sure that, even in that in which
all women are common, you would be distinguished
even though you might not have a manner of saying things which would render a cook-book interesting."

"You go quickly in friendship," said she with
her grave voice, which rendered d'Arthez serious
and disquieted.

The conversation changed, the hour advanced.
The poor man of genius went away in a contrite
frame of mind for having appeared curious, for having wounded this heart, and believing that this
woman had strangely suffered. She had passed her
life in amusing herself, she was a real female Don
Juan, with this difference only, that it was not to

supper that she would have invited the marble
statue, and certainly she would have gotten the better of the statue.

It is impossible to continue this recital without
saying a word of the Prince de Cadignan, better
known under the name of the Duc de Maufrigneuse;
otherwise, the salt in the miraculous inventions of
the princess would disappear, and strangers would
comprehend nothing of the frightful Parisian comedy
which she was going to play for a man. Monsieur
le Duc de Maufrigneuse, as a true son of the Prince
de Cadignan, is a man long and dry, with a most
elegant figure, full of graciousness, making charming speeches, who became colonel by the grace of
God and good soldier by luck; moreover, brave as a
Polander, on every occasion, without discernment,
and hiding the void in his head under the jargon oi
the *grande compagnie.* From the age of thirty-six
he was, by compulsion, of as complete an indifference to the fair sex as the King, Charles X., his
master; punished, like his master, for having, like
him, pleased too much in his youth. During eighteen years the idol of the Faubourg Saint-Germain,
he had, like all the sons of families, led a dissipated
life, filled only with pleasures. His father, ruined
by the Revolution, had recovered his position on the
return of the Bourbons, the government of a royal
château, salaries, pensions; but this factitious fortune the old prince had very soon devoured, remaining the grand seigneur which he had been before
the Restoration, so that, when the law of indemnity

arrived, the sums which he received were absorbed
by the luxury which he displayed in his immense
hôtel, the only property which he recovered, and
the largest part of which was occupied by his
daughter-in-law.   The Prince de Cadignan died
some time before the Revolution of July, at the age
of eighty-seven.   He had ruined his wife, and was
long in delicate relations with the Duc de Navarreins, who had married his daughter for his first
wife, and to whom he with difficulty rendered his
accounts.   The Duc de Maufrigneuse had had liaisons with the Duchesse d'Uxelles.   About 1814, at
the date when Monsieur de Maufrigneuse reached
his thirty-sixth birthday, the duchess, seeing him
poor, but very well received at Court, gave him her
daughter, who possessed about fifty or sixty thous-
and francs of income, in addition to that which she
might expect to receive from her.   Mademoiselle
d'Uxelles thus became also a duchess, and her
mother knew that she would have in all probability
the greatest liberty.   After having had the unhoped-for happiness of being presented with a son
and heir, the duke left his wife entirely free in her
actions, and went amusing himself from garrison to
garrison, passing the winters in Paris, contracting
debts which his father always paid, professing the
most complete conjugal indulgence, notifying the
duchess a week in advance of his return to Paris,
adored by his regiment, loved by the Dauphin, a
skilful courtier, something of a gambler, moreover
without any affectation; the duchess could never

persuade him to take an opera-dancer for appearance
sake and through regard for her, as she said pleasantly. The duke, who had the succession of the
office of his father, knew how to please the two
kings, Louis XVIII. and Charles X., which went to
prove that he made a very good use of his nullity;
but this conduct, this life, were all covered with a
most beautiful varnish,—language, nobility of manners, appearance, all offered in him their perfection; in short, the Liberals loved him. It was
impossible for him to continue the Cadignans who,
according to the old prince, were well known as
ruining their wives, for the duchess used up her
fortune herself. These details became so public in
the circle of the Court and in the Faubourg Saint-
Germain, that during the last five years of the
Restoration, any one who would have spoken of
them would have been laughed at, as if he wished
to relate the death of Turenne or that of Henry IV.
Thus there was not one woman who spoke of this
charming duke without eulogy,—his conduct toward
his wife had been perfect, it would be difficult for a
man to show himself as considerate as Maufrigneuse
had been for the duchess; he had left her the free
disposition of her fortune, he had defended her and
sustained her on every occasion. Whether it were
pride, or good nature, or chivalrousness, Monsieur
de Maufrigneuse had saved the duchess on more than
one occasion when any other woman would have
been lost, notwithstanding her connection, notwithstanding the credit of the old Duchesse d'Uxelles, of

the Duc de Navarreins, of her father-in-law and of
her husband's aunt.   To-day, the Prince de Cadignan passes for one of the finest characters of the
aristocracy.   Perhaps fidelity in need is one of the
very finest victories which the courtiers can win
over themselves.   The Duchesse d'Uxelles was
forty-five when she married her daughter to the
Duc de Maufrigneuse; she had looked for a long
time without jealousy and even with interest at the
success of her former friend.   At the time of her
marriage of her daughter and the duke, she maintained a conduct of great nobility, and one which
covered the immorality of this combination.   Nevertheless, the malice of persons at Court found matter
for jesting, and pretended that this fine conduct
had not cost the duchess very dearly, though for
about the last five years she had given herself up to
the devotion and repentance of a woman who has
much to be pardoned.

During several days, the princess showed herself
more and more remarkable for her literary attain-
ments.   She took up with the greatest hardihood
the most arduous questions, thanks to diurnal and
nocturnal readings pursued with an intrepidity
worthy of the highest eulogiums.   D'Arthez, stupefied and incapable of suspecting that Diane
d'Uxelles repeated in the evening what she had read
in the morning, as do a great many writers, held
her for a superior woman.   These conversations
increased the distance of Diane from her object, she
endeavored to place herself again on the footing of

D'ARTHEZ AND DIANE

———

"What troubles you?" said d'Arthez. "You appear disquieted."

"I have received a letter from Monsieur de Cadignan," she replied. "However grave may be his wrongs toward me, I reflected, after having read his letter, that he is exiled, without family, without his son, whom he loves."

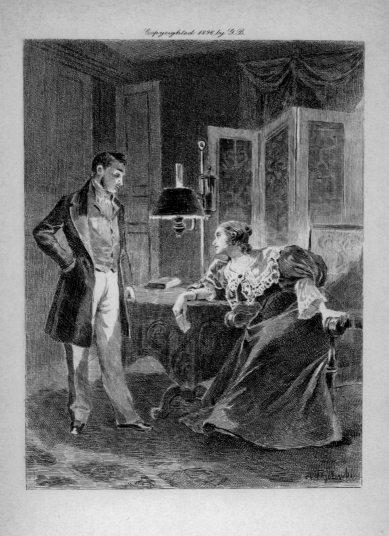

confidence from which her lover had prudently
retired; but it was not very easy to bring back to
this point a man of his temper who had once been
frightened off. Nevertheless, after a month of these
literary campaigns and fine Platonic discourses,
d'Arthez became more resolute and came every day
at three o'clock. He went away at six, and reappeared in the evening at nine, to remain until midnight or one o'clock in the morning, with the
regularity of a lover full of impatience. The princess was always dressed with more or less care at
the hour when d'Arthez presented himself. This
mutual fidelity, the care which they took of themselves, everything in them, expressed the sentiments
which they did not dare to avow, for the princess
divined marvelously well that this great child was
as much afraid of a contention as she was desirous
of it. Nevertheless, d'Arthez expressed in his constant, mute declarations a respect which pleased the
princess infinitely. Both of them felt themselves
each day so much more united that nothing conventional nor direct and open would arrest them in the
flow of their ideas, as when, between lovers, there
are on one side formal demands, and on the other a
defense sincere or coquettish. Like all those men
who are younger than their age would entitle them
to be, d'Arthez was a prey to those agitating irres-
olutions caused by the power of desires and by the
terror of displeasing, a situation of which a young
woman comprehends nothing when she shares it, but
to which the princess had too often given occasion

not to appreciate all its pleasures. Thus Diane
enjoyed these delicious childishnesses with so much
the more charm that she knew perfectly well how to
make them cease. She resembled a great artist
pausing over the indecisive lines of a sketch,
certain of being able to finish in an hour of inspiration the masterpiece still floating in the limbo of
creation. How many times, seeing d'Arthez ready
to advance, had she not pleased herself by arresting
him by an imposing air! She suppressed the secret
storms of this young heart, she stirred them up
again, pacified them by a look, in giving her hand
to be kissed or by insignificant words uttered in a
moved and tender voice. This management, coldly
arranged, but divinely played, engraved her image
still deeper in the soul of this spiritual writer,
whom she was pleased to render childlike, confiding,
simple and almost silly beside her; but she had
also occasional returnings upon herself, and it was
then impossible for him not to admire so much
grandeur mingled with so much innocence. This
play of a great coquette attached her insensibly
to her slave. Finally, Diane became impatient with
this amorous Epictetus, and, when she thought she
had brought him to the most entire credulity, she
gave herself as a duty the task of applying over his
eyes the very thickest bandage.

One evening, Daniel found the princess pensive,
an elbow on her little table, her beautiful blond
head bathed in the light from the lamp; she was
trifling with a letter which she made dance on the

table-cloth. When d'Arthez had seen this paper sufficiently, she finished by folding it and putting it in her girdle.

"What troubles you?" said d'Arthez. "You appear disquieted."

"I have received a letter from Monsieur de Cadignan," she replied. "However grave may be his wrongs toward me, I reflected, after having read his letter, that he is exiled, without family, without his son, whom he loves."

These words, pronounced in a voice full of soul, revealed an angelic sensibility. D'Arthez was moved to the last degree. The curiosity of the lover became, so to speak, a curiosity almost psychological and literary. He wished to know up to what point this woman was grand, for what injuries her pardon was required, how much these women of the world, accused of frivolity, of hardness of heart, of selfishness, could be angelic. Remembering that he had been already repulsed when he wished to know better this celestial heart, he himself had something like a trembling in his voice when, taking the transparent and slender hand, with tapering fingers, of the beautiful Diane, he said to her :

"Are we now sufficiently good friends for you to tell me what you have suffered? Your former griefs should be of influence in this revery."

"Yes," said she, whispering this syllable like the very softest note that had ever been sighed by the flute of Tulou.

She fell back again in her revery, and her eyes veiled themselves. Daniel remained waiting full of anxiety, penetrated by the solemnity of this moment. His poet's imagination caused him to see, as it were, the clouds which were dissipated slowly in discovering to him the sanctuary where he was about to see at the feet of God the blessed lamb.

"Well?—" said he, in a voice soft and calm.

Diane looked at the tender suitor; then she lowered her eyes slowly, displaying her eyelashes by a movement which revealed the most noble modesty. No one but a monster would have been capable of imagining any hypocrisy in the graceful undulation by which the malicious princess raised her pretty little head to plunge once more her glance in the desiring eyes of this great man.

"Can I? Should I?" she said, with an involuntary gesture of hesitation, looking at d'Arthez with a sublime expression of dreamy tenderness. "Men have so little faith in these things, they think themselves so little obliged to discretion!"

"Ah! if you doubt me, why am I here?" cried d'Arthez.

"Ah! my friend," she replied, giving to her exclamation the gracefulness of an involuntary avowal, "when she gives herself for life, does a woman calculate? It is not a question of my refusal —what can I refuse you?—but of the conception which you will have of me, if I speak. I could readily confide to you the strange situation in which I am at my age; but what would you think of a

woman who discovered the secret wounds of marriage, who would betray the secret of another? Turenne kept his word to the thieves; do I not owe to my executioners the probity of Turenne?"

"Have you given your promise to anyone?"

"Monsieur de Cadignan did not think it necessary to ask of me secrecy.   You wish, then, more than my soul?   Tyrant! you wish, then, that I bury in you my probity?" said she, throwing on d'Arthez a look by which she set a higher value on this false confidence than on her person.

"You make of me a man even less than common, if from me you fear anything whatever evil," he said, with a bitterness but thinly disguised.

"Forgive me, my friend," she replied, taking his hand, looking at it, taking it between her own and caressing it by drawing her fingers over it with a movement of the greatest gentleness. "I know all that you are worth.   You have related to me your whole life; it is noble, it is beautiful, it is sublime, it is worthy of your name; perhaps, in return, I owe you mine?   But I am afraid at this moment to fall in your view by recounting to you secrets which are not altogether mine.   Then, perhaps, you will not believe, you, a man of solitude and of poetry, in the horrors of the world.   Ah! you do not know that in inventing your dramas, they are surpassed by those which are really acted in families apparently the most united.   You are ignorant of the extent of certain gilded misfortunes."

"I know all," he cried.

"No," she resumed, "you know nothing. Should a daughter ever deliver up her mother?"

In hearing this word, d'Arthez found himself like a man lost in a black night on the Alps, and who, at the first light of day, perceives that he is on the edge of a bottomless precipice. He looked at the princess with a bewildered air, he had a chill in his back; Diane thought that this man of genius had a feeble spirit, but she saw a light in his eyes which reassured her.

"Finally, you have become for me almost a judge," she said, with a despairing air. "I can speak, in virtue of that right which everyone who has been slandered has to assert his innocence. I have been, I am still—so much so as anyone remembers a poor recluse forced by the world to renounce the world!—accused of so much lightness of conduct, of so many evil things, that it can be permitted to me to place myself in the heart in which I find an asylum in such a manner as not to be driven from it. I have always seen in self-justification a strong reflection on innocence, and for this reason have I always disdained to speak. To whom, moreover, could I address my speech? These cruel things can only be confided to God, or to some one who seems to us near to Him, a priest, or a second self. Well, if my secrets are not there," she said, placing her hand over d'Arthez's heart, "as they are here—" and the upper part of her corsage yielded to the pressure of her fingers—"you will not be the grand d'Arthez, I will have been deceived!"

A tear moistened the eye of d'Arthez, and Diane mastered this tear by a sidewise glance which did not cause the slightest movement of eyeball or eyelid. It was quick and neat as the stroke of a cat taking a mouse. D'Arthez, for the first time, after sixty days full of protocols, dared to take her warm and perfumed hand; he carried it to his lips, he impressed on it a long kiss trailed from the wrist to the nails with so delicate a voluptuousness that the princess inclined her head, auguring very favorably indeed of literature. She thought that men of genius might love with much more perfection than do the fops, the men of the world, the diplomats, and even the soldiers, who, however, have only that to do. She was a connoisseur, and knew that the amorous character signs itself in some way in nothings. An instructed woman can read her future in a simple gesture, as Cuvier could say, in seeing the fragment of a skeleton of a paw: "This belonged to an animal of such and such dimensions, with or without horns, carnivorous, herbivorous, amphibious, etc., so many thousand years old." Certain of encountering in d'Arthez as much imagination in love as he put in his literary style, she judged it necessary to make him arrive at the very highest degree of passion and of faith. She withdrew her hand quickly with a magnificent movement, full of emotions. She might have said: "Have done, you will make me die!" she would have spoken less energetically. She remained for a moment gazing at the eyes of d'Arthez, expressing all at once

happiness, prudishness, fear, confidence, languor, a vague desire and the shame of a virgin. She was but twenty years old! But, reflect that she had prepared for this hour of comic mendacity with an unheard-of art in her toilet; she was in her fauteuil like a flower which is about to expand at the first kiss of the sun. Deceiving or true, she intoxicated Daniel.

If I may be permitted to risk an individual opinion, let us admit that it would be delicious to be thus deceived for a long time. Certainly, Talma, before the footlights, has often been more convincing than nature. But was not the Princesse de Cadignan the greatest comedienne of her time? Nothing was lacking to this woman but an attentive audience. Unfortunately, in those epochs which are ravaged by political storms, women disappear like water-lilies which have need of a pure sky and the mildest zephyrs to flower before our delighted eyes.

The hour had come, Diane was about to enmesh this distinguished man in the inextricable lianas of a romance carefully prepared, and which he was about to listen to as a neophyte in the best days of the Christian faith would have listened to the epistle of an apostle.

"My friend, my mother, who is still living at Uxelles, married me at seventeen years of age, in 1814—you see how old I am!—to Monsieur de Maufrigneuse, not for love of me, but for love of him. She thus acquitted herself, with the only man whom

she had ever loved, for all the happiness which she
had received from him. Oh! you need not be
astonished at this horrible combination; it often
takes place. Very many women are more lovers
than mothers, as the greater number of them are
better mothers than wives. These two sentiments,
love and maternity, developed as they are by our
customs, often come into conflict in the hearts of
women; one of them necessarily has to succumb
when they are not equal in strength, a fact which
makes of some exceptional women the glory of our
sex. A man of your genius may readily comprehend these things, which astonish fools, but which
are none the less true, and, I will go still further,
which are justifiable by the differences of character,
of temperaments, of attachments, of situations.
Myself, for example, at this moment, after twenty
years of unhappinesses, of deceptions, of calumnies
endured, of heavy ennui, of hollow pleasures, would
I not be disposed to throw myself at the feet of a
man who would love me sincerely and forever?
Well, would I not be condemned by the world?
And yet, would not twenty years of suffering, would
they not furnish an excuse for giving to a holy and
pure love the dozen years which still remained to
me in which to be beautiful? This will not be, I am
not foolish enough to diminish my merits in the eyes
of God. I have borne the burden and heat of the
day unto the evening, I will finish my day's labor
and I shall have gained my reward—"

"What an angel!" thought d'Arthez.

12

"In short, I have never wished ill to the Duchesse d'Uxelles for having better loved Monsieur de Maufrigneuse than the poor Diane here present. My mother had seen very little of me, she had forgotten me; but she had behaved so badly towards me, as from one woman to another, that what is evil conduct from one woman to another becomes horrible from mother to daughter. Those mothers who lead a life like that of the Duchesse d'Uxelles keep their daughters at a distance from them, so that I only entered the world two weeks before my marriage. You may judge of my innocence! I knew nothing, I was incapable of suspecting the secret of this alliance. I had a fine fortune,—sixty thousand francs of income from forest land, in Nivernais, which the Revolution had forgotten to sell, or was not able to sell, and which appertained to the fine château d'Anzy; Monsieur de Maufrigneuse was riddled with debts. If, later, I learned what it is to have debts, I was then too completely ignorant of life to suspect it. The savings which had been effected on my fortune served to regulate the affairs of my husband. Monsieur de Maufrigneuse was thirty-eight years of age when I married him, but these years were like those of military campaigns, they should count double. Ah! he was indeed more than seventy-six. At forty, my mother still retained her pretensions, and I found myself between two jealousies. What a life did I lead during ten years! —Ah! if one knew what this poor little woman so much suspected had suffered! To be guarded by a

mother jealous of her daughter! God!—You, who
make dramas, you will never invent one as black,
as cruel, as this one. Usually, from the little that
I know of literature, a drama is a sequence of
actions, of discourse, of movements which hurry
themselves towards a catastrophe; but that of which
I speak to you is the most horrible catastrophe in
action! It is the avalanche which fell on you in the
morning, which falls again in the evening, and
which will fall again to-morrow. I am chilled at
this moment in which I speak to you and in which
I show you the cavern without exit, cold and dark,
in which I lived. If it is necessary to tell you
everything, the birth of my poor child, who, moreover, is all myself,—you must have been struck
with his resemblance to me? he has my hair, my
eyes, the shape of my face, my mouth, my smile,
my chin, my teeth,—well, his birth was a chance
or the result of a convention between my mother
and my husband. For a long time after my marriage I remained a young girl, all but abandoned the
next day, mother without being wife. The duchess
amused herself by prolonging my ignorance, and,
for this purpose, a mother has horrible advantages
over her daughter. I, poor little thing, brought up
in a convent like a *rose mystique,* knowing nothing
of marriage, developed very late, I found myself
very happy,—I took pleasure in the mutual understanding and the harmony of our family. In the
end I was entirely diverted from thinking of my
husband, who scarcely pleased me and who did

nothing to ingratiate himself, during my first joys
of maternity,—they were, moreover, so much the
more keen that I did not suspect that there were
others. I had had so constantly dinned in my ears
the respect that a mother owes to herself! And,
moreover, a young girl always likes to 'play
mamma.' At the age in which I then was, a child
replaces the doll. I was so proud of this beautiful
flower, for Georges was beautiful,—a marvel! How
be able to think of the world outside when one has
the happiness of nourishing and caring for a little
angel! I adore children when they are very little,
white and pink. I saw nothing but my son, I lived
with my son, I would not let his nurse clothe him,
unclothe him, change his linen. These cares, so
wearying for mothers who have regiments of children, were nothing but pleasure for me. But, after
three or four years, as I am not altogether stupid,
notwithstanding the care which was taken to bandage my eyes, the light finally reached them. Do
you see me undeceived, four years later, in 1819?
Les Deux Frères ennemis is a rose-water tragedy
compared with a mother and a daughter placed as we
were, the duchess and I; I braved them then, her and
my husband, by public coquetries which made the
world talk—God knows how much! You understand, my friend, that the men with whom I was
suspected of light conduct had for me the value of a
dagger which one makes use of to stab his enemy.
Absorbed in my vengeance, I was not conscious
of the wounds which I was inflicting on myself.

Innocent as a child, I passed for a perverse woman,
for the most wicked woman in the world, and I
knew nothing of it.   The world is very foolish, very
blind, very ignorant; it only penetrates those
secrets which amuse it, which serve its wickedness;
the greatest things, the most noble, it puts its hand
over its eyes not to see them.   But it seems to me
that, at that period, there must have been seen in
me glances, attitudes, of innocence in revolt, movements of pride which would have made fortunes for
the great painters.   I should have lit up the balls
by the tempests of my anger, by the torrents of my
disdain.   Poetry lost! these sublime poems are only
written in that indignation which seizes us at
twenty!   Later, one no longer gets indignant, one
is wearied; one is no longer astonished at vice, one
is cowardly, one is afraid.   I, I went on, oh! I went
on finely.   I played the part of the most foolish personage in the world,—I had all the costs of crime
without having the benefits.   I had so much pleasure in compromising myself!   Ah! I was guilty of
infantile malice.   I went to Italy with a young
scatterbrain whom I deposited there when he spoke
to me of love; but when I learned that he had compromised himself for me—he had committed a for-
gery to obtain money—I hastened to save him.   My
mother and my husband, who knew all these secrets,
restrained me like a prodigal woman.   Oh! this
time, I went to the king.   Louis XVIII., that man
without a heart, was touched—he gave me a hundred thousand francs from his privy purse.   The

Marquis d'Esgrignon, this young man whom you have perhaps met in society, and who finished by making a very rich marriage, was saved from the abyss into which he had plunged for me. This adventure, caused by my recklessness, made me reflect. I perceived that I was the first victim of my own vengeance. My mother, my husband, my father-in-law had the world on their side, they seemed to be protecting my follies. My mother, who knew me too proud, too grand, too much a d'Uxelles to be guilty of vulgar conduct, was then frightened at the evil which she had done. She was fifty-two years of age; she left Paris, she has gone to live at Uxelles. She now repents of her wrongs, she is expiating them by the most extravagant devotion and by a boundless affection for me. But, in 1823, she left me alone and face to face with Monsieur de Maufrigneuse. O, my friend, you other men, you can never know what it is to be a man of intrigues grown old. What a household is that of a man accustomed to the adoration of women of the world, who finds neither incense nor censer in his own house, when he is dead to everything, and all the more jealous for that! I desired, when Monsieur de Maufrigneuse was left alone with me, I desired to be a good wife; but I came into contact with all the asperity of a bitter spirit, with all the fantasies of impotence, with all the puerilities of silliness, with all the vanities of self-sufficiency, with a man who was, in short, the most wearying elegy in the world, and who treated me like a little girl, who

pleased himself with humiliating my self-respect on every occasion, with crushing me under the weight of his experience, with proving to me that I was ignorant of everything. He wounded me every moment. In short, he did everything to cause me to hold him in detestation and to give me the right to betray him; but I was the dupe of my own heart and of my desire to do well during three or four years! Would you know the infamous word which caused me to commit further follies? Would you ever invent the most sublime slander in the world? 'The Duchesse de Maufrigneuse has returned to her husband,' it was said. 'Bah! it is mere depravity; it is a triumph to reanimate the dead; she had done everything but that,' answered my best friend, a relative in whose house I had the happiness of meeting you."

"Madame d'Espard!" cried Daniel, making a gesture of horror.

" Oh! I have pardoned her, my friend. In the first place, the speech is excessively witty, and perhaps I have myself uttered crueler epigrams on poor women who were quite as pure as I was."

D'Arthez kissed again the hand of this saintly woman, who, after having served up to him a mother cut to pieces, after having made of the Prince de Cadignan, whom you know, an Othello of triple watchfulness, had hashed up her own character and accused herself of wrongs, in order to cover herself in the eyes of this ingenuous writer with that virginity which the most stupid of women endeavors at any price to offer her lover.

"You understand, my friend, that I re-entered society with a great display and in order to there make a display. I there encountered new struggles; it was necessary to conquer my independence and to neutralize Monsieur de Maufrigneuse. I accordingly led for other reasons a dissipated life. To distract myself, to forget real life in a fantastic life, I gave fêtes, I played the princess, and I made debts. For myself, I forgot everything in the sleep of fatigue; I woke again beautiful, gay, crazy for the world; but, in this melancholy combat of fancy against reality, I devoured my fortune. The revolt of 1830 arrived just at the moment when I encountered, at the end of this existence of the *Thousand and One Nights*, the pure and holy love which—I am frank!—I desired to know. Admit it, was it not natural for a woman whose heart, suppressed by so many causes and accidents, had re-awakened at the age in which a woman feels herself deceived, and at which I saw around me so many women happy and loving? Ah! why was Michel Chrestien so respectful? There was in this still another mockery for me. What would you have! in falling, I have lost everything, I had no longer any illusions whatever; I had tried everything excepting one fruit only for which I had no longer either taste or teeth. In short, I found myself disenchanted in the world at the period when it was necessary for me to quit the world. There is in this something providential, as in those insensibilities which prepare us for death."—She made a gesture full of religious

unction.—"Everything then served me," she resumed, " the disasters of the monarchy and its ruin
helped me to bury myself. My son consoles me for
very many things. Maternal love reimburses us for
all the other sentiments which have been deceived!
And the world is surprised at my retirement, but I
have here found happiness. Oh! if you could know
how happy here is the poor creature who is before
you! In sacrificing everything for my son, I forget
the happiness of which I am ignorant and of which
I shall always be ignorant. Who would be able to
believe that life has been, for the Princesse de Cadignan, only an evil marriage-night; and all the adventures that have been imputed to her only the
defiance of a young girl to two frightful passions?
No one. To-day, I have fear of everything. I
would repulse, doubtless, a true feeling, some true
and pure love, in remembering so many falsehoods,
so many misfortunes; just as the rich, imposed upon
by cheats who feign misfortune, repulse an honest
poverty, disgusted as they are with all benevolence.
All that is horrible, is it not? but, believe me, that
which I tell to you is the history of very many
women."

These last words were pronounced with the lightness and pleasantry of tone which recalled the elegant and mocking women of the world. D'Arthez
was stunned. In his eyes, those whom justice sends
to the galleys, for murder, for having stolen with ag-
gravating circumstances, for having made a mistake
of a signature on a note, are little saints compared

with the criminals of the great world. This
atrocious elegy, forged in the arsenal of deceit and
tempered in the waters of the Parisian Styx, had
been pronounced with the inimitable accent of
truth. The author contemplated for a moment this
adorable woman, sunk in the depths of her fauteuil,
and whose two hands hung over the two arms of
her seat like two dew-drops on the edge of a flower,
overwhelmed by this revelation, crushed in seeming
to have felt all the sorrows of her life again in relating them; in short, an angel of melancholy.

"And you may judge," said she, sitting up suddenly, lifting one of her hands and darting a swift
glance from her eyes in which twenty years of pretended chastity flamed, "you may judge what
impression must have made on me the love of your
friend; but, by an atrocious mockery of chance,—
or of God, perhaps,—for at that time, I avow it, a
man, that is a man worthy of me, would have found
me feeble, so much was I thirsting for happiness!
Well, he is dead, and dead in saving the life of
whom?—of Monsieur de Cadignan! Are you
astonished to find me thoughtful—"

This was the last stroke, and the poor d'Arthez
no longer restrained himself,—he fell on his knees,
he buried his head in the hands of the princess and
there wept; he poured on them those soft tears which
the angels shed,—if the angels weep. As Daniel
had his head thus, Madame de Cadignan could allow
to play around her lips a malicious smile of triumph,
such a smile as that with which the monkeys might

accompany a very superior trick,—if the monkeys laugh.

"Ah! I have him," she thought.

And she had him very much, in fact.

"But you are,—" said he, raising his handsome head and looking at her lovingly.

"—Virgin and martyr," she completed, smiling at the vulgarity of this old pleasantry, but giving it a charming meaning by this smile full of cruel gayety.

"If you see me smiling, it is that I think of the princess who knows the world so well, of this Duchesse de Maufrigneuse to whom they have given de Marsay, and the infamous de Trailles, a political ruffian, and that little fool d'Esgrignon, and Rastignac, Rubempré, ambassadors, ministers, Russian generals, who knows? Europe! They have put an evil meaning on this album which I had made, believing that those who admired me were my friends. Ah! it is frightful. I do not understand how I can permit a man at my feet: to scorn them all, such should be my religion."

She rose, went over to the window with a gait full of magnificent motifs.

D'Arthez remained on the chair where he had resumed his seat, not daring to follow the princess, but looking at her; he heard her wipe her pretty nose without blowing it. What can be said of the princess who blows her nose? Diane essayed the impossible in order to make her sensibility believed in. D'Arthez believed his angel in tears, he

hastened to her, took her round the waist, pressed her against his heart.

"No, leave me," she said, in a feeble and murmuring voice, "I have too many doubts to be worthy of anything. To reconcile me with life is a task beyond a man's strength."

"Diane! I will love you, I myself, for your whole lost life."

"No, do not speak to me thus," she replied. "In this moment I am ashamed and trembling as if I had committed the greatest sins."

She had entirely returned to the innocence of a young girl, and showed herself, nevertheless, august, great, noble, as much so as a queen. It is impossible to describe the effect of this management, so very skilful that it attained to pure truth, on a soul as new and fresh as that of d'Arthez. The great writer remained mute with admiration, passive in this window embrasure, waiting for a word, while the princess was waiting for a kiss; but she was too sacred for him. When she became cold, the princess went back to her fauteuil, her feet were frozen.

"It will take a long while," she thought, looking at Daniel, her forehead high and her head sublime in virtue.

"Is it a woman?" this profound observer of the human heart asked himself. "How must one act with her?"

Until two o'clock in the morning, they occupied themselves in repeating to each other those stupidities which women of genius, such as the princess

is, know how to render adorable. Diane pretended
to be too much destroyed, too old, too worn; d'Arthez proved to her, that of which she was well convinced, that she had the most delicate skin, the
most delicious to touch, the whitest to look at, the
most perfumed; she was young and in her flower.
They disputed beauty by beauty, detail by detail,
with the "Do you think so?—You are foolish!—It
is desire!—In two weeks, you will see me as I am.
—In fact, I am going on towards forty; can so old a
woman be loved?" D'Arthez's eloquence was impetuous and like that of a young scholar larded
with the most exaggerated epithets. When the
princess heard this witty and intelligent writer
uttering the sillinesses of an amorous sub-lieuten-
ant, she listened with an absorbed air, very tender,
but laughing inwardly.

When d'Arthez found himself in the street, he
asked himself if he might not have been a little less
respectful. He went over in his memory those
strange confidences which naturally have been very
much abridged here; they would have required an
entire volume to be rendered in all their mellifluous
abundance and with all the manners with which
they were accompanied. The retrospective per-
spicacity of this man, at once so natural and so profound, was deceived by the naturalness of this
romance, by its depth, by the accent of the princess.

"It is true," he said to himself, in his sleepless-
ness; "there are such dramas in the world; the

world covers such horrors under the flowers of its
elegance, under the embroidery of its slanders,
under the wit of its recitals. We never invent
anything but the truth. Poor Diane! Michel had
a presentiment of this enigma; he said that under
that layer of ice there were volcanoes! And Bianchon, Rastignac, were right,—when a man can be
able to combine the grandeurs of the ideal and the
pleasures of desire in loving a woman whose ways
are beautiful, full of wit, of delicacy, that should
indeed be a happiness without a name."

And he sounded in himself the depths of his love,
and he found it infinite.

The next day, about two o'clock, Madame d'Espard, who for more than a month had not seen the
princess, and had not received from her a single
traitorous word, came, drawn by an excessive curiosity. Nothing could have been more pleasant than
the conversation of these two fine adders during the
first half-hour. Diane d'Uxelles avoided speaking
of d'Arthez just as she would the wearing of a
yellow dress. The marchioness circled around this
question like a Bedouin around a rich caravan.
Diane was amusing herself, the marchioness was
becoming enraged. Diane waited; she wished to
utilize her friend and to make of her a hunting dog.
Of these two women so celebrated in the actual
world, one of them was stronger than the other.
The princess stood a head higher than the marchioness, and the marchioness recognized inwardly
this superiority. In this, perhaps, lay the secret of

this friendship.   The most feeble waited, crouching
in her false attachment, for the hour—so long
waited for by all feeble things—in which to leap at
the throat of the strong and to imprint upon it the
mark of a joyous bite.   Diane saw this clearly.
The whole world was the dupe of the cajoleries of
these two friends.   At the moment when the princess perceived an interrogation on the lips of her
friend, she said to her:

"Well, my dear, I owe to you a complete happiness, immense, infinite, celestial."

"What do you mean to say?"

"Do you remember what we were meditating on,
some three months ago, in this little garden, on the
bench in the sun, under the jessamine?   Ah! it is
only people of genius who know how to love.   I
would willingly apply to my grand Daniel d'Arthez
the speech of the Duc d'Albe to Catherine de
Medici: 'The head of one salmon is worth that of
all these frogs.'"

"I am not surprised that I have not seen you,"
said Madame d'Espard.

"Promise me, if you see him, not to say to him
one word about me, my angel," said the princess,
taking the hand of the marchioness.   "I am happy,
oh! but happy beyond all expression, and you know
how, in the world, a word, a pleasantry, will go a
great way.   A word kills, so well is it known how
to put venom in a word!   If you knew how, for the
last week, I have desired that you might have a
similar passion!   In fine, it is sweet, it is a

beautiful triumph for us women to complete our womanly life, to sink to rest in an ardent love, pure, devoted, complete, entire, above all when one has sought for it so long."

"Why do you ask me to be faithful to my best friend?" said Madame d'Espard. "You believe me, then, capable of playing you an evil trick?"

"When a woman possesses such a treasure, the fear of losing it arises so naturally that it makes one doubt everything. I am absurd; forgive me, my dear."

Some moments later the marchioness departed; and, as she saw her go, the princess said to herself:

"How she will serve me up! if she could but tell everything of me! But to spare her the trouble of drawing Daniel from here, I will send him to her."

At three o'clock, a few minutes later, d'Arthez came. In the midst of an interesting discourse, the princess cut his speech short and laid her handsome hand on his arm.

"Forgive me, my friend," she said, interrupting him, "but I will forget something which seems a foolishness, and yet which is of the utmost importance. You have not set your foot in the house of Madame d'Espard since the day, a thousand times happy, on which I met you there; go there, not for yourself, not for politeness, but for me. Perhaps you have made of her an enemy for me, if she has by chance learned that, since her dinner, you have not, so to speak, left my house. Moreover, my

friend, I should not like to see you abandon your relations in the world, nor your occupation and your works. I should be again strangely slandered. What would they not say? 'I keep you in leash, I absorb you, I fear comparisons, I wish to be talked about again, I take good care to preserve my conquest, well knowing that it is the last!' Who could guess that you are my only friend? If you love me as much as you say you love me, you will make it believed in the world that we are purely and simply brother and sister. Continue.''

D'Arthez was always disciplined by the ineffable sweetness with which this graceful woman arranged her robe so that it might fall in the most elegant manner. There was I know not what fineness and delicacy, in this discourse which touched him to tears. The princess came outside of all the ignoble and bourgeois conditions of women who disputed with each other and who quibble over coin after coin on the divans; she displayed an unheard-of grandeur; she had no need to say it, this union was nobly understood between them. It was neither yesterday, nor to-morrow, nor to-day; it would be whenever they wished it, one and the other, without the interminable fillets of that which common women call "a sacrifice;" doubtless, they are aware of all which they are likely to lose thus, whilst this fête is a triumph for those women certain of gaining by it. In this phrase, everything was vague as a promise, soft as a hope, and, nevertheless, certain as a right. Let us avow it, these sorts of

13

grandeurs appertain only to those illustrious and sublime deceivers, who remain royal there were other women become subjects. D'Arthez could then measure the distance which exists between these women and the others. The princess always showed herself worthy and beautiful. The secret of this nobility is perhaps in the art with which the great ladies know how to remove their veils; they succeed in being, in this situation, like antique statues; if they preserved a rag, they would be unchaste. The bourgeois women always endeavor to wrap themselves up.

Equipped with tenderness, sustained by the most splendid virtues, d'Arthez obeyed and went to call on Madame d'Espard, who displayed for him her most charming coquetry. The marchioness carefully avoided saying a word to d'Arthez about the princess; only she asked him to come to dinner on a near date.

D'Arthez met there a numerous company. The marchioness had invited Rastignac, Blondet, the Marquis d'Ajuda-Pinto, Maxime de Trailles, the Marquis d'Esgrignon, the two Vandenesses, Du Tillet, one of the richest bankers of Paris, the Baron de Nucingen, Nathan, Lady Dudley, two of the most perfidious attachés of embassies, and the Chevalier d'Espard, one of the most profound personages of this salon, the half of the politics of his sister-in-law.

It was laughingly that Maxime de Trailles said to d'Arthez:

"You see a great deal of the Princesse de Cadignan?"

D'Arthez answered this question only with a dry inclination of the head. Maxime de Trailles was a *bravo* of a superior order, without faith or law, capable of anything, ruining the women who were enamored of him, causing them to pawn their diamonds, but covering this conduct with a brilliant varnish, with charming manners and a wit that was satanic. He inspired in everyone a fear and a contempt that were equal; but, as no one was hardy enough to testify toward him any other sentiments than the most courteous ones, he could perceive nothing; or he lent himself to the general dissimulation. He owed to the Comte de Marsay the last degree of elevation to which he could arrive. De Marsay, who knew Maxime intimately, had judged him capable of filling certain secret and diplomatic functions which he gave him, and of which he acquitted himself marvelously. D'Arthez had been for some time sufficiently interested in political affairs to know this person to the bottom, and he alone perhaps had a sufficiently-elevated character to express openly that which everyone thought in secret.

"It ees toutless for her dat you neglegt la Jampre," said the Baron de Nucingen.

"Ah! the princess is one of the most dangerous women in whose house a man can put his foot," cried softly the Marquis d'Esgrignon; "I owe to her the infamy of my marriage."

"Dangerous?" said Madame d'Espard. "Do not speak thus of my best friend. I have never known nor seen anything in the princess which did not seem to me to partake of the most elevated sentiment."

"Let the Marquis speak," cried Rastignac. "When a man has been thrown by a fine horse, he finds him full of faults and he sells him."

Piqued at this speech, the Marquis d'Esgrignon looked at Daniel d'Arthez and said to him:

"Monsieur is not, I hope, on such terms with the princess as to prevent our speaking of her?"

D'Arthez kept silent. D'Esgrignon, who did not lack wit, made in reply to Rastignac an apologetic portrait of the princess, which put the table into good humor. As this jesting was excessively obscure for d'Arthez, he leaned over toward Madame de Montcornet, his neighbor, and asked of her the meaning of these pleasantries.

"But, excepting yourself only, to judge by the good opinion which you have of the princess, all the guests have been, it is said, in her good graces."

"I can assure you that there is nothing but what is false in that opinion," replied Daniel.

"However, there is Monsieur d'Esgrignon, a gentleman of Perche, who was completely ruined for her, some twelve years ago, and who, for her, nearly mounted the scaffold."

"I know all about that affair," said d'Arthez. "Madame de Cadignan saved Monsieur d'Esgrignon at the Court of Assizes, and we see how he rewards her to-day!"

Madame de Montcornet looked at d'Arthez with an astonishment and a curiosity that were almost stupid, then she turned her eyes on Madame d'Espard in indicating him to her, as if to say: "He is bewitched!"

During this short conversation, Madame de Cadignan had been defended by Madame d'Espard, whose protection resembled that of those lightning conductors which attract the lightning. When d'Arthez returned to the general conversation, he heard Maxime de Trailles launching this speech:

"In Diane, depravation is not an effect, it is a cause; perhaps she owes to this cause her exquisite naturalness; she does not seek, she invents nothing; she offers to you the most refined elegances as if they were an inspiration of the most naïve love, and it is impossible for you not to believe it."

This phrase, which seemed to have been prepared for a man of the capacity of d'Arthez, was so strong that it was like a conclusion. Every one left the princess, she seemed to be overwhelmed. D'Arthez looked at De Trailles and d'Esgrignon with a mocking air.

"The greatest fault of this woman is to come in competition with men," said he. "She dissipates like them all the wealth outside the jointures; she sends her lovers to the usurers, she devours dowries, she ruins orphans, she demolishes old châteaux, she inspires and, perhaps, also commits crimes; but—"

Of the two personages to whom d'Arthez was replying, neither had ever heard anything so strong.

With this *but,* the entire table was struck, each one
remained with his fork in the air, his eyes fixed
alternately on the courageous writer and on the
assassins of the princess, waiting for the conclusion
in a horrible silence.

"But," said d'Arthez, with a mocking lightness,
"Madame la Princesse de Cadignan has over men
an advantage,—when you have put yourself in danger for her, she saves you and speaks evil of none.
Why, among them all, can there not be found a
woman who will amuse herself with the men, as the
men amuse themselves with the women? Why is
it that the fair sex does not occasionally take its
revenge?—"

"Genius is stronger than wit," said Blondet to
Nathan.

This avalanche of epigrams was in fact like the
fire of a battery of cannon opposed to a fusillade of
musketry. Every one hastened to change the conversation. Neither the Comte de Trailles nor the
Marquis d'Esgrignon seemed disposed to quarrel
with d'Arthez. When the coffee was served,
Blondet and Nathan came up to the writer with an
air of earnestness which no one would dare to
imitate, so difficult was it to reconcile the admiration
inspired by his conduct and the fear of making two
powerful enemies.

"It is not to-day for the first time that we have
been convinced that your character is equal in
grandeur to your talent," said Blondet to him.
"You have conducted yourself, just now, not like a

man, but in a god-like fashion. Not to have allowed yourself to have been carried away, neither by your heart nor by your imagination; not to have taken up the defense of a loved woman, a fault which was expected of you, and which would have given a great triumph to this world so devoured with jealousy of literary celebrities—. Ah! permit me to say to you, this is to touch the sublime of private politics."

"Ah! you are a statesman," said Nathan. "It requires as much skill, as it is difficult to avenge a woman without defending her."

"The princess is one of the heroines of the Legitimiste party; is it not a duty for every man with a heart to protect her *in any case*? replied d'Arthez, coldly. "That which she has done for the cause of her masters would excuse the most frivolous life."

"He plays a close game," said Nathan to Blondet.

"Absolutely as if the princess were worth the trouble," replied Rastignac, who had joined them.

D'Arthez went to see the princess, who was waiting for him, a prey to the liveliest anxiety. The result of this experiment which Diane had brought about might be fatal to her. For the first time in her life, this woman felt a real suffering in her heart and a cold perspiration under her dress. She did not know what course to take in case d'Arthez should believe the world, which told the truth, instead of believing her, she who lied: for never had so fine a character, so complete a man, a soul so pure, a conscience so ingenuous, come

within her acquaintance. If she had concocted such cruel falsehoods, she had been driven to it by the desire of knowing veritable love. This love, she felt it dawning in her heart, she loved d'Arthez; she was condemned to deceive him, for she wished to remain for him all that he thought the sublime actress who had played her comedy before him. When she heard Daniel's step in the dining-room, she experienced a commotion, a thrill which agitated her in the very principles of her life. This movement, which she had never before experienced during an existence the most adventurous known for a woman of her rank, made her aware at this moment that she had gambled for her happiness. Her eyes, which looked into space, embraced d'Arthez in his entirety; she saw through his flesh, she read in his soul,—suspicion had not, then, even touched him with its bat's wing! The terrible *movement* of this fear was followed by its reaction, joy all but suffocated the happy Diane; for there is no creature which has not more strength to support trouble than to resist extreme happiness.

"Daniel, they have slandered me and thou hast avenged me!" she cried, rising and opening to him her arms.

In the profound astonishment produced in him by this word, the roots of which were invisible to him, Daniel permitted his head to be taken between two beautiful hands, and the princess kissed him in saintly fashion on the forehead.

"How did you know?—"

"Oh! illustrious ninny! seest thou not that I love thee foolishly?"

Since that day, there has no longer been any question of the Princesse de Cadignan nor of d'Arthez. The princess has inherited something of a fortune from her mother; she passes her summers at Geneva, in a villa, with the great writer, and returns to Paris for some months during the winter. D'Arthez only shows himself in the Chamber of Deputies. Finally, his publications have become excessively rare. Is this a dénouement? Yes, for the intelligent; no, for those who wish to know everything.

Aux Jardies, June, 1839.

SARRASINE

TO MONSIEUR CHARLES DE BERNARD DU GRAIL

SARRASINE

*

I was plunged in one of those profound reveries to which everybody is liable, even a frivolous man, in the midst of the most tumultuous festivals. Midnight had just sounded from the clock of the Élysée-Bourbon. Seated in the embrasure of a window and hidden behind the undulating folds of a curtain of moire, I was able to contemplate at my ease the garden of the hôtel in which I was passing the evening. The trees, partially covered with snow, detached themselves faintly against the grayish background formed by a cloudy sky, slightly whitened by the moon. Seen in the midst of this fantastic atmosphere, they bore a vague resemblance to spectres partially enveloped in their shrouds, a gigantic image of the famous *Dance of Death*. Then, turning toward the other side, I could admire the dance of the living! a splendid salon, with walls of silver and of gold, with sparkling candelabra, brilliant with tapers. There, crowded together, agitated and fluttered the most beautiful women in Paris, the richest, the highest-titled, splendid, pompous, blazing with diamonds! with flowers on their heads, on their breasts, in

their hair, scattered on their dresses, or in garlands at their feet. There were light shudderings, voluptuous steps which made the laces, the blonds, the gauze and the silk swirl around their delicate flanks. Here and there sparkled brilliant glances, eclipsing the lights, the fire of the diamonds, and which lent a new animation to hearts already too much on fire. There might be surprised also little attitudes of the head significant for the lovers, and negative attitudes for the husbands. The sudden outbursts of the voices of the players, at each unforeseen stroke, the clinking of gold, mingled with the music, with the murmur of the conversations; to complete the transport of this multitude—inebriated by all that the world can offer of seductions—a vapor of perfume and a general intoxication acted upon all these wandering imaginations. Thus, on my right, the sombre and silent image of death; on my left, the decent bacchanalians of life: here, nature cold, dull, in mourning; there, men in enjoyment. I myself, on the border of these two pictures so incongruous, which, a thousand times repeated in various manners, render Paris the most amusing city in the world and the most philosophical, I made for myself a sort of moral medley, half pleasant, half funereal. With the left foot I beat time to the music, and I seemed to have the other in a coffin. My leg was in fact chilled by one of those draughts of air which freeze one-half of your body whilst the other half feels the moist heat of the salons, an accident frequent enough at balls.

"It is not very long that Monsieur de Lanty has owned this hôtel?"

"Oh! yes. It is nearly ten years since the Maréchal de Carigliano sold it to him—"

"Ah!"

"These people must have an immense fortune?"

"I should say so."

"What a fête! It is of an insolent luxury."

"Do you think them as rich as Monsieur de Nucingen or Monsieur de Gondreville?"

"But you do not then know?—"

I put out my head and recognized the two interlocutors as belonging to that inquisitive class who, in Paris, occupy themselves exclusively with the *Whys? The Hows? Where did it come from? Who are they? What is there? What has she done?* They were talking in a low tone of voice, and went away to converse more at their ease on some solitary sofa. Never had a richer mine been opened to the searchers of mysteries. No one knew from what country came the family Lanty, nor from what commerce, from what spoliation, from what piracy, or from what inheritance proceeded a fortune estimated at several millions. All the members of this family spoke Italian, French, Spanish, English and German with such perfection as to make it seem probable that they had lived for a long time in these different countries. Were they Bohemians? Were they filibusters?

"If they were the devil!" said the young politicians, "they know how to receive marvelously well."

14

"Had the Comte de Lanty plundered some *Casbah*, I would marry his daughter all the same !" cried a philosopher.

Who would not have married Marianina, a young girl of sixteen, whose beauty realized the fabulous conception of the Oriental poets! Like the daughter of the Sultan in the tale of *The Wonderful Lamp,* she should have been kept veiled. Her singing made to pale their incomplete talents the Malibrans, the Sontags, the Fodors, in whom some dominant quality has always impaired the perfection of the ensemble; whilst Marianina knew how to unite in the same degree the purity of sound, the feeling, the justness of the movement and of the intonation, the soul and the science, the correctness and the sentiment. This girl was the type of that secret poetry, common bond of all the arts, and which always flies from those who seek it. Gentle and modest, learned and spirituelle, nothing could eclipse Marianina unless it were her mother.

Have you ever encountered one of those women whose overpowering beauty defies the attacks of age, and who seem, at thirty-six, more desirable than they could have been fifteen years earlier? Their countenance is a passionate soul, it sparkles; each feature is illuminated with intelligence; every detail possesses a particular brilliancy, especially in the light. Their seductive eyes attract, refuse, speak or keep silent; their gait is innocently knowing; their voice displays the melodious richness of tones, the most coquettishly soft and tender. Their

praises, by comparison, flatter the self-love of those most hard to please. A movement of their eyebrows, the least glance of the eye, their lip, which grows stern, all impress a sort of terror on those whose life and whose happiness depends on them. Inexperienced in love and docile to persuasion, a young girl may allow herself to be seduced; but for these women, a man should know how, like Monsieur de Jaucourt, not to cry out when, hiding himself in the back of a wardrobe, the femme de chambre crushes two of his fingers in the crack of a door. To love these puissant sirens, is it not to gamble with one's life? And this is why perhaps we love them so passionately! Such was the Comtesse de Lanty.

Filippo, the brother of Marianina, partook, like his sister, of the marvelous beauty of the countess. To say all in one word, this young man was a living image of the Antinous, with a form more slender. But how well these thin and delicate proportions accord with youth when an olive skin, strong eyebrows and the fire of a velvety eye, promise for the future male passions, generous thoughts! If Filippo lived in the hearts of all the young girls as a type, he lived equally in the regard of all the mothers as the best *parti* in France.

The beauty, the fortune, the wit, the graces of these two children came altogether from their mother. The Comte de Lanty was short, ugly, and pock-marked; sombre as a Spaniard, wearisome as a banker. He passed moreover for a profound politician, perhaps because he laughed but seldom, and

was always quoting Monsieur de Metternich or Wellington.

This mysterious family had all the attraction of a poem by Lord Byron, the difficulties of which were translated in a different manner by each person of the fashionable world,—a chant obscure and sublime from strophe to strophe. The reserve which Monsieur and Madame de Lanty preserved respecting their origin, their past existence and their relation with the four corners of the globe, was not for any great length of time a subject of astonishment in Paris. In no country perhaps is the axiom of Vespasian better comprehended. There, the écus, even though spotted with blood or with mud, betray nothing and represent everything. Provided that the upper classes of society know the figure of your fortune, you are classed among the sums which are equal to yours, and no one asks to see your parchments, because everybody knows how little they cost. In a city in which social problems are solved by algebraic equations, the adventurers have excellent chances in their favor. Even supposing that this family had been Bohemian in its origin, it was so rich, so attractive, that the upper circles of society could well afford to pardon it its little mysteries. But, unfortunately, the enigmatic history of the house of Lanty offered a perpetual interest of curiosity, similar enough to that of the romances of Anne Radcliffe.

The observers, those persons who make it a point to know in what shop you buy your candelabra, or

who ask you the amount of your rent when your
apartment pleases them, had remarked, from time
to time, in the midst of the fêtes, the concerts, the
balls, the routs given by the countess, the appearance of a strange personage. This was a man.
The first time that he showed himself in the hôtel,
was during a concert, where he seemed to have
been attracted to the salon by the enchanting voice
of Marianina.

"Within the last minute I have felt cold," said a
lady standing near the door, to her neighbor.

The unknown, who was near this lady, went
away.

"Here is something curious! I am too warm,"
said this woman after the departure of the stranger.
"And you will accuse me, perhaps, of being crazy,
but I cannot avoid the impression that my neighbor, that gentleman in black, who had just gone
away, made me cold."

Very soon, the exaggeration natural to people
in high society originated and accumulated the
most amusing ideas, the oddest expressions, the
most ridiculous stories concerning this mysterious
personage. Without being precisely a vampire, a
ghoul, an artificial man, a species of Faust or of
Robin des Bois, he partook, according to these
friends of the fantastic, of all these anthropomorphic
natures. There were to be met with here and
there certain Germans who took for truths these
ingenious mockeries of the Parisian slander.
The stranger was simply an *ancient man*. Several

of these young men, who were in the habit of
deciding the future of Europe every morning in a
few elegant phrases, determined to see in the unknown some great criminal, the possessor of immense riches. The romancers related the life of
this old man, and gave you truly remarkable details of the atrocities committed by him during the
time he was in the service of the prince of Mysore.
The bankers, a more positive class, set up a plausi-
ble fable.

"Bah!" said they, shrugging their great shoulders with a movement of pity, "this little old man
is a *tête génoise!*"

"Monsieur, if it is not an indiscretion, would
you have the kindness to explain to me what you
mean by a Genoese head?"

"Monsieur, it is a man upon the duration of whose
life repose enormous sums, and on his good health
depend doubtless the revenues of this family. I remember to have heard at Madame d'Espard's a
magnetizer proving, by very specious historical
considerations, that this old man, kept under glass,
was the famous Balsamo, called Cagliostro. According to this modern alchemist, the Sicilian adven-
turer had escaped death, and amused himself by
making gold for his grandchildren. And, finally,
the bailiff of Ferette pretended to have recognized
in this singular personage the Comte de Saint-
Germain."

These sillinesses, uttered in the light tone, with
the mocking air which, in our days, characterizes

a society without any faiths, gave rise to vague suspicions concerning the house of Lanty. Finally, by a singular combination of circumstances, the members of this family justified the conjectures of the world by a line of conduct sufficiently mysterious toward this old man, whose life was in some sort concealed from all investigation.

Should this personage cross the threshold of the apartment which he was reputed to occupy in the Hôtel Lanty, his appearance always caused a great sensation in the family. It could have been said to be an event of the highest importance. Filippo, Marianina, Madame de Lanty and an old domestic alone had the privilege of aiding the unknown to walk, to rise, to seat himself. Each one watched solicitously his slightest movements. It seemed as though this was an enchanted person on whom depended the happiness, the life or the fortunes of all. Was it fear or affection? The society people could not discover any indication which would aid them to solve this problem. Hidden for entire months in the depths of an unknown sanctuary, this familiar genius issued suddenly and, as it were, furtively, without being expected, and appeared in the midst of the salons like those fairies of other times who descended from their flying dragons to come and trouble those solemnities to which they had not been bidden. The most skilful observers could alone at these periods divine the inquietude of the masters of the household, who knew how to conceal their feeling with a singular skill. But,

sometimes, even while dancing in a quadrille, the too candid Marianina cast a glance of terror on the old man, whom she followed through the multitude. Or else Filippo hastened, slipping through the crowd, to join him, and remained near him, tender and attentive, as if the contact of men or the least breath would destroy this curious creature. The countess endeavored to approach him, without appearing to have the intention of rejoining him; then, in assuming a manner and a countenance as expressive of servility as of tenderness, of submission as of despotism, she said two or three words to which the old man nearly always deferred: he disappeared, led away, or, to speak more clearly, carried away, by her. If Madame de Lanty were not there, the count employed a thousand stratagems to reach him; but he had the appearance of making himself heard with difficulty and treated him like a spoiled child whose mother satisfies its caprices or dreads its unruliness. Some indiscreet persons have ventured to question rashly the Comte de Lanty, but this cold and reserved man had never appeared to be able to comprehend the interrogation of these curious ones. Thus, after a great many attempts, which the circumspection of all the members of this family had rendered fruitless, no one sought any longer to discover a secret so well guarded. The spies of good society, the open-mouthed and the politic ones, had finished, weary of the contest, by no longer occupying themselves with this mystery.

But, in this moment, there were perhaps in the

midst of these resplendent salons certain philosophers who, even while taking an ice, a sorbet, or in
setting down on a console their empty punch glass,
said to each other:

"I should not be surprised to learn that these people are sharpers. This old fellow, who hides himself and only appears at the equinoxes or at the
solstices, has to me quite the air of an assassin—"

"Or of a bankrupt—"

"It is very nearly the same thing. To kill a
man's fortune is sometimes worse than to kill him
himself."

"Monsieur, I have bet twenty louis; there are
forty coming to me."

"Faith, Monsieur, there are only thirty left on
the table."

"Well, there, you see how society is mixed here!
No one can play."

"That is true.—But here are now six months that
we have not seen the Spirit. Do you believe that
it is a living being?"

"Eh! eh! at the very most—"

These last words were uttered, near me, by unknown persons who went away at the moment in
which I resumed, in the last train of thought, my
reflections mingled with white and black, with life
and death. My fantastic imagination, as well as
my eyes, contemplated alternately the festivity
which had now reached its highest degree of splendor and the sombre picture of the gardens. I do not
know how long I had been meditating on these two

sides of the human medal; but suddenly the smothered laughter of a young woman recalled me to myself. I remained stupefied at the appearance of the
figure which presented itself before my eyes. By
one of the rarest caprices of nature, the half funereal thought which had been traversing my brain
had issued forth, it was there before me, personified,
living; it had sprung, like Minerva, from the head of
Jupiter, grand and strong; it had at once a hundred
years of age and twenty-two, it was living and dead.
Escaped from his chamber, like a maniac from his
cell, the little old man had doubtless slipped skilfully behind a hedge of persons listening to the
voice of Marianina, who was finishing the cavatina
of *Tancred.* He seemed to have issued from underground, pushed up by some theatrical mechanism. Motionless and sombre, he remained a
moment looking at this festival, the murmur of
which had perhaps reached his ears. His preoccu-
pation, almost somnambulic, was so concentrated on
certain things, that he found himself in the midst
of the world without seeing the world. He had
surged up without ceremony close to one of the
most ravishing women in Paris, a dancer elegant
and youthful, with delicate forms, one of those figures as fresh as that of a child, white and pink, and
so frail, so transparent, that it would seem as
though a man's glance could penetrate them, as the
rays of the sun traverse pure ice. They were
there, before me, both of them together, united and
so close together that the stranger touched the dress

of gauze and the garlands of flowers and the lightly crimped hair and the floating girdle.

I had brought this young woman to Madame de Lanty's ball. As this was the first time that she had been in this house, I forgave her her smothered laugh; but I made to her quickly some imperious sign, I do not know what, which filled her with confusion and inspired her with respect for her neighbor. She seated herself near me. The old man did not wish to quit this delicious creature, to whom he attached himself wilfully with that obstinacy, mute and without apparent cause, which is characteristic of the extremely aged, and which causes them to resemble children. In order to seat himself near the young lady, he was obliged to take a folding-chair. His least movements were marked by that cold heaviness, that stupid indecision which characterizes the gestures of a paralytic. He sat down slowly on his seat, with circumspection, and in mumbling some unintelligible words. His broken voice resembled the noise which a stone makes in falling into a well. The young woman pressed my hand closely, as if she sought to save herself from a precipice, and shuddered when this man, whom she was looking at, turned upon her two eyes without warmth, two glaucous eyes which could only be compared to tarnished mother-of-pearl.

"I am afraid," she said to me, leaning toward my ear.

"You can speak," I replied; "he hears with great difficulty."

"You know him, then?"

"Yes."

At this she took courage sufficiently to examine for a moment this creature without a name in human language, form without substance, being without life, or life without action. She was under the influence of that fearful curiosity which impels women to procure for themselves dangerous emotions, to see tigers chained, to look at boa-constrictors, while frightening themselves at being separated from them only by feeble barriers. Although the little old man was stoop-shouldered, like a laboring man, it could readily be seen that his figure must have been of ordinary height. His excessive meagreness, the delicacy of his limbs, proved that his proportions had always remained slender. He wore small-clothes of black silk which floated around his fleshless thighs in folds, like a furled sail. An anatomist could have promptly recognized the symptoms of a frightful phthisis on seeing the slight legs which served to sustain this strange body. You would have said they were two bones crossed on a tomb. A sentiment of profound horror for mankind seized the heart when a fatal attention had revealed to you the signs impressed by decrepitude on this fragile machine. The unknown wore a white waistcoat, embroidered with gold, in the ancient style, and his linen was of a dazzling whiteness. A jabot of English lace sufficiently yellowed, the richness of which would have been envied by a queen, formed yellow ruches on his chest; but, on

him, this lace was rather a rag than an adornment.
In the midst of this jabot a diamond of an incalcula-
ble value glittered, like the sun. This superannu-
ated luxury, this material richness without taste,
served to set off in still stronger fashion the countenance of this strange being. The frame was
worthy of the portrait. This dark visage was
angular and hollowed in every sense,—the chin
was hollow, the temples were hollow, the eyes were
lost in yellowish orbits. The maxillary bones,
rendered prominent by an indescribable meagreness, designed cavities in the middle of each cheek.
These gibbosities, more or less revealed by the
lights, produced curious shadows and reflections
which completed the want of resemblance between
this visage and the human countenance. Moreover,
the years had so closely fastened to the bone the
yellowish and fine skin of this visage that they had
there described everywhere a multitude of wrinkles,
either circular, like the ripples of water caused by a
stone thrown by a child, or star-shaped, like the
fracture of a window-pane, but always deep and as
close together as the edges of the leaves of a book.
There are old men who present to us more hideous
portraits; but that which contributed the most to
give the appearance of an artificial creation to the
spectre risen before us was the red and the white
with which he shone. The eyebrows of his mask
received from the lights a lustre which revealed a
painting very well executed. Happily for the sight
saddened by so many ruins, his cadaverous cranium

was concealed under a blond peruque, the innumerable curls of which betrayed an extraordinary pretension. For the rest, the feminine coquetry of this phantasmagoric personage was emphatically enough announced by the gold rings which hung in his ears, by the rings of which the wonderful stones glittered on his ossified fingers, and by a watch chain which scintillated like the brilliants of a necklace at the throat of a woman. Finally, this species of Japanese idol preserved on his bluish lips a fixed and arrested smile, a smile implacable and bantering, like that of a death's-head. Silent, motionless as a statue, it exhaled the musky odor of those old gowns which the heirs of a duchess exhume from her drawers during an inventory. If the old man turned his eyes toward the assembly, it seemed as though the movement of those globes, incapable of reflecting a light, were accomplished by an imperceptible artifice; and, when the eyes arrested themselves, he who examined them ended by doubting if they had moved. To see, near to this human débris, a young woman whose neck, whose arms and whose chest were naked and white; whose lines were full and redolent of beauty, whose hair rising admirably from an alabaster forehead inspired love, whose eyes did not receive but gave out light, who was soft, fresh, and whose vaporous curls, whose balmy breath, seemed too heavy, too hard, too powerful for this shadow, for this man in dust,—ah! it was certainly death and life, my revery, an imaginary arabesque, a

chimera half hideous, divinely female from the waist up.

"There are, however, such marriages, which take place with sufficient frequency in the world," I said to myself.

"He smells of the cemetery!" cried the terrified young woman, who pressed against me as if to assure herself of my protection, and whose tumultuous movements revealed to me the extremity of her fear.—"It is a horrible vision," she resumed.

"I cannot stay here any longer. If I look at it again I shall believe that death itself has come to seek me. But does it live?"

She put out her hand and touched the phenomenon with that hardihood of which women are capable in the violence of their desires; but a cold sweat broke out on her skin, for, as soon as she touched the old man, she heard a cry like that of a rattle. This sharp voice, if it were a voice, issued from a throat almost dried up. Then to this clamor succeeded quickly a little cough like a child's, convulsive and of a peculiar sonorousness. At this noise, Marianina, Filippo, and Madame de Lanty turned their looks upon us, and their glances were like lightning. The young woman could have wished herself at the bottom of the Seine. She took my arm, drew me off toward a boudoir. Men and women, everybody, made way for us. When we reached the end of the reception apartments, we entered a little semicircular cabinet. My companion

threw herself on a divan, palpitating with terror, without knowing where she was.

"Madame, you are distracted," I said to her.

"But," she answered, after a moment of silence during which I admired her, "is it my fault? Why does Madame de Lanty permit ghosts to wander about in her hôtel?"

"Come," I replied, "you imitate the silly ones. You take a little old man for a spectre."

"Keep silent," she replied, with that mocking and imposing air which all women know so well how to assume when they are determined to be right.— "What a pretty boudoir!" she cried, looking around her. "Blue satin always makes an admirable effect for hangings. How fresh it is! Ah! the beautiful picture!" she added, rising and going to take her stand before a magnificently framed canvas.

We remained for a moment contemplating this marvel, which seemed due to some supernatural brush. The picture represented Adonis reclining on a lion skin. The lamp suspended in the middle of the boudoir, and contained in an alabaster vase, illuminated this canvas with a soft light which permitted us to see all the beauties of the painting.

"Can so perfect a being exist?" she asked me, after having examined, not without a soft smile of contentment, the exquisite grace of the contours, the attitude, the color, the hair, everything in fact.

"He is too beautiful for a man," she added, after such a scrutiny as she would have given a rival.

Oh! how I then experienced the attacks of that

jealousy in which a poet had vainly endeavored to make me believe! the jealousy of engravings, of paintings, of statues, in which the artists exaggerate human beauty, carrying out the doctrine which leads them to idealize everything.

"It is a portrait," I replied to her. "It is a product of the talent of Vien. But this great painter never saw the original, and your admiration will be less lively, perhaps, when you learn that this academical study was painted from a statue of a woman."

"But who is it?"

I hesitated.

"I wish to know," she added, quickly.

"I think," I said to her, "that this *Adonis* represents a—a—a relative of Madame de Lanty."

I had the pain of seeing her absorbed in the contemplation of this figure. She seated herself in silence. I placed myself beside her and took her hand without her perceiving it! Forgotten for a portrait! At this moment, the slight sound of the step of a woman whose dress rustled was heard in the silence. We saw the young Marianina enter, still more brilliant by her expression of innocence than by her grace and by her fresh toilet; she was walking slowly, and leading with a maternal care, with a filial solicitude, the clothed spectre which had caused us to fly from the music-room; she conducted him, watching with a species of inquietude, the slow march of his debilitated feet. They both arrived with sufficient difficulty at a door

15

hidden in the tapestry. There Marianina knocked
softly. There immediately appeared, as if by
magic, a tall, dry man, a species of familiar genius.
Before confiding the old man to this mysterious
guardian, the beautiful child kissed respectfully the
walking skeleton, and her chaste caress was not
exempt from that graceful cajolery the secret of
which belongs to some privileged women.

"*Addio, addio!*" she said, with the most charming inflections of her young voice.

She even added to the last syllable a roulade
admirably executed, but in a low voice, and as if to
paint by a poetic expression the effusion of her
heart. The old man, suddenly struck by some
souvenir, remained on the threshold of this secret
retreat. We then heard, owing to a profound
silence, the heavy sigh which issued from his chest;
he drew off the richest of the rings with which his
skeleton fingers were loaded and placed it in Marianina's breast. The young girl commenced to
laugh, took the ring, slipped it over one of her gloved
fingers, and turned swiftly toward the salon, from
which might be heard at this moment the preludes
of a contradance. She perceived us.

"Ah! you were there!" she said, blushing.

After having looked at us as if to interrogate us,
she hastened to her partner with the careless petu-
lance of her age.

"What does it all mean?" asked of me my young
companion. "Is it her husband? I think I am
dreaming. Where am I?"

"You," I replied, "you, Madame, who are exalted, and who, comprehending so well the most imperceptible emotions, know how to cultivate in a man's heart the most delicate sentiments, without blighting them, without bruising them from the very first day; you who have pity for all the pains of the heart, and who, to the wit of a Parisienne, join a passionate soul worthy of Italy or of Spain—"

She saw clearly that my language was that of bitter irony; and, without appearing to pay any attention to it, she interrupted me:

"Oh! you make me according to your own ideas. What a singular tyranny! You would so have me that I should not be myself."

"Oh! I wish nothing," I cried, terrified at her severe attitude. "At least, is it true that you like to hear the recital of the histories of those vivid passions awakened in our hearts by the ravishing women of the South?"

"Yes. Well, then?"

"Well, then, I will come to see you to-morrow evening about nine o'clock, and I will reveal to you this mystery."

"No," she replied, with a mutinous air, "I wish to learn it immediately."

"You have not yet given me the right to obey you when you say: 'I wish.'"

"At present," she replied, with a coquetry that would drive a man to despair, "I have the greatest desire to know this secret. To-morrow I will not listen to you, perhaps—"

She smiled, and we separated, she even more proud, more forbidding, and I even more ridiculous at this moment than ever. She had the audacity to waltz with a young aide-de-camp, and I remained alternately vexed, pouting, admiring, loving and jealous.

"Till to-morrow," she said to me, near two o'clock in the morning, when she left the ball.

"I will not go," thought I, "and I abandon thee. Thou art more capricious, more fantastic a thousand times, perhaps—than my imagination."

The next evening, we were before a good fire, in an elegant little salon, seated both of us, she on a low sofa, I on a cushion, almost at her feet, and my eye under hers. The street was silent. The lamp shed a soft light. It was one of those evenings delightful to the soul, one of those moments which are never forgotten, one of those hours passed in peace and in desire,—and the charm of which is later always a subject of regret, even when we are more happy. What can efface the vivid impression of the first solicitations of love?

"Go on," she said, "I am listening."

"But I dare not commence. The adventure has some passages dangerous for the narrator. If I become enthusiastic, you will silence me."

"Speak."

"I obey."

"Ernest-Jean Sarrasine was the only son of a procurator of Franche-Comté," I resumed, after a pause. "His father had acquired with sufficient honesty

from six to eight thousand francs of income, a practitioner's fortune, which, formerly, in the provinces,
was considered colossal.   The old Maître Sarrasine,
having but one child, resolved to neglect nothing
for his education : he hoped to make of him a mag-
istrate, and to live long enough to see, in his old
days, the grandson of Mathieu Sarrasine, laborer in
the country of Saint-Dié, seated on his fleur-de-lys
and sleeping through the hearing for the greater
glory of justice; but Heaven did not reserve this joy
for the procurator.   The young Sarrasine, confided
at an early age to the Jesuits, gave proofs of an
uncommon turbulence.   He had the childhood of a
man of talent.   He would not study save as he
chose, was often in revolt, and remained sometimes
for hours plunged into confused meditation, occupied
sometimes in contemplating his comrades at their
play, sometimes in representing to himself the heroes
of Homer.   Then, when he did choose to divert
himself, he brought into his plays an extraordinary
ardor.   When a quarrel occurred between himself
and one of his comrades, it was but seldom that the
combat ended without bloodshed.   If he were the
weaker of the two, he bit.   Alternately acting or
passive, without aptitude or being too intelligent, his
singular character caused him to be feared by his
masters as much as by his comrades.   Instead of
acquiring the elements of the Greek language, he
made a drawing of the reverend father who
explained to them a passage of Thucydides; he
sketched the master of mathematics, the prefect, the

valets, the corrector, and covered all the walls with
shapeless outlines. Instead of chanting the praises
of the Lord in the church, he amused himself, during the service, with carving a bench; or, when
he had stolen a piece of wood, he sculptured some
figure of a saint. If he had no wood, nor stone, nor
crayon, he gave form to his ideas with soft bread.
Whether he was copying the figures in the paintings
which ornamented the choir, or whether he was
originating, he left always behind him gross
sketches, the licentious character of which filled
with horror the younger fathers; and the slanderers
pretended that the old Jesuits smiled over them.
Finally, if the chronicle of the college may be
believed, he was expelled for having, while waiting
his turn at the confessional on a Good Friday,
carved a large billet into the shape of Christ. The
impiety of this statue was too great not to draw
down chastisement on the artist. Had he not even
had the audacity to place on top of the tabernacle
this sufficiently cynical figure! Sarrasine came to
seek at Paris a refuge against the menaces of the
paternal malediction. Having one of those strong
wills which know no obstacles, he followed the
commands of his genius and entered the atelier of
Bouchardon. He worked throughout the day, and
in the evening begged for his livelihood. Bouchardon, surprised at the progress and at the intelligence
of the young artist, soon became aware of the poverty in which his pupil was living; he aided him,
took him into his affections and treated him as his

own child. Then, when the genius of Sarrasine had revealed itself by one of those works in which the dawning talent struggles against the effervescence of youth, the generous Bouchardon endeavored to restore him to the good graces of the old procurator. Before the authority of the celebrated sculptor the parental anger was appeased. All Besançon congratulated itself on having given birth to a future great man. In the first moments of ecstasy which his flattered vanity brought him, the avaricious practitioner enabled his son to again appear with advantage before the world. The long and laborious studies required by the art of sculpture kept for a long time in subjection the impetuous character and the wild genius of Sarrasine. Bouchardon, foreseeing the violence with which the passions would be unchained in this young soul, perhaps as vigorously constituted as that of Michael Angelo, smothered the energy under continual labors. He succeeded in maintaining within reasonable bounds the extraordinary impetuosity of Sarrasine, in forbidding him to work, in proposing some distraction when he saw him carried away by the fury of an idea or in confiding important works to him at the moment when he was about to deliver himself up to dissipation. But, upon this passionate soul, gentleness was always the most powerful of arms, and the master only assumed a great empire over his pupil when he excited his gratitude by a paternal kindness.

"At the age of twenty-two, Sarrasine was forcibly withdrawn from the salutary influence which

Bouchardon exercised over his manners and his habits. He carried off the fruits of his genius in gaining the prize in sculpture founded by the Marquis de Marigny, the brother of Madame de Pompadour, who did so much for the arts. Diderot extolled as a masterpiece the statue of Bouchardon's pupil. It was not without deep grief that the sculptor to the king saw depart for Italy a young man in whom, through principle, he had inculcated profound ignorance of the things of life. Sarrasine had been for six years of the household of Bouchardon. Fanatical in his art, as Canova was later, he rose at day-break, entered his atelier, from which he did not issue till night, and lived only with his Muse. If he went to the Comédie-Française, he was dragged there by his master. He felt himself so awkward in the house of Madame Geoffrin and in the great world in which Bouchardon endeavored to introduce him, that he preferred to remain alone, and repudiated the pleasures of this licentious epoch. He had no other mistresses than sculpture and Clotilde, one of the celebrities of the opera. But this intrigue did not last long. Sarrasine was sufficiently ugly, always badly dressed, and naturally so free, so little regular in his private life that the illustrious nymph, fearing some catastrophe, very soon returned the sculptor to the love of art. Sophie Arnould said a good thing on this subject that I have forgotten. She was astonished, I believe, that her comrade had been able to drag him away from the statues. Sarrasine departed for Italy in 1758.

During the journey, his ardent imagination took fire under a glowing sky and at the sight of the marvelous monuments with which the country of the arts is sown. He admired the statues, the frescoes, the paintings; and, full of emulation, he came to Rome a prey to the desire to inscribe his name between those of Michael Angelo and of Bouchardon; thus, during the first days, he divided his time between his work in the atelier and the examination of the works of art which abound in Rome. He had already passed two weeks in that state of ecstasy which seizes all young imaginations at the aspect of the queen of ruins, when, one evening, he entered the theatre of Argentina, before which a great crowd was gathered. He inquired the cause of this multitude and everybody answered him with two names:

" 'Zambinella!   Jomelli ! '

"He entered and took a seat in the parterre, crowded by two *abbati* notably fat; but he was fortunately placed near the stage. The curtain went up. For the first time in his life he heard that music of which Monsieur Jean-Jacques Rousseau had so eloquently praised the delights to him, during a soirée of the Baron d'Holbach. The senses of the young sculptor were, so to speak, lubricated by the accents of the sublime harmony of Jomelli. The languorous originalities of these Italian voices, skilfully commingled, plunged him into a ravishing ecstasy. He remained mute, motionless, not even feeling himself crowded by the two priests. His

soul passed into his ears and into his eyes. He
thought he listened by every one of his pores. All
at once, an outbreak of applause sufficient to bring
down the house welcomed the appearance on the
scene of the *prima donna*. She advanced coquettishly to the front of the scene and saluted the
public with an infinite grace. The lights, the enthusiasm of a whole audience, the illusion of the
scene, the attraction of her costume, which at that
period was sufficiently distinguished, all conspired
in favor of this woman. Sarrasine uttered cries of
pleasure. At that moment he was able to admire
that ideal beauty the perfections of which he had,
up to that moment, sought in vain throughout
nature, compelled to require from a model, often
ignoble, the roundness of a perfect leg; from such
another, the contours of a breast; from this one, her
white shoulders; reduced, in fact, to take the neck of
a young girl, and the hands of this woman, and the
polished knees of that infant, without ever finding
under the cold sky of Paris the rich and suave creations of antique Greece. These, La Zambinella
displayed to him all united in one figure, truly
living and delicate, those exquisite proportions of
feminine nature so ardently desired, of which a
sculptor is at once the judge the most severe and
the most enthusiastic. There was an expressive
mouth, loving eyes, skin of a dazzling whiteness.
And join to these details, which would have ravished
a painter, all the marvels of that Venus revered
and rendered by the chisel of the Greek. The

artist was never weary of admiring the inimitable grace with which the arms were joined to the chest, the bewitching roundness of the neck, the harmonious lines described by the eyebrows, by the nose; then the perfect oval of the visage, the purity of its living contour, and the effect of the heavy eyelashes, curled upward, which terminated the heavy and voluptuous eyelids. It was more than a woman, it was a *chef-d'œuvre*. There were to be found in this unhoped-for creation, love to ravish all men, and beauty worthy to satisfy a critic. Sarrasine devoured with his eyes the statue of Pygmalion, for him descended from its pedestal. When La Zambinella sang, it was a delirium. The artist grew cold; then he was conscious of a fire which sparkled suddenly in the depths of his inmost being, of that which we call the heart for want of a word! He did not applaud, he said nothing; he experienced a sensation of madness, a species of frenzy which only agitates us at that age in which desire has, I know not what, of terrible and of infernal. Sarrasine longed to spring upon the stage and to take possession of this woman. His strength, increased a hundred-fold by a moral depression impossible to explain, since these phenomena take place in a sphere inaccessible to human observation, had a tendency to project him forward with an unhappy violence. To see him, you would have taken him for a cold and stupid man. Glory, science, future, existence, crowns, everything crumbled.

" 'To be loved by her, or to die!' Such was the

judgment which Sarrasine pronounced upon himself.

"He was so completely intoxicated that he saw no longer either the theatre, or the spectators, or the actors; he heard no longer the music. Still more, no distance existed between him and La Zambinella; he possessed her, his eyes, fastened on her, took her for his own. A power almost diabolical permitted him to feel the breath of this voice, to respire the balmy powder with which her hair was impregnated, to see the details of this countenance, to count upon it the blue veins which marked the satin skin. And finally this voice, active, fresh and of a silvery tone, delicate as a thread to which the least breath of air gives a form, which it rolls and unrolls, develops and disperses, this voice attacked his soul so vividly, that he uttered more than once involuntary cries torn from him by the convulsive delights too rarely given by human passion. Presently he was obliged to leave the theatre. His trembling legs almost refused to sustain him. He was overwhelmed, weak as a nervous man who had delivered himself to some frightful anger. He had experienced so much pleasure, or perhaps he had suffered so much, that his life had flowed away from him like the water of a vase overturned by a shock. He felt within him a void, a swooning similar to those debilities which are the despair of convalescents recovering from a grave malady. A prey to an inexplicable sadness, he went and seated himself on the steps of a church.

There, his back against a column, he lost himself in a meditation confused as a dream. Passion had overwhelmed him. On his return to his lodging, he fell into one of those paroxysms of activity which reveal to us the presence of entirely new principles in our existence. A prey to this first fever of love which is connected as closely with pleasure as with sorrow; he wished to deceive his impatience and his delirium by designing La Zambinella from memory. It was a sort of material meditation. On this sheet of paper, La Zambinella was seen in that attitude, apparently calm and cold, favored by Raphaël, by Giorgione and by all the great painters. On such another, she turned her head with an appreciative delicacy, terminating a roulade, and seemed to be listening to herself. Sarrasine crayoned his mistress in all poses : he made her unveiled, seated, upright, lying, or chaste, or amorous, in realizing, thanks to the delirium of his crayon, all the capricious ideas which solicit our imagination when we think strongly of a mistress. But his furious thought went farther than his designing. He saw La Zambinella, he spoke to her, supplicated her, exhausted a thousand years of life and of happiness with her, placing her in all imaginable situations, in essaying—so to speak—the future with her. The next day, he sent his lackey to hire for the whole season a box near the stage. Then, like all young people in whom the soul is powerful, he exaggerated to himself the difficulties of his enterprise, and gave for first food to his passion the

happiness of being able to admire his mistress without obstacles. This golden age of love, during which we draw enjoyment from our own feeling and in which we find ourselves happy almost by ourselves, was not destined to endure long in the case of Sarrasine. Nevertheless, he was surprised by events while he was still under the charm of this springtime hallucination, as naive as it was voluptuous. During a week he lived a whole life, occupying his mornings with modeling the clay by the aid of which he succeeded in copying La Zambinella, despite the veils, the petticoats, the corsets and the knots of ribbon which hid her from him. In the evening, installed at an early hour in his box, alone, reclining on a sofa, he procured for himself, after the manner of a Turk intoxicated with opium, a happiness as fruitful, as prodigal as he could wish. At first, he familiarized himself gradually with the too vivid emotions which the song of his mistress occasioned him; then he subdued his eyes to see her, and finished by contemplating her without fearing the explosion of that dumb rage by which he had been animated on the first day. His passion became more profound as it became more tranquil. For the rest, the ferocious sculptor would not permit that his solitude, peopled with images, adorned with the fantasies of hope and full of happiness, should be troubled by his comrades. He loved with so much strength, and so ingenuously, that he had to submit to the innocent scruples with which we are assailed when we love for the first time. In

commencing to perceive that it would be necessary
very soon to act, to intrigue, to ask where La Zambinella lived, to know if she had a mother, an uncle,
a guardian, a family; in thinking, in short, on the
methods of seeing her, of speaking to her, he felt
his heart swell so strongly with such ambitious
ideas, that he put off all these cares till the morrow,
happy because of his physical sufferings as much as
of his intellectual pleasures."

"But," said Madame de Rochefide to me, interrupting me, "I do not see anything yet, either of
Marianina or of her little old man."

"You see nothing but him," I cried, impatient as
an author who had been compelled to spoil the effect
of his theatrical demonstration.

"For several days," I resumed after a pause,
"Sarrasine had come so faithfully to take his place
in his box, and his looks expressed so much love,
that his passion for the voice of Zambinella would
have been the news of all Paris if this adventure
had happened there; but, in Italy, Madame, at the
theatre each one is present on his own account,
with his own passions, with an interest of the heart
which excludes the spying of the lorgnettes. However, the frenzy of the sculptor was not destined to
long escape the observation of the singers and the
cantatrices. One evening, the Frenchman perceived that they were laughing at him in the side-
scenes. It would have been difficult to know to
what extremity he might not have been carried if
La Zambinella had not entered on the scene. She

threw upon Sarrasine one of those eloquent looks which often say much more than the women wish them to. This look was a complete revelation. Sarrasine was loved!

"'If it is only a caprice,' thought he, already accusing his mistress of too much ardor, 'she does not know the domination under which she is going to fall. Her caprice will endure, I hope, as long as my life.'

"At this moment, three blows lightly struck on the door of his box attracted the attention of the artist. He opened the door. An old woman entered mysteriously.

"'Young man,' said she, 'if you wish to be happy, have prudence. Wrap yourself up in a cape, pull down over your eyes a broad hat; then, about ten o'clock in the evening, place yourself in the Rue du Corso, before the Hôtel de *Spagna*.'

"'I will be there,' he replied, putting two louis in the withered hand of the duenna.

"He slipped out of his box, after having made a sign of intelligence to La Zambinella, who lowered timidly her voluptuous eyelids like a woman happy in being finally comprehended. Then he hastened home, in order to borrow from his toilet all the seductions which it could lend him. As he came out of the theatre, an unknown arrested him by the arm.

"'Take care of yourself, Seigneur Frenchman,' he said in his ear. 'It is a question of life or death. Cardinal Cicognara is her protector, and does not permit any frolics.'

"Though a demon should have opened between Sarrasine and La Zambinella the profundities of hell, in this moment he would have traversed them all with one stride.   Like the horses of the immortals, described by Homer, the love of the sculptor had passed over in the twinkling of an eye immense spaces.

"'Though death waited for me on coming out of the house, I would go still quicker,' he replied.

"'*Poverino!*' cried the unknown, as he disappeared.

"To speak of danger to a lover, is it not to sell him pleasures?   Never had Sarrasine's lackey seen his master so particular in matters of the toilet. His finest sword, a present from Bouchardon, the tie which Clotilde had given him, his gold embroidered coat, his waistcoat of silver brocade, his snuff-box, his jeweled watches, all were drawn from his coffers, and he adorned himself like a young girl who is about to present herself before her first lover.   At the appointed hour, drunk with love and boiling with hope, Sarrasine, his nose buried in his mantle, hastened to the rendezvous given by the old woman.   The duenna was waiting for him.

"'You are very late!' she said to him.   'Come.'

"She led the Frenchman through a number of little streets and stopped before a palace of a sufficiently handsome appearance.   She knocked, the door opened.   She conducted Sarrasine through a labyrinth of staircases, of galleries, and of apartments which were only lighted by the uncertain

16

gleams of the moon, and arrived presently at a door, between the wings of which escaped a bright light, through which issued the joyful sounds of several voices. Suddenly, Sarrasine was dazzled when, on a word from the old woman, he was admitted into this mysterious apartment and found himself in a salon as brilliantly lighted as it was sumptuously furnished, in the middle of which was placed a well-served table, charged with doubly-sacred bottles, with laughing flasks, the ruby facets of which sparkled in the light. He recognized the singers and the cantatrices of the theatre, mingled with charming women, all of them ready to commence an artistes' orgie which waited only for him. Sarrasine suppressed a movement of displeasure, and put on a good countenance. He had hoped for a chamber dimly lit, his mistress over a brazier, some jealous one within two steps, death and love, confidences exchanged in an undertone, heart-to-heart, perilous kisses, and the faces so close that the hair of La Zambinella should caress his forehead charged with desire, burning with happiness.

" *'Vive la folie!'* he cried.—'*Signori e belle donne,* you will permit me to take my revenge later, and to testify to you my gratitude for the manner in which you welcome a poor sculptor.'

"After having received the compliments, sufficiently hearty, of most of the persons present, whom he knew by sight, he endeavored to approach the couch on which La Zambinella was nonchalantly reclining. Oh! how his heart beat when he

perceived a delicate foot, shod in one of those slippers
which, permit me to say it, Madame, gave formerly
to the women's feet an expression so coquettish, so
voluptuous, that I do not know how the men were
able to resist. The white stockings, well fitting and
with green clocks, the short skirts, the pointed slippers and the high heels of the reign of Louis XV.
have perhaps contributed a little to demoralize
Europe and the clergy."

"A little," said the marchioness. "You have not,
then, read anything?"

"La Zambinella," I resumed, smiling, "had
saucily crossed her legs, swinging the one which was
on top, the attitude of a duchess, which suited very
well her species of capricious beauty, full of a certain engaging softness. She had discarded her
theatre costume, and wore a bodice which outlined
a slender figure and gave style to paniers and a
skirt of satin embroidered with blue flowers. Her
bust, whose treasures were hidden by lace with
a luxurious coquetry, shone with whiteness. Her
hair was dressed almost like that of Madame du
Barry, her face, although overshadowed by a large
bonnet, appeared none the less delicate, and the
powder suited her well. To see her thus, was to
adore her. She smiled graciously on the sculptor.
Sarrasine, quite discontented at being able to speak
to her only before witnesses, seated himself politely
near her, and conversed with her of music, praising
her extraordinary talent; but his voice trembled
with love, with fear and with hope.

" 'What are you afraid of?' Vitagliani, the most celebrated singer of the troupe, asked him. 'Go ahead; you have not a single rival to fear here.'

"After having spoken, the tenor smiled silently. The lips of all the guests repeated this smile, the expression of which had a hidden malice probably unperceived by a lover. The publicity of his love was like a dagger stroke which Sarrasine had suddenly received in his heart. Although endowed with a certain force of character, and though certainly no circumstances could master the violence of his passion, he had not yet, perhaps, reflected that Zambinella was almost a courtesan, and that he could not have in one being the pure delights which render the love of a young girl so delicious and the tempestuous transports by which a woman of the theatre causes to be purchased her perilous possession. He reflected and resigned himself. The supper was served. Sarrasine and La Zambinella placed themselves without ceremony by the side of each other. During half of the festival the artistes preserved some decorum, and the sculptor could converse with the cantatrice. He found in her wit and finesse; but she was of a surprising ignorance, and showed herself to be feeble and superstitious. The delicacy of her organs was reproduced in her intellectual apprehension. When Vitagliani uncorked the first bottle of champagne, Sarrasine read in the eyes of his neighbor a sufficiently lively fear of the little explosion produced by the release of the gas. The involuntary shudder of this feminine

organization was interpreted by the amorous artist
as the indication of an excessive sensibility. This
weakness charmed the Frenchman. There is so
much protection in the love of a man!

" 'You will dispose of my power as of a shield!'

"Is not this phrase written at the bottom of all
the declarations of love? Sarrasine, too passionate
to retail gallantries to the beautiful Italian, was,
like all lovers, alternately grave, laughing, or
thoughtful. Although he apppeared to listen to the
guests, he did not hear a word of what they said,
so much did he give himself up to the pleasure of
finding himself near her, of touching her hand, of
serving her. He was swimming in a secret joy.
Notwithstanding the eloquence of a few mutual
glances, he was astonished at the reserve which La
Zambinella maintained with him. She had indeed
been the first to commence to press his foot and to
incite him with the malice of a woman free and
amorous; but suddenly she enveloped herself in the
modesty of a young girl after having heard Sarrasine relate an incident which depicted the excessive
violence of his character. When the supper became
an orgie, the guests began to sing, inspired by the
peralta and the pedro-ximénès. There were ravishing duets, airs of Calabria, Spanish seguidillas,
Neapolitan canzonettes. Intoxication was in all
eyes, in the music, in the hearts and in the voices.
There broke out all at once an enchanting vivacity,
a cordial unreservedness, an Italian good nature,
of which nothing can give an idea to those who

know only the assemblies of Paris, the routs of
London, or the circles of Vienna. Jests and words
of love crossed each other, like balls in a battle,
through the laughter, the impieties, the invocations
to the Holy Virgin or *al Bambino.*   A man lay
down on a sofa and went to sleep.   A young girl
listened to a declaration without knowing that she
was spilling sherry on the table-cloth.   In the middle of this disorder, La Zambinella, as if struck
with terror, remained thoughtful.   She refused to
drink, ate perhaps a little too much; but gormandiz-
ing is, it is said, a grace in women.   While admiring the modesty of his mistress, Sarrasine was
making serious reflections upon the future.

"'She doubtless wishes to be married,' said he to
himself.

"Then he gave himself up to the delights of this
marriage.   His entire life seemed to him to be not
long enough to exhaust the spring of happiness
which he found in the bottom of his soul.   Vitagliani, his neighbor, filled his glass so often that,
towards three o'clock in the morning, without being
completely drunken, Sarrasine found himself unable
to resist his delirium.   In a moment of impetuosity
he seized and carried off this woman, taking refuge
in a sort of boudoir which communicated with the
salon, and to the door of which he had more than
once turned his eyes.   The Italian was armed with
a poniard.

"'If you approach,' she said, 'I shall be forced to
plunge this weapon in your heart.   Go! You would

despise me. I have conceived too much respect for your character to deliver myself thus. I do not wish to destroy the sentiment which you have for me.'

"'Ah! ah!' said Sarrasine, 'it is a bad way to extinguish a passion by exciting it. Are you already corrupted to such a point that, old in heart, you would act like a young courtesan, who sharpens the emotions of which she makes a commerce?'

"'But it is Friday to-day,' she replied, frightened at the violence of the Frenchman.

"Sarrasine, who was not devout, commenced to laugh. La Zambinella leaped like a young roebuck and fled into the supper room. When Sarrasine appeared running after her, he was welcomed by a laughter truly infernal. He saw La Zambinella fainting on a sofa. She was pale and as if exhausted by the extraordinary effort which she had just made. Although Sarrasine knew very little Italian, he heard his mistress saying in a low voice to Vitagliani:

"'But he will kill me!'

"This strange scene had the effect of quite confusing the sculptor. His reason returned to him. He remained at first motionless; then he recovered his speech, seated himself near his mistress and protested his respect for her. He found strength to transform his passion in proffering to this woman the most exalted discourse; and, to paint his love, he displayed the treasures of that magic eloquence, serviceable interpreter which women rarely refuse to believe. At the moment when the first gleams

of morning came to surprise the guests, a woman proposed to go to Frascati. Everybody welcomed with lively acclamations the idea of passing the day at the Villa Ludovisi. Vitagliani went down to hire some coaches. Sarrasine had the happiness of accompanying La Zambinella in a phaëton. Once out of Rome, the gayety, suppressed for a moment by the combats which each one had waged with sleep, suddenly reawakened. Men and women, all appeared accustomed to this strange life, to these continued pleasures, to this enthusiasm of the artiste which makes of life a perpetual festival, in which one laughs without any after-thought. The companion of the sculptor was the only one who appeared depressed.

" 'Are you unwell ?' said Sarrasine to her. 'Would you rather return to your own house ?'

" 'I am not strong enough to support all these excesses,' she replied. 'I am obliged to take great care of myself; but, by your side, I feel so well! Without you, I would not have stayed for that supper; a wasted night makes me lose all my freshness.'

" 'You are so delicate!' resumed Sarrasine, contemplating the refined features of this charming creature.

" 'The orgies ruin my voice.'

" 'Now that we are alone,' cried the artist, 'and that you have no longer to fear the effervescence of my passion, say to me that you love me.'

" 'Wherefore ?' she replied; 'for what purpose ? I

seem to you pretty. But you are French, and your feeling will pass away. Oh! you would not love me as I would like to be loved.'

" 'How?'

" 'Without any purpose of vulgar passion, purely. I abhor men still more perhaps than I hate women. I have need to take refuge in friendship. The world is a desert for me. I am an accursed creature, condemned to comprehend happiness, to feel it, to desire it, and, like so many others, obliged to see it flee away from me every hour. Remember, seigneur, that I would not have deceived you. I forbid you to love me. I can be a devoted friend for you, for I admire your strength and your character. I have need of a brother, of a protector. Be all that for me, but nothing more.'

" 'Not love you!' cried Sarrasine; 'but, dear angel, thou art my life, my happiness!'

" 'If I said one word, you would repulse me with horror.'

" 'Coquette! nothing can frighten me. Say to me that thou wilt cost me my future, that in two months I shall die, that I shall be damned for only having embraced thee—'

"He embraced her notwithstanding the efforts which La Zambinella made to avoid this passionate kiss.

" 'Say to me that thou art a demon, that thou wilt require my fortune, my name, all my celebrity! Wilt thou that I should not be a sculptor? Speak.'

" 'If I were not a woman?' asked La Zambinella, timidly, in a silvery and soft voice.

" 'What a fine pleasantry!' cried Sarrasine. 'Thinkest thou to deceive the eye of an artist? Have I not, for the last ten days, devoured, scrutinized, admired thy perfections? Only a woman could have this round and soft arm, these elegant contours. Ah! thou desirest compliments!'

"She smiled sadly, and said in a murmuring voice: " 'Fatal beauty!'

"She lifted her eyes to Heaven. At that moment her look had an unnamable expression of horror so powerful, so vivid, that Sarrasine shuddered at it.

" 'Seigneur Frenchman,' she resumed, 'forget forever an instant of madness. I esteem you; but, as to love, do not ask it of me; this feeling is smothered in my heart. I have no heart!' she cried, weeping. 'The theatre on which you have seen me, that applause, that music, that glory, to which I have been condemned, that is my life; I have no other. Within a few hours, you will no longer see me with the same eyes, the woman whom you love will be dead.'

"The sculptor did not reply. He was a prey to a dumb rage which oppressed his heart. He could only look at this extraordinary woman with ardent eyes which burned. This voice so full of weakness, the attitude, the manner, and the gestures of Zambinella, so expressive of sadness, of melancholy, and of discouragement, reawakened in his soul all the wealth of passion. Each word was another

goad. At that moment they arrived at Frascati. When the artist offered his arm to his mistress to help her to descend, he felt her shuddering all over.

"'What is the matter with you? You will cause me to die,' he cried, in seeing her turn pale, 'if you should have the least sorrow of which I am the cause, even innocently.'

"'A snake!', she said, indicating an adder which was sliding along the bottom of a ditch. 'I am afraid of those odious beasts.'

"Sarrasine crushed the head of the adder with his heel.

"'How can you have so much courage?' exclaimed La Zambinella, looking with a visible terror at the dead reptile.

"'Well,' said the artist, smiling, 'would you dare to pretend that you are not a woman?'

"They rejoined their companions and walked about in the woods of the Villa Ludovisi, which was then the property of Cardinal Cicognara. This morning passed away too quickly for the amorous sculptor, but it was filled with a crowd of incidents which revealed to him the coquetry, the weakness, the prettiness and delicacy of this soul soft and without energy. It was all the woman, with her sudden fears, her unreasonable caprices, her instinctive troubles, her audacities without cause, her bravadoes and her delicious nicety of sentiment. At one time, straying out into the country, the little company of joyful singers saw at a distance some men armed to the teeth and whose costume was in

no ways reassuring. At the exclamation: 'See!
the brigands!' each one hurried his steps to seek
refuge in the enclosure of the cardinal's villa. At
that critical moment Sarrasine perceived by the
pallor of La Zambinella that she no longer had
strength to walk; he took her in his arms and carried her, running for some distance. When he was
within a short distance of a neighboring vineyard,
he set his mistress on her feet again.

"'Explain to me,' he said to her, 'how this extreme weakness, which, in any other woman, would
displease me, would seem odious, and the least proof
of which would almost suffice to extinguish my
love, pleases me in you, charms me?—Oh, how I
love you!' he resumed. 'All your defects, your ter-
rors, your littlenesses, add an indescribable grace
to your soul. I feel that I should detest a strong
woman, a Sappho, courageous, full of energy, of
passion. O! frail and soft creature! how couldst
thou be otherwise? That voice of an angel, that
delicate voice, would be a contradiction if it issued
from any other body than thine.'

"'I cannot,' she said, 'give you any hope. Cease
to speak to me thus, for you are mocked. It is impossible for me to forbid you the entrance to the
theatre; but, if you love me or if you are wise, you
will come there no more. Listen, Monsieur,—' she
said, in a grave voice.

"'Oh! be silent,' said the intoxicated artist.
'Obstacles only increase the love in my heart.'

"La Zambinella remained in a graceful and

modest attitude; but she was silent, as if a terrible thought had revealed to her some misfortune. When it was time for them to return to Rome, she took her place in a four-seated berlin, and ordered the sculptor, with an imperiously cruel air, to return alone in the phaëton. On the road, Sarrasine resolved to carry off La Zambinella. He passed the whole day in forming plans, each one more extravagant than the other. At nightfall, as he left his house to inquire of someone the situation of the palace inhabited by his mistress, he encountered one of his comrades on the threshold of the door.

" 'My dear fellow,' said the latter to him, 'I am requested by our ambassador to invite you to come to his house this evening. He is giving a magnificent concert, and, when you know that Zambinella will be there—'

" 'Zambinella!' cried Sarrasine, in a delirium at this name; 'I am crazy for her!'

" 'You are like all the rest of the world,' replied his comrade.

" 'But, if you are my friends, you, Vien, Lauterbourg, and Allegrain, you will lend me your assistance for a fine stroke after the fête?' asked Sarrasine.

" 'There is not some cardinal to be killed?— some—?'

" 'No, no,' said Sarrasine, 'I ask nothing of you which honest people cannot do.'

"In a short time, the sculptor had arranged everything for the success of his enterprise. He was one of the last to arrive at the ambassador's, but he

came in a traveling carriage drawn by vigorous
horses driven by one of the most enterprising *vet-
turini* of Rome. The palace of the ambassador was
crowded; it was not without difficulty that the
sculptor, unknown to all the domestics, reached the
salon in which at that moment Zambinella was
singing.

" 'It is doubtless in consideration of the cardinals,
the bishops and the abbés who are here,' asked Sarrasine, 'that *she* is dressed like a man, that *she* has
her hair in a bag and frizzled and wears a sword?'

" 'She! What she?' replied the old seigneur to
whom Sarrasine spoke.

" 'La Zambinella.'

" 'La Zambinella!' replied the Roman prince. 'Of
what are you talking? Where do you come from?
Has there ever been a woman on the stage in the
theatres of Rome? And do you not know by what
kind of creatures the female parts are filled in the
States of the Pope? It is I, Monsieur, who gave
Zambinella his voice. I have paid everything for
that scamp, even his singing-master. Well, he has
so little gratitude for the service which I have rendered him, that he is never willing to set foot inside
my door. And yet, if he makes his fortune, he will
owe it to me entirely.'

"The Prince Chigi could certainly have spoken a
long time, Sarrasine did not hear him. A frightful
truth had penetrated his soul. He was struck as if
by a thunderbolt. He remained motionless, his eyes
fastened on this dubious singer. His flaming regard

had a sort of magnetic influence on Zambinella, for
the *musico* finally turned his eyes toward Sarrasine,
and then his celestial voice faltered. He trembled!
An involuntary murmur escaped the audience,
which he held spell-bound by his lips, and completed
his trouble; he discontinued his air and sat down.
The Cardinal Cicognara, who had seen out of the
corner of his eye the direction of the glance of his
protégé, perceived the Frenchman; he leaned over
toward one of his ecclesiastical aides-de-camp, and
seemed to demand the name of the sculptor.   When
he had obtained the desired response, he looked
very attentively at the artist and gave his order
to an abbé, who disappeared rapidly.   However, Zambinella, having recovered himself, recommenced the piece which he had interrupted so
capriciously; but he executed it badly, and refused,
notwithstanding all the insistence with which he
was surrounded, to sing any more.   This was the
first time that he exercised this capricious tyranny
which, later, rendered him not less celebrated than
his talent and his immense fortune, due, it was
said, not less to his voice than to his beauty.

" 'It is a woman,' said Sarrasine, thinking himself alone.   'There is underneath all this some
secret intrigue.   The Cardinal Cicognara deceives
the Pope and the whole city of Rome!'

"Whereupon, the sculptor left the salon, reassem-
bled his friends and ambuscaded them in the court-
yard of the palace.   When Zambinella was assured
of the departure of Sarrasine, he seemed to recover

some tranquillity. Toward midnight, after having
wandered through the salon like a man who is seeking an enemy, the *musico* left the assembly. At the
moment when he passed the door of the palace, he
was adroitly seized by men who gagged him with a
handkerchief and put him into the carriage hired by
Sarrasine. Frozen with horror, Zambinella remained in a corner without daring to make a movement. He saw before him the terrible figure of the
artist, who preserved the silence of death. The
journey was but short. Zambinella, carried up by
Sarrasine, soon found himself in an atelier, sombre
and bare. The singer, half dead, remained in a
chair, without daring to look at the statue of a
woman, in which he had recognized his own features. He did not offer a word, but his teeth chat-
tered; he was paralyzed with fear. Sarrasine
walked up and down with great strides. Suddenly
he stopped before Zambinella.

" 'Tell me the truth,' he demanded, in a dull and
changed voice. 'Thou art a woman? The Cardinal Cicognara—'

"Zambinella fell on his knees, and replied only by
bowing his head.

" 'Ah! thou art a woman,' cried the artist, in delirium; 'for even a—'

"He did not finish.

" 'No,' he resumed, *'he* would not have such
baseness.'

" 'Ah! do not kill me!' cried Zambinella, melt-
ing into tears. 'I only consented to deceive you

in order to please my comrades, who wished to laugh.'

" 'To laugh!' replied the sculptor, in a voice which had an infernal explosion. 'To laugh! to laugh! Thou hast dared to play with a man's passion, thou?'

" 'Oh, mercy!' replied Zambinella.

" 'I should put thee to death!' cried Sarrasine, drawing his sword with a violent movement. 'But,' he resumed, with a cold disdain, 'in searching all thy being with this blade, would I find in it a single sentiment to extinguish, one vengeance to satisfy? Thou art nothing. Man or woman, I would kill thee! but—'

"Sarrasine made a gesture of disgust which obliged him to turn his head, and then he looked at the statue.

" 'And that is an illusion!' he cried.

"Then, turning toward Zambinella:

" 'A woman's heart would be for me an asylum, a country. Hast thou sisters who resemble thee? No. Well, then, die!—But no, thou shalt live. To leave thee alive, is it not to devote thee to something worse than death? It is not my blood nor my existence that I regret, but the future and my heart's fortune. Thy debilitated hand has overthrown my happiness. What hope can I ravish from thee for all those which thou hast blighted? Thou hast dragged me down even to thy level. *To love, to be loved!* are henceforth words empty of meaning for me, as for thee. Without ceasing I

17

shall think of this imaginary woman in seeing a real woman.'

"He indicated the statue with a gesture of despair.

" 'I shall always have in memory a celestial harpy who will come to bury its claws in all my manhood sentiments, and who will stamp all other women with the seal of imperfection. Monster! thou who canst give life to nothing, thou hast unpeopled the earth of all its women.'

"Sarrasine seated himself in front of the terrified singer. Two great tears issued from his dry eyes, rolled down his manly cheeks and fell to the floor,— two tears of rage, two tears bitter and burning.

" 'No more love! I am dead to all pleasure, to all human emotions.'

"With these words, he seized a hammer and threw it at the statue with such extravagant force that he missed it. He thought he had destroyed this monument of his folly, and he then grasped his sword and brandished it to kill the singer. Zambinella uttered piercing cries. At this moment, three men entered, and the sculptor fell suddenly, pierced with three stiletto thrusts.

" 'From the Cardinal Cicognara,' said one of them.

" 'It is a good turn worthy of a Christian,' replied the Frenchman, as he expired.

"These sombre emissaries informed Zambinella of the uneasiness of his protector, who was waiting at the door, in a closed carriage, in order to carry him away as soon as he should be rescued."

FACINO CANE

FACINO CANE

*

I lived at that time in a little street which you
doubtless know, the Rue de Lesdiguiéres: it commences at the Rue Saint-Antoine, opposite a fountain near to the Place de la Bastille, and comes out
on the Rue de la Cerisaie. Love of science had
lodged me in a garret, where I worked during the
night, and I spent the day in a neighboring library,
that of MONSIEUR. I lived frugally, I had accepted all the conditions of the monastic life, so necessary
to workers. When the weather was fine, I permitted myself rarely to take a walk on the Boulevard Bourdon. One passion only drew me out of
my studious habits; but was not this also study? I
was interested in observing the manners and customs of the faubourg, its inhabitants and their characters. As poorly dressed as the workmen
themselves, indifferent to the proprieties, I did not
put them on their guard against me; I was able to
mingle with them, to see them concluding their bar-
gains, and quarreling amongst themselves at the
hour when they left their work. In me, the faculty
of observation had already become intuitive, it penetrated the soul without neglecting the body; or,

rather, it seized so promptly the exterior details, that it immediately went beyond them; it gave me the faculty of living the life of the individual on whom it was directed, in permitting me to substitute myself for him as the dervish of the *Thousand and One Nights* assumed the body and the soul of those persons over whom he pronounced certain words.

When, between eleven o'clock and midnight, I encountered a laborer and his wife returning together from the Ambigu-Comique, I amused myself by following them from the Boulevard du Pont-aux-Choux to the Boulevard Beaumarchais. These honest people talked at first of the piece which they had just seen; then they passed insensibly to their own affairs; the mother dragged her child along by the hand, without hearing either its complaints or its questions; the couple counted the money which would be paid to them the next day, they expended it in twenty different ways. Then there would be household details, lamentations over the excessive price of potatoes, or on the length of the winter and the dearness of fuel, energetic observations on the sum due to the baker; finally, discussions which became venomous, and in which each of them displayed his or her character in picturesque words. In hearing these poor folk, I was able to assume their life, I felt their rags on my back, I walked with my feet in their worn shoes; their desires, their needs, all passed into my soul, or my soul passed into theirs. It was the dream of a waking man. I grew

indignant, with them, at the overseers of the work-shops who tyrannized over them, or against the bad arrangements which made them return several times for their money. To quit one's daily habits, to become a being outside of yourself by the intoxications of the moral faculties, and to play this game at will, such was my distraction. To whom did I owe this gift? Is it a second sight? is it one of those qualities the abuse of which leads to madness? I had never sought for the causes of this power; I possess it and make use of it, that is all. Know only that, since that time, I have decomposed the elements of that heterogeneous mass called the people, that I have analyzed it in such a manner as to be able to value its good or its evil qualities. I knew already of what utility this faubourg could be made, this seminary of revolutions which encloses heroes, inventors, knowing practitioners, cheats, blackguards, virtues and vices all crowded together by poverty, smothered by necessity, drowned in wine, worn out by strong liquors. You could not possibly imagine how many lost adventures, how many forgotten dramas there are in this city of sorrow! How many horrible and beautiful things! Imagination will never discover the full truth which is hidden there and which no one can set out to discover; it is necessary to descend too low to find these admirable scenes, tragic or comic, master-pieces given birth to by chance. I do not know how I have so long kept untold the story which I am about to relate to you; it is one of those curious recitals

left in the sack from which memory draws them
capriciously like the numbers of the lottery: I have
many others quite as singular as this one, equally
hidden; but they will have their turn, believe me.

One day, my housekeeper, the wife of a workman, came to ask me to honor with my presence
the wedding of one of her sisters.   In order that you
may comprehend what this wedding could be, it is
necessary to tell you that I gave forty sous a month
to this poor creature, who came every morning to
make my bed, clean my shoes, brush my clothes,
sweep the chamber and prepare my déjeuner; the
rest of her time she spent in turning the handle of a
machine, and earned by this hard trade ten sous a
day.   Her husband, a cabinet-maker, earned four
francs.   But, as this household had three children,
it could with difficulty manage honestly to have
bread to eat.   I have never encountered more solid
honesty than that of this man and this woman.
Whenever I left the quarter, during five years, the
Mère Vaillant came to congratulate me on my fête,
bringing me a bouquet and some oranges, she who
never had ten sous of savings.   Poverty had brought
us close together.   I was never able to give her anything more than ten francs, often borrowed for this
purpose.   This may explain my promise to go to the
wedding, I counted on being able to envelop myself
in the happiness of these poor people.

The festival, the ball, all took place in the establishment of a wine merchant in the Rue de Charen-
ton, on the first floor, in a large room lit by lamps

with tin reflectors, ornamented with a dirty wall-
paper up to the height of the tables, and along the
walls of which there were wooden benches. In this
chamber, eighty persons in their best clothes, set
off with bouquets and ribbons, all of them animated
by the spirit of that lively quarter, la Courtille,
with flushed faces, danced as if the world were about
to end. The newly-married couple embraced each
other to the general satisfaction, and there were
the "Eh! eh!" the "Ah! ah!" very facetious, but
really less indecent than are the timid eye-glances
of well-bred young girls. All this company expressed a brutal contentment which had in it something inexpressibly contagious.

But neither the physiognomies of this assembly,
nor the wedding, nor anything of this company has
any relation to my story. Remember only the odd-
ness of the scene. Figure to yourself the ignoble
shop painted in red, smell the odor of the wine,
listen to the roarings of this joy, place yourself in
this faubourg, in the middle of these workpeople,
of these old men, of these poor women given over to
the pleasures of a night!

The orchestra was composed of three blind men
from the hospital of the Quinze-Vingts,—the first
was a violin, the second a clarionet, and the third a
flageolet. All three were paid a lump sum of seven
francs for the night. For that price, certainly,
they gave neither Rossini nor Beethoven; they
played what they would and what they could; no
one addressed them any reproaches, a charming

delicacy! Their music attacked the tympanum so
roughly, that after having looked at the general
assembly, I directed my observation to this blind
trio, and was immediately disposed to be indulgent
in recognizing their uniform. These artists were
placed in the embrasure of a window; to distinguish
their countenances it was necessary to be near
them.—I did not place myself there immediately,
but when I approached them, I do not know why,
everything was said, the wedding and its music
disappeared, my curiosity was excited to the highest
degree, for my soul passed into the body of the clarionet player. The violin and the flageolet had both
of them commonplace faces, the well-known countenance of the blind, full of intenseness, attentive
and grave; but that of the clarionet was one of
those phenomena which arrest suddenly the artist
and the philosopher.

Imagine to yourself the plaster mask of Dante, lit
up by the red light of the argand lamp, and sur-
mounted by a forest of hair of a silvery whiteness.
The bitter and dolorous expression of this magnificent head was increased by the blindness, for the
extinguished eyes were restored to life by thought;
it revealed itself in them like a burning light, produced by an unique and incessant desire, vigorously
inscribed on the arched forehead which was traversed by wrinkles like the courses on an old wall.
This old man blew in his instrument at hazard, without paying the least attention to the measure or the
air, his fingers were raised or lowered, manipulating

the old keys, mechanically; he did not give himself any trouble to make what is called in the language
of the orchestra the *canards*, the dancers did not perceive it any more than did the two acolytes of my
Italian; for I wished that he should be an Italian, and
he was an Italian. Something of grand and the des-
potic was to be encountered in this old Homer who
guarded in himself an Odyssey condemned to forgetfulness. It was a grandeur so real, that it
triumphed still over his abjection; it was a despotism so vivid that it dominated poverty. Not one of
the violent passions which conduct man to good as
to evil, which make of him a convict or a hero, was
lacking to this visage nobly modeled, of an Italian
lividness, shaded by grayish brows which projected
their shadows over profound cavities in which one
feared to see reappear the light of thought, as one
fears to see come to the mouth of a cavern brigands
armed with torches and poniards. There existed a
lion in that cage of flesh, a lion whose rage had
been uselessly exhausted against the iron of his barriers. The fire of despair was extinct in its cinders,
the lava had grown cold; but the furrows, the over-
turnings, a little smoke, still bore witness to the
violence of the eruption, the ravages of flame.
These ideas, called up by the aspect of this man,
were as heated in my soul as they were cold on his
countenance.

Between each contradance the violin and the
flageolet, seriously occupied with their glasses and
their bottle, hung their instruments to certain

buttons of their rusty coats, put out their hands to a little table placed in the embrasure of a window in which was their supply, and offered each time to the Italian a full glass, which he could not take himself, for the table was behind his chair; each time the clarionet thanked them by a friendly sign of the head.   Their movements were performed with that precision which is always so surprising among the blind of the Quinze-Vingts, and which makes it seem as though they saw.   I approached the three blind men to listen to them, but when I was near them, they studied me, failing to recognize doubtless one of the working-class, and kept silent.

"From what country are you, you who play the clarionet?"

"From Venice," replied the blind man, with a slight Italian accent.

"Were you born blind, or did you lose your sight by—?"

"By accident," he replied quickly, "a cursed *gutta serena.*"

"Venice is a beautiful city; I have always desired to go there."

The countenance of the old man became animated, his wrinkles were agitated, he was violently moved.

"If I were to go there with you, you would not lose your time," he said to me.

"Do not speak to him of Venice," said the violin to me, "or our Doge will go off again; all the more so that he already has put two bottles away, the prince!"

"Come, forward march, Père Canard," said the flageolet.

All three of them commenced to play; but, during the time which they took to execute the four parts of the contradance, the Venetian scented me; he guessed at the excessive interest which I took in him. His physiognomy lost its cold expression of sadness; I do not know what hope lit up his features, spread like a blue flame in his wrinkles; he smiled and wiped his forehead, that audacious and terrible forehead; in short, he became gay like a man who mounts his hobby-horse.

"How old are you?" I asked him.

"Eighty-two years."

"How long have you been blind?"

"For nearly fifty years," he replied, with an accent which revealed that his regrets were not only for the loss of his sight, but for some great power of which he had been deprived.

"Why do they, then, call you the Doge?" I asked him.

"Ah! a farce," said he: "I am a patrician of Venice, and I might have been Doge as well as any other."

"What is your name, then?"

"Here," he said to me, "the Père Canet. My name could never be inscribed in any other way on the registers; but, in Italian, it is *Marco Facino Cane, principe de Varese*."

"How! you are descended from the famous condottiere, Facino Cane, whose conquests passed to the Duke of Milan?"

"*E vero*," said he. "In those times, in order not
to be killed by the Visconti, the son of Cane took
refuge in Venice and caused his name to be inscribed on the Golden Book. But there is now no
longer any Cane nor any Book!"

And he made a terrifying gesture of extinguished patriotism and of disgust for all things
human.

"But, if you were Senator of Venice, you should
be rich; how have you been able to lose all your fortune?"

At this question, he raised his head toward me as
if to contemplate me with a movement truly tragic,
and replied to me:

"In misfortunes!"

He no longer cared to drink; he refused by a gesture a glass of wine which the old flageolet offered
him at this moment, then he lowered his head.
These details were not of a nature to extinguish
my curiosity. During the contradance which was
played by these three machines, I contemplated the
noble old Venetian with those sentiments which
take possession of a young man of twenty. I saw
Venice and the Adriatic, I saw it in ruins in this
ruined figure. I walked about in this city so dear
to its inhabitants; I went from the Rialto to the
Grand Canal, from the quay of the Schiavoni to the
Lido, I returned to its cathedral, so originally sublime, I looked at the windows of the Casa d'Oro,
the ornaments of each of which are different; I contemplated its old palaces so rich in marble, in short

all those marvels with which he who is wise sympathizes all the more that he colors them at his own will, and does not deprive his dreams of their poetry by the spectacle of reality.   I followed up the course of the life of this scion of the greatest of the condottieri, searching in it the traces of his misfortunes and the causes of that profound degradation, physical and moral, which rendered finer still the sparks of grandeur and of nobility reanimated in this moment.   Our thoughts were doubtless reciprocal, for I believe that blindness renders the intellectual communications much more rapid in prohibiting the attention from scattering itself on exterior objects. The proof of our sympathy was not long in manifesting itself.   Facino Cane ceased to play, rose, came to me and said to me "Let us go!" which produced on me the effect of an electric shock.   I gave him my arm and we went out.

When we were in the street, he said to me:

"Will you take me to Venice, conduct me there? Will you have faith in me?   You will be richer than are the ten richest houses of Amsterdam or of London, richer than the Rothschilds; in short, rich as the *Thousand and One Nights.*"

I thought that this man was mad; but he had in his voice a power which I obeyed.   I let him conduct me and he led me toward the ditches of the Bastille as if he had eyes.   He seated himself on a stone, in a very solitary locality, where since has been built the bridge by which the Canal Saint-Martin communicates with the Seine.   I placed

18

myself on another stone before this old man, whose white hair shone like silver threads in the light of the moon. The silence which was scarcely troubled by the stormy noise of the boulevard which reached us, the purity of the night, everything, contributed to render this scene truly fantastic.

"You speak of millions to a young man, and you think that he would hesitate to endure a thousand evils to possess them! Are you not mocking me?"

"May I die unconfessed," he said to me, violently, "if that which I am going to say to you is not true. I was twenty years of age, as you are at this moment. I was rich, I was handsome, I was noble; I commenced by the first of follies, love. I have loved as one no longer loves, even to the point of putting myself in a chest and risking being poniarded without having received anything but the promise of a kiss. To die for *her* seemed to me a whole life. In 1760, I fell in love with a Vendramini, a woman of eighteen, married to a Sagredo, one of the richest senators, a man of thirty, madly loving his wife. My mistress and I, we were as innocent as two cherubim, when the *sposo* surprised us talking love; I was without arms, he was armed, but he missed me; I sprang upon him, I strangled him with my two hands, twisting his neck like that of a pullet. I wished to depart with Bianca; she would not follow me. Such are women! I went away alone. I was condemned, my goods were sequestered for the benefit of my heirs; but I had carried off my diamonds, five pictures by Titian rolled up, and all

my gold. I went to Milan, where I was not disturbed: my affair did not interest the state.—A little observation before continuing," he said after a pause. "Whether the fancies of a woman have any influence or not on her child while she carries it or when she conceives it, it is certain that my mother had a passion for gold during her pregnancy. I have for gold a monomania, the satisfaction of which is so necessary to my life that, in all the situations in which I have found myself, I have never been without gold about me; I handle gold constantly; when young I always wore jewels and I had always about me two or three hundred ducats."

In saying these words, he drew two ducats from his pocket and showed them to me.

"I am sensitive to gold. Although blind, I stop before the jewelers' windows. This passion ruined me; I have become a gambler to play with gold. I was not a cheat; I was cheated, I was ruined. When I no longer had any fortune, I passionately longed to see Bianca again,—I returned secretly to Venice, I found her again; I was happy during six months, hidden by her, nourished by her. I thought deliciously to finish my life thus. She was sought by the Proveditor; he suspected a rival; in Italy, they smell them,—he spied on us, he surprised us in bed, the coward! Judge how fierce was our struggle: I did not kill him, I wounded him grievously. This adventure destroyed my happiness. Since that day, I have never found again a Bianca. I have had great pleasures, I have lived at the

Court of Louis XV., among the most celebrated
women; nowhere have I found the qualities, the
graces, the love of my dear Venetian. The Proveditor had his servants; he summoned them, the
palace was surrounded, invaded; I defended myself
so as to be able to die under the eye of Bianca, who
aided me in killing the Proveditor. This woman
had once not been willing to fly with me; but, after
six months of happiness, she wished to die with me,
and did receive several strokes. Taken in a great
cloak which was thrown over me, I was rolled
in it, carried to a gondola and transported to a
dungeon in the Wells. I was twenty-two years
of age; I held on so well to a fragment of my
sword that, to have taken it, it would have been
necessary to cut off my hand. By a singular chance,
or rather by a wise precaution, I hid this piece of
steel in a corner, as though it might be of use to
me. I was cared for. None of my wounds were
mortal. At twenty-two, one recovers from anything. As I was doomed to die decapitated, I pretended illness in order to gain time. I believed
myself in a dungeon near the canal; my project was
to escape by digging a hole through the wall and
swimming the canal, at the risk of drowning.

"These were the reasonings on which my hope
was founded.

"Every time that the jailer brought me food, I
read the indications written on the walls, such as
'To the Palace,' 'To the Canal,' 'To the Crypts,' and
I finally made out a plan the meaning of which

disquieted me but little, but which was explicable
by the actual condition of the ducal palace, not then
completed. With that inspiration which the desire
of regaining liberty gives, I succeeded in decipher-
ing, by feeling with the ends of my fingers, the
surface of a stone, an Arab inscription by which the
author of this work notified his successors that he
had detached two stones of the last course and exca-
vated eleven feet underground. To continue his
work, it would be necessary to spread on the floor
of the dungeon itself the pieces of stone and mortar
produced by the work of excavation. Even if the
guardians or the inquisitors had not been reassured
by the construction of the edifice, which required
only an exterior surveillance, the disposition of the
Wells, in which it was necessary to descend by several steps, permitted the gradual raising of the soil
without the guardians perceiving it. This immense
labor had been profitless, at least for the one who
had undertaken it, for its incompletion announced
the death of the unknown. In order that his devotion should not be forever lost, it was necessary
that a prisoner should understand Arabic, but I had
studied the Oriental languages at the Convent of
the Armenians. A phrase written behind the stone
revealed the destiny of this unfortunate, who had
died a victim to his immense wealth, which Venice
had coveted and of which she had taken possession.
A month's time was required to enable me to arrive
at a result. While I worked, and in those moments
in which fatigue overwhelmed me, I heard the sound

of gold, I saw gold before me, I was dazzled by diamonds!—Oh! wait.

"One night, my worn steel blade encountered wood. I sharpened my bit of sword, and made a hole in this wood. In order to work, I extended myself like a serpent on my stomach; I stripped myself naked to work like a mole, extending my hands in front of me and making of the stone itself a point of support. Two days before that in which I was to appear before my judges, during the night, I wished to make a last effort; I pierced the wood, and my steel encountered nothing beyond.

"Judge of my surprise when I applied my eye to this hole! I was in the roof of a cave in which a feeble light permitted me to perceive a mountain of gold. The Doge and one of the Ten were in this cavern; I heard their voices; their conversation informed me that this was the secret treasure of the Republic, the gifts of the Doges and a portion of booty called the *denier* of Venice, and taken from the product of expeditions.

"I was saved!

"When the jailer came, I proposed to him to aid me in my flight and to go with me, carrying off all that we could take. There was no question of hesitation; he accepted. A vessel was about to sail for the Levant, all precautions were taken. Bianca favored the plan which I dictated to my confederate. In order not to excite suspicion, Bianca was to rejoin us at Smyrna. In one night the hole was enlarged and we descended into the secret treasury of Venice.

What a night! I saw four casks full of gold. In the preceding room, the silver was also piled up in two heaps which left a path in the middle to traverse the chamber, where the coins in sloping piles rose to the height of five feet against the walls. I thought that the jailer would go crazy: he sang, he leaped about, he laughed, he gamboled in the gold; I threatened to strangle him if he wasted time or if he made a noise. In his joy, he did not see at first a table on which were the diamonds. I threw myself upon it cleverly enough to fill my sailor's jacket and the pockets of my pantaloons. My God! I did not take a third of them. Under this table were the ingots of gold. I persuaded my companion to fill with gold as many sacks as we could carry, telling him that this was the only means of avoiding detection in foreign countries.

" 'Pearls, jewels and diamonds would cause us to be recognized,' I said to him.

"With all our greediness we could only take two thousand pounds of gold, which necessitated six journeys through the prison to the gondola. The sentinel at the water-gate had been bribed by a sack of ten pounds of gold. As to the two gondoliers, they believed themselves serving the Republic. At day-break we departed. When we were in the open sea, and when I thought of this night; when I recalled to myself all the sensations which I had experienced, when I saw again this immense treasure, where, according to my valuation, I had left thirty millions in silver and twenty millions in gold,

several millions in pearls, diamonds and rubies, I felt in myself something like a sensation of madness. I had the fever of gold.

"We disembarked at Smyrna, and we took ship again immediately for France. As we went on board the French vessel, God did me the favor to relieve me of my confederate. At that moment I did not think of all the consequences of this chance evil, at which I so rejoiced. We were so completely unnerved that we remained stupefied, saying nothing to each other, while waiting till we should be in safety to enjoy ourselves at our ease. It is not surprising that this scamp lost his head. You will see how God punished me!

"I did not feel easy until I had sold two-thirds of my diamonds in London and in Amsterdam, and converted my gold-dust into commercial obligations. During five years I hid myself in Madrid; then, in 1770, I came to Paris under a Spanish name and led a most brilliant life. Bianca was dead. In the midst of my pleasures, while I was enjoying a fortune of six millions, I was struck with blindness. I do not doubt that this infirmity was the result of my sojourn in the cell, of my working in the stone, if, however, my faculty of seeing gold had not carried with it an abuse of the visual power which predestined me to lose my sight.

"At this time, I was in love with a woman to whom I thought to unite my fate. I had revealed to her the secret of my name: she belonged to a powerful family. I had great hopes in the favor which

Louis XV. accorded me; I had put all my confidence
in this woman, who was the friend of Madame du
Barry; she advised me to consult a famous oculist
in London; but after some months spent in that
city, I was abandoned there by this woman in Hyde
Park. She had stripped me of all my fortune without
leaving me any resource; for, obliged to conceal my
name, which would have delivered me to the vengeance of Venice, I could not invoke the assistance
of any one; I feared Venice. My infirmity was made
the most of by the spies with whom this woman had
surrounded me. I spare you the recital of adventures worthy of Gil Blas. Your Revolution arrived.
I was obliged to become an inmate of the Quinze-
Vingts, to which this creature caused me to be admitted after having kept me for two years at the
Bicêtre as a lunatic. I have never been able to kill
her. I could not see, and I was too poor to buy an
arm. If, before losing Benedetto Carpi, my jailer,
I had consulted him on the situation of my cell, I
would have been able to find again the treasury and
would have returned to Venice when the Republic was abolished by Napoléon—

"Nevertheless, notwithstanding my blindness, let
us go to Venice! I will find again the door of the
prison; I will see the gold through the walls, I will
smell it under the waters in which it is buried; for
the events which have overthrown the power of
Venice are such that the secret of this treasure must
have died with Vendramino, the brother of Bianca,
a Doge, who, I hoped, would have made my peace

with the Ten.   I sent letters to the First Consul, I
proposed a treaty to the Emperor of Austria; everywhere have I been refused as a madman! Come, let
us set out for Venice; we will depart beggars, we
will come back millionaires; we will re-purchase
my property and you shall be my heir, you shall be
Prince de Varese!"

Stupefied by this confidence, which in my imaginations took the proportions of a poem, at the aspect
of this whitened head, and before the black water
of the moat of the Bastille, a water as still as that
of the canals of Venice, I did not reply.   Facino
Cane thought, doubtless, that I judged him like all
the others, with a scornful pity; he made a gesture
which expressed all the philosophy of despair.

This recital had carried him back, perhaps, to his
happy days at Venice: he seized his clarionet and
began to play in a melancholy manner a Venetian
ballad, a barcarolle for which he found his early
skill, his talent of the amorous patrician.   It was
something like the *Super flumina Babylonis*. My eyes
filled with tears.   If some belated passers-by happened to pass along the Boulevard Bourdon, doubtless they lingered to hear this last prayer of the
banished, the last regret of a lost name, in which
was mingled the memory of Bianca.   But the gold
soon regained the ascendancy, and the fatal passion
extinguished the light of youth.

"This treasure," he said to me, "I see it everywhere, awakened as in a dream; I walk there, the
diamonds glitter before me; I am not so blind as you

think; the gold and the diamonds light up my night, the night of the last Facino Cane, for my title passes to the Memmi. My God! the punishment of the murderer commenced early! *Ave Maria*—"

He recited some prayers which I did not hear.

"We will go to Venice!" I said to him when he rose.

"I have then found a man!" he cried, his face lighting up.

I conducted him home, giving him my arm; he grasped my hand at the door of the Quinze-Vingts, at the moment when some of the guests at the wedding were returning and making a noise sufficient to waken the dead.

"Shall we set out to-morrow?" said the old man.

"As soon as we have a little money."

"But we can go on foot, I will ask alms.—I am robust, and one is young when one sees gold before him."

Facino Cane died during the winter, after having languished for two months. The poor man had a catarrh.

Paris, March, 1836.

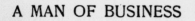

A MAN OF BUSINESS

A MAN OF BUSINESS

*

Lorette is a decent word invented to express the
state of a young girl or the young girl of a state
difficult to indicate, and which, in its modesty, the
French Academy has neglected to define, in consideration of the age of its forty members. When a
new name is applicable to a social case which cannot be otherwise expressed without periphrase, the
fortune of that word is made. Thus *la lorette* has
passed into all classes of society, even into those in
which a lorette herself will never pass. The word
was only made in 1840, doubtless owing to the
accumulation of these nests of swallows around the
church dedicated to Notre-Dame de Lorette. This
is only written for the etymologists. These gentlemen would not be so much embarrassed if the
writers of the Middle Ages had taken the pains to
describe manners and customs, as we do in these
times of analysis and of description. Mademoiselle
Turquet, or Malaga, for she is much better known
under her nom de guerre—see *The Pretended Mistress*
—is one of the first parishioners of this charming
church. This joyful and spirituelle young woman,
possessing as her fortune only her beauty, furnished,

at the moment of which this history relates, the
happiness of a notary who had in his notaress a
wife a trifle too devout, a trifle too stiff, a trifle too
dry to find happiness at home. Now, on an evening
of the Carnival, Maître Cardot had regaled, at
Mademoiselle Turquet's, Desroches the advocate,
Bixiou the caricaturist, Lousteau the feuilletonist,
and Nathan, whose illustrious names in LA COMÉDIE
HUMAINE render superfluous any kind of portrait.
The young La Palférine, notwithstanding his title
of *comte de vieille roche*, rock, alas! without any
vein of metal in it, had honored with his presence
the illegitimate domicile of the notary. If one does
not dine in the house of a lorette in order to eat
there the patriarchal beef, the meagre chicken of
the conjugal table and the family salad, neither is
one expected to hold there the hypocritical discourses
which take place in a salon furnished by virtuous
female bourgeoises. Ah! when will good manners
be attractive? when will the women of the fashionable world show a little less of their shoulders and a
little more of good humor or of wit? Marguerite
Turquet, the Aspasia of the Cirque-Olympique, is
one of those fresh and lively natures to whom everything is forgiven because of their candor in the fault
and their spirit in the repentance, to whom you say,
as did Cardot, clever enough, although a notary, to
say to her: "Cheat me cleverly!" Do not believe,
however, in any enormity. Desroches and Cardot
were two too good fellows and too old in the trade not
to be on a level with Bixiou, Lousteau, Nathan and

the young count. And these gentlemen, having
often had recourse to the two officers of the law,
knew them too intimately to, in lorette phrase,*"make
them pose."* The conversation, perfumed by the
fragrance of seven cigars, fantastic at first as a goat
at liberty, concentrated finally on that strategy which
creates at Paris the incessant battle waged between
the creditors and the debtors. Now, if you will
give yourself the trouble to remember the life and
the antecedents of the guests, you will recognize
that it would have been difficult to have found in
Paris persons better instructed in this matter, —
some *emeritus*, the others artists, they resembled
magistrates joking with the accused. A series of designs sketched by Bixiou on Clichy had been the
cause of the direction which the discourse had taken.
It was midnight. These personages, variously
grouped in the salon around the table and before the
fire, were discoursing in turns that not only are
comprehensible and possible only in Paris, but
which, still more, are only made and can only be
understood in the zone described by the Faubourg
Montmartre and by the Rue de la Chaussée-d'Antin,
between the heights of the Rue de Navarin and the
line of the boulevards.

In ten minutes, the profound reflections, the great
and the little moral, all the quibbles, were exhausted
on this subject, already exhausted about 1500 by
Rabelais. It was not of small merit to renounce
this display of fireworks terminated by this last
squib contributed by Malaga:

"All this turns to the profit of the bootmaker,"
said she. "I have left a milliner who failed me in
two hats. She came raging twenty-seven times to
demand of me twenty francs. She did not know
that we never have twenty francs. One has a
thousand francs, one sends to one's notary for five
hundred francs; but twenty francs, I have never had
them. My cook or my femme de chambre have
perhaps twenty francs between them. For myself,
I have only credit, and I should lose that in borrowing twenty francs. If I should ask for twenty francs,
nothing would any longer distinguish me from my
confrères who promenade along the boulevard."

"Has the milliner been paid?" said La Palférine.

"Ah, there! are you getting stupid, you there?"
she said to La Palférine, winking at him; "she
came this morning for the twenty-seventh time;
that is why I tell you about it."

"What did you do?" said Desroches.

"I took pity on her, and—I ordered of her the
little hat which I have ended by inventing in order
to get away from commonplace style. If Mademoiselle Amanda succeeds, she will ask nothing more
of me; her fortune is made."

"That which I have seen of the finest in this
species of contest," said Maitre Desroches, "paints,
it seems to me, Paris, for those who practice it,
much better than all the pictures which they are
forever painting of a fantastic Paris. You think
yourselves pretty strong, you others," he said,
looking at Nathan and Lousteau, Bixiou and La

Palférine; "but the king in this respect is a certain count who, at the present time, is occupying himself with coming to an end, and who, in his time, has passed for the most skilful, the most adroit, the most foxy, the most instructed, the most daring, the most subtle, the firmest, the most foreseeing of all the corsairs in yellow gloves, in cabriolets, with beautiful manners, who have navigated, navigate and will navigate on the stormy sea of Paris. Without faith or law, his private politics have been directed by the principles which direct those of the English cabinet. Up to the time of his marriage, his life was a continual warfare like that of—Lousteau," he said. "I have been and I am still his advocate."

"And the first letter of his name is Maxime de Trailles," said La Palférine.

"He has, moreover, always paid, has never wronged anyone," resumed Desroches; "but, as our friend Bixiou had just remarked, to pay in March that which you do not wish to pay till October is an attack on personal liberty. By virtue of an article of his particular code, Maxime considered as a swindling the mèans which one of his creditors employed to be paid immediately. For a long time the bill of exchange had been comprehended by him in all its consequences, immediate and mediate. A young man spoke of the bill of exchange in my place before him as: '*The Asses' Bridge!*' 'No,' said he, 'it is The Bridge of Sighs; one never returns.' Thus his science in matters of commercial jurisprudence was so complete that a procurator

could have taught him nothing. You know that at that time he possessed nothing; his carriage, his horses were hired; he lived with his valet de chambre, for whom, it is said, he will always be a great man, even after the marriage which he will make! A member of three clubs, he dined at one of them when he had no invitation out. Generally, he used his domicile so little—"

"He said to me, to me," cried La Palférine, interrupting Desroches: " 'my only fatuity is to pretend that I live in the Rue Pigalle.' "

"There is one of the two combatants," resumed Desroches; "now, then, here is the other. You have heard more or less spoken of a certain Claparon."

"He wears his hair in this way," cried Bixiou, making his hair stand on end.

And, gifted with the same talent that Chopin, the pianist, possessed in so high a degree, that of counterfeiting people, he represented the personage on the instant with a frightful truthfulness.

"He rolls his head this way in speaking; he has been a traveling salesman, he has tried all trades—"

"Well, he was born for traveling, for he is, at this moment while I am talking to you, on his way to America," said Desroches. "There is no other chance for him but that, for he will probably be condemned by contumacy for fraudulent bankruptcy at the coming Session."

"A man overboard," cried Malaga.

"This Claparon," resumed Desroches, "was during six or seven years the screen, the man of straw, the scapegoat, of two of our friends, Du Tillet and Nucingen; but, in 1829, his part was so well known that—"

"Our friends dropped him," said Bixiou.

"In short, they abandoned him to his destiny; and," resumed Desroches, "he rolled in the mud. In 1833, he associated himself to carry on business with a man named Cérizet—"

"What! he who in the matter of stock companies got up one with such a pretty combination that the sixth chamber knocked him over with two years in prison?" asked the lorette.

"The same," replied Desroches. "Under the Restoration, the trade of this Cérizet consisted, from 1823 to 1827, in signing intrepidly articles pursued inveterately by the public minister, and in going to prison. A man rendered himself illustrious cheaply at that time. The Liberal Party called its department champion THE COURAGEOUS CERIZET. This zeal was recompensed about 1828 by *the general interest*. The general interest is a species of civic crown awarded by the newspapers. Cérizet wished to discount the general interest; he came to Paris, where, under the patronage of the bankers of the Left, he made his debut by a business agency, combined with banking operations, with funds loaned by a man who had banished himself, a player too skilful, whose funds, in July, 1830, had foundered in company with the Ship of State—"

"Eh! it is that which we have surnamed the Method of the cards!—" cried Bixiou.

"Do not speak evil of that poor fellow," cried Malaga. "D'Estourny was a good boy!"

"You can understand the rôle which a ruined man might be expected to play in 1830 who was known, politically speaking, as the courageous Cérizet! He was sent into a very pretty sub-prefecture," resumed Desroches. "Unfortunately for Cérizet, authority has not as much ingenuity as have the parties, who, during the fight, make projectiles of everything. Cérizet was obliged to send in his resignation after three months of service. Had he not taken it into his head to wish to be popular! As he had not yet done anything to lose his title of nobility—the courageous Cérizet!—the government proposed to him, as an indemnity, to become director of an opposition journal which should be ministerial *in petto*. Thus it was the government who perverted this fine character. Cérizet, finding himself a little too much in his directorship like a bird on a rotten bough, launched himself into that pretty stock-company where he unluckily, as you have just said, caught two years in prison,—but in which the sharpest of them entrapped the public."

"We know the sharpest of them," said Bixiou; "do not slander that poor fellow, he is trapped! Couture let his cash be caught there; who would ever have thought it!"

"Cérizet is, moreover, an ignoble man, and one whom the evils of vulgar debauch have disfigured,"

resumed Desroches.   "Let us return to the promised
duel! Then, never did two traders of the worst
species, of the worst manners, more ignoble in
aspect, associate themselves together to carry on a
dirtier business.   For funds to provide for the running expenses, they counted on that species of slang
which is given by the knowledge of Paris, the
hardihood which is given by poverty, the trickery
which is given by the habits of business, the
science which is given by the knowledge of Parisian fortunes, of their origin, of their relations, the
acquaintances and intrinsic values of each one.
This association of two *carotteurs*, excuse the word,
the only one which can, in the slang of the Bourse,
describe them to you, was of short duration.   Like
two famished dogs, they fought over each bit of car-
rion.   The first speculations of the house of Cérizet
and Claparon were, however, sufficiently well con-
trived.   These two rogues associated themselves
with the Barbets, the Chaboisseaus, the Samanons
and other usurers from whom they bought doubtful claims.   The Claparon agency was then situated in a little entresol of the Rue Chabannais,
composed of five rooms, and the rent of which did
not amount to more than seven hundred francs.
Each partner slept in a little chamber which,
through prudence, was kept so carefully closed that
my master clerk was never able to penetrate them.
The offices consisted of an antechamber, a salon,
and a cabinet of which the furniture would not have
brought three hundred francs at the auctioneers'.

You know Paris well enough to be able to see the
arrangement of the two offices: haircloth chairs,
a table with a green cloth, a mean clock between
two candlesticks under glass which bored to look
at, before a little mirror with a gilded frame,
on a chimney-piece the fire-brands in which
were, according to my master clerk, two years old!
As to the cabinet, you can guess it: many paste-
board boxes and little business!—a common portfolio
for each partner; then in the middle the cylin-
drical desk empty as the cash-box! two working
chairs on each side of a chimney-piece with a coal
fire.   On the floor was laid a carpet, second-hand,
like the credits.   In short, it was that stuff
mahogany which is sold in our offices during
fifty years from predecessor to successor.   You are
now acquainted with each of the two adversaries.
Well, in the first three months of their association,
which was liquidated by blows of the fist at the end
of seven months, Cérizet and Claparon bought two
thousand francs' worth of paper signed Maxime—
since Maxime there is—and stuffed the two portfol-
ios full—judgment, appeal, decree, execution, report,
—in short, a credit of three thousand two hundred
francs and some centimes which they had for five
hundred francs by a conveyance under private signature, with special power of attorney to act in
order to avoid the costs.—At that time, Maxime,
already ripe, had one of those caprices peculiar to
men of fifty—"

"Antonia!" cried La Palférine, "that Antonia

whose fortune had been made by a letter in which I reclaimed a tooth brush from her!"

"Her real name is Chocardelle," said Malaga, whom this pretentious name vexed.

"That's the one," resumed Desroches.

"Maxime had committed this fault only this once in all his life; but, what would you have, vice is not perfect!" said Bixiou.

"Maxime was still ignorant of the life which one leads with a little girl of eighteen who wishes to throw herself, head first, out of her honest garret to fall into a sumptuous equipage," resumed Desroches, "and statesmen should know everything. At this epoch, De Marsay had just employed his friend, our friend, in the high comedy of politics. A man of great conquests, Maxime had known only titled women; and, at fifty, he certainly had the right to bite into a little fruit said to be wild, like a hunter who stops in a peasant's field under an apple tree. The count found for Mademoiselle Chocardelle a little literary establishment sufficiently elegant, a great opportunity, as always—"

"Bah! she did not stay there six months," said Nathan; "she was too handsome to keep a literary establishment."

"Are you the father of her child?—" said the lorette to Nathan.

"One morning," resumed Desroches, "Cérizet, who, since the purchase of Maxime's notes, had arrived by degrees at the style of the first clerk of a bailiff, was introduced, after seven unavailing

attempts, into the count's apartments. Suzon, the old valet de chambre, though expert, had come to take Cérizet for a solicitor who arrived to propose a thousand écus to Maxime if he would obtain for a young woman a shop for stamped paper. Suzon, without any suspicion of this little scamp, a real gamin of Paris with prudence drubbed into him by his condemnation by the correctional police, persuaded his master to receive him. Do you see this man of business, with an uneasy glance, thin hair, a bald forehead, with a little dry black coat, in muddy boots—"

"What an image of Credit!" cried Lousteau.

"—Before the count," resumed Desroches, "the image of the Debt insolent, in a dressing-gown of white flannel, in slippers embroidered by some marchioness, in pantaloons of beautiful white wool having on his black dyed hair a magnificent cap, displaying a dazzling shirt front, and playing with the tassels of his girdle?—"

"It is a Genre painting," said Nathan, "for those who know the pretty little waiting-room in which Maxime breakfasted, full of pictures of great value, hung with silk, in which one walked on a Smyrna carpet, whilst admiring cabinets full of curiosities, of rarities that would fill with envy a king of Saxony—"

"That is the scene," said Desroches.

With this word, the narrator obtained the most profound silence.

"'Monsieur le Comte,' said Cérizet, 'I am sent

by one Monsieur Charles Claparon, formerly a
banker.'

" 'Ah! what does he want with me, the poor
devil?—'

" 'Well, he has become your creditor for a sum of
three thousand two hundred francs seventy-five
centimes, in capital, interest, and costs—'

" 'The Coutelier claim,' said Maxime, who knew
all about his affairs as a pilot knows his coasts.

" 'Yes, Monsieur le Comte,' replied Cérizet bowing. 'I have come to know what are your intentions?'

" 'I shall not settle this obligation until it pleases
me,' replied Maxime, ringing for Suzon. 'Claparon
is very daring to buy a credit on me without consulting me! I am vexed on his account, he who for
so long had so well conducted himself as a *man of
straw* for my friends. I said of him 'Truly, he must
be an imbecile to serve for so little gain, and with so
much fidelity, men who are stuffed with miliions.'
Well, he gives me here a proof of his stupidity.—
Yes, men merit their fate! One is fitted with a
crown or a bullet! one is millionaire or porter, and
everything is just. What would you have, my dear
fellow! I—I am not a king, I maintain my principles. I am without pity for those who make costs
for me or who do not know their business of creditors.—Suzon, my tea!—You see, monsieur?' he said
to the valet de chambre. 'Well, you have let yourself be taken in, you poor old thing. Monsieur is a
creditor; you should have recognized it by his boots.

Neither my friends, nor the strangers who have
need of me, nor my enemies, come to see me on foot.
--My dear Monsieur Cérizet, you understand? You
will not wipe your boots on my carpet any more,'
said he, looking at the mud which whitened the
soles of his adversary. 'You will make my compliments to this poor boniface of a Claparon, for I
will put this affair in the Z.'

"All this was said in a tone of benevolence that
would have given the colic to a virtuous bourgeois.

"'You are wrong, Monsieur le Comte,' replied
Cérizet, taking a little peremptory tone; 'we will
be paid in full and in a manner which may be somewhat inconvenient to you. Therefore I have come
to see you amicably, as should be done by well-
bred people.'

"'Ah! you understand it that way?—' answered
Maxime, whom this last pretension of Cérizet
angered.

"In this insolence there was some of Talleyrand's
spirit, if you see clearly the contrast between the
two costumes and the two men. Maxime knit his
brows and fastened his looks upon the Cérizet,
who not only sustained this jet of cold rage but,
still more, who responded to it by that glacial
malice which distils from the fixed eyes of a cat.

"'Very well, monsieur, go—'

"'Very well; adieu, Monsieur le Comte. Before
the end of six months, we shall be even with each
other.'

"'If you can *steal* from me the amount of your

credit, which I recognize is legitimate, I shall be obliged to you, Monsieur,' replied Maxime; 'you will have taught me some new precaution to take.— I am truly your servant.'

" 'Monsieur le Comte,' said Cérizet, 'it is I who am yours.'

"This was neat, full of strength and of security on both sides.   Two tigers who regard each other before fighting, over some prey, would not be finer nor more wily than were these two natures as crafty one as the other, one in his impertinent elegance, the other in his filthy harness.—Which will you bet on?—" said Desroches, who looked at his audience surprised to find themselves so deeply interested.

"Well, that is one, that is a story!—" said Malaga. "Oh! go on, I beg you, my dear; that goes to my heart."

"Between two *dogs* of that strength, nothing common should have happened," said La Palférine.

"Bah! I will bet my furniture-maker's bill, and he worries me to death, that the little toad downed Maxime," cried Malaga.

"I will bet on Maxime," said Cardot; "no one ever took him napping."

Desroches made a pause while emptying a little glass which was presented to him by the lorette.

"The reading-room of Mademoiselle Chocardelle," he resumed, "was situated in the Rue Coquenard, two steps from the Rue Pigalle, in which Maxime lived.   The aforesaid Demoiselle Chocardelle

occupied a little apartment opening on a garden and separated from her shop by a large dark place in which she kept her books. Antonia had this estab-lishment kept by her aunt—"

"She already had her aunt?—" cried Malaga. "The devil! Maxime managed things well."

"It was, alas! a real aunt," resumed Desroches, "whose name was—wait a moment—"

"Ida Bonamy—," said Bixiou.

"Thus, Antonia relieved of a great deal of trouble by her aunt, rose late, went to bed late, and only appeared at her counter between two and four o'clock," resumed Desroches. "From the very first, her presence sufficed to bring customers to her reading-room; thither came several old gentlemen of the quarter, among others a former coach-maker named Croizeau. After having seen this miracle of feminine beauty through a window, the former coach-maker concluded to read the newspapers every day in this salon, an example which was fol-lowed by a former custom-house officer, named Denisart, a man with a decoration, in whom the Croizeau concluded to see a rival and to whom later he said: 'Môsieur, *you have certainly given me a practical lesson.*"

"This word should enable you to perceive the personage. The Sieur Croizeau belonged to that species of little old men who, since Henry Mon-nier, have been known as the species Coquerel, so well has he rendered the little voice, the little man-ners, the little queue, the little powder in the hair,

the little step, the little movements of the head, the little dry tone, in his character of Coquerel of *La Famille Improvisée*. This Croizeau said: 'Here, fair lady!' in passing his two sous to Antonia with a pretentious gesture. Madame Ida Bonamy, aunt of Mademoiselle Chocardelle, soon learned through the cook that the former coach-maker, a man of excessive ugliness, was taxed at forty thousand francs income in the quarter where he lived, Rue de Buffault. A week after the installation of the handsome circulator of romances, he was delivered of this pun:

"'You lend me *livres*, but I return you many francs—'

"Some days later he assumed a knowing little air to say:

"'I know that you are engaged, but my day will come: I am a widower.'

"Croizeau always appeared with beautiful linen, with a blue-bottle colored coat, a waistcoat in that silk known as *pou-de-soie*, black pantaloons, double-soled shoes tied with ribbons of black silk and creaking like those of an abbé. He carried always in his hand his fourteen-franc silk hat.

"'I am old and without children,' he said to the young person some days after the visit of Cérizet to Maxime. 'I have a horror of my collateral heirs. They are all peasants, made to cultivate the earth! Just imagine that I came from my village with six francs, and that I made my fortune here. I am not proud—. A pretty woman is my equal. Would it

20

not be better to be Madame Croizeau for some time
than to be the servant of a count during a year?—
You will be left, some day or other. And you
will then think of me. Your servant, fair lady!'

"All this was managed very quietly. The very
slightest gallantries are uttered secretly. No one
in the world knew that this spruce little old man
loved Antonia, for the prudent countenance of this
lover in the reading-room would have conveyed
nothing to a rival. Croizeau was suspicious for a
couple of months of the retired director of customs.
But towards the middle of the third month he had
grounds for recognizing the very slight foundations
of the suspicions. Croizeau exercised his ingenuity in keeping near to Denisart when in his company, then, taking his opportunity, he said to him:

" 'It is fine weather, Môsieur:—'

"To which the former functionary replied:

" 'The weather of Austerlitz, Monsieur: I was
there—, I was even wounded there; my cross is
because of my conduct on that fine day—'

"And, insensibly, from one thing to another,
step by step, through little confidences, an intimacy was developed between these two relics
of the Empire. The little Croizeau was connected with the Empire by his intimacy with the
sisters of Napoléon,—he had been their carriage-
maker, and he had often tormented them by his bills.
He therefore gave himself out as *having had relations
with the imperial family*. Maxime, informed by
Antonia of the propositions offered by the *agreeable*

old man, for such was the title given by the
aunt to the *rentier,* wished to see him. The declaration of war made by Cérizet had had the effect of
making this fine gentleman in yellow gloves study
his position on his chess-board and observe the least
important pieces. Now, apropos of this agreeable
old gentleman, he received the understanding that
stroke of the clock which announces to you a misfortune. One evening, Maxime placed himself in the
second dusky apartment, around which were arranged the shelves of the library. After having
examined by an opening between two green curtains
the seven or eight habitués of the salon, he gauged
with a look the soul of the little carriage-maker; he
appraised his passion, and was very well satisfied
to know that, at the moment when his fancy should
be over, a sufficiently sumptuous future would open
at command its varnished portals to Antonia.

" 'And that one,' he said, indicating the fine, large
old man decorated with the Legion of Honor; 'who
is he?'

" 'A former director of customs.'

" 'He has a disquieting appearance!' said Maxime,
admiring the style of the Sieur Denisart.

"In fact, this old soldier held himself straight as
a steeple; his head attracted attention by its pow-
dered and pomaded arrangement, almost similar to
that of the *postillons* of a masked ball. Under this
species of felt, modeled on an oblong head was
presented an old countenance, administrative and
military both at once, marked by a proud air, similar

enough to that which caricature has lent to the *Constitutionnel*. This former administrator, of an age, of a quality, of a curve of the back which permitted him to read nothing without glasses, maintained his respectable abdomen with all the pride of an old man with a mistress, and wore in his ears gold rings which recalled those of the old General Montcornet, the habitué of the Vaudeville. Denisart held blue in favor,—his pantaloons and his old frock-coat, very full, were of blue cloth.

"'How long has that old fellow been coming here?' asked Maxime, to whom the glasses appeared to have a suspicious aspect.

"'Oh! from the commencement,' replied Antonia. 'It is now nearly two months—'

"'Good; Cérizet came only about a month ago,' said Maxime to himself.—'Make him speak,' he said in Antonia's ear; 'I wish to hear his voice.'

"'Bah!' she replied, 'that would be difficult; he never says anything to me.'

"'Why does he come, then?—' asked Maxime.

"'For a queer enough reason,' replied the beautiful Antonia. 'In the first place, he has a passion, notwithstanding his sixty-nine years; but, because of his sixty-nine years, he is regulated like a clock-dial. This good man there goes to dine with his passion, Rue de la Victoire, at five o'clock every day.—There is an unlucky woman! He leaves her house at six o'clock, comes to read the newspapers for four hours, and returns there at ten o'clock. The papa Croizeau says he is acquainted with the

motives of Monsieur's conduct; he approves them;
and, in his place, he would act the same way.
Thus, I know my future! If ever I become Madame
Croizeau, from six to ten o'clock I shall be free.'

"Maxime consulted the *Almanach des 25,000
adresses;* he found there this reassuring line:

" 'DENISART *, former director of customs, Rue
de la Victoire.

"There was no further uneasiness. By degrees,
there were established between Monsieur Denisart
and the Sieur Croizeau certain confidences. Nothing unites men more than a certain conformity of
views respecting women. Papa Croizeau dined in
the house of her whom he called *La Belle de Monsieur Denisart.* Here I should insert a sufficiently
important observation. The reading-room had been
purchased by the count for a sum, half cash down
and half in notes signed by the aforesaid Demoiselle
Chocardelle. Rabelais' *quart d'heure* arrived, the
count found himself without funds. Whereupon,
the first of the three notes of a thousand francs
was paid in full by the agreeable coach-maker, whom
the old scoundrel of a Denisart counseled to secure
his loan by establishing for himself certain advantages of a privileged creditor upon the reading-room.

" 'I,' said Denisart, 'I have seen some beauties
among the fair sex!—Thus, in every case, even
when I have no longer my head about me, I
always take my precautions with women. This

creature for whom I am so crazy, well, she is not in
her own furniture; she is in mine.   The lease of the
apartment is in my name—'

"You know Maxime; he thought that the coach-
maker was very young!   The Croizeau could pay
the three thousand francs without having anything
to show for it for a long time, for Maxime found
himself more enamored than ever of Antonia—"

"I can well believe it," said La Palférine; "she
is the *Belle Imperia* of the Middle Ages."

"A woman who has a rough skin!" cried the lorette, "and so rough that she ruins herself in bran
baths."

"Croizeau spoke with a coach-maker's admiration
of the sumptuous furnishing which the amorous
Denisart had given for a setting-off to his Belle; he
described it with a satanic complacency to the ambitious Antonia," resumed Desroches.   "There
were coffers of ebony inlaid with mother-of-pearl
and gold wire, Belgian carpets, a mediæval bed of
the value of a thousand écus, a clock by Boulle; then,
in the dining-room, candelabra at the four corners,
curtains of China silk on which Chinese patience
had painted birds, and portières suspended from
cross-pieces much more valuable than the divided
portières.

" 'See what you should have, fair lady—, and
what I should be willing to offer you—,' said he in
conclusion.   'I know very well that you would love
me tolerably well; but, at my age, one is reasonable.   You may judge how much I love you, since

I have lent you a thousand francs. I can admit it
to you: in all my life nor in my days have I ever
lent so much!'

"And he tendered the two sous of his sitting
with the importance which a scientist attaches to a
demonstration.

"That evening, Antonia said to the count, at the
Variétés:

" 'It is pretty stupid all the same, a reading-room.
I don't feel any inclination for that sort of a business; I don't see any chance of fortune in that.
That is something for a widow who just wishes to
keep life together, or for a young woman who is
atrociously ugly and who thinks she may catch a
man by dressing a little.'

" 'That is what you asked of me,' replied the
count.

"At this moment, Nucingen, whom, from the
evening before, the king of the Lions, for the yellow
gloves had then become lions, had won a thousand
écus, came in to give them to him, and seeing the
astonishment of Maxime, he said to him:

" 'I haf receivet a brotest at the reguest of dat
tevil of a Glabaron—'

" 'Ah! that's their method!' cried Maxime; 'they
are not very clever, that lot—'

" 'All de zame,' replied the banker, 'bay dem, for
dey can attress demselves to others dan myself and
but you in de wrong—. I dake for widness dis
preddy voman dat I have baid you dis morning, even
bevore de brotest—'

"Queen of the spring-board," said La Palférine, smiling. "You will lose—"

"It has long happened," resumed Desroches, "that, in a similar case, but where the too honest debtor, frightened at having to make an affirmation in the courts of justice, did not wish to pay Maxime, we had roughly dragged in the protesting creditor by opposing protests *en masse*, so as to absorb the whole amount in expenses of contribution—"

"What's all that?"—cried Malaga. "Here are a lot of words which sound to me like gibberish. Since you have found the sturgeon excellent, pay me the value of the sauce in lessons in trickery."

"Well," said Desroches, "the amount which one of your creditors covers with a protest in the hands of one of your debtors may become the object of a similar protest on the part of all your other creditors. What, then, does the court, of whom all the creditors demand the authorization to be paid?—It divides legally the sum seized among them all. This division, made under the eye of justice, is called a contribution. If you owe ten thousand francs, and if your creditors seize by protest a thousand francs, they have each so much per cent of their claim, by means of a repartition *au marc le franc*, according to the terms of the Palais, that is to say, in a distribution pro rata of their amounts; but they only receive this by means of a legal paper called an *Extrait du Bordereau de Collocation*, which is delivered by the clerk of the court. You can imagine this work accomplished by a judge and prepared by

the advocates? it involves a great deal of stamped paper covered with empty and scattered lines, in which the figures are lost in columns of entire emptiness. The first thing to do is to deduct the cost. Now, the cost being the same for a sum of a thousand francs seized and for a sum of a million, it is not difficult to eat up a thousand écus, for instance, in costs, especially if one succeeds in stirring up contestants."

"An advocate always succeeds," said Cardot; "how many times has one of yours asked me: 'How much is there to get?'"

"They succeed above all," resumed Desroches, "when the debtor provokes you to eat up the sum in costs. Thus the count's creditors got nothing; they had only their running about to the advocates and their efforts. In order to be paid by a debtor as clever as the count, a creditor would be obliged to put himself in a legal situation excessively difficult to establish,—he would have to be at once his debtor and his creditor, for then one has the right, according to the law, to bring about the confusion—"

"Of the debtor?" said the lorette, who lent an attentive ear to this discourse.

"No, of the two qualities of creditor and debtor, and pay one's self by his hands," resumed Desroches. "The innocence of Claparon, who had only invented protests, had therefore the effect of tranquillizing the count. In taking Antonia home from the Variétés, he adopted the more readily the

idea of selling the reading-room in order to pay off
the last two thousand francs of the price, for he
feared the ridicule of being known as the silent
partner in such an enterprise. He therefore accepted
the plan of Antonia, who wished to enter the upper
sphere of her profession, to have a magnificent
apartment, a femme de chambre, a carriage, and to
enter the lists with our beautiful amphitryon, for
example—''

''She is not well enough made for that,'' cried the
illustrious beauty of the Cirque; ''but she well
rinsed out the little d'Esgrignon all the same!''

''Ten days later, the little Croizeau, perched upon
his dignity, used something like this language to the
beautiful Antonia,'' resumed Desroches:

'' 'My child, your literary shop is a hole, you are
becoming yellow in it, the gas will ruin your eyes;
you should get out of it, and here, now! let us profit
by the occasion. I have found for you a young
woman who asks nothing better than to purchase
your reading-room. She is a little woman, quite
ruined, who has nothing left but to throw herself in
the river; but she has four thousand francs in cash,
and it would be better to make use of them to nour-
ish and bring up two children—'

'' 'Well, you are very amiable, Papa Croizeau' ''
said Antonia.

'' 'Oh! I shall be much more amiable presently,'
replied the old coach-maker. 'Just imagine, that
that poor Monsieur Denisart has been so upset that it
has given him the jaundice—. Yes, that has

affected his liver, as is always the case with sensitive old men.   He was wrong to be so sensitive.   I
said to him: 'Be passionate if you like, good!
but sensitive,—stop there! one kills one's self—.'
I did not expect it, really, such an upsetting in a
man sufficiently strong, sufficiently wise to absent
himself while he was digesting from the house
of —'

   " 'But who is it?'—asked Mademoiselle Chocardelle.

   " 'That little creature with whom I dined left him
in the lurch, clean—. Yes, she forsook him without
notifying him in any other way than by a letter
without any spelling in it.'

   " 'See what it is, Papa Croizeau, to bore the
women!—'

   " 'It is a lesson! fair lady,' replied the affection-
ate Croizeau. 'Meanwhile, I have never seen a man
in such a state of despair,' said he. 'Our friend
Denisart can no longer tell his right hand from his
left; he no longer wishes to see that which he calls
the theatre of his happiness—.   He has so completely lost his senses, that he proposed to me to
buy for four thousand francs all the furniture of
Hortense—.   Her name is Hortense!'

   " 'A pretty name,' said Antonia.

   " 'Yes, it was that of the step-daughter of Napoléon.   I furnished her her equipages, as you know.'

   " 'Well, come, I will see,' said the clever Antonia;
'begin by sending me your young woman—'

   "Antonia hastened to see the furniture, returned

fascinated, and captivated Maxime by an enthusiasm
worthy of an antiquary.   That very evening the
count consented to the sale of the reading-room.
The establishment, you understand, was in the
name of Mademoiselle Chocardelle.   Maxime laughed
at the little Croizeau, who found him a pur-
chaser.   The firm of Maxime and Chocardelle lost
two thousand francs, it is true, but what was this loss
in presence of four beautiful notes of a thousand
francs each?—as the count said to me:

" 'Four thousand francs cash in hand!—there are
moments when one would sign eight thousand francs
of notes to have them!'

"The count went to see the furniture himself, on
the third day, having the four thousand francs about
him.   The sale had been consummated, thanks to
the diligence of the little Croizeau, who pushed at
the wheel; he had *enclaudé* the widow, as he said.
Concerning himself but little with this agreeable
old gentleman, who was going to lose a thousand
francs, Maxime wished to have all the furniture
carried immediately to an apartment taken in the
name of Madame Ida Bonamy, Rue Tronchet, in a
new house.   Thus he had furnished himself in advance with several large furniture vans.   Maxime,
enamored anew of the beauty of the furniture, which,
for an upholsterer, would have been worth six thous-
and francs, found the unhappy old man, yellow
with his jaundice, at the corner of the fire, his head
enveloped in two handkerchiefs and a cotton night-
cap over all, muffled up like a chandelier; collapsed,

not able to speak, in short, so dilapidated that the count was forced to negotiate with the valet de chambre. After having paid over the four thousand francs to the valet de chambre, who carried them to his master so that he might give a receipt for them, Maxime was about to order his people to bring up the furniture vans; but he heard at that moment a voice which sounded in his ears like a rattle, and which cried to him:

" 'It is unnecessary, Monsieur le Comte; we are even; I have six hundred and thirty francs and fifteen centimes to hand over to you!'

"And he was quite aghast to see Cérizet issue from his wrappings, like a butterfly from his larva, offering to him his cursed bundle of papers, and adding:

" 'In my misfortune I learned to play comedy, and I can equal Bouffé in the old men.'

" 'I am in the forest of Bondy!' cried Maxime.

" 'No, Monsieur le Comte, you are in the house of Mademoiselle Hortense, the friend of the old Lord Dudley, who concealed her from everybody; but she has the bad taste to love your servant.'

" 'If ever,' said the count to me, 'I had a desire to kill a man, it was at that moment; but what would you have! Hortense showed me her pretty head; it was necessary to laugh, and to preserve my superiority. I said to him, throwing him the six hundred francs: 'This is for the lady.'

" 'That is just like Maxime!' cried La Palférine.

" 'All the more so that it was the money of the little Croizeau,' said the profound Cardot.

"Maxime had a triumph," resumed Desroches, "for Hortense exclaimed: 'Ah! if I had known that it was thee!—'

"And there is one, *for* confusion," cried the lorette.—"Thou hast lost, milord," she said to the notary.

And it was thus that the furniture merchant to whom Malaga owed a hundred écus was paid.

Paris, 1845.

THE INVOLUNTARY COMEDIANS

TO MONSIEUR LE COMTE JULES DE CASTELLANE

THE INVOLUNTARY COMEDIANS

*

Léon de Lora, our celebrated landscape painter, is a member of one of the most noble families of Roussillon, Spanish in origin, and which, admirable as it is by the antiquity of the race, has for the last hundred years been devoted to the proverbial poverty of the Hidalgoes. Arrived light-footed in Paris from the department of the Pyrénées-Orientales, with the sum of eleven francs for his entire viaticum, he had there, in some measure, forgotten the sorrows of his childhood and of his family in the midst of the miseries which are never lacking to the struggling students of painting, whose entire fortune consists in an intrepid vocation. Then the cares of glory and those of success furnished additional causes for forgetfulness.

If you have followed the sinuous and capricious course of these Studies, perhaps you will remember Mistigris, pupil of Schinner, one of the heroes of *A Start in Life*—SCENES OF PRIVATE LIFE—and his appearances in some other Scenes. In 1845, the landscape painter, emulous of the Hobbemas, of the Ruysdaels, of the Lorrains, no longer resembles the

(323)

denuded and brisk *rapin* whom you have seen above.
An illustrious man, he now possesses a charming
house in the Rue de Berlin, not far from the Hôtel de
Brambourg, in which dwells his friend Bridau, and
near the house of Schinner, his first master.   He is a
member of the Institute and an officer of the Legion of
Honor; he is thirty-nine, he has an income of
twenty thousand francs, his canvases are purchased
at their weight in gold, and, that which seems to
him more extraordinary than to be invited sometimes to the Court balls, his name, thrown so often
for the last sixteen years by the press to the winds
of all Europe, has finally penetrated into the valley
of the Pyrénées-Orientales, where vegetate three
veritable Loras, his eldest brother, his father and an
old paternal aunt, Mademoiselle Urraca y Lora.

In the maternal line, there remained to the painter
only a cousin, a nephew of his mother, of the
age of fifty, the inhabitant of a little manufacturing
city of the department.   This cousin was the first
to remember Léon. In 1840, for the first time, Léon
de Lora received a letter from Monsieur Sylvestre
Palafox-Castel Gazonal, known simply as Gazonal,
to which he replied that it was indeed he, that is to
say, the son of the late Léonie Gazonal, wife of the
Comte Fernand Didas y Lora.

The cousin, Sylvestre Gazonal, went in the fine
season of 1841 to inform the illustrious unknown
family of the Loras that the little Léon had not
departed for the Rio de la Plata, as they believed;
that he was not dead, as they believed, and that he

was one of the finest geniuses of the French School,
which they did not believe.   The eldest son, Don
Juan de Lora, said to his cousin Gazonal that he
was the victim of some joker in Paris.

Now, the said Gazonal proposing to go to Paris in
order to follow up a legal process which, through a
contest, the prefect of the Pyrénées-Orientales had
wrested from the ordinary jurisdiction of the
province to carry it up to the Council of State, the
provincial promised himself to clear up the matter
and *to demand a reason* for his impertinence from
the Parisian painter.   It happened that Monsieur
Gazonal, putting up in *a poor lodging* in the Rue
Croix-des-Petits-Champs, was astonished to see the
palace in the Rue de Berlin.   When he learned that
the master was traveling in Italy, he renounced for
the moment his *demanding reason,* and doubted if
his maternal relationship would be recognized by
the celebrated man.

From 1843 to 1844 Gazonal followed his lawsuit.
This contest, which related to a question of the
course and of the height of the water, of the erection
of a dam, in which the administration was interested, sustained by the dwellers on the banks of the
river, menaced the very existence of the manufactory.   In 1845, Gazonal considered this case as
entirely lost, the secretary of the Maître des Requêtes charged with making the report having confided to him that this report would be opposed to his
contentions, and his advocate having confirmed it to
him.   Gazonal, though commandant in the National

Guard of his city and one of the most skilful manufacturers of his department, found so little in Paris,
he was so dismayed at the dearness of living and at
the least trifles, that he kept himself secluded in his
poor little hôtel. This Southerner, deprived of his
sun, execrated Paris, which he denominated a manufactory of rheumatisms. In counting up the
expenses of his lawsuit and of his sojourn, he promised himself that, when he returned, he would either
poison the prefect or he would make a cuckold of
him! In his moments of sadness he killed the prefect; in his moments of gayety, he contented himself with *minotaurising* him.

One morning, at the end of his déjeuner, fuming
and swearing, he took up furiously his newspaper.
These lines, which terminated an article, "Our
great landscape painter, Léon de Lora, who returned
from Italy a month ago, will exhibit several canvases
at the Salon; thus the exposition will be, as may
be seen, very brilliant,—" struck Gazonal as if that
voice which speaks to gamblers when they win had
sounded in his ear. With that promptness of action
which distinguishes the people of the South, Gazonal leaped from the hôtel into the street, from the
street into a cabriolet, and went to the Rue de Berlin, to see his cousin.

Léon de Lora sent word to his cousin Gazonal
that he invited him to déjeuner at the Café de *Paris*
for the next day, for he was at that moment occupied in such a manner that it would be impossible
for him to receive him. Gazonal, like a true man

of the South, related all his troubles to the valet de chambre.

The next morning, at ten o'clock, Gazonal, too well arrayed for the occasion—he had put on his blue-bottle coat with gilded buttons, a shirt with a jabot, a white vest and yellow gloves—waited for his amphitryon while walking up and down for an hour on the boulevard, after having learned from the *cafetier*—title of the café proprietors in the provinces—that these messieurs usually breakfasted between eleven o'clock and noon.

"About half-past eleven, two Parisians, like simple priests," he said, when he afterwards related his adventures to those of his locality, "and who had a general air of nothing at all, exclaimed on seeing me on the boulevard: 'Behold thy Gazonal!—"

This speaker was Bixiou, with whom Léon de Lora had provided himself to mystify his cousin.

" 'Do not disturb yourself, my dear cousin! I am yours,' cried the little Léon, clasping me in his arms," said Gazonal to his friends on his return. "The déjeuner was splendid. And I thought I saw double when I saw the number of gold pieces that it took to pay the bill. Those people must make their weight in gold, for my cousin gave thirty sols to the waiter, a day's wages."

During this monstrous breakfast, seeing that there were then consumed six dozen Ostende oysters, six cutlets à la Soubise, a chicken à la Marengo, a lobster mayonnaise, fresh peas, a croute aux

champignons, washed down with three bottles of Bordeaux, three bottles of champagne, plus the black coffee, the liqueurs, without counting the hors-d'œuvre, Gazonal was magnificent in his fury against Paris.   The noble manufacturer complained of the length of the four-pound loaves, of the height of the houses, of the indifference of the passers-by for each other, of the cold and of the rain, of the dearness of the hackney-coaches, and all that so cleverly, that the two artists conceived a lively friendship for Gazonal and got him to describe his lawsuit.

"My suit," said he, using his r's thickly and accenting everything provincially, "is something very simple: they want my manufactory.   I find here a beast of an advocate to whom I give twenty francs each time to keep his eye open, and I always find him asleep.—It is a snail which rolls in its carrriage and I go on foot.   They trrick me shamefully; I do nothing but run from one to the other, and I see that I shall have to take a carrriage—. No one pays attention here but to the people who hide themselves in their carrriages!—On the other hand, the Council of State is a pile of drones who let their work be done by some little scamps who are bribed by our prrefect—.   There is my case!—They want to get it, my manufactory; very well, they shall have it!—and they may come to terms with my workmen, of whom there are a hundred, and who will make them change their mind with a cudgel—"

"Come, cousin," said the landscapist, "how long hast thou been here?"

"Since two years!—Ah! this business of the prefect; he will pay dear for it; I will take his life and
I will give mine at the Court of Assizes—"

"Who is the Councilor of State who presides in
that section?"

"A former journalist, who is not worth ten sols,
and who calls himself Massol!"

The two Parisians looked at each other.

"The Rapporteur?—"

"Still bigger rogue! he is a Maître des Requêtes,
prrofessor of something or other at the Sorbonne,
who has written something in a review, and for
whom I prrofess a disesteem the most prrofound—"

"Claude Vignon?" said Bixiou.

"That is he,—" replied the Southerner; "Massol
and Vignon; there you have the social rright, without rright, the Trestaillons of my prrefect."

"There is some remedy," said Léon de Lora.
"Seest thou, cousin, everything is possible in
Paris, in good as in evil, just and unjust.   Everything is done there, everything is undone there,
everything is done over again there."

"To the devil if I stay ten seconds longer—; it is
the most tedious place in Frrance."

At this moment the two cousins and Bixiou were
promenading from one end to the other of that patch
of asphalt on which, between one and two o'clock,
it is difficult not to see passing some of those personages for whom Fame puts to her mouth one or
the other of her trumpets.   Formerly, it was the
Place Royale, then the Pont Neuf, which enjoyed

this privilege, acquired to-day by the Boulevard des Italiens.

"Paris," said the landscape painter to his cousin, "is an instrument on which it is necessary to know how to play; and, if we remain here ten minutes I will give you a lesson. There, now, look," said he to him, lifting his cane, designating a couple who came out of the Passage de l'Opéra.

"What is that?" asked Gazonal.

That was an old woman with a bonnet which had remained six months in stock, with a very pretentious gown, a shawl in faded plaid, who had evidently lived for twenty years in a damp lodge, whose greatly dilated *cabas* announced a social position no higher than that of an ex-portress; next a young girl, slender and thin, whose eyes, edged with black lashes, no longer showed innocence, whose complexion betrayed much weariness, but whose face, of a pretty outline, was fresh, and whose hair should be abundant; the forehead charming and audacious, the corsage thin; in two words, a green fruit.

"That," replied Bixiou to him, "is a rat ornamented with its mother."

"A rat?—what is that?"

"This rat," said Léon, who nodded in a friendly manner to Mademoiselle Ninette, "can gain for thee thy suit."

Gazonal started, but Bixiou held him by the arm since leaving the café, for he considered his face a trifle too much inclined to redness.

"This rat, which is coming out from a rehearsal at the Opera, goes home to get a thin dinner and will come back in three hours to dress itself, if it appears this evening in the ballet, for to-day is Monday. This rat is thirteen years old; it is a rat already old. In two years from now, this creature will be worth sixty thousand francs on the Exchange; she will be nothing or everything, a great danseuse or a *marcheuse*, a famous name or a common courtesan. She has been working since she was eight years old. Such as you see her, she is worn out with fatigue, she has broken her body this morning in the dancing-class; she is coming out from a rehearsal in which evolutions are as difficult as the combinations of a Chinese puzzle; she will come back this evening. The rat is one of the elements of the Opera, for she is to the première danseuse what the little clerk is to the notary. The rat, it is hope."

"Who produces the rat?" asked Gazonal.

"The porters, the poor, the actors, the dancers," replied Bixiou. "It is only the very deepest poverty which will advise a child of eight years to deliver her feet and her joints to the hardest torment, to remain virtuous till sixteen or eighteen, entirely through speculation, and to keep at her side a horrible old woman, as you put manure around a pretty flower. You are going to see file out, one after the other, all the talent little and great, artists in blade and in flower, who elevate, to the glory of France, that monument of all time called

the Opera, a reunion of the powers, the wills, the geniuses which are only found in Paris—"

"I have already seen the Opera," replied Gazonal, with a sufficient air.

"From the top of your bench at three francs, sixty centimes," replied the landscapist, "as you have seen Paris in the Rue Croix-des-Petits-Champs,— without knowing anything about it.—What were they giving at the Opera when you went there?"

" *William Tell.*"

"Good," returned the painter; "the grand duet of Matilda should have given you pleasure. Well, what, according to your ideas, would be the first thing the cantatrice would do on leaving the stage?"

"She would—, what?—"

"Sit down to eat two mutton cutlets nearly raw, which her servant kept ready—"

"Ah! *Bouffre!*"

"La Malibran sustained herself with brandy, and it was that which killed her.—Another thing! You have seen the ballet; you are going to see it go by here, in simple morning costume, without knowing that your suit depends on some of those legs?"

"My suit?—"

"There, cousin, see, what they call a *marcheuse.*"

Léon pointed out one of those superb creatures who, at twenty-five, have already lived sixty years, of a beauty so real and so sure to be cultivated, that they do not make it obvious. She was tall, walked well, had the assured look of a dandy and her toilet recommended itself by a ruinous simplicity.

"It is Carabine," said Bixiou, who made, as did the painter, a slight salutation with his head, to which Carabine replied with a smile.

"There is another who can shipwreck your prefect."

"A *marcheuzze!* but what is that?"

"The *marcheuse* is a rat of great beauty whom her mother, false or true, has sold the day on which she could not become either the first or the second or the third figure of the dance, and when she has preferred the state of coryphée to any other, for the great reason that after having employed her youth in it she could not take any other; she would be rejected at the little theatres where dancers are required; she would not have succeeded in the three cities of France in which ballets are given; she would not have had the money or the desire to go abroad, for, know it, the great Parisian school of the dance furnishes the entire world with dancers and danseuses. Thus, for a rat to become a *marcheuse*, that is to say, *figurante* of the dance, it is necessary that she should have had some solid attachment which detained her in Paris, a rich man whom she did not love, a poor youth whom she loved too much. This one whom you have just seen pass, who will change her costume perhaps three times this evening, as a princess, as a peasant woman, as a Tyrolean, etc., has some two hundred francs a month."

"She is better dressed than our prefect's wife—"

"If you go to see her," said Bixiou, "you will

find there a femme de chambre, cook and domestic; she occupies a magnificent apartment in the Rue Saint-Georges; in short, she is, in the proportions of the French fortunes of to-day with the ancient ones, the successor to the *fille d'Opéra* of the eighteenth century. Carabine is a power, she governs at this moment Du Tillet, a banker who is very influential in the Chambers—"

"And above these two steps of the ballet what else is there?" asked Gazonal.

"Look!" said his cousin to him, showing him an elegant calash which was passing at the end of the boulevard, in the Rue de la Grange-Batelière, "there is one of the *premiers sujets* of the dance, whose name on the poster attracts all Paris, who earns sixty thousand francs a year, and who lives like a princess: the price of your manufactory would not be enough to buy the right to say good-day to her thirty times."

"Eh! well, I can say it to myself; that will not be so dear!"

"Do you see," said Bixiou to him, "on the front of the calash that handsome young man? it is a viscount who bears a fine name; it is her first gentleman of the chamber, he who conducts her business with the newspapers, who carries the words of peace or war each morning to the director of the Opera, or who occupies himself with the applause which salutes her when she comes on the stage or when she leaves it."

"This, my dear Messieurs, is the final stroke; I knew nothing at all of Paris."

"Well, at least know all that can be seen in ten minutes, in the Passage de l'Opéra. Look!" said Bixiou.

Two persons came out from the passage at this moment, a man and a woman. The woman was neither pretty nor ugly, her dress had that distinction of form, of cut and of color which reveals an artist, and the man had sufficiently the air of a singer.

"There," said Bixiou to him, "is a baritone and a *second premier sujet* of the dance. The baritone is a man of immense talent, but being only an accessory to the score, he scarcely earns as much as the dancer earns. Famous before Taglioni and the Elssler appeared, the *second sujet* has preserved for us the character dance, the Mimic; if the two others had not revealed in the dance a poetry unperceived up to that time, this one would be a talent of the first order; but she is in the second rank to-day; nevertheless, she fingers her thirty thousand francs, and has for a faithful friend a peer of France, very influential in the Chamber. Ah! see, there is a danseuse of the third order, a danseuse who would not exist were it not for the all-powerfulness of a journal. If her engagement were not renewed, the Minister would have one enemy more on his back. The corps de ballet is to the Opera the great power,—therefore, is it of the very highest tone in the higher spheres of dandyism and of politics to have relations with the dance rather than with the singing. In the orchestra, where the

habitués of the Opera congregate, these words:
'Monsieur is for the singing,' are a sort of jest."

A little man, with a commonplace face, dressed
simply, passed by.

"Finally, see there the second half of the Opera's
receipts passing; it is the tenor.   There is no longer
any poem or any music or any theatrical representation possible without a celebrated tenor, whose
voice reaches a certain note.   The tenor, it is love,
it is the voice which touches the heart, which
vibrates in the soul, and which figures for a salary
more considerable than that of a minister.   A hundred thousand francs for a throat, a hundred thousand francs for a pair of heels, these are the two
financial burdens of the Opera."

"I am stupefied," said Gazonal, "at all the hundred thousand francs which promenade themselves
around here."

"You are going to be still more so, my dear
cousin; follow us.—We are going to take Paris as
an artist takes a violoncello, and make you see how
one performs on it; in short, how one amuses one's
self in Paris."

"It is a kaleidoscope seven leagues around!"
cried Gazonal.

"Before piloting Monsieur, I ought to see Gaillard," said Bixiou.

"But Gaillard may be useful to us for the cousin."

"What is this other machine?" asked Gazonal.

"It is not a machine! it is a machinist.   Gaillard
is one of our friends who has ended by becoming

the director of a newspaper, and of whom the character, as well as the cash, recommends itself by movements comparable to those of the tides. Gaillard can contribute to help you gain your suit."

"It is lost—"

"That is just the time to gain it!" replied Bixiou.

In the house of Théodore Gaillard, then lodged in the Rue de Ménars, the valet de chambre caused the three friends to wait in a boudoir, saying to them that Monsieur was in secret conference—

"With whom?" asked Bixiou.

"With a man who is selling to him the incarceration of an unseizable debtor," replied a magnificent woman who appeared in a delicious morning toilet.

"In that case, dear Suzanne," said Bixiou, "we can enter, we—"

"Oh! the beautiful creature!" cried Gazonal.

"It is Madame Gaillard," said Léon de Lora to him, speaking in his cousin's ear. "You see, my dear fellow, the most modest woman in Paris: she had all the public; she contents herself with her husband."

"*What would you have, messeigneurs?*" said the facetious director, seeing his two friends, and imitating Frédérick Lemaître.

Théodore Gaillard, formerly a man of wit, had ended by becoming stupid and in remaining in the same surroundings, a moral phenomenon which may be observed in Paris. His principal accomplishment consisted at this time in sprinkling his conversation with quotations taken from the theatrical

22

pieces then in favor and pronounced with the accent which was given them by the celebrated actors.

"We have come to humbug," replied Léon.

"*Again, young man!*"—Odry in *Les Saltimbanques*—.

"Finally, surely, we shall have him," said Gaillard's interlocutor, summing up.

"Are you very sure of it, Père Fromenteau?" asked Gaillard; "here are eleven times that we have had him in the evening and that you have missed him in the morning."

"What would you have! I have never seen a debtor like that one; he is a locomotive; he goes to sleep in Paris and wakes up in Seine-et-Oise. He is a *combination lock*."

Seeing a smile on the lips of Gaillard, he added:

"That is said also in our *partie*. To *pinch* a man, to *lock* a man, that is to arrest him. In the judiciary police, they speak otherwise. Vidocq said to his customer: '*You are served.*' That is droller, for it means the guillotine."

Under the jog with the elbow which Bixiou gave him, Gazonal became all eyes and all ears.

"Does Monsieur grease the palm?" asked Fromenteau, in a menacing tone, although a cold one.

"It is a question of *fifty centimes*"—Odry in *Les Saltimbanques*,—replied the director, taking a hundred sous and offering them to Fromenteau.

"And for the canaille?—" replied the man.

"Which?" asked Gaillard.

"Those whom I employ," replied Fromenteau, tranquilly.

"Are there any below?" asked Bixiou.

"Yes, Monsieur," replied the spy. "There are those who give information without knowing it and without being paid for it. I put the fools and the simpletons below the canaille."

"It is often fine and clever, the canaille!" cried Léon.

"You belong, then, to the police?" asked Gazonal, looking with an unquiet curiosity at this little dry man, impassible and dressed like the third clerk of a bailiff.

"Of which do you speak?" asked Fromenteau.

"There are, then, several of them?"

"There are as many as five of them," replied Fromenteau. "The judiciary police, the chief of which was Vidocq! The secret police, the chief of which is always unknown. The political police, that of Fouché. Then that of Foreign Affairs, and that of the Château—the Emperor, Louis XVIII., etc.,—which squabbled with that of the Quay Malaquais. That finished with Monsieur Decazes. I belonged to that of Louis XVIII. ; I was with it since 1793, with that poor Contenson."

Léon de Lora, Bixiou, Gazonal and Gaillard looked at each other, all expressing the same thought: "How many men's necks has he cut?"

"Nowadays, they want to go on without us, a stupidity!" resumed, after a pause, this little man, become so terrible in a moment. "At the Prefecture,

since 1830, they want honest people; I resigned and
I have made for myself a little *tran-tran* with
arrests for debt."

"It is the right arm of the guardians of commerce," said Gaillard in Bixiou's ear; "but you can
never know which pays it the most, the debtor or
the creditor."

"The more contemptible a trade is, the more it
must be honest," said Fromenteau, sententiously:
"I am for that one who pays me the most.   You wish
to recover fifty thousand francs and you come to an
agreement with the means of action.   Give me five
hundred francs, and to-morrow morning your man
is *arrested,* for we have him *spotted* since yesterday."

"Five hundred francs for you alone?" cried Théodore Gaillard.

"Lisette has no shawl," replied the spy, without
a muscle of his face moving; "I call her Lisette
because of Béranger."

"You have a Lisette and you remain in your vocation," cried the virtuous Gazonal.

"It is so amusing!   You may talk about the
charms of fishing and the chase; to hunt men in
Paris is a much more interesting occupation."

"In fact," said Gazonal, speaking aloud to himself, "they must have great talent—"

"If I were to enumerate to you the qualities which
make a man remarkable in our *partie,*" said Fromenteau to him, his rapid glance having enabled him
to take in the whole of Gazonal, "you would think

that I was speaking of a man of genius. Do we not have to have the eyes of the lynx!—Audacity! —to enter like bombs into the houses, to accost people as if one knew them, to propose villainies which are always accepted, etc.—Memory.—Sagacity.—Invention—to find schemes rapidly conceived, never the same, for the espionage is modified according to the character and the habits of each one; it is a heavenly gift.—Finally, agility, strength, etc. All these qualities, Messieurs, are inscribed on the door of the Gymnasium Amoros as being virtues! We have to possess all these under penalty of losing the allowance of a hundred francs a month which is given to us by the state, the Rue de Jérusalem, or the Garde de Commerce.''

"And you seem to me to be a remarkable man," said Gazonal to him.

Fromenteau looked at the provincial without replying to him, without giving any sign of emotion, and went out without saluting anybody. A trait of true genius!

"Well, cousin, you have seen the police incarnated," said Léon to Gazonal.

"It has had on me the effect of a digestive," replied the honest manufacturer, while Gaillard and Bixiou were conversing with lowered voices.

"I will give you an answer this evening at Carabine's," said Gaillard aloud, reseating himself at his desk, without seeing or saluting Gazonal.

"He is an impertinent!" exclaimed the Southerner on the threshold of the door.

"His paper has twenty-two thousand subscribers," said Léon de Lora. "It is one of the five great powers of the day, and he has not in the morning the time to be polite.—"

"If we are going to the Chamber, there to arrange his lawsuit, let us take the longest road," said Léon to Bixiou.

"Words said by great men are like spoons of silver-gilt which lose their gold by use: through being repeated they lose all their brilliancy," replied Bixiou; "but where are we going?"

"Near here, to our hatter's," replied Léon.

"Bravo," cried Bixiou. "If we continue thus, perhaps we shall have an amusing day."

"Gazonal," resumed Léon, "I am going to make him *pose* for you; only, be as serious as the king on a hundred-sou piece, for you are going to see gratis a proud original, a man whose importance has made him lose his head. To-day, my dear fellow, all the world wishes to cover itself with glory, and a great many cover themselves with ridicule; from thence come living caricatures entirely new—"

"When all the world shall have glory, how can anyone be distinguished?" asked Gazonal.

"Glory?—that would be to be a fool," replied Bixiou to him. "Your cousin is decorated, I am well dressed; it is I whom people look at—"

With this observation, which may explain why the orators and other great men of politics put nothing in the button-holes of their coats in Paris, Léon

caused Gazonal to read in letters of gold the illustrious name of VITAL, SUCCESSEUR DE FINOT, FABRICANT DE CHAPEAUX—and not *Chapelier* as formerly—whose advertisements bring as much money to the newspapers as those of three sellers of pills or of burnt almonds, and who, moreover, is the author of a little brochure on the hat."

"My dear fellow," said Bixiou to Gazonal, who was showing him the splendor of the front of the shop, "Vital has forty thousand francs income."

"And he remains a hatter!" cried the Southerner, twisting Bixiou's arm with a sudden movement.

"You are going to see the man," replied Léon. "You need a hat; you are going to have one gratis."

"Monsieur Vital is not in?" asked Bixiou, who did not see anyone at the counter.

"Monsieur is correcting his proofs in his office," replied a first salesman.

"Hein! what style!" said Léon to his cousin.

Then, addressing the first salesman:

"May we speak to him without injuring his inspirations?"

"Permit those gentlemen to enter," said a voice.

It was a bourgeois voice, a voice of an eligible, a powerful voice and one with a good income.

And Vital deigned to show himself, clothed all in black, decorated with a magnificent shirt, frilled and ornamented with a diamond. The three friends perceived a young and pretty woman seated in the office, working at embroidery.

Vital is a man of from thirty to forty years of

age, of a primitive joviality restrained under the pressure of his ambitious ideas. He enjoys a medium stature, a privilege of fine organizations. Sufficiently stout, he is careful of his person; his forehead is losing its hair, but he contributes to his baldness in order to give himself the air of a man devoured by thought. You may see, by the manner in which his wife looks at him and listens to him that she believes in the genius and in the fame of her husband. Vital loves the artists, not that he has any taste for the arts, but through confraternity; for he believes himself an artist and causes this to be made evident while protesting against his title of nobility, in placing himself with a constant premeditation at an enormous distance from the arts, in order that it may be said to him: "But you have elevated the hat to the height of a science."

"Have you at last found me a hat?" said the landscape-painter.

"How, monsieur, in two weeks?" replied Vital, "and for you!—But would it be enough to find the form which would be in consonance with your physiognomy in two months? See your lithograph, there it is; I have already studied you well! I would not give myself so much trouble for a prince; but you are more, you are an artist! and you comprehend me, my dear monsieur."

"Here is one of our greatest inventors, a man who would be as grand as Jacquart if he would let himself die a little," said Bixiou, presenting Gazonal. "Our friend, a cloth manufacturer, has discovered

a means of restoring the indigo of old blue coats, and
he has wished to see you as a great phenomenon, for
you have said: '*The hat, it is the man.*' This saying has delighted Monsieur.   Ah! Vital, you have
faith! you believe in something, you have an enthusiasm for your work."

Vital listened with difficulty; he had become pale
with pleasure.

"Rise, wife!—Monsieur is a prince of science."

Madame Vital rose at her husband's gesture,
Gazonal bowed to her.

"Shall I have the honor to serve you?" resumed
Vital, with a joyous obsequiousness.

"The same price as for me," said Bixiou.

"Certainly; I ask no other honorarium than the
pleasure of being occasionally quoted by you, Messieurs! Monsieur requires a picturesque hat, in the
style of that of Monsieur Lousteau," said he, looking at Bixiou with a magisterial air.   "I will reflect
upon it."

"You give yourself a great deal of trouble," said
Gazonal to the Parisian manufacturer.

"Oh! for some persons only, for those who know
how to appreciate the cost of my cares.   Why, in
the aristocracy there is only one man who has comprehended the hat, that is the Prince de Béthune.
How is it that men do not reflect, like women, that
the hat is the first thing which attracts attention in
the dress, and why do they not think to change the
actual system, which, let us say it, is ignoble?
But the Frenchman is, of all people, the one who

persists the longest in a stupidity! I know well the difficulties, Messieurs! I do not speak of my writings on this subject, in which I believe I have approached it in the spirit of philosophy, but merely as a hat-maker. I alone have discovered the means of giving a character to the infamous head-piece which France possesses until the moment when I shall succeed in overthrowing it."

He showed the frightful hat worn to-day.

"Here is the enemy, Messieurs," he resumed. " 'To say that the most brilliant people on the earth consent to wear on their head this piece of stovepipe!' has said one of our writers—. See all the inflections which I have been able to give to these frightful lines," he added, designating one by one *his creations.* "But, although I may know how to make them appropriate to the character of each one, as you see, for here is the hat of a physician, of a grocer, of a dandy, that of an artist, of a fat man, of a thin man, it is always horrible! Hold, grasp well all my thought!"

He took a hat, low in form and with a large rim.

"Here is the former hat of Claude Vignon, a great critic, a liberal man and a good liver.—He rallied to the support of the ministry; he is appointed professor, librarian; he works only for the *Débats,* he has been made *Maître des Requêtes;* he has sixteen thousand francs allowance, he earns four thousand francs on his journal; he is decorated.—Well, then, see his new hat!"

carry out this pleasantry, had brought home with him Léon and Gazonal; Madame Nourrisson found them as serious as authors whose collaboration *does not obtain all the success that it merits.*

"Madame," said the intrepid mystifier to her, showing her a pair of women's slippers, "here is something that belonged to the Empress Joséphine."

It was quite necessary to return to Madame Nourrisson the change for her guipure lace of the Princesse de Lamballe.

"That?—" she said. "Those were made this year; see this stamp on the soles?"

"Do you not guess that these slippers are a preface," replied Léon, "although they are usually the conclusion of a romance?"

"My friend, who is here," resumed Bixiou, designating the Southerner, "in some very important family interests wishes to learn if a young person, of a good, of a wealthy house, and whom he desires to marry, has committed a fault?"

"How much will Monsieur give?" she asked, looking at Gazonal, who was no longer surprised at anything.

"A hundred francs," replied the manufacturer.

"Thanks!" said she, embellishing her refusal with a grimace that might make a baboon despair.

"What is it you want, my little Madame Nourrisson?" asked Bixiou, taking her by the waist.

"In the first place, my dear Messieurs, since I have worked for my living I have never seen anyone, either man or woman, bargaining over happiness!

And, then, see here, you are three jokers," she
went on, permitting a smile to play around her
cold lips and reinforcing it with a look chilled by
a cat-like mistrust. "If it is not a question of your
happiness, it is one of your fortune; and, in the
high station in which you are placed, there is still
less bargaining over a dot.—Come, now," said she,
assuming an affected air, "what is it all about, my
lambs?"

"Of the house of Beunier & Co.," replied Bixiou,
well content to acquire some information concerning a person who interested him.

"Oh! for that," she answered, "a louis; that is
enough—"

"And why?"

"I have all the mother's jewels; and from one
three months to another she is mighty uncomfortable, I should say so! She has all she can do to pay
me the interest on that which I have lent her. You
wish to get married over there, ninny!—" said she.
"Give me forty francs, and I will talk for more than
a hundred écus."

Gazonal showed a forty-franc piece and Madame
Nourrisson launched herself into frightful details on
the secret poverty of certain women reputed *comme
il faut*. The dealer in old clothes, enlivened by the
conversation, revealed herself. Without betraying
any name, any secret, she made the two artists
shudder in demonstrating to them that there was
very little happiness in Paris which was not established on the vacillating basis of borrowing. She

held in her secret drawers souvenirs of late grand-mothers, of living children, of deceased husbands, of dead granddaughters, framed in gold and in brilliants! She learned frightful histories in setting her customers to talk of each other, in wresting their secrets from them in moments of passion, of quarreling, of anger, and in those soothing preparations which lead up to a loan for a conclusion.

"How did you come to engage in this business?" asked Gazonal.

"For my son," said she ingenuously.

Nearly always, these dealers in second-hand clothes justify their commerce by reasons full of fine motives. Madame Nourrisson pretended to have lost several suitors, three daughters who had taken to evil, all her illusions, in fact! She displayed as being among her most valuable effects, tickets from the pawnshops to prove how many evil chances there were in her business. She gave out that she would be much embarrassed on the thirtieth proximo. There was a great deal *stolen* from her, she said.

The two artists looked at each other on hearing this word, a little too strong.

"See here, my dears, I will show you how they *do us over again!* This is not my case, but that of my opposite neighbor, Madame Mahuchet, the ladies' shoemaker. I had lent some money to a countess, a woman who has too many passions considering her income. It is all putting on airs among beautiful furniture, in a magnificent apartment! It

23

is giving receptions, it is making, as we say, a devil of a spread. She owes, then, three hundred francs to her shoemaker, and there is a dinner given, a soirée, no later than the day before yesterday. The shoemaker, who learned this through the cook, came to see me; we got excited, she wished to make a scandal; I, I said to her: 'My little Mother Mahuchet, what good will that do? to get yourself hated. It would be much better to obtain good security. *To a liar, a liar and a half!* and you only save your bile—.' She insisted upon going there; asked me to back her up; we went there. 'Madame is not at home.' 'We know it!' 'We will wait for her,' said Mother Mahuchet, 'if I have to stay here till midnight.' And we settled ourselves in the antechamber and went to talking. Ah! you should have heard the doors which opened and shut, the little footsteps, the hushed voices—. For myself, that made me uncomfortable. The guests began to arrive for dinner. You can judge of the state of affairs which this made. The countess sent her femme de chambre to wheedle the Mahuchet. 'You shall be paid to-morrow!' In short, all the humbugs!—Nothing would work. The countess, fine as a Sunday, arrived at the dining-room. My Mahuchet, who heard her, opened the door and presented herself. Bless me! on seeing a table glittering with silver—the chafing-dishes, the chandeliers, everything shining like a jewel-box—she went off like a *sodavatre* and threw her bomb-shell: 'When one spends the money of others, one should be

temperate, and not give dinner parties! To be a countess and to owe a hundred écus to a poor woman-shoemaker who has seven children!—' You can imagine what a volley she poured forth, this woman has so little education. At a word of excuse—'No funds!'—of the countess, my Mahuchet cried: 'Eh! Madame, see the silver-ware, pawn your spoons and pay me!' 'Take them yourself,' said the countess, gathering up six covers and thrusting them into her hand. We tumbled down the stairs—ah, bah! like a success!—No, in the street, the Mahuchet began to cry, for she is a good woman; she took back the covers, making her excuses: she had understood the misery of this countess, they were in white metal!—"

"She remained *uncovered*," said Léon de Lora, in whom the ancient Mistigris often reappeared.

"Ah! my dear Monsieur," said Madame Nourrisson, enlightened by this pun, "you are an artist, you make the theatre pieces; you live in the Rue du Helder, and you were with Madame Antonia; you have the knacks that I know—. Come, now, you wish to have some rarity in the grand style, Carabine, or Mousqueton, Malaga or Jenny Cadine?"

"Malaga, Carabine! it is we who have made them what they are!—" cried Léon de Lora.

"I swear to you, my dear Madame Nourrisson, that we wished solely to have the pleasure of making your acquaintance and that we desire some information as to your antecedents, to know by what descent you slipped into your trade," said Bixiou.

"I was a confidential woman in the house of a marshal of France, the Prince d'Ysembourg," she said, taking a Dorine attitude. "One morning, there came one of the most topping countesses of the Imperial Court; she wished to speak to the marshal, and secretly. I, I placed myself immediately so that I could hear. My lady melted into tears, she confided to this booby of a marshal—the Prince d'Ysembourg, this Condé of the Republic, a booby!—that her husband, who was serving in Spain, had left her without a thousand-franc note; that, if she did not have one or two immediately, her children would be without bread, she would have nothing to eat to-morrow—. My marshal, sufficiently generous at that time, drew two thousand-franc notes from his secretary. I watched this fine countess from the stairway without her being able to see me; she was laughing with a contentment that seemed so little maternal that I slipped out under the peristyle, and I heard her say in a very low voice to her footman: 'To Leroy's!' I hastened there. My materfamilias entered the shop of this famous merchant, in the Rue de Richelieu, you know—. She ordered and paid for a dress fifteen hundred francs; at that time a dress was settled for when it was ordered. Two days later she was able to appear at an ambassador's ball, adorned as a woman should be to please at the same time all the world and some one in particular. From that day, I said to myself: 'I have a business! When I shall be no longer young, I will lend money on their apparel to the great

ladies, for passion does not calculate and pays blindly.' If it is subjects for vaudeville that you are seeking, I will sell them to you—"

She went off on this tirade, in which each of the phases of her previous life had left its color, leaving Gazonal as much aghast at this confidence as at five yellow teeth which she had shown in endeavoring to smile.

"And what are we going to do?" asked Gazonal.

"Notes!—" said Bixiou, who whistled for his porter, "for I have need of money, and I will let you see what the porters are for; you think that they are to pull the cords of the front door,—they are to pull out of embarrassment vagabond people like myself, artists whom they take under their protection; thus some day, mine will have the prize Montyon."

Gazonal opened his eyes in such a manner as to make comprehendable this phrase,—an *œil-de-bœuf*.

A middle-aged man, half lackey and half office-boy, but more oily and more oiled, the hair greasy, the stomach plump, the complexion pale and damp like that of the Superior of a convent, shod with cloth slippers, clothed in a vest of blue cloth and grayish pantaloons, suddenly appeared.

"What will you have, Monsieur?—" said he, with an air which partook at once of the protector and of the subordinate.

"Ravenouillet—, his name is Ravenouillet," said Bixiou, turning toward Gazonal, "have you our bill-book?"

Ravenouillet drew from his side pocket the most glutinous note-book that Gazonal had ever seen.

"Write in it, at three months, these two notes for five hundred francs each which you will sign for me."

And Bixiou presented two notes already drawn to his order by Ravenouillet, which Ravenouillet signed on the spot, and which he put down in the greasy note-book in which his wife recorded the debts of the lodgers.

"Thanks, Ravenouillet," said Bixiou.   "Well, now, here is a box for the Vaudeville."

"Oh! my daughter will have a good time this evening," said Ravenouillet, going away.

"We are here seventy-one tenants," said Bixiou; "the average of what is owed to Ravenouillet is about six thousand francs a month, eighteen thousand francs every three months, for advances and carrying letters, without counting the rents due. It is a Providence—at thirty per cent, which we give to him without his ever having asked for anything—"

"Oh! Paris, Paris—" cried Gazonal.

"When we go away," said Bixiou, who pocketed the notes, "for I am going to take you, cousin Gazonal, to see again a comedian who is going to play gratuitously a charming scene—"

"Where?" interrupted Gazonal.

"At a usurer's—. As we go, I will relate to you the début of friend Ravenouillet in Paris."

As they passed before the porter's lodge, Gazonal

saw Mademoiselle Lucienne Ravenouillet, who was studying a solfeggio; she was a pupil of the Conservatoire; the father was reading a newspaper, and Madame Ravenouillet held in her hand letters to be sent up to the lodgers.

"Thanks, Monsieur Bixiou," said the little one.

"It is not a rat," said Léon to his cousin, "it is a chrysalis of a grasshopper."

"It appears," said Gazonal, "that the friendship of the lodge is obtained, like that of all the rest of the world, by *les loges*—the lodges—"

"Which is developed in our society!" cried Léon, charmed with the pun.

"This is the history of Ravenouillet," resumed Bixiou when the three friends found themselves on the boulevard. "In 1831, Massol, your Councilor of State, was a journalist-advocate who wished at that time only to be Keeper of the Seals, he deigned to leave Louis-Philippe on the throne; but his ambition will have to be forgiven, he was from Carcassonne. One morning he saw a young countryman enter, who said to him: 'You know me very well, *Monsu* Massol, I am the little one of your neighbor, the grocer; I have just come from down there, for they say to us that in coming here each one will find his place—' On hearing these words Massol was taken with a shudder, and said to himself that, if he had the misfortune to oblige this compatriot, who was otherwise perfectly unknown to him, the whole department would come tumbling in upon him; that he would lose a great many bell-actions,

eleven bell-cords, his carpets; that his only valet would leave him; that he would have difficulties with his landlord concerning the stairway, and that the other tenants would complain of the odor of garlic and of the commotion caused throughout the house. Therefore, he looked at this solicitor as a butcher looks at his sheep before cutting its throat; but although the peasant had received this glance or this knife-thrust, he went on in this way, as Massol told us: 'I am ambitious just like any other, and I do not wish to return to the country in any other way but rich, if I do return; for Paris is the antechamber of paradise. It is said that you who write in the journals, you make here rain and fair weather; that it is enough for you to ask to obtain no matter what from the government; but, if I have any abilities, like all of us, I know myself, I have no education; even if I had the means I would not know how to write, and that is a misfortune, for I have ideas; I do not, then, think to rival you; I judge myself, I would not succeeed; but, as you can manage anything, and as we are almost brothers, having played together during our childhood, I count on your giving me a start and your protecting me—. Oh! it is necessary; I want a situation, a place which is suitable to my means, to what I am, and where I can make my fortune—.' Massol was about to put his *pays* out of the door brutally, throwing in his face some brutal phrase, when the countryman concluded thus: 'I do not ask, then, to enter the administration, where one gets on like tortoises,

where your cousin has remained traveling comptroller for twenty years—.   No, I wish only to come out—.' 'At the theatre?—' said Massol to him, happy at this termination.   'No, I have, well enough, the gesture, the face, the memory; but there is too much pulling; I wish to make my début in the career—of a porter.' Massol kept his gravity and said to him: 'There will be still more pulling in that, but at least you will see the lodges full.' And he obtained for him, as Ravenouillet says, his first cordon.''

"I am the first," Léon said, "who has seriously occupied himself with the species *portier*. There are sharpers of morality, buffoons of vanity, modern sycophants, *septembriseurs* * caparisoned with gravity, inventors of questions palpitating with actuality which preach the emancipation of the negroes, the amelioration of petty thieves, benevolence toward liberated convicts, and who leave their porters in a state worse than that of the Irish, in prisons more frightful than dungeons, and who give them less money to live on than the state gives for a convict—. I have only done one good action in my life, that is the lodge of my porter.''

"If," continued Bixiou, "a man having built great cages, divided into a thousand apartments like the cells of a bee-hive or the cages of a menagerie, and destined to receive creatures of every species and of every avocation, if this animal in the figure of an

* *Septembriseurs*—the name given to those who took part in the massacre of September, 1792.

owner should come to consult a scientist and say to
him: 'I want an individual of the genus *bimana*
who can live in a sink full of old shoes, pestiferous
with rags, and ten feet square; I want him to live
there all his life, to sleep there, to be happy there,
to have children as pretty as Loves; that he shall
work there; that he shall do his cooking there; that
he shall promenade himself there; that he shall cultivate flowers there; that he shall sing there, and
that he shall not go out; that he shall not see clearly
there, and that he shall perceive everything that
goes on outside!—' assuredly, the scientist would
not have been able to invent the porter; it required
Paris to create him, or, if you like, the devil—"

"Parisian industry has gone still farther into the
impossible," said Gazonal, "there are the workpeople—. You do not know all the products of industry, you who display them. Our industry combats that of the continent by misfortunes as, under
the Empire, Napoléon combated Europe with regiments."

"Here we are at the house of my friend Vauvinet,
the usurer," said Bixiou. "One of the greatest
faults committed by the people who depict our manners is to repeat the old portraits. To-day, every
profession has been renewed. The grocers become
peers of France, the artists capitalize, the vaude-
villistes have incomes in Rentes. If some rare
figures remain that which they formerly were, in
general, the professions no longer have their special
costume, nor their ancient manner. If we have had

Gobseck, Gigonnet, Chaboisseau, Samanou, the last of the Romans, we are in the enjoyment to-day of Vauvinet, the good-fellow usurer, little fop who haunts the side-scenes, the lorettes, and who takes the air in a little low coupé with one horse—. Observe my man well, friend Gazonal, you are going to see the comedy of money, the cold man who wishes to give nothing, the hot man who suspects a profit; listen to him, above all.''

And, all three of them entered the second story of a house of a very fine appearance situated on the Boulevard des Italiens, and there found themselves surrounded by all the luxuries then in fashion. A young man of about twenty-eight came to meet them with an almost laughing air, for he saw Léon de Lora first. Vauvinet gave a hand-clasp, in appearance the most friendly, to Bixiou, saluted Gazonal with a cold air, and caused them to enter into a cabinet, where all the tastes of the bourgeois might be divined under the artistic appearance of the furnishing, and, despite the statuettes *à la mode*, the thousand little things appropriated to our little apartments by the modern art, which has made itself as little as the consumer. Vauvinet was gotten up, like the young people who occupy themselves with business, with an excessive care, which, for very many of them, is a species of prospectus.

"I have come to you to get some money,'' said Bixiou, laughing, presenting his note.

Vauvinet assumed a serious air which made Gazonal smile, so much difference was there between

the smiling visage and that of a discounter officially occupied.

"My dear fellow," said Vauvinet, looking at Bixiou, "I would oblige you with the greatest pleasure, but at this moment I have no money."

"Ah, bah!"

"Yes, I've given everything, you know to whom. —That poor Lousteau has associated himself for the management of a theatre with an old vaudevilliste very much protected by the minister—, Ridal; and they had to have thirty thousand francs yesterday. I am cleaned out, and so cleaned out that I have sent for some money to Cérizet to pay a hundred louis lost at lansquenet this morning, at Jenny Cadine's—"

"It must be that you are very much cleaned out not to oblige this poor Bixiou," said Léon de Lora, "for he has a very short tongue when he finds himself *by the side*—"

"But—" said Bixiou, "I cannot say anything but good of Vauvinet; he is full of good—"

"My dear fellow," resumed Vauvinet, "it would be impossible for me, even if I had the money, to discount for you, were it at fifty per cent, notes signed by your porter.—The Ravenouillet is not in demand. It is not like the Rothschild. I warn you that this endorsement is quite worn out; it will be necessary for you to invent another banking-house. Look out for an uncle! for, the friend who signs notes for us, that is no longer to be had, the positivism of the century makes horrible progress."

"I have," said Bixiou, indicating Léon's cousin, "I have Monsieur,—one of our most illustrious cloth manufacturers of the Midi, named Gazonal.—He is not very well *coiffé*," he resumed, looking at the luxuriant and upright head of hair of the provincial; "but I am going to take him to Marius, who will relieve him of this resemblance to a poodle, so injurious to his consideration and to ours."

"I do not believe much in the securities of the Midi, be it said without offence to Monsieur," replied Vauvinet, who rendered Gazonal very well content, for he was not in the least vexed at this insolence.

Gazonal, in his character of an excessively shrewd man, believed that the painter and Bixiou intended, in order to make him acquainted with Paris, to make him pay a thousand francs for the *déjeuner* of the *Café de Paris;* for the son of the Roussillon had not abandoned that prodigious suspicion which in Paris fortifies the man from the provinces.

"How would you have me have business relations at two hundred and fifty leagues from Paris, in the Pyrenees?" added Vauvinet.

"Then that is all?" replied Bixiou.

"I have twenty francs about me," said the young discounter.

"I am sorry for you," replied the joker. "I thought that you were worth a thousand francs," he added, dryly.

"You are worth a hundred thousand francs,"

replied Vauvinet, "sometimes even you are inestimable,—but I am cleaned out."

"Well," replied Bixiou, "let us say no more about it—. I would have arranged for you this evening, at the Carabine's, the best affair that you could have wished,—you know?"

Vauvinet winked in looking at Bixiou, a grimace of the horse dealers which says between themselves: "Let us not play sharp with each other."

"You no longer remember having taken me around the waist, exactly like a pretty woman, and wheedling me with looks and with words," replied Bixiou, "when you said to me: 'I will do anything for you if you can procure me at par shares of the railroad which Du Tillet and Nucingen put on the market.' Well, my dear fellow, Maxime and Nucingen are coming to Carabine's, who is receiving this evening a great many men in political life. You are losing there, my old fellow, a beautiful opportunity. Come, good day, dabbler!"

And Bixiou arose, leaving Vauvinet sufficiently unmoved in appearance, but really dissatisfied, like a man who is conscious of having committed a folly.

"My dear fellow, a moment,—" said the discounter; "if I have no money, I have credit.—If your notes are worth nothing I can keep them and give you in exchange securities in bills—. Afterwards, we can come to an arrangement about the railway shares; we will divide, in a certain proportion, the profits of this operation, and I will then make you a remittance on account of the prof—"

"No, no," replied Bixiou, "I must have some money; it is necessary that I should use my Ravenouillet—"

"Ravenouillet is otherwise very good," said Vauvinet; "he deposits in the savings-bank, he is excellent—"

"He is better than you," said Léon to him, "for he does not keep a lorette; he has no rent to pay; he does not embark in speculations fearing all the time the rise or the fall—"

"You think to amuse, great man?" replied Vauvinet, suddenly become jovial and caressing; "you have got out the quintessence of La Fontaine's fable, *The Oak and the Reed.*—Come, *Gubetta, my old confederate,*" said Vauvinet, taking Bixiou by the waist, "you must have some money? very well, I can just as well borrow three thousand francs from my friend Cérizet, instead of two thousand.—And *we will be friends, Cinna!*—Give me your two giant cabbage-leaves. If I refused you, it was because it was very hard for a man who can only carry on his poor business by depositing his securities with the Bank, to keep your Ravenouillet in his bureau drawer,—it is hard, it is very hard.—"

"And what will you take for discount?" asked Bixiou.

"Almost nothing," replied Vauvinet. "That will cost you, at three months, fifty unhappy francs—."

"As Émile Blondet said formerly, you will be my benefactor," replied Bixiou.

"Twenty per cent and interest!" said Gazonal in

Bixiou's ear, who replied to him by a great poke with his elbow in the region of the œsophagus.

"Wait," said Vauvinet, opening the drawer of his bureau; "I see here, my good fellow, an old note of five hundred which has stuck to the band and I did not know myself so rich, for I find for you a bill receivable due very soon, of four hundred and fifty. Cérizet will lend it to you without much *rebate,* and there is your sum made up.   But no joking, Bixiou?—.   Hein! this evening, I will go to Carabine's—you swear to me"

"Are we not *re*-friends?" said Bixiou, who took the five-hundred-franc bill and the note for four hundred and fifty francs; "I give you my word of honor that you will see this evening Du Tillet and a number of other people who wish to make their way, —railway, with Carabine."

Vauvinet conducted the three friends as far as the landing, wheedling Bixiou.   Bixiou remained serious until upon the threshold of the door; he was listening to Gazonal, who endeavored to enlighten him upon this operation and who proved to him that, if the confederate of Vauvinet, this Cérizet, lent him at twenty francs of discount on a note of four hundred and fifty francs it was money at forty per cent.—On the asphalt of the pavement, Bixiou froze Gazonal by the laugh of the Parisian mystifier, this silent and cold laugh, a sort of labial north-easter.

"The adjudication of the railway will be positively adjourned in the Chamber," he said; "we know it since yesterday through that *marcheuse* at whom

we have smiled.—And, if I gain this evening five or six thousand francs at lansquenet, what are seventy francs of loss for having the wherewithal to stake!"—

"Lansquenet is still one of the thousand facets of Paris as it is," resumed Léon. "Thus, cousin, we count on presenting you in the house of a duchess of the Rue Saint-Georges, where you will see the aristocracy of the lorettes and where you can gain your lawsuit. Now, it is impossible to show you with your Pyrenean hair; you have the appearance of a hedgehog; we are going to conduct you near here in the Place de la Bourse, to Marius, another of our actors—"

"Who is this new actor?"

"Here is the anecdote," replied Bixiou. "In 1800, a Toulousian named Cabot, a young peruke-maker devoured with ambition, came to Paris, and there *lifted* a shop—I adopt your slang.—This man of genius—he enjoys twenty-four thousand francs income at Libourne, where he has retired—comprehended that this common and ignoble name would never attain to fame. Monsieur de Parny, whom he served, gave him the name of Marius, infinitely superior to the Christian names of Armand and of Hippolyte, under which hid themselves the patronymic names attacked with the Cabot-disease. All the successors of Cabot are called Marius. The present Marius is Marius V.; his name is Mougin. This is the custom in many trades, as for the eau de Botot, for the ink de la Petite-Vertu. At Paris,

24

a name becomes a commercial property and ends by constituting a sort of sign of nobility. Marius, who moreover has pupils, has created, he says, the first school of coiffure in the world."

"I have already seen, in traveling through France," said Gazonal, "a number of signs on which might be read these words: 'SUCH A ONE, Pupil of Marius.'"

"These pupils must wash their hands after each curling and dressing," replied Bixiou; "but Marius does not admit them indiscriminately; they must have handsome hands and not be ugly. The most remarkable in address, in appearance, serve their customers in their own houses; they return very much fatigued. Marius himself only leaves his establishment for women with titles; he has a cabriolet and a groom."

"But this is after all only a *merlan!* (journeyman hair-dresser)," cried Gazonal, indignantly.

"*Merlan!*" replied Bixiou; "remember that he is a captain in the National Guard and that he is decorated for having been the first to leap a barricade in 1832."

"Take care; this is neither a coiffure nor a perruquier, this is a director of salons of coiffure," said Léon, as they mounted a stairway with a crystal balustrade, with a mahogany rail, and the steps of which were covered with a sumptuous carpet.

"Ah, there! do not go and compromise us," said Bixiou to Gazonal: "In the antechamber, you will

find lackeys who will relieve you of your coat, your hat, to brush them, and who will accompany you to the door of one of the salons de coiffure, to open and shut it. It is well to tell you this, my friend Gazonal," added Bixiou, slyly, "for you might cry out: 'Help, thieves!'"

"These salons," said Léon, "are three boudoirs in which the director has assembled all the inventions of modern luxury. At the windows are lambrequins; everywhere are jardinières, luxurious divans, on which you can await your turn while reading the papers, when all the attendants are occupied. When you enter you may feel for your purse, thinking that at least five francs will be demanded of you; but there is extracted from every species of pocket only ten sous for a *frisure*, and twenty sous for a *coiffure* with cutting the hair. Elegant dressing-tables are interspersed among the jardinières, and the water flows from them through brass taps. Everywhere enormous mirrors reflect the figures. Therefore, do not show any astonishment. When the *client*—such is the elegant word substituted by Marius for the ignoble word *customer* —when the client appears on the threshold, Marius gives him a glance and he is gauged,—for him, you are *a head* more or less worthy of his attention. For Marius, there are no longer any men, there are only *heads*."

"We are going to let you hear Marius in all the tones of his gamut," said Bixiou, "if you know how to imitate our methods."

As soon as Gazonal appeared, the rapid glance of Marius was favorable to him, and he exclaimed:

"Regulus! that head for you! clip it first with the little scissors."

"Pardon," said Gazonal to the pupil, at a gesture from Bixiou, "I desire to have my head dressed by Monsieur Marius himself."

Marius, very much flattered by this preference, came forward, leaving the head on which he was operating.

"I am at your service; I am finishing, do not be uneasy; my pupil will prepare you; I alone, I will decide on the cut."

Marius, a little pock-marked man, the hair frizzled like that of Rubini, black as jet, and dressed all in black with ruffles, the jabot of his shirt ornamented with a diamond, then recognized Bixiou, whom he saluted as a power equal to his own.

"It is an ordinary head," he said to Léon, indicating the gentleman with whom he was then occupied, "a grocer!—. What will you have! if one were occupied with nothing but art, one would die in the Bicêtre, mad!—"

And he returned with an inimitable gesture to his client, after having said to Regulus:

"Attend to Monsieur; he is evidently an artist."

"A journalist," said Bixiou.

At this word, Marius gave two or three touches with the comb to the commonplace head, and threw himself on Gazonal, taking Regulus by the arm at

the moment when he was about to commence operations with his little scissors.

"I will take charge of Monsieur.—See, Monsieur,"
said he to the grocer, "look at yourself in the large
mirror, if the mirror will permit.—Ossian!"

The lackey entered and took possession of the
client to dress him.

"You will pay the cashier, Monsieur," said
Marius to the stupefied customer, who had already
produced his purse.

"Is it very advantageous, my dear fellow, to proceed with this operation of the little scissors?" said
Bixiou.

"No head comes to me until it has been cleansed,"
replied the illustrious coiffeur; "but for you, I will do
that of Monsieur altogether. My pupils make the
preliminary sketch, for I do not attend to that. The
phrase of all the world is yours: 'To be *coiffé* by
Marius!' I can only give the finishing touch.—On
what journal is Monsieur engaged?"

"In your place, I would have three or four Mari-
uses," said Gazonal.

"Ah! Monsieur, I see, is a feuilletonist?" said
Marius. "Alas! in hairdressing, in which one is
obliged to act personally, it is impossible—.
Pardon!"

He left Gazonal to go and oversee Régulus, who
was preparing a newly-arrived head. By striking
his tongue against the palate he produced a little
disapproving sound which might be translated by
"titt titt, titt!"

"Come, bon Dieu! that is not square enough; your scissors are cutting jaggedly—. Wait—see! Régulus, it is not a question of clipping poodles, but of men who have their own character; and, if you continue to look at the ceiling instead of dividing yourself between the mirror and the face, you will dishonor *my house.*"

"You are severe, Monsieur Marius."

"I owe to them the secrets of the art—"

"It is, then, an art?" said Gazonal.

Marius, indignant, looked at Gazonal in the mirror and stood motionless, the comb in one hand, the scissors in the other.

"Monsieur, you speak about it like a—child! and yet, by your accent, you appear to be of the South, the land of men of genius."

"Yes, I know that it requires a sort of taste," replied Gazonal.

"Oh! keep silent, Monsieur! I expected better things of you. That is to say that a coiffeur, I do not say a good coiffeur, for one is or one is not a coiffeur,—a coiffeur,—it is more difficult to find— than—, what is it that I can best say?—than a, I do not know what, a minister—keep your place—no, for one cannot judge of the value of a minister, the streets are full of ministers—. A Paganini?—no, that is not enough!—A coiffeur, Monsieur, a man who divines your soul and your habits in order to arrange your hair according to your physiognomy, it is necessary for him to have that which constitutes a philosopher. And the women, then!—. Ah!

the women appreciate us; they know what we are
worth to them,—it is we who bring the conquest
which they wish to make the day on which they
have their hair arranged to carry off a victory;—
that it to say that a coiffeur, one does not know
what he is. Hold, I who speak to you, I am nearly
that which might be found of—, without praising
myself, I am known—. Eh! well, no, I find that
there should be something better—. The execution, that is the thing! Ah! if the women would
only give me *carte blanche,* if I could execute all
the ideas that come to me!—for I have, do you see,
an infernal imagination!—but the women do not
lend themselves to it; they have their plans, they
will stick you their fingers or their comb, when you
have gone, into our delicious edifices, which should
remain grave and reserved, for our works, Monsieur,
only endure for a few hours—. A great coiffeur,
eh! that would be something like Carême and Ves-
tris, in their parts—. The head this way, there,
if you please, *I am doing the faces;* good.—Our profession is spoiled by the bunglers who comprehend
neither their epoch nor their art—. There are
dealers in wigs and in washes to make the hair
grow,—they see in it only so many bottles to sell
you!—that is pitiful!—that is business. These
miserables cut the hair or they dress it anyway
they can!—. I, when I arrived here from Toulouse,
I entertained the ambition to succeed to the great
Marius, to be a true Marius, and to illustrate the
name, in myself alone, more than the four others.

I said to myself, 'To conquer or die'—There, hold
yourself straight, I am about to finish you off.—
It was I who, first, employed elegance. I have rendered my salons an object of curiosity. I disdain
advertising, and that which advertising costs, I
will put it, Monsieur, in comfort, in embellishment.
Next year, I will have in a little salon a quartette;
they will furnish music, and of the best. Yes, it
is necessary to charm the weariness of those who
are having their hair dressed. I do not conceal
from myself the discomforts of the operation.—Look
at yourself.—To have one's hair dressed, it is
fatiguing, perhaps as much so as to *pose* for one's
portrait; and Monsieur knows perhaps that the
famous Monsieur de Humboldt—I knew how to
make the most of the little hair that America had
left him; science has this in common with the
savage, that it scalps its man very well—this illustrious scientist has said that after the pain of being
hanged—*se faire pendre*—, there was that of going
to be painted—*se faire peindre;*—but, according to
certain women, I should place that of having the
hair dressed before that of being painted. Well,
Monsieur, I wish that people might come to have
their hair dressed for pleasure.—You have a lock of
hair which should be kept in place.—A Jew proposed to me Italian cantatrices who, between the
acts, should attend to the hair of the young men of
forty; but they are all to be found in the condition
of young girls at the Conservatoire, of teachers of
the piano in the Rue Montmartre. There you are,

Monsieur, dressed as a man of talent should be.—
Ossian," said he to his lackey in livery, "brush
Monsieur and show him out.—Whose turn next?"
he added with pride, looking at the persons who
were waiting.

"Do not laugh, Gazonal," said Léon to his cousin
as they reached the bottom of the stairway, from
which his eye wandered over the Place de la
Bourse, "I see down there one of our great men,—you
will be able to compare his speech with that of this
workman, and you can tell me, after having heard
him, which of these two is the more original."

"Do not laugh, Gazonal," said Bixiou, repeating
facetiously Léon's intonation.   "In what do you
think Marius is occupied?"

"In hair-dressing."

"He has acquired," replied Bixiou, "the monopoly of the sale of hair in bulk, as any dealer in provisions who comes to sell us a dish for an écu
claims for himself that of the sale of truffles; he discounts the paper of his business; he lends on security to his clients when they are embarrassed; he
deals in annuities, he gambles at the Bourse; he is
a shareholder in all the fashion journals; finally, he
sells, through a druggist, an infamous remedy
which, for his share, gives him thirty thousand
francs a year, and which costs a hundred thousand
francs in advertising."

"Is it possible?" cried Gazonal.

"Retain this in your memory," said Bixiou,
gravely.   "In Paris, there is no small business;

everything enlarges itself, from the sale of rags up to that of matches. The lemonade-seller who, with a napkin under his arm, sees you enter his shop, may have an income of fifty thousand francs; a waiter in a restaurant is an eligible elector, and such a man whom you would take for a very poor one, to see him passing in the street, carries in his waistcoat a hundred thousand francs' worth of diamonds to have them mounted, and does not steal them—''

The three inseparables, for this day at least, went along under the direction of the landscape-painter in such a manner that they ran against a man of about forty, wearing a decoration, who came from the boulevard by the Rue Neuve-Vivienne.

"Well," said Léon, "what are you dreaming of, my dear Dubourdieu? of what fine symbolic composition?—My dear cousin, I have the pleasure of presenting to you our illustrious painter Dubourdieu, not less celebrated by his talent than by his humanitarian convictions.—Dubourdieu, my cousin Palafox!"

Dubourdieu, a little man with a pale complexion, with a melancholy blue eye, slightly saluted Gazonal, who bowed before the man of genius.

"You have then nominated Stidmann in the place of—?"

"What would you have! I was not in it," replied the great landscapist.

"You bring the Academy into disesteem," replied the painter. "To choose such a man, I do not wish to speak evil of him, but he makes it a

trade!—. To what point would you conduct the first of the arts, that of which the works are the most durable, which portrays the nations after the world has lost all trace of them, even their memory, —which consecrates the great men? It is a priesthood, sculpture; it resumes the thoughts of an epoch, and you want to recruit it with a maker of images and of chimneys, an ornamentalist, one of the hawkers in the Temple! Ah! as Chamfort said, it is necessary to commence the day by swallowing a viper every morning in order to support life in Paris.—At least, art remains to us; we cannot be hindered from cultivating it."

"And then, my dear fellow, you have a consolation which few artists possess, the future is yours," said Bixiou. "When the world shall be converted to our doctrine, you will be at the head of your art, for you bring to it ideas which will be comprehended when they shall have been generalized! In fifty years from now you will be for all the world what you are now only for a few, a great man! Only, it is a question of going that far!"

"I am going," replied the artist, whose countenance dilated as does that of a man whose hobby is flattered, "to finish the allegorical figure of Harmony, and if you will come to see it you will readily comprehend how it is that I have been able to spend two years upon it. There is in it everything! At the very first glance, you will perceive the destiny of the globe. The queen holds a pastoral staff in one hand, symbol of the aggrandizement

of the races useful to mankind; she wears on her head the liberty cap, her breasts are sextuple in the Egyptian fashion, for the Egyptians anticipated Fourier; her feet rest upon two joined hands which embrace the globe as the sign of the fraternity of the human races; she tramples upon cannon, broken to signify the abolition of war, and I have endeavored to make her express the serenity of triumphant agriculture.—I have, moreover, placed near her an enormous curled colewort which, according to our master, is the image of concord. Oh! it is not one of the least of Fourier's titles to veneration that he has restored meanings to plants, he has re-united all things in creation by the reciprocal signification of things and also by their special language. In a hundred years, the world will be much greater than it is—"

"And how, Monsieur, will that be done?" said Gazonal, stupefied to hear a man speak in this manner outside of an insane asylum.

"By the extent of production. If one were willing to apply THE SYSTEM, it would not be impossible to react upon the stars—"

"And what would then become of painting?" asked Gazonal.

"It would be greater."

"And would we have greater eyes?" said Gazonal, looking at his two friends with a significant air.

"Man would become that which he was before his degeneracy; our men of six feet would then be dwarfs—"

"Your picture," said Léon, "is it finished?"

"Entirely finished," replied Dubourdieu. "I have endeavored to see Hiclar to have him compose a symphony; I would that in seeing this composition one should hear music like Beethoven's which should develop the ideas expressed in it in order to bring them to the level of intelligent comprehension by two methods. Ah! if the government would lend me one of the halls of the Louvre—"

"But I will speak of it, if you wish, for nothing should be neglected to attract attention—"

"Oh! my friends are preparing some articles, but I am afraid that they will go too far—"

"Bah!" said Bixiou, "they will not go so far as the future—"

Dubourdieu looked at Bixiou askance, and continued on his way.

"But he is crazy," said Gazonal; "it is the moon that guides him."

"He has the hand, he has the knowledge,—" said Léon; "but Fourierism has killed him. You may see there, cousin, one of the effects of ambition on artists. Too often, at Paris, in the desire to arrive more quickly than by the natural way at that celebrity which is for them fortune, the artists borrow wings from circumstances; they think to make themselves greater in making themselves the men of one thing, in becoming the sustainers of a system, and they hope to change a clique into a public. Such a one is Republican, such another was Saint-Simonian, such a one is aristocratic, such a one is

Catholic, such a one just medium, such a one mediæval, or German, by deliberate choice. But, if
the opinion does not give the talent, it always ruins
it; witness the poor fellow whom we have just seen.
The opinion of an artist should be the faith in his
works,—and his only means of success, work, when
nature has given him the sacred fire."

"Let us escape," said Bixiou, "Léon is moraliz-
ing."

"And this man acts in good faith?" exclaimed
Gazonal, still stupefied.

"In very good faith," replied Bixiou; "as sincere
as was just now the king of the *merlans.*"

"He is crazy!" said Gazonal.

"And he is not the only one whom Fourier's ideas
have rendered crazy," said Bixiou. "You know
nothing of Paris. Ask of it a hundred thousand
francs to realize the most useful idea for the human
species, to try something like the steam engine,
you will die there like Salomon de Caus, in the
Bicêtre; but, if it is a question of a paradox, you
will let yourself be killed for it, you and your
fortune. Well, here, it is with systems as it is
with things. The impossible publications brought
out here have devoured millions within the last
fifteen years. That which renders your case so
difficult to gain is that you are right, and that
there are, according to you, secret reasons for the
prefect."

"Do you imagine that when he has once comprehended the moral aspect of Paris, a man of

intelligence could live elsewhere?" said Léon to his cousin.

"If we take Gazonal to the Mère Fontaine," said Bixiou, who made a sign to a closed public coach to come forward, "that would be to pass from the severe to the fantastic?—Coachman, Rue Vieille-du-Temple."

And they all three rolled away in the direction of the Marais.

"What are you going to show me?" asked Gazonal.

"The proof of that which Bixiou said to you," replied Léon, "by showing you a woman who makes twenty thousand francs a year by exploiting an idea."

"A fortune-teller!" said Bixiou, who could not refrain from interpreting as an interrogation the Southerner's air. "Madame Fontaine passes, among those who seek to know the future, for being wiser than was the late Mademoiselle Lenormand."

"She ought to be very rich!" exclaimed Gazonal.

"She has been the victim of her idea, as long as the lottery existed," replied Bixiou; "for, at Paris, there are no great receipts without great expenses. All the strong heads come to grief in this way, as if to give a safety-valve to their steam. All those who earn a great deal of money have vices or fancies, doubtless to establish an equilibrium."

"And now that the lottery is abolished?—" asked Gazonal.

"Well, she has a nephew for whom she saves."

Once arrived, the three friends perceived, in one of the oldest houses of this street, a staircase with shaky steps, having the upright of each step rough with mud, which conducted them, in the half-light and through an evil odor peculiar to houses in alleys, up to the third floor, to a door which a design alone could justly render; literature would lose too many nights in endeavoring to paint it suitably.

An old woman, in harmony with the door, and who, perhaps, was the door animated, introduced the three friends into a room serving as antechamber, where, notwithstanding the warm atmosphere which flooded the streets of Paris, they felt the icy cold of the most profound crypts. There came into it a damp air from an interior court-yard which resembled a vast breathing-hole of a dungeon, the daylight was gray, and on the sill of the window was a little garden full of unhealthy plants. In this room, plastered with a greasy and sooty substance, the chairs, the table, everything had a miserable air. The floor sweated like a water-cooler. In short, the least accessory was here in harmony with the frightful old woman with a hooked nose, a pale face, and clothed in decent rags, who told the consultors to seat themselves, informing them that only one at a time could go in to see MADAME.

Gazonal, affecting intrepidity, entered bravely and found himself before one of those women forgotten by Death, who, doubtless, forgets them purposely in order to leave some exemplars of himself among the living. It was a dried face, in which

glittered two gray eyes of a fatiguing immobility;
an indented nose, smeared with tobacco; with two
small bundles of bones very well covered by muscles
sufficiently like them and which, under the pretext
of being hands, were nonchalantly shuffling the
cards, like a machine, the movement of which is
about to stop. The body, a species of broom-
handle, decently covered with a gown, enjoyed all
the advantages of still life; it did not move in the
least. Over the forehead rose a head-dress of black
velvet. Madame Fontaine, it was a real woman,
had a black hen at her right, and at her left an immense toad called Astaroth, which Gazonal did not
see at first.

The toad, of surprising dimensions, was less terrifying in himself than by two topazes, large as fifty-
centime pieces and which threw two lights like a
lamp. It is impossible to sustain this look. As
was said by the late Lassailly, who, lying out in the
country, wished to get the best of a toad by which
he was fascinated, the toad is an unexplained being.
Perhaps the animal creation, man included, is
summed up in him; for, said Lassailly, the toad lives
indefinitely; and, as is known, it is the one of all
created animals whose marriage endures the longest.

The black hen had her cage at two steps from the
table, which was covered with a green cloth, and
reached it by a board which served as a drawbridge
between the cage and the table.

When this woman, the most unreal of the creatures which furnished this Hoffmannesque den,

25

said to Gazonal "Cut!—" the honest manufacturer felt an involuntary shudder. What renders these creatures so formidable, is the importance of that which we wish to know. One wishes to buy from them hope, and they know it very well.

The grotto of this sibyl was much more sombre than the antechamber, the color of the paper could not be distinguished. The ceiling, blackened by smoke, far from reflecting the little light which came through the window obstructed by a meagre and pale vegetation, absorbed the greater part of it; but this half-light lit fully the table at which the sorceress was seated. This table, the arm-chair of the old woman and that in which Gazonal sat composed all the furniture of this little apartment, cut in two by a loft, in which doubtless Madame Fontaine slept. Through a little door partly opened, Gazonal heard a peculiar murmur of a pot boiling over the fire. This sound of cooking, accompanied with a composite odor in which preponderated that of a sink, mingled incongruously the ideas of the necessities of actual life with the ideas of a supernatural power. It was disgust in curiosity. Gazonal perceived a step of white wood, the last doubtless of the interior stairway which led to the loft. He took in all these details with one glance, and he was nauseated. It was frightful in a very different way from the recitals of the romancers and the scenes in the German dramas; it was of a suffocating veracity. A heaviness that induced vertigo disengaged itself from the air, the obscurity

ended by irritating the nerves. When the South-erner, stimulated by a species of fatuity, looked at the toad, he felt something like the heat of an emetic in the pit of his stomach, in experiencing a terror similar enough to that of a criminal before the gendarme. He endeavored to recomfort himself by examining Madame Fontaine, but he encountered two eyes almost white, the motionless and freezing eyeballs of which were to him insupportable. The silence then became frightful.

"What will you have, Monsieur," said Madame Fontaine to Gazonal, "the deal of five francs, the deal of ten francs, or the grand deal?"

"The deal of five francs is already sufficiently dear," replied the Southerner, who was making un-heard-of efforts within himself not to allow himself to be affected by his surroundings. At the moment when Gazonal was endeavoring to gather himself together, an infernal voice made him leap in his chair: the black hen cackled.

"Go away, my daughter, go away; Monsieur does not wish to expend more than five francs."

And the hen seemed to have comprehended her mistress, for, after having come to within a step of the cards, she returned gravely to her place.

"What flower do you like?" asked the old woman, in a voice made hoarse by the humors which inces-santly ascended and descended in her bronchial tubes.

"The rose."

"What color do you like the best?"

"Blue."

"What animal do you prefer?"

"The horse.   Why these questions?" asked Gazonal in his turn.

"Man is connected with all forms by his anterior states," said she, sententiously; "from these come his instincts, and his instincts dominate his destiny. —What do you eat with the most pleasure? fish, game, cereals, butchers' meat, sweets, vegetables or fruits?"

"Game."

"In what month were you born?"

"September."

"Put out your hand."

Madame Fontaine studied very attentively the lines in the hand which was presented to her.   All this was done seriously, without any premeditation of sorcery, and with a simplicity which a notary would have assumed in inquiring the intentions of a client before drawing up a deed.   When the cards were sufficiently shuffled, she requested Gazonal to cut them, and to make himself three packs.   She took the packs, spread them out one above the other, examined them as a player examines the thirty-six numbers of the roulette before risking his stake. Gazonal felt his bones chilled, he no longer knew where he was; but his astonishment mounted higher and higher as this frightful old woman in a green capote, greasy and flat, of which the false elevation showed much more of black ribbons than of hair, frizzled into points of interrogation, went on to retail to him in her voice charged with phlegm all the

particulars, even the most secret, of his former life, recounted to him his tastes, his habits, his character, even the ideas of his childhood; all that could have had influence upon him, his intended marriage, why it had failed, with whom, the exact description of the woman whom he had loved, and finally, from what country he had come, his lawsuit, etc.

Gazonal believed at first in a mystification prepared by his cousin; but the absurdity of this conspiracy revealed itself to him as soon as the idea presented itself, and he rested open-mouthed before this power truly infernal, the incarnation of which borrows from humanity that which, in all times, the imagination of painters and poets has regarded as the most frightful thing,—an atrocious little old woman, short-winded, toothless, with cold lips, with a flat nose, with white eyes. The eyeball of Madame Fontaine had become animated, there passed into it a ray sprung from the profundities of the future or of hell. Gazonal asked mechanically, in interrupting the old woman, of what use were the toad and the hen.

"To be able to predict the future. The *consultor* himself throws some grains at hazard on the cards, Cleopatra comes to pick them up; Astaroth drags himself over to seek his nourishment which the client offers him, and these two admirable intelligences are never deceived: would you wish to see them at work, you will know your future? It is a hundred francs."

Gazonal, frightened at the look of Astaroth,

precipitated himself into the antechamber, after having saluted the terrible Madame Fontaine. He was all wet, and as if under the infernal incubation of the evil spirit.

"Let us go!—" he said to the two artists. "Have you ever consulted this sorceress?"

"I do nothing important without making Astaroth speak," said Léon, "and I have always been recompensed."

"I am waiting for the honest fortune which Cleopatra has promised me," said Bixiou.

"I am in a fever," cried the Southerner; "if I believe in what you tell me, I should then believe in sorcery, in a supernatural power?"

"That can only be natural," replied Bixiou. "The third of the lorettes, a quarter of the statesmen, half the artists consult Madame Fontaine, and a minister is known to whom she served as an Egeria."

"Did she tell you your future?" asked Léon.

"No, I had enough of it with my past. But, if she can, with the aid of her frightful collaborators, predict the future," said Gazonal, seized with an idea, "how is it that she loses at the lottery?"

"Ah! there you put your finger upon one of the greatest mysteries of the occult sciences," replied Léon. "As soon as that species of interior mirror in which is reflected for them the future or the past becomes obscure under the breath of a personal sentiment, of any idea whatever foreign to the active power which they exercise, sorcerers or sorceresses no longer see anything, in the same way that an

artist who sullies art by a political or systematic combination loses his talent. It is not so long ago that a man endowed with a gift of divination by the cards, a rival of Madame Fontaine, and who was addicted to criminal practices, was not able to cut the cards for himself and to foresee that he would be arrested, judged and condemned in the Court of Assizes. Madame Fontaine, who predicts the future eight times out of ten, has never been able to foretell that she would lose her stake in the lottery."

"It is so in magnetism," observed Bixiou. "No one is able to magnetize himself."

"Good! now for magnetism!" cried Gazonal. "Ah, there! you are then acquainted with everything?—"

"Friend Gazonal," replied Bixiou, gravely, "in order to be able to laugh at everything, it is necessary to be acquainted with everything. As for myself, I have been in Paris since my childhood, and my pencil enables me to live here by ridicule, five caricatures a month—. I thus very often mock at an idea in which I have faith!"

"Let us go on to other exercises," said Léon; "let us go to the Chamber, and we will arrange the cousin's affair."

"This," said Bixiou, imitating Odry and Gaillard, "is in the realms of high comedy, for we will make the first orator whom we meet in the audience-hall *pose* for us, and you will recognize there as everywhere else the Parisian language, which has never but two rhythms: interest and vanity."

As they took their carriage again, Léon perceived in a cabriolet which passed rapidly a man, to whom, with a sign of the hand, he communicated his desire to speak a word to him.

"It is Publicola Masson," said Léon to Bixiou; "I am going to ask him for a sitting this evening, at five o'clock, after the Chamber. The cousin will have the most curious of all the originals—"

"Who is it?" asked Gazonal while Léon was speaking to Publicola Masson.

"A pedicure, author of a treatise on *Corporistique,* who will treat your corns by subscription, and who, if the Republicans triumph in the next six months, will certainly become immortal."

"In a carriage?" cried Gazonal.

"But, friend Gazonal, it is only the millionaires who have sufficient leisure to go on foot in Paris."

"To the Chamber," cried Léon to the coachman.

"Which one, Monsieur?"

"Of Deputies," replied Léon, after exchanging a smile with Bixiou.

"Paris begins to confound me," said Gazonal.

"In order to make you acquainted with its immensity, moral, political and literary, we are doing at this moment like the Roman cicerone, who shows to you at St. Peter's the thumb of the statue which you thought of the size of life; you find it a foot long. You have not yet measured one of the great toes of Paris!—"

"And notice, Cousin Gazonal, that we take what we meet; we are not making a selection."

"This evening, you will sup as they used to feast with Belshazzar, and you will see our Paris, intimately, playing at lansquenet, and risking a hundred thousand francs on a stake, without winking."

A quarter of an hour later, the coach stopped at the foot of the steps to the Chamber of Deputies, at that end of the Pont de la Concorde which leads to discord.

"I thought the Chamber unattainable?—" said the Southerner, surprised to find himself in the middle of the great *Salle des Pas Perdus.*

"That is according to circumstances," replied Bixiou; "materially speaking, it costs thirty sous for carriage hire; politically, one expends something more. The swallows think, says a poet, that the Arc de Triomphe de l'Étoile was built for them; we think, we artists, that this monument here has been built to compensate us for the deficiencies of the Théâtre-Français and to make us laugh; but these comedians cost a much higher price, and do not always give us the worth of our money."

"Let us then see the Chamber!—" repeated Gazonal.

And he strode around the hall, in which there happened to be at this moment some ten persons, looking at everything with an air which Bixiou engraved in his memory for one of those celebrated caricatures in which he contested the supremacy with Gavarni.

Léon went to speak with one of the doorkeepers who came and went constantly from this hall into

that of the sittings, with which it communicated by
the corridor in which were stationed the stenogra-
pher of the *Moniteur* and some persons attached to
the Chamber.

"As to the minister," replied the doorkeeper to
Léon at the moment when Gazonal approached them,
"he is there; but I do not know if Monsieur Giraud
is still there; I will go and see—"

When the doorkeeper opened one of the wings
of the swing door by which entered only the
deputies, the ministers or the commissioners from
the king, Gazonal saw come out a man who
appeared to him still young, although he was forty-
eight years of age, and to whom the doorkeeper
pointed out Léon de Lora.

"Ah, you are here!" said he, giving a grasp of the
hand to Léon and to Bixiou. "Ah! you rogues!
what are you doing here in the sanctuary of Law?"

"*Parbleu!* we come here to learn to talk nonsense," said Bixiou; "without that, one would get
rusty."

"Let us then go into the garden," replied the
young man, not thinking that the Southerner was of
the company.

On seeing this unknown well dressed, all in black,
and without any decoration, Gazonal did not know
in what political category to classify him, but he
followed him into the garden adjoining the hall and
which extends along the quay formerly called Quai
Napoléon. Once in the garden, the ci-devant young
man gave utterance to a laugh which he had been

suppressing since his entrance into the *Salle des Pas Perdus.*

"What is it that amuses you?—" said Léon de Lora to him.

"My dear friend, in order to be able to establish the sincerity of the constitutional government, we are compelled to utter frightful falsehoods with an incredible assurance. But, for myself, I work by the day. If there are days in which I lie like a programme, there are others in which I cannot be serious. This is my day of hilarity. Now, at this moment, the head of the cabinet, summoned by the opposition to reveal diplomatic secrets which it would refuse to reveal if it itself were the ministry, is in the act of going through his exercises in the tribune; and, as he is an honest man, as he does not lie on his own account, he whispered to me before mounting to the assault: 'I do not know what to retail to them!—' When I saw him there, I had a wild desire to laugh, and I came out, for you cannot laugh on the bench of the ministers, where my youthfulness sometimes returns to me tempestuously."

"At last!" cried Gazonal, "I find an honest man in Paris! You must be a very superior man!" said he, looking at the unknown.

"Ah, now! who is monsieur?" said the ci-devant young man, examining Gazonal.

"My cousin," replied Léon, quickly. "I answer for his silence and for his honesty as for my own. It is he who brings us here, for he has an

administrative process which depends upon your minister; his prefect wishes quite simply to ruin him, and we have come to see you to hinder the Council of State from consummating an injustice—"

"Who is the *Rapporteur?*—"

"Massol."

"Good!"

"And our friend Giraud and Claude Vignon are in the section," said Bixiou.

"Say a word to them, and they will come this evening to Carabine's, where Du Tillet is giving a fête under pretext of the railways, for they are robbing more than ever now on the roads," added Léon.

"Ah, there! but this is in the Pyrenees?—" asked the young man, suddenly become serious.

"Yes," said Gazonal.

"And you did not vote for us in the elections?—" said the statesman, looking at Gazonal.

"No; but, after what you have just said before me, you have corrupted me: on the word of a commandant in the National Guard, I will cause your candidate to be nominated—"

"Well, will you still guarantee your cousin?—" asked the young man of Léon.

"We will form him,—" said Bixiou, in a profoundly funny tone.

"Well, I will see—," said this personage, leaving his friends and returning hastily into the Chamber.

"Well, now, who is that?" asked Gazonal.

"Well, the Comte de Rastignac, the minister of the department in which is your case—"

"A minister!—it is no more than that?—"

"But he is an old friend of ours. Has three hundred thousand livres income; he is peer of France, the king has made him count; he is the son-in-law of Nucingen, and he is one of the two or three statesmen to whom the Revolution of July gave birth; but power wearies him sometimes and he comes to laugh with us—"

"Ah, there! you did not tell us that you were in the opposition down there?—" said Léon, taking Gazonal by the arm. "Are you stupid? Whether there is a deputy the more or the less in the Left or in the Right, will that furnish you with better cloths?"

"We are for others—"

"Let them alone," said Bixiou, quite as comically as Monrose would have said it; "they have Providence on their side; he will bring them out all right without you and despite themselves—. A manufacturer should be a fatalist."

"Good! there is Maxime with Canalis and Giraud!" cried Léon.

"Come, friend Gazonal, the promised actors arrive on the stage," said Bixiou to him.

And all three of them moved toward the persons indicated, who seemed to be sufficiently disengaged.

"Have they sent you out to take a walk, that you go about like that?" said Bixiou to Giraud.

"No: while they are voting on the secret ballot," replied Giraud, "we came out to take the air—"

"And how did the chief of the Cabinet acquit himself?"—

"He was magnificent!" said Canalis.

"Magnificent!" repeated Giraud.

"Magnificent!" said Maxime.

"Well, now! the Left, the Right, the Centre, are unanimous?"

"We have each of us a different idea," observed Maxime de Trailles.

Maxime was a ministerial deputy.

"Yes," replied Canalis, laughing.

Although Canalis had already been a minister, he was sitting at this period in the neighborhood of the Right.

"Ah! you have just had a fine triumph!" said Maxime to Canalis, "for it is you who forced the minister to mount the tribune."

"And to lie like a charlatan," replied Canalis.

' A fine victory!" said the honest Giraud. "In his place, what would you have done?"

"I would have lied."

"That is not called lying," said Maxime de Trailles, "that is called covering the crown."

And he led Canalis some paces away.

"He is a really fine orator!" said Léon to Giraud, indicating Canalis.

"Yes and no," replied the Councillor of State; "he is hollow, he is sonorous; it is rather an artist in words than an orator. In fact, it is a fine instrument, but it is not music; thus he has not and never will have *the ear of the Chamber*. He believes

himself necessary to France; but in no case can he ever be *the man of the situation.*"

Canalis and Maxime returned to the group at the moment when Giraud, deputy of the Left Centre, had pronounced this verdict. Maxime took Giraud by the arm and led him away from the others to make to him, perhaps, the same confidences that he had just done to Canalis.

"What an honest and worthy fellow!" said Léon, indicating Giraud to Canalis.

"It is those honesties which kill governments," replied Canalis.

"In your opinion, is he a good orator?—"

"Yes and no," replied Canalis; "he is verbose, he is fine-drawn. He is a workman in reasoning, he is a good logician; but he does not comprehend the great logic, that of events and of affairs: thus he has not and he never will have *the ear of the Chamber—*"

At the moment in which Canalis issued this verdict on Giraud, the latter returned with Maxime to the group; and, forgetting the presence of a stranger whose discretion was not known to them as was that of Léon and of Bixiou, he took the hand of Canalis in a significant fashion.

"Well," said he, "I consent to the proposition of Monsieur le Comte de Trailles, I will make the interpellation to you, but with a great severity."

"We will then have the Chamber with us in this question; for a man of your capacity and of your eloquence *has always the ear of the Chamber,*"

replied Canalis. "I will reply,—but promptly, to crush you."

"You may be able to bring about a change in the Cabinet, for you can bring about on such a ground whatever you wish of the Chamber, *and you will become the man of the situation—*"

"Maxime has hoodwinked both of them," said Léon to his cousin. "That rascal there finds himself in the intrigues of the Chamber like a fish in the water."

"Who is it?" asked Gazonal.

"An ex-rogue on the way to become an ambassador," replied Bixiou.

"Giraud!" said Léon to the Councillor of State, "do not go away without having asked of Rastignac that which he promised me to say to you in relation to a case which you will judge the day after to-morrow and which relates to my cousin here; I will come to see you to-morrow on this subject, in the morning."

And the three friends followed the three men of politics at a distance, directing their steps toward the *Salle des Pas Perdus.*

"Look, cousin, see those two men," said Léon to Gazonal, showing to him a former minister, very celebrated, and the chief of the Left Centre, "there are two orators who have the ear of the Chamber and who have been facetiously surnamed the ministers of the departments of the Oppositions; they have so well the ear of the Chamber, that they pull it very often."

"It is four o'clock, let us return to the Rue de Berlin," said Bixiou.

"Yes, you have just seen the heart of the government; it is necessary to show you the helminths, the ascarides, the tœnia, the Republican, since it is necessary to call it by its name," said Léon to his cousin.

When the three friends were installed in their fiacre, Gazonal looked mischievously at his cousin and at Bixiou, like a man who is about to launch a flood of oratorical and Meridional bile.

"I was strongly suspicious of this great drab of a city, but since this morning, I despise it! The poor province, so shabby, is an honest girl; but Paris, it is a prostitute, greedy, lying, an actress, and I am very well content not to have left any more of my skin here—"

"The day is not ended," said Bixiou, sententiously, winking at Léon.

"And why do you complain stupidly," said Léon, "of a pretended prostitution to which you are going to owe the winning of your suit?—Do you believe yourself more virtuous than we are and less of a comedian, less grasping, less prompt to descend any path whatever, less vain than all those with whom we have played as with jumping-jacks?"

"Suppose you try me—"

"Poor fellow!" said Léon, shrugging his shoulders, "have you not already promised your electoral influence to Rastignac?—"

26

"Yes, because he is the only one who has laughed at himself."

"Poor fellow!" repeated Bixiou, "you suspect me, I who have done nothing but laugh!—You are like a little cur wearying a tiger. —Ah! if you had seen us ridiculing anyone!— Do you know that we can drive out of his wits a man of perfectly sound judgment?—"

This conversation conducted Gazonal to the house of his cousin, where the sight of the rich furnishings cut short his speech and put an end to this debate. The Southerner perceived, but later, that Bixiou had already made him *pose*.

At half-past five, at the moment when Léon de Lora finished his toilet for the evening, to the stupefaction of Gazonal, who enumerated the thousand and one superfluities of his cousin and who admired the serious air of the valet de chambre in full function, the *pedicure of Monsieur* was announced.

Publicola Masson, a little man, fifty years old, whose face recalled that of Marat, entered, depositing a little box of instruments and placing himself on a low chair in front of Léon, after having saluted Gazonal and Bixiou.

"How are affairs?" asked Léon of him, abandoning to him one of his feet already preparatively washed by the valet de chambre.

"Oh! I have been obliged to take two pupils, two young persons who, despairing of making their fortune, have abandoned chirurgery for the

corporistique; they were dying of hunger, and yet they have talent—"

"Oh! I was not speaking to you of pedestrian affairs, I am asking you where you are in your political affairs—"

Masson threw at Gazonal a look more eloquent than any species of interrogation.

"Oh! speak, he is my cousin, and he is almost one of yours; he thinks himself Legitimist."

"Well, we are getting on! we are marching! In five years from now, Europe will be all ours!—Switzerland and Italy have been zealously worked, and, when the occasion arrives, we are ready. Here, we have fifty thousand men armed, without counting the two hundred thousand citizens who are penniless—!"

"Bah!" said Léon, "and the fortifications?"

"Pie crusts, which will be swallowed," replied Masson. "In the first place, we will not allow the cannon to be brought; and then we have a little machine more powerful than all the forts in the world, a machine invented by a doctor who has cured more people than the doctors have killed during the whole period in which they have been operating."

"How you go on!—" said Gazonal, who shuddered at the sight of Publicola.

"Ah! it is necessary! we come after Robespierre and Saint-Just; it is to do better; they were timid, for you see what has happened to us,—an emperor, the elder branch and the younger branch! The Montagnards did not sufficiently prune the social tree."

"Ah, there! you who are going to be, as it is said, Consul or something like Tribune, do not forget," said Bixiou, "that I have been demanding your protection for the last twelve years."

"Nothing will happen to you, for we shall want loustics,* and you can take Barère's trade," replied the pedicure.

"And I?" said Léon.

"Ah! you, you are my client; it is that which will save you; for genius is an odious privilege to which too much has been granted in France, and we shall be obliged to demolish some of our great men in order to teach the others to learn to be simple citizens—"

The pedicure spoke with an air half-serious, half-waggish, which made Gazonal shiver.

"So," said the Southerner, "there will be no more religion?"

"No more religion *of the State*," replied the operator, emphasizing the last three words, "each one will have his own. It is very fortunate that at this moment they are protecting the convents; it is there that we are preparing the capital of our government. Everything is conspiring for us. Thus, all those who pity the people, who *bawl* on the question of proletariats and of wages, who work against the Jesuits, who occupy themselves with the amelioration of, no matter what,—the communist, the humanitarian, the philanthropist, you understand, all those people are our advance-guard. While we are

---

* Loustics—buffoons in the Swiss regiments formerly in the service of France; professional jesters

gathering the powder, they are weaving the fuse to which the spark of a circumstance will set fire."

"Ah, so! what is it you wish then for the happiness of France?" asked Gazonal.

"Equality for the citizens, the cheapness of all commodities—we wish that there shall no longer be those who are in want of everything and millionaires, blood-suckers and victims!"

"That is it! the *maximum* and the *minimum*?" said Gazonal.

"You have said it," replied the pedicure, decisively.

"No more manufacturers?"—asked Gazonal.

"There will be manufactories for the benefit of the State, we shall all be usufructuaries of France—. Each one will have his ration as on a vessel, and everyone will work then according to his capacity."

"Good!" said Gazonal, "and, while waiting till you can cut off the heads of the aristocrats—"

"I pare their nails," said the radical Republican, who put away his tools and who finished the jest himself.

He bowed very politely and went out.

"Is it possible? in 1845—" cried Gazonal.

"If we had the time, we would show you," replied the landscape-painter, "all the personages of 1793; you could talk with them all. You have just seen Marat; well, we know also Fouquier-Tinville, Collot-d'Herbois, Robespierre, Chabot, Fouché, Barras, and there is even a magnificent Madame Roland."

"Come, in this theatrical representation, the tragedy has not been missing," said the Southerner.

"It is six o'clock: before we take you to see *Les Saltimbanques*, which Odry plays this evening," said Léon to his cousin, "it is necessary to go and pay a visit to Madame Cadine, an actress who cultivates a good deal your *Rapporteur* Massol, and to whom you will have this evening to pay assiduous court."

"As it is necessary for you to conciliate this power, I am going to give you some instructions," added Bixiou. "Do you employ workwomen in your manufactory?"

"Certainly," replied Gazonal.

"That is all I wish to know," said Bixiou; "you are not married, you are a great—"

"Yes!" cried Gazonal, "you have guessed my strong point, I love women—"

"Well, if you will execute the little manœuvre which I am going to prescribe to you, you will know, without expending a liard, the charms which one tastes in the intimacy of an actress."

When they arrived in the Rue de la Victoire, in which the celebrated actress lived, Bixiou, who was meditating a trick upon the suspicious Gazonal, had barely finished indicating his rôle to him; but the Southerner had, as will be seen, comprehended it at the first word.

The three friends mounted to the second story of a handsome enough house, and found Jennie Cadine finishing her dinner, for she was playing in the

second piece on the boards of the Gymnase. After the presentation of Gazonal to this fair puissance, Léon and Bixiou, in order to leave him alone with her, invented a pretence of going to see a new piece of furniture; but, before leaving the actress, Bixiou said to her, aside:

"It is Léon's cousin, a manufacturer worth millions, and who, to gain his suit before the Council of State against the prefect, thinks it worth while to seduce you, in order to have Massol on his side."

All Paris knows the beauty of this young première; the stupefaction of the Southerner on seeing her may then be readily understood. Received almost coldly at first, he soon became the object of the good graces of Jennie Cadine during the few minutes that they remained alone.

"How," said Gazonal, looking with disdain at the furniture of the salon through the door which his confederates had left partially open, and in computing that it was about equal to that of the dining-room, "how is it that a woman like you is left in such a dog-kennel?"

"Ah! see!—what would you have! Massol is not rich, I am waiting till he becomes a minister—"

"What a lucky man!" cried Gazonal, giving vent to the sigh of a provincial.

"Good!" said the actress to herself, "my furniture will be renewed—I can then rival Carabine!"

"Well," said Léon, re-entering, "my dear child, you are coming to Carabine's this evening, are you

not? One will sup there, one will play lans-quenet."

"Will Monsieur be there?" said Jennie, gracefully and ingenuously.

"Yes, Madame," said Gazonal, dazzled with this rapid success.

"But Massol will be there," rejoined Bixiou.

"Well, what does that matter?" retorted Jennie. "But let us go, my jewels, I must be off to my the-atre."

Gazonal gave his hand to the actress down to the closed carriage which was waiting for her, and he pressed it so tenderly that Jennie Cadine replied, shaking her fingers:

"Eh, I have no spare ones!"

When they were in the carriage, Gazonal under-took to take Bixiou by the waist, exclaiming:

"She has bitten!—. You are a fine scoundrel—"

"So the women say—" replied Bixiou.

At half-past eleven, after the theatre, a carriage conveyed the three friends to the house of Made-moiselle Séraphine Sinet, better known under the name of Carabine, one of those *noms de guerre* which the illustrious lorettes take or which is given to them, and which was derived perhaps from the fact that she has always killed her pigeon.

Carabine, who had become almost a necessity for the famous banker Du Tillet, deputy of the Left Centre, was living at this time in a charming house in the Rue Saint-Georges. There are in Paris houses the destinies of which does not vary, and

IN THE RUE DE LA VICTOIRE

Gazonal gave his hand to the actress down to the closed carriage which was waiting for her, and he pressed it so tenderly that Jennie Cadine replied, shaking her fingers:

"Eh, I have no spare ones!"

When they were in the carriage, Gazonal undertook to take Bixiou by the waist, exclaiming:

"She has bitten!— You are a fine scoundrel—"

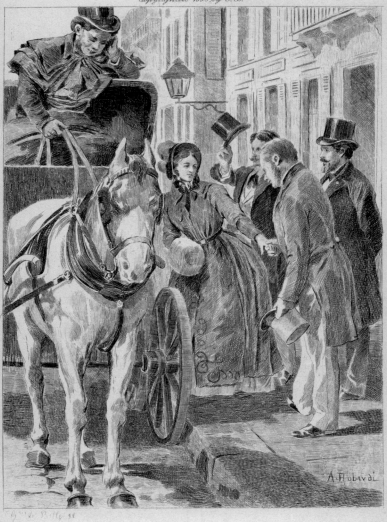

this one had already seen seven occupations by courtesans. A stock-broker had lodged there, about 1827, Suzanne du Val-Noble, since become Madame Gaillard. The famous Esther there caused the Baron de Nucingen to commit the only follies of which he had been guilty. Florine, and she who was facetiously named *the late Madame* Schontz, had alternately shone there. Wearied of his wife, Du Tillet had acquired this little modern house and had installed in it the illustrious Carabine, whose lively wit, whose cavalier manners, whose brilliant dissoluteness, formed a counter-weight to the works of his domestic, political and financial life. Whether Du Tillet and Carabine were or were not at home, the table was served, and splendidly, for ten plates every day. The artists, the literary people, the journalists, habitués of the house, dined there. In the evening there was play. More than one member of each of the Chambers came to seek there that which is bought in Paris at its weight in gold, pleasure. The eccentric women, those meteors of the Parisian firmament which are classified with such difficulty, brought there the richness of their toilets. One could there be very witty, for everything could be said there, and everything was said there. Carabine, rival of the not less celebrated Malaga, had thus come to inherit the salon of Florine, become Madame Nathan; of that of Tullia, become Madame du Bruel; of that of Madame Schontz, become Madame la Présidente du Ronceret. On entering, Gazonal only said one word, but it was at

once legitimate and Legitimist: "It is finer than at the Tuileries—" The satin, the velvet, the brocades, the gold, the objects of art which abounded there so occupied the eyes of the provincial that he did not at first perceive Jennie Cadine in a toilet to inspire respect and who, hidden behind Carabine, watched the entrance of the pleader while conversing with her friend.

"My dear child," said Léon to Carabine, "this is my cousin, a manufacturer who fell on me from the Pyrenees this morning; he knows nothing yet of Paris, he has need of Massol for an action before the Council of State; we have then taken the liberty of bringing to you Monsieur Gazonal for supper, recommending to you to leave him all his reason—"

"As Monsieur pleases; wine is dear," said Carabine, who surveyed Gazonal and saw nothing remarkable in him.

Gazonal, dazed by the toilets, the lights, the gold and the chatter of the various groups who, he thought, were occupied with him, could only stammer these words:

"Madame—, Madame—is—very good."

"What do you manufacture?—" asked the mistress of the household, smiling.

"Laces! And offer guipure laces to her!—" whispered Bixiou in Gazonal's ear.

"*Des—dent—, des—*"

"You are a dentist!—Say, Cadine? a dentist! you are *plundered*, my little one."

"*Des dentelles,*—" returned Gazonal, comprehending that it would be necessary for him to pay for his supper. "I will do myself the greatest pleasure in offering you a dress,—a scarf,—a mantilla of my manufacturing."

"Ah, three things? Well, you are nicer than you appear," replied Carabine.

"Paris has pinched me!" said Gazonal to himself, perceiving Jennie Cadine and going to speak to her.

"And I, what shall I have?—" asked the actress of him.

"Why—my whole fortune," replied Gazonal, who reflected that to offer everything was to give nothing.

Massol, Claude Vignon, Du Tillet, Maxime de Trailles, Nucingen, Du Bruel, Malaga, Monsieur and Madame Gaillard, Bauvinet, a crowd of persons, entered.

After a conversation apart with the manufacturer concerning his case, Massol, without promising anything, said to him that the report was yet to be made, and that the citizens could confide in the intelligence and in the independence of the Council of State. At this cold and dignified answer, Gazonal, despairing, believed it necessary to seduce the charming Jennie Cadine, with whom he was desperately in love. Léon de Lora and Bixiou left their victim in the hands of the most roguish of the women of this bizarre society, for Jennie Cadine is the only rival of the famous Déjazet. At the table,

where Gazonal was fascinated by the silverware of that modern Benvenuto Cellini, Froment-Meurice, and of which the contents were worthy of the interest of that which contained them, the two jokers were careful to place themselves at some distance from him; but they followed with a sly eye the progress of the witty actress, who, instigated by the insiduous promise of the renewal of her furniture, gave herself for a theme the winning over of Gazonal. And, never did a lamb of the Corpus-Christi allow itself to be conducted with more complacency by its St. John the Baptist than did Gazonal in obeying this siren.

Three days later, Léon and Bixiou, who had not seen Gazonal again, came to seek him at his hôtel about two o'clock in the afternoon.

"Well, cousin, a decree of the Council gives you your case—"

"Alas! it is useless, cousin," said Gazonal, lifting to the two friends a melancholy eye, "I have become Republican—"

"What is that?" said Léon.

"I have no longer anything, not even to pay my lawyer," replied Gazonal. "Madame Jennie Cadine has notes of mine for more money than I have goods—"

"The fact is that Cadine is a little dear, but—"

"Oh! I have had it for my money," replied Gazonal. "Ah! what a woman!—Well, the province cannot contend with Paris; I am going to retire to the Trappist Monastery."

"Good!" said Bixiou; "you are reasonable. Now, then, recognize the majesty of the Capital—"

"And of capital!" exclaimed Léon, offering to Gazonal his notes.   Gazonal looked at these papers with a stupid air.

"You will not say that we do not understand hospitality: we have instructed you and saved you from poverty, regaled, and—amused," said Bixiou.

"And *gratis!*" added Léon, making the gesture of the street gamins when they wish to express the action of *pilfering*.

Paris, November, 1845.

LIST OF ETCHINGS

VOLUME IX